Seventh Edition

Medical Pharmacology

As per the latest

CBME Guidelines |

Competency Based Undergraduate Curriculum
for the Indian Medical Graduate

Seventh Edition

Medical Pharmacology

As per the latest
CBME Guidelines |
Competency Based Undergraduate Curriculum for the Indian Medical Graduate

Padmaja Udaykumar MD
Professor and Head
Department of Pharmacology
Fr Muller Medical College
Mangalore, Karnataka

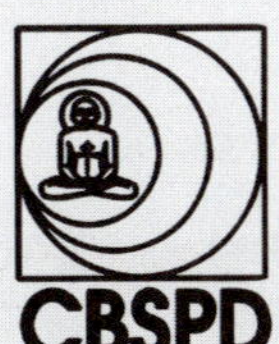

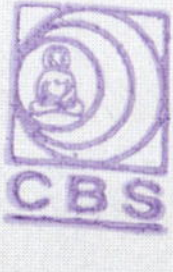

CBS Publishers & Distributors Pvt Ltd
New Delhi • Bengaluru • Chennai • Kochi • Kolkata • Lucknow • Mumbai
Hyderabad • Jharkhand • Nagpur • Patna • Pune • Uttarakhand

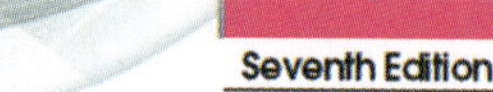

Medical Pharmacology

ISBN: 978-81-947082-8-5

Seventh Edition: 2021
Reprint: 2022, 2023, **2024**
First Edition: 2004
Second Edition: 2006
Third Edition: 2011
Fourth Edition: 2013
Reprint: 2015
Fifth Edition: 2017
Reprint: 2017, 2019
Revised Fifth Edition: 2020
Sixth Edition: 2021

Disclaimer

Science and technology are constantly changing fields. New research and experience broaden the scope of information and knowledge. The author has tried her best in giving information available to her while preparing the material for this book. Although, all efforts have been made to ensure optimum accuracy of the material, yet it is quite possible some errors might have been left uncorrected. The publisher, the printer and the author will not be held responsible for any inadvertent errors, omissions or inaccuracies.

Published by Satish Kumar Jain and produced by Varun Jain for
CBS Publishers & Distributors Pvt Ltd
4819/XI Prahlad Street, 24 Ansari Road, Daryaganj, New Delhi 110 002, India.
Ph: 011-23289259, 23266861 Website: www.cbspd.com
e-mail: delhi@cbspd.com

Corporate Office: 204 FIE, Industrial Area, Patparganj, Delhi 110 092
Ph: 011-4934 4934 Fax: 011-4934 4935 e-mail: publishing@cbspd.com; publicity@cbspd.com

Branches

- Bengaluru: Seema House 2975, 17th Cross, KR Road, Banasankari 2nd Stage, Bengaluru 560 070, Karnataka, India
  Ph: +91-80-26771678/79 Fax: +91-80-26771680 e-mail: bangalore@cbspd.com
- Chennai: 7, Subbaraya Street, Shenoy Nagar, Chennai 600 030, Tamil Nadu, India
  Ph: +91-44-26680620, 26681266 Fax: +91-44-42032115 e-mail: chennai@cbspd.com
- Kochi: 42/1325, 1326, Power House Road, Opp KSEB, Power House, Ernakulum, Kochi 682 018, Kerala, India
  Ph: +91-484-4059061–67 Fax: +91-484-4059065 e-mail: kochi@cbspd.com
- Kolkata: 147, Hind Ceramics Compound, 1st Floor, Nilgunj Road, Belghoria, Kolkata 700 056, West Bengal, India
  Ph: +91-33-25633055/56 e-mail: kolkata@cbspd.com
- Lucknow: Basement, Khushnuma Complex, 7 Meerabai Marg (behind Jawahar Bhawan), Lucknow 226 001, UP, India
  Ph: +91-522-4000032 e-mail: tiwari.lucknow@cbspd.com
- Mumbai: PWD Shed, Gala no. 25/26, Ramchandra Bhatt Marg, Next to JJ Hospital Gate no. 2, Opp. Union Bank of India, Noorbaug, Mumbai 400 009, Maharashtra, India
  Ph: +91-22-66661880/89 e-mail: mumbai@cbspd.com

Representatives

- Hyderabad 0-9885175004
- Jharkhand 0-9811541605
- Nagpur 0-9421945513
- Patna 0-9334159340
- Pune 0-9923910676
- Uttarakhand 0-9716462459

Printed at Goyal Offset Works Pvt. Ltd., Haryana (INDIA)

to

my dear students

Preface to the Seventh Edition

"Change is the only constant thing in life"—as we keep delving into the depth of this saying, one cannot help appreciating how true it is in everyone's life.

Perceived as one of the biggest changes in medical education in recent times, the new CBME syllabus was received with much enthusiasm and expectations by the medical fraternity though it meant more efforts to be put in by everyone. Implementation of it needed training right from terminology to planning examinations. Just as the air of confusion was getting cleared and the first batch was settling well, the COVID-19 pandemic barged in. It had a say in almost everything and played havoc in the lives of millions.

Implementation of CBME has brought out the need to tailor the contents of the *Medical Pharmacology* book. All competencies have been covered. Some new topics which were earlier not taught in pharmacology classes—like pesticides, national health programs, occupational and environmental poisoning, dietary supplements, nutraceuticals and so on have been added.

More flowcharts, tables, figures and mnemonics have been done. Attempt has been made to do justice to the subject and the new syllabus, keeping in mind the reduced time frame.

Hope this book reduces the burden of the students and the faculty alike.

Please mail your valuable feedback to padmajaudaykumar@gmail.com

Padmaja Udaykumar

Acknowledgements

I owe my sincere thanks to my husband Prof Udaykumar K, Medical Superintendent, Fr Muller Medical College Hospital, for his constant encouragement, suggestions, help and guidance in bringing out this book.

My sincere thanks are due to the below mentioned doctors who have helped me with this book:

- Dr Prabhakar H, Cardiologist, for reviewing and for guiding me in writing Clinical Pharmacology of the Cardiovascular System.
- Dr Krishna Prasad (Oncologist), Dr Sujaya V Rao (Gynecologist), Dr Sudeep K (Endocrinologist), Dr Raghavendra BS (Neurologist) and Dr Saurabh Kumar (Community Medicine) for reviewing chapters in their respective specialization.
- Dr Bhavani, Professor of Pharmacology, Shadan Medical College, Hyderabad, and Dr P Rama Mohan, Professor of Pharmacology, Narayana Medical College, Nellore, for their inputs in updating the chapter "Antiarrhythmics".
- Dr KL Bairy, Prof DR Kulkarni, Dr Jagdish K, Dr Vijayaraghavan, Prof Kumar, Prof Nataraj KV, and my colleagues Dr Vijayalakshmi, Dr Nicole Periera, Dr Chandralekha, Dr Vinita K for their feedback and postgraduates for their encouragement and support.
- Dr Nanette Suares and Dr P Bharati for their assistance in framing some mnemonics.

I offer my grateful acknowledgements to the following peers for providing source material:

1. Dr Skandashree, Assistant Professor, Dept of Pharmacology, Fr Muller Medical College, Mangalore; Topic: Occupational and Environmental Pesticides, Food Adulterants, Pollutants and Insect Repellents.
2. Dr Pratibha Periera, Professor and Head, Dept of Geriatrics, JSS Medical College, Mysore; Topic: Geriatric Pharmacology.

For contributing a chapter each:

1. Dr Sudhir Prabhu, Associate Professor, Dept of Community Medicine, Pharmacology, Fr Muller Medical College, Mangalore. Chapter—National Health Programs.
2. Dr Rashmi Rasquina, Nutrition Therapist KMC and ENT surgeon, Mangalore. Topic: Dietary Supplements and Nutraceuticals.
3. Dr Skandashree, Assistant Professor, Dept of Pharmacology, Fr Muller Medical College, Mangalore. Topic: Herbal Medicines.

My acknowledgements are due to the below mentioned peers for their feedback:

- Dr Saurabh Patel, Tutor, Dept of Pharmacology, BJ Medical College, Ahmedabad
- Dr Sandeep Rao Koradkal and Mr Abhishek Sharma, Fr Muller Medical College, Mangalore.

I thank the management of Father Muller Medical College, Rev Fr Richard Coelho, Director; Rev Fr Rudolph Ravi D'Sa Administrator; Rev Fr Ajith Menezes, Administrator; Rev Fr Nelson Pais, Assistant Administrator; Dr JP Alva, Dean and Dr B Sanjeev Rai, Chief of Research for their encouragement.

I thank my children, Chirag and daughter-in-law Prateeksha, for their support and Dr Anurag for his feedback and suggestions.

I also thank Mr YN Arjuna Senior Vice President, Mrs Ritu Chawla Gerneral Manager and the team for their dedicated work, meticulous editorial and DTP work and Mr SK Jain CMD, CBS Publishers & Distributors, New Delhi, for bringing out this book.

Padmaja Udaykumar

Contents

Unit III: Autacoids and Related Drugs

Unit IV: Anaesthetics

Unit V: Central Nervous System

Unit VI: Drugs Acting on the Kidney

Unit VII: **Blood**

Unit VIII: **Cardiovascular System**

Unit IX: **Respiratory System**

Unit X: **Gastrointestinal Tract**

Unit XI: **Drugs used in Haematological Disorders**

Unit XII: **Drugs used in Endocrine Disorders**

Unit XIII: Chemotherapy

Unit XIV: **Immunopharmacology**

Unit XV: **Toxicology**

Unit XVI: **Miscellaneous Topics**

Competencies

Code	Competency	Chapter	Page no
PH 1.1	Define and describe the principles of pharmacology and pharmacotherapeutics.	1	3
PH 1.2	Describe the basis of evidence-based medicine and therapeutic drug monitoring.	1, 2	3, 6, 38
PH 1.3	Enumerate and identify drug formulations and drug delivery systems.	1	7
PH 1.4	Describe absorption, distribution, metabolism and excretion of drugs.	2	18
PH 1.5	Describe general principles of mechanism of drug action.	3	40
PH 1.6	Describe principles of pharmacovigilance and ADR reporting systems.	4	60
PH 1.7	Define, identify and describe the management of adverse drug reactions (ADR).	4	60
PH 1.8	Identify and describe the management of drug interactions.	4	66
PH 1.9	Describe nomenclature of drugs, i.e. generic, branded drugs.	5	69
PH 1.10	Describe parts of a correct, complete and legible generic prescription. Identify errors in prescription and correct appropriately.	5	76
PH 1.11	Describe various routes of drug administration, e.g. oral, SC, IV, IM, SL.	1	9
PH 1.12	Calculate the dosage of drugs using appropriate formulae for an individual patient, including children, elderly and patient with renaldysfunction.	63	736, 739, 742
PH 1.13	Describe mechanism of action, types, doses, side effects, indications and contraindications of adrenergic and anti-adrenergic drugs.	6	82
PH 1.14	Describe mechanism of action, types, doses, side effects, indications and contraindications of cholinergic and anticholinergic drugs.	7	109
PH 1.15	Describe mechanism/s of action, types, doses, side effects, indications and contraindications of skeletal muscle relaxants.	8	127
PH 1.16	Describe mechanism/s of action, types, doses, side effects, indications and contraindications of the drugs which act by modulating autacoids, including: Anti-histaminics, 5-HT modulating drugs, NSAIDs, drugs for gout, anti-rheumatic drugs, drugs for migraine.	9–11	139–175
PH 1.17	Describe the mechanism/s of action, types, doses, side effects,indications and contraindications of local anesthetics.	12	179
PH 1.18	Describe the mechanism/s of action, types, doses, side effects, indications and contraindications of general anaesthetics, and pre-anesthetic medications.	13	187
PH 1.19	Describe the mechanism/s of action, types, doses, side effects,indications and contraindications of the drugs which act on CNS (including anxiolytics, sedatives and hypnotics, anti-psychotic, anti-depressant drugs, anti-manics, opioid agonists and antagonists,drugs used for neurodegenerative disorders, anti-epileptics drugs).	14–19	199–269
PH 1.20	Describe the effects of acute and chronic ethanol intake.	20	270
PH 1.21	Describe the symptoms and management of methanol and ethanol poisonings	20	270
PH 1.22	Describe drugs of abuse (dependence, addiction, stimulants, depressants, psychedelics, drugs used for criminal offences).	21	275
PH 1.23	Describe the process and mechanism of drug deaddiction.	21	275
PH 1.24	Describe the mechanism/s of action, types, doses, side effects, indications and contraindications of the drugs affecting renal systems including diuretics, antidiuretics–vasopressin and analogues.	22	283

Code	Competency	Chapter	Page no
PH 1.25	Describe the mechanism/s of action, types, doses, side effects, indications and contraindications of the drugs acting on blood, like anticoagulants, antiplatelets, fibrinolytics, plasma expanders.	23	301
PH 1.26	Describe mechanisms of action, types, doses, side effects, indications and contraindications of the drugs modulating the renin angiotensin and aldosterone system.	24	321
PH 1.27	Describe the mechanisms of action, types, doses, side effects,indications and contraindications of antihypertensive drugs and drugs used in shock.	26	335
PH 1.28	Describe the mechanisms of action, types, doses, side effects, indications and contraindications of the drugs used in ischemic heart disease (stable, unstable angina and myocardial infarction), peripheral vascular disease.	28	362
PH 1.29	Describe the mechanisms of action, types, doses, side effects, indications and contraindications of the drugs used in congestive heart failure.	27	351
PH 1.30	Describe the mechanisms of action, types, doses, side effects, indications and contraindications of the antiarrhythmics.	29	374
PH 1.31	Describe the mechanisms of action, types, doses, side effects, indications and contraindications of the drugs used in the management of dyslipidemias.	30	384
PH 1.32	Describe the mechanism/s of action, types, doses, side effects, indications and contraindications of drugs used in bronchial asthma and COPD.	31	395
PH 1.33	Describe the mechanism of action, types, doses, side effects, indications and contraindications of the drugs used in cough (antitussives, expectorants/mucolytics).	31	406
PH 1.34	Describe the mechanism/s of action, types, doses, side effects, indications and contraindications of the drugs used as below:		
	1. Acid-peptic disease and GERD	32	413
	2. Antiemetics and prokinetics	33	424
	3. Antidiarrhoeals		
	4. Laxatives	34	431
	5. Inflammatory bowel disease		
	6. Irritable Bowel Disorders, biliary and pancreatic diseases		
PH 1.35	Describe the mechanism/s of action, types, doses, side effects, indications and contraindications of drugs used in hematological disorders like: 1. Drugs used in anemias 2. Colony stimulating factors	35	443
PH 1.36	Describe the mechanism of action, types, doses, side effects, indications and contraindications of drugs used in endocrine disorders:		
	• Thyroid disorders and	37	460
	• Diabetes mellitus	42	504
	• Osteoporosis	43	519
PH 1.37	Describe the mechanisms of action, types, doses, side effects, indications and contraindications of the drugs used as sex hormones, their analogues and anterior pituitary hormones.	36, 39 41	453, 479 500
PH 1.38	Describe the mechanism of action, types, doses, side effects, indications and contraindications of corticosteroids.	38	468
PH 1.39	Describe mechanism of action, types, doses, side effects, indications and contraindications the drugs used for contraception.	39	488
PH 1.40	Describe mechanism of action, types, doses, side effects, indications and contraindications of: 1. Drugs used in the treatment of infertility, and 2. Drugs used in erectile dysfunction	39	494, 495
PH 1.41	Describe the mechanisms of action, types, doses, side effects, indications and contraindications of uterine relaxants and stimulants.	40	496

Abbreviations

Ang I/II/III	Angiotensin I/II/III
AC	Adenylyl cyclase
ACE	Angiotensin II converting enzyme
ACh	Acetylcholine
AChE	Acetylcholinesterase
ACT	Artemisinin-based combination therapy
ACTH	Adrenocorticotropic hormone
AD	Alzheimer's disease
ADH	Antidiuretic hormone
ADP	Adenosine diphosphate
Adr	Adrenaline
ADR	Adverse drug reaction
AF	Atrial fibrillation
AFl	Atrial flutter
AHG	Antihaemophilic globulin
AIDS	Acquired immunodeficiency syndrome
AMP	Adenosine monophosphate
AMPA	α-aminohydroxy methylisoxazole propionic acid
ANC	Acid neutralizing capacity
ANP	Atrial natriuretic peptide
ANS	Autonomic nervous system
ARS	Anti-rabies serum
5-ASA	5-amino salicylic acid
ATG	Antithymocyte globulin
ATP	Adenosine triphosphate
ATS	Antitetanus serum
AZT	Zidovudine
BAL	British anti-Lewisite
BD	Twice daily
BPH	Benign prostatic hypertrophy
BMD	Bone mineral density
BMR	Basal metabolic rate
BNP	Brain natriuretic peptide
BP	Blood pressure
BSA	Body surface area
BZD	Benzodiazepine
CCB	Calcium channel blocker
CD	Collecting duct
ChE	Cholinesterase
Chy. rem	Chylomicron remnants
CHF	Congestive heart failure
CCF	Congestive cardiac failure
CL	Clearance
CMV	Cytomegalovirus
CNS	Central nervous system
C.O.	Cardiac output
COMT	Catecol-O-methyl transferase
COX	Cyclo-oxygenase
CPZ	Chlorpromazine
CSF	Cerebrospinal fluid
CTZ	Chemoreceptor trigger zone
CV	Cardiovascular
CVS	Cardiovascular system
DA	Dopamine
DAD	Delayed after depolarization
DAG	Diacyl glycerol
DAM	Diacetyl monoxime
DEC	Diethyl carbamazine citrate
DHE	Dihydroergotamine
DHFA	Dihydro folic acid
DHFR	Dihydrofolate reductase
DM	Diabetes mellitus
DI	Diabetes insipidus
DMPA	Depot medroxyprogesterone acetate
DNA	Deoxyribonucleic acid
DOCA	Desoxy corticosterone acetate
dopa	Dihydroxyphenyl alanine
DOPAA	3,4-Dihydroxyphenyl acetic acid
DOSS	Dioctyl sulfosuccinate
DOTS	Directly observed treatment short course
DPT	Diphtheria–Pertussis–Tetanus triple antigen
DRC	Dose-response curve
DT	Distal tubule
DUB	Dysfunctional uterine bleeding
EACA	Epsilon aminocaproic acid
EAD	Early after depolarization
ECG	Electrocardiogram
ECT	Electroconvulsive therapy
ED	Erectile dysfunction
EEG	Electroencephalogram
ENS	Enteric nervous system
EPO	Erythropoietin
EPS	Extrapyramidal symptoms
EPSP	Excitatory postsynaptic potential
ER	Estrogen receptor
ESR	Erythrocyte sedimentation rate
FFA	Free fatty acid
FSH	Follicle stimulating hormone
5-FU	5-Fluorouracil

GABA	Gamma aminobutyric acid
GC	Guanylyl cyclase
GCP	Good clinical practice
G-CSF	Granulocyte colony stimulating factor
GDP	Guanosine diphosphate
GERD	Gastroesophageal reflux disease
GFR	Glomerular filtration rate
GH	Growth hormone
GHRH	Growth hormone releasing hormone
GHRIH	Growth hormone release inhibitory hormone
GIT	Gastrointestinal tract
GITS	Gastrointestinal therapeutic system
GLUT	Glucose transporter
GMCSF	Granulocyte macrophage colony stimulating factor
GnRH	Gonadotropin releasing hormone
G6PD	Glucose-6-phosphate dehydrogenase
GTCS	Generalised tonic-clonic seizures
GTN	Glyceryl trinitrate
GTP	Guanosine triphosphate
H	Isoniazid
HAART	Highly active antiretroviral therapy
Hb	Haemoglobin
HBV	Hepatitis B virus
HCG	Human chorionic gonadotropin
HDL	High density lipoprotein
5-HIAA	5-hydroxyindole acetic acid
HIV	Human immunodeficiency virus
HMG-CoA	Hydroxymethyl glutaryl coenzyme A
HMW	High molecular weight
HPA axis	Hypothalamopituitary adrenal axis
hr	Hour
HR	Heart rate
HRT	Hormone replacement therapy
5-HT	5-hydroxytryptamine
HVA	Homovanilic acid
IBD	Inflammatory bowel disease
IBS	Irritable bowel syndrome
ID	Intradermal (injection)
Ig	Immunoglobulin
IGF	Insulin-like growth factor
IL	Interleukin
IM/im	Intramuscular
INH	Isonicotinic acid hydrazide
INR	International normalized ratio
IOP	Intraocular pressure
IP	Inositol triphosphate
IPSP	Inhibitory postsynaptic potential
ISA	Intrinsic sympathomimetic activity
IU	International unit
IV/iv	Intravenous
JAK	Janus-kinase
JNC	Joint National Committee
KTZ	Ketoconazole
LA	Local anaesthetic
LDL	Low density lipoprotein
LES	Lower esophageal sphincter
LH	Luteinizing hormone
LL	Lepromatous leprosy
LMW	Low molecular weight
LOX	Lipoxygenase
LSD	Lysergic acid diethylamide
LT	Leukotriene
LVF	Left ventricular failure
MAC	*Mycobacterium avium* complex
MAO	Monoamine oxidase
MDR	Multidrug resistant
MI	Myocardial infarction
MIC	Minimal inhibitory concentration
MLCK	Myosin light chain kinase
MMF	Mycophenolate mofetil
6-MP	6-Mercaptopurine
MPTP	4-methyl-4-phenyltetrahydropyridine
Mtx	Methotrexate
MW	Molecular weight
NA	Noradrenaline
NADP	Nicotinamide adenine dinucleotide phosphate
NAG	N-acetyl glucosamine
NAM	N-acetyl muramic acid
NANC	Nonadrenergic noncholinergic
NET	Norepinephrine transporter
NMDA	N-methyl-D-aspartate
NNRTI	Non-nucleoside reverse transcriptase inhibitor
NSAID	Nonsteroidal anti-inflammatory drug
NSTEMI	Non-ST-segment elevation myocardial infarction
NTG	Nitroglycerine
NTS	Nucleus tractus solitarius
NVBDCP	National Vector-Borne Disease Control Programme
OCD	Obsessive-compulsive disorder
OD	Once daily
OPV	Oral poliomyelitis vaccine
ORS	Oral rehydration salt (solution)
ORT	Oral rehydration therapy

PABA	Para-aminobenzoic acid
PAE	Post-antibiotic effect
PAF	Platelet activating factor
PAS	Para-aminosalicyclic acid
PBPs	Penicillin binding proteins
PBL	Paucibacillary leprosy
PD	Parkinson's disease
PDE	Phosphodiesterase
PG	Prostaglandin
PGI_2	Prostacyclin
PI	Protease inhibitor
PLA	Phospholipase A
PLC	Phospholipase C
PnG	Penicillin G
POMC	Pro-opio melanocortin
PP	Partial pressure
PPA	Phenyl propanolamine
PPAR	Paroxisome proliferator-activated receptor
PPH	Post-partum haemorrhage
PPI	Proton pump inhibitor
PPNG	Penicillinase producing *N. gonorrhoeae*
PSVT	Paroxysmal supra-ventricular tachycardia
PT	Proximal tubule
PTCA	Percutaneous transluminal coronary angioplasty
PTH	Parathyroid hormone
PTP	Post-tetanic potentiation
QID	Four times a day
R	Rifampin (Rifampicin)
RAS	Renin-angiotensin system
RBC	Red blood cells
REM	Rapid eye movement (sleep)
RNA	Ribonucleic acid
RNTCP	Revised National Tuberculosis Control Programme
RP	Refractory period
RyR	Ryanodine receptor
SA	Sinoatrial (node)
SAARD	Slow acting antirheumatic drug
SBE	Subacute bacterial endocarditis
sc/SC	Subcutaneous
SCh	Succinylcholine
SERDs	Selective estrogen receptor down-regulators
SERM	Selective estrogen receptor modulator
SERT	Serotonin transporter
SL	Sublingual
SMON	Subacute myelo-optic neuropathy
SNRI	Serotonin and noradrenaline reuptake inhibitor
SOS	As required
SPF	Sun protection factor
SR	Sustained release
SRS- A	Slow reacting substance of anaphylaxis
STAT	Signal transducer and activator transcription
STEMI	ST-segment elevation myocardial infarction
Susp	Suspension
Syr	Syrup
t½	Half life
tab	Tablet
TBG	Thyroxine binding globulin
TCAs	Tricyclic antidepressants
TDM	Therapeutic drug monitoring
TDS	Three times a day
TG	Triglyceride
6-TG	6-Thioguanine
THC	Tetrahydrocannabinol
THFA	Tetrahydrofolic acid
TIAs	Transient ischaemic attacks
TNF-α	Tumor necrosis factor-α
t-PA	Tissue plasminogen activator
TRH	Thyroid releasing hormone
TSH	Thyroid stimulating hormone
TTS	Transdermal therapeutic system
U	Unit
UDP	Uridine diphosphate
UTI	Urinary tract infection
VF	Ventricular fibrillation
VIP	Vasoactive intestinal peptide
Vit	Vitamin
VLDL	Very low density lipoprotein
VMA	Vanilyl mandelic acid
VMC	Vasomotor centre
VRSA	Vancomycin resistant *Staphylococcus aureus*
VT	Ventricular tachycardia
vWF	von Willebrand factor
WBC	White blood cells
WHO	World Health Organization
WPW	Wolff-Parkinson-White syndrome
XDR-TB	Extensively drug resistant-TB
Z	Pyrazinamide

Unit I

General Pharmacology

1. Principles of Pharmacology, Evidence-based Medicine and Routes of Drug Administration
2. Pharmacokinetics
3. Pharmacodynamics
4. Adverse Drug Reactions, Pharmacovigilance and Drug Interactions
5. Drug Nomenclature, Drug Development, Drug Regulations, Essential Medicines, Prescriptions and Related Topics

Principles of Pharmacology, Evidence-based Medicine and Routes of Drug Administration

CHAPTER 1

Competency achievement: The student should be able to:

PH 1.1 Define and describe the principles of pharmacology and pharmacotherapeutics.[1]

PH 1.2 Describe the basis of evidence-based medicine and therapeutic drug monitoring.[2]

Pharmacology is the science that deals with the study of drugs and their interaction with the living systems. The word pharmacology is derived from the Greek word—*Pharmacon* meaning an active principle and *logos* meaning a discourse.

HISTORICAL ASPECTS

The useful and toxic effects of many plant and animal products were known to man since ancient times. In fact, there has been a quest for drugs and remedies since the existence of mankind itself.

In early days, there was a close relationship between religion and the treatment of diseases. The knowledge of the use of drugs often rested with the priest or holyman. Drugs were thought to be magical in their actions. Several cultures like the Chinese, Greek, Indian, Roman, Persian, European and many others contributed a great deal to the development of medicine in early times. The drug prescriptions included preparations from herbs, plants, animals and minerals. However, written information on remedies used in early times is lacking.

The Indian and the Chinese writings are amongst the oldest written material in medicine. India's earliest pharmacological writings are from the 'Vedas'. Rigveda (3000 BC) has description of some medicines. An ancient Indian physician Charaka, and then, Sushruta and Vagbhata, described many herbal preparations included in **'Ayurveda'** (meaning the science of life). Indians practiced vaccination as early as 550 BC.

'Pen Tsao' the Chinese materia medica was written as early as 1700 BC and it contained classification of medicinal plants and some preparations of plants, metals and animals.

The Egyptian medical papyri (1600 BC) described several preparations. The largest of them, Ebers Papyrus lists some 800 preparations.

The Greeks studied the toxic effects of various plant extracts. Their contribution to the growth of modern medicine is significant. **Hippocrates** (460–377 BC), a Greek physician, studied the cause of disease and wrote on the ethics of medicine and recommended judicious use of drugs. Galen (130–201 BC), also a Greek physician, practiced in Rome and put forth a doctrine that diseases are due to an imbalance of fluids—blood, phlegm, black bile and yellow bile. He believed that drugs had some properties like warmth, coldness, dryness or humidity and also thought that it is beneficial to use a combination of drugs to obtain these effects.

In the Middle Ages, many herbal gardens were cultivated by the monasteries. **Paracelsus** the **'Grandfather of Pharmacology'** born in Switzerland was the son of a physician. He opined that complicated mixture of drugs should not be used and also wrote, "all drugs are poisons—it is only the dose which makes a thing a poison." This statement holds good even today.

Though medicine developed simultaneously in several countries, the spread of knowledge was limited because of poorly developed communication across the world. By the beginning of the first century, it was realized that there was a need to standardize the method of obtaining uniform medical preparations.

James Gregory (1735–1821 AD) recommended certain dangerous measures like blood letting, use of emetics and purgatives in the treatment of diseases—such measures were often fatal. He meant to induce other suffering to relieve pain/suffering and this was probably the basis of the word '**allopathy**' meaning 'the other suffering'. This word, still being used for the modern system of medicine, is a misnomer. **Homeopathy** meaning 'similar suffering' was introduced by **Samuel Hahnemann.** The principles of this system include 'like cures like' and 'dilution enhances the potency of drugs'. Various traditional systems of medicine were practiced in different parts of the world like Homeopathy, Ayurveda, Unani, Siddha system and Allopathy.

Thus several systems of medicine were introduced, of which only a few survived. The basic reason for the failure of these systems is that man's concepts about diseases were incorrect and baseless in those days. By the end of the 17th century, the importance of experimentation, observation and scientific methods of study became clear. **Francois Magendie** and **Claude Bernard** popularized the use of animal experiments to understand the effects of drugs. Simultaneous development of other branches of science, viz. botany, zoology, chemistry and physiology helped in the better understanding of pharmacology.

By the nineteenth century, methods for isolation of drugs were developed. **Rudolph Bucheim** (1820–1879) set up the first laboratory in his home at Dorpat Estonia in 1847 exclusively meant for research on drugs. **Oswald Schmiedeberg** (1838–1921), a student of Bucheim, conducted extensive research on drugs, trained 120 students and wrote a medical textbook. He has been called '**Father of Pharmacology**' for his contribution and was the most prominent pharmacologist of the 19th century.

With the growth of science and the development of scientific methods of research, treatment of diseases now relies largely on scientific evidence. Well-designed multicentric trials involving a fair number of participants are required to prove the safety and benefits of a drug in a given condition before it can be used in general population making the modern system **evidence-based medicine** (*see* page 6).

The last century has seen a rapid growth of the subject with several new drugs, new concepts and techniques being introduced. We now know much more about receptors and molecular mechanisms of action of many drugs. Several diseases, which were considered incurable and fatal, can now be completely cured with just a few tablets.

TERMINOLOGY

Drug (*Drogue*—a dry herb in French) is a substance used in the diagnosis, prevention or treatment of a disease. **WHO definition**, "A drug is any substance or product that is used or intended to be used to modify or explore physiological systems or pathological states for the benefit of the recipient."

Pharmacokinetics is the study of the absorption, distribution, metabolism and excretion of drugs, i.e. what the body does to the drug (in Greek *Kinesis = movement*).

Pharmacodynamics is the study of the effects of the drugs on the body and their mechanisms of action, i.e. what the drug does to the body.

Therapeutics deals with the use of drugs in the prevention and treatment of disease.

Pharmacoeconomics deals with the cost, i.e. economic aspects of drugs used therapeutically.

Pharmacogenetics (and pharmacogenomics) is the science that deals with the study of genetic basis for variation in drug responses (*see* page 54).

Pharmacoepidemiology is the study of both the useful and adverse effects of drugs on large number of people.

Pharmacovigilance is related to the detection, assessment, understanding and prevention of adverse effects of drugs (*see* page 65).

Toxicology deals with the adverse effects of drugs and also the study of poisons, i.e. detection, prevention and treatment of poisoning *(Toxicon = poison in Greek)*.

Chemotherapy is the use of drugs and chemicals for the treatment of infections. The term now also includes the use of chemical compounds to treat malignancies.

Essential medicines are those that satisfy the healthcare needs of majority of the population and should be available at all times in adequate amounts and in the appropriate dosage forms (*see* page 74) as defined by the WHO.

Orphan drugs are drugs to be used for prevention and treatment of rare diseases.

Pharmacopoeia is the official publication containing information on drugs (*see* page 72).

Pharmacy is the science of identification, compounding and dispensing of drugs. It also includes collection, isolation, purification, synthesis and standardization of medicinal substances.

Chronopharmacology is the science that involves the correlation of drug effects to the circadian rhythm to obtain optimum therapeutic effect and minimize the adverse effects, e.g. bronchospasm usually occurs at night. Blood pressure rises at dawn and dusk and is the lowest at midnight (*see* page 73). **Chronotherapy** is the administration of drugs to match the circadian rhythm. ***Chronobiotics*** are drugs that can be used to modify or reset the circadian rhythm. They find application mostly in conditions like sleep disorders and jet lag.

SOURCES OF DRUGS

The sources of drugs could be natural, or synthetic and biotechnology.

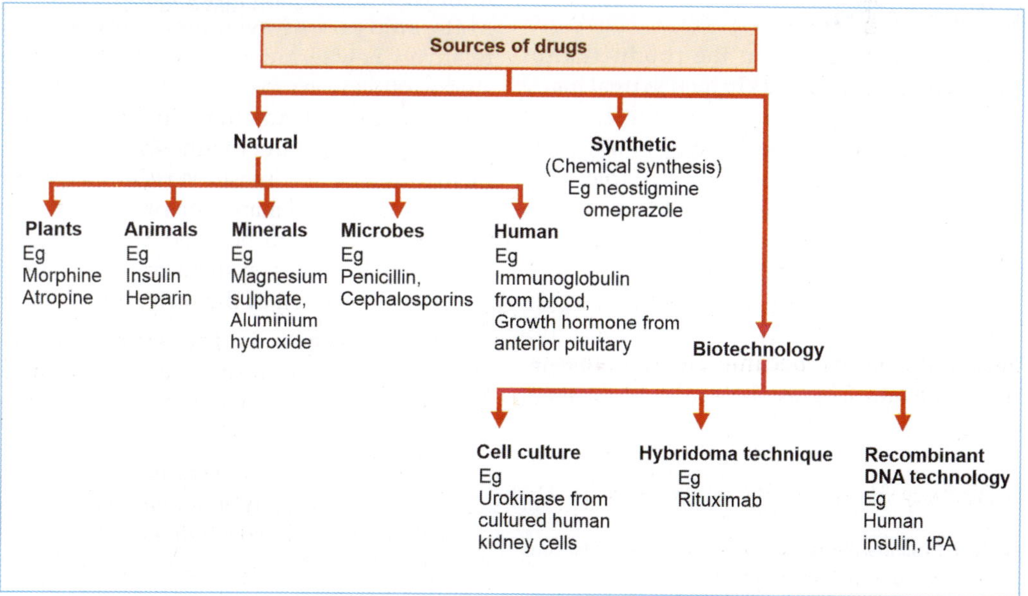

A. Natural Sources

Drugs can be obtained from:

1. *Plants*, e.g. atropine, morphine, quinine, digoxin, pilocarpine, and physostigmine.
2. *Animals*, e.g. insulin, heparin, gonadotrophins and antitoxic sera.
3. *Minerals*, e.g. magnesium sulphate, aluminium hydroxide, iron, gold, sulphur and radioactive isotopes.
4. *Microorganisms*—antibacterial agents are obtained from some bacteria and fungi, e.g. penicillin, cephalosporins, tetracyclines.
5. *Human*—some drugs are obtained from human source, e.g. immunoglobulins from blood, growth hormone from anterior pituitary and chorionic gonadotrophins from the urine of pregnant women.

B. Synthetic

Most drugs used now are synthetic. They may be manufactured in large quantities and therefore can be less expensive, e.g. quinolones, omeprazole, sulfonamides, pancuronium and neostigmine.

C. Biotechnology

Use of biotechnology in the production of drugs and biologicals has helped to treat many ailments which were once incurable. It has been possible to synthesize many congeners with minor modifications. For example:

- By **cell cultures,** e.g. urokinase from cultured human kidney cells.
- By **recombinant DNA technology,** e.g. human insulin, tissue plasminogen activator, haematopoietic growth factors like erythropoietin, filgrastim and sargramostim.
- By **hybridoma technique,** e.g. monoclonal antibodies like rituximab.

Competency achievement: The student should be able to:

PH 1.2 Describe the basis of evidence-based medicine and therapeutic drug monitoring.[3]

Evidence-based Medicine (EBM)

With the growth of science and the development of scientific methods of research, treatment of diseases now relies largely on scientific evidence obtained from studies.

Definition: EBM is applying the best evidence that can be found in the medical literature to medical practice, resulting in the best possible patient care.

Need for EBM: There is high degree of variation in medical practice despite doctors being trained with the same curriculum. With the medical care getting more complex and expensive, it is important to know the best possible care and whenever possible cost-effective treatment.

EBM has 3 components—acquiring information, critical analyse of it and then applying the information to patient care.

Searching the medical literature for best evidence requires good searching skills using medical informatics. It can be time consuming, but many database providers are developing search engines to quickly find reliable and valid information.

The most complex part of the process of EBM is the critical analysis of the medical literature. **Meta-analysis or systematic review** is a relatively new technique that combines many studies on a given topic and analyses them. The **TRIP** database can be used for a systematic search of nearly 100 evidence-based databases including Medline and Cochrane library and can provide a summary of the results.

Steps in EBM

Frame a Question (what is the information wanted)
↓
Search the databases for answers
↓
Analyse the evidence
↓
If found appropriate, apply to practice
↓
Assess the outcome

Lastly, effectiveness of the practice should also be evaluated before it is incorporated into routine practice.

EBM is a relatively new concept but is now largely popular. Evidence based practices can be more or less expensive than current practices, but they are better.

Therapeutic Drug Monitoring is the use of plasma drug levels to guide treatment (*see* page 38).

Competency achievement: The student should be able to:
PH 1.3 Enumerate and identify drug formulations and drug delivery systems.[4]

DRUG FORMULATIONS AND DOSAGE FORMS

Drug formulation is the drug dosage form in which the drug is administered. The right dosage form is important to deliver the drug to the site of action. Drugs may be administered in solid or liquid dosage forms (Table 1.1).

Drug Delivery Systems

Appropriate drug delivery systems are important to attain right drug levels at the site of action. In order to improve drug delivery, to prolong the duration of action and thereby improve patient compliance, **special drug delivery systems** are being tried. Drug targeting, i.e. to deliver drugs at the site where it is required to act is also being aimed at, particularly for anticancer drugs. Some such systems are:

***a. Ocusert*:** Ocusert systems are thin elliptical units that contain the drug in a reservoir which slowly releases the drug through a membrane by diffusion at a steady rate, e.g. pilocarpine ocusert used in glaucoma is placed under the lid and can deliver pilocarpine for 7 days.

***b. Progestasert*:** Progestasert is inserted into the uterus where it delivers progesterone constantly for over one year.

c. Transdermal adhesive units: *See* page 15

***d. Prodrug*:** Prodrug is an inactive form of a drug which gets metabolized to the active derivative in the body. Using a prodrug may overcome some of the disadvantages of the conventional forms of drug administration, as follows:

Advantages

1. *Increase availability at the site*, e.g. dopamine does not cross the BBB; levodopa, a prodrug, crosses the BBB and is then converted to dopamine in the CNS.
2. *Prolong duration of action:* Prodrugs may be used to achieve longer duration of action, e.g. bacampicillin (a prodrug of ampicillin) is longer-acting than ampicillin.
3. *Improve tolerability*, e.g. cyclophosphamide, an anticancer drug, gets converted to its active metabolite aldophosphamide in the liver. This allows oral administration of cyclophosphamide without causing much gastrointestinal toxicity.
4. *Drug targeting:* Zidovudine is taken up by the virus infected cells and gets activated in these cells. This results in selective toxicity to infected cells.
5. *Improve stability:* A prodrug may be more stable at gastric pH, e.g. aspirin is converted to salicylic acid which is the more stable active drug and aspirin is also better tolerated than salicylic acid.
6. *Reduce side effects:* Prodrug could be used to lower side effects—for example, bacampicillin, a prodrug of ampicillin, is better absorbed and therefore causes less diarrhoea.

Disadvantages

1. Prodrugs are likely to have a slower onset of action and therefore are not suitable in emergencies.
2. In presence of liver diseases prodrugs may not be activated to attain therapeutic levels (Mnemonic *see* page 17).

***e. Osmotic pumps*:** These are small tablet-shaped units containing the drug and an osmotic substance in two different chambers. The tablet is coated with a semipermeable membrane in which a minute laser-drilled hole is made. When the tablet is swallowed

Table 1.1: Drug formulations and dosage forms

Drug dosage forms

Solids

Powders are solid dosage forms in a finely divided state. They may be used for internal administration or for external application. e.g: Neomycin powder

Capsules are solid dosage forms in which the drug is enclosed in a tasteless, hard or soft soluble shell made up of a suitable form of gelatin. They may be spherical, ovoid or cylindrical; Spherical capsules are known as 'pearls'.

Tablets are solid dosage forms of medicaments prepared by molding or by compression.

Lozenges are solid dosage forms meant for slow dissolution in the mouth.

Dry syrups are powders which are to be made into solution before use. Drugs which are not stable in solution are dispensed as dry syrups, eg: Antibiotics including amoxicillin, erythromycin, cephalexin, ampicillin.

Liquids

Solutions are liquid dosage forms prepared by dissolving a solute in a solvent. eg: Potassium permanganate solution.

Mixture is a liquid preparation containing two or more substances intended for oral administration.

Elixirs are clear, pleasantly flavored, sweetened liquid preparations for oral administration. eg: Chlorpheniramine elixir, paracetamol elixir.

Syrups are sweet, viscous, aqueous preparations of sugars in an aqueous vehicle.

Suspensions are liquid dosage forms in which finely divided solid particles (0.5 to 5.0 microns) are suspended in a liquid or semisolid vehicle using a suspending agent. Eg: Barium sulphate suspension, kaolin suspension

Linctuses are sweet, viscous liquid preparations used for the treatment of cough. Linctuses are swallowed slowly in small doses without addition of water, eg: Codeine linctus, noscapine linctus.

Gargles and mouthwashes: Gargles are aqueous solutions used for the prevention or treatment of throat infections. Mouthwashes are aqueous solutions for deodorizing and refreshing the oral cavity.

Tinctures are alcoholic liquid preparations prepared by dissolving the corresponding liquid extract in solvents, eg: Belladonna tincture, opium tincture.

Emulsions are liquid dosage forms in which two immiscible liquids are made miscible with the help of an emulsifying agent. Labeled with 'shake the bottle before use. Examples: Phenolphthalein emulsion.

Liniments are liquid or semiliquid preparations meant for external application to the skin with friction but should not be applied to the broken skin.

Lotions are liquid suspensions meant for external application without friction.

Others

1. **Aerosols:** Pressurized dosage forms in which the liquid or solid drugs are dissolved or suspended in gas. They bring about fine dispersion of liquid (mist) or solid particles of size less than 50 microns in diameter, eg: Drugs for bronchial asthma, deodorant sprays, cosmetic hair sprays.

2. **Semisolids:** Ointments are soft semisolid preparations meant for external application to the skin or mucous membrane. Creams are viscous semisolid emulsions meant for application to skin. Creams are lighter than ointments.

3. **Enemas** are aqueous or oily solutions or suspensions intended for introduction into the rectum.

4. **Injections** are liquid preparations containing one or more medicaments dissolved or suspended in a suitable vehicle and are meant for introduction into the body tissues with the help of a syringe and needle, eg: Ampicillin injection, dextrose intravenous infusion.

5. **Suppositories** are special shaped solid dosage forms for insertion into body cavities other than mouth. They may be inserted into rectum, vagina or urethra, eg: Clotrimazole suppository.

and reaches the gut, water enters into the tablet through the semipermeable membrane. The osmotic layer swells and pushes the drug slowly out of the laser-drilled orifice. This allows slow and constant delivery of the drug over a long period of time. It is also called **gastrointestinal therapeutic system** (GITS). Some drugs available in this formulation are iron and prazosin.

f. Computerised miniature pumps: These are programmed to release drugs at a definite rate either continuously as in case of insulin or intermittently in pulses as in case of GnRH.

Various methods of drug targeting are tried especially for anticancer drugs to reduce toxicity.

g. Targeted drug delivery systems: In the last decade, efforts have been made to deliver drugs to the site of action. Such drug targeting is the dream of any pharmacologist, since it would mean a remarkable progress in therapeutics. Drug targeting largely reduces the adverse drug reactions because the required amount of the drug will be delivered at the required site of action.

Some of the targeted delivery systems currently available are:

(i) *Liposomes* are phospholipids suspended in aqueous vehicles to form minute vesicles. They are used as carriers for both water-soluble and lipid-soluble substances as they can be entrapped in the aqueous spaces or within the lipid layer itself. For example, a lipid is hydrated with an aqueous solution of the drug.

Though liposomes can be given both orally and parenterally, IV route is the most common. Small liposomes are taken up by the reticuloendothelial cells while larger ones are deposited in the lungs and are also concentrated in malignant tumours. Thus site-specific delivery of drugs may be possible with the help of liposomes. Liposomes are used in the treatment of cancers, systemic fungal infections, diabetes mellitus and in heavy metal poisoning. Examples of some liposomes available are doxorubicin, cytarabin, cisplatin and irinotecan.

(ii) *Monoclonal antibodies* against the tumour-specific antigens are used to deliver anticancer drugs to specific tumour cells.

(iii) *Nanoparticles:* The drug is encapsulated or dissolved in the nanoparticle (NP) matrix to obtain nanocapsules or nanoparticles. The size of the nanoparticles vary from 10 to 1000 nm and are biogradable. They can be used to deliver the anticancer drugs to the cancer tissue in order to improve efficacy and reduce toxicity.

(iv) *Polymer-based drug delivery:* Polymers have been used in transdermal drug delivery systems. Polymers are used for coating as in enteric-coated capsules and drug eluting stents. Drugs are also designed to be delivered directly to the colon in ulcerative colitis and inflammatory bowel disease.

(v) *Drug eluting stents* are devices consisting of a metallic stent (tubular mesh-like device) coated with a drug on a polymer coating. The drug may be sirolimus or paclitaxel. The drug is gradually released over 4–6 weeks and prevents the proliferation of vascular smooth muscles and endothelial cells over the stent placed.

ROUTES OF DRUG ADMINISTRATION

Competency achievement: The student should be able to:

PH 1.11 Describe various routes of drug administration, e.g. oral, SC, IV, IM, SL .[5]

Drugs may be administered by various routes. The choice of the route in a given patient depends on the properties of the drug and the patient's requirements. A knowledge of the advantages and disadvantages of the different routes of drug administration is essential for appropriate use of drugs.

The routes can be broadly divided into:

- Systemic routes
- Local/topical routes.

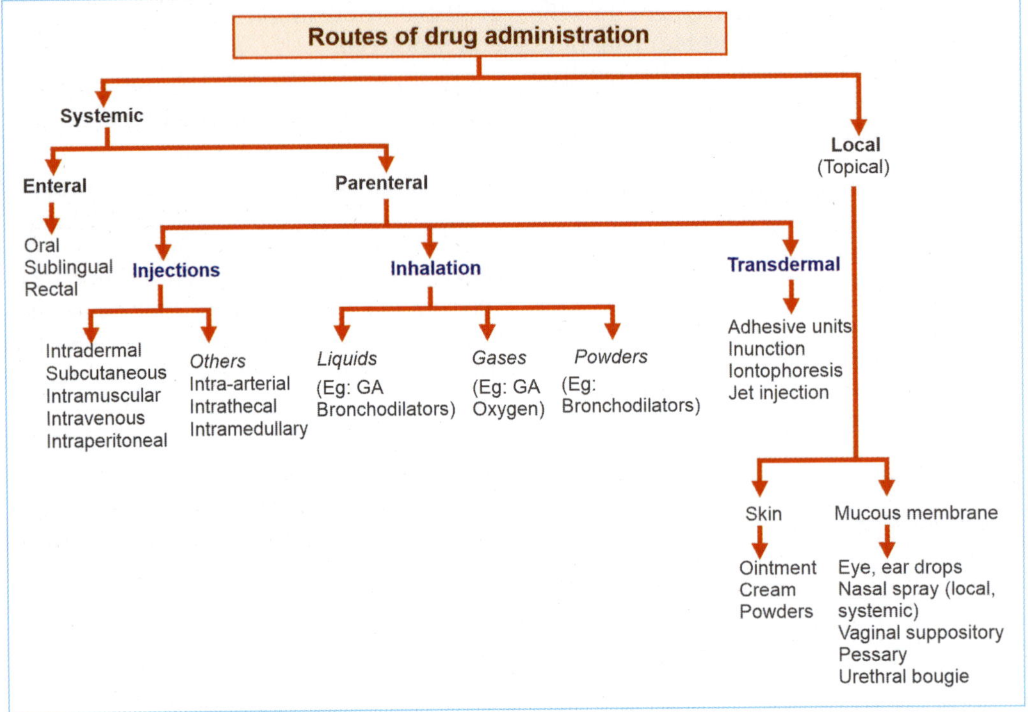

SYSTEMIC ROUTES

Enteral Routes

Enteral routes include oral, sublingual and rectal routes.

1. Oral route is the most commonly used, oldest and safest route of drug administration. The large surface area of the gastrointestinal tract, the mixing of its contents and the differences in pH at different parts of the gut facilitate effective absorption of the drugs given orally.

However, the acid and enzymes secreted in the gut and the biochemical activity of the bacterial flora of the gut can destroy some drugs before they are absorbed.

Advantages

- Safest route
- Most convenient
- Most economical
- Drugs can be self-administered
- Non-invasive route.

Disadvantages

- ***Slow action:*** Onset of action is slower as absorption needs time—hence particularly not suitable for emergencies.
- ***Drug properties:*** Irritant and unpalatable drugs cannot be administered.
- ***Poor absorption:*** Some drugs may not be absorbed due to certain physical and chemical characteristics, e.g. streptomycin is not absorbed orally.
- ***GI irritation:*** Irritation to the gastrointestinal tract may lead to vomiting.
- ***Unpredictable absorption:*** There may be irregularities in absorption.
- ***Metabolism:*** Some drugs may be destroyed by gastric juices, e.g. insulin.

- ***Unsuitable situations:*** Oral preparations cannot be given to unconscious and uncooperative patients.
- ***First pass effect:*** Some drugs may undergo extensive first pass metabolism in the liver.

To overcome some of the disadvantages, irritants are given in capsules, while bitter drugs are given as sugar-coated tablets. Sometimes drugs are coated with substances like synthetic resins, gums, sugar, colouring and flavouring agents, making them more acceptable.

Enteric-coated Tablets

Some tablets are coated with substances or polymers like cellulose-acetate, phthalates, gluten, shellac, etc. which are not digested by the gastric acid but get disintegrated in the alkaline juices of the intestine. The choice of the polymer and the thickness of coating influence the dissolution of the coat in the intestines. Enteric coating will:

- Prevent gastric irritation
- Avoid destruction of the drug by the stomach
- Provide higher concentration of the drug in the small intestine
- Retard the absorption, and thereby prolong the duration of action.

However, if the coating is inappropriate, the tablet may be expelled without being absorbed at all.

Similarly, controlled-release or sustained-release preparations are designed to prolong the rate of absorption and thereby the duration of action of the drugs (Fig. 1.1). This is useful for short-acting drugs. In newer controlled release formulations, the tablet is coated with a semipermeable membrane through which water enters and displaces the drug out.

Advantages

- Frequency of administration may be reduced.

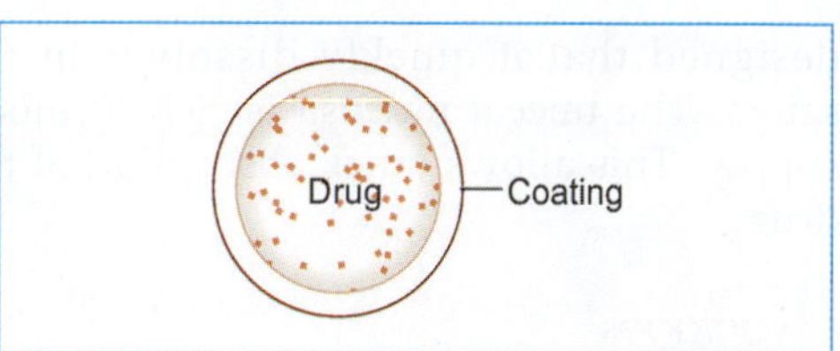

Fig. 1.1: Sustained release preparation. Dissolution of coating depends on the thickness and stability of the coat

- Therapeutic concentrations may be maintained specially when nocturnal symptoms are to be treated.

Disadvantages

- There may be 'failure of the preparation' resulting in release of the entire amount of the drug in a short time, leading to toxicity.
- Enteric coated tablets are more expensive.

Certain precautions are to be taken during oral administration of drugs—capsules and tablets should be swallowed with a glass of water with the patient in upright posture either sitting or standing. This facilitates passage of the tablet into the stomach and its rapid dissolution. It also minimises the chances of the drug getting into the larynx or behind the epiglottis. Recumbent patient should not be given drugs orally as some drugs may remain in the oesophagus due to the absence of gravitational force facilitating the passage of the drug into the stomach. Such drugs can damage the oesophageal mucosa, e.g. iron salts, tetracyclines.

2. Sublingual

Here, the tablet or pellet containing the drug is placed under the tongue. As the drug dissolves, it is absorbed across the sublingual mucosa, e.g. nitroglycerin, nifedipine, buprenorphine. The tablet may also be crushed in the mouth but not swallowed and the contents are absorbed across the buccal mucosa. The formulation should be so designed that it quickly dissolves in the saliva. The buccal mucosa is rich in blood supply. This allows quick absorption of the drug.

Advantages

- Absorption is rapid—within minutes the drug reaches the circulation.
- First pass metabolism is avoided because the drug directly reaches the systemic circulation.
- After the desired effect is obtained, the drug can be spat out to avoid the unwanted effects.

Disadvantages

- Buccal ulceration can occur.
- Lipid-insoluble drugs, drugs of higher molecular weight, irritant and unpalatable drugs cannot be given by this route.

3. Rectal

Rectum has a rich blood supply and drugs can cross the rectal mucosa to be absorbed for systemic effects. Drugs absorbed from the upper part of the rectum are carried by the superior haemorrhoidal vein to the portal circulation (can undergo first pass metabolism), while that absorbed from the lower part of the rectum is carried by the middle and inferior haemorrhoidal veins to the systemic circulation. Drugs like indomethacin, chlorpromazine, diazepam and paraldehyde can be given rectally.

Some irritant drugs are given rectally as suppositories.

Advantages

- Gastric irritation is avoided.
- Can be administered by unskilled persons.
- Useful in geriatric patients; patients with vomiting, those unable to swallow and after gastrointestinal surgery.
- Also useful in unconscious patients.

Disadvantages

- Irritation of the rectum can occur.
- Absorption may be irregular and unpredictable.

Drugs may also be given by rectal route as enema.

Enema is the administration of a drug in a liquid form into the rectum. Enema may be evacuant or retention enema.

Evacuant enema: In order to empty the bowel, about 600 ml of soap water is administered per rectum. Water distends and thus stimulates the rectum while soap lubricates. Enema is given prior to surgeries, obstetric procedures and radiological examination of the gut.

Retention enema: The drug is administered with about 100 ml of fluids and is retained in the rectum for local action, e.g. prednisolone enema in ulcerative colitis.

Parenteral Routes

Routes of administration other than the enteral (intestinal) route are known as parenteral routes. Here the drugs are directly delivered into the tissue fluids or blood.

Advantages

- Action is more rapid and predictable than oral administration.
- These routes can be employed in an unconscious or uncooperative patient.
- Gastric irritants can be given parenterally and, therefore, irritation to the gastrointestinal tract can be avoided.
- It can be used in patients with vomiting or those unable to swallow.
- Digestion by the gastric and intestinal juices and the first pass metabolism are avoided.

Therefore, in emergencies, parenteral routes are very useful for drug administration as the action is rapid and predictable and are useful even in unconscious patients.

Disadvantages

- Asepsis must be maintained
- Injections may be painful
- More expensive, less safe and inconvenient
- Injury to nerves and other tissues may occur.

Parenteral routes include:

1. Injections
2. Inhalation
3. Transdermal route

1. Injections

Injections are given with the help of syringe and needle.

Intradermal

The drug is injected:

- Into the layers of the skin raising a bleb, e.g. BCG vaccine, tests for allergy.
- By multiple punctures of the epidermis through a drop of the drug, e.g. smallpox vaccine. Only a small quantity can be administered by this route and it may be painful.

Subcutaneous (SC) Injection

Here the drug is deposited in the SC tissue, e.g. insulin, heparin. As this tissue is less vascular, absorption is slow and largely uniform, making the drug long-acting. It is reliable and patients can be trained for self-administration. Absorption can be enhanced by the addition of the enzyme hyaluronidase.

Disadvantages

- As SC tissue is richly supplied by nerves, irritant drugs cannot be injected because they can cause severe pain.
- In shock, absorption is not dependable because of vasoconstriction.
- Repeated injections at the same site can cause lipoatrophy resulting in erratic absorption.

Hypodermoclysis is the subcutaneous administration of large volumes of saline employed in paediatric practice.

Drugs can also be administered subcutaneously as:

i. *Dermojet:* In this method, a high velocity jet of drug solution is projected from a fine orifice using a 'gun'. The solution gets deposited in the SC tissue from where it is absorbed. As needle is not required, this method is painless. It is suitable for vaccines.

ii. *Pellet implantation:* Small pellets packed with drugs are implanted subcutaneously. The drug is slowly released for weeks or months to provide constant blood levels, e.g. testosterone, desoxycorticosterone acetate (DOCA).

iii. *Sialistic implants:* The drug is packed in sialistic tubes and implanted subcutaneously. The drug gets absorbed over months to provide constant blood levels, e.g. hormones and contraceptives. The empty non-biodegradable implant has to be removed.

Intramuscular (IM)

Aqueous solution of the drug is injected into one of the large skeletal muscles—deltoid, triceps, gluteus or rectus femoris. Absorption into the plasma occurs by simple diffusion. Larger molecules enter through the lymphatic channels. As the muscles are vascular, absorption is rapid and quite uniform. Drugs are absorbed faster from the deltoid region than gluteal region especially in women. The volume of injection should not exceed 10 ml. For infants, rectus femoris is used instead of gluteus because gluteus is not well-developed till the child starts walking. If the drug is injected as oily solution or suspension, absorption is slow and steady and can have prolonged effect. Soluble substances, mild irritants, depot preparations, suspensions and colloids can be injected by this route.

Advantages

- Intramuscular route is reliable.
- Absorption is rapid.

Disadvantages

- Intramuscular injection may be painful
- May even result in an abscess. Local infection and tissue necrosis are possible.
- Nerve injury should be avoided—irritant solutions can damage the nerve, if injected near a nerve.
- In case of some drugs, absorption by IM route is slower than oral, e.g. diazepam, phenytoin.
- For some drugs, IM route should be avoided, e.g. heparin, calcium gluconate, diazepam, and tetracycline.

Intravenous (IV)

Here, the drug is injected into one of the superficial veins so that it directly reaches the circulation and is immediately available for action. Drugs can be given IV as:

1. *A bolus:* Where an initial large dose (loading dose) is given, e.g. heparin. The drug is dissolved in a suitable amount of the vehicle and injected slowly.
2. *Slow injection*—over 15–20 minutes, e.g. aminophylline.
3. *Slow infusion*—when constant plasma concentrations are required, e.g. oxytocin in labour or when large volumes have to be given, e.g. dextrose, saline. Generally, about one litre of solution is infused over 3 to 4 hours. However, the patient's condition and the drug factors like the onset and duration of action of the drug dictate the rate of infusion.

Advantages

- Most useful route in emergencies as the drug is immediately available for action.
- Provides predictable blood concentrations with 100% bioavailability.
- Large volumes of solutions can be given.
- Irritants can be given by this route as they get quickly diluted in blood.
- Rapid dose adjustments are possible—if unwanted effects occur, infusion can be stopped; if higher levels are required, infusion rate can be increased—specially for short-acting drugs.

Disadvantages

- Once injected, the drug cannot be withdrawn.
- Irritation of the veins may cause thrombophlebitis.
- Extravasation of some drugs may cause severe irritation and sloughing.
- Only aqueous solutions can be given IV but not suspensions, oily solutions and depot preparations.
- Self-medication is difficult.
- Risk of embolism—though rare.

Intraperitoneal

Peritoneum offers a large surface area for absorption. Fluids are injected intraperitoneally in infants. This route is also used for peritoneal dialysis.

Other Injections

Intrathecal: Drugs can be injected into the subarachnoid space for action on the CNS, e.g. spinal anaesthetics. Some antibiotics and corticosteroids are also injected by this route to produce high local concentrations. Strict aseptic precautions are a must.

Drugs are also given extradurally. Morphine can be given epidurally to produce analgesia. Direct intraventricular administration of drugs may be employed in brain tumors.

Intra-articular: Drugs are injected directly into a joint for the treatment of arthritis and other diseases of the joints, e.g. in rheumatoid arthritis, hydrocortisone is injected into the affected joint. Strict aseptic precautions are required.

Intra-arterial: Intravenous and intra-arterial are intravascular routes. In intra-arterial route, the drug is injected directly into the arteries. It is used only in the treatment of:

1. Peripheral vascular diseases
2. Local malignancies
3. Diagnostic studies like angiograms.

Intramedullary: Injection into a bone marrow—now rarely used.

2. Inhalation

Lungs offer a large surface area for absorption of drugs. Volatile liquids and gases are given by inhalation, e.g. general anaesthetics. In addition, drugs can be administered as solid particles, i.e. solutions of drugs can be atomised and the fine droplets are inhaled as aerosol, e.g. salbutamol. These inhaled drugs and vapours may act locally on the pulmonary epithelium and mucous membranes of the respiratory tract or may also be absorbed through these membranes. The drug delivery by this route is influenced by the particle size and the breathing pattern. Drugs for inhalation are available as metered dose inhalers (MDI), dry powder inhalers (DPI) and nebulizers. In a metered dose inhaler, a solution containing multiple doses of particles of the drug, along with a propellant is stored under high pressure in a container. When the inhaler is activated, a fixed amount of the drug jets out of an orifice as a mist. In a dry powder inhaler, the drug is stored in a dry powder form. Nebulizers have the advantages that they do not require a propellant and the drug is delivered as small droplets which are breathed into the lungs.

Advantages

- Almost instantaneous absorption of the drug is achieved because of:
  - The large surface area of the lungs
  - Thin alveolar membrane
  - High vascularity
- In pulmonary diseases, inhalation serves almost as a local route as the drug is delivered at the desired site making it more effective and less harmful.
- Because the drug is directly delivered, smaller dose is needed and, therefore, toxicity is much less.
- Hepatic first pass metabolism is avoided.
- Blood levels of volatile anaesthetics can be conveniently controlled as their absorption and excretion through the lungs are governed by the laws of gases.

Disadvantages

- Irritant gases may enhance pulmonary secretion—should be avoided.
- Drug particles may induce cough, e.g. cromolyn sodium.

This is an important route of entry of certain drugs of abuse.

3. Transdermal

Highly lipid-soluble drugs can be applied over the skin for slow and prolonged absorption, e.g. nitroglycerine ointment in angina pectoris. Adhesive units, inunction, iontophoresis and jet injection are some forms of transdermal drug delivery.

***Adhesive units*:** Transdermal adhesive units (transdermal therapeutic systems) are adhesive patches (Fig. 1.2) of different sizes and shapes made to suit the area of application. The drug is held in a reservoir between an outer polymer layer and a porous membrane. The under surface of the membrane is smeared with an adhesive to hold on to the area of application. The drug slowly diffuses through the membrane and percutaneous absorption takes place. The rate of absorption is constant and predictable. Highly potent drugs (because small quantity is sufficient) and short-acting drugs (because

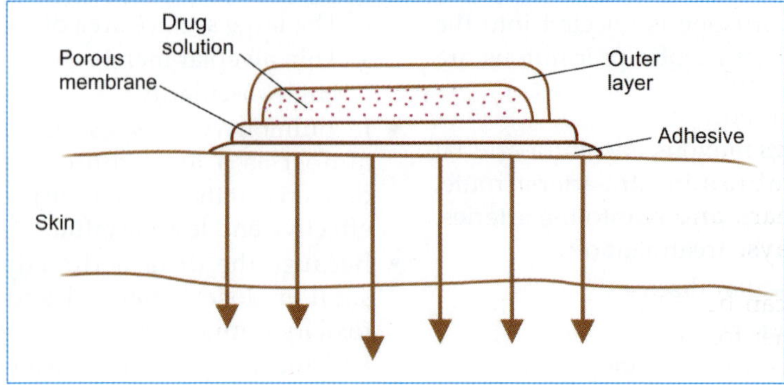

Fig. 1.2: Transdermal adhesive unit

effect terminates quickly after the system is removed) are suitable for use in such systems.

Sites of application depend on the indication—they may be applied over the chest, abdomen, upper arm, back or mastoid region; testosterone patch is applied over the scrotum.

For examples: Hyoscine, nitroglycerin, testosterone, oestrogen, nicotine and fentanyl transdermal patches (Table 1.2).

Advantages

- Duration of action is prolonged
- Provides constant plasma drug levels
- Patient compliance is good.

Disadvantages

- Large doses of the drug cannot be loaded into the system
- Can cause irritation to the skin
- Expensive.

Inunction: The route where a drug rubbed into the skin gets absorbed to produce systemic effects is called inunction.

Iontophoresis: Since flow of electricity enhances the permeability of the skin, in this procedure, galvanic current is used for bringing about penetration of lipid-insoluble drugs into the deeper tissues where their action is required, e.g. salicylates. Fluoride iontophoresis is used in the treatment of dental hypersensitivity.

Jet injection: As absorption of the drug occurs across the layers of the skin, dermojet may also be considered as a form of transdermal drug administration.

Table 1.2: Transdermal therapeutic system—some examples

Drug	*Site*	*Indication*
Nitroglycerin	Chest	Angina pectoris
Scopolamine	Mastoid region	Travelling sickness
Estrogen	Waist	Post-menopausal syndrome
Nicotine	Forearm/arm	To stop smoking
Testosterone	Scrotum, back, thigh	Deficiency
Fentanyl	Upper arm/back	Analgesic

LOCAL/TOPICAL APPLICATION

Drugs may be applied on the skin for local action as ointment, cream, gel, powder, paste, etc. Drugs may also be applied on the mucous membrane as in the eyes, conjunctiva, ears and nose as ointment, drops and sprays.

***Nasal*:** Drugs can be administered through nasal route either for systemic absorption or for local effects.

For example, for systemic absorption, oxytocin spray is used.

For local effect—decongestant nasal drops, e.g. oxymetazoline; budesonide nasal spray for allergic rhinitis.

Many drugs are administered as **suppository** for rectum, **bougie** for urethra and **pessary** and douche for vagina. Pessaries are oval-shaped tablets to be placed in the vagina to provide high local concentrations of the drug at the site, e.g. antifungal pessaries in vaginal candidiasis.

Douche is an aqueous solution used for rinsing a body cavity. Though the word 'douche' is generally used for vaginal solutions, it can also be used for solutions meant for bladder or the rectum.

Mnemonic for advantages and disadvantages of prodrugs.

TATA Safari for Long Drive

T—↑ Tolerability
A—↑ Availability
T—Targeting possible
A—↓ ADR
S—Stability better
L—in Liver disease—not activated
D—↑ Duration of action

1–5 From Medical Council of India, *Competency based Undergraduate Curriculum for the Indian Medical Graduate*, 2018;1:136–144.

CHAPTER 2

Pharmacokinetics

Competency achievement: The student should be able to:

PH 1.4 Describe absorption, distribution, metabolism and excretion of drugs.[1]

Pharmacokinetics is the study of the absorption, distribution, metabolism and excretion of drugs, i.e. the movement of the drugs into, within and out of the body. For a drug to produce its specific response, it should be present in adequate concentrations at the site of action. This depends on various factors apart from the dose. Once the drug is administered, it is absorbed, i.e. enters the blood, is distributed to different parts of the body, reaches the site of action, is metabolised and excreted (Fig. 2.1). All these processes involve passage of the drug molecules across various barriers—like the intestinal epithelium, cell membrane, renal filtering membrane, capillary barrier and so on. To cross these barriers, the drug has to cross the cell membrane or pass in-between the epithelial or endothelial cells.

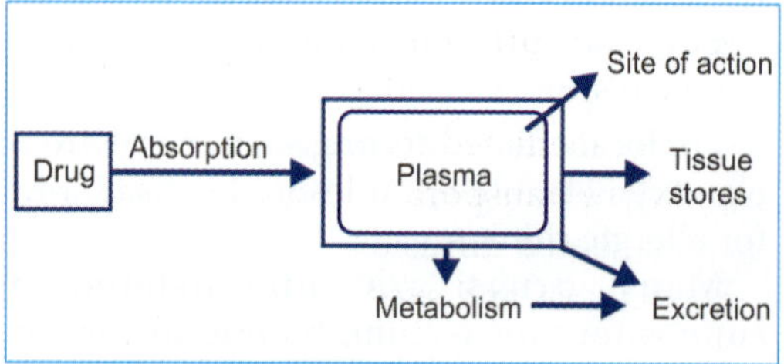

Fig. 2.1: Schematic representation of movement of drug in the body

The cell membrane/biological membrane is made up of two layers of phospholipids with intermingled protein molecules (Fig. 2.2). All lipid-soluble substances get dissolved in the cell membrane and readily permeate into the cells.

The junctions between adjacent epithelial or endothelial cells have pores through which

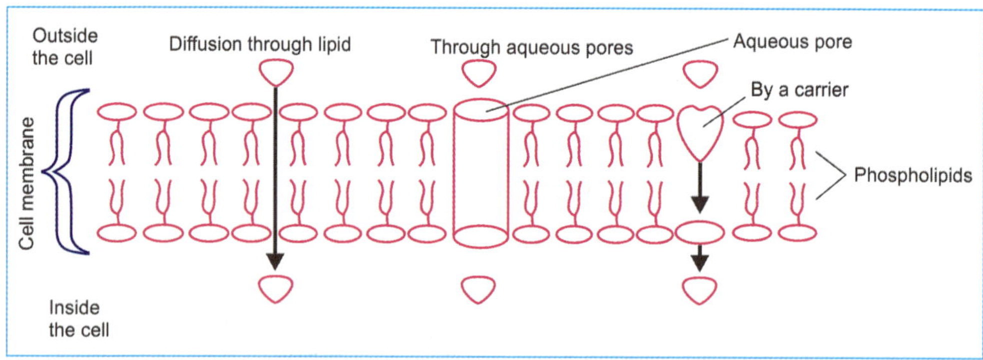

Fig. 2.2: Movement of drugs across biological membrane

small water-soluble molecules can pass. Movement of some specific substances is regulated by special carrier proteins. The passage of drugs across biological membranes or drug permeation involves processes like passive (filtration, diffusion) and active transports.

TRANSPORT OF DRUGS ACROSS BIOLOGICAL MEMBRANES

1. Passive transfer
   - Simple diffusion
   - Filtration
2. Carrier-mediated transport
   - Active transport
   - Facilitated diffusion
3. Endocytosis and exocytosis

Passive Transfer

The drug moves across a membrane without any need for energy.

Simple Diffusion

Simple diffusion is the transfer of a drug across the membrane in the direction of its concentration gradient. The speed of diffusion depends on the degree of concentration gradient, lipid solubility and ionisation. Higher the concentration gradient, faster is the diffusion across the membrane. Lipid-soluble, unionized drugs are rapidly transferred across membranes by simple diffusion—after dissolving in the lipids of the cell membrane (also called lipid diffusion). Most drugs follow simple diffusion.

Filtration

Filtration is the passage of drugs through aqueous pores in the membrane. Water-soluble drugs with molecular size (mol. wt. <100) smaller than the diameter of the pores (7Å) cross the biological membranes by filtration or aqueous diffusion. The movement is along the concentration gradient, e.g. urea.

The capillaries in certain tissues, like the brain and testes, lack the aqueous pores and may also contain efflux pumps. Thus many drugs do not reach them and are called **'sanctuary sites'**.

Carrier-mediated Transport

Transport of certain substances, which cannot move by diffusion, is aided by specific carriers.

Active Transport

Active transport is the transfer of drugs against a concentration gradient and needs energy. It is carried by a specific carrier protein. Only drugs related to natural metabolites are transported by this process, e.g. levodopa, iron, sugars and amino acids. The compound binds to a specific carrier on one side of the membrane and moves across the cell. At the other side of the cell, the complex dissociates and the carrier moves back to transport another molecule. Other substances competing for the same mechanism for transport may interfere with drug movement because this process is saturable, e.g. when penicillin and probenecid are administered together, the duration of action of penicillin is prolonged because both of them compete for renal tubular secretion.

Facilitated Diffusion

Facilitated diffusion is a unique form of carrier transport which differs from active transport in that it is not energy dependent and the movement occurs in the direction of the concentration gradient. The carrier facilitates diffusion and is highly specific for the substance, e.g. uptake of glucose by cells, vitamin B_{12} from intestines.

Endocytosis and Exocytosis

Endocytosis is the process where small droplets are engulfed by the cell membrane and carried into the cell as a vesicle. The vesicular membrane is then broken down to release the substances. Some proteins and vitamin B_{12} with the help of intrinsic factor are taken up by this process (like pinocytosis in amoeba). This process is currently being tried for delivery of some anticancer drugs to the tissues. The reverse process—exocytosis is responsible for secretion of many substances from cells, e.g. neurotransmitters stored in nerve endings.

ABSORPTION

Absorption is defined as the passage of the drug from the site of administration into the circulation. For a drug to reach its site of action, it must pass through various membranes depending on the route of administration. Absorption occurs by one of the processes described above, i.e. passive diffusion or carrier-mediated transport. Thus except for intravenous route, the drug needs to be absorbed from all other routes of administration. The rate and extent of absorption varies with the route of administration.

Absorption from the Gut

Medication taken orally may be absorbed from any part of the gut. Highly lipid-soluble drugs may be absorbed from the buccal cavity from where it directly enters the systemic circulation. Acidic drugs are absorbed from the stomach, while basic drugs get ionised in the stomach and are not absorbed from the stomach (*see* below).

Intestines have a large surface area and most drugs are absorbed from the proximal part of the jejunum. Basic drugs are absorbed from the intestines because of the favourable pH. Various factors, like intestinal motility and pH, influence absorption from the gut. Absorption from the large intestine is negligible.

It has now been found that certain drugs may be transported out from the cells of the intestinal wall back into the gut lumen. This is done with a reverse transporter or efflux transporter P-glycoprotein.

Factors Influencing Drug Absorption

Several factors influence the rate and extent of absorption of a drug given orally (Fig. 2.3).

A. *Pharmaceutical factors*

1. **Disintegration and dissolution time:** The drug taken orally should break up into individual particles (disintegrate) to be absorbed. It then has to dissolve in the gastrointestinal fluids and the rate at which it dissolves influences absorption. In case of drugs given subcutaneously or intramuscularly, the drug molecules have to dissolve in the tissue fluids. Liquids are absorbed faster than solids. Delay in disintegration and dissolution as with poorly water-soluble drugs like aspirin, results in delayed absorption.
2. **Formulation:** Pharmaceutical preparations are formulated to produce desired absorption. Inert substances used with drugs as diluents like starch and lactose may sometimes interfere with absorption.
3. **Particle size:** Small particle size is important for better absorption of drugs. Drugs like corticosteroids, griseofulvin, digoxin, aspirin and tolbutamide are better absorbed when given as small particles. On the other hand, when a drug has to act on the gut and its absorption is not desired, then particle size should be kept large, e.g. anthelmintics like bephenium hydroxynaphthoate.

B. *Drug factors*

4. **Lipid solubility:** Lipid-soluble drugs are absorbed faster and better by dissolving in the phospholipids of the cell membrane.
5. **pH and ionisation:** Ionised drugs are poorly absorbed while unionised drugs are lipid-soluble and are well absorbed. Strong electrocytes are almost completely ionised at both acidic and alkaline pH. However, most drugs are weak electrolytes and exist in both ionised and unionised forms. The degree of ionisation depends on the pH of the medium. Thus acidic drugs remain unionised in acidic

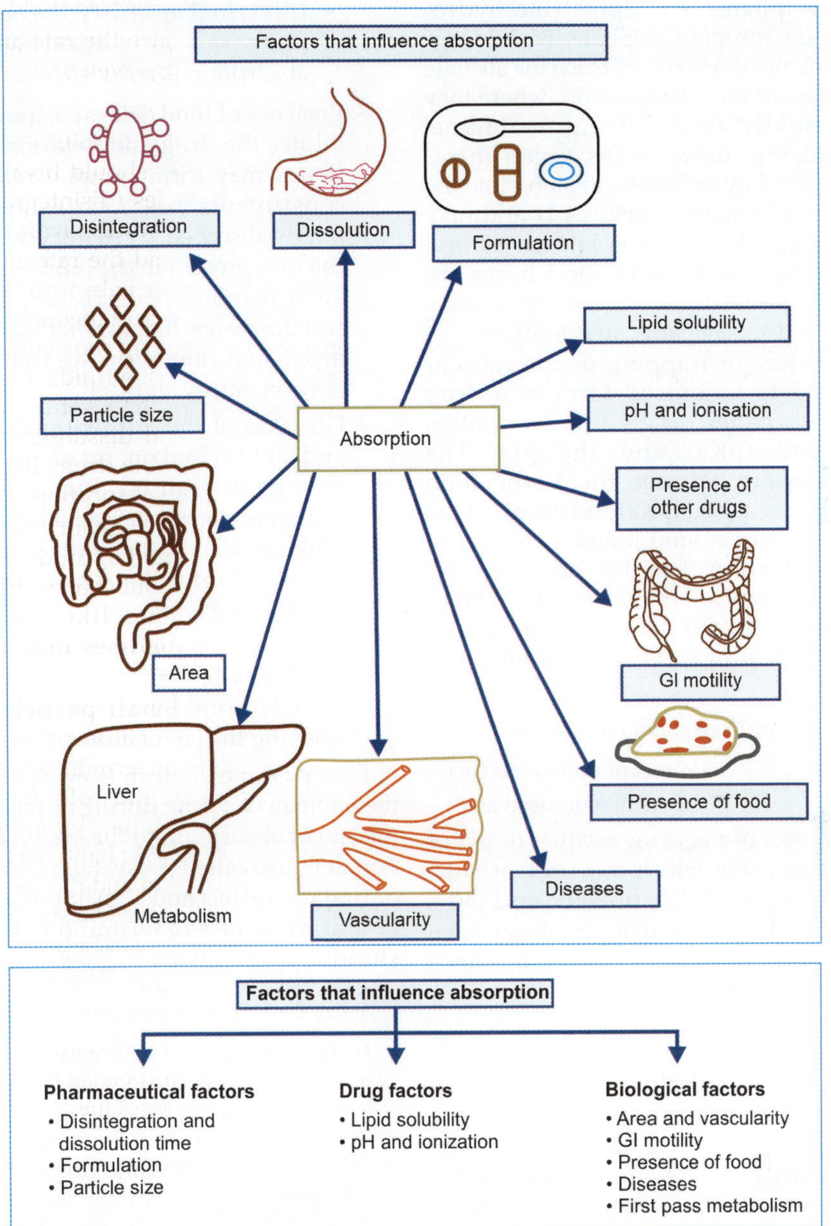

Fig. 2.3: Factors affecting absorption of drugs

medium of the stomach and are rapidly absorbed from the stomach, e.g. aspirin, barbiturates. Weakly acidic drugs form salts with bases and are available for use as sodium or potassium salts, e.g. phenobarbitone sodium, potassium penicillin-V. Weakly basic drugs form salts with acids and thus we have their hydrochlorides and sulphates, e.g. ephedrine hydrochloride, atropine sulphate. Basic drugs are unionised when they reach the alkaline medium of the intestine from where they are rapidly absorbed, e.g. pethidine, ephedrine. Basic drugs given intravenously may diffuse from blood into the stomach because of acidic pH and may ionise quickly. This is known as 'ion trapping'. Strong acids and bases are highly ionised and, therefore, poorly absorbed, e.g. heparin, streptomycin.

The extent of trapping or the ratio of ionised to unionised form of a drug depends on the drug's acid dissociation constant (pKa) and the pH. The relationship between the dissociation constant of a drug (pKa) and the pH of the environment around it and the extent of its ionisation can be obtained by **Henderson-Hasselbalch equation**. From the equation, the ratio of the unionised form of the drug to its ionised form can be obtained.

Henderson-Hasselbalch equation

$$pKa = pH + \log \frac{\text{Concn. of nonionised acid}}{\text{Concn. of ionised acid}}$$

when pKa of the drug is equal to pH of the medium in which it is present, then the drug is 50% ionised and 50% unionised. In general, acidic drugs have low pKa (2.5–6), while basic drugs have higher pKa (8–10).

C. *Biological factors*

6. **Area and vascularity of the absorbing surface:** The larger the area of the absorbing surface and more the vascularity—better is the absorption. Thus most drugs are absorbed from the small intestine.

7. **Gastrointestinal motility**
   - Gastric emptying time—if gastric emptying is faster, the passage of the drug to the intestines is quicker and hence absorption is faster.
   - Intestinal motility—when highly increased as in diarrhoeas, drug absorption is reduced.

8. **Presence of food** delays gastric emptying, dilutes the drug and delays absorption. Drugs may form complexes with food constituents and such complexes are poorly absorbed, e.g. tetracyclines chelate calcium present in the food—hence their bioavailability is decreased. Moreover, certain drugs like ampicillin, roxithromycin and rifampicin are well absorbed only on empty stomach.

9. **Diseases** of the gut like malabsorption and achlorhydria result in reduced absorption of drugs. Particularly acidic drugs are poorly absorbed in presence of achlorhydria. In the absence of intrinsic factor, vitamin B_{12} is not absorbed in pernicious anemia.

10. **First pass metabolism:** Some drugs may be degraded in the GI tract, e.g. nitroglycerine, insulin (*see* below) before reaching the circulation.

First pass metabolism (Key Box 2.1) is the metabolism of a drug during its passage from the site of absorption to the systemic circulation. It is also called **presystemic metabolism** or **first pass effect** and is an important feature of oral route of administration. Such drugs should be given in higher doses or by

 **Key Box 2.1:** First pass metabolism

- First pass metabolism is the metabolism of a drug during its first passage through the gut wall and liver to the systemic circulation
- Reduces bioavailability
- Extent of metabolism depends on the drug and individuals
- *Examples:* Morphine, chlorpromazine, nitroglycerin, verapamil, testosterone, insulin, lignocaine, salbutamol
- Measures to compensate first pass effect
  - Dose has to be increased for some drugs like propranolol
  - Route has to be changed for some others like hydrocortisone, insulin.

alternative routes. Drugs given orally may be metabolised in the gut wall and in the liver before reaching the systemic circulation. The extent of first pass metabolism differs from drug to drug and among individuals from partial to total inactivation.

Clinical Significance

When it is partial, it can be compensated by giving higher dose of the particular drug, e.g. nitroglycerine, propranolol, salbutamol. For drugs that undergo complete first pass metabolism, the route of administration has to be changed, e.g. isoprenaline, hydrocortisone, insulin.

Bioavailability of many drugs is increased in patients with liver disease due to reduction in hepatic metabolism.

Extent of first pass metabolism may vary between individuals and fixing the dose may be a problem.

Absorption from Parenteral Routes

On **intravenous administration,** the drug directly reaches the circulation (Fig. 2.4). On **intramuscular injection,** the drug is deposited in the muscles and the drug molecules should dissolve in the tissue fluids and then be absorbed. Since muscles have a rich blood supply, absorption is fast. Drug molecules diffuse through the capillary membrane and reach the circulation. Lipid-soluble drugs are absorbed faster.

Absorption from **subcutaneous administration** is slower but rate of absorption is somewhat steady. Hyaluronidase increases rate of absorption.

Inhaled drugs are rapidly absorbed from the pulmonary epithelium particularly the lipid-soluble ones.

On topical application, highly lipid-soluble drugs are absorbed from the intact skin, e.g. nitroglycerine; but absorption is relatively slow because of the multiple layers of closely-packed cells in the epidermis. Most drugs are readily absorbed from the mucous membranes.

BIOAVAILABILITY

Definition: Bioavailability is the fraction (F) of the administered drug that reaches the

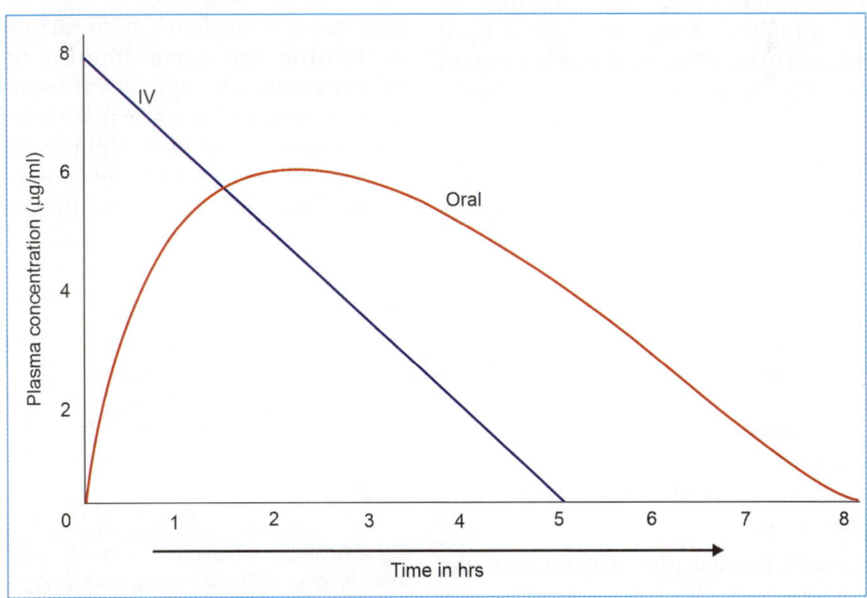

Fig. 2.4: Plasma concentration–time curve of a drug following a single oral and IV dose

systemic circulation in unchanged form following administration by any route.

Thus, when a drug is given intravenously, the bioavailability is 100%. On IM/SC injection and sublingual administration, drugs are almost completely absorbed (bioavailability >75%) while by oral route, bioavailability may be low due to incomplete absorption and first pass metabolism, e.g. bioavailability of chlortetracycline is 30%, carbamazepine—70%, chloroquine—80%, minocycline and diazepam almost 100%.

Transdermal preparations are absorbed systemically and may have 80–100% bioavailability while for rectal administration it may be 30% to almost 100%. Large bioavailability variations of a drug, particularly when it is unpredictable, can result in toxicity or therapeutic failure as in case of halofantrine.

Factors that influence bioavailability: In fact, all the ten factors which influence the absorption of a drug including the pharmaceutical factors, drug factors and biological factors also alter bioavailability. Drugs which undergo extensive first pass metabolism have a low bioavailability. In general, unionised drugs with good lipid solubility and of small particle size have good bioavailability since they are well absorbed.

Determining bioavailability: The drug is injected intravenously and its plasma concentration is measured at one hourly intervals. The plasma concentration is plotted against time on a graph paper. Similarly plasma concentration–time graph is also obtained, after oral administration of the same dose of the drug. Once these curves are obtained, the area under the curve (AUC) is measured (Fig. 2.5). From such a curve, we know the maximum concentration attained following absorption (E_{max}), the time taken for it (T_{max}) and the extent of absorption from area under the curve.

Bioavailability is calculated by the formula:

$$\text{Bioavailability (F)} = \frac{\text{AUC (oral)} \times 100}{\text{AUC (IV)}}$$

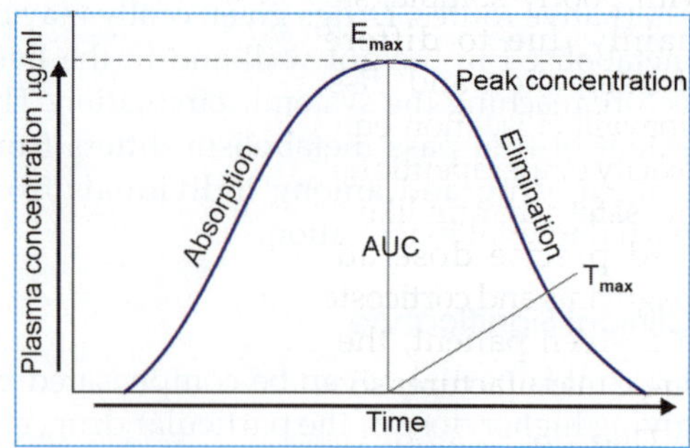

Fig. 2.5: Graph showing peak plasma concentration (E_{max}), time to peak plasma concentration (T_{max}) and area under the curve (AUC) which are the parameters of bioavailability

EQUIVALENCE

1. Chemical equivalence: If two-dosage forms of a drug contain the same amount of the drug, they are said to be chemically equivalent.

2. Bioequivalence: If two formulations of a drug have the same bioavailability, they are bioequivalent.

Comparison of bioavailability of different formulations of the same drug is the study of bioequivalence. If two drug formulations have the same bioavailability and rate of absorption, they are bioequivalent. Often oral formulations containing the same amount of a drug (pharmaceutically equivalent) from different manufacturers may result in different plasma concentrations, or may differ in the rate of absorption, i.e. there is no bioequivalence among them (Fig. 2.6). Such differences occur

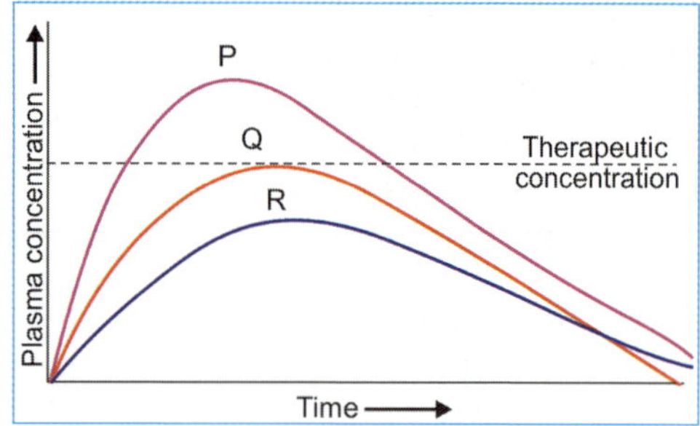

Fig. 2.6: Study of bioequivalence—three different oral formulations—P, Q and R of the same drug yield different bioavailability values. The area under each curve gives the bioavailability of the respective formulation

with poorly soluble, slowly absorbed drugs, mainly due to differences in the rate of disintegration and dissolution. Variation in bioavailability (non-equivalence) can result in toxicity or therapeutic failure of drugs that have low safety margin like digoxin and drugs that need precise dose adjustments like anticoagulants and corticosteroids. For such drugs, in a given patient, the preparations from a single manufacturer should be used.

3. Therapeutic equivalence: If two drugs produce the same therapeutic response, they are said to be therapeutically equivalent. For example, if drug A and drug B can produce the same degree of diuresis, they are said to be therapeutically equivalent.

DISTRIBUTION

After a drug reaches the systemic circulation, it gets distributed to other tissues. It should cross several barriers before reaching the site of action. Like absorption, distribution also involves the same processes, i.e. filtration, diffusion and specialized transport. Various factors determine the rate and extent of distribution, viz. lipid solubility, ionization, blood flow and binding to plasma proteins and cellular proteins. Unionized lipid-soluble drugs are widely distributed throughout the body.

Plasma Protein Binding

On reaching the circulation, most drugs bind to plasma proteins; acidic drugs bind mainly albumin and basic drugs to alpha-acid glycoprotein. The free or unbound fraction of the drug is the only form available for action, metabolism and excretion while the protein bound form serves as a reservoir (Fig. 2.7). The extent of protein binding varies with each drug, e.g. warfarin is 99% and morphine is 35% protein bound while binding of ethosuximide and lithium is 0%, i.e. they are totally free (Table 2.1).

Some drugs also bind to tissue proteins (*see* as follows) and specific carrier proteins (e.g. corticosteroids to transcortin, iron to ferritin).

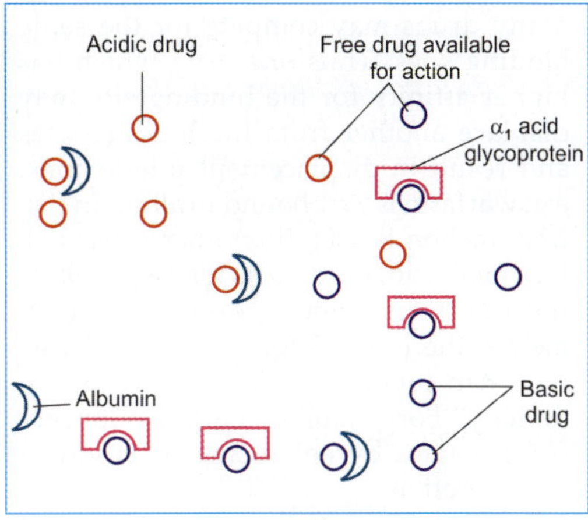

Fig. 2.7: Plasma protein binding

Table 2.1: Some highly protein bound drugs

Warfarin	Tolbutamide	Phenytoin
Frusemide	Clofibrate	Sulfonamides
Diazepam	Salicylates	Phenylbutazone
Indomethacin		

Some drugs not bound to plasma proteins

Isoniazid	Lisinopril
Lithium	Ethosuximide
Metformin	

Clinical Significance of Plasma Protein Binding

1. Only free fraction is available for action, metabolism and excretion. When the free drug levels in the plasma fall, bound drug is released. Thus protein binding may delay the drug reaching the site of action.
2. Protein binding serves as a store (reservoir) of the drug and the drug is released when free drug levels fall.
3. Protein binding prolongs the half-life and thereby the duration of action of the drug because the bound form is protected from metabolism and excretion. Bound form is not filtered at the glomerulus and the excretion is therefore delayed. Highly protein bound drugs are generally long-acting.

4. Many drugs may compete for the same binding sites. Thus one drug which has higher affinity for the binding site may displace another from the binding sites and result in displacement interactions, e.g. warfarin is 99% bound to albumin (i.e. free fraction is 1%). If another drug, like indomethacin, reduces its binding to 95%, the free form then becomes 5% which means, there is a 5-fold increase in free warfarin levels which could result in toxicity. Fortunately, the body largely compensates by enhancing metabolism and excretion.
5. Protein binding sites may get saturated with repeated administration of the drug and thereafter more and more drug will remain in the free form.
6. *Low albumin:* Nephrotic syndrome, chronic renal failure and chronic liver disease result in hypoalbuminaemia with reduced protein binding of drugs leading to raised levels of free drug. The normal plasma albumin concentration is 0.6 mm/litre. Highly protein bound drugs should be carefully used in such patients because even therapeutic doses of such drugs can result in toxicity and may require dose reduction.
7. In pregnancy, there is an increase in thyroxine binding protein levels resulting in reduced free thyroxine levels.
8. In acute inflammatory states, alpha 1 acid glycoprotein levels may rise resulting in more extensive binding and thereby lower free drug levels—hence, higher doses may be needed.

Tissue Binding

Some drugs get bound to certain tissue constituents because of special affinity for them as given in Key Box 2.2.

Tissue binding delays elimination and thus prolongs duration of action of the drug. For example, lipid-soluble drugs are bound to adipose tissue. Tissue binding also serves as a **reservoir** of the drug.

Key Box 2.2: Special affinity of drugs for tissues

Tissue	*Binding drugs*
Adipose tissue	Thiopentone sodium, benzodiazepines
Muscles	Emetine
Bone	Tetracyclines, lead
Retina	Chloroquine
Thyroid	Iodine

Redistribution

When some highly lipid-soluble drugs are given intravenously or by inhalation, they get rapidly distributed into highly perfused tissues like the brain, heart and kidney. But soon they get redistributed into less vascular tissues like the muscle and fat resulting in termination of the action of these drugs. The best example is the intravenous anaesthetic thiopental sodium which induces anaesthesia in 10–20 seconds but the effect ceases in 5–15 minutes due to redistribution.

BloodñBrain Barrier (BBB)

The endothelial cells of the brain capillaries lack intercellular pores and instead have tight junctions. Moreover, glial cells envelope the capillaries and together these form the BBB. Drugs have to pass through the cells to cross the barrier (Key Box 2.3). Only lipid-soluble, unionised drugs can cross this BBB. During inflammation of the meninges, the barrier becomes more permeable to drugs, e.g. penicillin readily penetrates during meningitis. The barrier is weak at some areas like CTZ, posterior pituitary and parts of hypothalamus and allows some compounds to diffuse. Since the pH of CSF is 7.35, weakly basic drugs concentrate in it more than the acidic drugs.

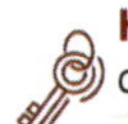

Key Box 2.3: Sites which are 'difficult to enter' for drugs

- CSF
- Lymph
- Ocular fluids
- Pleural fluids
- Synovial fluid

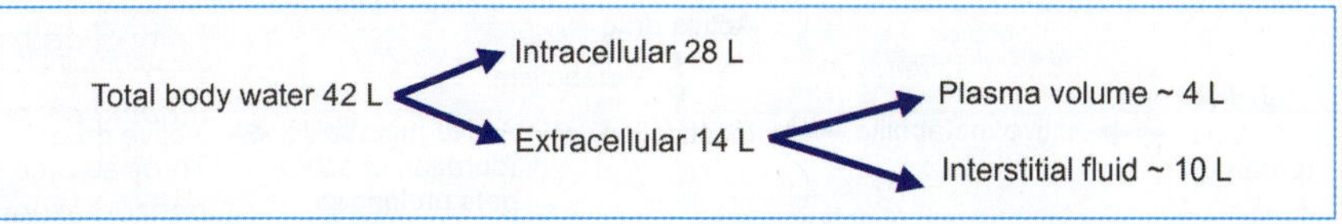

Placental Barrier

Lipid-soluble, unionised drugs readily cross the placenta while lipid-insoluble drugs cross to a much lesser extent. Thus drugs taken by the mother can cause several unwanted effects in the foetus. Lipid-soluble drugs with molecular weight of about 200–500 can easily cross the placenta while those with large molecular size (mol.wt >1000) can hardly cross the placenta. These require transporters for crossing the placenta.

VOLUME OF DISTRIBUTION (V)

For the purpose of pharmacokinetic studies, body can be considered as a single compartment into which drugs are distributed uniformly. Each drug actually follows its own pattern of distribution from plasma to other body fluids and tissues.

Apparent Volume of Distribution

Apparent volume of distribution is a hypothetical concept. This is defined as the volume necessary to accommodate the entire amount of the drug administered, if the concentration throughout the body is equal to that in plasma. It can also be defined as the volume in which the drug can be evenly distributed, if the concentration attained was equal to that in plasma. It is called 'apparent' as the volume here is 'apparently' needed to hold the drug and the uniform distribution of the drug is presumed. It relates the amount of the drug in the body to the concentration (C) of the drug in plasma. The volume so calculated can be more than the total body water and is therefore called the 'apparent' volume of distribution. It is calculated as:

$$V = \frac{\text{Amount of drug in the body}}{\text{Plasma concentration (C)}}$$

e.g. if the dose of a drug given is 500 mg and it attains a uniform concentration of 10 mg/litre of plasma in the body, its $V = 50$ litres.

Important facts about V are:

- If a drug is retained mostly in the plasma, its *V* is small (e.g. aspirin, aminoglycosides) while if it is distributed widely in tissues, then its *V* is large (e.g. pethidine). *V* may vary with changes in tissue permeability and protein binding as seen in some diseases.
- Highly lipid-soluble drugs that get sequestered in the adipocytes have a large *V* (e.g. chloroquine ~13000 L). Drugs with

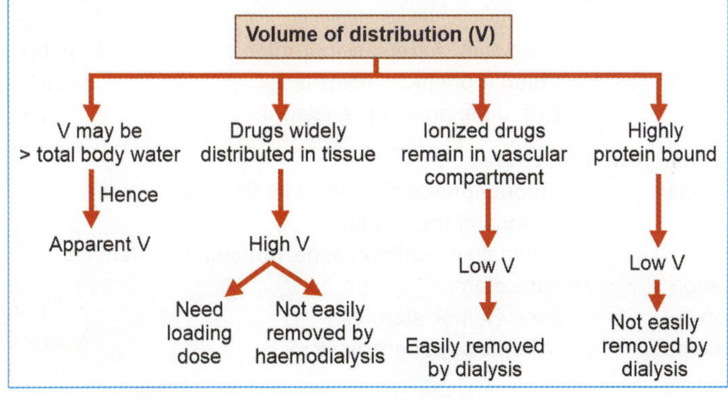

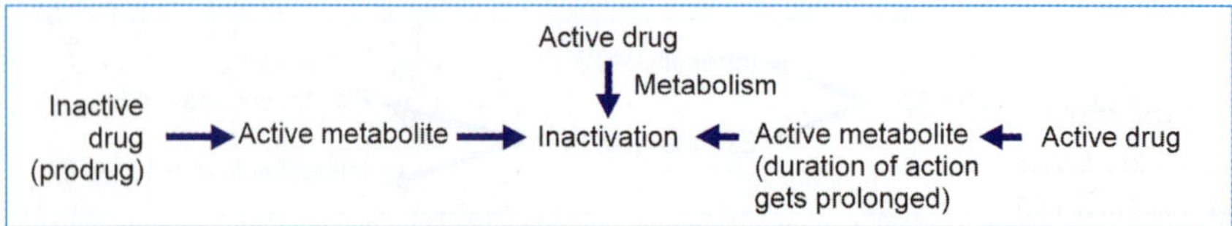

Fig. 2.8: Biotransformation

large *V* need to be given as loading dose (e.g. chloroquine) to attain therapeutic concentration. Drugs extensively bound to plasma proteins have a low *V* (~3L), e.g. phenylbutazone and are not easily removed by hemodialysis.

- Ionised drugs have a low 'V' as they remain in the vascular compartment. Low *V* drugs may have a larger *V* in presence of oedema or ascites due to increased ECF volume.
- In conditions like CCF, uraemia and cirrhosis, *V* could change since reduced perfusion of tissues would lead to reduced *V*.
- The knowledge of *V* of drugs is clinically important in the treatment of poisoning. Drugs with large *V* like pethidine are not easily removed by haemodialysis because such drugs are widely distributed in the body. **Factors affecting *V***—plasma protein binding, pKa of the drug, lipid solubility (directly proportional to V) special affinity for the tissues and diseases like cirrhosis and CCF.

BIOTRANSFORMATION (METABOLISM)

Biotransformation is the process of biochemical alteration of the drug in the body. Body treats most drugs as foreign substances (called xenobiotics) and tries to inactivate and eliminate them by various biochemical reactions. These processes convert the non-polar, lipid soluble drugs into more polar, water-soluble compounds so that they are easily excreted through the kidneys and not reabsorbed. Some drugs may be excreted largely unchanged in the urine, e.g. frusemide, atenolol (Figs 2.8, 2.9 and Table 2.2)

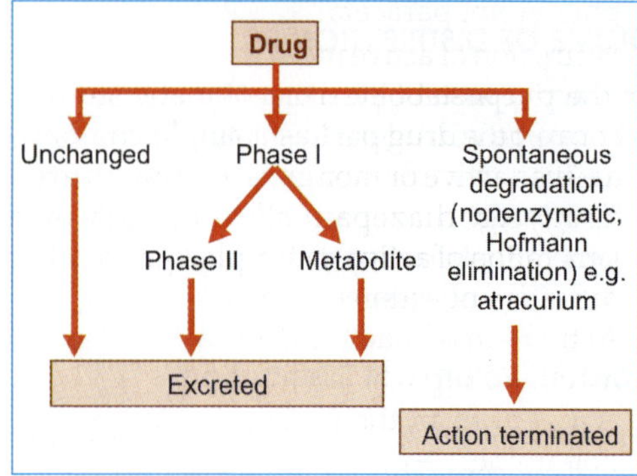

Fig. 2.9: Phases in metabolism of drugs. A drug may be excreted as phase I metabolite or as phase II metabolite. Some drugs may be excreted as such

Table 2.2: Important drug biotransformation reactions

Reactions	*Examples of drugs*
Phase I reactions	
Oxidation	Phenytoin, diazepam, ibuprofen, amphetamine, chlorpromazine, dapsone
Reduction	Chloramphenicol, halothane
Hydrolysis	Pethidine, procaine, enalapril
Phase II reactions (conjugation reactions)	
Glucuronide conjugation	Chloramphenicol, morphine, diazepam, aspirin
Acetylation	Sulfonamides, isoniazid
Methylation	Adrenaline, noradrenaline, dopamine, histamine
Glutathione conjugation	Paracetamol
Sulphate conjugation	Paracetamol, steroids
Amino acid conjugation	Salicylic acid, benzoic acid

Site

The most important organ of biotransformation is the liver. Drugs are also metabolised though to a small extent by the kidney, gut mucosa, lungs, blood and skin.

Consequences of Biotransformation

Though biotransformation generally inactivates the drug, some drugs may be converted to metabolites which are also active or more active than the parent drug.

Biotransformation reactions may result in any or all of the following (Table 2.3)

1. **Inactivation**—Largely biotransformation inactivates the drug and most drugs are converted to inactive metabolites, e.g. phenytoin, paracetamol, phenobarbitone.
2. Formation of active metabolite—(active drug to active metabolite) biotransformation may convert the drug partly to metabolites which are also active or more active than the parent drug, e.g. diazepam to oxazepam; such generation of active metabolites prolongs the duration of action of the drug.
3. Activation of inactive drug—prodrug is an inactive drug which gets converted into an active drug in the body, e.g. Levodopa to dopamine
4. Formation of toxic metabolite—in case of some drugs, the active metabolite may be toxic. For example, paracetamol is converted to N-acetyl-p-benzoquinoneimine (NAPQI) which causes hepatotoxicity; cyclophosphamide is converted to acrolein which causes bladder toxicity.

Some drugs may be converted to epoxides which are short acting but highly reactive molecules. They bind to cells and tissues resulting in toxicity. Epoxide-induced liver damage is countered to a large extent by glutathione conjugation.

Enzymes in Biotransformation

The biotransformation reactions are catalysed by specific enzymes located either in the liver microsomes (microsomal enzymes) or in the cytoplasm and mitochondria of the liver cells and also in the plasma and other tissues (non-microsomal enzymes).

Microsomal enzymes are a mixed function oxidase system or mono-oxygenases and require nicotine adenine dinucleotide phosphate (NADPH) and oxygen. Microsomal enzymes cytochrome P450 (CYP) are important in the oxidation reduction reactions. There are several isoforms of the P450 enzymes. Several CYP gene families are known, of which the first three—CYP1, CYP2 and CYP3—are important groups. Some isozymes are CYP1A2, CYP2A6, CYP2B6, CYP2C9, CYP2C19, CYP3A4 and are the most important enzymes involved in biotransformation in the liver. CYP3A4 alone is found to metabolise nearly 50% of the drugs degraded in the liver. For naming the enzymes, e.g. in CYP1A2—1-Family; A-Subfamily, 2-Gene.

The chemical reactions of biotransformation can take place in two phases (Fig. 2.9):

1. Phase I (non-synthetic reactions)
2. Phase II (synthetic reactions).

Table 2.3: Consequences of biotransformation with examples

Active drug to inactive metabolite	*Active drug to active metabolite*	*Inactive drug to active metabolite (prodrug)*
Examples	Examples	Examples
• Phenobarbitone → hydroxy phenobarbitone	• Primidone ▸ Phenobarbitone	• Levodopa ▸ Dopamine
• Phenytoin → hydroxyphenytoin	• Digitoxin ▸ Digoxin	• Prednisone ▸ Prednisolone
	• Diazepam ▸ Oxazepam	• Enalapril ▸ Enalaprilat
	• Allopurinol ▸ Alloxanthine	• Bacampicillin ▸ Ampicillin

Phase I Reactions

Phase I reactions convert the drug to a more polar metabolite by oxidation, reduction or hydrolysis.

1. Oxidation is the process of addition of oxygen (or a negatively charged radical) to a drug molecule or removal of hydrogen (or a positively charged radical) from a drug molecule. Oxidation reactions are the most important metabolizing reactions, mostly catalyzed by mono-oxygenases present in the liver (Table 2.4). They are carried on by a system which includes cytochrome P450, NADPH and molecular oxygen. There are several types of oxidation reactions like:

A. *Microsomal oxidation*

i. S-oxidation (sulfoxidation)
 Cimetidine → cimetidine sulfoxide

ii. N-oxidation
 Dapsone → hydroxylamine dapsone

ii. Dealkylation
 Imipramine → desmethylimipramine
 Codeine → morphine

iii. Hydroxylation
 Salicylic acid → gentisic acid
 Phenytoin → hydroxy phenytoin

iv. Deamination
 Amphetamine → Benzyl methyl ketone

B. *Non-microsomal oxidation*

Oxidation can also be catalysed by non-microsomal enzymes like monoamino oxidase, xanthine oxidase, alcohol dehydrogenase and aldehyde dehydrogenase.

Example: Ethyl alcohol → CO_2 + H_2O

2. Reduction may be catalysed by microsomal or non-microsomal enzymes. Microsomal reduction reactions include

i. Nitro reduction
 e.g. Chloramphenicol → Arylamine

ii. Keto reduction
 e.g. Cortisone → hydrocortisone

Disulfiram and nitrites are reduced by **non-microsomal enzymes** (Fig. 2.10).

3. Hydrolysis is the process where a drug molecule is 'split' by the addition of a molecule of water (both microsomal and non-

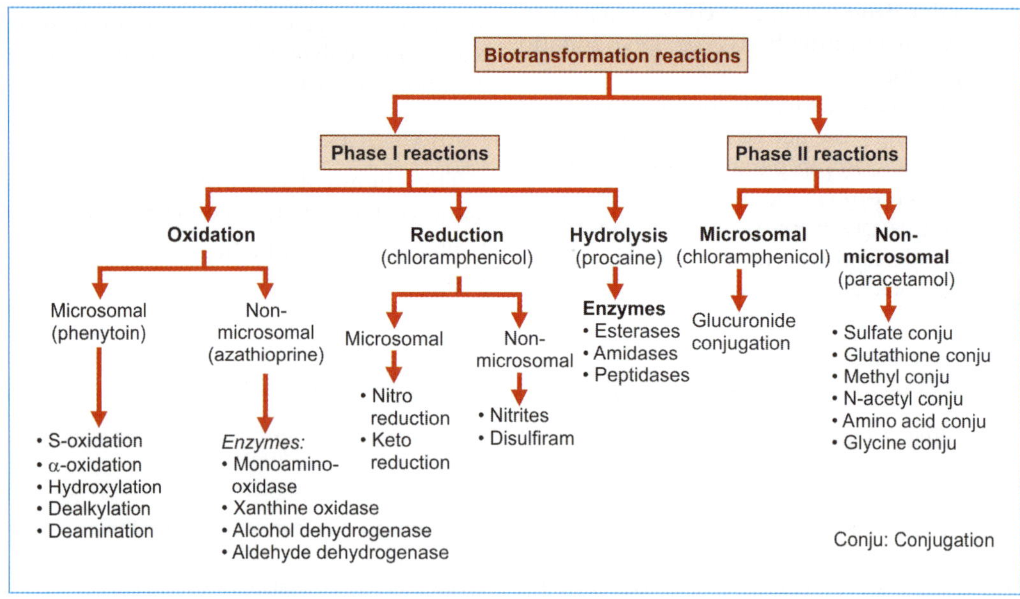

Fig. 2.10: Types of biotransformation reactions with examples

microsomal enzymes may be involved). Esterases, amidases and peptidases catalyze hydrolytic reactions are non-microsomal enzymes.

For example:

Acetylcholine + $H_2O \rightarrow$ Choline + Acetic acid

Other drugs like lignocaine, procaine, atropine, pethidine and neostigmine are metabolized by hydrolysis.

If the metabolite of phase I reaction is not sufficiently polar to be excreted, it undergoes phase II reactions.

Phase II Reactions

In phase II reactions, endogenous water-soluble substances like glucuronic acid, sulfuric acid, glutathione or an amino acid combine with the drug or its phase I metabolite to form a highly polar conjugate which is inactive and gets readily excreted by the kidneys. Large molecules are excreted through the bile. **Conjugation** results invariably in inactivation of the drug. Some products of conjugation are glucuronides, ethereal sulphates and amino acid conjugates.

Microsomal conjugation reaction

Glucuronide conjugation is the most common type of metabolic reaction. Endogenous substances like bilirubin and steroid hormones also undergo conjugation.

The drug or its phase I metabolite undergoes conjugation with uridine diphosphate glucuronic acid (UDPGA) followed by transfer of glucuronic acid to the drug. The reaction is catalysed by the enzyme UDP glucuronyl transferase and the drug—glucuronide conjugate formed is polar, inactive and can be readily excreted through the kidneys.

$$\text{Drug + UDPGA} \xrightarrow[\text{transferase}]{\text{Glucuronyl}} \text{Drug glucuronide + UDP}$$

$$\downarrow$$

Excreted

e.g.

Morphine + Glucuronic acid $\rightarrow$ Morphine glucuronide

The enzyme glucuronyl transferase is not adequately formed in the neonate. Hence bilirubin levels increase and result in **neonatal jaundice**. Grey baby syndrome—an adverse effect to high doses of chloramphenicol seen in neonates is also because of the lack of UDP glucuronyl transferase.

Several endogenous substances involved in conjugation are supplied by the diet. Hence nutrition is also important for conjugation and thereby detoxification of the drugs.

Non-microsomal conjugation reactions

i. **Acetylation (acetyl conjugation):** Drugs like sulfonamides and isoniazid undergo conjugation with acetylcoenzyme A. This acetylation is catalysed by N-acetyl-transferase found in the cytoplasm.
ii. **Methylation (methyl conjugation):** Catecholamines, like adrenaline and dopamine, undergo methyl conjugation or methylation catalyzed by the enzyme transmethylase. The methyl group is donated by methionine and cysteine. The following are other conjugation reactions.
iii. **Glutathione conjugation:** Though a minor pathway of metabolism, glutathione conjugation inactivates highly reactive intermediates formed during the metabolism of drugs like paracetamol. Many epoxides and drugs with nitrate groups undergo glutathione conjugation with the help of the enzyme glutathion-S-transferase.
iv. **Amino acid conjugation** is a minor pathway for metabolism of certain acidic drugs like aspirin, for example: Benzoic acid + glycine $\rightarrow$ Hippuric acid
v. **Sulfate conjugation** is catalyzed by sulfo-transferases, e.g steroids, chloramphenicol, methyldopa. Sulfation can also result in the conversion of minoxidil, a prodrug into its active metabolite.
vi. **Glycine conjugation** though also a minor metabolic pathway, drugs like salicylates are conjugated with glycine.

Hofmann Elimination

Some drugs undergo a unique type of metabolism—they are metabolised by spontaneous degradation due to spontaneous molecular rearrangement in plasma and tissues, e.g. atracurium and cisatracurium—called Hofmann degradation which adds to their short action.

ENZYME INDUCTION

Microsomal enzymes are located in the microsomes that line the smooth endoplasmic reticulum of the liver cells. The **synthesis** of these microsomal enzymes, mainly cytochrome P450, can be enhanced by certain drugs and environmental pollutants. This is called **enzyme induction** and this process speeds up the biotransformation of the inducing drug itself and also other drugs metabolised by the same microsomal enzymes, e.g. phenobarbitone, rifampicin, alcohol, cigarette smoke, DDT (environmental pollutants), griseofulvin, carbamazepine, phenytoin and many antiretroviral drugs like nevirapine and efavirenz are enzyme inducers.

Enzyme induction may be selective for some particular enzymes (as with DDT) or may be nonselective as with phenobarbitone which could induce most microsomal enzymes. Enzyme induction may be blocked by drugs that inhibit protein synthesis. Enzymes are induced gradually and take about 1–2 weeks for peak effect and induction continues till the drug is administered. However, it is reversible and the enzyme levels return to initial levels in about 1–3 weeks. Enzyme induction can enhance drug metabolism by 2–4 times. However, it can also result in toxicity if the metabolite is toxic.

Clinical Relevance of Microsomal Enzyme Induction

1. *Drug interactions*
   a. ***Therapeutic failure:*** By speeding up metabolism, enzyme induction may reduce the duration of action of some other drugs which can result in therapeutic failure, e.g. failure of oral contraceptives in patients taking rifampicin.

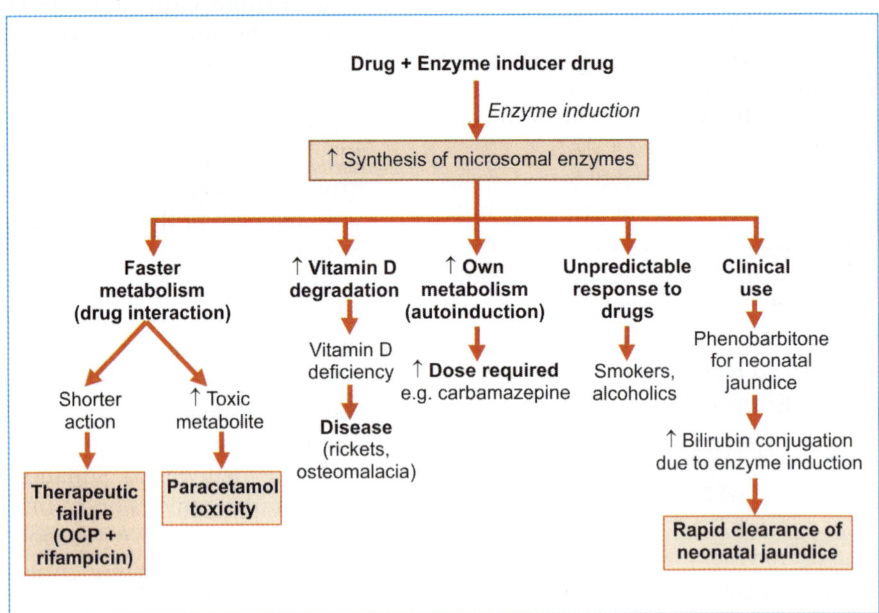

Fig. 2.11: Clinical significance of enzyme induction

b. ***Toxicity:*** Enzyme induction may result in toxicity due to production of higher amounts of the toxic intermediate metabolites, e.g. a patient undergoing treatment with rifampicin is likely to develop hepatotoxicity with paracetamol because a higher amount of the toxic intermediate metabolite of paracetamol is formed due to enzyme induction.

2. *Tolerance to drugs* may develop as in case of carbamazepine since it induces its own metabolism called **autoinduction**.
3. *Result in disease:* Antiepileptics enhance the breakdown of vitamin D resulting in osteomalacia on long-term administration.
4. *Variable response:* In chronic smokers and alcoholics, enzyme induction may result in failure to achieve the expected response to some drugs metabolised by the same enzymes.
5. *Therapeutic application of enzyme induction:* Neonates are deficient in both microsomal and non-microsomal enzymes. Hence their capacity to conjugate bilirubin is low which results in jaundice. Administration of phenobarbitone, an enzyme inducer, helps in rapid clearance of the jaundice in the neonates by enhancing bilirubin conjugation.

Enzyme Inhibition

Some drugs inhibit cytochrome P450 enzyme activity. Drugs like cimetidine bind to cytochrome P450 and competitively inhibit the metabolism of endogenous substances like testosterone and other drugs given concurrently. Enzyme inhibition by drugs is the basis of several drug interactions. Chloramphenicol, erythromycin, ketoconazole, cimetidine, ciprofloxacin and verapamil are some enzyme inhibitors. With some drugs, the binding of enzymes may be irreversible—leading to inactivation of the enzyme. Such substrates are called **suicide inhibitors**, e.g. selegiline, ticlopidine, clopidogrel and prophylthiouracil.

Many of the antiretroviral drugs used in AIDS are enzyme inhibitors.

Drugs could also inhibit other enzymes, i.e. **non-microsomal enzymes**. Such inhibition could be competitive or non-competitive inhibition.

Competitive enzyme inhibitors are structurally similar to the natural substrates and thereby compete for binding to the enzyme. This type of enzyme inhibition may be reversed by higher substrate concentration. For example, xanthine oxidase inhibition by allopurinol. However, if the binding takes place by covalent bonds, then it could be irreversible like organophosphates inhibiting acetylcholinesterase.

Competitive Inhibitors

Drugs	Enzyme inhibited
Captopril	Angiotensin converting enzyme
Allopurinol	Xanthine oxidase
Sulfonamide	Folic acid synthetase
Meclobemide	MAO-A
Neostigmine, organophosphates	Acetylcholinesterase

Non-competitive inhibition: Here there is no structural similarity and the inhibition is generally irreversible because such drugs prevent the formation of enzyme substrate complex by altering the structure of the enzyme. New enzymes need to be synthesized to resume activity. For example, statins inhibiting HMG-CoA reductase.

Non-competitive Inhibitors

Drugs	Enzymes inhibited
Disulfiram	Aldehyde dehydrogenase
Isocarboxazid	Monoamino-oxidase
Statins	HMG-CoA reductase
Digoxin	Na^+-K^+-ATPase
Sildenafil	Phosphodiesterase

Factors that Influence Biotransformation

- *Genetic variation* results in altered metabolism of drugs, e.g. succinylcholine is metabolised very slowly in people with defective pseudocholinesterase resulting in prolonged apnoea.
- *Environmental pollutants,* like cigarette smoke, cause enzyme induction.
- *Age:* At extremes of age, the activity of metabolic enzymes in the liver are low and hence there is increased risk of toxicity with drugs.
- *Diseases of the liver:* Markedly affect metabolism of drugs.

EXCRETION

Drugs are excreted from the body after being converted to water-soluble metabolites while some are directly eliminated without metabolism. The major organs of excretion are the kidneys, the intestine, the biliary system and the lungs. Drugs are also excreted in small amounts in the saliva, sweat and milk.

Renal Excretion

Kidney is the most important organ of drug excretion. The three processes involved in the elimination of drugs through kidneys are glomerular filtration, active tubular secretion and passive tubular reabsorption.

Glomerular Filtration

The rate of filtration through the glomerulus depends on GFR, concentration of free drug in the plasma and its molecular weight. Ionised drugs of low molecular weight (<10,000) are easily filtered through the glomerular membrane.

Active Tubular Secretion

Cells of the proximal tubules actively secrete acids and bases by two transport systems. Thus acids like penicillin, salicylic acid, probenecid, frusemide; bases like amphetamine and histamine are so excreted. Drugs may compete for the same transport system resulting in prolongation of action of each other, e.g. penicillin and probenecid.

Passive Tubular Reabsorption

Passive diffusion of drug molecules can occur in either direction in the renal tubules depending on the drug concentration, lipid solubility and pH. As highly lipid-soluble drugs are largely reabsorbed, their excretion is slow. Acidic drugs get ionised in alkaline urine and are easily excreted while bases are excreted faster in acidic urine. This property is useful in the treatment of poisoning. In poisoning with acidic drugs like salicylates and barbiturates, forced alkaline diuresis (diuretic + sodium bicarbonate + IV fluids) is employed to hasten drug excretion. Similarly, elimination of basic drugs, like quinine and amphetamine, is enhanced by forced acid diuresis.

Faecal and Biliary Excretion

Unabsorbed portions of the orally administered drugs are eliminated through the faeces. Liver transfers acids, bases and unionised molecules into bile by specific acid transport processes. Large water-soluble conjugates are excreted in the bile. Some drugs may get reabsorbed in the lower portion of the gut and are carried back to the liver. Such recycling is called enterohepatic circulation and it prolongs the duration of action of the drug; examples are chloramphenicol, tetracycline, oral contraceptives and erythromycin.

Pulmonary Excretion

The lungs are the main route of elimination for gases and volatile liquids, viz. general anaesthetics and alcohol. The drug is eliminated with the expired air and is dependent on the rate of respiration and the blood flow to the lungs. This also has legal implications in medicolegal practice as the breath analyser is used to measure alcohol levels in the expired air in vehicle drivers.

Other Routes of Excretion

Small amounts of some drugs are eliminated through the sweat and saliva. Excretion in saliva may result in a unique taste of some drugs like phenytoin, clarithromycin; metallic

Table 2.4: Example of drugs that could be toxic to the suckling infant when taken by the mother

Sulphasalazine	Doxepin
Theophylline	Amiodarone
Anticancer drugs	Primidone
Salicylates	Ethosuximide
Chloramphenicol	Phenobarbitone
Nalidixic acid	Phenothiazines

taste with metronidazole, metoclopramide and disulfiram. Drugs like iodide, rifampicin and heavy metals are excreted through sweat.

The excretion of drugs in the milk is in small amounts and is of no significance to the mother. However, for the suckling infant, it may be sometimes important especially because of the infant's immature metabolic and excretory mechanisms. Though most drugs can be taken by the mother without significant toxicity to the child, there are a few exceptions (Table 2.4).

CLINICAL PHARMACOKINETICS

The knowledge of pharmacokinetics is clinically useful for several purposes including selection and adjustment of the dosage regimen, and to obtain optimum effects from a drug. The three most important pharmacokinetic parameters are bioavailability (*see* page 23), volume of distribution (*see* page 27) and clearance.

Clearance (CL)

Clearance is the volume of plasma freed completely of the drug in unit time. It can be calculated by the ratio of the rate of elimination to the plasma concentration.

$$\text{Thus, CL} = \frac{\text{Rate of elimination}}{\text{Plasma concentration}}$$

Clearance is expressed as ml/litre/unit time.

Clearance is the most important factor determining drug concentration and should be considered when any drug is intended for long-term administration.

Drugs are metabolised/eliminated (elimination kinetics) from the body by:

1. First order kinetics: In first order kinetics (linear kinetics), a constant fraction of the drug is metabolised/eliminated per unit time. Most drugs follow first order kinetics and the rate of metabolism/excretion is dependent on their concentration in the body, i.e. it is exponential (Fig. 2.12). It also holds good for absorption of drugs.

2. Zero order kinetics (saturation kinetics or nonlinear kinetics): Here a constant amount of the drug present in the body is metabolised/eliminated per unit time. The amount remains same and does not increase with increase in dose. The metabolic enzymes get saturated and hence with increase in dose, the plasma drug level increases disproportionately resulting in toxicity. Such elimination is known as zero order kinetics.

Some drugs like phenytoin and warfarin are eliminated by both processes, i.e. by first order initially and by zero order at higher concentrations (**mixed order kinetics or Michaelis-Menten kinetics**). Hence, at higher doses, there is accumulation of the drug.

Examples of drugs that follow zero order kinetics:

- Alcohol
- Phenytoin
- Aspirin
- Heparin
- Phenylbutazone.

Plasma Half-life (t½)

Plasma half-life (t½) is the time taken for the plasma concentration of a drug to be reduced to half its value (Fig. 2.13). For example, if a particular dose of a drug is injected intravenously and its plasma concentration is found to be 100 µg/ml and the plasma concentration is estimated every hour and at the end of four hours it falls to 50 µg/ml, then the plasma half-life of the drug is four hours. Four to five half-lives are required for the complete elimination of a drug. Each drug has its own t½ and is an important pharmacokinetic parameter that guides the dosing

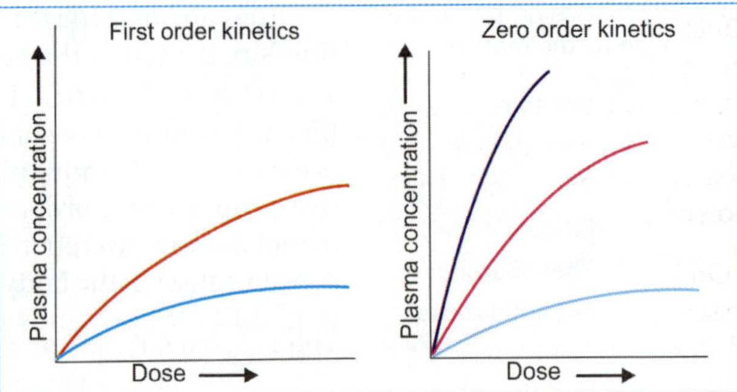

Fig. 2.12: First order kinetics: As the plasma concentration rises, metabolism and excretion proportionately increase. **Zero order kinetics:** In higher doses, the drug accumulates and the plasma concentration rises resulting in toxicity

Comparison between first order and zero order kinetics

Parameter	*First order*	*Zero order*
Definition	A constant fraction of drug is metabolized/eliminated per unit time	A constant amount of drug is metabolized per unit time
t½	Constant	Short at low and longer at high concentrations
Metabolism	Proportional to plasma concentration	Independent of plasma concentration
Higher doses	More drug gets metabolized → safer	Drug accumulates → toxicity
Drugs following	Most drugs	Few drugs, e.g. phenytoin, alcohol, aspirin

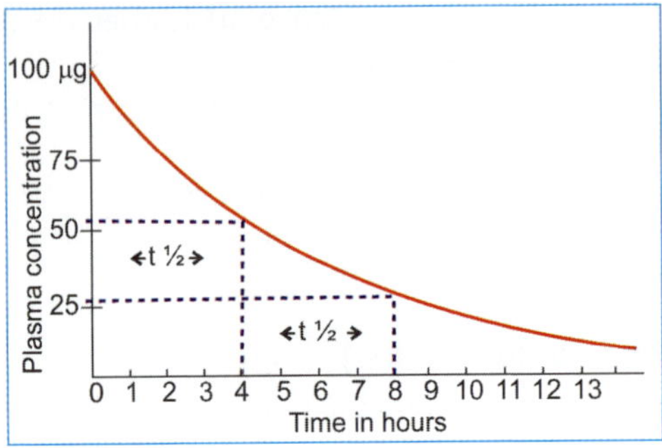

Fig. 2.13: Plasma concentration: Time curve following intravenous administration of a drug. Plasma t½ of the drug = 4 hours

regimen, e.g. esmolol has a t½ of 10 minutes, zolpidem 2 hours, aspirin 4 hours and chloroquine 10–24 days.

Significance of Plasma t½

Plasma t½ is necessary to know:

- The duration of action of the drug
- The frequency of administration
- The time needed for attainment of steady state concentration (SSC)—longer the t½, longer is the time needed to attain SSC.
- To calculate the loading and maintenance doses of the drug.

Factors Influencing Plasma t½

1. Plasma protein binding—drugs which are extensively bound to plasma proteins have a longer t½.
2. Enterohepatic circulation—increases the t½ of the drug.
3. Metabolism—faster the metabolism of a drug, shorter is its plasma t½.
4. Tissue storage—drugs which are sequestered in the tissues have a longer t½.
5. Clearance of the drug—drugs which are cleared faster have a shorter t½.

Biological half-life is the time required for total amount of drug in the body to be reduced to half.

Biological effect half-life is the time required for the biological effect of the drug to reduce to half. With some drugs, like propranolol, the pharmacological effect of the drug may last much longer, i.e. even after its plasma levels fall. In such drugs, biological effect half-life gives an idea of the duration of action of the drug.

Terminal half-life: On long-term use, certain drugs may remain in secondary compartments and they get gradually released into the circulation as the plasma concentration of drugs fall, e.g. terminal t½ of chloroquine is 30 to 60 days.

Steady-state concentration (SSC)

If a drug is administered repeatedly at short intervals before complete elimination, the drug accumulates in the body and reaches a 'state' at which the rate of elimination equals the rate of administration. This is known as the **'steady-state' or plateau level** (Fig. 2.14). After attaining this level, the plasma concentration fluctuates around an average steady level. It takes 4–5 half-lives for the plasma concentration to reach the plateau level. A drug with t½ >24 hr, if given daily, accumulates on prolonged use and could lead to toxicity. Hence for such drugs, once the SSC is attained, the dose given should be equal to the dose eliminated everyday. Steady-state plasma concentration (C_{pss}) can be obtained as follows:

$$C_{pss} = \frac{\text{Dose rate}}{\text{Clearance}}$$

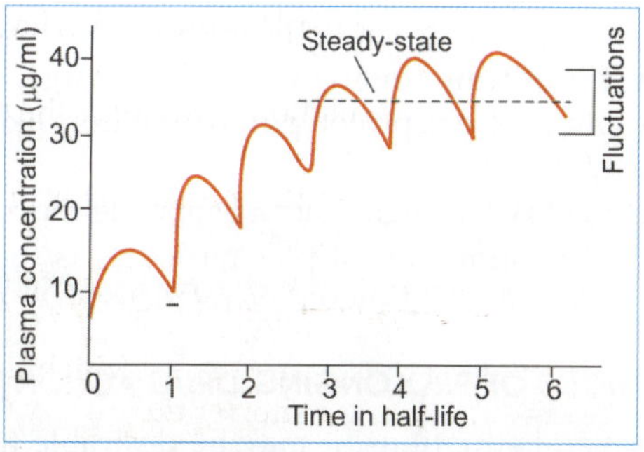

Fig. 2.14: Drug accumulation and attainment of steady-state concentration on oral administration

DRUG DOSAGE

Depending on the patient's requirements and the characteristics of the drug, drug dosage can be of the following kinds:

Fixed dose: In case of reasonably safe drugs, a fixed dose of the drug is suitable for most patients, e.g. analgesics like paracetamol—500 to 1000 mg 6 hourly is the usual adult dose.

Individualised dose: For some drugs especially the ones with low safety margin, the dose has to be 'tailored' to the needs of each patient, e.g. anticonvulsants, antiarrhythmic drugs.

Loading dose: In situations when target plasma concentrations have to be attained rapidly, a loading/bolus dose of the drug is given at the beginning of the treatment. A loading dose is a single large dose or a series of quickly repeated doses given to rapidly attain target concentration, e.g. heparin given as 5000 IU bolus dose. Once the target level is reached, a maintenance dose is sufficient to 'maintain the drug level' and to balance the elimination. Drugs with large V (e.g. chloroquine) and drugs with long t½ (e.g. digitoxin) need a long time to attain SSC and, therefore, need a loading dose. In emergencies, loading dose is often used to rapidly attain SSC for many drugs including the short t½ ones. Loading dose is calculated by:

$$\text{Loading dose:} \frac{\text{Target } C_p \times V}{F}$$

where, C_p is plasma concentration, *V* is volume of distribution and F is bioavailability.

The disadvantage with the loading dose is that the patient is rapidly exposed to high concentrations of the drug which may result in toxicity.

Maintenance dose is the dose given at constant intervals after the target C_{pss} is attained to maintain the steady state. The dose should be calculated to balance elimination, that is, the rate of administration should be equal to the rate at which it is eliminated.

Fixed Dose Combinations

When two or more drugs are combined to be given as a single preparation, it is called fixed dose combination (FDC). In these, both the drugs and the doses are fixed. There are hundreds of such FDCs available in the market. The rationale for giving any two drugs in a single formulation include:

1. Convenience of single pill and thereby better patient compliance, e.g. antitubercular drugs/antiretroviral drugs in a single tablet
2. Synergistic effect, e.g. cotrimoxazole, levodopa + carbidopa
3. To reduce adverse effects—thiazides with potassium sparing diuretics
4. Prevent development of resistance—antitubercular drugs.

Disadvantages

1. Reduced flexibility in dose adjustment
2. Difficulty to assess side effects
3. Increased risk of toxic effects—due to both drugs especially if there are overlapping side effects, e.g. hepatotoxicity due to INH, rifampicin and pyrazinamide.

Several rational and approved FDCs are available to improve patient compliance. They may be used in suitable patients, particularly when dose adjustments of individual drugs are not needed. However, hundreds of such FDCs are being marketed which are irrational, wasteful and often harmful. Use of such irrational FDCs should be avoided. For example:

- Amoxicillin + cloxacillin for staphylococcal infection
- Norfloxacin + metronidazole for diarrhoea
- Enalapril + losartan for hypertension.

Competency achievement: The student should be able to:

PH 1.2 Describe the basis of evidence-based medicine and **therapeutic drug monitoring.**[2]

THERAPEUTIC DRUG MONITORING

The response to a drug generally depends on the plasma concentration attained in the patient. This in turn depends on the bioavailability, volume of distribution and clearance. As these parameters vary among individuals, there is a wide variation in the plasma concentration attained from patient to patient. In some situations, it may be necessary to monitor treatment by measuring plasma drug concentrations. TDM may be done for such drugs in which plasma concentration correlates well with the effect. It should be done after steady state concentration is reached.

TDM is required for the following:

1. While using drugs with low safety margin to avoid therapeutic failure, e.g. digoxin, theophylline, lithium.
2. To reduce the risk of toxicity particularly when nephrotoxic drugs are used in renal failure, e.g. aminoglycosides.
3. When there are no reliable methods to assess benefit, e.g. antidepressants (TCAs).
4. To treat poisoning
5. When there is unexplainable therapeutic failure
6. To check patient compliance.

Therapeutic drug monitoring is **not required** for:

1. Drugs whose response can be easily measured chemically, e.g. blood pressure for antihypertensives.
2. 'Hit and run' drugs, whose effect persist for a long time even after the drug is eliminated, e.g. proton pump inhibitors like pantoprazole.
3. Drugs to which significant tolerance develops.
4. When estimation of plasma levels is too expensive, TDM should be restricted.

METHODS OF PROLONGING DRUG ACTION

In several situations, it may be desirable to use long-acting drugs, e.g. to avoid repeated

Table 2.5: Methods of prolonging duration of action of drugs

Processes	*Methods*	*Examples*
Pharmaceutical modification		
1. *Oral*	Sustained release preparations, controlled release preparation, coating with resins, etc.	Iron, deriphylline, diclofenac
2. *Parenteral*	1. Reducing solubility—oily suspension	Procaine + penicillin, benzathine penicillin
	2. Altering particle size	Depot progestins Insulin zinc suspension as large crystals that are slowly absorbed
	3. Pellet implantation—sialistic capsules	DOCA Testosterone
	4. Combining with protein	Protamine + zinc + insulin
	5. Chemical alteration—esterification	Estrogen, testosterone
3. *Topical*	Transdermal adhesive patches, ointments	Scopolamine, nitroglycerin
	Ocuserts (transmucosal)—used in eye	Pilocarpine
Pharmacokinetic intervention		
1. Absorption	Reducing vascularity of absorbing surface	Adrenaline + lignocaine (vasoconstrictor)
2. Distribution	Choosing more protein bound member of the group	Sulfonamides like sulfamethoxypyridazine
3. Metabolism	• Inhibiting the metabolising enzyme cholinesterase	Physostigmine—prolongs action of acetylcholine
	• By inhibiting the enzyme peptidase in renal tubular cells	Cilastatin—prolongs action of imipenem
4. Excretion	Competition for same transport system—for renal tubular secretion	Probenecid—prolongs the action of penicillin and ampicillin

doses and to avoid too much fluctuations in plasma concentration. When such drugs are not available, the duration of action of the available drugs may be prolonged (Table 2.5).

The duration of action of drugs can be prolonged by pharmaceutical intervention or by interfering with the pharmacokinetic processes, i.e. by:

1. Slowing absorption
2. Using a more plasma protein bound derivative
3. Inhibiting metabolism
4. Delaying excretion.

[1–2] From Medical Council of India, *Competency based Undergraduate Curriculum for the Indian Medical Graduate*, 2018;1:136–144.

CHAPTER 3

Pharmacodynamics

Competency achievement: The student should be able to:

PH 1.5 Describe general principles of mechanism of drug action.[1]

Pharmacodynamics is the study of actions of the drugs on the body and their mechanisms of action, i.e. to know what drugs do and how they do it.

Drugs produce their effects by interacting with the physiological systems of the organisms. By such interaction, drugs merely modify the rate of functions of the various systems. Drugs cannot bring about qualitative changes, i.e. they cannot change the basic functions of any physiological system. Thus drugs act by:

1. Stimulation
2. Depression
3. Irritation
4. Replacement
5. Anti-infective or cytotoxic action
6. Modification of immune status

Stimulation is the increase in activity of the specialised cells, e.g. adrenaline stimulates the heart.

Depression is the decrease in activity of the specialised cells, e.g. quinidine depresses the heart; barbiturates depress the central nervous system. Some drugs may stimulate one system and depress another, e.g. morphine depresses the CNS but stimulates the vagus.

Irritation can occur on all types of tissues in the body and may result in inflammation, corrosion and necrosis of cells.

Replacement: Drugs may be used for replacement when there is deficiency of natural substances like hormones, metabolites or nutrients, e.g. insulin in diabetes mellitus, iron in anaemia, vitamin C in scurvy.

Anti-infective and cytotoxic action: Drugs may act by specifically destroying infective organisms, e.g. penicillins, or by cytotoxic effect on cancer cells, e.g. anticancer drugs.

Modification of immune status: Vaccines and sera act by improving our immunity while immunosuppressants act by depressing immunity, e.g. glucocorticoids.

MECHANISMS OF DRUG ACTION

Most drugs produce their effects by binding to specific target proteins like receptors, enzymes and ion channels. Drugs may act on the cell membrane, inside or outside the cell to produce their effect. Drugs may act by one or more complex mechanisms of action. Some of them are yet to be understood. The fundamental mechanisms of drug actions may be:

1. Through receptors
2. Through enzymes and pumps
3. Through ion channels
4. Through transporters and symporters
5. By physical action
6. By chemical interaction
7. By altering metabolic processes.

1. *Through receptors:* A large number of drugs act by interacting with specific receptors in the body (*see* as follows).

2. *Through enzymes and pumps:* A large number of drugs act by inhibition of various enzymes, thus altering the enzyme-mediated reactions, e.g. allopurinol inhibits the enzyme xanthine oxidase;
   - Acetazolamide inhibits carbonic anhydrase;
   - Enalapril inhibits angiotensin-converting enzyme;
   - Aspirin inhibits cyclo-oxygenase, neostigmine inhibits acetylcholinesterase.

   Methotrexate binds DHFR with high affinity and inhibits it. Sildenafil inhibits phosphodiesterase-5 to cause vasodilatation. Several enzymes are influenced by drugs and this forms one of the common models of drug action.

   Membrane pumps, like H^+-K^+-ATPase may be inhibited by omeprazole and Na^+-K^+-ATPase by digoxin.
3. *Through ion channels:* Drugs may interfere with the movement of ions across specific channels either by opening or closing them. Such channels may be voltage-gated, ligand-gated or G-protein regulated channels, e.g.
   i. *Ca^{++} channels:*
      - Calcium channel blockers like verapamil block the voltage-sensitive L-type Ca^{++} channels in the myocardium.
      - Ethosuximide blocks T type Ca^{++} channels in thalamic neurons.

   ii. *K^+ channels:*
      - Nicorandil opens K^+ channels in the heart and vascular smooth muscles.
      - Sulfonylureas close the ATP sensitive K^+ channels in the pancreatic β cells to promote insulin release.

   iii. *Sodium channels:*
      - Lignocaine blocks the Na^+ channels to depress nerve conduction
      - Phenytoin blocks the Na^+ channels to stabilize neuronal membrane for antiepileptic activity.

   iv. *GABA-gated chloride channels:* Diazepam acts through $GABA_A$ receptor to increase the frequency of chloride channel opening in the neurons to cause CNS depression.
4. *Through transporters and symporters:* Many of the endogenous substances are transported across the biological membrane with the help of carriers. The action of several of the neurotransmitters is terminated by reuptake into the presynaptic nerve terminal. Drugs may act by blocking or inhibiting the movement of these transporters, symporters or antiporters. They are explained in detail in the respective chapters.

   Antidepressant imipramine acts by binding to transporters SERT and NET to inhibit the reuptake of serotonin and norepinephrine. Most diuretics act by influencing the movement of ions across the cells in the nephron by action on the symporters and transporters—thiazides inhibit Na^+-Cl^- symporter and furosemide inhibits Na^+-K^+-2Cl cotransporter.
5. *By physical action:* The action of a drug could result from its physical properties like:
   - Adsorption—*Activated charcoal in poisoning*
   - Mass of the drug—*bulk laxatives like psyllium, bran*
   - Osmotic property—*osmotic diuretics like* mannitol

     Osmotic purgatives like magnesium sulphate
   - Radioactivity—^{131}I
   - Radio-opacity:
     - *Barium sulphate*
     - *Contrast media.*
6. *By chemical interaction:* Drugs may act by chemical reaction.
   - Antacids—neutralise gastric acids
   - Oxidising agents—potassium permanganate and germicidal
   - Chelating agents—bind heavy metals making them nontoxic.
7. *By altering metabolic processes:* Drugs like antimicrobials alter the metabolic pathway in the micro-organisms resulting in destruction of the micro-organism, e.g. sulfonamides interfere with bacterial folic acid synthesis.

RECEPTOR

The works of **Langley** and **Ehrlich** put forth the concept of a 'receptor substance.' In the late 19th century, Langley noted that curare could oppose contraction of skeletal muscles caused by nicotine but did not block the contraction due to electrical stimulation. Paul **Ehrlich** observed that some organic chemicals had antiparasitic activity while others with slightly different structures did not have such activity. **Clark** put forward a theory to explain the drug action based on the drug-receptor occupation.

Last three decades have seen an explosion in our knowledge of the receptors. Various receptors have been identified, isolated and extensively studied.

Definition: A receptor is a macromolecular site on the cell with which an agonist binds to bring about a change.

Affinity: Affinity is the ability of a drug to bind to a receptor.

Intrinsic activity or efficacy: Intrinsic activity is the ability of a drug to elicit a response after binding to the receptor.

Agonist: An agonist is a substance that binds to the receptor and produces a response. It has both affinity and intrinsic activity, e.g. adrenaline is an agonist at α and β adrenergic receptors; morphine is an agonist at mu(μ) opioid receptors.

Antagonist: An antagonist is a substance that binds to the receptor and prevents the action of agonist on the receptor. It has affinity but no intrinsic activity. An antagonist has a structural similarity to the natural ligand for the receptor because of which the receptor identifies the antagonist as its ligand. Naloxone is an antagonist at μ opioid receptors. It binds to the receptor, has no effect by itself, but blocks the action of the opioid agonists like morphine. Tubocurarine is an antagonist at the nicotinic receptors. It blocks the receptors and prevents the action of acetylcholine on the receptors.

Partial agonist: A partial agonist binds to the receptor but has low intrinsic activity. Pentazocine is a partial agonist at μ opioid receptors, pindolol is a partial agonist at β-adrenergic receptors. A partial agonist occupies the receptor and brings about weak effects. It also blocks the action/binding of the full agonists. Thus a partial agonist is also called agonist–antagonist.

Inverse agonist: Some drugs, after binding to the receptors produce actions opposite to those produced by a pure agonist. They are known as inverse agonists, e.g. diazepam acting on benzodiazepine receptors produces sedation, anxiolysis, muscle relaxation and controls convulsions, while the inverse agonists β-carbolines bind to the same receptors to cause arousal, anxiety, increased muscle tone and convulsions.

Ligand: Ligand is a molecule which binds selectively to a specific receptor.

Spare receptors: In an experiment using adrenaline on rabbit aortic strips, Furchgott showed that the agonist occupied only a small percentage of receptors to produce maximum contraction. Some experiments showed that high concentration of an agonist can still produce maximal response in the presence of an irreversible antagonist and this was because of the presence of **'spare' or reserve receptors.** Thus it is possible to stimulate the myocardium even when 90% of the cardiac β-adrenergic receptors are blocked by an irreversible β-blocker.

Silent receptors: These are receptors to which an agonist binds but does not produce a response. Presence of such silent receptors may explain the phenomenon of tolerance. Plasma proteins that bind drugs are considered to act as silent receptors as they just bind the drug and the drug is not available for action.

Site: The receptors may be present in the cell membrane, in the cytoplasm or on the nucleus.

Nature of receptors: Receptors are proteins.

Synthesis and lifespan: Receptor proteins are synthesized by the cells. They have a definite lifespan after which the receptors are degraded by the cell and new receptors are synthesized.

Functions of receptors: The two functions of receptors are:

1. Recognition and binding of the ligand.
2. Propagation of the message.

For the above functions, the receptor has two functional domains (areas):

1. A ligand-binding domain (LBD)—the site to bind the drug molecule or ligand.
2. An effector domain—which undergoes a change to propagate the message.

Several theories have been proposed to explain drug–receptor interaction. Drug–receptor interaction has been considered to be similar to **'lock and key'** relationship where the drug specifically fits into the particular receptor (lock) like a key. The **rate theory** proposes that the magnitude of response depends on the rate of agonist–receptor association and dissociation. The rate of receptor-binding is more initially but after it reaches the peak, there is a decrease.

The **occupation theory** suggests that the magnitude of drug response depends on the proportion of the receptors occupied by the drug. As per this theory, the response will progressively increase till a steady state is reached.

Receptor model: Currently, the drug–receptor interaction is explained by a 'two-state' model of the receptor. According to this, a receptor exists in two states, namely *resting or inactive (Ri)* and *activated (Ra)*. A drug with greater affinity for the activated state will function as a full agonist while that with moderate affinity for the activated state will be a partial agonist.

Interaction of the agonist with the receptor brings about changes in the receptor which in turn conveys the signal to the **effector system.** The final response is brought about by the effector system through **second messengers.** The agonist itself is the first messenger. The entire process involves a chain of events triggered by drug–receptor interaction. The transduction process which links the binding of the receptor and the actual response is called 'coupling'.

Receptor classification: International Union of Pharmacologists (IUPHAR) has setup expert working groups to classify receptors based on different criteria. For example, they have classified adrenergic and cholinergic receptors.

Receptor families: On stimulation of a receptor, the time required to elicit the response varies largely from a fraction of a second in some receptors to hours and days in others. This difference is because of the variation in mechanisms involved in linking the receptor and the effector systems (transduction mechanisms). Based on this, 5 types or super families of the cell surface receptors are identified. They are best understood with the help of Fig. 3.1.

The receptor types are:

1. G-protein-coupled receptors (metabotropic receptor)
2. Ion channel receptors (ionotropic receptor)
3. Transmembrane enzymatic receptors (kinase-linked receptor)
4. Transmembrane non-enzymes (cytokine and TLR).
5. Nuclear receptors (transcription factors or receptors that regulate gene transcription).

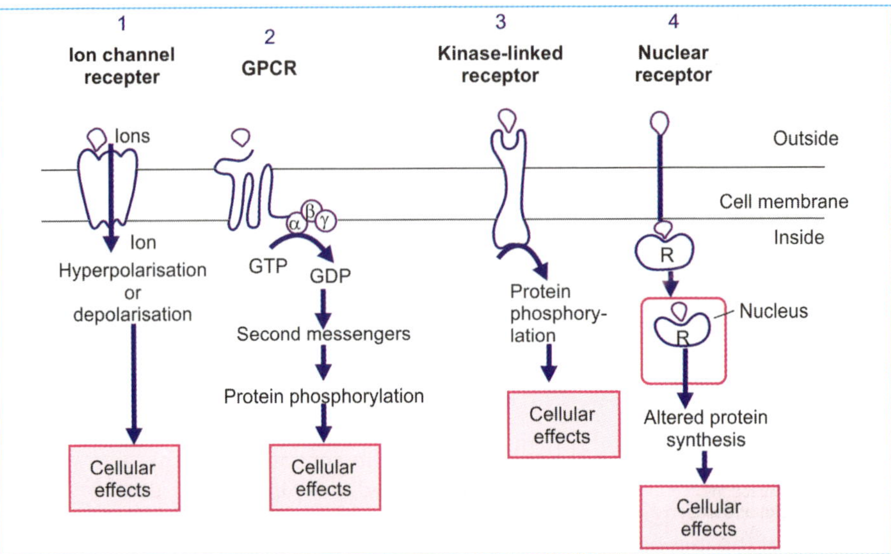

Fig. 3.1: Type 1: Binding of the agonist directly regulates the opening of the ion channel. Type 2: Agonist binding activates the receptor linked to an effector system by a G protein (G). Type 3: Agonist binding to extracellular domain activates enzymatic activity of its intracellular catalytic domain. Type 4: Agonist binds to the intracellular receptor, the complex moves to the nucleus and directs protein synthesis

Receptor Families and their Signal Transduction Mechanisms (Flowchart 3.1)

1. **Ion channel receptors or receptor channels or ionotropic receptors** are proteins present on the cell surface or cell membrane. Binding of the agonist opens the channel allowing ions to cross the membrane. These are called **ligand-gated ion channels** and the ion channel acts as the target for the drug. Depending on the ion and the channel, depolarisation/hyperpolarisation occurs, e.g. nicotinic cholinergic receptor channel permits passage of Na^+ ions resulting in depolarisation while the benzodiazepines bind the GABA receptor-chloride channel complex and facilitate the opening of the channel. The chloride ions flow into the neurons and cause hyperpolarisation. Some examples are given in Table 3.1.

2. **G-protein-coupled receptors (GPCR)** are receptors that signal through G proteins and form a family of transmembrane proteins, present across the plasma membrane. The receptor consists of 7α helices (Fig. 3.1). The G proteins are bound to the inner face of the plasma membrane and form a complex with (coupled to) the receptor. They are called G proteins because of their interaction with guanine nucleotides GTP and GDP. G proteins act as signal transducers, that is, they convey the information to the effector system when

Table 3.1: Drugs acting through ion channel receptors

Ion channels	*Drug*	*Action*
Na^+ channel	Lignocaine	Blockade
	Quinidine	Blockade
	Acetylcholine	Opening
Ca^{++} channel	Nifedipine	Blockade
	Verapamil	
K^+ channel	Sulfonylureas	Blockade
	Nicorandil	Opening
Cl^- channel	Diazepam	Opening
	Barbiturates	Opening

Flowchart 3.1: Receptor families and their transduction mechanisms

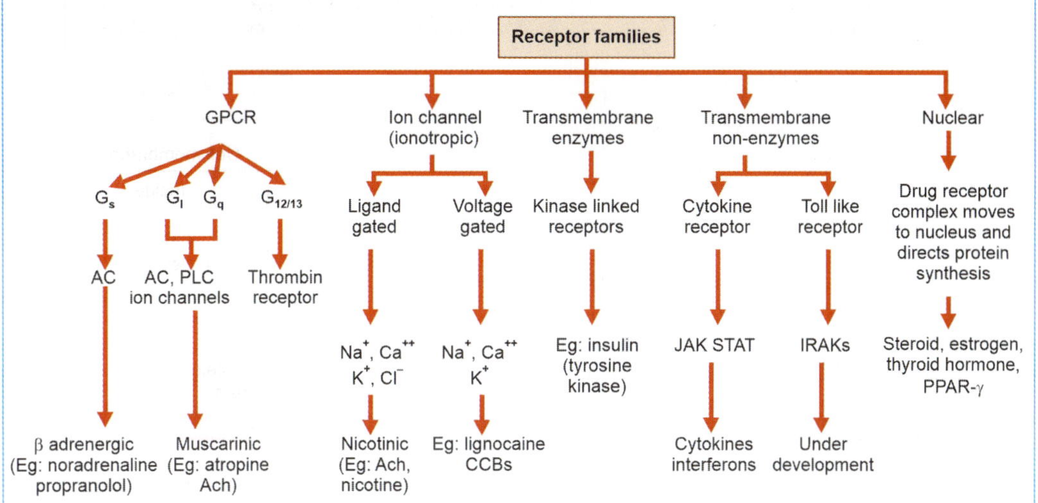

an agonist binds to the GPCR. The G-proteins consist of three subunits, viz. α, β and γ (called heterotrimer meaning 3 different subunits) with GDP bound to a subunit (Fig. 3.2a). The G proteins act as signal transducers, i.e. they convey the information to the effector system. When a ligand binds to the G-protein-coupled receptor, the associated G-protein gets activated. This in turn activates adenylyl cyclase or phospholipase C to generate the respective second messengers. These second messenger systems are called effector pathways. The second messengers include cAMP, IP_3, DAG, Ca^{++} and cGMP. G-proteins acting through second messengers, bring about a chain of intracellular changes. Thus G-proteins act as links or mediators between the receptor and the effector systems. The α subunit possesses GTPase activity. G-proteins are of different classes like G_s, G_i, G_q, G_o and $G1_{12/13}$. G_s is stimulatory and G_i is inhibitory. For example, G_s activation opens Ca^{++} channels in myocardium and skeletal muscles while Gi opens K^+ channels in the heart and smooth muscles. Adrenergic receptors and muscarinic cholinergic receptors are examples of G-protein-coupled receptors.

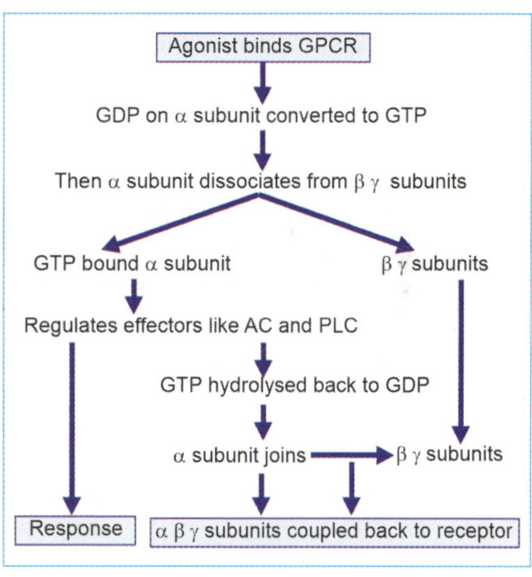

Fig. 3.2a: Functioning of GPCRs

Effector pathways through which the G-protein-coupled receptors work are:

- Adenylyl cyclase/cAMP pathway
- Phospholipase C/IP_3-DAG pathway
- Ion channel regulation.

Second messenger pathways for some GPCRs

Pathway	*Second messenger*	*Receptors*
Adenylyl cyclase	↑cAMP	β, D1, H2, V2
	↓cAMP	α_2, D2, M2, μ, 5HT1
PLC	IP3-DAG	α_1, M1, M2, 5HT2
Ion channels	↑Ca^{++}	β_1
	↓Ca^{++}	D2, κ opioid
	↑K^+	α_2, D2, $GABA_B$, δ opioid

- *Adenylyl cyclase pathway* (Fig. 3.2b): Stimulation of adenylyl cyclase results in the formation and accumulation of cAMP within the cell. This cAMP acts through protein kinases which phosphorylate various proteins to regulate the cell function. The response may be contraction, relaxation, lipolysis or hormone synthesis.
- *Phospholipase C/IP_3-DAG pathway* (Fig. 3.3): Activation of phospholipase C (PLC) results in the formation of second messengers IP_3 and DAG from the membrane phospholipids phosphoinositol pyrophosphate (PIP_2). IP_3 mobilises Ca^{++} from intracellular depots and this Ca^{++} mediates responses like secretion, contraction, metabolism and hyperpolarization. DAG activates protein kinase C (PKC) which regulates cell function.

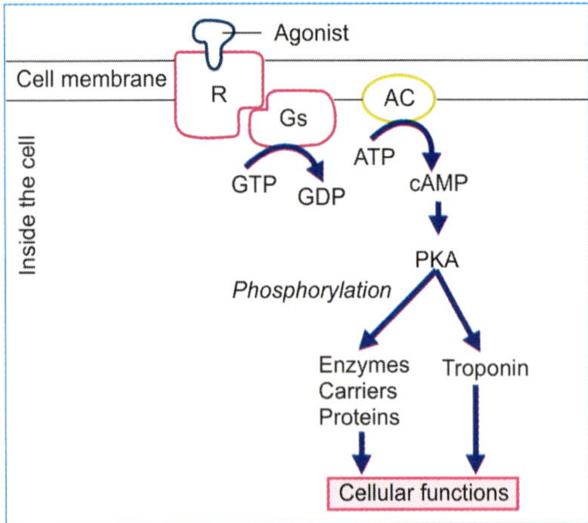

Fig. 3.2b: G-protein-coupled receptor—transduction through adenylyl cyclase pathway with cAMP as second messenger. R = Receptor, G_s = G-protein (stimulatory)

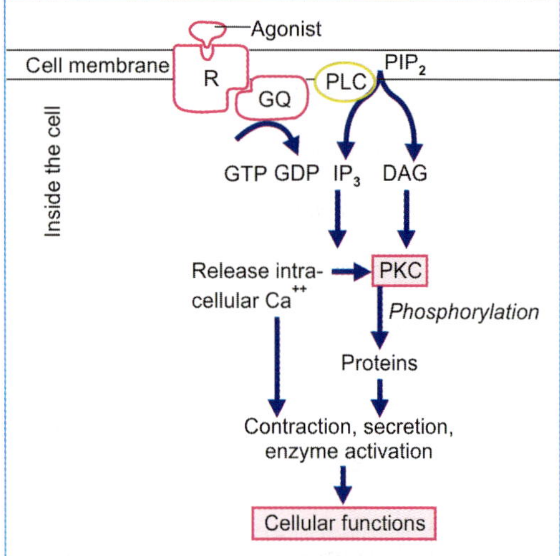

Fig. 3.3: G-protein-coupled receptor acting through the second messengers IP_3 and DAG. CaM-calmodulin

- *Ion channel regulation:* The activated G-proteins can also directly (without the help of second messengers) convey the signal to some ion channels of calcium and potassium causing opening or closing of the channels. The resulting responses include depolarisation/hyperpolarisation.

3. **Enzymatic receptors** are transmembrane proteins with an extracellular domain (site) for ligand binding and intracellular domain to carry out the catalytic activity and the two domains are linked by a single peptide chain. They are protein kinases and hence are also known as **kinase-linked receptors**. Binding of the agonist to the ligand binding domain results in autophosphorylation of the intracellular domain. This in turn triggers phosphorylation of various intracellular proteins resulting in the characteristic response, e.g. receptors of insulin, leptin and growth factors including epidermal growth factors and platelet-derived growth factors.
4. A type of non-enzymatic receptor is the **JAK-STAT binding receptor**. When an agonist binds to the extracellular domain, it activates the intracellular domain (which

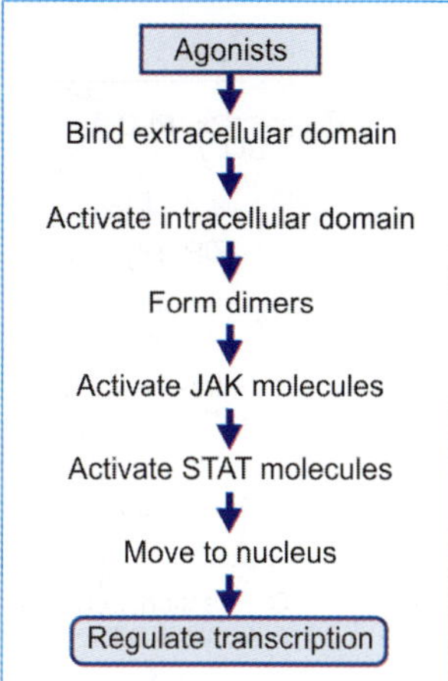

forms dimers, i.e. groups of two) and mobile JAK (Janus kinase) molecules are activated. These molecules in turn activate signal transducers and activation of transcription-molecules (STAT-molecules). STAT-molecules move to the nucleus and regulate transcription, e.g. growth hormones, cytokines, interferons.

5. **Receptors that regulate gene transcription** are also called transcription factors or nuclear receptors. They are intracellular proteins which are in an inactive state. Binding of the agonist activates the receptor. The agonist-receptor complex moves to the nucleus where it interacts with DNA, regulates gene transcription and thereby directs the synthesis of specific proteins to regulate the activity of target cells. Examples are receptors for steroidal hormones, thyroid hormones, vitamin D and retinoids.

Receptor Regulation

The number of receptors (density) and their sensitivity can be altered in many situations. Denervation or prolonged deprivation of the agonist or constant action of the antagonist, all result in an increase in the number and sensitivity of the receptors. This phenomenon is called **upregulation.** Prolonged use of a β adrenergic antagonist, like propranolol, results in upregulation of β adrenergic receptors.

On the other hand, continued stimulation of the receptors causes desensitisation and a decrease in the number of receptors—known as **downregulation** of the receptors.

Clinical Consequences and Implications of Receptor Regulation

Upregulation: After prolonged administration, a receptor antagonist should always be tapered. For example, if propranolol, a β adrenoceptor blocker is suddenly withdrawn after long-term use, it precipitates angina. This

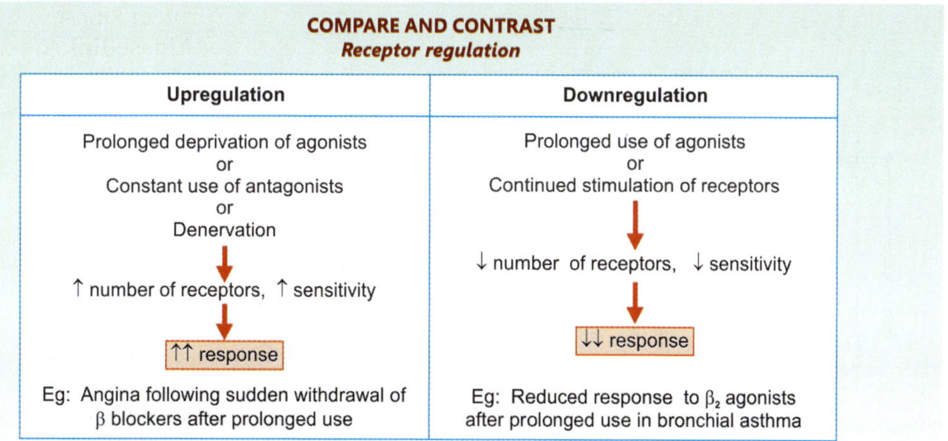
COMPARE AND CONTRAST
Receptor regulation

Upregulation	Downregulation
Prolonged deprivation of agonists or Constant use of antagonists or Denervation ↓ ↑ number of receptors, ↑ sensitivity ↓ ↑↑ response Eg: Angina following sudden withdrawal of β blockers after prolonged use	Prolonged use of agonists or Continued stimulation of receptors ↓ ↓ number of receptors, ↓ sensitivity ↓ ↓↓ response Eg: Reduced response to β_2 agonists after prolonged use in bronchial asthma

is because of upregulation of β receptors. Normal amounts of noradrenaline released during any stress can stimulate the heart and cause angina. This is because of upregulation of beta receptors. Normal amounts of noradrenaline released during any stress can stimulate the heart and cause angina.

Downregulation: Constant use of β adrenergic agonists in bronchial asthma results in reduced therapeutic response due to down-regulation of β_2 receptors develop tolerance.

DOSE RESPONSE RELATIONSHIP

The clinical response to the increasing dose of the drug is defined by the shape of the dose response curve (DRC). Initially, the extent of response increases with increase in dose till the maximum response is reached.

There are 2 types of dose response relationships, viz. **graded dose response relationship** and **quantal dose response relationship**. The graded dose response curve has the shape of a rectangular **hyperbola** (Fig. 3.4). After the maximum effect has been obtained, further increase in doses does not increase the response. If the dose is plotted on a logarithmic scale, the curve becomes **sigmoid** (Fig. 3.5).

Advantages of plotting log DRC are:

1. Wide range of doses can be displayed on the graph.

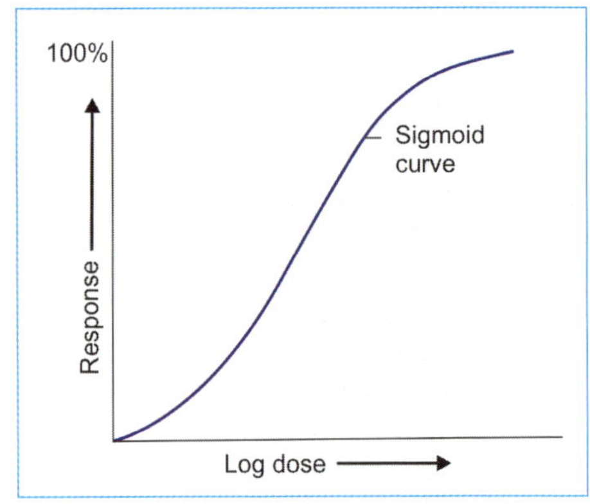

Fig. 3.5: Log dose response curve

2. Easy to compare agonists and study antagonists.

The slope of DRC (Fig. 3.6) has clinical significance. A steep slope indicates that a small increase in dose produces a large increase in response, e.g. loop diuretics. Such drugs are more likely to cause toxicity and, therefore, individualisation of dose is required. A relatively flat DRC indicates that with an increase in dose, there is little increase in the response, e.g. thiazide diuretics. For such drugs, standard doses can be given to most patients.

Quantal DRC: Certain responses can only be all-or-none (e.g. vomiting) and when represented on the dose response curve, the curve appears bell-shaped (*see* Fig. 2.5, page 24) and it indicates the percentage of responders.

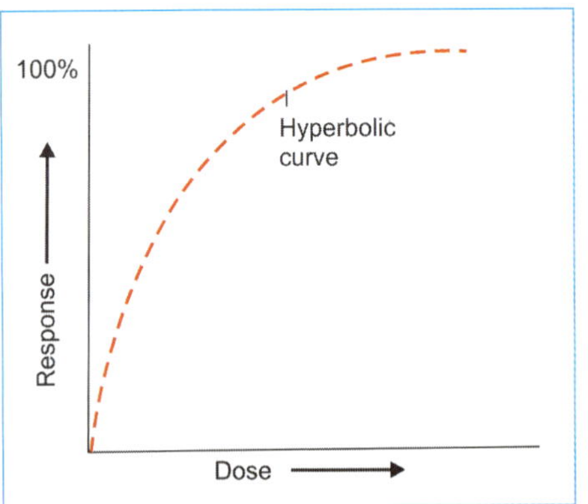

Fig. 3.4: Dose response curve

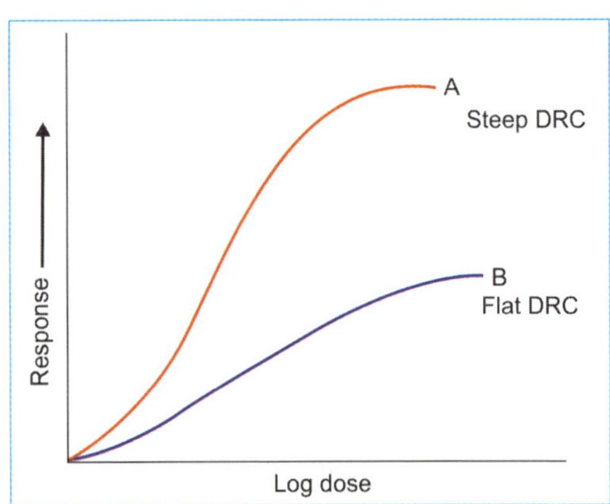

Fig. 3.6: Steep and flat dose response curves

Drug Potency

The amount of drug required to produce a response indicates the potency. For example, 1 mg of bumetanide produces the same diuresis as 50 mg of frusemide. Thus bumetanide is more potent than frusemide. In Fig. 3.7, drugs A and B are more potent than drugs C and D, drug A being the most potent and drug D the least potent. Hence higher doses of drugs C and D are to be administered as compared to drugs A and B. Generally, potency is of little clinical significance unless very large doses of the drug needs to be given due to low potency.

Maximal Efficacy

Efficacy indicates the maximum response that can be produced by a drug, e.g. frusemide produces powerful diuresis, not produced by any dose of amiloride. In Fig. 3.7, drugs B and C are more efficacious than drugs A and D. Drug A is more potent but less efficacious than drugs B and C. Such differences in efficacy are of great clinical importance.

Therapeutic Index

The dose response curves for different actions of a drug could be different. Thus salbutamol may have one DRC for bronchodilation and another for tachycardia. The distance between beneficial effect DRC and unwanted effect DRC indicates the safety margin of the drug (Fig. 3.8).

Median lethal dose (LD_{50}): Dose which is lethal to 50% of the population.

Median effective dose (ED_{50}): Dose that produces a desired effect in 50% of the test population.

Therapeutic index (TI) in experimental animals is obtained by the ratio of the median lethal dose to the median effective dose.

$$\text{Therapeutic index} = \frac{LD_{50}}{ED_{50}}$$

- TI gives an idea about the safety of the drug.
- The higher the therapeutic index, the safer is the drug.
- TI varies from species to species.
- For a drug to be considered reasonably safe, its TI must be >1.
- Penicillin, amoxicillin, diazepam, and atenolol have a high TI and their dose response curve is relatively flat.
- Llithium, digoxin, theophylline, barbiturates and carbamazepine have low TI and their DRC is steep.

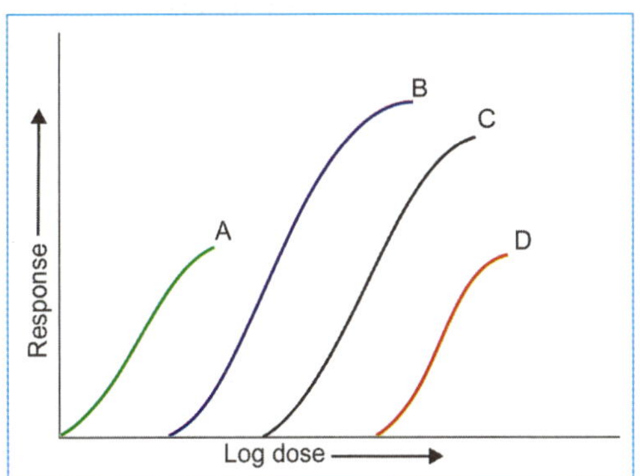

Fig. 3.7: Dose response curves of four drugs showing different potencies and maximal efficacies. Drug A is more potent but less efficacious than B and C. Drug D is less potent and less efficacious than drugs B and C

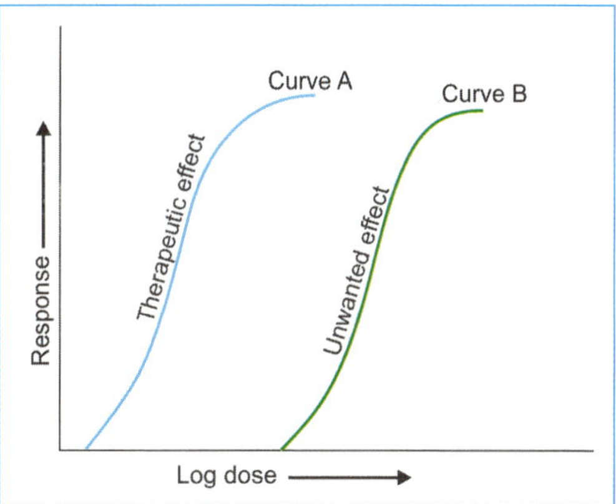

Fig. 3.8: The distance between the curves A and B indicates safety margin or therapeutic index (TI) of the drug. The greater the distance, more selective is the drug

- TI may be different for each action of a drug. For example, TI of aspirin used for headache is different from its TI for inflammation.

Limitations of Therapeutic Index

Therapeutic index does not consider idiosyncratic responses that result in toxicity. Moreover, the data is based on animal studies which may be difficult to apply on human beings and considers only 50% of a given set of animals. To get a more certain idea about safety, the drug should be effective in 99% and lethal to 1% of the test population. Such an index is called **certain safety factor.**

Thus, certain safety factor = $\frac{LD_1}{ED_{99}}$.

In human population, LD_{50} cannot be obtained and, therefore, ED_{50} is considered.

Therapeutic Window

Therapeutic window is the range of plasma concentrations below which the drug is ineffective and above which toxicity appears (therapeutic range). Hence, it is desirable to have the plasma concentration of drugs within this optimal therapeutic range in order to derive therapeutic effect without significant toxic effects. Therapeutic index quantifies the therapeutic window, i.e. if therapeutic window is small, TI is also small. Drugs with low therapeutic index have a narrow therapeutic window, e.g. the plasma drug levels of digoxin is 0.8–1.2 ng/ml, lithium 0.5–1.3 mEq/l, carbamazepine 3–10 µg/ml and clonidine 0.2–2 ng/ml. Imipramine produces optimum therapeutic effect only when its plasma levels are maintained between 50 and 200 ng/ml. Doses of such drugs must be titrated carefully.

DRUG SYNERGISM AND ANTAGONISM

When two or more drugs are given concurrently, the effect may be additive, synergistic or antagonistic.

Additive Effect

The effect of two or more drugs get added up and the total effect is equal to the sum of their individual actions.

Examples

Ephedrine + theophylline in bronchial asthma; nitrous oxide + ether as general anaesthetics.

Synergism

When the action of one drug is enhanced or facilitated by another drug, the combination is synergistic. In Greek, *ergon* = work; *syn* = with. Here, the total effect of the combination is greater than the sum of their independent effects. It is often called 'potentiation' or 'supra-additive' effect.

Examples

- Acetylcholine + physostigmine
- Levodopa + carbidopa.

Thus additive effect can be understood as 2 + 2 = 4 while synergistic effect is 2 + 2 = 5!

Antagonism

One drug opposing or inhibiting the action of another is antagonism. Based on the mechanisms, antagonism can be (Fig. 3.9):

1. Chemical Antagonism

Two substances interact chemically to result in inactivation of the effect, e.g. chelating agents inactivate heavy metals like lead and mercury to form inactive complexes; antacids like aluminium hydroxide neutralize gastric acid.

2. Physiological Antagonism

Two drugs act at different sites to produce opposing effects. For example, histamine acts on H_1 receptors to produce bronchospasm and hypotension while adrenaline reverses these effects by acting on adrenergic receptors.

Insulin and glucagon have opposite effects on the blood sugar level.

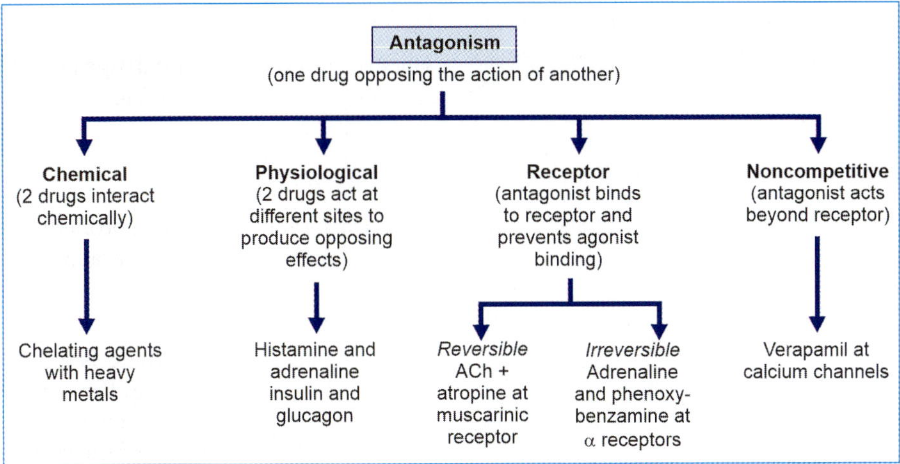

Fig. 3.9: Types of antagonism with examples

3. Antagonism at the Receptor Level

The antagonist binds to the receptor and inhibits the binding of the agonist to the receptor. Such antagonism may be reversible or irreversible.

Reversible or competitive antagonism: The agonist and antagonist compete for the same receptor. When a fixed concentration of an agonist is employed and the dose of the antagonist is progressively increased, the response to the agonist is progressively diminished. However, by increasing the concentration of the agonist, the antagonism can be overcome. It is thus reversible antagonism. The same maximal response can still be obtained by increasing the dose of the agonist. It is also called **surmountable** or **equilibrium type** of antagonism. This is the most common type of antagonism. Acetylcholine and atropine compete at muscarinic receptors. The antagonism can be overcome by increasing the concentration of acetylcholine at the receptor. Tubocurarine and acetylcholine compete for the nicotinic receptors at the neuromuscular junction. The dose response curve of the agonist shifts to the right (Fig. 3.10) in the presence of competitive antagonists.

Clinical significance: When an antagonist is used therapeutically, it should be borne in mind that the extent of inhibition brought about by a reversible antagonist depends on the concentration of the agonist. Therefore, the dose of the antagonist should be adjusted to get the optimum response, e.g. propranolol is used to block β adrenergic receptors. An increased amount of the endogenous agonists noradrenaline and adrenaline are released in stress and the dose of the antagonist (propranolol) needed would also be more in such situations.

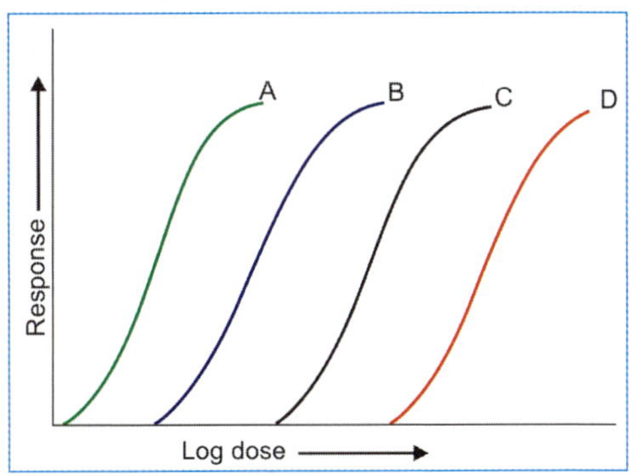

Fig. 3.10: Dose response curves of an agonist: A in the absence of competitive antagonist; B, C and D in the presence of increasing doses of a reversible competitive antagonist

Irreversible antagonism: The antagonist binds by covalent bonds to the receptor and it binds so firmly that it dissociates very slowly or not at all. Thus it blocks the action of the agonist and the blockade cannot be overcome by increasing the dose of the agonist and hence it is irreversible antagonism. In this type of antagonism, the duration of action is usually long since the effect remains till the new receptors are synthesized, e.g. adrenaline and phenoxybenzamine at alpha adrenergic receptors. This antagonism is also called **non-equilibrium** type of antagonism.

There is progressive flattening of the dose response curve (Fig. 3.11).

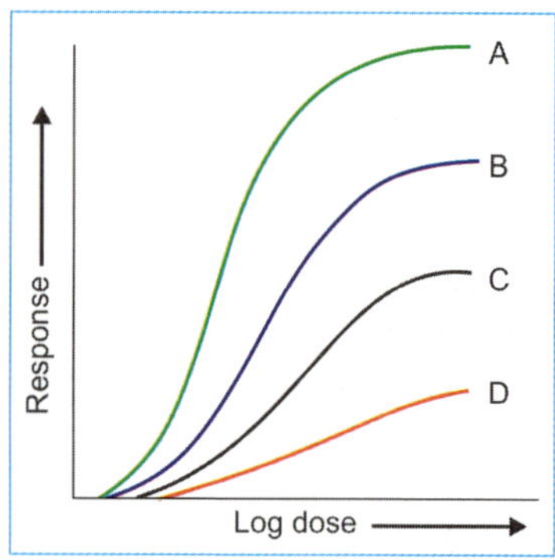

Fig. 3.11: Dose response curves of an agonist A, in the absence of antagonist, B, C, and D in the presence of increasing doses of an irreversible antagonist

4. Noncompetitive Antagonism

The antagonist blocks at the level of the receptor–effector linkage, i.e. at a different site beyond the receptor and not on the receptor. There is flattening as well as some rightward shift of the dose response curve (Fig. 3.12). For example, verapamil blocks the cardiac calcium channels and inhibits the entry of Ca^{++} during depolarisation. It thereby antagonises the effect of cardiac stimulants like isoprenaline and adrenaline. Since non-competitive antagonism is often confused with irreversible antagonism, they are compared in the table (below).

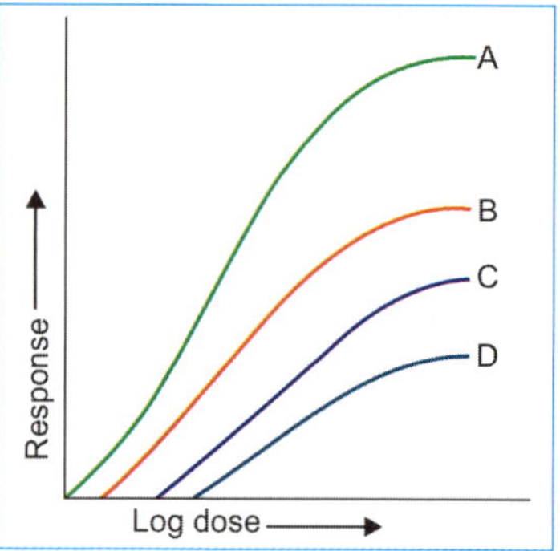

Fig. 3.12: Non-competitive antagonism—there is flattening as well as some rightward shift of DRC

FACTORS THAT MODIFY THE EFFECTS OF DRUGS

The same dose of a drug can produce different degrees of response in different patients and even in the same patient under different situations. Various factors modify the response to a drug. They are:

1. Body weight: The recommended dose is calculated for medium built persons. For the obese and underweight persons, the dose has to be calculated individually. Though body surface area is a better parameter for more accurate calculation of the dose, it is inconvenient and hence not generally used.

COMPARE AND CONTRAST

Parameter	*Irreversible antagonism*	*Non-competitive antagonism*
Receptor binding	Yes	Not involved
Mode of action	Binding irreversible or very long lasting	Binding at a different site than receptor
Example	Phenoxybenzamine at α receptors	Verapamil at Ca^{++} channels
DRC	Progressive flattening	Flattening and rightward shift

Formula:

$$\text{Dose} = \frac{\text{Body weight (kg)} \times \text{average adult dose}}{70}$$

2. Age: The pharmacokinetics of many drugs change with age resulting in altered response in extremes of age.

Newborn and infants: In the newborn, the liver and kidneys are not fully mature to handle the drugs, e.g. chloramphenicol can produce grey baby syndrome. The blood–brain barrier is not well-formed and drugs can easily reach the brain. The gastric acidity is low, intestinal motility is slow, skin is delicate and is permeable to drugs applied topically. Hence calculation of the appropriate dose, depending on the body weight is important to avoid toxicity. Also pharmacodynamic differences could exist, e.g. barbiturates which produce sedation in adults may produce excitation in children.

Formula for calculation of dose for children.

1. *Young's formula*

$$\text{Child's dose} = \frac{\text{Age (years)}}{\text{Age} + 12} \times \text{Adult dose}$$

2. Dilling's formula

$$\text{Child's dose} = \frac{\text{Age}}{20} \times \text{Adult dose}$$

In the elderly, the capacity of the liver and kidney to handle the drug is reduced and they are more susceptible to adverse effects. Hence, lower doses are recommended, e.g. elderly are at a higher risk of ototoxicity and nephrotoxicity by streptomycin.

3. Sex: There are no gross gender differences in response to drug. However, the hormonal effects and smaller body size may influence the drug response in women. Special care is necessary while prescribing for pregnant and lactating women and during menstruation. For example, purgatives cause pelvic congestion and if they are administered during menstruation, they may increase the menstrual blood loss.

Adult male rats metabolize drugs at a much faster rate than their female counterparts.

4. Species and race: Response to drugs may vary with species and race. For example, rabbits are resistant to atropine. Such variation makes it difficult to extrapolate the results of animal experiments. Variation in response to drugs is also noted among different races. Blacks need higher doses of atropine to produce mydriasis. The antipsychotic clozapine may cause a higher incidence of agranulocytosis in people of Finland. Hence most countries now approve a drug to be used in their country only after it has undergone trials on its own population.

5. Diet and environment: Food interferes with the absorption of many drugs and such drug–food interactions should be borne in mind. For example, tetracyclines form complexes with calcium present in the food and are poorly absorbed.

Polycyclic hydrocarbons present in the cigarette smoke may induce microsomal enzymes resulting in enhanced metabolism of some drugs. Examples of drug–food interactions:

Absorption increased by food—spironolactone, chloroquine, riboflavin, lithium, albendazole.

Absorption reduced by food—ampicillin, rifampicin, tetracycline, INH.

6. Route and time of administration: Occasionally route of administration may modify the pharmacodynamic response, e.g. magnesium sulphate given orally is a purgative. But given IV it causes CNS depression and has anticonvulsant effects for which it is used in eclampsia of pregnancy. Applied topically (poultice), it reduces local oedema. Hypertonic magnesium sulphate retention enema reduces intracranial tension.

N-acetylcysteine is another similar example. When given orally and IV it acts as an antidote in paracetamol overdosage—acetylcysteine replenishes glutathione stores in the liver. If inhaled as a solution, it acts as a mucolytic while if irrigated into the urinary bladder, it counters cystitis caused by cyclophosphamide.

Time of administration: There are several diurnal variations in the body and the time of drug administration is important to obtain the benefit of such variations. For example, secretion of glucocorticoids is highest in the morning. Hence, if exogenous glucocorticoids are also administered in the morning, the HPA axis suppression is much less. The study of such correlation of drug effects to the circadian rhythm has emerged as chronopharmacology (*see* page 73).

7. Genetic factors: Variations in an individual's response to drugs could be genetically mediated. **Pharmacogenetics** is the study of genetically mediated variations in drug responses. Variation in nucleotide sequences could result in differences in response to drugs.

Competency achievement: The student should be able to:

PH 1.60 Describe and discuss pharmacogenomics and pharmacoeconomics.[2]

Pharmacogenomics and pharmacogenetics are often used to mean the same (as synonyms) but difference is pharmacogenetics deals with monogenetic variants while pharmacogenomics involves the entire spectrum of genes that could modify drug response.

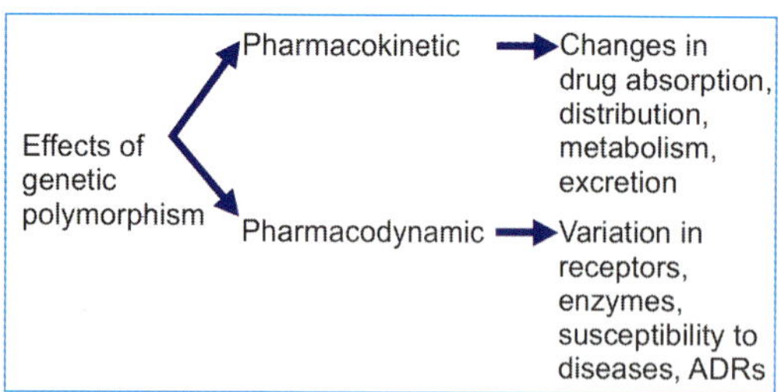

Genetic **polymorphisms/variations** could result in changes in pharmacokinetics or pharmacodynamics.

i. ***Pharmacokinetic variations:*** Production of drug metabolizing enzymes is genetically controlled and variations are common.

Examples

a. *Oxidation of drugs* genetic polymorphism in cytochrome P450 enzymes result in variation in the rate of metabolism (oxidation, hydroxylation) of drugs metabolised by these enzymes, e.g. SSRIs, phenytoin, warfarin.
b. *Acetylation of drugs:* The rate of drug acetylation differs among individuals who may be fast or slow acetylators, e.g. INH, sulfonamides, hydralazine, procainamide and dapsone are metabolized by acetylation. Slow acetylators treated with hydralazine are more likely to develop lupus erythematosus.
c. *Atypical pseudocholinesterase:* Succinylcholine is metabolised by the enzyme pseudocholinesterase. Some people inherit an atypical pseudocholinesterase which cannot quickly metabolise succinylcholine. When succinylcholine is given to such people, they develop a prolonged apnoea due to persistant action of succinylcholine.

ii. ***Pharmacodynamic variations:*** Variations in receptor, enzymes, susceptibility to ADRs and diseases:

a. *G6PD deficiency:* Deficiency of G6PD in RBCs leads to NADPH deficiency resulting in accumulation of glutathion. Exposure of such RBCs to drugs like primaquine, sulphones, and quinolones leads to hemolysis.
b. *Malignant hyperthermia:* Halothane and succinylcholine can trigger malignant hyperthermia in some genetically predisposed individuals (*see* pages 131, 190).
c. *Hepatic porphyrias:* Some people lack an enzyme required for haeme synthesis, and this results in accumulation of porphyrin-containing haeme precursors. Some drugs,

like barbiturates, griseofulvin and carbamazepine, induce the enzyme required for porphyrin synthesis resulting in accumulation of porphyrins. In both the above cases, neurological, gastrointestinal and behavioural abnormalities can occur due to excess porphyrins.

8. **Dose:** It is fascinating that the response to a drug may be modified by the dose administered. Generally as the dose is increased, the magnitude of the response also increases proportionately till the 'maximum' is reached. Further increases in doses may with some drugs produce effects opposite to their lower-dose effect, e.g.
   i. In myasthenia gravis, neostigmine enhances muscle power in therapeutic doses, but in high doses it causes muscle paralysis.
   ii. Physiological doses of vitamin D promotes calcification while hypervitaminosis D leads to decalcification.

Pharmacoeconomics *see* page 73.

9. **Diseases:** Presence of certain diseases can influence drug responses, e.g.

- *Gastrointestinal diseases:* Drugs are poorly absorbed in malabsorption syndrome.
- *Liver diseases:* Rate of drug metabolism including first pass metabolism is reduced due to dysfunction of hepatocytes. Also protein binding is reduced due to low serum albumin, because albumin is synthesized in the liver and blood levels of the free form of the drug increases in liver failure.
- *Cardiac diseases:* In CCF, there is oedema of the gut mucosa and decreased perfusion of liver and kidneys. These may result in cumulation and toxicity of drugs like propranolol and lignocaine.
- *Renal dysfunction:* Drugs mainly excreted through the kidneys are likely to accumulate and cause toxicity, e.g. streptomycin, amphotericin B. Doses of such drugs need to be reduced. Several drugs are totally eliminated unchanged only by the kidneys and such drugs can cause more toxicity. Also, the diseased kidneys are more susceptible to the toxic effects of nephrotoxic drugs like gold, penicillamine and aminoglycosides.
- *Endocrine diseases:* Hypothyroid patients are more sensitive to the effects of certain drugs like CNS depressants. Patients with benign prostatic hypertrophy are more susceptible to urinary retention with anticholinergics and tricyclic antidepressants.

10. **Repeated dosing:** Repeated dosing can result in:

a. Cumulation
b. Tolerance
c. Tachyphylaxis
d. Resistance

a. *Cumulation:* Drugs like digoxin which are slowly eliminated may cumulate resulting in toxicity.

b. *Tolerance:* It is the requirement of higher doses of a drug to produce a given response. Tolerance may be natural or acquired.

- *Natural tolerance:* The species/race shows less sensitivity to the drug, e.g. rabbits show tolerance to atropine; black race are tolerant to mydriatics.
- *Acquired tolerance* develops on repeated administration of a drug. The patient who was initially responsive becomes tolerant, e.g. tolerance develops to barbiturates, opioids, nitrites.

Tolerance may develop to some actions of the drug and not to others, e.g. morphine—tolerance develops to analgesic and euphoric effects of morphine but not to its constipating and miotic effects. Barbiturates—tolerance develops to sedative but not antiepileptic effects of barbiturates.

Table 3.2: Compilation of some useful examples

Drugs that are almost completely absorbed on oral ingestion (~100% bioavailability)

- Diazepam
- Chlordiazepoxide
- Lithium
- Salicylic acid
- Digitoxin
- Minocycline
- Valproic acid
- Indomethacin
- Phenobarbitone
- Linezolid

Drugs that undergo extensive first pass metabolism

- Propranolol
- Lignocaine
- Verapamil
- Pentazocine
- Nitroglycerin
- Testosterone
- Hydrocortisone
- Metoprolol
- Chlorpromazine
- Morphine
- Pethidine
- Insulin
- Isoprenaline
- Levodopa

Drugs that are highly bound to plasma proteins

- Warfarin
- Diazepam
- Phenylbutazone
- Indomethacin
- Clofibrate
- Phenytoin
- Sulfonamides
- Salicylates
- Tolbutamide
- Frusemide

Absorption increased by fatty food

- Halofantrine
- Albendazole
- Atovaquone
- Griseofulvin
- Efavirenz
- Posaconazole

Apparent volume of distribution (V_d)

Low V_d drugs

- Heparin
- Warfarin
- Aminoglycosides
- Aspirin
- Furosemide
- Ampicillin
- Amoxicillin

High V_d drugs

- Pethidine
- Digoxin
- Chloroquine
- Nortriptyline
- Fluoxetine
- Haloperidol
- Amiodarone

Some microsomal enzyme inducers

- Phenobarbitone
- Rifampicin
- Tolbutamide
- Phenylbutazone
- DDT
- Carbamazepine
- Phenytoin
- Griseofulvin
- Metronidazole
- Cigarette smoke
- Alcohol

Some microsomal enzyme inhibitors

- Cimetidine
- Erythromycin
- Omeprazole
- Grape fruit juice
- Allopurinol
- Fluoxetine
- Quinidine
- Ketoconazole
- Chloramphenicol

Some folate antagonists

- Sulfonamides
- Trimethoprim
- Methotrexate
- Pemetrexed
- Pyrimethamine
- Proguanil
- Dapsone

Prodrugs

- Levodopa → Dopamine
- Prednisone → Prednisolone
- Enalapril → Enalaprilat
- Bacampicillin → Ampicillin
- Cortisone → Hydrocortisone
- Azathioprine → Mercaptopurine
- Cyclophosphamide → Aldophosphamide
- Zidovudine → Zidovudine triphosphate

Hit and run drugs

- Reserpine
- Omeprazole

Drugs metabolised by zero-order kinetics

- Alcohol
- Salicylates
- Phenylbutazone
- Phenytoin
- Heparin

Drugs that undergo enterohepatic recycling

- Tetracyclines
- Doxorubicin
- Mefloquine
- Indomethacin
- Estradiol
- Amphetamine
- Metronidazole
- Morphine
- Phenytoin

Drugs available as transdermal patches

- Nitroglycerin
- Fentanyl
- Testosterone
- Hyoscine
- Estrogen

Drugs to which tolerance develops easily

- Nitrates
- Barbiturates
- Hydralazine
- Opioids

Agents which exhibit tachyphylaxis

- Ephedrine
- 5-HT
- Amphetamine
- Tyramine

Drugs which need tapering (after long-term use)

- β-blockers
- Antiepileptics
- Sedatives
- Antipsychotics
- Glucocorticoids
- Clonidine
- Antidepressants

Contd...

Table 3.2: Compilation of some useful examples (*contd...*)

Drugs with very short t½ (2–10 min)
- Dobutamine
- Dopamine
- Esmolol
- Adenosine
- Sodium nitroprusside
- Alteplase
- 5-Fluorouracil

Drugs with long t½

Drug	t½ in days
• Chloroquine	10–24
• Etanercept	3–4
• Phenylbutazone	3–4
• Mefloquine	16–24
• Gold salts	7
• Suramin	90

Some haemodialysable drugs
- Isoniazid
- Barbiturates
- Methaqualone
- Phenytoin
- Theophylline
- Ethyl and methyl alcohol
- Amphetamines
- Lithium
- Salicylates

Histamine liberators
- Morphine
- Pentamidine
- Hydralazine
- Tubocurarine
- Vancomycin
- Amphetamine

Drugs that colour urine

Orange red
- Rifampicin
- Phenazopyridine
- Daunorubicin
- Vitamin B complex (yellow)
- Nitazoxanide (green)

Nitric oxide donors
- Sodium nitroprusside
- Nitrates
- Nitrites

Drugs with low therapeutic index
- Digoxin
- Theophylline
- Lithium
- Quinidine

Drugs which need plasma concentration monitoring
- Lithium
- Digoxin
- Aminoglycosides
- Carbamazepine
- Theophylline

Some teratogenic drugs
- Thalidomide
- Sodium valproate
- Carbamazepine
- Lithium
- Androgens
- Progestins
- Anticancer drugs
- Tetracyclines
- Phenytoin
- Phenobarbitone
- Glucocorticoids
- Oestrogens
- Antithyroid drugs

Drugs to be used with caution in renal failure
- Aminoglycosides
- Cyclosporine
- Foscarnet
- Ifosfamide
- ACE inhibitors
- Anticancer drugs like cisplatin, methotrexate
- Amphotericin
- Acyclovir
- Pentamidine
- NSAIDs
- Sulphonamides
- Penicillamine

Drugs that can produce gingival hyperplasia
- Phenytoin
- Calcium channel blockers
- Cyclosporin

Drugs that can induce haemolysis in G6PD deficient patients
- Sulfonamides
- Nitrofurans
- Vitamin K analogs
- Some vegetables
- Primaquine
- NSAIDs
- Dapsone

Drugs excreted in saliva
- Clarithromycin
- Phenytoin
- Metoclopramide
- Metronidazole
- Disulfiram

Mechanisms: The mechanisms of development of tolerance could be of two types:

Tolerance
- Pharmacokinetic mechanisms
- Pharmacodynamic causes

Pharmacokinetic: Changes in absorption, distribution, metabolism and excretion of drugs may result in reduced concentration of the drug at the site of action and is also known as **dispositional tolerance**, e.g. barbiturates induce microsomal enzymes and enhance their own metabolism.

Pharmacodynamic: Changes in the target tissue, may make it less responsive to the drug. It is also called **functional tolerance**. It could be due to downregulation of receptors as in opioids or due to compensatory mechanisms of the body, e.g. blunting of response to some antihypertensives due to salt and water retention.

Cross tolerance is the development of tolerance to pharmacologically related drugs, i.e. to drugs belonging to a particular group. Thus chronic alcoholics also show tolerance to barbiturates and general anaesthetics.

c. ***Tachyphylaxis:*** It is the rapid development of tolerance. When some drugs are administered repeatedly at short intervals, tolerance develops rapidly and is known as tachyphylaxis or acute tolerance, e.g. ephedrine, amphetamine, tyramine and 5-hydroxytryptamine. This is thought to be due to depletion of noradrenaline stores as the above drugs act by displacing noradrenaline from the sympathetic nerve endings. Other mechanisms involved may be slow dissociation of the drug from the receptor thereby blocking the receptor. Thus ephedrine given repeatedly in bronchial asthma may not give the desired response.

d. ***Resistance:*** Repeated administration of an antibiotic can result in reduced or no response to it and this could lead to life-threatening infections (*see* page 533).

11. Psychological factor: The doctor–patient relationship influences the response to a drug often to a large extent by acting on the patient's psychology. The patient's confidence in the doctor may itself be sufficient to relieve a suffering, particularly the psychosomatic disorders. This can be substantiated by the fact that a large number of patients respond to placebo. **Placebo** is the inert dosage form with no specific biological activity but only resembles the actual preparation in appearance (dummy medication).

Placebo = 'I shall be pleasing' (in Latin).

Placebo medicines are used in:

i. Clinical trials as a control to compare and assess whether the new compound is significantly better than the placebo.
ii. To benefit or please a patient psychologically when he does not actually require an active drug as in mild psychosomatic disorders and in chronic incurable diseases.

In fact all forms of treatment including physiotherapy and surgery have some placebo effect. The effect of placebo is influenced by the **personality** of the treating doctor, personality of the **patient** and the **formulation** of placebo used. Placebo can release endorphins in the brain to provide analgesia. The ability of the doctor to instill confidence in the patient itself carries enough weightage and the skill should be developed right from the student days as part of medical education. Some people are more likely to respond to placebo and are called **placebo reactors**. The formulation given as placebo should appear 'impressive'. **Injections** seem to have more pronounced 'placebo effect' than oral preparations. Substances used as placebo include **lactose**, **some vitamins**, **minerals** and **distilled water injections**. Placebo can **release endorphins** in the brain produce analgesia. However, the effect of placebo may not be consistant or could be temporary.

Nocebo: When an established drug fails to produce its known therapeutic effect, it is often referred to as 'nocebo' effect which means it is opposite to that of 'placebo'. It could be because the patient lacks faith in the drug or doctor.

Psychological factor thus plays an important role in therapeutics.

12. Presence of other drugs: The concurrent use of two or more drugs can influence the response of each other (*see* Drug Interactions, page 66).

Patient Compliance

For the success of any treatment, good patient compliance is essential.

Patient compliance is considered 'good' when the patient strictly follows the treatment related instructions given by the doctor. It may vary from partial compliance to total noncompliance. Compliance is an important factor which influences treatment.

Various factors which determine the patient compliance are:

1. Inadequate education—unable to understand the instructions, particularly complex regimen
2. Adverse effects—particularly disturbing ADRs
3. Polypharmacy (multiple drugs)—some drugs may be missed.
4. Lack of confidence in doctors
5. Financial—may be unable to afford
6. Disease—psychiatric illness or false belief

Directly observed treatment short course (DOTS) is a strategy to ensure good compliance to antitubercular drugs where a health worker supervises the tablet being swallowed.

[1–2] From Medical Council of India, *Competency based Undergraduate Curriculum for the Indian Medical Graduate*, 2018;136–144.

CHAPTER 4

Adverse Drug Reactions, Pharmacovigilance and Drug Interactions

Competency achievement: The student should be able to:

PH 1.6 Describe principles of pharmacovigilance and ADR reporting systems.[1]

PH 1.7 Define, identify and describe the management of adverse drug reactions (ADR).[2]

ADVERSE DRUG REACTIONS

All drugs can produce unwanted effects. WHO has defined an adverse drug reaction as "any response to a drug that is noxious and unintended and that occurs at doses used in man for prophylaxis, diagnosis or therapy." All drugs can cause adverse effects. Some patients are more likely to exhibit adverse effects to drugs.

Adverse drug reactions are classified (Fig. 4.1) as follows:

Type A (or augmented) reactions are related to the known pharmacological effects of the drug and are **predictable**, dose-related and quantitative adverse effects. For example, hypotension following alpha-blockers, insulin-induced hypoglycaemia, bleeding following anticoagulants. Most ADRs are of this category and are mostly reversible by dose reduction or stopping the drug. Type A

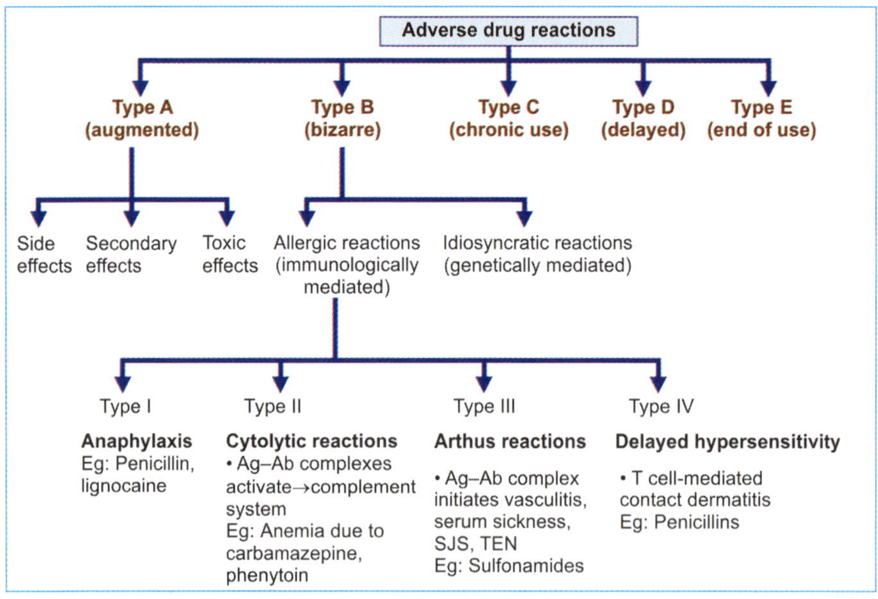

Fig. 4.1: Classification of ADRs

reactions include side effects, secondary effects and toxic effects.

a. *Side effects:* Side effects are unwanted effects of a drug that are an extension of the pharmacological effects and are seen with the therapeutic dose of the drug. They are predictable, common and can occur in all people, e.g. hypoglycaemia due to insulin; hypokalaemia following frusemide.
b. *Secondary effects:* Secondary effects are the indirect consequences of a primary drug action. Examples include superinfection on treatment of a primary infection by broad-spectrum antibiotics.
c. *Toxic effects:* Toxic effects are seen with higher doses of the drug and can be serious, e.g. morphine causes respiratory depression in overdosage which can be fatal (*see* Toxicology, Chapter 60).

Type B (bizarre) reactions are unrelated to the primary pharmacological effects of the drug and are, therefore, not predictable. They are less common, not tolerated and are an abnormal reaction to the drug. They could be idiosyncratic (genetically mediated) reactions or allergic reactions (immunologically mediated).

- **Idiosyncrasy** is a genetically determined abnormal reaction to a drug, e.g. primaquine and sulfonamides induce haemolysis in patients with G6PD deficiency; some patients show excitement with barbiturates. In addition, some responses like chloramphenicol-induced agranulocytosis, where no definite genetic background is known, are also included under idiosyncrasy. In some cases, the person may be highly sensitive even to low doses of a drug (e.g. a single dose of quinine can produce cinchonism in some) or highly insensitive even to high doses of the drug.
- **Allergic reactions** to drugs (*see* below) are immunologically-mediated reactions which are not related to the therapeutic effects of the drug. The drug or its metabolite acts as an antigen to induce antibody formation. Subsequent exposure to the drug may result in allergic reactions. The manifestations of allergy are seen mainly on the target organs, viz. skin, respiratory tract, gastrointestinal tract, blood and blood vessels.

Type C (continuous or chronic use) reactions occur on prolonged use of drugs and both dose and duration of drug use influence these ADRs. For example, chloroquine retinopathy, Cushing's syndrome, analgesic nephropathy.

Type D (delayed effects)—occur long after stopping treatment, sometimes after years. For example, leukaemia following treatment of Hodgkin's lymphoma; teratogenic effects.

Type E (end of use): These effects are due to sudden discontinuation of a drug after prolonged use. For example, acute adrenal insufficiency after sudden cessation of glucocorticoids, angina after sudden withdrawal of atenolol. Withdrawal syndrome to opioids and other drugs of abuse also are categorized as type E ADRs.

Pharmacovigilance

See page 65.

DRUG ALLERGY

Drugs can induce allergic reactions which could range from mild itching to anaphylaxis. They can induce both types of allergic reactions, viz. humoural and cell-mediated immunities. Mechanisms involved in Types I, II and III reactions are humoural immunity while Type IV reactions are due to cell-mediated immunity.

Types of Allergic Reactions and their Mechanisms

Type I (anaphylactic) reactions: The drug induces the synthesis of IgE antibodies which are fixed to the mast cells. On subsequent exposure, the antigen–antibody complexes cause degranulation of mast cells releasing the mediators of inflammation like histamine, leukotrienes, prostaglandins and platelet-activating factor. These are responsible for the characteristic signs and symptoms of anaphylaxis like bronchospasm, laryngeal oedema and hypotension which could be fatal. Allergy develops within minutes and is called immediate hypersensitivity reaction, e.g. penicillins. Skin tests may predict this type of reactions. Penicillins, cephalosporins, lignocaine, procaine, iron dextran and streptomycin are some drugs known to cause anaphylaxis.

Type II (cytolytic) reactions: The drug binds to a protein and together they act as antigens and induce the formation of antibodies. The antigen–antibody complexes activate the complement system resulting in cytolysis causing thrombocytopenia, agranulocytosis and aplastic anemia. Examples are carbamazepine, phenytoin, sulfonamides and phenylbutazone. Mismatched blood transfusion reactions are also cytolytic reactions.

Type III (Arthus) reactions: The antigen binds to circulating antibodies and the complexes are deposited on the vessel wall where it initiates the inflammatory response resulting in vasculitis. Rashes, fever, arthralgia, lymphadenopathy, serum sickness and Stevens-Johnson syndrome are some of the manifestations of arthus type reaction. **Serum sickness** is characterized by fever, arthritis, nephritis, oedema and skin rashes. Penicillins, sulfonamides, phenytoin, streptomycin and heparin can cause serum sickness. **Stevens-Johnson syndrome** (SJS) is characterized by severe bullous erythema multiforme particularly in the mucous membranes with fever and malaise. **Toxic epidermal necrolysis** (TEN) is the most serious form of drug allergy with mucocutaneous reactions that can be fatal. Aminopenicillins, sulfonamides, sulfones, phenytoin, barbiturates, carbamazepine, phenylbutazone and quinolones are the drugs associated with SJS and TEN. Both SJS and TEN involve mucocutaneous manifestations but the extent of involvement is greater in TEN.

Type IV (delayed hypersensitivity) reactions: This type of reactions is mediated by T lymphocytes and macrophages. The antigen reacts with receptors on T lymphocytes which produce lymphokines leading to a local allergic reaction, e.g. contact dermatitis in nurses and doctors handling penicillins and local anaesthetics.

Prevention of allergic reactions: In order to prevent allergic reactions, it is important to take history of drug allergy. If such a history is present, the drug as well as its chemically related drugs should be avoided. For drugs which are known to cause allergy like penicillins and cephalosporins, sensitivity skin test should be done before administering the full therapeutic dose.

Drugs Likely to Cause Allergy

Penicillins	Sulphonamides (and
Cephalosporins	other sulpha drugs)
	Salicylates
Radio contrast media (with iodine)	Quinolones
Antisera	Local anesthetics

Desensitization: Hyposensitization or desensitization is required for some drugs like penicillin G when there are not many alternatives available. To start with, very small doses of the drug is given repeatedly at short intervals to desensitize and the dose is then gradually increased as the patient gets desensitized.

Other forms of adverse drug reactions:

1. *Drug intolerance:* Drug intolerance is the inability of a person to tolerate a drug even in therapeutic doses and is unpredictable. It could be quantitative or qualitative. Quantitative intolerance is when patients show exaggerated response to even small doses of the drug, e.g. vestibular dysfunction after a single dose of streptomycin may be seen in some patients. Intolerance could

also be qualitative, e.g. idiosyncrasy and allergic reactions.

2. *Iatrogenic diseases (physician-induced):* These are drug-induced diseases. Even after the drug is withdrawn, its toxic effects can persist, e.g. isoniazid-induced hepatitis; chloroquine-induced retinopathy. Drugs that can induce parkinsonism are chlorpromazine, haloperidol and other phenothiazines, metoclopramide and reserpine.
3. *Photosensitivity:* Drugs could sensitize the skin to sunlight and the UV rays of the sun.
4. *Drug dependence:* Drugs that influence the behaviour and mood are often misused to obtain pleasurable effects. Repeated use of such drugs results in dependence. Several words, like drug abuse, addiction and dependence, are used confusingly. Drug dependence is a state of compulsive use of drugs in spite of the knowledge of the risks associated with their use. It is also referred to as drug addiction. Dependence could be 'psychologic' or 'physical' dependence. Psychologic dependence is compulsive drug-seeking behaviour to obtain its pleasurable effects, e.g. cigarette smoking. Physical dependence is said to be present when withdrawal of the drug produces adverse symptoms. The body undergoes physiological changes to adapt itself to the continued presence of the drug in the body. Stopping the drug results in 'withdrawal syndrome.' The symptoms of withdrawal syndrome are disturbing and the person then craves for the drug, e.g. alcohol, opioids and barbiturates (*see* page 277).

   Mild degree of physical dependence is seen in people who drink too much of coffee.
5. *Teratogenicity:* Teratogenicity is the ability of a drug to cause foetal abnormalities when administered to a pregnant woman. *Teratos* in Greek means monster. The sedative thalidomide taken during early pregnancy for relief from morning sickness resulted in thousands of babies being born with phocomelia (seal limbs). This thalidomide disaster (1958–61) opened the eyes of drug licensing authorities and various nations made it mandatory to conduct strict teratogenicity tests before a new drug is approved for use.

   Depending on the stage of pregnancy during which the teratogen is administered, it can produce various abnormalities.
   - Conception to 16 days—usually resistant to teratogenic effects. If affected, abortion occurs.
   - Period of organogenesis (17 to 55 days of gestation): Most vulnerable period; major physical abnormalities occur.
   - Foetal period (56 days onwards)—period of growth and development—hence developmental and functional abnormalities result.

   Therefore, in general, drugs should be avoided during pregnancy specially in the first trimester. The type of malformation also depends on the drug, e.g. thalidomide causes phocomelia; tetracyclines cause deformed teeth; sodium valproate causes spina bifida. Drugs are categorised based on their teratogenic potential as given in Table 4.1.
6. *Carcinogenicity and mutagenicity:* Some drugs can cause cancers and genetic abnormalities. For example, anticancer drugs can themselves be carcinogenic; other examples are radioactive isotopes and some hormones.
7. *Organ toxicities:* Drugs can also cause toxicity to various **organ systems** (Table 4.2).

Hepatotoxicity: Liver is the major organ of drug metabolism and most drugs are metabolized by it. Drug-induced hepatotoxicity is a serious problem accounting for nearly 10% of all cases of hepatitis. It is also a common cause of acute hepatic failure. Hepatotoxicity can complicate treatment because it can result in reduced metabolism of drugs, which in turn increases their plasma levels, further worsening toxicity.

Drug-induced hepatotoxicity could be:

1. *Dose dependent:* Hepatocellular, e.g. a metabolite of paracetamol generates free

Table 4.1: Teratogenicity risk categories (general interpretation in brackets for simplification)

Category	*Features*
A	Studies in women have failed to demonstrate risk to the fetus, e.g. chloroquine (safe)
B	Risk not confirmed in humans (animal studies do not show teratogenic potential), e.g. paracetamol, amoxicillin (mostly safe)
C	Teratogenic in animal studies but inadequate human data. Drug used only if benefits outweigh risk to fetus, e.g. glucocorticoids (likely to be safe)
D	Evidence of risk in humans but benefit in mother may need the drug as in life-threatening disease, e.g. phenytoin (likely to be teratogenic)
X	Evidence of risk; drug contraindicated in pregnancy, e.g. thalidomide, isotretinoin (teratogenic)

radicals which in small amounts will be detoxified by glutathione conjugation. In larger doses glutathione stores get depleted and toxic metabolites get accumulated loading to liver cell injury. Toxic doses of paracetamol cause fatal fulminant hepatic failure.

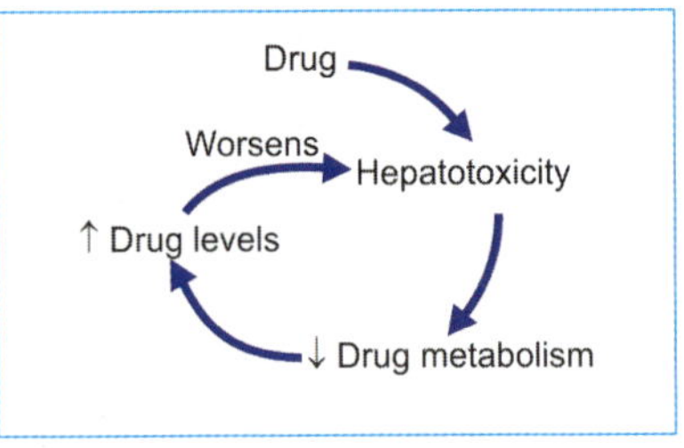

2. *Non-dose-dependent hepatocellular damage:* Drugs like halothane, isoniazid, NSAIDs, ethambutol, antiepileptics like valproic acid and phenytoin and many other drugs are known to cause liver toxicity which is not dose related and could be an idiosyncratic reaction.
3. *Fatty liver:* Chronic alcoholism and drugs like glucocorticoids, methotrexate, indomethacin, bleomycin and tamoxifen can cause fatty liver. Triglycerides get accumulated in the liver which may lead to inflammation called steatohepatitis.
4. *Chronic active hepatitis:* Drugs like isoniazid, paracetamol, nitrofurantoin, halothane and hydralazine can cause prolonged hepatitis with altered liver enzymes. This could be due to autoantibodies against the antigens specific to the liver in genetically

Table 4.2: Examples of drugs affecting various organ systems

Organ system affected	*Examples*
1. Hepatotoxicity	Isoniazid, pyrazinamide, paracetamol, chlorpromazine, 6-mercaptopurine, halothane, ethanol, phenylbutazone
2. Nephrotoxicity	Analgesics, aminoglycosides, cyclosporine, cisplatin, cephalexin, penicillamine, gold salts
3. Ototoxicity	Aminoglycosides, frusemide
4. Ocular toxicity	Chloroquine, ethambutol
5. Gastrointestinal system	Opioids, broad-spectrum antibiotics
6. Cardiovascular system	Digoxin, doxorubicin
7. Respiratory system	Aspirin, bleomycin, busulfan, amiodarone, methotrexate
8. Musculoskeletal system	Corticosteroids, heparin
9. Behavioural toxicity	Corticosteroids, reserpine
10. Neurological system	INH, haloperidol, ethambutol, quinine, doxorubicin vincristine
11. Dermatological toxicity	Doxycycline, sulfonamides, gold, d-penicillamine
12. Electrolyte disturbances	Diuretics, mineralocorticoids
13. Hematological toxicity	Chloramphenicol, sulfonamides
14. Endocrine disorders	Methyldopa, oral contraceptives
15. Sexual dysfunction	Prazosin, reserpine, anticholinergics, barbiturates, methyldopa, tricyclic antidepressants

predisposed individuals. If not treated on time, it may progress to cirrhosis.

5. *Cholestasis:* Obstruction to the secretion of bile from the liver may result in jaundice. It may be seen following use of estrogen, anabolic steroids, glibenclamide and rifampicin. Long-term cholestasis may lead to cholestatic hepatitis with hepatocellular damage. *Examples:* Erythromycin, carbamazepine, some NSAIDs and sulphonamides.

Signs and Symptoms

Raised liver enzymes, jaundice, hepatomegaly and vomiting

Examples of drugs	*Hepatotoxic effect*
Paracetamol	Hepatic necrosis
Erythromycin, rifampicin	Cholestatic jaundice
Pyrazinamide, isoniazid, halothane	Hepatitis
Alcohol	Cirrhosis

Factors Contributing to Hepatotoxicity

1. Age—more common in infants and elderly patients.
2. Gender—women are more at risk of hepatotoxicity due to drugs like methyldopa, erythromycin (in pregnancy).
3. Genetics and race—variations in the drug metabolizing enzymes may be responsible for some races being at risk of drug-induced hepatotoxicity. For example, people could be fast acetylators (INH t½ 1 hr) or slow acetylators (INH t½ 3–5 hours) of INH, based on their genetic inheritance. Slow acetylators respond better to INH but hepatotoxicity is more likely in them.
4. Dose and duration of use—higher the dose and longer the use, risk of hepatotoxicity is higher.
5. Pre-existing liver disease—patients who are suffering from liver diseases are more likely to be affected by hepatotoxic drugs.

Precautions

- Drugs which are known to cause hepatotoxicity should be used carefully.
- Lowest effective dose should be used.
- Combination of 2 or more hepatotoxic drugs should be avoided.
- Liver function tests should be done at regular intervals to monitor the status.

TREATMENT OF DRUG OVERDOSAGE

See Chapter 60.

PHARMACOVIGILANCE

Competency achievement: The student should be able to:
PH 1.6 Describe principles of pharmacovigilance and ADR reporting systems.[3]

Definition: Pharmacovigilance is the science and activities relating to the detection, assessment, understanding and prevention of adverse effects or any other drug-related problems.

It deals with the epidemiologic study of adverse drug effects.

The aim of pharmacovigilance is to ensure safe and rational use of medicines. Since clinical trials are done on a limited number of patients, many potential adverse effects go undetected. Hence reporting adverse reactions is the **duty of all medical professionals**. The adverse reactions reported and related data is collected and assessed by the pharmacovigilance system consisting of ADR reporting centres, regional and national pharmacovigilance centres which in turn report to the Uppsala Monitoring Centre at Sweden.

In India, the Central Drugs Standard Control Organization (CDSCO) in collaboration with Indian Pharmacopoeia Commission, located at Ghaziabad has initiated a pharmacovigilance programme of India **(PVPI)**, which consists of peripheral, regional and zonal centres for coordinating the activity. Under the ADR monitoring centre, various medical colleges and hospitals function to report ADRs. The data collected is uploaded into the pharmacovigilance software **Vigiflow**. Effective pharmacovigilance activity and awareness of toxic effects of drugs has resulted in the withdrawal of several potential toxic drugs from the market (Fig. 4.2).

ADR analysis: The reported ADRs are assessed to know whether they were actually drug induced. Several scales are available for the purpose but the most preferred are the Naranjo's scale and WHO scale.

Haemovigilance: Adverse reactions associated with transfusion of blood and blood products is haemovigilance. It also needs to be reported through the software 'haemovigil'.

Materiovigilance is ADRs to biological devices.

Medication errors: Medication errors are errors that occur in the process of prescribing, dispensing and administration of drugs. They could occur at the level of doctors, pharmacists, nurses or patients. Adequate care should be taken to avoid them.

Look-alike Sound-alike (LASA) Drugs

LASA drugs are also referred to as **SALA** (sound-alike look-alike) drugs particularly in India! These are drugs which have similar names or look similar due to packaging and should be dealt with extra care since they can be confusing and result in medication errors. Drugs like clotrimazole and cotrimoxazole are likely to be easily mistaken. Precautions are to be taken to avoid such errors like writing the names in capital letters. Several brand names also sound similar. Look-alike drugs should be stored in separate racks or cupboards to avoid dispensing errors.

Some examples of sound-alike drugs are:

Amiodarone – Amantadine
Amlodipine – Amiloride
Buspirone – Bupropion
Cycloserine – Cyclosporine
Hydroxyzine – Hydralazine
Lamotrigine – Lamivudine

Over-the-counter (OTC) Drugs

Drugs which are considered safe for use by general public without a prescription are called 'over-the-counter' drugs or non-prescription drugs. Directions for their use can be easily understood by the patients and are mentioned on the information sheet dispensed along with the drugs. Drugs that can be dispensed as OTC drugs are chosen by the regulatory agency and include drugs for common ailments like cough, influenzae, diarrhoea, vomiting, allergy and gastric hyperacidity. However, OTC drugs also carry the risk of side effects and inappropriate use. History of OTC drug intake is essential since they could result in adverse effects and drug interactions.

Off-label use of drugs: When a drug is used for indications other than the approved ones, it is called 'off-label' use of drugs. The drug may be used for a different disease, indicated by a different route of administration or in a different dose. Examples: Clonidine is also used in attention deficit hyperactivity disorder. Diazepam from ampoule for injection is used rectally in febrile convulsions and status epilepticus. Azathioprine used topically for psoriasis, atopic dermatitis; erythromycin for gastroparesis, SSRIs for fibromyalgia and pathologic gambling.

COUNTERFEIT DRUGS

Counterfeit drugs are fake drugs. They are drugs or pharmaceutical products that contain inadequate dose or the inappropriate drug itself. The labelling, packaging or other information provided may be inappropriate with the intention of misleading the consumers. These spurious drugs may contain hazardous adulterants, beyond expiry date drugs, fake brand name drugs, or substandard drugs. Such counterfeit drugs can be harmful to the consumers.

DRUG INTERACTIONS

Competency achievement: The student should be able to:

PH 1.8 Identify and describe the management of drug interactions.[4]

Definition

Drug interaction is the alteration in the duration or magnitude of the pharmacological effects of one drug by another drug.

When two or more drugs are given concurrently, the response may be greater or lesser than the sum of their individual effects. Such responses may be beneficial or harmful. For example, a combination of drugs is used in hypertension—hydralazine + propranolol for their beneficial interaction. However, drug interactions may also result in severe toxicity. Such interactions can be avoided by adequate knowledge of their mechanisms and by judicious use of drugs. Some important drug interactions are mentioned in Appendix 1.

Site

Drug interactions can occur:

1. *In vitro* in the syringe before administration—mixing of drugs in syringes can cause chemical or physical interactions—such drug combinations are incompatible in solution, e.g. penicillin and gentamicin should never be mixed in the same syringe.
2. *In vivo,* i.e. in the body after administration.

Pharmacological Basis of Drug Interactions

The two major mechanisms of drug interactions include pharmacokinetic and pharmacodynamic interactions.

Pharmacokinetic Mechanisms

Alteration in the extent or duration of response may be produced by influencing absorption, distribution, metabolism or excretion of one drug by another.

Absorption of drugs from the gut may be affected by:

1. *Binding:* Tetracyclines chelate iron and antacids resulting in reduced absorption. Cholestyramine is a bile acid binding resin which also binds many drugs.
2. *Altering gastric pH:* Antacids raise gastric pH and interfere with the absorption of drugs like iron and anticoagulants.
3. *Altering GI motility:* Atropine and morphine slow gastric emptying and delay the absorption of drugs. Purgatives reduce the absorption of riboflavin.

Distribution: Competition for plasma protein or tissue binding results in displacement interactions, e.g. warfarin is displaced by phenylbutazone from protein binding sites.

Metabolism: Hepatic microsomal enzyme induction and inhibition can both result in drug interactions (*see* page 31), e.g. phenytoin, phenobarbitone, carbamazepine and rifampicin are enzyme inducers while chloramphenicol and cimetidine are some enzyme inhibitors.

Excretion: When drugs compete for the same renal tubular transport system, they prolong each other's duration of action, e.g. penicillin and probenecid.

Pharmacodynamic Mechanisms

Drugs acting on the same receptors or physiological systems result in additive, synergistic or antagonistic effects. Many clinically important drug interactions have this basis. Examples are:

- Atropine opposes the effects of physostigmine.
- Naloxone antagonises morphine.
- Antihypertensive effects of β-blockers are reduced by ephedrine or other vasoconstrictors present in cold remedies.
- Many diuretics produce hypokalaemia which potentiate digitalis toxicity.
- Organic nitrates (used in angina) act by increasing cGMP activity. Sildenafil inhibits phosphodiesterase which inactivates cGMP and thereby potentiates the effects of nitrates. Hence the combination can cause severe hypotension and even deaths have been reported.

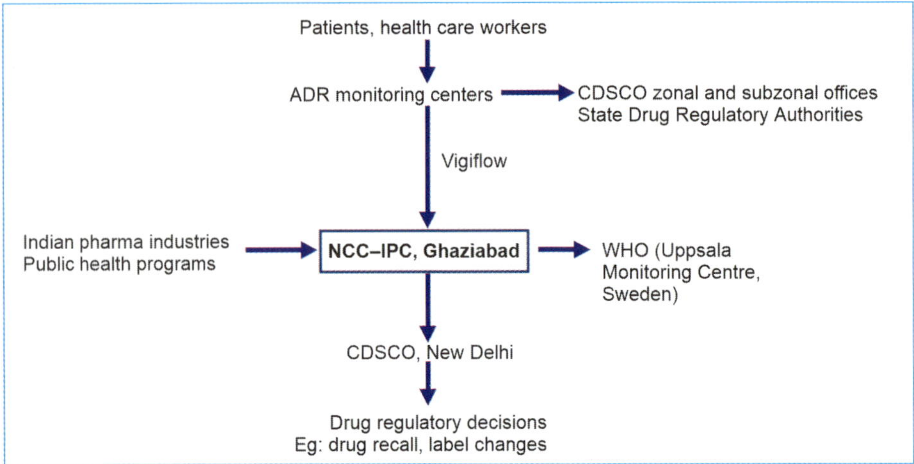

Fig. 4.2: Flow of ADR information and working of PvPI

NCC: National Co-ordination Centre, PvPI: Pharmacovigilance Program of India

- Aspirin inhibits platelet aggregation and enhances the risk of bleeding due to oral anticoagulants like warfarin.
- Many antihistamines produce sedation which may be enhanced by alcohol intake.

Drug–Food Interactions

Simultaneous intake of food and drugs could result in some interactions. Presence of food itself interferes with the absorption of several drugs like rifampicin, roxithromycin which need to be given on an empty stomach.

- Drugs also interact with constituents of food like milk (tetracycline, iron) and reduce the bioavailability of these.
- Tender coconut water and fruits (e.g. sweet lime) rich in potassium can add up to the hyperkalaemia caused by ACE inhibitors.
- Cheese reaction—consumption of tyramine-containing foods like cheese, beer, wines, yeast, buttermilk and fish by patients receiving MAO inhibitors results in hypertension—termed cheese reaction. Inhibition of MAO by drugs leads to raised tyramine levels which displaces NA from the adrenergic nerve terminals resulting in hypertension.
- Grapefruit is an enzyme inhibitor and thereby raises the levels of phenytoin.

Databases for drug interactions: Since memorizing drug interactions is a great challange, help of software may be needed often to ensure patient safety when multiple drugs are used. Many softwares are available for the purpose on the internet some of which are free.

[1–4] From Medical Council of India, *Competency based Undergraduate Curriculum for the Indian Medical Graduate*, 2018;1:136–144.

Drug Nomenclature, Drug Development, Drug Regulations, Essential Medicines, Prescriptions and Related Topics

CHAPTER 5

Competency achievement: The student should be able to:
PH 1.9 Describe nomenclature of drugs, i.e. generic, branded drugs.[1]

DRUG NOMENCLATURE

A drug can have four names:

1. **Code name:** When a new drug is synthesized/discovered, it is given a **code name** at the time of development. It consists of letters and numbers like AMG 785. Once the drug is approved for use, the code name is no more used (Table 5.1).

2. **Chemical name:** The *chemical name* gives the chemical description of the drug, e.g. 3, (10, 11-dihydro-5H-dibenz (b,f)-azepin-5-yl) propyldimethylamine. This is lengthy, complex and unsuitable for prescribing.

3. **Generic name (non-proprietary)** is given by a competent recognized official agency like WHO and is internationally accepted, i.e. the drug has the same generic name all over the world. It is called International Non-proprietary Name (INN). The INN system came into effect in 1953 and was initiated at a resolution by World Health Assembly. It gives a clue to the class of the drug, because drugs in a group sound similar as they end with the same letters, e.g. propranolol, atenolol, esmolol, metoprolol—all are β-blockers and cimetidine, ranitidine, famotidine, and roxatidine are all H_2 receptor blockers. It is convenient and the drug is sometimes cheaper when prescribed by generic name. The nonproprietary name of the above example given under chemical name is imipramine.

4. **Brand name (proprietary)** is the trade name given by the manufacturer. Hence each drug may have many brand names, e.g. Crocin, Metacin, Pacemol, Calpol are different brand names of paracetamol. The main advantage in using brand name is the consistency of the product especially bioavailability. Hence, for drugs with low therapeutic index like digoxin and antiepileptics, prescribing the same brand name is beneficial. Certain guidelines are laid by the concerned authorities in giving brand names to pharmaceutical products in each country and the name has to be approved by the authority before being marketed by the company.

DRUG DEVELOPMENT

Competency achievement: The student should be able to:
PH 1.64 Describe overview of drug development, Phases of clinical trials and Good Clinical Practice.[2]

The last few decades have seen the development of several new drugs which have

Table 5.1: Drug names

Code name	Generic name	Chemical name	Brand names
RU-486	Mifepristone	11beta17alpha(1propynyl)estra-4,9-dien-17beta-01-3-one	UNDO, MT-PILL, UNWANTED

revolutionised the practice of medicine. The discovery and development of a new drug is a time-consuming and expensive procedure.

A new drug may be identified by the following processes:

1. Chemical modification of a known drug.
2. Random screening of natural and synthetic chemicals to detect useful activity.
3. Rational drug designing based on the chemical structure.

After identification, the structure of the new compound and its purity are determined by the analytical chemist. The compound is screened for the presence of any useful biological activity by a series of tests like bioassays, molecular and cellular studies. If the compound is found to be promising, then it is subjected to preclinical evaluation in animals and then clinical trials in humans.

Preclinical Studies

Preclinical studies involve both *in vitro* and *in vivo* studies in different animal species. Testing the compounds in animals involves phamacodynamic, pharmacokinetic and toxicity studies. At the end of it (i) the maximum recommended starting dose for use in humans should be found out. (ii) Therapeutic index should be obtained.

Toxicity studies are done to study the potential toxic effects of drugs. At least 2 species of animals—a rodent and a non-rodent are used because there are differences in response to drugs among different species. Toxicity studies can be acute, subacute and chronic toxicity studies.

Acute toxicity study is usually a single dose test to study the gross effects on behaviour and to know the lethal and toxic dose. Subacute toxicity studies with graded doses are done to study the toxicity on target organ and to establish maximum therapeutic dose. Chronic toxicity studies involve 3 dose levels and may go on for 6 months to 2 years.

Clinical Trials

When the drug is found to be reasonably safe in animals, it is subjected to clinical trials in human beings after obtaining permission from the regulatory agency. Clinical trials are conducted to compare the therapeutic efficacy of a new drug with an existing drug or a placebo.

Good clinical practice: For the conduct of clinical trials, certain regulatory guidelines are laid down in order to ensure safety of the subjects and transparency in the trial activities. The guidelines for good clinical practice and ethics are formulated by certain regulatory bodies. For the conduct of clinical trials in India, the guidelines by International Conference on Harmonization (ICH) Food and Drug Administration USA (USFDA), New Drug and Clinical Trials rules (NDCT-2019), Good Clinical Practice (GCP) guidelines of India, and the guidelines by WHO and ethical guidelines by Indian Council of Medical Research (ICMR) are followed. These guidelines aim to protect human rights and ensure that authentic and credible clinical trial data is generated.

Ethical clearance: After obtaining permission from the concerned regulatory authorities to conduct the trial in a given setting, permission should be obtained from the local institutional ethics committee (IEC) or institutional review board (IRB). The IEC looks into the ethical aspects of the trial and ensures that the trial is conducted ethically and the rights of the study participants are protected.

Informed consent: For enrolling a subject into a clinical trial, he/she should be informed in detail about the trial including the risks involved and the subject should willingly consent to participate in the study. He should sign the informed consent form and should also be made aware that he is free to withdraw from the study whenever he wants to. This is to ensure that the participation in the study is purely voluntary and not by force.

Table 5.1: Phases of clinical trials

Phases	*Number of subjects*	*Objectives*	*Conducted by*
Phase 0	10–15	Explore pharmacokinetics and pharmacodynamics	Clinical pharmacologist
Phase I	20–50 normal volunteers	To establish safety, to know biological effects, pharmacokinetic profile and to design a safe dose	Clinical pharmacologist
Phase II	100–300 patients	To establish efficacy, detect adverse effects and pharmacokinetics	Clinical pharmacologists and clinical investigators
Phase III	250 to >1000 selected patients	To establish efficacy, safety, to identify latent side effects, tolerance, design ideal dose-range, and to compare with existing drugs	Clinical investigators
Phase IV (Post-marketing surveillance)	2000 to >10,000 patients	Long-term safety and efficacy; to identify other possible therapeutic uses	Medical practitioners

Phases of Clinical Trials

Clinical trials are generally conducted in 4 phases though phase 0 is also included in some situations (Table 5.1):

Phase 0: Phase 0, also called **microdosing**, is a recent approach in clinical trials to cut cost in drug development. It is conducted in a small number of subjects (10–15) for a short duration (<7 days). A very small dose is used to evaluate the pharmacodynamics and pharmacokinetics in human beings (the first exposure in humans) and are exposed to the drug for a short period. Analysis is done by highly sensitive methods like accelerated mass spectrometry and positron emission tomography (PET).

Phase I: Less than 50 normal healthy volunteers are given the drug to establish safety, to know the actions, determine pharmacokinetic profile and to design a safe dose for further use.

Phase II: If phase I is successful, the compound undergoes phase II evaluation in order to establish efficacy, to detect any adverse effects, appropriate dose and detailed pharmacology of the chemical in 100–300 patients suffering from diseases for which the drug under trial has therapeutic prospects.

Phase III: If the phase II establishes that the drug is useful and generally safe, phase III clinical trials are undertaken. A large number of selected patients is given the drug to establish the benefits of the drug in the target disease, to identify the latent side effects, susceptibility to tolerance and to design ideal dosage regimen for different groups of patients.

Phase IV: Postmarketing surveillance—If phase III studies are satisfactory, the new drug is marketed. Since the earlier phases involve a relatively smaller number of patients (3000) for short periods (<1 year), they cannot be expected to provide full safety information. Thus postmarketing surveillance is done for systematic detection and evaluation of long-term safety of the drug. It is done by collection and evaluation of data based on information sent by medical practitioners prescribing the drug. Phase IV trials are thus conducted by medical practitioners.

Clinical Trials Registry

With the progress in research, several new molecules have been synthesized all over the world. With the growing public awareness about drugs and diseases, information on newer drugs and upcoming medication is

> **Meta-analysis**
>
> Data from several clinical trials or studies are combined and the results are analysed (each study should have followed the same procedure). This is known as meta-analysis and helps to obtain more accurate results as a larger number of subjects are considered.

sought both by doctors as well as public. In order to make the drug development transparent, accountable and data accessible, **Clinical Trial Registry of India (CTRI)** has been set up by the joint efforts of Indian Council of Medical Research (ICMR), Department of Science and Technology (DST) and World Health Organisation (WHO). All clinical trials being conducted in India should be registered in CTRI. Though the registration is voluntary and free of cost, registration has several benefits for the investigators, like—it is possible to publish data from clinical trials because, for the publication of data from clinical trials, CTRI registration is required. The details registered are freely accessible to all including general public.

Orphan Drugs

Orphan drugs are drugs to be used for prevention and treatment of rare diseases. Such drugs are not readily developed and marketed because they are not profitable to the manufacturer. Example: Acetylcysteine used for paracetamol overdosage, 4 methylpyrazole in poisoning due to methanol or ethylene glycol, 4-aminosalicylic acid in the treatment of ulcerative colitis. Such rare diseases are also called **orphan diseases**. The Orphan Drugs Act provides incentives to the drug manufacturers for the development of orphan drugs.

DRUG INFORMATION SOURCES

Information on drugs can be obtained by:

- *Primary source:* Original research published in journals and information from clinical trials.
- *Secondary source:* Data from research analysed, compiled and published, e.g. in medline, index medicus, etc.
- *Tertiary source*—include drug compendia.

Drug Compendia

Books that are sources of information on drugs, i.e. pharmacopoeia and formularies are together known as drug compendia. The third one is e-source, i.e. the medline

1. **Official compendia**
   - Pharmacopoeia
   - Drug formulary
2. **Non-official compendia**
   - Textbooks
   - Journals
   - Periodicals
3. **Medline**

1. Official compendia are recognized by the government of that country as 'legal standard'.

Pharmacopoeia: Pharmacopoeia is the official publication of a list of drugs and medicinal preparations. In Greek 'Pharmacon' means drug and 'poeia' is to make. It contains a list of drugs and related substances that are approved for use, their source, formulae and other information needed to prepare the drugs, their physical properties, tests for their identity, purity and potency. Each country may follow its own pharmacopoeia. We thus have Indian Pharmacopoeia, British Pharmacopoeia, United States Pharmacopoeia, USSR and Japanese Pharmacopoeia. The European Pharmacopoeia was published by the Public Health Committee and the European Pharmacopoeia Commission. The International Pharmacopoeia is published by WHO in many languages like English, French, Spanish and Russian.

The first pharmacopoeia of India was published in 1868. But later under the British rule, the British Pharmacopoeia was followed. After independence, a committee was set up and Indian Pharmacopoeia was released in 1955. Experts from pharmaceutical industry, drug control laboratories and research and teaching institutions helped the committee.

Pharmacopoeia is revised at regular periods to delete old, useless drugs and to include newly introduced ones.

Drug formulary: The National Formulary contains information on therapeutically used formulations. It is prepared by the National Formulary Committee set up by the Ministry of Health, Government of India. Expert opinion is also taken from medical associations, hospitals, teaching institutions and pharmaceutical industry in preparing this book.

2. Non-official compendia: These are books other than the official compendia and include textbooks of pharmacology, journals and periodicals.

3. Medline: Medline or medical literature analysis and retrieval system online is a literature database of life sciences and biomedical information.

PHARMACOECONOMICS

Competency achievement: The student should be able to:
PH 1.60 Describe and discuss pharmacogenomics and **pharmacoeconomics.**[2]

Pharmacoeconomics is the science that compares the cost of various treatment modalities to the outcome. It helps to know which treatment is less expensive and effective. This information will be useful to effectively use the funds and resources to improve healthcare. It aims to effectively use the resources to improve healthcare and also pays attention to quality of life in healthcare policies—'value-for-money' approach.

In recent years extensive research in **pharmacoeconomics** is undertaken.

Goals of pharmacoeconomics research are:

1. To know which healthcare alternatives provide the best outcome for the money spent
2. To improve allocation of funds

Whenever possible the doctor needs to consider cheaper and effective alternatives for the treatment of all ailments. Pharmacoeconomics studies aim to provide such information.

Types of Pharmacoeconomics Analysis

1. *Cost minimization analysis:* This aims to find out the best treatment alternative with minimum cost. For example, comparing 2 generic drugs.
2. *Cost effectiveness analysis:* In this the health benefits can be measured in units and is the most commonly used pharmacoeconomics analysis. It compares therapies where the outcome is common and can help in the identification of a preferred choice among alternatives. For example, number of years of life prolonged following treatment.
3. *Cost-benefit analysis:* This compares the cost and the outcome of alternative regimens. For example, cost and outcome of surgery vs pharmacotherapy for coronary heart disease.
4. *Cost utility analysis:* Here the outcome of treatment is measured in terms of quality of life or QALY (quality adjusted life years). For example, comparing the quality of life while using two different antihypertensives.

Pharmacogenomics—see page 54.

CHRONOPHARMACOLOGY

Chronopharmacology deals with the correlation of drug effects to the circadian rhythm.

Association of Diseases with Circadian Rhythm

- Higher incidence of MI and stroke is seen early in the morning.
- Intraocular pressure variations are seen throughout the day.
- BP is highest during the afternoon and gradually decreases to reach lowest levels at night.
- Symptoms of allergic rhinitis is worst in the morning.

Application of Chronopharmacology in Therapeutics

Morning: Glucocorticoids and testosterone are administered in the morning to mimic the natural secretion.

Evening: Statins are given in the evening.

Night:

- Aspirin is administered at night to prevent platelet aggregation which is more likely in the morning.
- For allergic rhinitis, antihistamines are given at night to prevent allergic response the next morning.
- Diuretics are given in the morning to reduce hypokalemia.

ESSENTIAL MEDICINES

Competency achievement: The student should be able to:
PH 1.59 and 3.7 Prepare a list of essential medicines for a healthcare facility.[1]

WHO has compiled the list of medicines that is required to meet the primary healthcare needs of majority of the population and are called essential drugs. Essential medicines have been defined by WHO as those that satisfy the healthcare needs of majority of the population and should, therefore, be available at all times in adequate amounts and in the appropriate dosage forms. The original list has undergone revisions and updating from time to time to meet the changing requirements. Based on the WHO guidelines for selection of essential drugs and by referring its model list, each country puts forth its national list of essential drugs.

- Adoption of the list has resulted in greater coordination in healthcare development.
- The list serves as a guideline for indenting and stocking essential drugs.
- The concept has also helped in the development of national formularies.
- A short list is compiled for community health workers to aid in providing primary healthcare.
- The use of essential medicines list has also emphasised the need for drug research and development, e.g. safety and efficacy of a new drug should be established for it to be included in the essential medicines list.

India's first National **Essential Medicines** List consisting of about 300 drugs was formulated in 1996. 21st model list of essential medicines was brought out by WHO in June 2019.

RATIONAL DRUG USE

Once a patient is diagnosed to have a particular disease and needs to be treated with drugs, the specific **therapeutic objective** should be defined. For example, in hypertension, the objective is to bring down the BP to a particular level in order to prevent complications of prolonged hypertension. Once the objective is clear, the **choice of drugs** should be made. Various aspects should be considered while choosing the drug. When many drugs are available for the treatment of the particular condition, the right choice should be carefully made. For example, hyperacidity and mild gastritis may be managed with antacids. When not controlled, an H_2 receptor blocker like ranitidine helps. Only more severe cases require to be treated with omeprazole. Patient factors including age, presence of other diseases, renal and liver function, other drugs being administered and cost of therapy should be considered. Newer drugs are all expensive. When less expensive older drugs are available, they should be preferred to the newer ones. Though human insulin is the rational choice for all diabetics who need insulin, majority of patients in the developing countries like India cannot afford such an expensive medication for the rest of their lives. Hence conventional insulins are still preferable in them—unless contraindicated.

The **dose and the duration** of treatment should be determined. When long-term treatment is required, the regular review and monitoring of treatment should be planned. The therapeutic end point should be defined.

When a **combination of drugs** is to be administered, the guidelines like better therapeutic benefit, avoiding drugs with overlapping adverse effects and cost of therapy should be borne in mind. Equally important is to avoid irrational combination of drugs. The flourishing drug industry often comes out with absurd combinations of drugs. They serve no useful purpose, are more expensive and unnecessary, but are vigorously promoted and unfortunately often prescribed by doctors. Some such examples are:

1. *Amoxicillin (250 mg) with cloxacillin (250 mg):* Combined with the view that cloxacillin can destroy the penicillinase producing *Staphylococcus aureus* (PPSA) while amoxicillin can help, if the infection is with other bacteria. But, in fact, if the infecting organism is PPSA, 250 mg cloxacillin is an underdosage. If it is not PPSA, 250 mg of amoxicillin is an underdosage. It should be noted that cloxacillin is not an efficient antibiotic in infections other than PPSA while amoxicillin is of no use in PPSA. Therefore, the combination is totally irrational.
2. *Ibuprofen with paracetamol:* Either of them can be given based on the requirement. Combination serves no useful purpose.
3. *Diclofenac + nimesulide:* Either of them can be given based on the requirement. Combination serves no useful purpose. Nimesulide is now banned in most of the countries.
4. *Ciprofloxacin + tinidazole:* The combination is used in diarrhoea. It is claimed that it helps in diarrhoea due to both gram-negative bacteria and amoeba. In reality, the diarrhoea is due to either of the organisms and not both. Using the combination only exposes the patient to the risk of toxicity from the other antimicrobial agent and also adds to the cost of therapy.

P-DRUGS

Pharmacology has grown to an extent where it extensively taxes the memory of any human brain to remember all the drugs described in the books. In daily practice, however, a physician needs to be proficient in using fewer drugs (40–60). For any illness, if there are many drugs in a group, the physician may choose some primary drugs which need to be used routinely and be thorough with their pharmacology. Such a choice of drugs called **P** or **personal drugs** are used to prescribe regularly. The doctor needs to also know the dose, formulations, duration of treatment, drug interactions and precautions in using such P-drugs.

P-treatment: For any given illness, the treatment of first choice is the P-treatment. It depends on the therapeutic objective, safety, efficacy and cost of treatment.

When a patient has to be treated with drugs, the question of 'selection of the right drug' arises. WHO provides certain guidelines for **good prescribing**. When a patient is seen by a doctor, the steps of approach would be to establish the diagnosis and then to specify the therapeutic objective. For example, if an infection is to be treated, the objective would be to cure the infection; in some of the cancers, the objective would be palliation. Having defined the objective, the P-drugs have to be chosen and their suitability for the particular patient verified. The treatment is then started where caution is to be taken to avoid overprescribing or under treatment. The strength, precautions for use, right dose for the right length of time and the relevant information to the patient regarding the drugs including its mode of action, adverse effects and dosage instructions are to be given. Once the patient is on treatment, monitoring is required. **Monitoring** is done to ensure if the treatment was effective, safe, to look for any adverse effects and if the compliance was good. Monitoring may be passive where the patient is instructed about the outcome of treatment and is told what to do if there is toxicity or no response. Active monitoring may be needed for most conditions where the doctor has to check, if the treatment was effective.

Hence, every doctor needs to do his best for his patients with the right drug, the right dose and for the right duration of treatment based on his judgement and guided by his experience. He has to update his knowledge regularly and revise his list of P-drugs from time to time rather than blindly following the directions of the seniors in his field.

DRUG REGULATIONS

Competency achievement: The student should be able to:
PH 1.63 Describe drug regulations, acts and other legal aspects.[4]

In 1940, The Drugs Act was passed to control the manufacture, sale and distribution of allopathic drugs. Later the Act was amended several times and it now also includes Ayurvedic, Unani, Siddha and Homeopathic drugs. An amendment was made in 1962 to include cosmetics and the title changed to the **Drugs and Cosmetics Act.** Under the Act, clear rules have been framed for the import, manufacture, sale, labelling and packing of drugs.

Drug schedules: Some important schedules controlling manufacture, distribution and sale of drugs in India are given in Table 5.2.

Some Recent Concepts in Pharmacology

Reverse pharmacology is the science of integrating drug development by subjecting clinical hits to experimentation to know their mechanism of action and other pharmacological aspects. The safety of many of the routinely used traditional medicines like ayurvedic drugs are well known. They are subjected to experimentation to scientifically detect and prove their therapeutic benefits. It helps to understand the mechanisms of action and other pharmacological aspects of these drugs. Here regular approach of the drug discovery course from 'lab to clinics' is reversed to 'clinics to labs'. Examples of drugs which were successfully proved to be useful are—artemisinin and reserpine.

- *Conventional method*
  Molecule → mice → man
- *Reverse pharmacology path*
  Man → mice → molecule

Translational medicine is the application of laboratory research to patient care, i.e. from the bench to bedside. Translational medicine involves closer collaboration between the industry and academics, that is, transfer of advances in basic scientific research to treatment of diseases in a shorter time.

PRESCRIPTION WRITING

Competency achievement: The student should be able to:
PH 1.10 Describe parts of a correct, complete and legible generic prescription. Identify errors in prescription and correct appropriately.[5]

The Prescription is a written order by a physician to the pharmacist to prepare and/or dispense specific medication for a specific patient. A specific pattern should be followed in writing prescriptions, in order to avoid errors and to safeguard the interests of the patient. Moreover, the fact that it is a medicolegal document makes it all the more important to be accurate and precise.

The following points should be remembered in writing a prescription:

1. The writing should be legible. The drug names should be in capital letters so that they are legible.
2. Indelible ink should be used in writing.
3. Abbreviations should be avoided.
4. Generic names of drugs should be written below the brand names.
5. In writing quantities, decimals should be avoided; when inevitable, zero should be used—0.1 for .1.
6. Less than 1 g should be written as milligrams, e.g. 200 mg and not 0.2 g. No abbreviation should be used for micrograms and units.

Table 5.2: Important drug schedules

Schedule	*Features*	*Examples*
Schedule H drugs—to be sold under "prescription only"	• Warning to be given on the label: Schedule H drug. Warning: To be sold on the prescription of registered medical practitioner only • Symbol R_x should be printed prominently on the left hand top corner of the label • If the drug is covered under Narcotic Drugs and Psychotropic Substances Act, symbol NR_x should be printed instead of R_x • The rules for sale are same as for schedule X drugs	Acyclovir Alprazolam Amitriptyline Atenolol Azathioprine Bacampicillin Barbiturates Antibiotics
Schedule X: Psychotropic drugs	• The label should contain the warning: "Schedule X drug" • Symbol X R_x in red letters on left hand top corner • Warning: To be sold on presciption of a registered medical practitioner only • Schedule X drugs should be stored under lock and key • Drugs should not be dispensed more than once unless such an instruction is given in the prescription • No substitute or alternative drug should be given • The prescription should be in duplicate and a copy should be retained for at least 2 years • On the cash bill, the purchaser's signature should be taken.	Amphetamine Barbiturates Methaqualone Glutethimide
NDCT-2019	Describes requirements and guidelines for new drug and clinical trials	
Other important drug schedules:		
Schedule C	Includes biological and special (intravenous) products Druggists require separate license for sale of these drugs	Insulin, adrenaline
Schedule E	Includes poisons and drugs under Ayurvedic, Siddha and Unani systems of medicine. It applies to the storage and sale of such drugs.	
Schedule F, F1	Include vaccines and sera	
Schedule G	For these drugs, label should have the warning—'Caution: It is dangerous to take this preparation except under medical supervision'. Containers should be labelled in red bottles against white background	Ethosuximide; anticancer drugs like bleomycin; hormones antidiabetics like insulin, glibenclamide
Schedule S	Prescribes standards for cosmetics	

7. Blank space should be avoided between direction and the signature of the doctor. If blank space is present, it should be striked off to avoid misuse of the space to obtain drugs illegally.

PARTS OF THE PRESCRIPTION

1. Date of writing the prescription.
2. Address of the prescriber—preferrably prescriptions are written on the letter pad with doctor's name and address printed at the top.
3. Name, age, sex and address of the patient.
4. Superscription—the symbol R_x meaning 'take thou' is also considered as an invocation to the Greek Gods of healing—Jupitor and Horus.
5. Drug name and strength. This is the body of the prescription—also called inscription. Abbreviations should never be used.

Model Prescription

Dr Vaidya
Highland
Mangalore

July 10, 2001

Telephone no.........................

Ramu, Male, Age: 35 years
Address: No. 7, Kankanady
Mangalore 575002

R_x
Tab ROXITHROMYCIN 150 mg
Dispense 10 tablets

Directions: Take 1 tab orally twice a day, 30 minutes before food for 5 days.

Signature
Regn. No.

Some commonly used Latin abbreviations in prescriptions

Abbreviation	*Latin derivation*	*Meaning in English*
o.d.	onus in die	once a day
b.d.	bis in die	twice a day
b.i.d.	bis in die	twice a day
t.i.d.	ter in die	three times a day
t.d.s.	ter die sumendum	three times a day
q.i.d.	quarter in die	four times a day
h.s.	hora somni	at bedtime
stat	statim	at once
s.o.s.	si opus sit	if necessary
q.s.	quantum sufficit	a sufficient amount
p.o./po	per os	by mouth
ung	unguentum	ointment
caps	capsula	capsules
Tab	Tabella	tablet
a.c.	ante cibum	before food

6. Directions to the pharmacist (subscription)—consists of instructions for compounding if any and the quantity to be supplied.
7. Directions to the patient—should be clear and should indicate the quantity, frequency, time, route of administration and other information relevant to the preparation. If a drug is meant only for external application or needs to be shaken well or mixed before using—such instructions should be mentioned.
8. Signature of the prescriber—the prescriber should sign along with registration number.

TYPES OF PRESCRIPTIONS

1. *Precompounded prescription*—orders for a drug manufactured by a pharmaceutical company, has a trade name and is available for use.
2. *Compounded or extemporaneous prescription*—the physician directs the pharmacist to compound a preparation. The ingredients, their quantity and the form of preparation (like mixture, powder or ointment) is chosen by the physician and instructed accordingly.

[1–5] From Medical Council of India, *Competency based Undergraduate Curriculum for the Indian Medical Graduate*, 2018;1:136–144.

Unit II

Autonomic Nervous System

6. Adrenergic Agonists and Antagonists
7. Cholinergic and Anticholinergic Drugs
8. Skeletal Muscle Relaxants

CHAPTER 6

Adrenergic Agonists and Antagonists

OVERVIEW

The nervous system is divided into central and peripheral nervous systems (Fig. 6.1). The peripheral nervous system consists of autonomic and somatic nervous systems. The autonomic nervous system (ANS) is **not under voluntary control** and, therefore, was so named by Langley (*Autos* = self, *nomos* = governing—in Greek). The ANS innervates the **heart**, the **smooth muscles**, the **glands** and the **viscera** and controls the functions of these organs (Fig. 6.2).

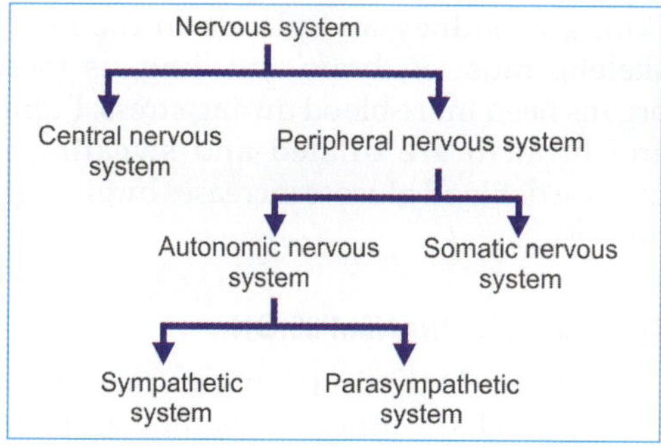

Fig. 6.1: Nervous system

The centres for autonomic reflexes are present in the hypothalamus, medulla and spinal cord. Hypothalamus coordinates the autonomic activity.

The ANS consists of two major divisions—the **sympathetic** and the **parasympathetic** (Fig. 6.4). Most of the viscera have both sympathetic and parasympathetic innervation. ***The two divisions have opposing effects and normally their effects are in a state of equilibrium.*** The prime function of the sympathetic

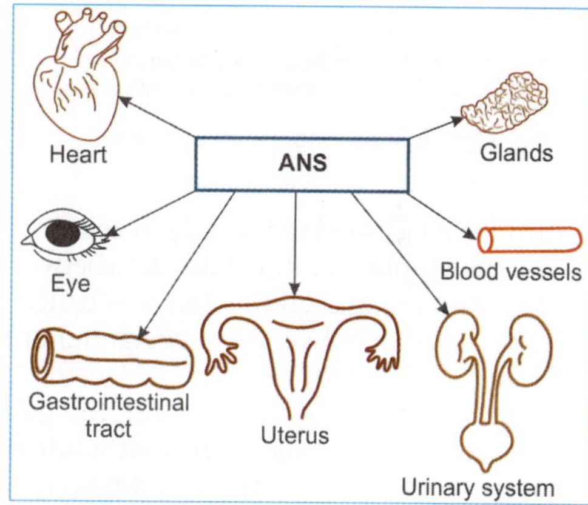

Fig. 6.2: Structures under the control of autonomic nervous system

system is to help a person to adjust to stress and prepare the body for **fight or flight reactions**, while the parasympathetic mainly participates in **tissue building reactions.** Man can survive and remain alive without sympathetic system (if maintained stress-free) but not without parasympathetic.

AUTONOMIC INNERVATION

Like the somatic nervous system, autonomic innervation also has an afferent, a center and an efferent.

Autonomic afferents: The autonomic afferents (Fig. 6.3) are carried in visceral nerves through nonmyelinated fibres. For example, the parasympathetic afferents are carried by the 9th and 10th cranial nerves. The autonomic efferent innervation consists of a myelinated preganglionic fibre which synapses with the postganglionic fibre. The postganglionic fibre

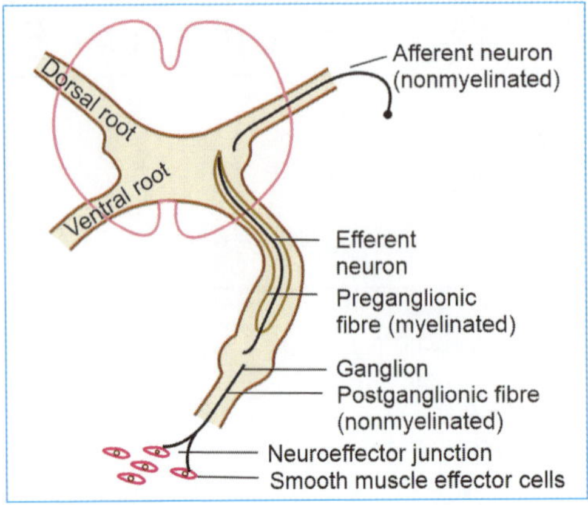

Fig. 6.3: Autonomic innervation

in turn forms a junction with the receptors of the organs supplied by it. The junction between the pre- and postganglionic fibres is called a *ganglion* and that between the postganglionic fibre and the receptors is the *neuroeffector junction*. The travelling of an impulse along the nerve fibre is known as *conduction* while its passage across a synapse is known as *transmission*.

Autonomic efferents: The autonomic efferents are divided into sympathetic and parasympathetic divisions. The parasympathetic efferents are carried through the craniosacral outflow. The parasympathetic ganglia are located close to the innervated structures and, therefore, their postganglionic fibres are short. The preganglionic fibres of the parasympathetic system are long and postganglionic fibres are short while in sympathetic system, the preganglionic fibres are short and postganglionic fibres are long. The sympathetic efferents extend from 1st thoracic to 2nd or 3rd lumbar segments (T_1–L_3) of the spinal cord. The sympathetic ganglia are found at three sites—**paravertebral, prevertebral** and **terminal**. Postganglionic fibres arising from sympathetic ganglia innervate the head, neck and the viscera of the thorax and abdomen. Adrenal medulla is also considered a sympathetic ganglion and differs from other sympathetic ganglia in that the principal catecholamine that is released is **adrenaline**.

Neurotransmitters: For the transmission of an impulse across a synapse, a neurohumoral transmitter substance is released into the synaptic cleft. In the ANS, the neurotransmitters released are **acetylcholine, noradrenaline, dopamine** and in adrenal medulla, it is **adrenaline** and noradrenaline.

Competency achievement: The student should be able to:

PH 1.13 Describe mechanism of action, types, doses, side effects, indications and contraindications of adrenergic and anti-adrenergic drugs.[1]

The prime function of the adrenergic or sympathetic nervous system is to help the human being to adjust to stress and prepare the body for fight or flight reactions. When exposed to stress, the heart rate and stroke volume increase with the resultant increase in cardiac output. The blood is shifted from the skin, gut, kidney and glands to the heart, skeletal muscles, brain and lung, as these organs need more blood during stress. Pupils and bronchi are dilated and sweating is increased. Blood glucose increases by glycogenolysis.

ADRENERGIC TRANSMISSION

The sympathetic division consists of the thoracolumbar outflow extending from 1st thoracic to 2nd or 3rd lumbar segments. The sympathetic ganglia are paravertebral, prevertebral and terminal ganglia and adrenal medulla.

Neurotransmitters

Neurotransmitters of the sympathetic system are noradrenaline (NA, norepinephrine) and dopamine (DA). Adrenaline (epinephrine) is the major hormone secreted by the adrenal medulla which contains 85% adrenaline (15% NA).

Synthesis, Storage and Release of Catecholamines

The three endogenous catecholamines—NA, adrenaline and DA are synthesized from the amino acid phenylalanine (Fig. 6.4).

The sympathetic postganglionic nerve fibres that synthesize, store and release NA are called **adrenergic**. Noradrenaline is stored in small vesicles in the adrenergic nerve terminals (Fig. 6.5). In response to nerve impulse, NA is released into the synaptic cleft by a process called **exocytosis**. This NA binds to adrenergic receptors located on the postsynaptic membrane to produce the response. A small portion of NA is metabolized by the enzyme COMT. A large portion (nearly 80%) is however, taken back into the nerve terminals by an energy dependent active transport process termed **uptake 1**, which is responsible for termination of the action of NA. The nerve terminal takes up NA with the help of an amine pump norepinephrine transporter (NET). Of this, a fraction is metabolised by MAO present on mitochondria and the remaining NA is then transferred to the storage vesicles (Fig. 6.5). This utilizes another amine pump called vesicular monoamine transporter 2 (VMAT2). Some part of NA released into the synaptic cleft penetrates into the effector cells and is known as **uptake 2** with the help of another amine pump called extraneuronal amine transporter (ENT).

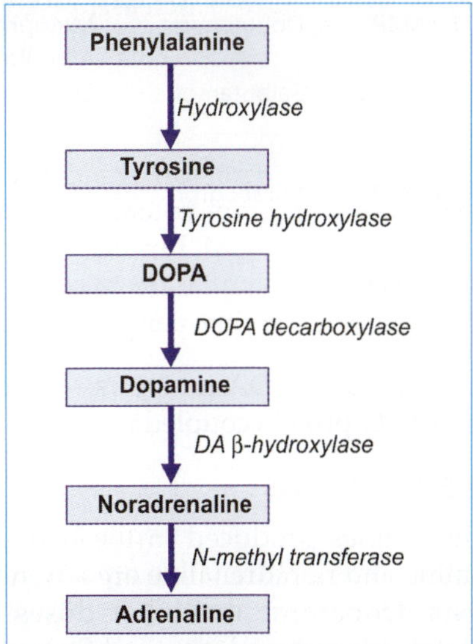

Fig. 6.4: Biosynthesis of catecholamines

Adrenergic Receptors

Ahlquist classified adrenergic receptors into 2 types: α and β. With the availability of newer, synthetic, selective drugs, these are further classified into subdivisions. We now know α_1 α_2, three subtypes each with α_{1A}, α_{1B}, α_{1D}, and α_{2A}, α_{2B} and α_{2C}. β receptors are of 3 subtypes: β_1, β_2 and β_3 adrenergic receptors.

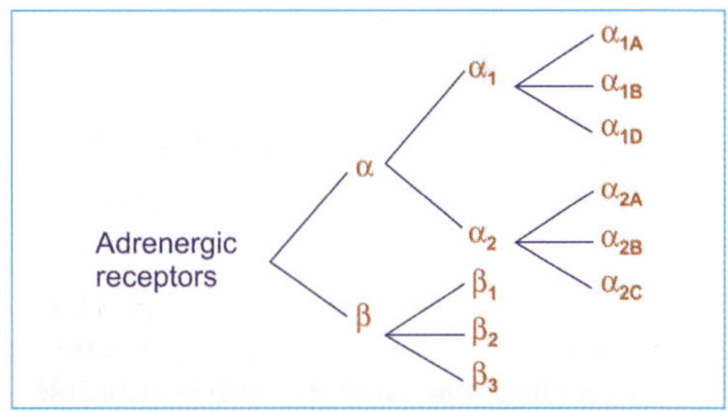

The stimulation of α receptor mainly produces excitatory effects (exception—GIT); β stimulation causes mainly inhibitory effects (exception—heart). The characteristics of these receptors are given in Table 6.1. α_2 receptors are located on the presynaptic membrane (Fig. 6.6). Stimulation of presynaptic α_2 receptors inhibits the further release of NA. Thus, α_2 receptors exert a negative feedback on NA release. α_2 receptors are also present postsynaptically in the pancreatic islets, platelets and brain.

Mechanism of Action

Both α and β adrenergic receptors are G-protein coupled receptors. Stimulation of α receptors activates phospholipase C in the cell membrane which acts through generation of second messengers inositol triphosphate (IP_3) and diacylglycerol (DAG) and increase intracellular calcium.

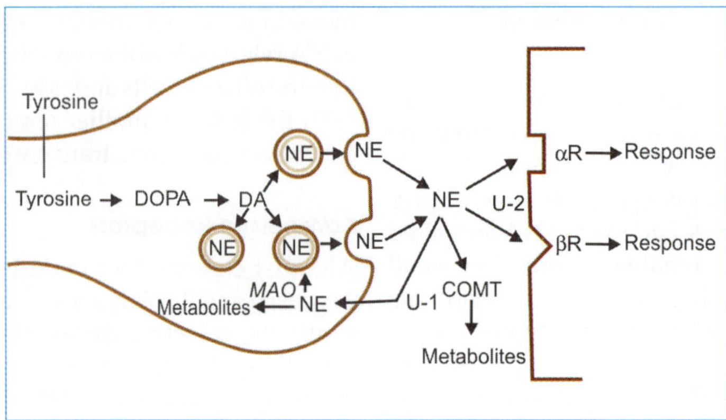

Fig. 6.5: Synthesis, storage, release and metabolism of noradrenaline. DA: Dopamine, NE: Norepinephrine, U-1: Uptake 1, U-2: Uptake 2, MAO: Monoamine oxidase, COMT: Catechol-O-methyltransferase, αR: α receptor, βR: β receptor

Table 6.1: Characteristics of adrenergic receptors

Receptor type	*Location*	*Response*	*Second messengers*	*Selective agonist*	*Selective antagonist*
α_1	Vascular smooth muscle	Contraction	↑ IP_3, DAG	Phenylephrine	Prazosin
	Gut	Relaxation	Ca^{++}	Mephentermine	Terazosin
	Genitourinary smooth muscle	Contraction		Methoxamine	
	Liver	Glycogenolysis			
α_2	Pancreatic β cells	↓ Insulin release	↓ cAMP	Clonidine	Yohimbine
	Platelets	Aggregation			
	Nerve terminals	↓ NE release			
β_1	Heart	↑ FOC, ↑ HR ↑ AV cond. vel.	↑ cAMP	Dobutamine	Metoprolol Atenolol
β_2	Smooth muscle—vascular, bronchial, gut and genito-urinary	Relaxation	↑ cAMP	Salbutamol	Butoxamine
β_3	Adipose tissue	Lipolysis	↓ cAMP	Mirabegron	–
	Bladder	Detrusor relaxation			

FOC: Force of contraction; HR: Heart rate; Cond. vel.: Conduction velocity

Stimulation of β receptors activates an enzyme adenylyl cyclase resulting in increased intracellular cyclic AMP levels. This second messenger acts through various intracellular proteins to bring about the response.

Dopamine Receptors

Dopamine acts on the dopamine receptors which are widely distributed in the body. There are five subtypes of DA receptors—D_1 to D_5. They are all G-protein coupled receptors.

ADRENERGIC DRUGS

Catecholamines produced in the body, *viz.* adrenaline and noradrenaline are adrenergic agonists. Dopamine in higher doses also stimulates adrenergic receptors. Sympathomimetics are drugs whose actions mimic that

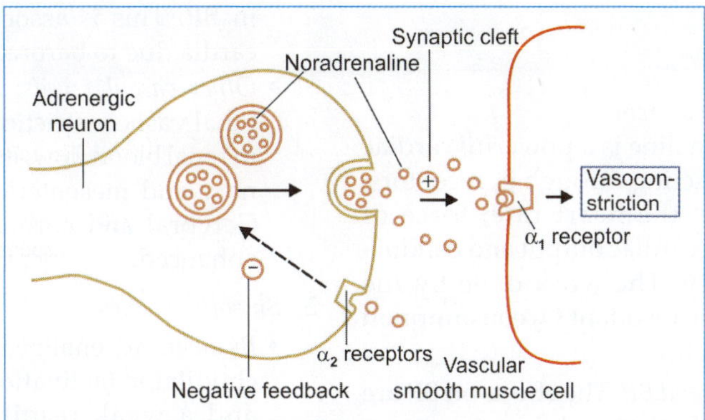

Fig. 6.6: α_1 and α_2 receptors stimulation: NA binds to α_1 receptors and stimulates it to produce response like vasoconstriction. Presynaptic α_2 receptor stimulation inhibits the further release of NA from the storage vesicles

of sympathetic stimulation. Catecholamines and sympathomimetics or adrenergic drugs may be classified in various ways depending on the presence/absence of catechol nucleus, mode of action and therapeutic indications as given in classification.

Classification

I. *Chemical classification*—based on the presence/absence of catechol nucleus
1. ***Catecholamines***
   Noradrenaline, adrenaline, dopamine
   Synthetic—isoprenaline, dobutamine, dopexamine, dipivefrine
2. ***Non-catecholamines***
   Ephedrine, amphetamine

II. *Depending on the mode of action*
1. Directly acting sympathomimetics (by interacting with adrenergic receptors)
   Noradrenaline, adrenaline, dopamine, isoprenaline, phenylephrine, salbutamol, xylometazoline, methoxamine
2. Indirectly acting sympathomimetics (by releasing NA from nerve terminals)
   Amphetamine, tyramine
3. Mixed action amines (both direct and indirect actions)
   Ephedrine, pseudoephedrine, phenylpropanolamine
4. Catecholamine reuptake inhibitors
   Atomoxetine, reboxetine, duloxetine, sibutramine

III. *Therapeutic or clinical classification*
1. Vasopressors
   Noradrenaline, dopamine, phenylephrine, methoxamine, mephentermine, metaraminol
2. Cardiac stimulants
   Adrenaline, dopamine, dopexamine, dobutamine, fenoldopam, isoprenaline, ephedrine
3. CNS stimulants
   Amphetamine, dexamphetamine, ephedrine
4. Bronchodilators
   Adrenaline, isoprenaline, salbutamol, terbutaline, salmeterol, perbuterol, fenoterol, formoterol
5. Nasal decongestants
   Ephedrine, pseudoephedrine, phenylpropanolamine, phenylephrine, oxymetazoline, xylometazoline, naphazoline
6. Appetite suppressants (anorectics)
   Fenfluramine, dexfenfluramine, sibutramine (banned)
7. Uterine relaxants
   Salbutamol, terbutaline, isoxsuprine, ritodrine

ADRENALINE

Actions

1. *Cardiovascular system*
   - *Heart:* Adrenaline is a powerful cardiac stimulant. Acting through β_1 receptors, it increases the heart rate, force of contraction, cardiac output and conduction velocity. The work done by the heart and the resultant O_2 consumption are increased.
   - *Blood vessels and BP:* The effects on BP are complex as both α and β receptors are stimulated by adrenaline. Blood vessels of the skin and mucous membrane are constricted (α_1) and that of the skeletal muscles are dilated (β_2) by adrenaline. Since adrenaline causes cutaneous vasoconstriction, it is used to prolong the duration of action of local anaesthetics.

     Small doses of (0.1 mg/kg) adrenaline given by infusion produce a fall in blood pressure because of vasodilation of the blood vessels in the skeletal muscles. This is because β_2 receptors are sensitive even to this small dose of adrenaline.

     Moderate doses of adrenaline given IV produce a rapid increase in BP followed by a fall—a biphasic response. The systolic rises due to α_1 mediated vasoconstriction and β_1 mediated increase in heart rate, force of contraction and (thereby) cardiac output. Action on β receptors is more persistent and as the action on α receptors wears off, the action on β_2 receptors gets unmasked resulting in decreased BP due to a fall in the diastolic. Sir Henry Dale demonstrated that when α receptors are blocked (with ergot alkaloids), adrenaline produces only a fall in BP and this is named after him as Dale's vasomotor reversal (or Dale's phenomenon).

     Noradrenaline is mainly an alpha agonist and therefore brings about a rise in BP. This is associated with bradycardia due to baroreceptor stimulation.
   - *Other vascular beds:* Adrenaline causes renal vasoconstriction resulting in a fall in renal blood flow; it also causes pulmonary and mesenteric vasoconstriction. Cerebral and coronary blood flow is enhanced.
2. *Smooth muscles*
   - *Bronchi:* Adrenaline is a powerful bronchodilator (activation of β_2 receptors) and a weak respiratory stimulant. Pulmonary vasoconstriction (α) relieves bronchial congestion. All these result in an increase in vital capacity.
   - *Uterus*
     - Nonpregnant uterus—contracts
     - Last month of pregnancy—relaxes.
   - *Gut:* Smooth muscle is relaxed, but weak and transient action.
   - *Splenic capsule:* Contracts resulting in the release of RBCs into the circulation.
   - *Pilomotor muscles* of the hair follicle contract.
   - *Bladder:* Detrusor is relaxed (β_3 receptors) while trigone is contracted, thereby increasing the holding capacity of the bladder.
3. *Eye:* Adrenaline causes mydriasis due to active contraction of the radial muscles (a_1) of the iris—**active mydriasis** (*see* Compare and Contrast—active and passive mydriases); it also reduces intraocular pressure. The exact mechanism is not known, but it is thought that adrenaline reduces both the production of aqueous humor (b) and improves its drainage (a receptor).
4. *Metabolic effects:* Adrenaline increases the blood sugar level by enhancing hepatic glycogenolysis. It also inhibits insulin release. By enhancing the breakdown of triglycerides in the adipose tissue, more free fatty acids are made available in the plasma by action on β_3 receptors in adipocytes.

COMPARE AND CONTRAST

Active mydriasis and Passive mydriasis

Features	*Active mydriasis*	*Passive mydriasis*
Produced by	Sympathomimetics—like adrenaline, ephedrine, phenylephrine	Anticholinergics—like homatropine, eucatropine, tropicamide
Mechanism of action	Stimulation of dilator pupillae—active contraction of dilator	Relaxation of sphincter pupillae
Receptor involved	α_1 (stimulation)	M_3 (blockade)
Light reflex	Retained (because constrictor not affected)	Lost (because constrictor is relaxed and cannot contract in response to light)
Cycloplegia	Absent	Present

5. *Skeletal muscles:* Catecholamines facilitate neuromuscular transmission by action on both α and β receptors, they enhance the amount of ACh released.

Pharmacokinetics

As catecholamines are rapidly inactivated in the gut and the liver, they are not given orally. Adrenaline and NA are metabolised by COMT and MAO.

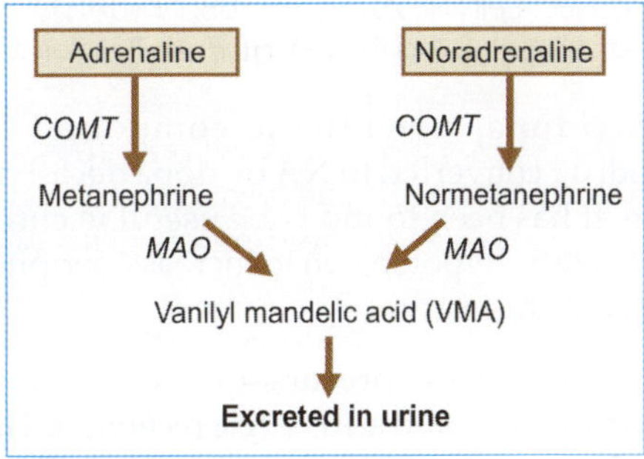

Preparations

Adrenaline 1:1000, 1:10,000 and 1:1,00,000 solutions are available for injection. Adrenaline is given SC/IM; intracardiac in emergencies. ADRENA® 2 mg/ml inj. NALINE® 1 mg/ml inj. Adrenaline aerosol for inhalation and 2% ophthalmic solution are also available.

Adverse Reactions

Anxiety, palpitation, weakness, tremors, pallor, dizziness, restlessness and throbbing headache may follow adrenaline/NA administration. In patients with ischemic heart disease, both adrenaline and NA can precipitate anginal pain. Rapid IV injection can cause sudden sharp rise in BP which may precipitate arrhythmias, subarachnoid hemorrhage or hemiplegia.

Uses of Adrenaline

1. *Anaphylactic shock:* Adrenaline is the drug of choice (0.3–0.5 ml of 1:1000 solution IM).

   Rationale

   - Adrenaline is physiological antagonist of histamine.
   - It promptly reverses hypotension, laryngeal oedema and bronchospasm and is lifesaving in anaphylactic shock.

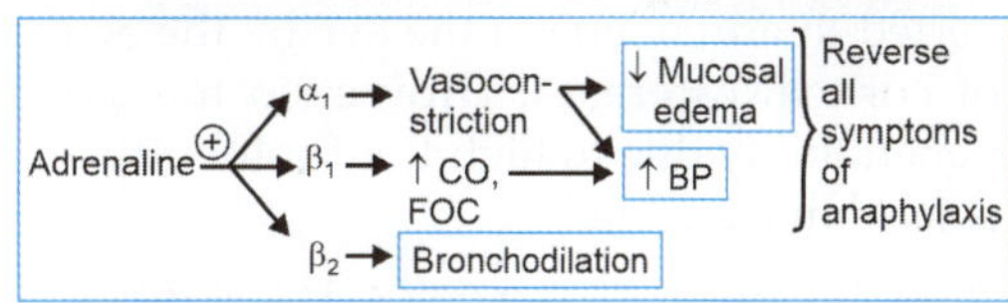

   Adrenaline is also life-saving in angioneurotic oedema of the larynx. IM route is preferred as absorption by SC route is not reliable in shock.

2. *Cardiac arrest:* Sudden cardiac arrest due to drowning, electrocution, etc. are treated with cardiopulmonary resuscitation (CPR). Intravenous or intracardiac adrenaline (1 mg) (into 4th or 5th intercostal space, 2–3 inches from the sternum) is tried but before injecting, ensure that the tip of the needle is in the heart. If the piston of the syringe is withdrawn, blood should

enter the syringe, however, intracardiac not preferred now.

3. *Control of hemorrhage:* Adrenaline in 1:10,000 to 1:20,000 concentration is used as a topical haemostatic to control bleeding. Bleeding stops due to vasoconstriction. Adrenaline packs are used for bleeding after tooth extraction and in epistaxis.
4. *With local anesthetics* (*see* page 180): Injected with LA, adrenaline produces vasoconstriction and reduces the rate of absorption of LA. By this it prolongs the action and reduces systemic toxicity of LA. 1:10,000 to 1:2,00,000 adrenaline is used.
5. *Acute bronchial asthma:* Though SC/inhalation adrenaline produces bronchodilation, it is not preferred as more selective drugs are available.
6. *Glaucoma* (*see* page 106) Adrenaline decreases IOP and can be used in glaucoma, but it has the disadvantages of being:
   i. Poorly absorbed.
   ii. Short acting as it is quickly metabolised in the eye.

Dipivefrin is a prodrug which gets converted to adrenaline in the eye by the action of corneal esterases. Dipivefrin has good penetrability due to high lipid solubility and is used in glaucoma.

Dose: PROPINE 0.1% eye drops; 1 drop BD.

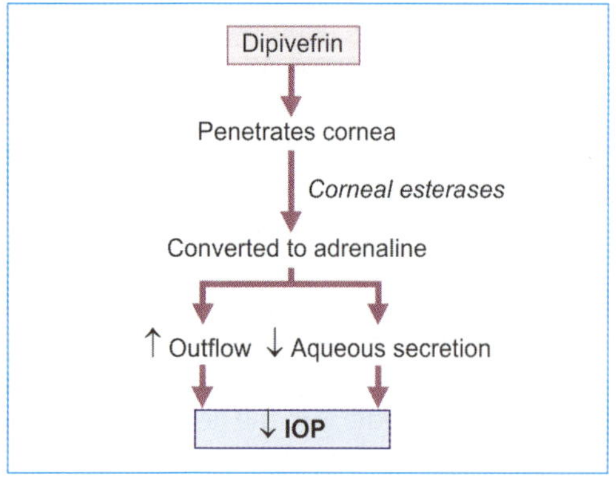

Contraindications

Adrenaline is contraindicated in patients with angina pectoris, hypertension and in patients on β blockers.

Other Catecholamines

Noradrenaline is used in shock to increase BP. It is commonly used by the intensive care specialists—2–4 μg/min IV.

Dose: ADRONIS, NOR-S 2 mg/ml inj.

Isoprenaline (isoproterenol, isopropyl arterenol) is a synthetic catecholamine with predominantly β receptor stimulant action and negligible α actions. It has cardiac stimulant and smooth muscle relaxant properties. Due to vasodilation BP falls; it is a potent bronchodilator. Adverse effects include palpitation, angina, headache and flushing.

Isoprenaline is used in heart block and shock for its cardiac stimulant actions. It can also be used in bronchial asthma.

Dose: NEO-EPININE 20 mg tab SUBLINGUAL; ISOPRIN 2 mg/ml inj. 1–2 mg IM, 5–10 μg/min IV infusion.

Droxidopa, a synthetic compound is a prodrug converted to NA by dopa decarboxylase. It has been found to be useful in chronic orthostatic hypotension to increase peripheral vascular resistance.

Dopamine is the precursor of NA. It acts on dopaminergic and adrenergic receptors. There are 5 subtypes of dopamine receptors: D_1–D_5. Dopamine is a central neurotransmitter. Low doses stimulate vascular D_1 receptor in renal, mesenteric and coronary beds causing vasodilatation in these vessels. D_2 receptor stimulation in the sympathetic nerve terminals and in cardiovascular centres also results in **renal vasodilation**. Hence, renal blood flow and GFR increase. Higher doses cause cardiac stimulation through β_1 receptors resulting in an increase in the force of contraction with a relatively minor increase in the heart rate. In high doses α_1 receptors are activated resulting in vasoconstriction and ↑BP.

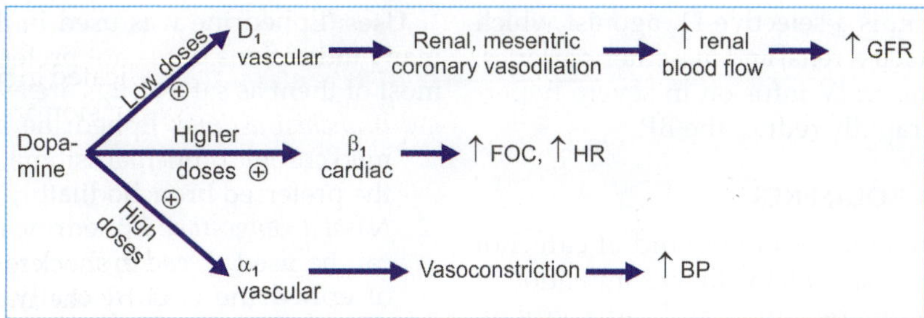

Dopamine does not cross the BBB, hence it has no CNS effects. It is given IV. It is short acting and the infusion rate can be adjusted to get the appropriate effect by monitoring BP. Dopamine is metabolised by COMT and MAO. **Epinine** (Ibopamine) is an ester of methyldopamine which acts like dopamine.

Adverse effects: Nausea, vomiting, palpitation, headache, angina and sudden rise in BP may occur.

Uses: Dopamine is used in the treatment of shock—cardiogenic, hypovolaemic and septic. It is specially useful when there is renal dysfunction and low cardiac output because

a. DA ↑renal blood flow and thereby GFR
b. DA stimulates the heart—↑FOC, ↑cardiac output and BP.
c. DA is short-acting and therefore the response can be easily controlled by modifying the infusion rate.

Dose: 2–5 μg/kg/min. DOPACARD, DOPAMINE, 40 mg/ml inj.

Dopexamine is a synthetic analog of dopamine acting on D_1, D_2 and β_2 receptors. It is found to have beneficial effects in CCF.

Dobutamine, a derivative of dopamine, is a relatively selective β_1 agonist. Though it also activates α_1 receptors, in therapeutic doses the only dominant action is an increase in the force of contraction of the heart without a significant increase in the heart rate. Hence, the increase in myocardial demand is milder when compared to dopamine and is therefore more useful than dopamine in **cardiogenic shock.** Dobutamine is used in patients with **CCF** or acute myocardial infarction or following cardiac surgery when there may be **pump failure.**

Dose: 2–15 μg/kg/min. CARDIFORCE, DOBICARD, 250 μg/20 ml inj.

COMPARE AND CONTRAST

Adrenaline and Noradrenaline

Features	***Adrenaline***	***Noradrenaline***
Chemistry	Catecholamine	Catecholamine
On adrenergic receptors	Agonist	Agonist
Receptor selectivity	Both α and β	Predominantly α agonist
Effect on BP	• Biphasic • ↑ in systolic • ↓ in diastolic	• Monophasic • ↑ in systolic, diastolic and mean BP
Dale's vasomotor reversal	Yes	No
Clinical uses	Many	Rarely used
Major indications	• Anaphylactic shock • Cardiac arrest • Local hemostatic	• Used to reverse hypotension

Fenoldopam is a selective D_1 agonist which dilates coronary, renal and mesenteric arteries. It is used as an IV infusion in severe hypertension to rapidly reduce the BP.

NONCATECHOLAMINES

Noncatecholamines are devoid of catechol nucleus, they act both by direct stimulation of the adrenergic receptors and indirectly by releasing NA. In contrast to catecholamines, they are effective orally, relatively resistant to MAO and therefore are longer-acting; they cross the blood–brain barrier and have CNS effects.

Ephedrine is an alkaloid obtained from the plants of the genus *Ephedra* and has been used in China for more than 2000 years. Ephedrine acts by direct stimulation of α and β receptors and indirectly through release of NA. Ephedrine raises BP by peripheral vasoconstriction and by increasing the cardiac output. Repeated administration at short intervals results in tachyphylaxis. Like adrenaline it relaxes smooth muscles—it is a bronchodilator (β_2); it is a CNS stimulant and produces insomnia, restlessness, anxiety, tremors and increased mental activity. Ephedrine has good oral bioavailability and a t½ of 4–6 hr (*see* Compare and Contrast: Noradrenaline and Ephedrine).

Adverse effects include gastric upset, insomnia, tremors, difficulty in micturition, anxiety and restlessness.

Uses: Ephedrine was used in the past for many indications but is not preferred now in most of them as safer drugs are available.

1. *Bronchial asthma:* Ephedrine is useful in mild chronic bronchial asthma, but it is not the preferred bronchodilator.
2. *Nasal decongestion:* Ephedrine nasal drops can be used. *Pseudoephedrine*—an isomer of ephedrine is used orally for decongestion. It causes vasoconstriction in the skin and mucous membrane but its effects on the CNS and the heart are milder. Hence, it is preferred over ephedrine.
3. *Mydriasis:* Ephedrine eye drops are used to produce mydriasis without cycloplegia.
4. *Hypotension:* For prevention and treatment of hypotension during spinal anesthesia, IM ephedrine is used.
5. *Narcolepsy:* It is a condition with an irresistible desire and tendency to sleep. As ephedrine is a CNS stimulant, it is useful in narcolepsy.
6. *Nocturnal enuresis* (bed-wetting): In children may be treated with ephedrine as it increases the holding capacity of the bladder. Drugs should be used only when non-pharmacological measures have failed.
7. *Stokes Adam's syndrome:* As an alternative to isoprenaline.

Amphetamine is a synthetic compound with actions similar to ephedrine; tachyphylaxis can occur on repeated use.

COMPARE AND CONTRAST

Catecholamines and Noncatecholamines

Features	*Catecholamines*	*Noncatecholamines*
Chemistry	Have catechol nucleus	No catechol nucleus
Route	Not effective orally	Effective orally
Metabolised by	MAO, COMT (hence not effective orally)	Relatively resistant to MAO, COMT
Duration of action	Short acting	Longer acting
BBB	Does not cross	Crosses
CNS effects	No	Yes
Action	By direct stimulation of α and β receptors	Indirectly by release of NA

Mechanism of action: Amphetamine produces most of its effects indirectly by promoting the release of noradrenaline from the central noradrenergic nerve terminals. It also releases some DA and in high doses serotonin in the CNS.

Actions

CNS: Amphetamine readily crosses the BBB to reach the CNS. It is a potent CNS stimulant; it produces increased mental and physical activity, alertness, increased concentration and attention span, elation, euphoria and increased capacity to work. It also increases initiative and self-confidence, postpones fatigue, sleep and improves physical performance (temporarily) as seen in athletes. All these properties make amphetamine a drug of dependence and abuse. Higher doses produce confusion, delirium and hallucinations. On long-term use tolerance develops.

Respiration: Amphetamine stimulates respiratory center, it is an analeptic.

Suppression of appetite: Acting on the feeding centre in the hypothalamus, amphetamine reduces hunger and suppresses appetite. However, tolerance develops rapidly.

Other effects: Amphetamine also has weak anticonvulsant and analgesic properties. Amphetamine increases the tone of bladder sphincter.

Adverse effects include restlessness, tremors, insomnia, palpitation, anxiety, confusion and hallucinations. Prolonged use may precipitate psychosis.

Dependence: Amphetamine causes addiction and dependence. Long-term use results in psychosis and other behavioural abnormalities.

Toxicity: High doses cause headache, nausea, vomiting, abdominal cramps, flushing, angina, delirium, arrhythmias, hypertension, restlessness, suicidal or homicidal tendencies, acute psychosis, followed by coma and death due to convulsions. Treatment includes acidification of urine with ammonium chloride to promote urinary excretion of amphetamine; sedatives, α blockers/sodium nitroprusside to control the BP and chlorpromazine to control the psychosis. Peritoneal dialysis may be needed.

Uses

1. *Attention deficit hyperactivity disorder (ADHD)* in children is characterised by decreased ability to concentrate and hold attention, aggressive behaviour and hyperactivity; Amphetamine increases attention span in such children and improves performance in school. However, reduced appetite and other side effects including addiction limit the use of amphetamine for this purpose.
2. *Narcolepsy:* Though amphetamine is preferred over ephedrine for this purpose, dependence liability and side effects make these drugs less used. Other drugs used in narcolepsy include **methylphenidate** and **modafinil**. Methylphenidate is an indirectly acting sympathomimetic like amphetamine. Modafinil is a centrally acting CNS stimulant which may act by stimulating α_1 adrenoceptors. In addition, it also influences GABA and serotonin receptors. It is better tolerated with fewer adverse effects than amphetamine.
3. *Obesity:* Though appetite is suppressed, due to risk of dependence and other side effects, amphetamine should not be used for this purpose.
4. *Epilepsy:* Amphetamine has been used in the past as an adjuvant and to counter the sedation due to antiepileptics.

Dose: 5–10 mg oral.

Methamphetamine has more prominent central than peripheral actions and is a drug of dependence.

Methylphenidate (*see* page 277) phenmetrazin and pemoline are other amphetamine-

COMPARE AND CONTRAST

Noradrenaline and Ephedrine

Features	*Noradrenaline*	*Ephedrine*
Source	Endogenous	Exogenous (from plants of the genus Ephedra)
Chemistry	Monoamine	Non-catecholamine
Structure	Has catechol nucleus	No catechol nucleus
Mode of action	Directly stimulates adrenergic receptors	Acts both i. Directly on adrenergic receptors ii. Indirectly through release of NA
BBB	Does not easily cross	Easily crosses
Action on CNS	Only in very high doses	CNS stimulation in therapeutic doses
Role in CNS	Central neurotransmitter	Not formed in the body
Action on adrenoceptors	Predominantly α agonist	Stimulates both α and β receptors
t½	Short (minutes)	Long (hrs)
Oral use	Not effective orally	Effective orally
Topical use	Not used	Used as eyedrops—mydriasis Nasal drops—decongestion

like drugs with actions and abuse potential similar to amphetamine.

VASOPRESSORS

These are α_1 agonists and include noradrenaline, dopamine, metaraminol, mephentermine, midodrine, phenylephrine and methoxamine. They cause contraction of vascular smooth muscles by activating the α_1 receptors in them. They increase the BP by increasing total peripheral resistance (TPR) or cardiac output (CO) or both. The rise in BP is associated with reflex bradycardia. Vasopressors are given parenterally with constant monitoring of BP. Hypovolaemia if any should be corrected before administration of vasopressors. Tachyphylaxis may develop. BP should be constantly monitored to avoid sudden hypertension.

Uses: Vasopressors are used to raise the BP in hypotension as seen in cardiogenic or neurogenic shock and during spinal anaesthesia.

Metaraminol is an alpha stimulant and also acts indirectly by NA release. CO is increased. It is also a nasal decongestant.

Mephentermine acts both directly and indirectly on both α and β receptors to ↑TPR and ↑CO and thereby raises BP. It is orally effective. Pressor effect is accompanied by bradycardia. Mephentermine may be used to prevent hypotension following spinal anaesthesia and in hypotension due to other causes.

Dose: 10–20 mg oral, IM, IV INFUSION, MEPHENTINE 10 mg tab, 15, 30 mg/ml amp.

Phenylephrine is a selective α_1 stimulant; it is a vasopressor and also a nasal decongestant. Reflex bradycardia is prominent. It produces mydriasis without cycloplegia and therefore used to attain only mydriasis when cycloplegia is not needed. Phenylephrine is used as a vasopressor, nasal decongestant and a mydriatic.

Dose: 5–10 mg oral; 2–5 mg IM and 30–60 mcg/min IV Infusion, FRENIN 10 mg/ml inj, SINAREST. Phenylephrine 10 mg with paracetamol 500 mg, chlorpheniramine 2 mg and caffeine 30 mg tab.

Methoxamine has actions similar to phenylephrine and is a drug of dependence.

Midodrine is an orally effective prodrug converted to the active metabolite desglymidodrine. It contracts both arterial and venular smooth muscles and is useful in controlling orthostatic hypotension particularly in autonomic imbalance. Peak effect is seen in about 60 minutes and the action is sustained for 4–6 hr. Midodrine can cause hypertension in supine position which can be avoided by elevating the head-end of the bed.

Dose: 2.5–10 mg thrice daily.

NASAL DECONGESTANTS

Nasal decongestants are α_1 agonists.

Mechanism of action: Nasal decongestants act by stimulating the α_1 receptors present in the blood vessels of the nasal mucosa.

They bring about vasoconstriction of the nasal mucosa, resulting in its shrinkage and decreased volume of the mucosa. Thus they relieve nasal congestion and decrease resistance to airflow through the nose. They also reduce nasal secretion. The nasal decongestants thus provide only symptomatic relief in rhinitis due to allergy and upper respiratory infections.

They may be used

1. *Orally* Ephedrine, pseudoephedrine, phenylephrine
2. *Topically (as nasal drops)* Oxymetazoline, xylometazoline naphazoline, phenylephrine, mephentermine, metaraminol

Ephedrine hydrochloride in normal saline relieves congestion and the effect lasts up to 6 hrs. Pseudoephedrine is a component of several cold remedies given orally. Topically acting agents may also be used but the patient should be warned against overuse.

Adverse Effects

1. *When orally used,* ephedrine and pseudoephedrine can cause insomnia, tremors and irritability.
2. Topical agents can cause nasal irritation. Most disadvantages result from long-term use. They can get absorbed from the nasal mucous membrane and cause systemic toxicity.
3. *Prolonged use can cause*
   - Atrophy of the nasal mucosa due to intense vasoconstriction.
   - Recongestion or 'after congestion' may result when the drug is stopped (due to vasodilatation).
   - Loss of efficacy or tolerance due to desensitization of the receptors.
   - Nasal decongestants should be used carefully in patients with hypertension.
   - Phenylpropanolamine (PPA) was widely used in cold remedies and as an anorexiant. Its use is associated with an increased risk of haemorrhagic stroke and is therefore **banned** now.

Uses

- Rhinitis in upper respiratory infections.
- Allergic and vasomotor rhinitis and sinusitis.
- Blocked eustachian tubes.

α_2 AGONISTS

Clonidine, apraclonidine, brimonidine are selective α_2 agonists. Clonidine is used in hypertension (*see* page 338). Apraclonidine reduces intraocular pressure and is used topically in the treatment of glaucoma and other situations like post-trabeculoplasty and post-iridotomy to lower the IOP. It is preferred over clonidine in these. Brimonidine also lowers IOP when applied topically. It can be used in the treatment of glaucoma. **Guanfacine** and **guanabenz** are central α_2 agonists like clonidine and effectively lower blood pressure (*see* page 340).

BRONCHODILATORS AND UTERINE RELAXANTS (SELECTIVE β_2 STIMULANTS)

Selective β_2 stimulants include orciprenaline, salbutamol, terbutaline and the newer ones include salmeterol, perbuterol, bitolterol, fenoterol, carmoterol and formoterol. These are smooth muscle relaxants which produce bronchodilatation, vasodilation and uterine relaxation without significant cardiac stimulation.

Table 6.2: Uses of adrenergic agonists

Indications	*Sympathomimetic used*
I. Cardiac	
1. Cardiac arrest	– Adrenaline
2. Hypotension	– Methoxamine, mephentermine
3. Chronic orthostatic hypotension	– Droxidopa
4. Hypertension	– Clonidine, fenoldopam
5. Cardiogenic shock	– Dopamine, dobutamine
6. Cardiac decompensation	– Dobutamine
7. A-V block	– Isoprenaline
II. Hypersensitivity	
8. Anaphylactic shock	– Adrenaline
9. Severe allergic reactions (bee sting, food and drug allergy, angioneurotic edema—larynx)	– Adrenaline
III. Local vasoconstriction	
10. To arrest local bleeding	– Adrenaline pack
11. To prolong local anesthesia	– Adrenaline (mixed with LA)
12. Nasal decongestion	– Oxymetazoline, xylometazoline, ephedrine, pseudoephedrine
IV. CNS	
13. Narcolepsy	– Amphetamine, ephedrine
14. Attention deficit hyperactivity disorder	– Amphetamine (not preferred), atomoxetine, reboxitine, methylphenidate
15. Obesity	– Fenfluramine, amphetamine
V. Respiratory	
16. Bronchial asthma	– Salbutamol, terbutaline, salmeterol, ibuterol
VI. Ocular	
17. Glaucoma	– Adrenaline, dipivefrine, apraclonidine, brimonidine
18. Mydriasis for fundoscopy	– Phenylephrine
VII. Genitourinary	
19. Uterine relaxants	– Isoxsuprine, terbutaline (β_2 agonist)
20. Overactive bladder	– Mirabegron (β_3 agonist)

Selective β_2 agonists are used in:

i. Bronchial asthma—they can be given by inhalation.

ii. As uterine relaxants to delay premature labour.

Side effects include muscle tremors, palpitation and arrhythmias.

Isoxsuprine is a selective β receptor stimulant used as uterine relaxant in premature labour, threatened abortion and dysmenorrhoea.

β_3 AGONIST

Mirabegron is a selective β_3 agonist used to treat overactive bladder symptoms with repeated urgency, increased frequency of micturition and incontinence. Since β_3 agonists promote lipolysis, they may also have a role in the treatment of obesity.

ANORECTIC AGENTS (ANOREXIANTS)

Though **amphetamine** suppresses appetite, it is not recommended for the treatment of obesity due to its central stimulant effects. Many amphetamine like drugs which suppress appetite are **fenfluramine, dexfenfluramine, mazindol, phenylpropanolamine and phenmetrazine** but due to risk of abuse, drowsiness and depression, most of them are withdrawn. Phenylpropanolamine is now **banned** because of the risk of stroke. Sibutramine (*see* below).

CATECHOLAMINE REUPTAKE INHIBITORS

Several drugs inhibit the uptake of noradrenaline and dopamine by inhibiting the amine transporters that influence adrenergic transmission. **Atomoxetine** and **reboxetine** selectively inhibit the norepinephrine reuptake transporter and thereby potentiate noradrenergic transmission. They improve the attention span in attention deficit hyperactivity disorder. Noradrenaline reuptake inhibitors like **duloxetine** are also used in depression. Sibutramine inhibits the uptake of NA and 5HT and was used in obesity but is now withdrawn (*see* page 392).

Clinical Pharmacology

- On administration of adrenaline, watch for arrhythmias and ischemia of the limbs.
- Adrenaline should be avoided in patients with ischaemic heart disease.
- Intracardiac adrenaline is rarely used as in cardiac arrest. The piston of the syringe should be withdrawn to make sure that the tip of the needle is in the heart.
- NA, DA and vasopressin are commonly used as vasopressors in clinical practice.
- Ephedrine and amphetamine are now not in common use.

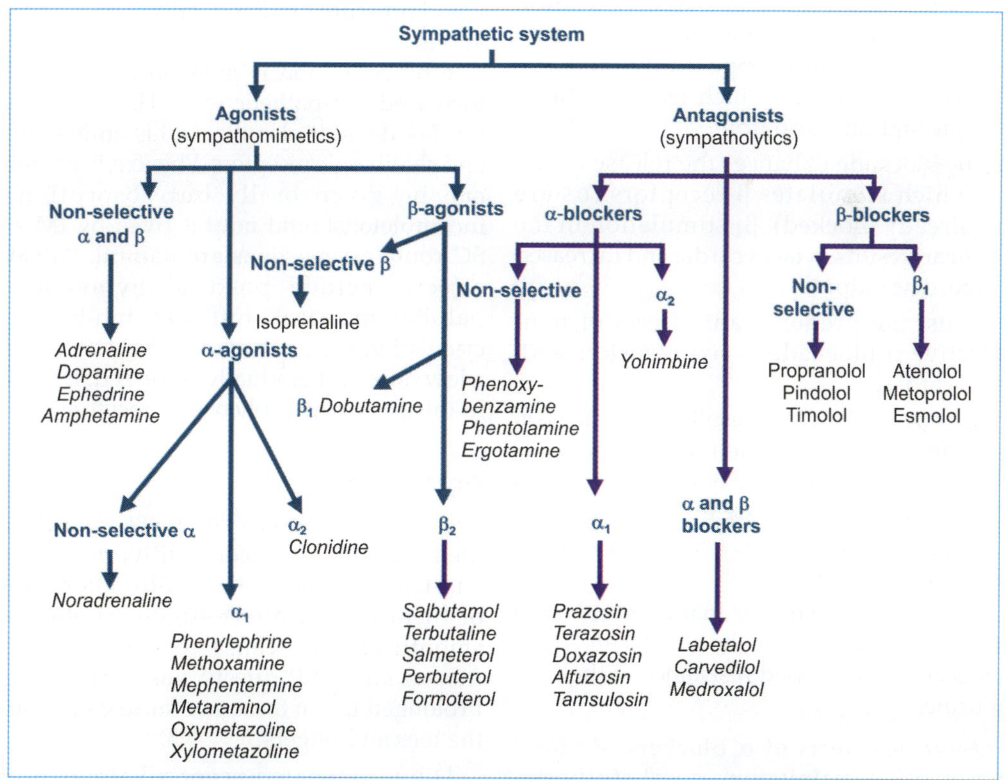

Fig. 6.7: Few examples of drugs acting on sympathetic nervous system

ADRENERGIC ANTAGONISTS

Adrenergic blockers bind to the adrenergic receptors and prevent the action of adrenergic drugs. They may block α or β receptors or both.

α ADRENERGIC BLOCKING AGENTS

α receptor antagonists block the adrenergic responses mediated through α adrenergic receptors. Some of them have selectivity for α_1 or α_2 receptors.

Actions

The important effects of α receptor stimulation are α_1 mediated vasoconstriction and α_2 (presynaptic) receptor mediated inhibition of NA release. The result of α-blockade by α-antagonists (*see* Fig. 6.6) is:

1. α_1-blockade inhibits vasoconstriction leading to vasodilation and thereby ↓BP. This fall in BP is opposed by the baroreceptor reflexes which tend to ↑heart rate and cardiac output.
2. α_2-blockade enhances the release of NA which stimulates β receptors (αs are already blocked). β_1 stimulation in the heart results in tachycardia and increased cardiac output.

Thus, the predominant effects of non-selective α-blockade is hypotension with tachycardia.

Selective α_1-blockade results in hypotension without significant tachycardia. This is because α_2 receptors are not blocked which means there is no increase in NA release.

Selective α_2-blockade: ↑NA release resulting in hypertension.

α-blockade also results in miosis and nasal stuffiness. α-blockade in the bladder and prostate leads to decreased resistance to the flow of urine.

Adverse effects of α blockers: Postural hypotension, palpitation, nasal stuffiness, miosis, impaired ejaculation and impotence.

α blockers are classified as follows

1. Non-selective
- a. *Non-competitive blocker*
  Phenoxybenzamine
- b. *Competitive blockers*
  Ergot alkaloids (ergotamine), tolazoline, phentolamine, chlorpromazine

2. Selective
- a. *α_1 blockers*
  Prazosin, terazosin, trimazosin, doxazosin, tamsulosin, alfuzosin, indoramin
- b. *α_2 blocker*
  Yohimbine, idazoxan

Phenoxybenzamine

Phenoxybenzamine binds covalently to α-receptors causing irreversible blockade or non-equilibrium type of blockade. Given IV, blood pressure gradually falls over 1–2 hours and is associated with tachycardia and ↑CO. The BP reduction is more in patients with increased sympathetic tone. The action lasts for 3–4 days. It also blocks histamine, 5-HT and cholinergic receptors. Phenoxybenzamine can be given orally but absorption is incomplete; should not be given by IM and SC route as injections are painful. Adverse effects include postural hypotension, palpitation, nasal stuffiness, inhibition of ejaculation and depression, hence started with a low dose and gradually increased. It is used in the treatment of pheochromocytoma.

Ergot Alkaloids

Ergotamine (*see* page 147), ergotoxine and their derivatives are competitive antagonists and the blockade is of short duration. Some of them have a direct stimulant effect on smooth muscles cause contraction of the uterus and ↑BP due to vasoconstriction. Prolonged use of these can cause gangrene of the toes and fingers.

Dihydrogenated ergot alkaloids block α receptors and also depress the VMC.

Flowchart 6.1: Effects of nonselective and selective α blockade

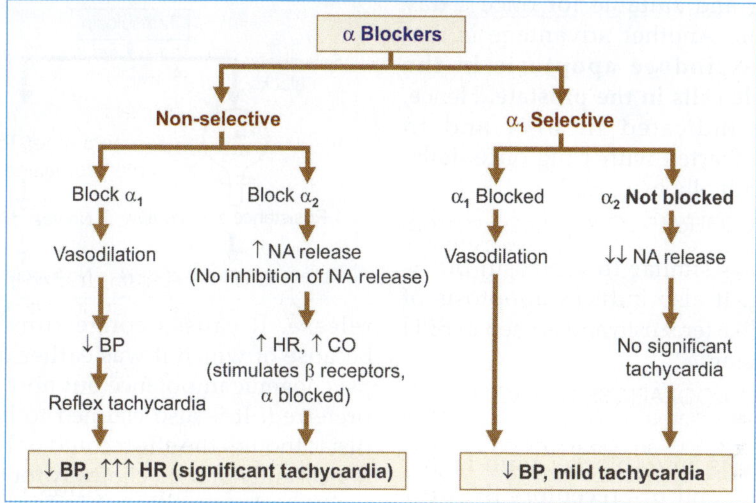

Phentolamine and Tolazoline

Phentolamine and tolazoline are imidazoline derivatives. They are competitive α blockers. In addition, they also block 5-HT receptors, stimulate gut motility and ↑gastric secretion. Hence, they can cause vomiting and diarrhoea in addition to the effects of α-blockade.

SELECTIVE α_1 BLOCKERS

Prazosin

Prazosin is a potent, highly selective, α_1 blocker with 1000 times greater affinity for α_1 receptors. Arterioles and venules are dilated resulting in decreased peripheral vascular resistance and cardiac output. Cardiac output falls because of reduced preload which is due to venodilation. There is no significant tachycardia (as α_2 receptors are spared, there is no ↑in NA release). In addition, it may decrease central sympathetic outflow. Prazosin also inhibits phosphodiesterase, the enzyme that degrades cAMP resulting in ↑cAMP which also contributes to vasodilation (*see* Compare and Contrast—Phenoxybenzamine and Prazosin).

Other Actions

- Prazosin and its congeners are found to ↓LDL and triglycerides and ↑HDL cholesterol.
- They also relax the urinary bladder neck and the prostatic capsule because of which they are useful in prostatic hypertrophy.

Prazosin is orally effective, has an oral bioavailability of 60%, is extensively bound to plasma proteins (about 97%) and is metabolised in the liver. Its duration of action is 8–10 hr.

Dose: 1–4 mg BD-TDS. PRAZOPRES 0.5, 1, 2 mg tab.

Adverse Effects

First dose phenomenon—one hour after the initial dose, marked postural hypotension occurs which may lead to fainting. To avoid this, prazosin should be started with a low dose (0.5 mg) and taken at bedtime. Other side effects include headache and dizziness.

Congeners of prazosin include **terazosin, doxazosin, alfuzosin and tamsulosin**. Others are **indoramin and urapidil.**

Terazosin is highly selective for α_1 receptors, is more water soluble, has higher bioavailability (>90%) than prazosin; it is also longer acting and suitable for once a day administration. Another advantage is that terazosin may **induce apoptosis in the smooth muscle cells in the prostate.** Hence, terazosin is indicated in BPH and in hypertension. Started with 1 mg once daily, the dose is gradually increased.

Dose: 2–10 mg OD. TERALFA, OLYSTER 1, 2, 5 mg tab.

Doxazosin is similar to terazosin but is longer acting. It also induces apoptosis of prostate cells like terazosin and is used in BPH and hypertension.

Dose: 1–8 mg OD. DOXAPRESS, DOXACARD 1, 2, 4 mg tab.

Tamsulosin is an α_1 blocker with higher activity on α_{1A} and α_{1D} receptors than α_{1B} subtype. α_{1A} is abundant in the bladder and prostate while α_{1B} in the blood vessels. Therefore, tamsulosin relieves the symptoms of BPH without a significant fall in BP (which is mediated by α_{1B} receptors). Hence, it is **preferred** in BPH. Tamsulosin has a high bioavailability and t½ of 9–15 hr but its duration of action is increased in the extended release preparations. Tamsulosin can cause abnormal ejaculation (Flowchart 6.2).

Dose: 0.4 mg OD. Contiflo OD, 0.4 mg cap.

Flowchart 6.2: Tamsulosin in BPH

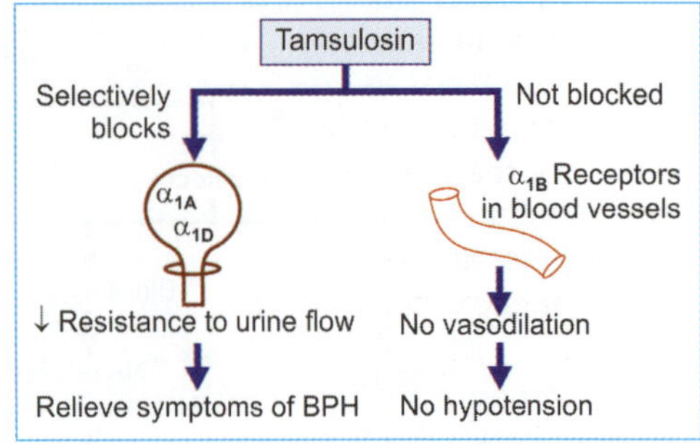

α_2 BLOCKER

Yohimbine

Yohimbine is a relatively selective α_2 blocker which increases BP and heart rate due to ↑NA release. It causes congestion of genitals because of which it was earlier used to treat psychogenic impotence but now sildenafil is preferred. It is also claimed to be an aphrodisiac though the effect could only be psychological and not used clinically for the purpose.

Other drugs with α blocking properties: Several drugs block α-receptors. **Ergot alkaloids** have complex actions and some of them act as partial agonists or antagonists of α receptors. Neuroleptics like chlorpromazine and haloperidol block the α receptors in addition to dopamine receptors. Ketanserin, a serotonin antagonist, has additional α blocking properties.

Uses of α blockers

1. *Hypertension*
   - Selective α_1 blockers like prazosin are used in the treatment of hypertension (*see* page 341).
   - Phenoxybenzamine or phentolamine can be used in hypertensive crisis.

COMPARE AND CONTRAST

Phenoxybenzamine and Prazosin

Features	***Phenoxybenzamine***	***Prazosin***
Chemistry	β-haloalkylamine	Quinazoline
Receptors blocked	α-adrenergic	α-adrenergic
Receptor subtype selectivity	Both α_1 and α_2 (non-selective)	α_1-selective
Type of blockade	Non-equilibrium	Equilibrium
Effect of α_2 blockade	↑ NA release	Does not increase
Reflex tachycardia	Significant	Negligible
Postural hypotension	Significant	Less
Primary use	Pheochromocytoma	Hypertension

2. *Pheochromocytoma* is an adrenal medullary tumour which secretes large amounts of catecholamines resulting in hypertension. The tumour has to be removed surgically. Phenoxybenzamine and phentolamine are used for the preoperative management of the patient and during the surgery. Inoperable cases are put on long-term treatment with phenoxybenzamine.
3. *Peripheral vascular diseases* like Raynaud's phenomenon may be benefited by α blockers which afford symptomatic relief (*see* page 371).
4. *Congestive cardiac failure:* Because of its vasodilator action, prazosin is useful in CCF, but ACE inhibitors are preferred.
5. *Benign prostatic hypertrophy (BPH):* Though BPH is common in men, it is fortunately not a precancerous condition. Enlargement of the prostate gland results in lower urinary tract symptoms like incomplete voiding, hesitancy, straining to pass urine, often associated with nocturia, urgency and occasional incontinence. Blockade of α_1 receptors in the bladder, prostate and urethra, decreases the tone of smooth muscles and thereby reduces the resistance to urine outflow. Prazosin, terazosin, doxazosin, tamsulosin and alfuzosin are useful in patients who cannot be operated upon. Of these, tamsulosin is preferred because of its selective activity on α_{1A} receptors.

Congeners of prazosin

- Congeners are longer acting—given once daily.
- Highly selective for α_1 receptors.
- Postural hypotension is milder than with prazosin.
- No significant effect on cardiac function.
- ↓LDL and ↑HDL cholesterol
- **Tamsulosin** has selective activity on α_{1A} receptors and relieves the symptoms of benign prostatic hypertrophy (BPH) with milder fall in BP. Hence it is preferred in BPH (uroselective)
- **Alfuzosin** is also useful in BPH.
- **Terazosin** and **doxazosin** are used in hypertension.
- **Urapidil** has α_1 and β_1 (weak) blocking properties. It is used in hypertension and BPH.
- **Indoramin** is a selective α_1 blocker. It is used in the treatment of benign prostatic hypertrophy.

6. *Erectile dysfunction:* A combination of phentolamine with papaverine injected directly into the corpora cavernosa is used as an alternative to sildenafil in erectile dysfunction.

β-ADRENERGIC BLOCKING AGENTS

β-blockers are drugs that block the actions of catecholamines mediated through the β receptors.

$$\text{C}_{10}\text{H}_7\text{-OCH}_2\text{-CH(OH)-CH}_2\text{NHCH(CH}_3)_2$$

Structure of propranolol

Classification

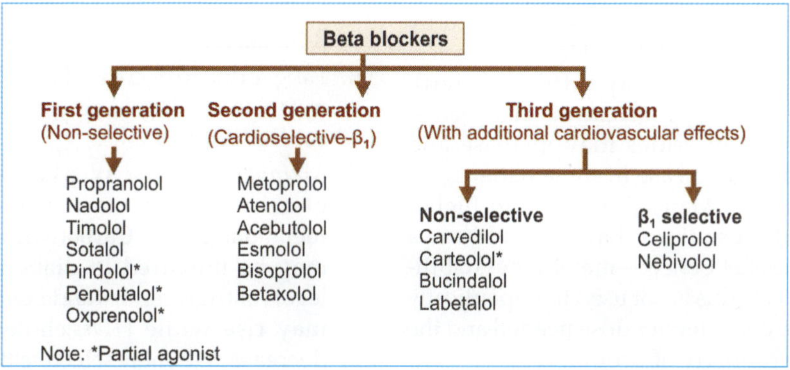

Pharmacological Actions

1. *CVS*
   - **Heart:** β blockers decrease heart rate, force of contraction and cardiac output. Blood pressure falls. The effect is more pronounced in presence of increased sympathetic tone than in a normal situation.

   AV conduction is delayed due to blockade of β receptors in the AV node. Myocardial oxygen requirement is reduced due to reduced cardiac work.

   β-blockers also improve exercise tolerance in angina patients. They prevent the exercise-induced increase in heart rate and force of contraction.

   High doses produce membrane-stabilizing activity like quinidine, causing direct depression of the heart.

   Blood vessels—β-blockers reduce BP. On long-term use, β-blockers reduce peripheral vascular resistance in hypertensive patients. They reduce renin release, decrease central sympathetic outflow, reduce cardiac output and thereby reduce blood pressure.
2. *Respiratory tract:* Blockade of β_2 receptors in the bronchial smooth muscle causes an increase in airway resistance may precipitate acute attack in asthmatics.
3. *Eye:* Many β-blockers reduce intraocular pressure by decreased secretion of aqueous humour.
4. *Metabolic* β-antagonists block lipolysis and glycogenolysis (β_2 mediated) induced by sympathetic stimulation. Hence, nonselective β-blockers may interfere with recovery from hypoglycaemia in diabetics. Plasma triglycerides may increase and HDL levels decrease in some patients.
5. *Other effects:* Many β-blockers in higher doses block sodium channels and have a local anesthetic effect—**membrane- stabilizing** effect. This is not used therapeutically because of the higher dose needed and the irritant property of propranolol.

Pharmacokinetics

Though well absorbed on oral administration (propranolol almost completely absorbed), some β-blockers like propranolol undergo extensive first pass metabolism which reduces the bioavailability to ~25%; food improves the bioavailability of propranolol. Most of the β-blockers have short t½ and are metabolised in the liver. The plasma levels of propranolol increase disproportionately in overdosage because its hepatic metabolism is saturable.

Dose: 40–160 mg/day in divided doses. INDERAL, CIPLAR 10, 40, 80 mg tab: BETALOC 10, 40 mg tab.

Adverse Reactions

1. *Bradycardia* is common. Patients with AV conduction defects may develop arrhythmias and heart block with β-blockers.
2. *CCF:* In patients with impaired myocardial function, sympathetic activity supports the heart. β-blockade eliminates this compensatory effect and may precipitate CCF and acute pulmonary oedema.
3. *Cold extremities* may be seen especially in patients with peripheral vascular disease.
4. β-blockers can precipitate **acute asthmatic attack** in asthmatics and is contraindicated in them. They can worsen COPD.
5. *CNS:* Insomnia, depression and rarely hallucinations can follow the use of β-blockers.
6. *Fatigue* due to decreased blood flow to the muscles during exercise and reduced cardiac output.
7. *Metabolic effects:* Weakness, reduced exercise capacity may be seen due to its metabolic effects. Carbohydrate tolerance may be impaired in diabetics. Plasma levels of triglycerides and LDL cholesterol may rise while HDL cholesterol may decrease with non-selective β-blockers.

8. Abrupt withdrawal of β-blockers after prolonged use can cause **rebound hypertension** and precipitate anginal attacks. This is due to upregulation of β receptors. Hence, β-blockers should be gradually tapered.
9. β-blockers can also cause **dizziness**.
10. *Topical:* Timolol eye drops can sometimes cause burning and dryness of the eyes.

Some important drug interactions

1. *Propranolol + insulin:* When diabetics on insulin also receive propranolol:
   i. β-blockade masks tachycardia which is the first warning signal of hypoglycemia.
   ii. β-blockade delays the recovery from hypoglycaemia by preventing glycogenolysis induced by sympathetic stimulation (acting through β_2 receptors). This may be avoided by using a β_1-selective blocker.
2. *Propranolol + verapamil:* Since both cause myocardiac depression, profound depression may result when both are used together. Hence, the combination should be avoided.
3. *β-blockers + catecholamines:* In patients on non-selective β-blockers, blockade of vascular β-receptors could predispose peripheral vessels to intense vasoconstriction (receptor upregulation) from even small doses of adrenaline used with LAs. Hence, it is safer to use plain local anaesthesia in such patients.
4. *β-blockers,* digitalis and verapamil: All cause depression of AV conduction and together may cause cardiac arrest.
5. *Enzyme inducers:* Like rifampicin can hasten the metabolism and reduce the plasma levels of propranolol.
6. *NSAIDs* counter the antihypertensive effects of β-blockers.

Some Individual β-blockers

First-generation β-blockers: Include non-selective β-blockers and **propranolol** is the prototype. Being highly lipid soluble, propranolol readily crosses the BBB. Plasma t½ is 4 hr. Sustained release preparations are available. Though the t½ is short, the effects of β-blockade are much longer.

Nadolol

- Long acting β-blocker (t½ 20 hr OD dose)
- Used in hypertension, angina, oesophageal varices, migraine prophylaxis and in tremors.

Timolol

- Non-selective, short-acting.
- Used in glaucoma as eye drops (*see* page 106).
- Used orally in hypertension, angina and MI.

Dose: Oral 10–40 mg 0.5% eye drops. TIMOPTAL, GLUCOMOL 0.25, 0.5% eye drops.

Pindolol, Oxprenolol and Penbutalol

- Non-selective
- Partial agonists at β_1, β_2 receptors
- **Penbutolol** in addition has weak intrinsic sympathomimetic activity, *see* below.

Advantages

- Milder bradycardia
- Milder myocardiac depression
- Better tolerated in asthmatics
- Milder effect on lipid profile
- Less chances of rebound hypertension on withdrawal.

Table 6.3: Doses of some β-blockers

Drug	*Total daily dose (mg)*	*Frequency*
Propranolol	40–240	6–12 hr
Metoprolol	50–200	12–24 hr
Atenolol	25–100	Once daily
Pindolol	10–45	6 hourly
Acebutolol	200–400	12–24 hr

Disadvantage: Not suitable for prophylaxis of migraine and myocardial infarction.

Doses
- Pindolol 10–30 mg. PINADOL 5 mg tab.
- Oxprenolol 40–80 mg. TRASICOR 40, 80 mg tab.
- Penbutolol 20–80 mg. LEVATOL 20, 40 mg.

Partial Agonists

Some of them, for example, pindolol, oxprenolol, and penbutolol, have intrinsic sympathomimetic activity due to their partial β-agonistic property. As a result, bradycardia and myocardiac depression are less marked. They are therefore preferred in patients with low cardiac reserve or those who are likely to have severe bradycardia.

Second-generation β-blockers (cardioselective β-blockers)

For example, atenolol, metoprolol, esmolol.

These drugs
- Selectively block β_1 receptors, β_2-blockade is weak.
- Bronchospasm is less/negligible.
- Inhibition of glycogenolysis is lower, hence safer in diabetics.
- Exercise performance is impaired to a lesser degree.
- Lesser chances of peripheral vascular disease.

Atenolol
- Selective β_1-blocker
- Longer acting—given once daily
- Less lipid soluble—does not cross BBB, hence no CNS side effects
- No side effects on lipid profile
- Very commonly used in hypertension and angina where it is preferred to propranolol because of the above advantages (*see* Compare and Contrast: Propranolol and Atenolol).

Dose: 25–100 mg daily. BETACARD, ATEN, BETA 25, 50, 100 mg tab.

Metoprolol
- Selective β_1-blocker
- Well absorbed but undergoes significant first pass metabolism
- Given twice daily
- Used in hypertension and angina pectoris.

Dose: 50–200 mg OD-BD. BETALOC, Met-XL 25, 50, 100 mg tab.

Esmolol
- Selective β_1-blocker
- Ultra short-acting—t½–8 minutes
- Rapid acting
- Used IV
- Safer (due to short action) in critically ill patients and useful in emergencies (due to rapid action) when immediate β-blockade is needed.
- Used in supraventricular and other arrhythmias, perioperative hypertension, and to reduce myocardial work done and tide over acute myocardial ischemia.

Dose: 0.1–0.2 mg/kg/min infusion. ESOCARD, BREVIBLOCK 10 mg/ml inj.

Acebutolol
- β_1 selective with some partial agonistic effects
- Less likely to cause bradycardia because of partial agonistic activity on β_1 receptors.
- Converted to active metabolite.
- May be used in hypertension and arrhythmias.
- 400 mg/day in one or two divided doses.

Dose: 200–400 mg OD, 20–30 mg IV. SECTRAL 200, 400 mg tab.

Betaxolol is used in glaucoma, hypertension and angina pectoris.

Third-generation β-blockers

Include carteolol, carvedilol, labetalol, bucindolol, celiprolol and nebivolol. These are β-blockers with **additional vasodilatory properties**. Some of them, viz. celiprolol and nebivolol, selectively block β_1 cardiac receptors.

Carteolol is a non-selective β-blocker with partial agonistic activity at the β_1 receptors and, therefore, may cause less bradycardia.

Carvedilol blocks β_1, β_2 and α_1 receptors. It also has membrane-stabilizing and anti-inflammatory properties.

Nebivolol

- A highly selective β_1-blocker.
- Also causes vasodilation through nitric oxide production.
- No myocardial depression.
- Reduce BP by reducing vascular resistance.

Dose: 2.5–5 mg OD. NEBICARD, NEBISTAR 2.5, 5 mg tab.

Labetalol

Labetalol blocks α_1, β_1 and β_2 receptors and is useful in pheochromocytoma and hypertension in the elderly.

Butoxamine

Butoxamine is a selective β_2-blocker but therapeutic applications are not known.

Uses of β-blockers

A. Cardiovascular

1. *Hypertension:* β-blockers are useful in the treatment of mild to moderate hypertension. β-blocker can be used alone or with other antihypertensives (*see* page 341). They are particularly suitable for combination with drugs that produce tachycardia.
2. *Angina pectoris:* β-blockers are useful in the prophylaxis of exertional angina. Both the severity and frequency are reduced (*see* page 367). They reduce both cardiac work and O_2 demand.
3. *Cardiac arrhythmias:* β-blockers are useful in the treatment of both ventricular and supraventricular arrhythmias. Sotalol has additional anti-arrhythmic effects (*see* page 379). Depression of AV conduction and membrane-stabilizing effects help.
4. *Myocardial infarction:* Intravenous β-blockers in acute MI may limit the size of the infarct and also prevent ventricular arrhythmias. In patients who have recovered from MI, long-term treatment with β blockers prolongs survival (*see* page 369).
5. *Congestive cardiac failure:* Earlier experience had shown that β-blockers can worsen CCF because of their negative inotropic effect (*see* page 357). However, several recent studies have shown that when judiciously used in selected patients, β-blockers can be beneficial in CCF. They reduce the risk of sudden death and prolong survival on long-term use. The exact mechanism is not known. Sympathetic system is stimulated in CCF which may infact be deleterious to the heart in many ways and even contribute to cardiac remodelling. Blocking the β receptors may help to improve cardiac function and prevent cardiac remodelling.
6. *Obstructive cardiomyopathy:* β-blockers are found to be beneficial.
7. *Pheochromocytoma:* Propranolol is given with α-blockers before surgery to control hypertension.
8. *Dissecting aneurysm of the aorta:* Propranolol helps by reducing aortic pulsations.

***Mnemonic:* HAC My COPD**

B. Non-Cardiac Uses

9. *Thyrotoxicosis:* Propranolol controls symptoms like palpitation, tremors and affords symptomatic relief in thyrotoxicosis; it is used as an adjuvant. Propranolol can also be used in thyrotoxic crisis or thyroid storm as it quickly affords symptomatic relief. It also impairs conversion of T_4 to T_3.
10. *Glaucoma:* Timolol used topically is the first line treatment in glaucoma.

COMPARE AND CONTRAST

Propranolol and Atenolol

Features	***Propranolol***	***Atenolol***
Receptors blocked	Both β_1 and β_2	β_1 selective
Lipid solubility	High	Low
First pass metabolism	High	Not significant
Protein binding	Extensive (>90%)	Poor (<5%)
BBB	Crosses	Does not cross
Adverse effects on CNS	Significant	No significant effects
Excretion through kidneys	Negligible (0.5%)	Major route (85%)
Plasma t½	3–6 hr	6–8 hr
Features	Prop	Ateno
Frequency of administration	2–4 times a day	Once a day
Duration of action	Short (6–12 hr)	Long (12–24 hr)
In asthmatic and chronic bronchitis patients	Contraindicated	Not contraindicated
In diabetics and peripheral vascular diseases	Avoided	Can be used with caution
Local anaesthetic action	Yes	No

Betoxalol, levobunalol, carteolol and metipranolol can also be used in glaucoma. The fall in IOP is sustained and even if 1 or 2 doses are missed, there is no sudden rise in IOP.

11. *Prophylaxis of Migraine:* Propranolol reduces the frequency and severity of migraine headache; used for prophylaxis.
12. *Anxiety:* Propranolol prevents the acute panic symptoms seen in public speaking, examination and other such anxiety-provoking situations. Performance in musicians can be improved when taken prophylactically. Tremors, tachycardia and other symptoms of sympathetic overactivity are alleviated.
13. *Cirrhosis:* β-blockers may help by reducing the portal venous pressure by about 40%.
14. *Esophageal varices:* In patients who have bleeding varices, a combination of nadolol and isosorbide mononitrate has been shown to prevent rebleeding by inducing splanchnic vasoconstriction and reducing cardiac output.
15. *Alcohol withdrawal:* β-blockers help to overcome some of the symptoms in alcohol withdrawal by reducing the central sympathetic overactivity.

Mnemonic: **CAT GAME** (**c**irrhosis, **a**nxiety, **t**hyrotoxiosis, **g**laucoma, **a**lcohol withdrawal, **m**igraine, **e**sophageal varices)

Contraindications to β-blockers

- **CCF:** β-blockers prevent an increase in the heart rate and cardiac output. These effects may be dangerous in patients with CCF. They should be used cautiously and only in selected patients with CCF.
- **Bradycardia:** β-blockers should be avoided in patients with bradycardia.
- β-blockers are contraindicated in patients with heart block because they depress AV conduction.
- They are to be avoided in patients with bronchial asthma and COPD. If needed, a cardioselective β-blocker may be used with caution.

- β-blockers should be avoided in diabetics because they mask the initial symptoms of hypoglycaemia as discussed under drug interactions.

α- AND β-ADRENERGIC BLOCKERS

Labetalol, carvedilol and medroxolol block alpha (α_1) and beta receptors (β_1 and β_2). *See* under 3rd generation β-blockers.

Clinical Pharmacology

- While administering β-blockers, watch for bradycardia especially, if the patient is on digoxin or amiodarone.
- Atenolol, propranolol, metoprolol are commonly used β-blockers while esmolol (IV) is used in emergencies.
- β-blockers even as eye drops (timolol) can precipitate bronchospasm in asthmatics.
- β-blockers reduce the hepatic blood flow by about 30% and thereby delay the hepatic metabolism of some drugs.
- Postural hypotension and sexual dysfunction may reduce the utility of α blockers but these effects are milder with α_1-selective blockers.
- β-blockers, particularly metoprolol and carvedilol use, have shown reduced morbidity and mortality in CCF.
- Most β-blockers do not block the β_3 receptors and thereby have no significant effect on lipolysis.

DRUGS USED IN TREATMENT OF GLAUCOMA

Glaucoma is a chronic, progressive optic neuropathy often associated with increased intraocular pressure. Constant rise in IOP can damage the optic nerve and if untreated optic nerve degenerates leading to permanent blindness. The rise in IOP (called **ocular hypertension)** may be due to increased formation or impaired drainage of aqueous humors. Aqueous humors is secreted by the ciliary body and it drains through the canal of Schlemm. In most cases, the drainage is affected and sustained ocular hypertension can result in irreversible damage. Glaucoma is one of the common causes of blindness. Hypertension, myopia and family history of glaucoma are risk factors.

Glaucoma may be

- Open angle (wide angle, chronic simple) glaucoma
- Narrow angle (acute congestive, closed angle) glaucoma
- Congenital glaucoma
- Secondary glaucoma—secondary to some eye diseases.

Open angle glaucoma is a slow onset chronic ocular disease seen often in genetically predisposed individuals. Trabecular meshwork may lose patency gradually. Intraocular pressure may be raised but may be normal too. It needs long-term treatment.

Two categories of drugs may be used in the treatment of open angle glaucoma. They are:

I. *Drugs that increase the drainage of aqueous humor*
   - **PG analogs**
     Latanoprost, bimatoprost, travoprost, unoprostone.
   - **Cholinergic drugs**
     Carbachol, pilocarpine, physostigmine, echothiophate.

II. *Drugs that decrease the formation of aqueous humor*
   - **β-blockers**
     Timolol, betaxolol, levobunolol, carteolol.

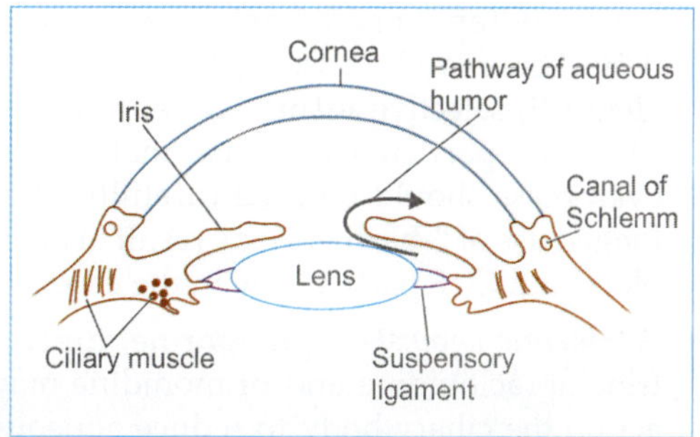

Fig. 6.8: Schematic diagram showing pathway for the drainage of aqueous humor

- **Adrenergic agonists**
  Adrenaline, dipivefrine, apraclonidine, brimonidine.
- **Carbonic anhydrase inhibitors**
  Acetazolamide, dorzolamide.

III. *Others:* Osmotic agents.

Drugs used in glaucoma are summarised in Table 6.4.

- *Prostaglandin analogs:* These are now considered the first line drugs. **Latanoprost** is a prostaglandin analog—a prodrug of $PGF_{2\alpha}$. It increases the outflow of aqueous humor probably by relaxing the ciliary muscle. It can be used as an adjuvant to other drugs. Bimatoprost, travoprost and unoprostone are similar to latanoprost. PG analogs are all expensive.
- *Cholinergic drugs:* Miotics like pilocarpine and physostigmine improve drainage of aqueous humor by constricting the pupil and opening the iridocorneal angle. They may be used in acute congestive glaucoma for short periods to lower the IOP. However, miotics are not the preferred drugs in open angle glaucoma.
- *β-blockers* like timolol are the first line drugs in glaucoma. They reduce aqueous humor formation by blocking the β_2 receptors in the ciliary body. Since they do not cause miosis, there is no associated headache or browache which are due to spasm of the iris and the ciliary muscles. The reduction in IOP is smoother and constant. However, even when used as eye drops, β-blockers may be absorbed systemically. Hence, β_1-selective agents like betaxolol are preferred particularly in asthmatics and even these should be used carefully. Prolonged use of β-blockers may result in heart block and CCF particularly in the elderly.
- *Adrenergic agonists:* Epinephrine, dipivefrine apraclonidine and brimonidine may act on the ciliary body to reduce aqueous humor formation or act by reducing ciliary blood flow (α_1). They also reduce uveoscleral outflow. Corneal penetration of adrenaline is poor, not preferred. It can also cause conjunctival blanching followed by hyperemia. **Dipivefrine,** a prodrug of adrenaline penetrates cornea and is converted to adrenaline. It is better tolerated and longer acting than adrenaline—used as adjuvant. **Apraclonidine** is an analog of clonidine which has higher topical than systemic activity. It is used following surgical corrections like iridotomy. **Brimonidine** is more α_2 selective and has higher lipophilicity than apraclonidine. Ocular side effects (α_1) are milder. Used as an alternative to other drugs and as an adjuvant.
- *Carbonic anhydrase inhibitors:* Production of aqueous humor requires active transport of bicarbonate ions. Inhibition of carbonic anhydrase decreases aqueous humor formation by enhancing bicarbonate loss. Acetazolamide and methazolamide are given orally but are poorly tolerated. Topical agents like dorzolamide eye drops are now available. These can also be combined with β-blockers and miotics.
- *Osmotic agents:* 20% mannitol/10% glycerol injected IV exert osmotic effects and draw fluid from the eye. These are used for rapid reduction of IOP in acute congestive glaucoma along with other drugs.

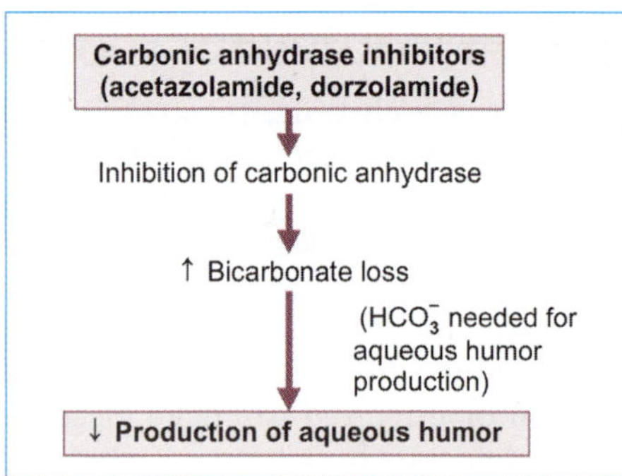

Narrow angle glaucoma also called closed angle glaucoma as it occurs in people with narrow irido-corneal angle. The intraocular pressure rises rapidly and requires immediate

Table 6.4: Drugs used in glaucoma

Drugs	Mode of action	Adverse effects	Route of administration and comments
1. **PG analogs** Latanoprost, Bimatoprost Trovaprost	↑ Uveoscleral outflow	Conjunctival redness, discomfort, dryness and burning sensation; darkening of the eye lashes and iris; allergic reactions	Topical: First line drugs; good efficacy; once a day; well tolerated, superior to timolol in reducing IOP
2. **Cholinergics** • Pilocarpine, Carbachol • Physostigmine, Echothiophate	Miosis, opens trabecular meshwork , ↑ drainage	Corneal oedema, spasm of accommodation, browache, Myopia, browache, cataract, retinal detachment	Used with β-blockers; inconvenient due to frequent dosage and adverse effects Echothiophate—quaternary ammonium compound—not absorbed
3. **β-blockers** Timolol, Betaxolol Carteolol, Levobunolol	↓ Aqueous secretion from ciliary epithelium	Conjunctival irritation, redness and discomfort, Bronchospasm in asthmatics	Topical: First line drugs; smooth control of IOP; No miosis, hence no headache, browache or visual disturbances; CI in asthmatics; Betaxolol β_1 selective but less efficacious may be tried in asthmatics
4. **Adrenergic agonists** • Dipivefrine, Adrenaline	↓ Aqueous formation, ↑ outflow	Conjunctival redness, photosensitivity, allergic reactions	Second line drugs may be combined with β blockers
• α_2-adrenergic agonists Apraclonidine	↓ Secretion	Conjunctival redness, photosensitivity, dryness of mouth	Higher topical activity than clonidine, do not cross BBB—no CNS effects; used after trabeculoplasty
Brimonidine	↓ Aqueous formation, ↑ uveoscleral outflow	Dry mouth, sedation, ocular effects milder than apraclonidine	As an alternative to other drugs or as an adjuvant
5. **Carbonic anhydrase inhibitors** Acetazolamide (oral) Methazolamide, Dorzolamide	↓ Aqueous formation	Hypokalemia, anorexia, drowsiness	Second line drugs; acetazolamide given orally; dorzolamide fewer side effects; topical preparation better tolerated
6. **Osmotic agents** Mannitol (20% IV) Glycerol (10% IV)	Draw fluid from eye into systemic circulation by osmotic activity	Headache, nausea, vomiting, allergic reactions	Used in acute congestive glaucoma for rapid ↓ of IOP

CI: Contraindicated *SR: Slow release* *IOP: Intraocular pressure* treatment as delay can lead to blindness. Objective is to quickly reduce the IOP till surgery or other measures like laser iridotomy are available. A combination of drugs is preferred (Table 6.3).

- Injection mannitol (20%)—1.5–2 g/kg or glycerol (10%) act by osmotic activity to reduce the IOP
- Acetazolamide a carbonic anhydrase inhibitor 0.5 g IV—reduces formation of aqueous humor
- Cholinergic drugs—miotics open the trabecular meshwork and increase the drainage of aqueous humor.
  Pilocarpine 4% with physostigmine (anticholinesterase) is used as eye drops.
- β-blocker—timolol/betaxolol eye drops are used every 12 hours
- α agonists—additional apraclonidine 1% eye drops may be needed.
- PG analog—latanoprost eye drops may be added.

[1] From Medical Council of India, *Competency based Undergraduate Curriculum for the Indian Medical Graduate*, 2018;1:136–144.

CHAPTER 7

Cholinergic and Anticholinergic Drugs

Competency achievement: The student should be able to:

PH 1.14 Describe mechanism of action, types, doses, side effects, indications and contraindications of cholinergic and anticholinergic drugs.[1]

Cholinergic Transmission

Acetylcholine (ACh), an ester of choline, is the neurotransmitter of the parasympathetic system. The nerves that synthesize, store and release ACh are called *cholinergic*.

The **sites** of release of acetylcholine are (Fig. 7.1):

1. Ganglia—all the preganglionic fibres of ANS, i.e. at both the sympathetic and parasympathetic ganglia.
2. The postganglionic parasympathetic nerve endings.
3. Sweat glands—the sympathetic postganglionic nerve endings supplying the sweat glands.
4. Skeletal muscles—somatic nerve endings supplying skeletal muscles.
5. Adrenal medulla.
6. CNS—brain and spinal cord.

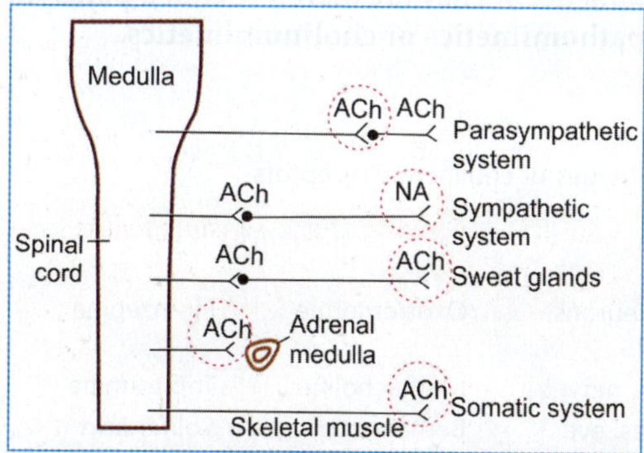

Fig. 7.1: Sites of release of neurotransmitters—acetylcholine and noradrenaline in the peripheral nervous system

Muscarinic receptors are more abundant in the brain while nicotinic receptors are more in the spinal cord.

Synthesis of Acetylcholine

Acetylcholine is synthesized from acetyl CoA and choline, choline enters into the cholinergic neuron by a carrier mediated transport.

Structure of Acetylcholine

$$(CH_3)_3\overset{+}{N}CH_2\,CH_2\,O\overset{\overset{O}{\|}}{C}CH_3$$

It reacts with acetyl CoA and the reaction is (Fig. 7.2) catalysed by an enzyme choline acetyltransferase. This ACh so formed is stored in small oval vesicles in the cholinergic nerve terminals.

Transmission of an impulse: When an action potential reaches the presynaptic membrane, ACh is released into the synaptic cleft (Fig. 7.2). This ACh binds to and activates the cholinergic receptor on the postsynaptic membrane leading to depolarization of this membrane. Thus, the impulse is transmitted across the synapse. ACh released intothe synaptic cleft is rapidly destroyed by the enzyme acetylcholinesterase (AChE). Then the postsynaptic membrane is repolarized.

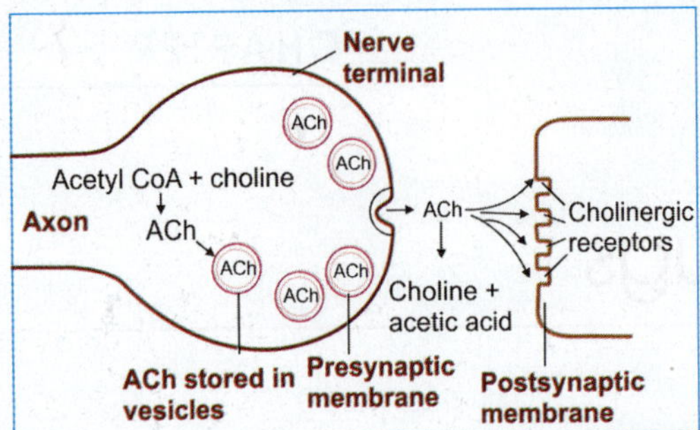

Fig. 7.2: Cholinergic transmission—schematic representation

Cholinesterases

Acetylcholine is hydrolysed to choline and acetic acid by the enzymes cholinesterases. Two types of cholinesterases are present:

1. **True cholinesterase** (Acetylcholinesterase)—at neurons, ganglia and neuromuscular junction.
2. **Pseudocholinesterase** (butyrylcholinesterase)—in plasma, liver and other organs. It hydrolyses many other esters apart from acetylcholine.

Cholinergic Receptors

There are two classes of cholinergic receptors—**muscarinic** and **nicotinic**.

Muscarinic receptors are present in the heart, smooth muscles, glands, eyes and CNS. Five subtypes of muscarinic receptors, M_1–M_5 are recognised (Table 7.1).

COMPARE AND CONTRAST

Cholinesterases

	Acetyl cholinesterase	***Butyryl cholinesterase***
Synonym	True cholinesterase	Pseudo cholinesterase
Distribution	Neurons, ganglia NMJ	Plasma, liver, intestines
Hydrolysis of ACh	Fast (in micro-seconds)	Slow
Methacholine	Hydrolysed	Resistant—not hydrolysed

Muscarinic receptors are all G protein coupled receptors.

Nicotinic receptors are present in the neuromuscular junction, autonomic ganglia and adrenal medulla. Nicotinic receptors are ion channels—five subunits (2α, 1β, 1γ and 1δ) enclose the channel (Fig. 7.3). Binding of acetylcholine to α subunits opens the channel allowing the entry of Na^+ into the cell. Two subtypes of nicotinic receptors are identified (Table 7.1). N_M receptors are present at the skeletal muscle end plate and N_N receptors at the autonomic ganglia and adrenal medulla.

CHOLINERGIC DRUGS

Cholinergic drugs are chemicals that act at the same site as acetylcholine and thereby mimic its actions. They are therefore called **parasympathomimetics or cholinomimetics.**

Table 7.1: Features of important subtypes of cholinergic receptors

Subtypes	*Receptor family*	*Location*	*Agonist*	*Antagonists*
M_1	G_q	Gastric gland, enteric neurons, autonomic ganglia, CNS	Oxotremorine	Pirenzepine
M_2	G_i	Heart, smooth muscles, nerves	Methacholine	Tripitramine
M_3	G_q	Glands, smooth muscles, eye	Bethanechol	Solifenacin
N_M	Ion channels	Neuromuscular junction	Nicotine	Tubocurarine
N_N	Ion channels	Autonomic ganglia, adrenal medulla, CNS	Nicotine	Hexamethonium Trimethaphan

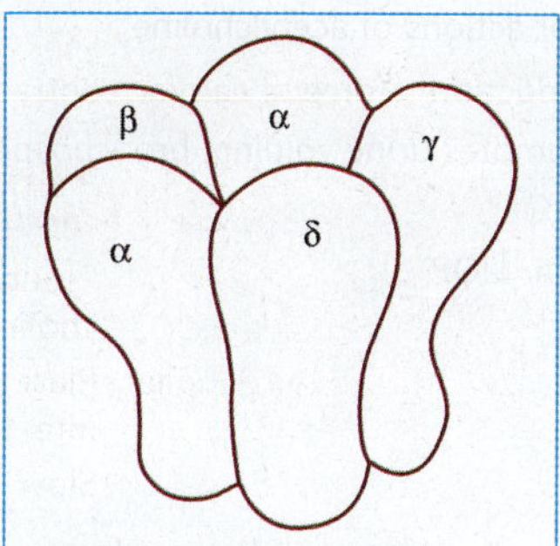

Fig. 7.3: Nicotinic receptor contains 5 subunits—2α + β + γ + δ. Acetylcholine binds to the sites on α subunits resulting in opening of the channel

Cholinergic drugs may be classified as

Classification

I. Directly acting

1. Esters of choline
Acetylcholine
Methacholine
Carbachol
Bethanechol

2. Cholinomimetic alkaloids
Pilocarpine
Muscarine, arecoline

II. Indirectly acting
Anticholinesterases

1. Reversible *(carbamates)*

Neostigmine	Physostigmine
Pyridostigmine	Ambenonium
Edrophonium	Galantamine

2. Irreversible

A. Organophosphorus compounds
Echothiophate
Malathion
Parathion
Sumithion
Dyflos
Diazinon
Toxic nerve gases: Sarin, Tabun

B. Carbamate insecticides
Carbaryl
Propoxure
Aldicarb

Directly Acting Cholinergic Drugs

Acetylcholine is taken as the prototype of parasympathomimetic drugs.

Actions of Acetylcholine

Muscarinic actions: Muscarinic actions resemble the actions of the alkaloid muscarine found in some mushrooms. These actions result from the stimulation of the muscarinic receptors by acetylcholine.

1. *Heart:* The actions of acetylcholine are similar to that of vagal stimulation. It depresses the SA node and thereby reduces the heart rate and force of contraction. In larger doses, AV conduction is depressed and partial to total AV block may be produced.
2. *Blood vessels:* ACh relaxes the vascular smooth muscles and dilates the blood vessels of almost all vascular beds including pulmonary and coronary vessels and of the skin (causing flushing) and mucous membrane. The BP falls due to a fall in total peripheral resistance. The vasodilator effect is mediated by stimulation of endothelial NO production. Vasodilation may also be due to an indirect effect by inhibition of noradrenaline release from the adrenergic nerve endings by acetylcholine.
3. *Smooth muscle:* ACh increases the tone of all other (nonvascular) smooth muscles.
   - *Gastrointestinal tract*: Tone and peristalsis is enhanced, sphincters are relaxed, resulting in rapid forward propulsion of intestinal contents.
   - *Urinary bladder:* Detrusor contracts and trigonal sphincter relaxes—promotes voiding of urine.
   - *Bronchial smooth muscle:* Contracts resulting in bronchospasm.
4. *Secretory glands:* Acetylcholine **increases** the secretions of all glands; salivary, lacrimal, nasopharyngeal, tracheobronchial, gastric and intestinal secretions are increased. Sweating is also increased. Enhanced bronchial secretions and

Table 7.2: Effects of cholinergic stimulation or actions of acetylcholine

CVS	Vasodilation, ↓BP, ↓HR, ↓AV conduction, ↓force of cardiac contraction
Non-vascular smooth muscle	Contraction, ↑gut peristalsis, promotes urine voiding, bronchospasm
Glands	↑Secretion
Eye	Miosis, spasm of accommodation, ↓IOP
NMJ	Muscle contraction
Ganglia	Stimulation

bronchospasm result in severe dyspnoea.

5. *Eye:* Cholinergic stimulation brings about constriction of pupil (miosis) by contracting the circular muscles of the iris. Stimulation of the muscarinic receptors (M_3) presents in the sphincter pupillae results in miosis. Drainage of aqueous humor is facilitated and intraocular pressure falls. Ciliary muscle contracts resulting in spasm of accommodation.

Nicotinic actions: These effects resemble the actions of the alkaloid nicotine and are brought about by stimulation of nicotinic receptors by acetylcholine.

1. *NMJ:* ACh brings about contraction of skeletal muscles by stimulating the N_M receptors present in the neuromuscular junction. Large doses cause persistent depolarisation of skeletal muscles resulting in paralysis.
2. *Autonomic ganglia:* ACh stimulates the sympathetic and parasympathetic ganglia and the adrenal medulla.
3. *CNS:* ACh is a neurotransmitter at several sites in the CNS. ACh injected IV cannot cross the BBB and has no central effects.

The important effects of cholinergic stimulation are summarised in Table 7.2.

Uses: Acetylcholine is rapidly destroyed in the gut when given orally. On intravenous administration, it is rapidly metabolised by pseudocholinesterases in the plasma and by true cholinesterase at the site of action. Therefore, it is **not used therapeutically except** occasionally as 1% eye drops to rapidly produce miosis that is required during some eye surgeries.

Esters of choline are effective orally; **carbachol and bethanechol** are resistant to both cholinesterases and have a longer duration of action. Their muscarinic actions are prominent with a sustained effect on GI smooth muscles and urinary bladder. **Methacholine** is resistant to pseudocholinesterase but is rarely used. Carbachol (eye drops) is used in glaucoma. **Bethanechol may be used in:**

- Hypotonia of the bladder.
- Hypotonia of the gastrointestinal smooth muscles and in congenital megacolon.
- Some cases of postoperative paralytic ileus.
- Urinary retention and neurogenic bladder.
- Xerostomia as an alternative to pilocarpine.

Bethanechol dose: 10–40 mg oral, 2.5–5 mg SC.
UROTONIN 25 mg tab.

Adverse effects include diarrhoea, flushing, salivation, sweating, bradycardia, hypotension, syncope and bronchospasm.

CHOLINOMIMETIC ALKALOIDS

Pilocarpine is an alkaloid obtained from the leaves of *Pilocarpus microphyllus*. Like ACh it stimulates cholinergic receptors, but its muscarinic actions are prominent. It is a tertiary amine, crosses BBB and can cause CNS effects.

Its actions on the eye are important—when applied to the eye it causes miosis, contraction of the ciliary muscle, spasm of accommodation and a fall in intraocular tension. It also increases sweat **(diaphoretic)** and salivary secretions **(sialogogue).** Pilocarpine lowers the

BP in therapeutic doses but may cause hypertension and tachycardia in higher doses.

PILOCAR 1%, 2%, 4% eye drops. PILODROPS, CARPIN 0.5% eye drops.

Adverse effects: When used as eye drops, burning sensation and painful spasm of accommodation, browache and corneal edema can occur. Long-term use can cause retinal detachment. Following systemic use, salivation, sweating, bradycardia, diarrhea and bronchospasm can occur.

Uses

1. **Glaucoma** as pilocarpine causes miosis and reduces IOP, it is used in **glaucoma** as a 0.5–4% eye drops. Pilocarpine ocusert is available and can deliver pilocarpine constantly at 20 µg/hr for 7 days.
2. Pilocarpine is also used alternately with mydriatics like homatropine **to break the adhesions between the iris and the lens.**
3. It is used to **counter the dryness of mouth** that is seen following radiation of head and neck.
4. **Sjögren's syndrome** is characterised by dryness of mouth and lack of tears. Pilocarpine being a sialogogue is useful.

Cevimeline, a derivative of ACh, directly stimulates the muscarinic receptors and can be used to increase salivary secretions in Sjögren's syndrome and radiation induced xerostomia.

Muscarine: Muscarine is an alkaloid present in several species of the mushrooms of Amanita and Inocybe species. It is responsible for the symptoms of poisoning when mushrooms are consumed (Table 7.3).

Arecoline: Arecoline found in areca nut (*Areca catachu*) has both muscarinic and nicotinic actions but is of no therapeutic value.

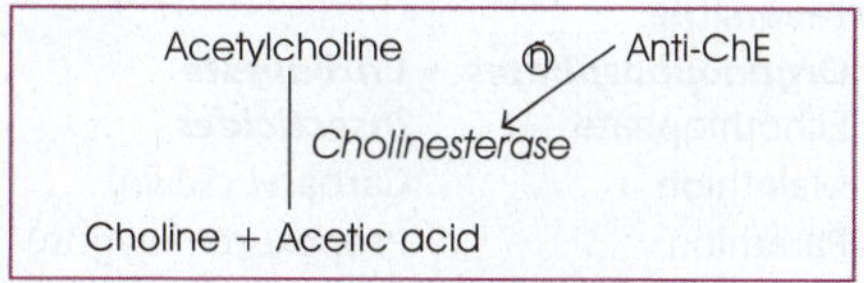

INDIRECTLY ACTING CHOLINERGIC DRUGS

Anticholinesterases

Anticholinesterases (anti-ChEs) or cholinesterase inhibitors are drugs which inhibit the enzyme cholinesterase. They primarily inhibit acetyl ChE but also target butyryl ChE. Anticholinesterases are either esters of carbamic acid (carbamates) or derivatives of phosphoric acid (organophosphates). They may be:

Mechanism of Action

As the structure of anticholinesterases resembles that of ACh, they bind to AChEs and inactivate them. Thus, ACh is not hydrolysed and it accumulates. The actions of all these drugs are due to this accumulated ACh. Hence, the actions are similar to cholinergic agonists.

Table 7.3: Mushroom poisoning

Mushroom poisoning can be of three types

Early onset	***Hallucinogen***	***Late onset***
Caused by Inocybe and related species. The symptoms of poisoning appear in 30–60 minutes of mushroom ingestion and resemble muscarinic stimulation (salivation, nausea, vomiting, bronchospasm, abdominal colic, diarrhea, bradycardia and hypotension). Symptoms respond to atropine (1–2 mg IM every 30 minutes)	Due to *Amanita muscaria* and related species—restlessness, hallucinations, ataxia and delirium (symptoms like atropine poisoning). No specific antidote. Treatment is supportive. Atropine is contraindicated	Due to *Amanita phalloides* is the most serious type and can be fatal. Symptoms develop after several hours and are because of cell death in the liver, kidney and gastrointestinal mucosa. May be treated with thiotic acid or penicillin

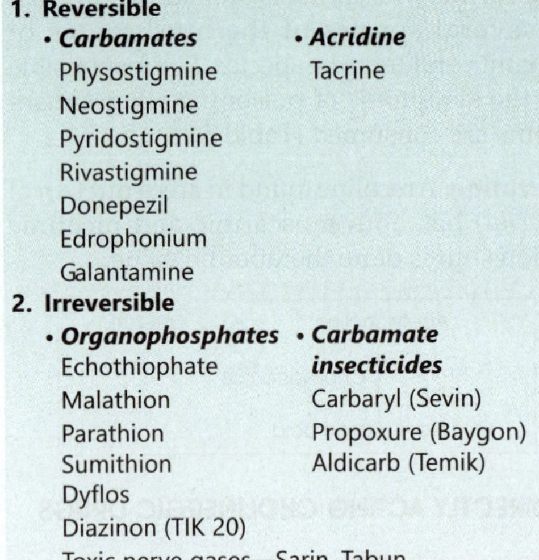

1. **Reversible**
   - ***Carbamates***
     Physostigmine
     Neostigmine
     Pyridostigmine
     Rivastigmine
     Donepezil
     Edrophonium
     Galantamine
   - ***Acridine***
     Tacrine
2. **Irreversible**
   - ***Organophosphates***
     Echothiophate
     Malathion
     Parathion
     Sumithion
     Dyflos
     Diazinon (TIK 20)
     Toxic nerve gases—Sarin, Tabun
   - ***Carbamate insecticides***
     Carbaryl (Sevin)
     Propoxure (Baygon)
     Aldicarb (Temik)

The structure of AChE contains an anionic site and an esteratic site (Fig. 7.4). Reversible anticholinesterases except edrophonium bind to both anionic and esteratic sites. Edrophonium binds only to anionic site and the binding is quickly reversible in minutes, hence it is very short acting. Organophosphates (OP) bind only to the esteratic site but the enzyme is phosphorylated (by covalent bonds) and the binding is stable. With some OPs the binding takes many days to be reversed while with others it is not fully reversible at all.

Pharmacological actions: The actions are similar to that of cholinergic stimulation as they cause accumulation of ACh.

The quaternary ammonium compounds like neostigmine are poorly absorbed from the gut, do not cross the CNS and have mostly peripheral effects (on the skeletal muscles). The lipid soluble compounds like physostigmine and organophosphates are well absorbed, reach the CNS and have both central and peripheral effects.

Anticholinesterases stimulate both sympathetic and parasympathetic ganglia. On the CVS, the parasympathetic effects predominate leading to bradycardia, hypotension, negative inotropic effects and the cardiac output falls.

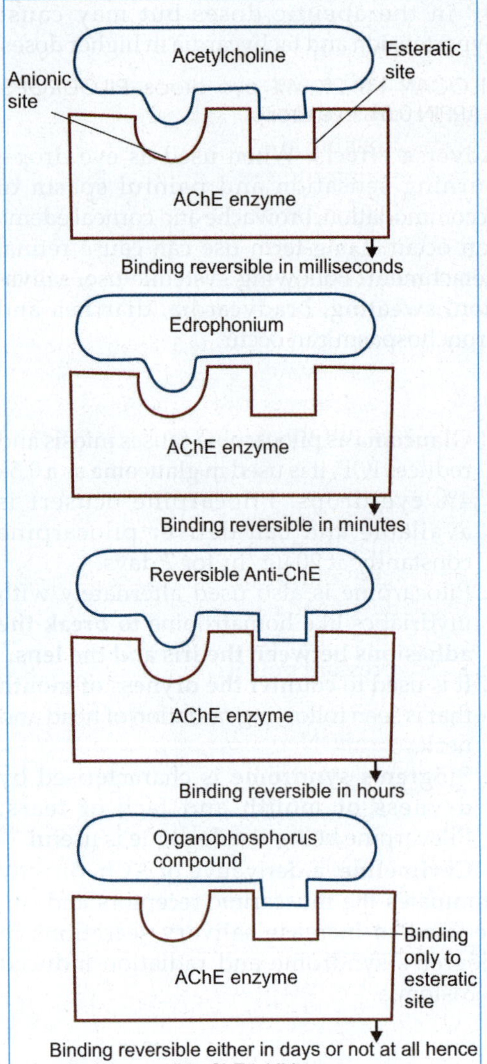

Fig. 7.4: Acetylcholine and reversible anticholinesterases bind to both anionic and esteratic sites of the acetylcholinesterase (AChE) enzyme. Edrophonium binds only the anionic site and is short acting because the binding is rapidly reversible. OP compounds bind only the esteratic site but exception is echothiophate which binds both anionic and esteratic sites.

In higher doses the BP increases due to stimulation of the sympathetic ganglia. The effect on gastrointestinal tract, respiratory tract and eye are all similar to cholinomimetics. In higher doses anti-ChE can cause convulsions followed by coma and respiratory arrest.

At the NMJ, low doses increase the force and strength of contraction with fibrillations and fasciculations but higher doses cause persistent depolarization and may result in paralysis.

Physostigmine: Physostigmine (eserine) is an alkaloid obtained from the plant *Physostigma venenosum* (Calabar bean). It is a lipid soluble, tertiary ammonium compound, hence has better penetration into tissues and also crosses the BBB. It is available for IV injection, as 0.1–1% eye drops and in combination with pilocarpine nitrate 2%.

Uses

- *Glaucoma:* Physostigmine is used in glaucoma: Its use as eye drops can cause browache and on long-term use, retinal detachment and cataract.
- *Poisoning:* In atropine and tricyclic antidepressant poisoning: 0.5–1 mg oral or 0.5 mg IV.

Neostigmine: Neostigmine is a synthetic quaternary ammonium compound—poorly absorbed from the gut; it does not cross the BBB. Neostigmine enhances the skeletal muscle strength and force of contraction in myasthenia gravis—by anticholinesterase activity, by direct stimulation of nicotinic N_M receptors and by enhancing the amount of ACh released during each action potential. It is used in myasthenia gravis (*see* below), post-operative paralytic ileus and atony of the urinary bladder (*see* ***Compare and contrast:*** Physostigmine and neostigmine).

Dose: 15–30 mg TDS-QID. PROSTIGMIN, MYOSTIGMINE 15 mg tab 0.5 mg/ml inj.

Pyridostigmine is similar to neostigmine but is longer acting and is used in myasthenia gravis.

Dose: 60–180 mg TDS. MYESTIN 60 mg tab.

Ambenonium is also a longer acting congener of neostigmine.

Edrophonium is a quaternary ammonium compound and binds only to the anionic site; it is rapid and short acting (10–20 mins). It is used in the diagnosis of myasthenia gravis, and intravenously in snakebite and in curare poisoning.

Rivastigmine is a longer acting carbamate that somewhat selectively binds to the AChE in the brain. Being highly lipid soluble, rivastigmine is rapidly absorbed and reaches the brain and augments cholinergic transmission in the brain. It is used in the treatment of mild to moderate Alzheimer's disease. Started with 1.5 mg BD the dose may be gradually increased at 2-week intervals to a maximum of 6 mg BD.

EXELON 1.5, 3, 4, 5 and 6 mg tab.

Donepezil is another reversible anticholinesterase with longer duration of action—given once daily. It was shown to produce improvement in the symptoms of Alzheimer's disease.

Dose: 5–10 mg OD. DONECEPT 5, 10 mg tab.

COMPARE AND CONTRAST

Physostigmine and Neostigmine

Features	***Physostigmine***	***Neostigmine***
Source	Natural (*Physostigma venenosum*)	Synthetic
Intestinal absorption	Good	Poor
Chemistry	Tertiary ammonium compound	Quaternary ammonium compound
Absorption	Absorbed orally	Not absorbed
Tissue penetration	Good	Poor
BBB	Crosses BBB-has both CNS and peripheral effects	Does not cross BBB—only peripheral effects
Primary use	In glaucoma	Myasthenia gravis
Use in poisoning	Used in atropine poisoning	Used in curare poisoning

Tacrine, a lipophilic acridine, enhances ACh levels in the brain and has been used in Alzheimer's disease. It is hepatotoxic, and therefore, not used.

Galantamine is similar to rivastigmine with good oral bioavailability of ~ 90%. Dose 8–16 mg BD in Alzheimer's disease.

GALAMER 4 mg tab.

Uses of Reversible Anticholinesterases

1. ***As a miotic:*** Physostigmine causes miosis, spasm of accommodation and a decrease in IOP. It is used:
   a. In **glaucoma**—physostigmine (0.1%) can be used with pilocarpine for better effect.
   b. **Alternately with a mydriatic** to break the adhesions between the iris and the lens.
   c. **To reverse the effect of mydriatics** as they cause blurring of vision and photophobia.
2. ***Myasthenia gravis:*** Anticholinesterases improve muscle strength and bring about symptomatic improvement (*see* page 118).
3. ***Poisoning due to anticholinergic drugs:*** Physostigmine is used in atropine poisoning and in toxicity due to other drugs with anticholinergic activity like phenothiazines, tricyclic antidepressants and antihistamines. Since physostigmine crosses the BBB, it reverses all the symptoms of atropine poisoning including CNS effects.
4. ***Curare poisoning:*** Skeletal muscle paralysis caused by curare can be antagonised by anti-ChEs. The neuromuscular paralysis due to neuromuscular blockers used along with anesthesia may be reversed using reversible anti-ChEs. Neostigmine and pyridostigmine can be used. Though edrophonium is faster acting, it is less effective than neostigmine specially in severe poisoning.
5. ***Postoperative paralytic ileus and urinary retention:*** Neostigmine may be useful—given 0.5–1 mg subcutaneously.
6. ***Cobra bite:*** Cobra venom, a neurotoxin, causes skeletal muscle paralysis. Specific treatment is antivenom. Intravenous edrophonium prevents respiratory paralysis.
7. ***Alzheimer's disease:*** To overcome the deficient cholinergic neurotransmission, rivastigmine, donepezil and galantamine are tried in Alzheimer's disease. Tacrine is another reversible anticholinesterase tried in this disease—but tacrine causes hepatotoxicity because of which it is not preferred (*see* page 233).

Irreversible Anticholinesterases

Organophosphorus (OP) compounds are powerful inhibitors of AChE enzyme; binding with the enzyme is stable by covalent bonds. They bind only the esteratic site (Fig. 7.4) and the enzyme is phosphorylated. Effects are similar to that of cholinergic stimulation as ACh accumulates in the tissues. All organophosphates except echothiophate are highly lipid soluble and hence are absorbed from all routes including intact skin. This makes OP poisoning possible even while insecticides are used for spraying the plants.

Uses

Glaucoma—echothiophate eye drops are sometimes used in glaucoma.

Organophosphorus Poisoning

Acute toxicity: As organophosphates are used as agricultural and domestic insecticides, poisoning by them is quite common. Poisoning may be occupational—as while spraying insecticides, accidental or suicidal. Symptoms result from muscarinic, nicotinic and central effects; muscarinic effects: vomiting, abdominal cramps, diarrhea, miosis, sweating, increased salivary, tracheobronchial and gastric secretions and bronchospasm; hypotension; nicotinic effects: muscular twitchings, weakness; central effects: convulsions and coma. Death is due to respiratory paralysis.

Treatment (Flowchart 7.1)

1. If poisoning is through skin, remove clothing and wash the skin with soap and water; if consumed by oral route thorough gastric lavage must be given.
2. Patient should be put in prone position to avoid aspiration of secretions.
3. Maintain BP and patent airway.
4. Drug of choice is **atropine** IV 2 mg every 10 minutes till pupil dilates. Maximum dose can be anything from 50 to 100 mg or much more depending on the severity of the poisoning. Treatment should be carefully monitored because of the risk of reappearance of symptoms due to delayed absorption of the OP compounds. Atropine administration may often be needed for 3–4 weeks.
5. Cholinesterase reactivators: **Pralidoxime, obidoxime, diacetylmonoxime.** These oxime compounds combine with cholinesterase organophosphate complex, release the binding and set free AChE enzyme. Thus, they reactivate the cholinesterase enzyme. They should be given within minutes after poisoning preferably immediately, because the complex undergoes ***'ageing'*** and the enzyme cannot be released. The complex becomes more stable by loss of a chemical group and this is responsible for 'ageing' and it is difficult to break the complex. Cholinesterase reactivators are not useful in poisoning due to carbamate compounds because these compounds do not have a free site (anionic site) for the binding of oximes. Moreover, pralidoxime itself has weak anticholinesterase activity particularly at higher doses. The rate at which ageing occurs varies from a few minutes to several hours with different compounds.

Flowchart 7.1: Treatment of organophosphorus poisoning

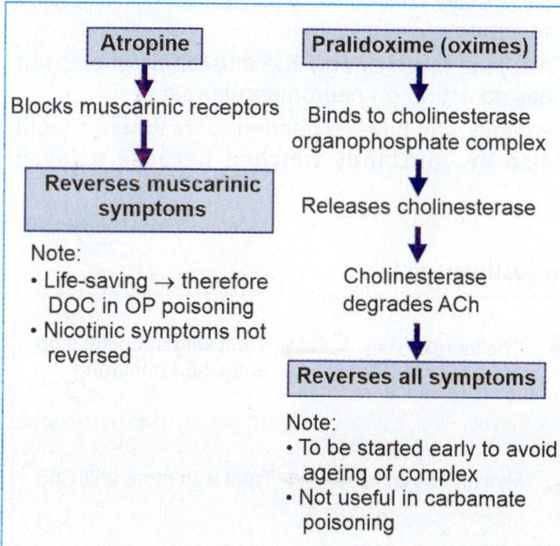

In severe poisoning 1–2 g of IV pralidoxime given within five minutes (before ageing takes place) of poisoning gives best results. In practice, it is rather uncommon for a patient to get such quick treatment within minutes particularly in the rural setup and cholinesterase reactivators are tried up to a few hours (maximum 6 hours) after poisoning.

Diacetylmonoxime (DAM) is lipid soluble and, therefore, crosses the BBB and regenerates the cholinesterase in the brain.

Chronic Organophosphate Toxicity

Some OP compounds can produce neurotoxicity (polyneuropathy) several days after exposure to the compound. This toxicity came to light when thousands of people developed paralysis in America after consuming "Jamaica ginger" which contained small amounts of triorthocresyl phosphate (TOCP). The symptoms include weakness, fatigue, ataxia, sensory disturbances, muscle twitching and in severe cases flaccid paralysis, which may last for several years.

Treatment of Myasthenia Gravis

Myasthenia gravis is a chronic autoimmune disease characterised by progressive weakness with rapid and easy fatigability of the skeletal muscles. Antibodies to nicotinic receptors are formed, which may act as follows:

i. Bind to the receptor and inhibit the action of acetylcholine.
ii. Cause cross-linking of nicotinic receptors and stimulate their degradation, thereby

resulting in a decrease in the number of these receptors at the NMJ.

iii. Damage (cause lysis of) the post-synaptic membrane.

The symptoms resemble that of neuromuscular paralysis produced by tubocurarin-eptosis, diplopia, dysphagia and difficulty in speaking (dysarthria) with weakness of the extremities. In later stages the disease involves all skeletal muscles.

Treatment

Anticholinesterases: Anti-ChEs enhance ACh levels at NMJ by preventing its destruction. They thus increase the force of contraction and improve muscle power by more frequent activation of the existing nicotinic receptors. Anticholinesterases bring about only symptomatic relief and do not alter the cause. In advanced disease anti-ChEs are not effective because the available nicotinic receptors are very few.

The adverse effects are due to concurrent muscarinic receptor stimulation—salivation, miosis, abdominal cramps and diarrhea. These may be blocked by atropine. In addition to its anti-ChE activity, neostigmine directly stimulates the nicotinic receptors and increases the amount of ACh released during each nerve impulse. Neostigmine (15 mg 4 hrly) pyridostigmine (60 mg 6 hrly)/ambenonium or a combination of these may be given. Edrophonium (2 mg) is used IV for the diagnosis.

Factors like infection, surgery and stress can result in severe muscle weakness called *myasthenic crisis*. However, severe weakness may also result from an excess dose of an anticholinesterase drug (flaccid paralysis due to more of acetylcholine) called *cholinergic crisis*.

These two crises can be differentiated by 2 mg IV edrophonium—the patient immediately improves if it is myasthenic crisis but the weakness worsens if it is cholinergic crisis (Flowchart 7.2).

Treatment of cholinergic crisis is with atropine while myasthenic crisis requires a higher dose of or an alternative anticholinesterase drug.

Other Drugs Used in Myasthenia Gravis

Glucocorticoids: Inhibit the production of antibodies to the nicotinic receptors. These are used when anticholinesterases alone are not adequate.

Immunosuppressants: Azathioprine and cyclosporine can be used as alternatives to prednisolone in advanced myasthenia gravis. They inhibit the production of antinicotinic receptor antibodies by inhibiting the proliferation of B lymphocytes. The clinical response however is delayed.

Clinical Pharmacology

- Organophosphorus poisoning is quite common due to easy availability of the compounds as insecticides. Patient should be put in prone position and airway cleared as OP compounds increase all secretions.

  Atropine reverses only the muscarinic effects but has no action on neuromuscular paralysis.
- Patients who have responded to treatment should also be constantly watched because delayed

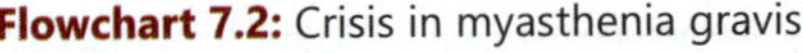
Flowchart 7.2: Crisis in myasthenia gravis

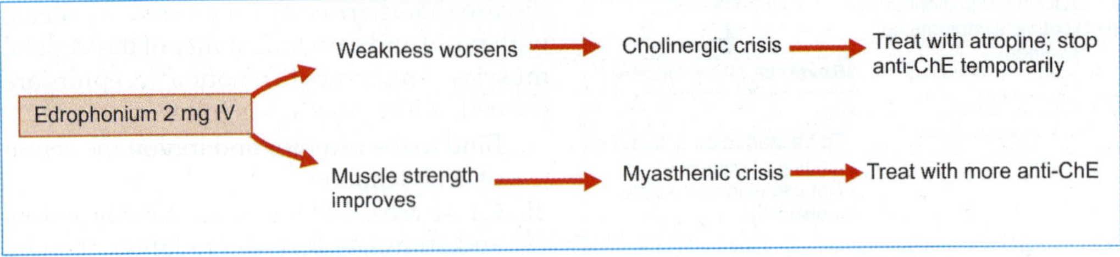

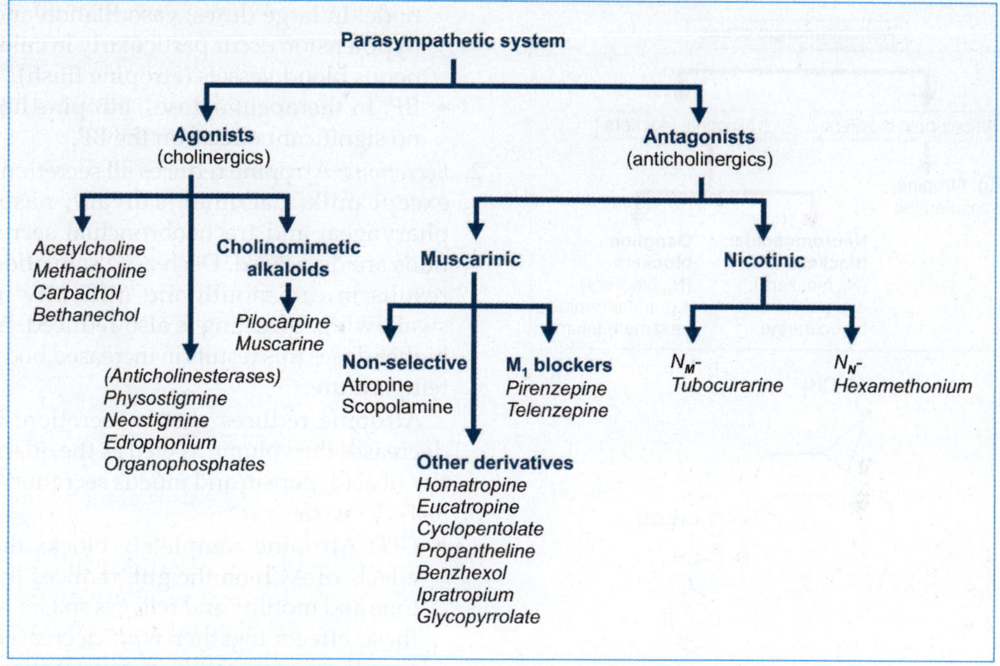

Fig. 7.5: Few examples of drugs acting on parasympathetic nervous system

absorption of OP compounds can lead to recurrence of symptoms and even sudden death.

- Return of plasma cholinesterase levels to normal would require several weeks.
- Acetylcholine is not used clinically (except rarely as eye drops) due to its rapid degradation.
- In myasthenia gravis, pyridostigmine and ambenonium are now preferred to neostigmine because of their longer action.

ANTICHOLINERGIC DRUGS

Anticholinergic drugs are agents which block the effects of acetylcholine on cholinergic receptors but conventionally **antimuscarinic drugs** are referred to as anticholinergic drugs. They are also called cholinergic blocking or parasympatholytic drugs. Drugs that block the nicotinic receptors are ganglion blockers and neuromuscular blockers.

Anticholinergic drugs include atropine and related drugs—atropine is the prototype.

Atropine is obtained from the plant *Atropa belladonna*. Atropine and scopolamine (hyoscine) are the **Belladonna Alkaloids**. They compete with acetylcholine for muscarinic receptors and block these receptors—they are muscarinic antagonists.

Mechanism of Action

Atropine and scopolamine bind to muscarinic receptors and block the effects of acetylcholine (and other cholinergic agonists) on these receptors. These are competitive antagonists and the antagonism is reversible by increasing the concentration of the agonist. Atropine and scopolamine are non-selective antagonists and block all the subtypes (M_1 to M_5) of muscarinic receptors.

Actions

The actions of atropine and scopolamine are similar except that atropine is a CNS stimulant

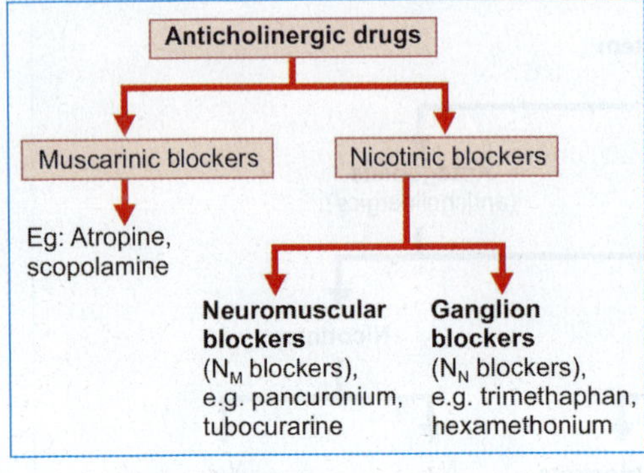

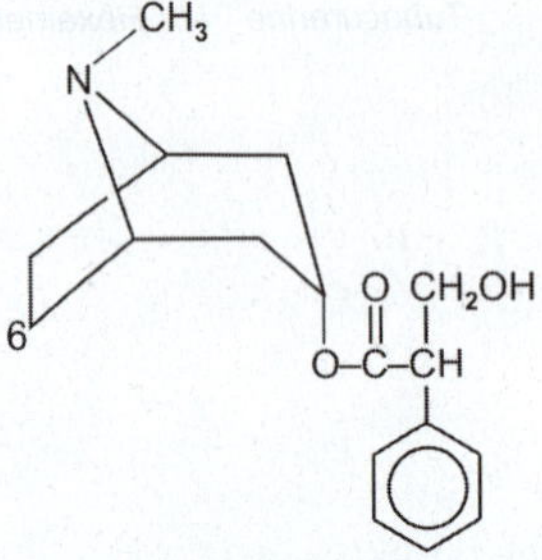

Structure of atropine

Classification

1. **Natural alkaloids**
   Atropine, hyoscine (scopolamine)
2. **Semisynthetic derivatives**
   Homatropine, atropine methonitrate, ipratropium bromide, tiotropium bromide
3. **Synthetic substitutes**
   - Mydriatics
     Eucatropine, cyclopentolate, tropicamide
   - Antispasmodic–antisecretory
     Propantheline, methantheline, dicyclomine, oxyphenonium, glycopyrrolate, pirenzepine, telenzepine, propiverine
   - Antiparkinsonian
     Benzhexol (trihexyphenidyl), benztropine, biperiden
   - Vasicoselective
     Oxybutynin, tolterodine, roterodine, flavoxate, trospium, solifenacin.

while scopolamine is a CNS depressant and causes sedation.

1. *CVS:*
   - Heart: Atropine increases the heart rate by blockade of M_2 receptors in the SA node. In large doses, vasodilation and hypotension occur particularly in cutaneous blood vessels (atropine flush).
   - *BP:* In therapeutic doses, atropine has no significant effects on the BP.
2. *Secretions:* Atropine reduces all secretions except milk. Lacrimal, salivary, nasopharyngeal and tracheobronchial secretions are decreased. Decreased salivation results in dry mouth and difficulty in swallowing. Sweating is also reduced. In higher doses this results in increased body temperature.

   Atropine reduces gastric secretion, it decreases the volume as well as the quantity of acid, pepsin and mucus secretions.
3. *Smooth muscle*
   - *GIT*: Atropine completely blocks the effects of ACh on the gut, reduces the tone and motility and relieves spasm → these effects together with decreased secretions may result in constipation. As atropine reduces the tone of the intestines it is used as an antispasmodic.
   - *Biliary tract*: Smooth muscles are relaxed; biliary spasm is relieved.
   - *Bronchi:* Atropine causes bronchodilatation. As the secretions are also reduced and mucociliary clearance is interrupted, mucus plugs may be formed which are a source of concern in these patients. Atropine affords symptomatic relief in bronchial asthma and COPD patients.
   - *Genitourinary tract:* Atropine relaxes ureters and the urinary bladder which may cause **urinary retention** particularly in the elderly men since they may already have prostatic hypertrophy.
4. *Eye:* On local instillation, atropine produces mydriasis by blocking the muscarinic receptors in the sphincter pupillae. The sphincter pupillae relaxes resulting in **passive mydriasis** (*see* page 87: Compare and Contrast). The ciliary muscle is

COMPARE AND CONTRAST

Atropine and Scopolamine

Features	*Atropine*	*Scopolamine (hyoscine)*
Chemistry	Both are belladonna alkaloids and tertiary ammonium compounds	
Mechanism of action	Both block the muscarinic receptors	
Source	*Atropa belladonna*	*Hyoscyamus nigra*
BBB	Does not readily cross—higher doses are needed to reach CNS	Readily crosses—even low doses produce CNS effects
Principal effect on CNS	CNS stimulation	CNS depression
Prominent actions on CNS	Confusion, excitement, hallucinations	Sedation, drowsiness, ataxia, amnesia
Use in motion sickness	Not used	Used
Duration of action	Longer	Shorter
Use as cardiac vagolytic	Can be used	Not used

paralysed resulting in cycloplegia or paralysis of accommodation. Because of mydriasis, the iris may block the drainage of aqueous humor—IOP increases and may precipitate glaucoma in some patients.

5. *CNS:* In higher doses atropine stimulates the CNS resulting in restlessness, disorientation, hallucinations and delirium. In contrast, scopolamine produces sedation and drowsiness. It can also cause euphoria (*see* Compare and Contrast: *Atropine and Scopolamine*).

Pharmacokinetics: Atropine and hyoscine are well-absorbed, cross the BBB and are metabolised in the liver. Atropine has a t½ of 3–4 hours. Hyoscine is absorbed even through the intact skin and is therefore used also as a transdermal patch. Atropine and its tertiary amines like pirenzepine, dicyclomine and benztropine are widely distributed in the body.

Dose: 0.6–2 mg IM/IV ATROPINE SULPHATE 1–2% eye drops, 0.6 mg/ml inj.

Adverse effects: Adverse effects are common but not serious and include blurring of vision, dry mouth, dysphagia, dry skin, fever, constipation and urinary retention. Skin rashes may appear.

Belladonna poisoning: Overdose of atropine or belladonna alkaloids or Datura can be fatal.

- High doses cause hyperthermia, palpitation, flushing, restlessness, delirium, hallucinations, psychosis, convulsions and coma. In toxic doses, CNS stimulation is followed by depression with circulatory collapse and respiratory failure.
- Treatment is symptomatic. If the poison is taken orally, gastric lavage should be done. Hyperthermia should be controlled with cold water sponging; respiratory support may be needed. **Physostigmine** 1–3 mg slow IV (repeated after 1–2 hr) can reverse both central and peripheral effects but many toxicologists prefer to treat symptomatically. Diazepam may be used to control seizures.
- Children are more susceptible to the toxic effects of atropine and it can be rapidly fatal in them.

Uses of Belladonna Alkaloids

1. *As antispasmodics*
   - In diarrhoea and dysentery, atropine relieves colic and abdominal pain. It is generally combined with loperamide.
   - In renal and biliary colic—atropine is used with morphine. Atropine partly overcomes the spasm of the sphincter of Oddi.
2. *As mydriatic and cycloplegic*
   - *Diagnostic* for testing error of refraction and fundoscopic examination of the eye.

Symptoms of atropine poisoning have been described by Cohen as

Hot as a hare: Body temperature is increased because of inhibition of sweating.

Red as a beet: The skin is hot and red or flushed like a beetroot because of cutaneous vasodilation called atropine flush.

Blind as a bat: Blurring of vision and photophobia due to mydriasis and cycloplegia.

Dry as a bone: As atropine inhibits sweating, the skin and mucous membrane get dry.

Mad as a wet hen: Atropine delirium, confusion, excitement, disorientation and restlessness resemble that of a wet hen.

- *Therapeutic*
  i. To provide rest to the iris in iritis, iridocyclitis and keratitis and after iridectomy.
  ii. Mydriatics are used alternately with miotics to break the adhesions between the iris and the lens in uveitis and iritis. They can be used both for the treatment and prevention of adhesion formation. For prevention, longer acting agents like homatropine are preferred.

3. *As pre-anesthetic medication:* When administered 30 mins before anesthesia, atropine reduces salivary and respiratory secretions and prevents laryngospasm, bradycardia and aspiration pneumonia during surgery. Its bronchodilator action is of additional value. Glycopyrrolate is preferred for this use (*see* below).
4. *In poisoning*
   - *Organophosphorus poisoning:* Atropine is lifesaving in OP poisoning (*see* page 117).
   - *Mushroom poisoning:* Atropine is used in poisoning due to some mushrooms (Inocybe family).
   - *Atropine is used along with neostigmine in curare poisoning:* Used to block the muscarinic effects of neostigmine.
5. *Bronchial asthma*
6. *Peptic ulcer*
7. *Parkinsonism*

} Atropine derivatives are preferred over atropine (*see* below)

8. *In cardiovascular disorders:* Atropine may be of help in some patients with bradycardia or partial heart block due to excessive vagal tone as seen in myocardial infarction. It should be used carefully to avoid tachycardia which could be dangerous in myocardial infarction patients.
9. *Motion sickness:* Hyoscine given 30 minutes before the journey prevents travelling sickness. The exact mode of action is not known but scopolamine could act as a vestibular sedative by blocking the muscarinic receptors. Muscarinic transmission may be involved in vestibular pathway. Transdermal hyoscine patches are available to be applied behind the ear for a prolonged action.
10. *Urinary disorders:* Since muscarinic receptors are present in the epithelial cells lining the urinary tract, atropine and its derivatives have clinical application in urinary disorders like in overactive bladder, urinary incontinence and in nocturnal eneuresis in children—atropine reduces urinary frequency (*see* below).
11. *Labour:* Hyoscine can also be used during labour to produce sedation and amnesia (twilight sleep).

Drug Interactions

When anticholinergics are given with other drugs that also have anticholinergic properties like antihistaminics, phenothiazines and tricyclic antidepressants, the anticholinergic side effects get added up.

ATROPINE SUBSTITUTES

Belladonna alkaloids produce a wide range of effects, most of which are of therapeutic value. However, these can also result in various side effects since they lack selectivity. Hence, several semisynthetic and synthetic derivatives have been introduced some of which have selective actions (Tables 7.4 and 7.5).

Table 7.4: Atropine substitutes

Indications	*Derivatives used*
1. On the eye—mydriatics and cycloplegics	Homatropine, eucatropine, cyclopentolate, tropicamide
2. As antispasmodics	Propantheline, methantheline, dicyclomine, flavoxate hydrochloride, oxybutynin chloride, oxyphenonium, glycopyrrolate, clidinium
3. Peptic ulcer	Pirenzepine, telenzepine
4. Bronchial asthma	Ipratropium, tiotropium
5. Preanesthetic medication	Glycopyrrolate
6. Urinary disorders	Oxybutynin, tolterodine, propiverine, trospium, dicyclomine, darifenacin
7. Antiparkinsonism drugs	Benzhexol, benztropine, biperiden

1. *Derivatives used on the eye:* Mydriasis and cycloplegia produced by atropine last for 7–10 days. The derivatives homatropine, eucatropine, cyclopentolate have shorter action (6–24 hours), tropicamide being the shortest acting (4–6 hours). Some can selectively produce either prominent mydriasis or cycloplegia.
2. *Antispasmodics* or *spasmolytics* are used to relieve spasms of the gastrointestinal tract, biliary tract, ureter and uterus. They are also found to be useful in irritable bowel syndrome. Some of them in addition reduce gastrointestinal motility.
3. *Peptic ulcer:* Pirenzepine and telenzepine are selective M_1 blockers which inhibit gastric secretion at doses that do not affect other functions. Pirenzepine also does not cross the BBB, hence has no CNS effects. They are tried in peptic ulcer.
4. *Bronchial asthma:* When used in bronchial asthma atropine thickens the bronchial secretions and interferes with the movement of cilia, thus favoring the formation of mucus plugs. **Ipratropium and tiotropine** are bronchodilators that do not affect mucociliary activity. When given as inhalation, they act only on the airways and do not produce any significant systemic effects because they are poorly absorbed. Tiotropium is longer acting and can be given once daily since it is bound to M_3 receptors for a longer time. They are used in bronchial asthma and COPD.
5. *Glycopyrrolate* is an antisialogogue (reduces salivary secretions). This will prevent the development of laryngospasm and aspiration pneumonia by decreasing salivary secretions.
   - It also prevents bradycardia during surgery.
   - Its bronchodilator action is of additional value.
   - It is a quaternary ammonium compound does not cross the BBB, therefore no effects on the CNS.
   - It is given IM as preanaesthetic medication (*see* page 197) and is the most commonly used atropine derivative for this purpose.
6. Benztropine, benzhexol, and biperiden are the derivatives used in drug-induced parkinsonism (*see* page 232). They are effective in drug-induced parkinsonism due to their anticholinergic effects. They control tremors and rigidity.
7. Urinary disorders—atropine substitutes **tolterodine, fesoterodine and oxybutynin** are used to reduce urinary urgency and frequency, to relieve bladder spasm and improve bladder capacity in urinary

Key Box 7.1: Some drugs that have anticholinergic properties

- Antihistamines, e.g. diphenhydramine
- Antipsychotics, e.g. chlorpromazine
- Tricyclic antidepressants, e.g. imipramine
- Atropine derivatives, e.g. glycopyrrolate

Table 7.5: Salient features of atropine derivatives

	Derivative	Preparations and dose	Indications	Comments
1.	Homatropine	HOMIDE 1, 2% eye drops; 1–2 drops	For fundoscopy and in iritis to produce mydriasis, it also produces cycloplegia	Duration of mydriasis 1–3 days
2.	Cyclopentolate	CYCLOMID 0.5, 1% eye drops; 1–2 drops	To produce cycloplegia	Mydriasis up to 24 hrs
3.	Tropicamide	TROPICAMET, TROMIDE 0.5, 15% eye drops 1–2 drops	Mydriasis for fundoscopy	Mydriasis 3–6 hrs—shortest acting
4.	Propantheline	PROBANTHINE 15 mg tab; 15–30 mg TDS	Peptic ulcer	Gastric emptying is delayed
5.	Oxyphenonium	ANTRENYL 5, 10 mg tab; 5–10 mg	Peptic ulcer, GI hypermotility	Delays gastric emptying; NM blockade in higher dose
6.	Clidinium	NORMAXIN 2.5 mg with dicyclomine 10 mg + chlordiazepoxide 5 mg; 2.5–5 mg oral	Peptic ulcer, colic, IBS	May be combined with BZD for dyspepsia
7.	Glycopyrrolate	PYROLATE 0.2 mg/ml, 1 ml amp, 10 ml vial; 0.1 –0.3 mg IM; 1–2 mg oral	Preanaesthetic medication	Does not cross BBB – No CNS effects
8.	Dicyclomine	CYCLOPAM 20 mg with paracetamol 500 mg; 20 mg/ml inj. 10–20 mg TDS	Motion sickness, morning sickness, antispasmodic in dysmenorrhoea, IBS	Also has antiemetic properties
9.	Valethamate	EPIDOSIN 10 mg tab, 8 mg inj.; 10 mg oral, 8 mg IM	Spasmolytic, dilatation of cervix	—
10.	Oxybutynin	OXYSPASS, OXYBUTIN 2.5, 5 mg tab; 5 mg BD-TDS	Urinary disorders—to increase bladder holding capacity	Can also be instilled directly into bladder or applied transdermally
11.	Tolterodine	TORQ 1, 2 mg tab; 2 mg BD	Urinary disorders—to reduce urinary urgency and frequency	Dose to be reduced in patients receiving microsomal enzyme inhibitors
12.	Flavoxate	URISPAS 200 mg tab; 200 mg TDS	Urinary disorders—to reduce urinary urgency and frequency as in cystitis, urethritis and prostatitis	Also has local anesthetic and analgesic properties
13.	Darifenacin	DARITEN 7.5 mg OD	Over active bladder	—
14.	Benzhexol	ARTANE, PACITANE 2 mg tab; 2–12 mg/day	Drug-induced EPS	FDC with antipsychotics available
15.	Ipratropium	IPRAVENT 20 µg and 40 µg/puff; 20–40 µg 3–4 times a day inhalation	COPD, bronchial asthma	More useful in COPD than asthma
16.	Tiotropium	TIOVA 18 µg ROTACAPS; 18 µg OD	COPD, bronchial asthma	Longer acting than ipratropium

IBS: Irritable bowel syndrome FDC: Fixed dose combination
EPS: Extrapyramidal symptoms NM: Neuromuscular

Atropine: Please Act Longer

A 28-year-old medical representative attempted suicide and he chose an organophosphorous compound to poison himself. He was found lying on his bed with saliva drooling from his mouth and was brought to the district government medical college hospital. He responded to treatment and was shifted to the ward. On day 3 the postgraduate came for rounds in the morning to see the patient dead. This was because of the delayed absorption of the poison—more careful monitoring and a more frequent atropine dose were needed.

disorders and following urologic surgeries. They are also tried in nocturnal enuresis in children as they reduce urinary frequency. Oxybutynin is almost selective for M_3 receptor in the bladder and can relieve bladder spasm, increase bladder holding capacity and reduce involuntary voiding. It can be given orally or instilled into the bladder cavity or applied transdermally. **Tropium** is similar to oxybutynin. **Darifenacin (most M3 selective), solifenacin, tolterodine** and **fesoterodine** are more M_3 selective and, therefore, anticholinergic side effects are negligible.

Contraindications

- Antimuscarinic drugs are contraindicated in glaucoma—particularly narrow angle glaucoma.
- Atropine and other antimuscarinic drugs should be avoided in elderly men as they may cause urinary retention in them because most of them have prostatic hypertrophy.

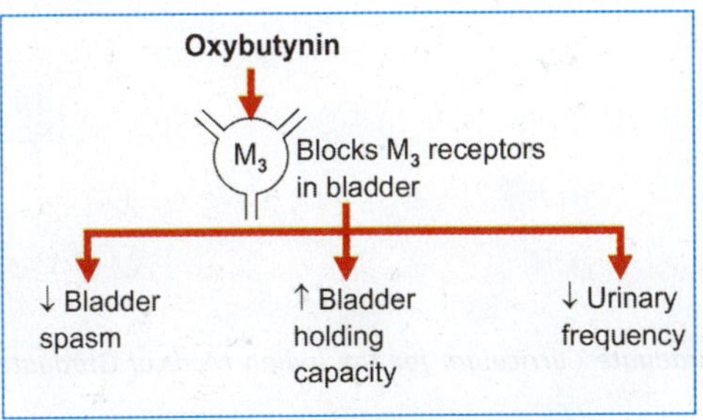

Drugs Acting on Autonomic Ganglia

Acetylcholine is the principal neurotransmitter at both the sympathetic and parasympathetic ganglia. N_N type of nicotinic receptors are abundant in the ganglia. Neurotransmission at the ganglia is a complex process.

Ganglion stimulants: Nicotine, lobeline, acetylcholine and anticholinesterases can stimulate the ganglia.

Ganglion stimulants are of no therapeutic value. Nicotine the tobacco alkaloid is used as a transdermal patch to de-addict chronic smokers.

Ganglion blockers: Hexamethonium, mecamylamine, trimethaphan block the autonomic ganglia.

Ganglion blockers were earlier used in the treatment of hypertension but since they block both sympathetic and parasympathetic ganglia, a wide range of adverse effects are seen. Moreover, selective antagonists which act at particular receptor subtypes are now available. Hence, ganglion blockers are not in clinical use except:

i. **Trimethaphan** is short-acting and is used intravenously to produce transient hypotension during certain surgeries. It reduces bleeding during surgery and in dissecting aneurysm of the aorta.
ii. **Mecamylamine** has been tried along with transdermal nicotine in smokers trying to quit smoking. It blocks central nicotinic receptors and may reduce nicotine craving.

Clinical Pharmacology

- Several drugs like antihistamines, many antipsychotics and some antidepressants have anticholinergic properties.
- Common anticholinergic side effects include dryness of mouth, constipation, diplopia and urinary retention.
- Elderly men are more susceptible to urinary retention. Drugs with atropinic effects should be avoided in them.
- In overdosage, infants and children are at a higher risk of toxic effects of anticholinergic drugs.
- Atropine should be used cautiously in patients with chronic pulmonary diseases because its drying effect may sometimes be troublesome.
- Atropine derivatives may be preferred to atropine whenever the derivatives are available.
- Since atropine causes tachycardia, it should be used with caution in patients with CCF.

[1] From Medical Council of India, *Competency based Undergraduate Curriculum for the Indian Medical Graduate*, 2018;1:136–144.

CHAPTER 8

Skeletal Muscle Relaxants

Competency achievement: The student should be able to:

PH 1.15 Describe mechanism/s of action, types, doses, side effects, indications and contraindications of skeletal muscle relaxants .[1]

Skeletal muscle relaxants (SMRs) are drugs that reduce the muscle tone either by acting peripherally at the neuromuscular junction (neuromuscular blockers) or centrally in the cerebrospinal axis or directly on the contractile mechanism. They reduce the spasticity in a variety of neurological conditions and are also useful in surgeries.

Skeletal muscle relaxants may be classified as given in Flowchart 8.1.

Structure of d-Tubocurarine

Flowchart 8.1: Classification of skeletal muscle relaxants

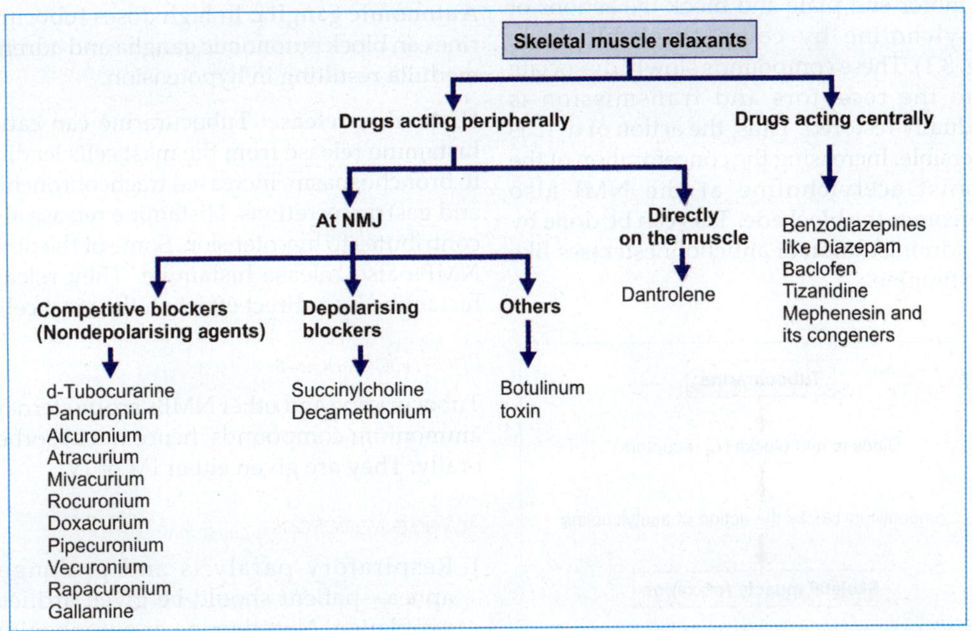

1. PERIPHERALLY ACTING SKELETAL MUSCLE RELAXANTS

Neuromuscular Blockers (NMB)

A. Competitive Blockers

d-Tubocurarine: Curare was used by the South American Indians as arrow poison for hunting wild animals because curare paralysed the animals. On extensive research, the active principle from curare, **tubocurarine** was identified.

d-Tubocurarine (d-Tc) is the dextrorotatory quaternery ammonium alkaloid obtained from the plant *Chondrodendron tomentosum* and plants of the *Strychnos* species (l-tubocurarine is less potent). Several synthetic agents have been developed. All these are quaternary ammonium compounds because of which they are not well absorbed, do not cross the BBB and are quickly excreted.

Mechanism of Action

Non-depolarising blockers bind to N_M nicotinic receptors (*see* Fig. 7.3, page 111) on the motor end plate and block the actions of acetylcholine by competitive blockade (Fig. 8.1). These compounds slowly dissociate from the receptors and transmission is gradually restored. Thus, the action of d-Tc is reversible. Increasing the concentration of the agonist acetylcholine at the NMJ also overcomes the blockade. This can be done by the administration of anticholinesterases like neostigmine.

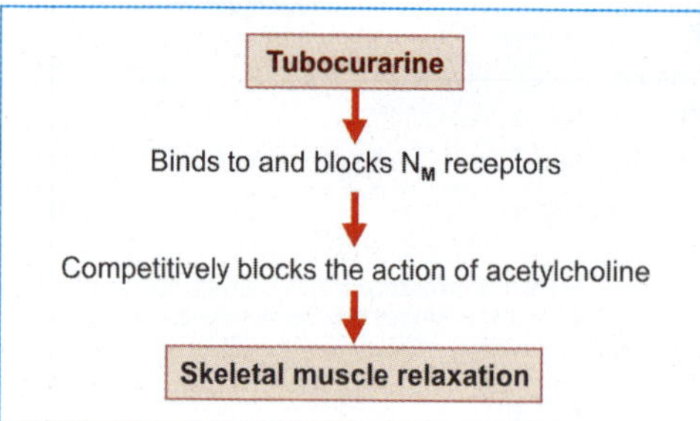

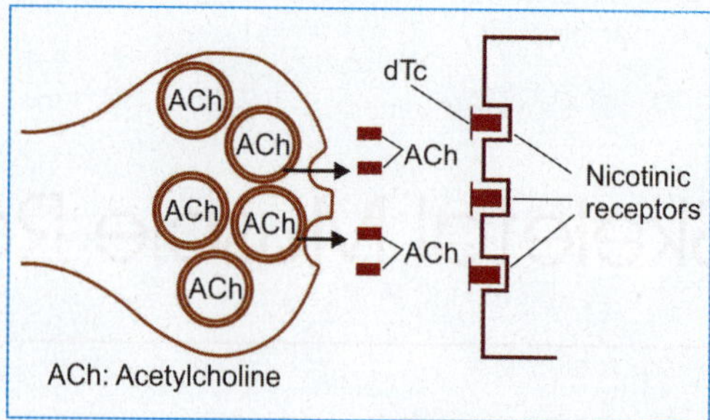

Fig. 8.1: d-Tc molecules bind to nicotinic receptors and prevent the binding of ACh on these receptors

Pharmacological Actions

Skeletal muscle: On parenteral administration, tubocurarine initially causes muscular weakness followed by flaccid paralysis. Small muscles of the eyes and fingers are the first to be affected, followed by those of the limbs, neck and trunk. Later the intercostal muscles and finally the diaphragm are paralysed and respiration stops. Consciousness is not affected throughout. Recovery occurs in the reverse order, i.e. the diaphragm is the first to recover. The effect lasts for 30–60 minutes (Table 8.1).

Autonomic ganglia: In high doses tubocurarine can block autonomic ganglia and adrenal medulla resulting in hypotension.

Histamine release: Tubocurarine can cause histamine release from the mast cells leading to bronchospasm, increased tracheobronchial and gastric secretions. Histamine release also contributes to hypotension. Some of the other NMBs also release histamine. They release histamine by a direct effect on the mast cells.

Pharmacokinetics

Tubocurarine and other NMBs are quaternary ammonium compounds, hence not absorbed orally. They are given either IM or IV.

Adverse Reactions

1. Respiratory paralysis and prolonged apnea—patient should be given artificial ventilation. Neostigmine or edrophonium

Table 8.1: Duration of action of competitive neuromuscular blockers

Drug	*Onset (min) of action*	*Duration (min)*
	Long acting	
Tubocurarine	5	35–60
Gallamine	5	35–60
Pancuronium	2–4	35–80
Doxacurium	5	90–120
Pipecuronium	2–4	80–100
	Intermediate acting	
Atracurium	2–4	20–35
Vecuronium	2–4	20–35
Rapacuronium	1–2	15–30
Rocuronium	1–2	30–60
	Short acting	
Mivacurium	2–4	12–18

may be used to reverse the skeletal muscle paralysis.

2. Hypotension is due to ganglion blockade and histamine release.
3. Flushing and bronchospasm due to histamine release by tubocurarine; this is not seen with newer agents.

Treatment of toxicity: Neostigmine and **edrophonium** reverse the skeletal muscle paralysis and are the antidotes in curare poisoning. **Antihistamines** should be given to counter the effects of histamine. **Neostigmine/edrophonium** may be used to reverse the N_M blockade after the surgical procedure is completed.

An antidote **sugammadex** has been introduced for overdosage of rocuronium and vecuronium. Sugammadex binds to rocuronium, chelates and quickly reverses its effects. The complex is excreted in the urine. It can also chelate other NMBs like pancuronium to some extent.

Synthetic Competitive Blockers

Pancuronium, atracurium, vecuronium, gallamine, doxacurium, mivacurium, pipecuronium, rapacuronium, rocuronium are synthetic NMBs. They have the following advantages over tubocurarine:

- Less histamine release
- Do not block autonomic ganglia, hence cause less hypotension
- Spontaneous recovery takes place with most of these drugs
- Some are more potent than tubocurarine
- The newer agents ***rapacuronium*** and ***rocuronium*** have a rapid onset of action. Hence, they can be used as alternatives to succinylcholine for muscle relaxation. When so used, rapacuronium can cause severe bronchospasm before endotracheal intubation.
- ***Rocuronium*** does not cause hypotension, tachycardia and is fast acting.
- ***Atracurium*** can be safely used in patients with renal impairment because it is degraded spontaneously by a non-enzymatic hydrolysis by ***Hofmann elimination*** and to a small extent by plasma esterases and does not depend on the kidney for excretion. It is partly metabolised in the liver. **Laudanosine,** a metabolite of atracurium, can cause seizures and increases the requirement of the anaesthetics.

  Cisatracurium is an isomer of atracurium.
  Advantages:
  – Forms lesser laudanosine
  – Lesser histamine release when compared to atracurium.

Therefore, cisatracurium is **now preferred** over atracurium.

- **Mivacurium** is a short-acting neuromuscular blocker with a slow onset of action. It is rapidly metabolised by plasma cholinesterases, hence short acting. It causes significant histamine release.
- Tubocurarine, doxacurium and gallamine have a slow onset (about 5 minutes) but long duration of action (30–120 mins). Pancuronium, vecuronium, atracurium and cisatracurium have intermediate onset (2–4 minutes) while rapacuronium and rocuronium have fast onset of action (1–2 minutes) (*see* Compare and Contrast—*Tubocurarine and Succinylcholine*).
- **Gantacurium** is a new non-depolarising neuromuscular blocker under clinical

COMPARE AND CONTRAST
Tubocurarine and Succinylcholine

Features	***Tubocurarine***	***Succinylcholine***
Mechanism	Competitive blockade	Persistent depolarisation
Type of blockade	Nondepolarising	Depolarising
Phases of blockade	Single	Dual block
Anticholinesterases	Reverse blockade	Does not reverse
Initial fasciculations	Nil	Present
Metabolism	Only partly metaoblised in the liver	By pseudocholinesterase
Onset of action	Slow	Fast
Duration of action	Long (1–2 hr)	Short (10 mins)

development that has a rapid (~1½ min) and short action (~10 mins). Its actions can be completely reversed by administration of cysteine since it is metabolised by adduction to cysteine. It appears to be a promising NMB. Transient hypotension, tachycardia and flushing are related to histamine release which is dose dependent.

- **Tubocurarine** causes histamine release, ganglion blockade (resulting in hypotension) and its muscle relaxant effect needs to be reversed with drugs. Hence, it is not used now. The synthetic compounds are preferred. Alcuronium and gallamine are also not used.

B. *Depolarising Blockers*

Succinylcholine (SCh, suxamethonium) is a quaternary ammonium compound with the structure resembling two molecules of acetylcholine joined together.

Mechanism of Action

The neuromuscular effects of SCh are like those of ACh. SCh stimulates the N_M nicotinic receptors and depolarises the skeletal muscle membrane. However, unlike ACh which gets metabolised in a fraction of a second, SCh is destroyed very slowly by pseudocholinesterase (in about 5 minutes). Thus, continued presence of the drug causes persistent depolarisation resulting in flaccid paralysis. This is phase I block. In high doses SCh produces a dual block—initial depolarising block followed by non-depolarising block. The membrane gets slowly repolarised but cannot be depolarised again. The mechanism is not clearly known (Fig. 8.2).

Pharmacological Actions

Skeletal muscle: On intravenous administration, onset of action is very rapid—within 1 minute. Initial transient muscular fasciculations and twitchings, mostly in the chest and abdominal regions, are followed by skeletal muscle paralysis.

The fasciculations are maximum in 2 minutes and subside in 5 minutes. They are due to stimulation of the muscle fibres by the discharge of action potentials in them. SCh is a short-acting muscle relaxant and the effect lasts for 5–10 minutes. Hence, it has to be given continuously as an infusion for longer effect.

Succinylcholine!—Not an analgesic ☹

A young lady doctor in the pink of her health underwent a minor cosmetic surgery. She was recovering from anesthesia in the postoperative room. The nurse came smiling, wished the patient and loaded the syringe. She was supposed to give an analgesic injection. She instead administered succinylcholine. Within minutes the patient went into total muscular paralysis and cerebral anoxia resulting in brain death. The lady survived on ventilator for a few weeks and finally succumbed to it—*a fatal medication error.*

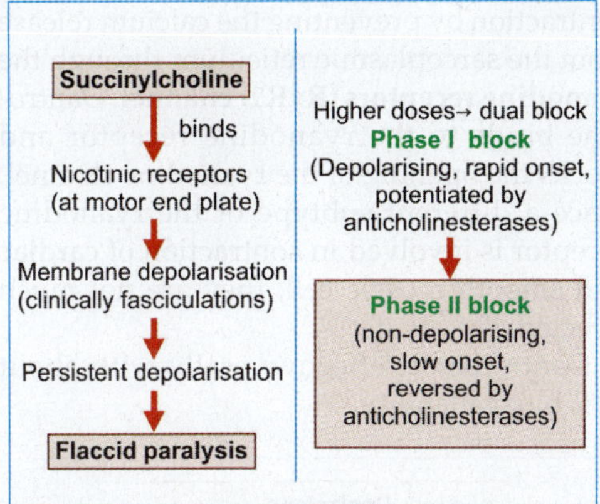

Fig. 8.2: Mechanism of action of succinylcholine

CVS: Initially hypotension and bradycardia may result from stimulation of vagal ganglia. This is followed by hypertension and tachycardia due to stimulation of sympathetic ganglia. Higher doses can cause cardiac arrhythmias. SCh can also cause histamine release, if injected rapidly.

Pharmacokinetics

Succinylcholine is rapidly hydrolysed by pseudocholinesterase, hence it is short-acting (about 5 minutes). Some people (1 in 2000) have an **abnormal (atypical) pseudocholinesterase enzyme**, a hereditary defect. In such people, SCh does not get metabolised and even the usual dose results in prolonged apnea and paralysis which may last for several hours. Artificial ventilation and fresh blood transfusion are needed to supply pseudocholinesterase.

Adverse Reactions

1. ***Postoperative muscle pain*** is a common adverse effect of SCh. It may be due to the damage to muscle fibres that occur during initial fasciculations.
2. ***Hyperkalemia:*** Succinylcholine can cause hyperkalemia due to sudden release of K^+ from the intracellular sites which could be due to fasciculations. This can be dangerous particularly in patients with CCF. It may result in cardiac arrest in patients with burns, nerve injuries and neuromuscular disease.
3. ***Cardiac arrhythmias:*** SCh can cause cardiac arrhythmias. It stimulates the nicotinic receptors in the ganglia and cardiac muscarinic receptors.
4. ***Malignant hyperthermia*** is a rare genetically determined condition where there is a sudden increase in the body temperature and severe muscle spasm due to release of intracellular Ca^{++} from the sarcoplasmic reticulum. Metabolic acidosis and tachycardia may be present. Certain drugs like halothane, isoflurane, sevoflurane and succinylcholine can trigger the process which can be fatal. Combination of these general anesthetics and SCh is the most common triggering factor. Intravenous dantrolene (1 mg/kg repeated if required) is life-saving in malignant hyperthermia. Oxygen inhalation, treatment of acidosis and immediate cooling of the body also help.
5. ***Others:*** Succinylcholine administration may result in *increased intraocular and intragastric pressure.* The increased intragastric pressure due to fasciculations would lead to regurgitation which in turn may result in aspiration of gastric contents particularly in muscular patients.

Uses of Peripherally Acting Skeletal Muscle Relaxants

Inappropriate use of peripherally acting SMRs can be fatal. Hence, they should be given only by qualified anesthetists or adequately trained doctors and the brand names therefore are not given in this chapter.

1. *Adjuvant to anesthesia:* Adequate muscle relaxation is essential during surgeries. Skeletal muscle relaxants are used as adjuvants to general anesthesia. Short-acting SMRs like succinylcholine are used during endotracheal intubation.

2. *In minor procedures:* SMRs are also useful in laryngoscopy, bronchoscopy, oesophagoscopy, tracheal intubation and in orthopedic procedures like reduction of fractures and dislocations.
3. *In electroconvulsive therapy:* SMRs protect the patient from convulsions and trauma during ECT.
4. *In spastic disorders:* SMRs are used to overcome the spasm of tetanus and athetosis.
5. *In status epilepticus:* When convulsions cannot be controlled by anticonvulsants alone, sometimes a NMB is used to control the muscular component of convulsions. However, they do not cross the BBB and have no central effects.
6. *In patients on ventilator:* To reduce the resistance of the chest wall and enhance thoracic compliance and to facilitate artificial ventilation, NMBs are used in intensive care units.

C. Other Drugs Acting at NMJ

Botulinum toxin is produced by the anaerobic bacterium *Clostridium botulinum.* The toxin inhibits the release of acetylcholine at the cholinergic synapses resulting in flaccid paralysis of skeletal muscles.

Botulinum toxin is useful (local injection) in the treatment of dystonias, including sports or writer's cramps, muscle spasms, tremors, cerebral palsy and in rigidity seen in extrapyramidal disorders. It is commonly used to relieve blepharospasm. Botulinum toxin is also gaining popularity in **cosmetic therapy** for the removal of facial lines and wrinkles by local injection.

2. DIRECTLY ACTING MUSCLE RELAXANTS

Dantrolene is a phenytoin analog that acts directly on the skeletal muscle.

Mechanism of Action

Dantrolene directly affects the skeletal muscle contractile mechanism. It inhibits the muscle contraction by preventing the calcium release from the sarcoplasmic reticulum through the **ryanodine receptors (RyR1) channel**. Dantrolene binds to the ryanodine receptor and blocks the opening of the ryanodine channel. Since a different subtype of the ryanodine receptor is involved in contraction of cardiac and smooth muscle cell, they are not much affected.

Dantrolene is effective orally with about 30% bioavailability.

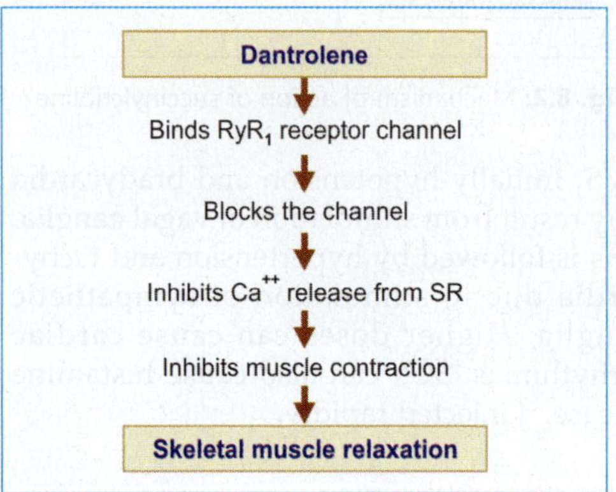

Adverse effects include drowsiness, dizziness, fatigue, diarrhoea, muscle weakness and rarely hepatotoxicity. Liver function tests should be done to look for hepatotoxicity.

Uses

- Dantrolene is used in spastic disorders like hemiplegia and paraplegia, multiple sclerosis and spinal cord injury.
- Dantrolene is the drug of choice in malignant hyperthermia. Dantrolene prevents the release of Ca^{++} from the sarcoplasmic reticulum and relieves muscle spasm in malignant hyperthermia.
- Dantrolene has also been found to be useful in malignant neuroleptic syndrome.

Quinine: The antimalarial quinine is a skeletal muscle relaxant. It is a sodium channel blocker, it reduces the excitability of the motor end plate. Quinine is used in myotonia congenita and in nocturnal muscle cramps.

3. CENTRALLY ACTING MUSCLE RELAXANTS

These drugs act on higher centres and cause muscle relaxation without loss of consciousness. They also have sedative properties. Drugs in this category are:

$GABA_A$ agonists: Benzodiazepines like diazepam

$GABA_B$ agonist: Baclofen

Central α_2 agonist: Tizanidine

Mephenesin and congeners: Carisoprodol, chlorzoxazone, chlormezanone, methocarbamol

Others: Thiocolchicoside, riluzole, gabapentin, progabide.

Most of these drugs are used in the treatment of muscle spasms and spasticity. In spasticity the basal muscle tone itself is elevated with flexor muscle spasm. The pathology involves tonic stretch reflexes as well as higher centres in the CNS. Centrally acting muscle relaxants that depress the polysynaptic reflex arc have been used in spasticity.

Mechanism of Action

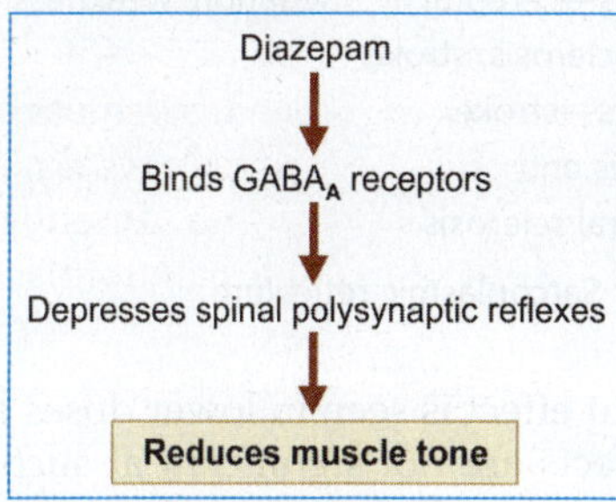

Centrally acting muscle relaxants depress the spinal polysynaptic reflexes. These reflexes maintain the muscle tone. By depressing these spinal reflexes, centrally acting muscle relaxants reduce the muscle tone.

Diazepam has useful antispastic activity. It can be used in relieving muscle spasm of almost any origin including that of local muscle trauma. Started with a low dose of 4 mg/day, the dose is gradually increased. Of the BZDs, diazepam is the most commonly used for this purpose (*see* page 203).

Baclofen is an analog of the inhibitory neurotransmitter GABA. It is a **$GABA_B$ agonist.** It depresses the monosynaptic and polysynaptic reflexes in the spinal cord.

It relieves painful spasms including flexor and extensor spasms and may also improve bladder and bowel functions in patients with spinal lesions. Normal tendon reflexes are not affected. Baclofen also inhibits the release of substance P which could contribute to pain relief.

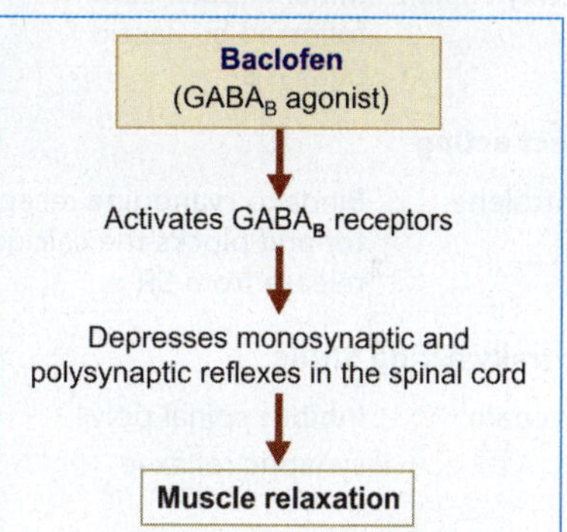

Baclofen is generally given orally. It is rapidly and completely absorbed. It should be gradually withdrawn after prolonged use because abrupt withdrawal can cause anxiety, palpitations and hallucinations. Side effects include drowsiness (which is milder than diazepam and tolerance develops), weakness and ataxia (Table 8.2).

Dose: 10–50 mg BD. LIOFEN 10, 25 mg tab.

Other Uses

a. Severe low back pain
b. Reduces craving in chronic alcoholics may be used in alcohol deaddiction.

Mephenesin is not preferred due to its side effects. A number of related drugs like **carisoprodol, methocarbamol, chlormezanone, chlorzoxazone** are used in acute muscle spasm caused by local trauma. All of them also cause sedation. Carisoprodol also has weak analgesic, antipyretic and anticholinergic properties.

Dose: 350 mg TDS CARISOMA, SANOMA 350 mg tab.

Table 8.2: Some important features of skeletal muscle relaxants

SMR	*MOA*	*Indications*	*Remarks*
Peripherally acting SMRs			
Pancuronium	Blocks N_M receptors—competitive antagonist of acetylcholine	Surgical procedures	Tubocurarine not in use; atracurium undergoes Hofmann's elimination
Cisatracurium	Blocks N_M receptors—competitive antagonist of acetylcholine	To facilitate ventilation in patients on ventilators	Cisatracurium, rocuronium can be used in patients with renal impairment
Succinylcholine	Initial depolarization followed by flaccid paralysis	Tracheal intubation Status epilepticus	Short acting (5 mins); metabolized by pseudocholinesterase
Direct acting			
Dantrolene	Binds to ryanodine receptor and blocks the calcium release from SR	Spastic disorders, malignant hyperthermia, malignant neuroleptic syndrome	Hepatotoxicity, sedation
Centrally acting SMRs			
Diazepam	Inhibits spinal polysynaptic reflexes	Acute and chronic spastic disorders–cerebral palsy, stroke, spinal cord injury, local muscle spasm, tetanus, fracture reduction	Sedation may be a problem.
Baclofen	$GABA_B$ agonist	Spastic disorders—cerebral palsy, multiple sclerosis, stroke	Sedation, weakness
Tizanidine	Central α_2 agonist	Spastic disorders—stroke, multiple sclerosis and amyotropic lateral sclerosis	

SMR: Skeletal muscle relaxant; MOA: Mechanism of action; SR: Sarcoplasmic reticulum

Methocarbamol can be given orally and parenterally.

Dose: 500 mg TDS 100 mg/ml IV/IM ROBINAX 500 mg tab, 100 mg/ml inj.

Chlormezanone also has antianxiety effects.

Dose: 100–200 mg TDS WINTRAC 100 mg tab.

Chlorzoxazone is better tolerated and longer acting.

Dose: 300–600 mg TDS DUODIL CHLORZOXAZONE 250 + PARACETAMOL 300 mg.

Tizanidine is a congener of clonidine. It is a central α_2 agonist like clonidine. It increases the presynaptic inhibition of motor neurons and reduces muscle spasms. The muscle relaxant effect is seen in lower doses and the CV effects are not significant at such doses. Adverse effects include drowsiness, weakness, hypotension and dry mouth. Tizanidine is used in the treatment of spasticity due to stroke, multiple sclerosis and amyotropic lateral sclerosis.

Dose: 2 mg TDS. TIZAN 2, 4 mg tab. BRUZEN MR IBUPROFEN 400 mg + TIZANIDINE 2 mg.

Other centrally acting spasmolytic agents include **riluzole, gabapentin** and **progabide**. Riluzole and **idrocilamide** have both presynaptic and postsynaptic effects. They inhibit glutamate release in the CNS. They are well tolerated with minor adverse effects like nausea and diarrhea. Riluzole is used to reduce spasticity in amyotropic lateral sclerosis. **Thiocolchicoside** related to colchicine acts as a GABA mimetic and is used in combination with NSAIDs for painful muscle spasms. **Cyclobenzaprine** has anticholinergic effects and can therefore cause dryness of mouth, drowsiness and dizziness.

Many of them are available in combination with NSAIDs. Muscle spasms which could be due to inflammation can be relieved by NSAIDs.

Uses of Centrally Acting Muscle Relaxants

1. *Musculoskeletal disorders* like muscle strains, sprains, myalgias, cervical root syndromes, herniated disc syndromes, low backache, dislocations, arthritis, fibrositis and bursitis all cause painful muscle spasms. Muscle relaxants are used with analgesics in these conditions.
2. *Spastic neurological disorders* like cerebral palsy, multiple sclerosis, poliomyelitis, hemiplegia and quadriplegia are treated with diazepam or baclofen.
3. *Tetanus:* Diazepam is given IV.
4. *ECT:* Diazepam is given along with peripherally acting SMRs.
5. *Orthopaedic procedures* like fracture reduction may be done after administering diazepam.

Drug Interactions with SMRs

1. General anaesthetics augment the action of SMRs (stabilize post synaptic membrane).
2. Aminoglycosides, quinine and calcium channel blockers potentiate the action of SMRs.
3. Succinylcholine and halothane together increase the risk of malignant hyperthermia.
4. Anticholinesterases like neostigmine reverse the action of competitive blockers.

Contraindication of SMRs

1. Myasthenia gravis
2. Severe hepatic and renal dysfunction
3. Alcohol to be avoided
4. Allergy to a specific SMR

Clinical Pharmacology

- Skeletal muscle relaxants must be used only by trained doctors because inadvertent use can prove fatal.
- Peripherally acting SMRs do not affect the consciousness, hence awareness may be a horrifying experience to the patient—adequate precautions should be taken.
- Vecuronium, pancuronium and atracurium are the commonly used SMRs in India.
- Cisatracurium is not yet available in India.
- People belonging to certain communities like the Vysya community and Chettiar community of Tamil Nadu are known to inherit the atypical pseudocholinesterase. Proper history is therefore vital before administration of succinylcholine in all patients.
- Dibucaine number indicates the ability of a person to metabolize succinylcholine. Dibucaine inhibits normal pseudocholiesterase upto 80% and pseudoChE by 20%.
- Succinylcholine should be avoided in patients with muscular dystrophies, paraplegia, spinal cord injuries, ocular injuries and in rhabdomyolysis.
- Though dantrolene is the drug of choice in malignant hyperthermia, its high cost is a disadvantage.

[1] From Medical Council of India, *Competency based Undergraduate Curriculum for the Indian Medical Graduate*, 2018;1:136–144.

Unit III

Autacoids and Related Drugs

CHAPTER 9

Drugs Modulating Autacoids

Competency achievement: The student should be able to:

PH 1.16 Describe mechanism/s of action, types, doses, side effects, indications and contraindications of the drugs which act by modulating autacoids, including: antihistaminics, 5-HT modulating drugs, NSAIDs, drugs for gout, anti-rheumatic drugs, drugs for migraine.[1]

Autacoids are substances formed in various tissues, have complex physiological and pathological actions and act locally at the site of synthesis. They have a brief action and are destroyed locally. Hence they are called *'local hormones'*. They differ from true hormones which are produced by specific cells and reach their target tissues through circulation. The word autacoid is derived from Greek: *autos* = self *akos* = remedy.

Autacoids are grouped as:

- **Amines**
  Histamine, 5-hydroxytryptamine
- **Peptides**
  Angiotensin, kinins
- **Phospholipid derived autacoids**
  Prostaglandins, leukotrienes, platelet-activating factor (PAF)

HISTAMINE

Histamine (tissue amine, *Histos* = tissue) is a biogenic amine formed in many tissues. It is also found in the venoms of bees, wasps and other stinging secretions.

Synthesis, Storage, Distribution and Degradation

In humans, histamine is formed by the decarboxylation of the amino acid histidine. Large amounts of histamine are found in the lungs, skin and intestines. It is stored in the granules of the mast cells and basophils in an inactive form. Degranulation of the mast cells releases histamine which is quickly degraded by deamination and methylation. Non-mast cell histamine found in brain serves as a neurotransmitter. Non-mast cell histamine is also found in many other tissues. The enterochromaffin cells (ECL) in the fundus of the stomach release histamine which in turn activates the H_2 receptors on the gastric parietal cells to stimulate acid secretion.

Mechanism of Action

Histamine produces its effects by acting on the histamine receptors. Four subtypes H_1–H_4 are known. These are all G-protein-coupled receptors.

Receptor Location

H_1 Smooth muscle, endothelium, lungs, blood vessels, gut, brain
H_2 Stomach, heart muscle, brain
H_3 Presynaptic—in the brain, myentric plexus, neurons
H_4 Eosinophils, neutropils, CD4 cells.

H_1 receptors are present in the smooth muscles and mediate a variety of actions of

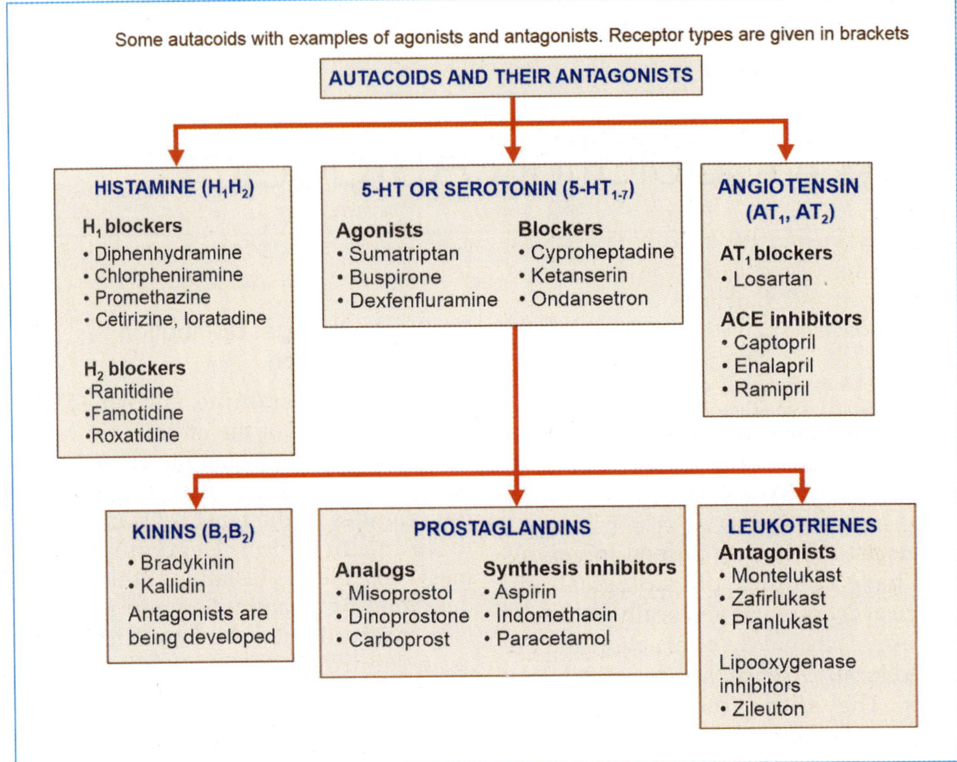

histamine in the body. H_1 antagonists block many of the actions of histamine related to allergy and inflammation.

H_2 receptors present in the gastric glands mediate gastric acid secretion by the parietal cells.

H_3 receptors are presynaptic autoreceptors which control histamine release from the neurons in the brain.

H_4 receptors present on leukocytes, CD4 cells and mast cells have recently been cloned. H_4 blockers seem to have therapeutic application in chronic inflammatory conditions.

Actions

1. **CVS:** Histamine dilates small blood vessels resulting in hypotension accompanied by reflex tachycardia. Cerebral blood vessels dilate producing severe throbbing headache.

Triple response: Intradermal injection of histamine elicits triple response comprising of:

- *Red spot at the site* (flush)—due to local capillary dilation.
- *Flare*—redness surrounding the 'flush' due to arteriolar dilatation.
- *Wheal*—local edema due to the escape of fluid from the capillaries.

This response is accompanied by pain and itching.

2. **Smooth muscle:** Histamine causes contraction of the nonvascular smooth muscles. Thus bronchospasm and increased intestinal motility are produced.

Actions on other visceral smooth muscles like uterus are insignificant in humans.

3. **Glands:** Histamine is a powerful stimulant of the gastric acid secretion—acts through H_2

receptors (*see* page 416). It also stimulates pepsin and intrinsic factor secretion.

4. **CNS:** Histamine functions as a neurotransmitter in the CNS.

5. **Nerve endings:** Histamine stimulates sensory nerve endings causing pain and itching.

Adverse reactions include hypotension, flushing, tachycardia, headache, wheal, bronchospasm and diarrhea.

Uses

Histamine is of **no therapeutic value**. It is occasionally used in some diagnostic tests like:

1. *Testing gastric acid secretion:* To test the acid secreting ability of the stomach. Now pentagastrin is preferred for this purpose.
2. *Diagnosis of pheochromocytoma:* Histamine releases catecholamines and raises BP—now not used.
3. *Pulmonary function:* To test for bronchial hyper-reactivity.

Histamine Substitutes

Betazole is H_2 agonist and can be used in gastric function tests. *Betahistine* is an H_1 agonist that may be used to control vertigo in Ménière's disease.

HISTAMINE ANTAGONISTS (ANTIHISTAMINES)

Drugs that competitively block H_1 histamine receptors are conventionally called the ***antihistamines***.

Actions

1. *Blockade of actions of histamine:* H_1 receptor antagonists bind to and block the actions of histamine on H_1 receptors. They block the histamine-induced effects on smooth muscles of the gut, bronchi, blood vessels and triple response.
2. *Sedation:* First generation antihistamines cause CNS depression; sedation, dizziness, inability to concentrate and disturbances of coordination are common. Alcohol and other CNS depressants potentiate this action. The extent of sedation varies with each drug and some second generation antihistamines do not produce sedation. In toxic doses, antihistamines may cause CNS stimulation and sometimes even convulsions. Some patients may experience tremors, restlessness and insomnia.
3. *Antimotion sickness and antiemetic effects:* Several first generation antihistamines like promethazine, diphenhydramine and meclizine prevent motion sickness and vomiting due to other labyrinthine disturbances. Some of them also control **vomiting of pregnancy** and **doxylamine** was used for this purpose often in combination with pyridoxine.
4. *Antiparkinsonian effects:* Some of them like diphenhydramine and promethazine suppress tremors, rigidity and sialorrhoea probably due to their anticholinergic properties.
5. *Anticholinergic actions:* Many of the first generation H_1 blockers have anticholinergic properties. This accounts for both useful and adverse effects. Such antihistaminics have antisecretory (used in rhinorrhoea), antiemetic and antiparkinsonian effects but they also have anticholinergic side effects like urinary retention and dryness of mouth. The second generation agents do not block the muscarinic receptors.

Classification

First-generation (sedative) antihistamines	Second-generation (non-sedative) antihistamines
Diphenhydramine, dimenhydrinate, promethazine, pheniramine, chlorpheniramine, cyclizine, meclizine, buclizine, mepyramine, tripelennamine.	Desloratadine, loratadine, cetirizine, levocetirizine, fexofenadine, acrivastine, azelastine, mizolastine, levocabastine, mequitazine.

6. *Other actions:*
   - Antihistamines also have **local anesthetic effects** in high doses. They block the sodium channels in excitable tissues.
   - Some of them also **block α_1-adrenergic** and **5-HT receptors**.
   - Few antihistamines also block the **potassium channels** resulting in cardiac arrhythmias.
   - Some antihistaminics, like cetirizine, inhibit the release of histamine from the mast cells which could be of help in the treatment of allergies. H_4 receptor blockade is thought to be responsible for this action.
   - Some antihistamines, like chlorpheniramine, inhibit the P-glycoprotein transporter because of which they may reverse the resistance in cancer cells and chloroquine resistance in malaria.

Pharmacokinetics

Antihistamines are well-absorbed on oral administration, widely distributed in the body, metabolised in the liver and are excreted in the urine. Dose, route of administration and preparations are given in Table 33.1.

Adverse Reactions

Adverse reactions are mild and on continued use tolerance develops.

Sedation, dizziness, motor incoordination and inability to concentrate make driving dangerous while on antihistamines. Anticholinergic effects like dryness of mouth, blurred vision, constipation and urinary retention may be troublesome. Epigastric distress, allergic reactions and headache can also occur. Many of them are teratogenic.

Drug Interactions

1. Drugs that can produce sedation and CNS depression like alcohol, barbiturates, clonidine, benzodiazepines and antidepressants should not be combined with sedative antihistamines because sedation gets added up.
2. Antimuscarinic effects of older antihistamines get added up when combined with other drugs having antimuscarinic effects.

Second-generation Antihistamines or Non-sedative Antihistamines

Newer non-sedative antihistamines have the following **advantages over first-generation antihistamines:**

1. They are selective H_1 blockers.
2. No sedation because they poorly cross the blood–brain barrier.
3. No anticholinergic side effects as these agents are pure H_1 blockers and do not block cholinergic receptors.
4. Some of them are long-acting—given OD.

Disadvantages

1. Therapeutic uses of these agents are limited to **allergic disorders** like allergic rhinitis and chronic urticaria.

COMPARE AND CONTRAST

Diphenydramine and Loratadine

Features	*Diphenydramine*	*Loratadine*
Receptors blocked	H_1 histamine, M_1 muscarinic	H_1
t½	4–6 hr	16–18 hr
Ability to cross BBB	Present	Absent
Sedation	Yes	No
Anticholinergic effects	Yes	No
In rhinorrhoea	Useful	Not useful
Route of administration	Oral and parenteral	Oral

2. They are ineffective in motion sickness, cough, rhinorrhoea, vomiting and to produce sedation.
3. They are more expensive.

Loratadine is a selective H_1 blocker with longer duration of action because a metabolite is also active. Absence of cardiac toxicity has made it a commonly prescribed antihistamine for allergic disorders. **Desloratadine**, a metabolite of loratadine, is safer and more potent. **Cetirizine** is a metabolite of hydroxyzine. Though considered nonsedative, cetirizine can cause some sedation in many when compared to other second generation agents. Cetirizine also inhibits the release of histamine and other mediators which may be of additional benefit in the treatment of allergies. **Levocetirizine** is more potent and better tolerated. **Fexofenadine**, is a weak K^+ channel blocker-should be avoided in patients with prolonged QT interval. Fexofenadine is rapidly absorbed and has a long duration of action of 24 hr. Dose: 120–180 mg OD. **Azelastine** is a newer second generation antihistamine which also inhibits the release of histamine and other mediators of allergy; given **intranasally**, it reduces hypersensitivity of the airways as it has good topical antiallergic activity. Onset of action is within 30 minutes.

Salient features of individual agents are given in Table 9.1.

Other Drugs

Doxepin, a tricyclic antidepressant, also blocks H_1 receptors. Hydroxyzine is a good antipruritic and has a long duration of action—it is used in skin allergies—but it causes significant sedation. **Cyproheptadine** blocks both H_1 histamine and 5-HT_2 receptors (*see* page 147).

Uses of Antihistamines

1. *Allergic reactions:* Antihistamines are useful for the prevention and treatment of symptoms of allergic reactions. They are effective in allergic rhinitis, allergic conjunctivitis, hay fever, urticaria, pruritus, some allergic skin rashes and pollinosis. They also relieve the pain, itching and other symptoms in ivy sting, insect bite and other similar conditions.

   Though they prevent bronchospasm induced by histamine, antihistamines are *not* useful in bronchial asthma because many other mediators are also involved in the pathogenesis of bronchial asthma. Moreover, antihistamines render the respiratory secretions more thick making it difficult to be coughed out.
2. *Common cold:* Antihistamines reduce rhinorrhoea and afford symptomatic relief in common cold because of their antimuscarinic properties. Sedation also helps. The nonsedative antihistamines lack anticholinergic activity and are not useful in reducing rhinorrhoea or producing sedation.
3. *Motion sickness:* Given 30–60 minutes before journey, antihistamines prevent motion sickness—promethazine, dimenhydrinate, flunarizine, meclizine and cyclizine are useful. They may be combined with ephedrine or amphetamine for better efficacy in the treatment of motion sickness.
4. *Vertigo:* Antihistamines are also useful in treating vertigo of Meniere's disease and other vestibular disturbances—dimenhydrinate, meclizine and cinnarizine are preferred.
5. *Antiemetic:* Promethazine is used to prevent drug-induced and postoperative vomiting. Some of them have also been used in 'morning sickness'. **Doxylamine** has been particularly used for this purpose.
6. *Preanesthetic medication:* For the sedative, anticholinergic and antiemetic properties, promethazine has been used as preanesthetic medication.

Table 9.1: Dose, route, preparations and salient features of some antihistamines

Antihistamine	*Dose and route*	*Trade name*	*Salient features*
First-generation antihistamines			
Diphenhydramine HCl	25–50 mg oral, 10 mg IM	BENADRYL 25, 50 mg cap, 12.5 mg/ml Syr	Sedation +++, antimuscarinic
Dimenhydrinate	25–50 mg oral, IM	DRAMAMINE 16 mg/5 ml Syr, 50 mg tab	Sedation, effective in motion sickness
Promethazine	25–50 mg oral, IM	PHENERGAN 10, 25 mg tab, 5 mg/ml elixer, 25 mg/ml inj.	Sedation, antiemetic, alpha blocking activity
Promethazine chlortheophyllinate	25–75 mg oral	AVOMINE 25 mg Tab	Sedation, effective in motion sickness
Pheniramine maleate	25–50 mg oral, IM	AVIL 25, 50 mg tab, 15 mg/5 ml Syr, 22.5 mg/ml inj.	Sedation, antimuscarinic
Hydroxyzine	25–50 mg oral IM	ATARAX 10, 25 mg tab, 10 mg/5 ml Syr, 6 mg/ml drops, 25 mg/ml inj.	Sedation +++
Chlorpheniramine	4–20 mg oral, IM	PIRITON, ZEET 4 mg tab, Syr, Inj	Sedation, mild antimuscarinic ++
Cyclizine HCl	50 mg oral	MAREZINE 50 mg tab	Sedation mild, effective in motion sickness
Meclizine HCl	25–50 mg oral	DIGIGAN 12.5 mg +, ANCOLAN, NIACIN 50 mg tab	Sedation mild, effective in motion sickness
Buclizine	25–50 mg oral	LONGIFENE 25 mg tab, Syr 6 mg/5 ml Syr	Sedation mild, effective in motion sickness
Cinnarizine	25–50 mg oral	STUGERON, VERTIGON 25 and 75 mg tab.	Sedation mild, effective in vertigo
Second-generation (nonsedative) antihistamines			
Loratadine	10 mg oral	LORFAST, LORIDIN, 10 mg tab, 5 mg/5 ml Syr.	No sedation, longer acting, no antimuscarinic effects
Desloratadine	5 mg oral	DESLOR, DEZIT 5 mg tab.	Metabolite of loratadine, long acting, no CVS side effects, safer.
Cetirizine	10 mg oral	ALERID, CETZINE, 10 mg	Also inhibits release of histamine and other mediators.
Levocetirizine	5–10 mg oral	LEVOCET, LEVORID, 5, 10 mg tab.	Less sedation
Azelastine	4 mg, 0.28 mg nasal spray	A2EP nasal spray 0.14 mg/puff	For allergic rhinitis; has good topical activity
Fexofenadine	20 mg oral	ALLEGRA, FEXO 20, 80 mg tab	Not arrhythmogenic, longer acting—once daily dose.
Acrivastine	8 mg oral	SEMPREX 8 mg	Bronchodilator, once daily dose
Mizolastine	10 mg oral	ZEHIST, ELINA 10 mg tab	No sedation, once daily dose

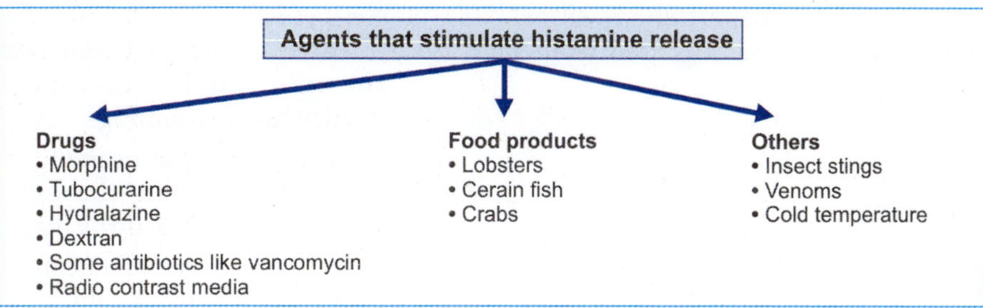

7. *Hypnotic:* The sedative antihistamines are sometimes used to induce sleep. Hydroxyzine has been used as an anxiolytic.
8. *Parkinsonism:* Diphenhydramine, orphenadrine, and promethazine are useful in drug-induced parkinsonism due to their anticholinergic action.
9. *Cough:* Due to postnasal drip can be controlled by antihistamines like diphenhydramine. Antihistamines have also been used in many cough syrups. Cough due to allergy may respond. In productive cough, drying up of secretions may infact thicken the sputum and cause further difficulty in coughing out.
10. *Dystonia:* H_1 blockers with prominent anticholinergic activity like promethazine may be used to relieve acute dystonia due to antipsychotic drugs.

H_2 Receptor Antagonists

H_2 blockers (cimetidine, ranitidine, famotidine) are used in the treatment of peptic ulcer (*see* page 416).

H_3 Receptor Antagonists

H_3 receptors are presynaptic receptors present mostly in the neurons. On activation, they inhibit the release of histamine from the nerve terminals. H_3 receptor agonists and antagonists modulate the histaminergic neurotransmission in the brain. Drugs that selectively act on H_3 receptors have application in obesity, sleep disorders, neuropsychiatric disorders and in cognitive functions. **Thioperamide** and **clobenpropit** are H_3 blockers known presently and tiprolisant is an H_3 receptor inverse agonist.

H_4 Receptor Antagonists

H_4 receptors are present mostly on mast cells, eosinophils and basophils and to a small extent in the intestines. H_4 antagonists have therapeutic application in **chronic inflammatory conditions** like **asthma** and **rheumatoid arthritis**. Clobenpropit is a partial agonist at H_4 receptors.

5-HT MODULATING DRUGS

5-HYDROXYTRYPTAMINE

5-Hydroxytryptamine **(serotonin)** was isolated in 1948 and has been of great pharmacological interest. It is found in various plant and animal tissues including banana, pineapple, wasp and scorpion sting.

Distribution, Synthesis and Degradation

In human body, 90% of 5-HT is present in the intestines and the remaining mostly in platelets and brain. 5-HT is synthesized and stored by the enterochromaffin cells of the gastrointestinal mucosa. It is synthesized from the amino acid tryptophan and stored in granules in serotonergic neurons. After it is released into the serotonergic synapses, serotonin is taken up by an amine pump called serotonin transporter (SERT) into the serotonergic nerve endings where it is stored in vesicles. 5-HT is taken up into platelets from circulation by active transport and is stored in secretory granules. It is degraded mainly by MAO.

Tryptophan
↓
5-Hydroxytryptophan
↓
5-HT $\xrightarrow{\text{MAO}}$ 5-Hydroxy indole acetic acid

5-HT Receptors

The actions of serotonin are mediated through its receptors. Four types of 5-HT receptors with further subtypes of each are presently known. Many receptors—selective agonists and antagonists are being developed. 5-HT_1, 5-HT_2 and 5-$HT_{4–7}$ are G-protein-coupled receptors while $5HT_3$ is a ligand-gated ion channel through which sodium and potassium ions move.

Actions

1. **CVS:** The action on blood vessels is complex. Large vessels are constricted while arterioles dilate. A characteristic triphasic response is seen on blood pressure following IV injection:
   - *Initial fall in BP* is due to increased vagal activity.
   - *Rise in BP* due to vasoconstriction of large vessels, followed by
   - *Fall in BP* due to arteriolar dilation.
2. **Gastrointestinal tract:** The enterochromaffin cells of the gut store a major part of body's serotonin. It increases GI motility and contraction resulting in diarrhoea. Activation of 5-HT_4 receptors in the gut promotes ACh release resulting in a prokinetic effect. Cisapride acts as a prokinetic agent by stimulation of 5-HT_4 receptors.
3. **Other actions:** Behaviour—5-HT is a neurotransmitter at several sites in the CNS and is involved in the control of behaviour, mood and emotion. Selective serotonin reuptake inhibitors (SSRIs) are used in the treatment of depression (*see* page 245).
   i. *Emesis:* 5-HT plays an important role in emesis. 5-HT_3 receptors present in the gut and in vomiting centre participate in vomiting.
   ii. *Platelets:* Serotonin promotes platelet aggregation acting through 5-HT_2 receptors. It is taken up by the platelets.
   iii. *Respiratory system:* 5-HT causes weak bronchoconstriction which could be mediated by 5-HT_{2A} receptors.
   iv. *Stimulation of sensory nerve endings:* Serotonin causes pain, if injected into the skin.
   v. *Skeletal muscles:* Though 5-HT receptors are present on skeletal muscles, their role is not exactly known. In 'serotonin syndrome' hyper-reflexia and increased muscle contractions are noted.

Physiological and Pathophysiological Role

5-HT is postulated to be having a role in peristalsis, vomiting, platelet aggregation, behaviour, homeostasis and inflammation. It is also thought to initiate the vasoconstriction in migraine.

Drugs Acting on 5-HT Receptors

Serotonin has no therapeutic uses. However, its receptor agonists and antagonists have been used in various conditions.

Serotonin Agonists

Sumatriptan a 5-$HT_{1D/1B}$ agonist is effective in the treatment of acute migraine and cluster headache. It stimulates the 5-$HT_{1D/1B}$ receptors on presynaptic trigeminal nerve endings and blocks the release of vasodilator peptides. The triptans also constrict the cerebral blood vessels and may prevent the stretching of pain nerve endings.

Given orally/SC at the onset of an attack, sumatriptan relieves headache and also suppresses nausea and vomiting of migraine. Bioavailability is ~14% and is short-acting—t½ 2 hr.

Triptans are the first-line drugs in acute migraine attacks except in patients with coronary artery disease. **Short duration of action is a disadvantage** with most triptans.

Adverse effects include dizziness, altered sensations, weakness, chest discomfort and neck pain. It is contraindicated in coronary artery disease.

Zolmitriptan, almotriptan, frovatriptan, rizatriptan, naratriptan and eletriptan are other triptans. Specific advantages include better bioavailability, longer action and ability to cross BBB to reach the CNS. They also seem to have lower cardiac side effects.

Other Agonists

Buspirone (*see* page 242) is a 5-HT_{1A} agonist–antagonist used as an antianxiety agent.

Cisapride, a 5-HT_4 agonist, is a prokinetic agent.

Tegaserod is a 5-HT_4 agonist used in irritable bowel syndrome.

Dexfenfluramine is used as an appetite suppressant.

Selective serotonin reuptake inhibitors (SSRIs), like fluoxetine, inhibit the reuptake of serotonin and are used in the treatment of depression.

Serotonin Antagonists

Cyproheptadine blocks 5-HT_2, H_1 histamine and cholinergic receptors. It increases appetite and is used to promote weight gain especially in children but the weight gained is also lost after withdrawing the drug. It is also used in carcinoid tumors, serotonin syndrome and post-gastrectomy dumping syndrome. Cyproheptadine is often prescribed in pruritus and seasonal allergy where it could help due to its H_1 receptor blocking effects.

Cyproheptadine can cause some drowsiness, dryness of mouth, dizziness and ataxia.

Ketanserin blocks 5-HT_2 receptors and antagonises the vasoconstriction and platelet aggregation promoted by 5-HT. Ketanserin is used in hypertension. It also blocks alpha1 receptors and this action contributes to its hypotensive effects.

Retanserin is another 5-HT_2 blocker devoid of alpha-blocking actions but alters platelet function.

Lorcaserin is an agonist at 5-HT_{2C} receptors and is approved for use in obesity as it decreases appetite.

Ondansetron is a 5-HT_3 antagonist (*see* page 425) used in the prevention and treatment of vomiting due to radiation and cancer chemotherapy.

Clozapine: The atypical antipsychotic clozapine is an antagonist at 5-$HT_{2A/2C}$ receptors.

Many other drugs including some antihistamines, phenoxybenzamine also block serotonin receptors.

ERGOT ALKALOIDS

Ergot alkaloids are produced by *Claviceps purpurea,* a fungus that infects rye, millet and other grains. Consumption of such grains results in 'ergotism' manifested as gangrene of the hands and feet, hallucinations and other CNS effects. Barger and Dale isolated ergot alkaloids in 1906.

Natural ergot alkaloids include **ergometrine, ergotamine** and **ergotoxine**. The semisynthetic dehydrogenated derivatives are also available.

Actions

Ergot alkaloids have agonist, partial agonist and antagonistic actions at 5-HT and alpha adrenergic receptors and agonistic actions at CNS dopamine receptors. Thus their actions are complex. Some of them are powerful hallucinogens, e.g. lysergic acid diethylamide (LSD). They cause stimulation of smooth muscles—some stimulate mainly vascular smooth muscles and others mainly uterine smooth muscles. The vasoconstrictor effect is responsible for gangrene.

Adverse effects like nausea, vomiting and diarrhoea are common. Prolonged use results in gangrene due to persistent vasospasm. Methysergide causes retroperitoneal and mediastinal fibrosis.

Uses (Table 9.2)

1. Migraine (*see* below)
2. Postpartum haemorrhage—ergometrine is used (*see* page 497) for the prevention and treatment of postpartum hemorrhage but is not preferred now.

DRUGS USED IN THE TREATMENT OF MIGRAINE

Migraine is a common disorder characterised by severe, throbbing and unilateral headache often associated with nausea, vomiting, giddiness and fatigue lasting for several hours. In the classical migraine, a brief 'aura' of visual disturbances occurs prior to the headache. An attack is triggered by factors like stress, anxiety, excitement, food (like chocolate and cheese) and hormonal changes. These triggering factors stimulate the release of vasoactive substances from nerve endings which are responsible for the events that follow. The peptide neurotransmitters released, the most important of which is calcitonin gene-related peptide (CGRP) is a powerful vasodilator. However, the exact pathophysiology is not understood and several hypotheses have been put forward.

Drugs used in Acute Attacks

Analgesics: Aspirin, paracetamol or other analgesics are effective for mild cases. Analgesics should be taken at the initiation of attack. For moderate to severe migraine, ibuprofen, diclofenac, naproxen or mefenamic acid may be used. They may be given in combination with caffiene, because caffiene also has anlagesic effect and promotes the absorption of NSAIDs. Severe migraine may not respond to NSAIDs and may require ergotamine or sumatriptan along with antiemetics.

Antiemetics: Metoclopramide can be combined with aspirin as it is an antiemetic, promotes gastric emptying and also speeds up absorption of aspirin. In presence of vomiting, paracetamol and metoclopramide may be needed.

Ergotamine given orally (or sublingual/rectal when vomiting is present) is an effective alternative.

MIGRANIL Paracetamol 250 mg + Ergotamine 1 mg + Caffiene 100 mg + Belladonna dry extract 10 mg.

Sumatriptan is very effective but short-acting. The dose needs to be repeated, if pain recurs.

Dose: 50–100 mg at the onset of migraine. SUMINAT, SUMITREX, 25, 50, 100 mg Tab, 12 mg/ml Inj.

Zolmitriptan and other tryptans are longer acting and may be used.

Prophylaxis

When the attacks are frequent (2–3 per month) and severe, prophylaxis is needed to prevent them. Drugs used for the prophylaxis are:

1. **β-adrenergic blockers:** Propranolol reduces the frequency and severity of attacks. The initial dose is 40 mg twice daily and is gradually increased to a maximum of 160 mg twice daily. The mechanism of action is not exactly known but is the most commonly used drug for the prophylaxis of migraine. To be avoided in asthmatics.
2. **Calcium channel blockers:** Flunarizine may be useful. It has weak Ca^{++} channel blocking properties and is thought to be selective for the CNS. Adverse effects include hypotension, flushing, dry mouth, constipation and sedation.

   Dose: 10–20 mg OD FLUNARIN 5, 10 mg cap.
3. **Pizotifen and cyproheptadine** block 5-HT and H_1 histamine receptors; may be used as alternatives but cause sedation and weight gain.
4. **Tricyclic antidepressants:** Amytriptyline may be tried but it is associated with many adverse effects. It may be considered in patients who also have depression.

Table 9.2: Drugs influencing serotonergic activity

	Receptors	*Uses*	*Comments*
Agonists			
Sumatriptan	5-$HT_{1B,\ 1D}$ agonist	• Acute migraine • Cluster headache	Short-acting; may need repetition of dose
Buspirone	5-HT_{1A} (partial agonist)	Anxiolytic	No drowsiness
Lorcaserin	5HT_{2C} agonist	Weight loss	Hallucinogenic at higher doses
Antagonists			
Cyproheptadine	5-$HT_{2A\ 2C}$; H_1 histamine and muscarinic receptors	• Appetite stimulant • Carcinoid tumors • Post gastrectomy dumping syndrome	—
Ketanserin	5-HT_1, 5-$HT_{2A\ 2C}$, α-adrenergic	Hypertension	Also antagonises platelet aggregation promoted by 5-HT
Ondansetron	5-HT_3	Antiemetic	Powerful antiemetic
Ergot alkaloids			
Ergotamine	5-HT_1 partial agonist/antagonist	Migraine prophylaxis	—
Ergometrine	5-HT_1 partial agonist/antagonist	Postpartum haemorrhage	—
Methysergide	5-HT_2 partial agonist/antagonist	• Acute migraine • Vascular headaches	Not preferred due to risk of retroperitoneal and mediastinal fibrosis
Others			
SSRIs– Fluoxetine Sertraline	5-HT	Depression Chronic neuralgias	Commonly used
Antipsychotics			
Clozapine Risperidone	5-HT	Schizophrenia Psychoses	Commonly used

5. **Antiepileptics:** Sodium valproate and gabapantin have prophylactic value in migraine. **Topiramate,** a newer antiepileptic drug, has also been found to reduce the frequency of attacks. Started with 25 mg OD, the dose is gradually increased up to 50 mg once or twice a day. Topiramate can be used as an alternative to beta blockers.
6. **Methysergide blocks** 5-HT receptors but due to adverse effects like retroperitoneal fibrosis, it is not preferred.

OTHER AUTACOIDS

Cytokines

Cytokines are also considered as autacoids. They are peptides released from the inflammatory cells. They are classified into 5 families.

- Interleukins
- Colony-stimulating factors
- Chemokines
- Growth factor and tumour necrosis factors
- Interferons.

Cytokines stimulate specific receptors to bring about their effects. IL-1 and TNF-alpha are involved in inflammation—they are pro-inflammatory cytokines while IL-4, IL-10 and IL-13 inhibit inflammatory activity—they are antiinflammatory cytokines. The interferons alpha and beta have antiviral activity (*see* page 619). While interferon γ has immunoregulatory activity and is used in multiple sclerosis.

Kinins

Kinins (*see* page 327) are vasodilator peptides synthesized from kininogen with the help of the enzymes kallikriens. Kinins include bradykinin and kallidin.

Angiotensin

Drugs influencing angiotensin are described in Chapter 24.

EICOSANOIDS

Eicosanoids are 20-carbon (*eicosa* referring to 20 in Greek) unsaturated fatty acids derived mainly from arachidonic acid in the cell membrane. The principal eicosanoids are **prostaglandins** (PG), **prostocyclin** (PGI_2), **thromboxanes** (TX), and the **leukotrienes** (LT).

Biosynthesis

Eicosanoids are synthesized locally in most tissues from arachidonic acid. The pathway for synthesis is shown in Fig. 9.1.

The cyclo-oxygenase (COX) pathway generates PGs and TXs while lipoxygenase (LOX) pathway generates LTs. There are 2 cyclo-oxygenase isozymes, *viz.* COX-1 and COX-2. COX-1 is present in almost all cells and prostanoids (PGs and TXs) obtained from COX-1 mainly take part in physiological functions. COX-2 is induced by inflammation in the inflammatory cells and the prostanoids produced by COX-2 are involved in inflammatory and pathological changes. All products of COX pathway are metabolised by oxidation and excreted in urine.

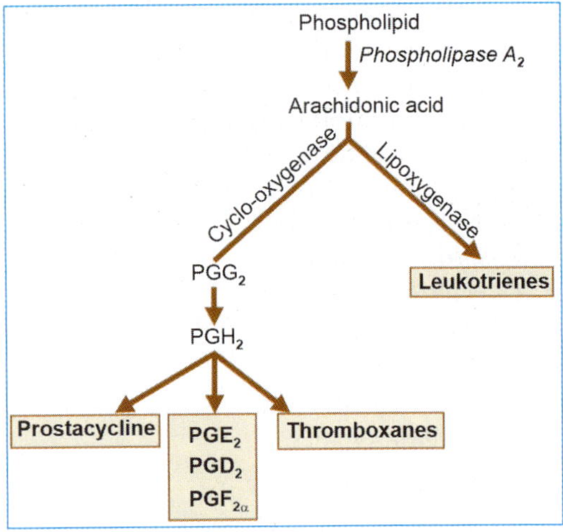

Fig. 9.1: Biosynthesis of eicosanoids

PROSTAGLANDINS AND THROMBOXANES

In 1930s, it was found that human semen contains a substance that contracts uterine smooth muscle. As this substance was thought to originate in the prostate, they called it 'Prostaglandin' but it was later found to be produced in many tissues.

Prostanoid Receptors

The prostanoids bring about their effects by acting on prostanoid receptors, which are all G-protein-coupled receptors. Some of them act through cAMP and others via inositol triphosphate pathway. There are five classes of prostanoid receptors. They are:

- DP (for PGD_2)—subtypes DP_1 and DP_2
- EP (for PGE_2)—subtypes EP_1 to EP_4
- FP (for $PGF_{2\alpha}$)
- IP (for PGI_2)
- TP (for TXA_2)

Actions

The prostanoids act on many tissues to bring about the following effects:

1. **CVS:** Prostacyclin and PGE_2 cause vasodilation while TXA_2 causes vasoconstriction. PGE_2 and $PGF_{2\alpha}$ are weak cardiac stimulants. The vasodilator prostaglandins PGE_2 and PGI_2 are produced in the ductus arteriosus during foetal life which could be responsible for maintaining the patency of the ductus arteriosus during this period.
2. **GIT:** Most PGs and TXs stimulate gastrointestinal smooth muscle resulting in colic and watery diarrhea. PGE_2 inhibits gastric acid secretion and enhances mucus production. Thus they have a protective effect on gastric mucosa.
3. **Airways:** PGE_2 and PGI_2 relax bronchial smooth muscle while TXA_2 and $PGF_{2\alpha}$ contract them. They may have a role in the pathophysiology of bronchial asthma.

4. **Platelets:** TXA_2 induces platelet aggregation while PGI_2 inhibits platelet aggregation. In low concentrations, PGE_2 enhances platelet aggregation but in higher concentrations it inihibits platelet aggregation. TXA_2 biosynthesis in the platelets is irreversibly inhibited by long-term administration of low dose aspirin.
5. **Reproductive system**

   Female reproductive system
   - *Uterus:* PGE_2 and $PGF_{2\alpha}$ contract human uterus which is more sensitive to PGs during pregnancy.

     They also soften the cervix. Thus PGs may be involved in the initiation and progression of labour. PGs are produced by foetal tissues during labour.
   - They also play a role in dysmenorrhoea and menorrhagia.

   Male reproductive system
   - PGs present in the semen may facilitate movement of sperms and fertilization by coordinating the movement of the uterus.
   - A large amount of PGs are found in the seminal vesicle and a small amount in the prostate and testes.
   - PGs also have a role in penile erection as they relax the smooth muscle of the corpora cavernosa.
6. **Kidneys:** PGE_2 and PGI_2 cause renal vasodilation and have a diuretic effect. PGs also oppose the action of ADH. PGs are synthesized both in the medulla and the cortex and regulate the renal function particularly during states of renal impairment. PGs also play an important role in maintaining the BP. They regulate the excretion of sodium and water. They enhance renal blood flow and also have direct effects on renal tubules which are responsible for most of their actions on the kidney. PGE_2 also stimulates renin release. NSAIDs inhibit PG synthesis and their long-term use can result in renal dysfunction.
7. **Central and peripheral nervous system:**
   - PGs increase body temperature when administered into cerebral ventricles. PGD_2 also induces sleep.
   - *Nerves:* PGs sensitize sensory nerve endings to pain and on intradermal injection cause pain. They enhance the excitability of the nerve membrane and also modulate pain centrally.
   - PGs inhibit the release of the neurotransmitter noradrenaline from the sympathetic nerve endings.
8. **Inflammation and immunity:** PGs have a major role in the genesis of inflammation—they enhance the blood flow in the inflamed area, facilitate leukocyte infiltration and development of edema. They also suppress lymphocyte function, proliferation and cytokine release to inhibit the immunologic response.
9. **Bone:** PGs stimulate bone resorption and formation through osteoclastic and osteoblastic activities.
10. **Endocrine system:** PGs stimulate the release of insulin and growth hormone, has thyrotropin like effects on the thyroid and also stimulate the production of steroids by the adrenals.
11. **Eye:** $PGF_{2\alpha}$ reduces the intraocular pressure probably by facilitating the drainage of aqueous humour through the uveoscleral pathway.
12. **Cancer:** PGs may have a role in the genesis of cancer. PGE_2 is considered the pro-oncogenic prostanoid and is found to promote the growth and metastasis of cancers. Use of NSAIDs particularly COX-2 inhibitors has shown to restrict tumour formation.

Adverse Effects

Adverse effects depend on the type of PG, dose and route. Diarrhoea, nausea, vomiting, fever, hypotension and pain due to uterine contractions are common.

Uses

1. **Gynaecological and obstetrical**
   - *Abortion:* For I and II trimester abortion and ripening of the cervix during abortion, PGE_2 and $PGF_{2\alpha}$ are used. They are also used with mifepristone to ensure complete expulsion of the products of conception in early pregnancy. **Dinoprostone,** a synthetic PGE_2 analog, has been used as a vaginal pessary for second trimester abortion.
   - *Facilitation of labour:* As an alternative to oxytocics in patients with renal failure, PGE_2 is used for induction of labour as it does not cause fluid retention. PGE_2 may be used intravaginally for this purpose.
   - *Cervical priming:* Intravaginal PGE_2 is used as a gel to soften the cervix and make it more compliant.
   - *Postpartum hemorrhage:* $PGF_{2\alpha}$ (IM) is used as an alternative to ergometrine.
2. **Gastrointestinal**
   - *Peptic ulcer:* PGE_1 (analog—misoprostol) and PGE_2 (analog—enprostil) are used for the prevention of peptic ulcer in patients on high dose NSAIDs (*see* page 422). Misoprostol Dose: 200 µg QID oral.

Prostaglandins

- 20-carbon unsaturated fatty acids synthesized from arachidonic acid through cyclo-oxygenase pathway.
- PGI_2 causes vasodilation while TXA_2 causes vasoconstriction.
- PGs contract GI and bronchial (TXA_2, $PGF_{2\alpha}$) smooth muscles. TXA_2 induces platelet aggregation (PGI_2 inhibits); PGE_2 and $PGF_{2\alpha}$ contract uterus. PGs stimulate bone turnover and sensitize the nerve endings to pain.
- Uses: Abortion, facilitation of labour, cervical priming, PPH, to maintain the patency of ductus arteriosus, for prevention of platelet aggregation, pulmonary hypertension, open-angle glaucoma and peptic ulcer.

3. **Cardiovascular**
   - *Patent ductus arteriosus:* Patency of fetal ductus arteriosus depends on local PG synthesis and at birth the ductus arteriosus closes. In neonates with some congenital heart diseases, patency of the ductus arteriosus needs to be maintained even after birth and is maintained with PGs until surgical correction is done. Alprostadil is given as an IV infusion.
   - To prevent platelet aggregation during hemodialysis and cardiopulmonary bypass.
4. **Glaucoma:** $PGF_{2\alpha}$ analog **latanoprost** is the first-line drug to lower the intraocular pressure in glaucoma. It is available as eye drops to be used once or twice a day (*see* page 105). **Bimatoprost, travoprost and unoprostone** are other PG analogs used in glaucoma.
5. **Peripheral vascular diseases:** PGs are used in some peripheral vascular diseases—PGI_2 or PGE_1 given as IV infusion brings about vasodilation and provides relief from pain in intermittent claudication and in Raynaud's disease. However, further studies are needed to confirm the benefit.
6. **Pulmonary hypertension:** Epoprostenol (PGI_2) has been used to lower pulmonary hypertension because it reduces pulmonary resistance (also decreases peripheral and coronary resistance). Epoprostenol has a short t½ of 3–5 min and is given as infusion. Longer acting analogs iloprost (inhalation/IV infusion) and treprostinil (SC/IV infusion) are now available.
7. **Erectile dysfunction:** 2.5–5 µg of alprostadil injected into the cavernosa or as urethral suppository is used as an alternative to sildenafil in erectile dysfunction (*see* page 495). Drugs inhibiting PG synthesis (NSAIDs) are described in Chapter 10.

LEUKOTRIENES

Leukotrienes (LT) are products of arachidonic acid metabolism synthesized by the lipoxygenase pathway and are found in

Table 9.3: Preparations, routes and uses of prostaglandin analogs

PG analog	*PG type*	*Preparations and routes of administration*	*Uses*
Misoprostol	PGE_1	MISO 200 μg tab 2 tabs oral	Abortion (along with mifepristone)
Gemeprost	PGE_1	CERVAGEM 1 mg vaginal pessary	Cervical priming, midtrimester abortion
Alprostil	PGE_1	2.5–25 μg intra-cavernosal inj/ intraurethral pessary	Erectile dysfunction, to maintain patency of ductus arteriosus
Dinoprostone	PGE_2	0.5 mg vaginal gel, cervical gel, vaginal tab Extra-amniotic solution, IV inj PROSTIN-E, CERVIPRIME	Induction/facilitation of labour, midterm abortion
Dinoprost	$PGF_{2\alpha}$	PROSTIN $F_{2\alpha}$ 5 mg/ml intra-amniotic inj	Midterm abortion, induction of labour
Latanoprost	$PGF_{2\alpha}$	LATOPROST 0.005% eye drops—	Glaucoma
Bimatoprost }	$PGF_{2\alpha}$	1 drop every evening	
Epoprostanol }	PGI_2	FLOLAN 0.5 mg inj, IV infusion	• To prevent platelet aggregation in cardiopulmonary bypass
Iloprost	PGI_2	VENTAVIS inhalation	• Pulmonary hypertension

Rioplast—PGE_1 analog and enprostil—PGE_2 analog preparations are not available in India at present.

the lungs, platelets, mast cells and white blood cells. ('Leuko'—because they are found in white cells; 'trienes'—they contain three double bonds). LTA_4 is the precursor from which LTB_4, LTC_4, LTD_4, LTE_4 and LTF_4 are derived. LTC_4, LTD_4 and LTE_4 are together known as slow reacting substances (SRS-A) of anaphylaxis. The LTs produce their effects through specific receptors.

Actions

Leukotrienes cause vasoconstriction, alter vascular permeability leading to edema, increase airway mucus secretion and are potent bronchiolar spasmogens. Given subcutaneously they cause wheal and flare. Leukotrienes have a role in inflammation including rheumatoid arthritis, psoriasis and ulcerative colitis. They also contribute to bronchial hyper-responsiveness in bronchial asthma.

Drugs that inhibit lipoxygenase like zileuton and thus block the synthesis of leukotrienes are useful in the treatment of bronchial asthma and allergic rhinitis.

Leukotriene Receptor Antagonists

Montelukast, zafirlukast and **pranlukast** block the actions of LTC_4 and LTD_4 on the bronchial and vascular smooth muscles. They are useful as adjuvants in bronchial asthma (*see* page 404). They are all effective orally.

PLATELET ACTIVATING FACTOR

Platelet activating factor (PAF) is an important mediator in acute and chronic, allergic and inflammatory phenomena. PAF is a lipid released from inflammatory cells on stimulation and acts on specific receptors. It causes local vasodilatation resulting in edema, hyperalgesia and wheal formation. It is a potent chemotaxin for leukocytes and a spasmogen on bronchial and intestinal smooth muscles. It is a mediator of inflammation.

[1] From Medical Council of India, *Competency based Undergraduate Curriculum for the Indian Medical Graduate*, 2018;1:136–144.

CHAPTER 10

Nonsteroidal Anti-inflammatory Drugs (NSAIDs)

Competency achievement: The student should be able to:

PH 1.16 Describe mechanism/s of action, types, doses, side effects, indications and contraindications of the drugs which act by modulating autacoids, including: anti-histaminics, 5-HT modulating drugs, **NSAIDs**, drugs for gout, anti-rheumatic drugs, drugs for migraine.[1]

Nonsteroidal anti-inflammatory drugs are aspirin-type or non-narcotic or non-opioid analgesics. In addition, they have anti-inflammatory, antipyretic and uricosuric properties—without addiction liability. **They act by inhibiting prostaglandin synthesis.**

The medicinal effects of the bark of the willow tree have been known since centuries. The active principle 'salicin' was isolated from the willow bark. This salicin is converted to glucose and salicylic acid in the body. In 1875, sodium salicylate was first used in the treatment of rheumatic fever. After its anti-inflammatory and uricosuric properties were established, efforts were made to synthesize derivatives which were less expensive and aspirin was introduced in 1899. Now the synthetic compounds have replaced the natural ones in the market.

COOH

$OCOCH_3$

Aspirin

Mechanism of Action of NSAIDs

During inflammation, arachidonic acid liberated from membrane phospholipids is converted to prostaglandins (PGs), catalysed by the enzyme cyclo-oxygenase (COX). These prostaglandins produce hyperalgesia—they sensitize the nerve endings to pain caused by other mediators of inflammation like bradykinin and histamine.

NSAIDs inhibit the PG synthesis by inhibiting the enzyme cyclo-oxygenase and is the major mechanism responsible for pharmacological effects of aspirin.

Aspirin is an irreversible inhibitor of COX (acetylates COX) while the others are reversible competitive COX inhibitors. There are two forms of cyclo-oxygenase, viz. COX-1

Classification

A. Nonselective COX inhibitors

1. **Salicylates**
   Aspirin
2. **Para-aminophenol derivatives**
   Paracetamol
3. **Propionic acid derivatives**
   Ibuprofen, fenoprofen, ketoprofen, flurbiprofen, oxaprozin, naproxen
4. **Acetic acid derivatives**
   Ketorolac, tolmetin, indomethacin, sulindac
5. **Fenamates (anthranilic acids)**
   Mefenamic acid, meclofenamic acid
6. **Pyrazolone derivatives**
   Phenylbutazone, azapropazone
7. **Oxicams** (Enolic acid derivatives)
   Piroxicam, tenoxicam

B. Preferential COX-2 inhibitors
Diclofenac, aceclofenac, etodolac, meloxicam, nabumetone, nimesulide

C. Selective COX-2 inhibitors
Celecoxib, parecoxib, etoricoxib

Mnemonic (for groups): **S**aw **P**retty **P**riyanka, she's **A F**antastic **POP S**inger.

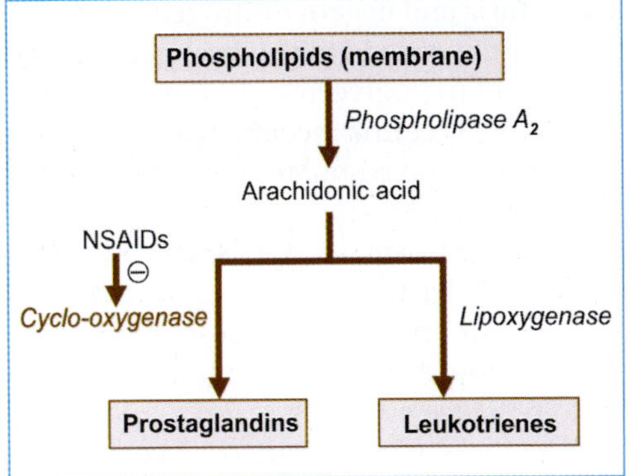

and COX-2 (*see* page 150). COX-1 is found in most of the normal cells (constitutive) and is involved in maintaining tissue homeostasis. COX-2 is induced in the inflammatory cells by cytokines and other mediators of inflammation. This COX-2 catalyzes the synthesis of prostanoids which are the mediators of inflammation. Most NSAIDs inhibit both COX-1 and COX-2 while some newer agents like celecoxib and rofecoxib selectively inhibit only COX-2.

1. SALICYLATES

Salicylates are salts of salicylic acid, e.g. methyl salicylate, sodium salicylate, acetylsalicylic acid (aspirin). Aspirin is taken as the prototype.

Pharmacological Actions

1. **Analgesia:** Aspirin is a good analgesic and relieves pain of inflammatory origin. This is because PGs are formed during inflammation and they sensitize the tissues to pain and aspirin inhibits PG synthesis. Pain originating from the integumental structures like muscles, bones, joints, and pain in connective tissues is relieved. But in vague visceral pain, aspirin is relatively ineffective.

   The pain is relieved without euphoria and hypnosis. Hence there is no development of tolerance and dependence. But aspirin is a weaker analgesic when compared to morphine.

2. **Antipyretic action:** In presence of fever, salicylates bring down the temperature to normal level. But, in normal individuals, there is no change in temperature.

   In fever, pyrogen, a protein, circulates in the body and this increases the synthesis of PGs in the hypothalamus, thereby raising its temperature set point. The thermostatic mechanism in the hypothalamus is thus disturbed. Aspirin inhibits PG synthesis in the hypothalamus and resets the thermostat at the normal level bringing down the temperature.

   Enhanced sweating and cutaneous vasodilatation promote heat loss and assist in the antipyretic action.

3. **Anti-inflammatory action:** At higher doses of 4–6 g/day, aspirin acts as an anti-inflammatory agent. Signs of inflammation like tenderness, swelling, erythema and pain are all reduced or suppressed. But, the progression of the disease in rheumatoid arthritis, rheumatic fever or osteoarthritis is not affected.

   Once again the mechanism involved is PG synthesis inhibition—PGs present in inflammatory tissues are responsible for edema, erythema and pain. In addition, aspirin also interferes with the formation of chemical mediators of the kallikrein system. As a result, it decreases the adherence of granulocytes to the damaged vasculature, stabilizes lysosomes and decreases the migration of the polymorphonuclear leukocytes and macrophages into the site of inflammation.

4. **Respiration:** In therapeutic doses of 4–6 g/day, salicylates increase consumption of oxygen by skeletal muscles. As a result, there is increased CO_2 production. This increased CO_2 stimulates the respiratory centre. Salicylates also directly stimulate the medullary respiratory centre. Both these actions increase the rate and depth of respiration. These effects are dose-dependent.

As a result of this stimulation of respiration, plasma CO_2 is washed out leading to respiratory alkalosis. With toxic doses, the respiratory centre is depressed leading to respiratory failure.

5. **Acid–base and electrolyte balance:** In anti-inflammatory doses, salicylates produce significant respiratory stimulation—more CO_2 is washed out resulting in respiratory alkalosis; pH becomes alkaline. This is compensated by increased excretion of HCO_3^- in the urine accompanied by Na^+, K^+ and water. pH then returns to normal. This stage is known as compensated respiratory alkalosis.

   With toxic doses, salicylates depress the respiratory centre directly. As a result, CO_2 accumulates because more CO_2 is produced than is exhaled. Thus plasma CO_2 rises and pH decreases. Since the concentration of HCO_3^- is already low due to enhanced renal excretion, the change results in uncompensated respiratory acidosis. This is superimposed by metabolic acidosis caused by accumulation of acids.

   Toxic doses also depress vasomotor centre. This vasomotor depression impairs renal function resulting in accumulation of strong acids of metabolic origin like lactic, pyruvic and acetoacetic acids.

   The above effects are accompanied by dehydration due to:

   - Water lost in urine with HCO_3^-, Na^+ and K^+
   - Increased sweating
   - Water lost during hyperventilation.

   Thus there is severe dehydration with acidosis.

6. **Metabolic effects:** Salicylates enhance the cellular metabolism due to uncoupling of oxidative phosphorylation. More of O_2 is used and more CO_2 is produced, especially in skeletal muscles, leading to increased heat production.

   In toxic doses, hyperpyrexia, increased protein catabolism with resultant aminoaciduria and negative nitrogen balance are seen. Enhanced utilization of glucose leads to mild hypoglycemia. But in toxic doses, hyperglycemia occurs due to central sympathetic stimulation which increases adrenaline levels.

7. **Gastrointestinal tract:** Aspirin is a gastric irritant. Irritation of the gastric mucosa leads to epigastric distress, nausea and vomiting. Aspirin also stimulates the CTZ to produce vomiting.
   Erosive gastritis, mucosal congestion, gastric ulceration and GI bleeding resulting in malaena and occasionally haematemesis can occur particularly in higher doses.

   Mechanism

   i. In the acidic pH of the stomach, salicylates remain unionised. These drug particles adhere to the mucosa producing irritation. These particles also diffuse into the gastric mucosal cells. Inside the cells, as the pH is alkaline, the drug particles get ionised and the ions cannot move back into the lumen **ion trapping**—resulting in more toxicity.
   ii. The ions promote local back diffusion of acid.
   iii. PGs are cytoprotective to gastric mucosa because they reduce acid secretion, increase mucus production and mucosal blood flow. As aspirin inhibits synthesis (irreversible inhibitor of COX), the defence mechanism of PGs is lost.
   iv. Antiplatelet effect of aspirin may result in increased bleeding if there is any gastric erosion.

   The above actions make aspirin ulcerogenic. With soluble aspirin, gastric irritation is less. The selective COX-2 inhibitors cause less gastric irritation because gastric epithelial cells have COX-1.

8. **CVS:** In therapeutic doses, no significant cardiovascular effects are seen. In toxic

doses, it depresses the VMC and thus depresses the circulation.

9. **Immunological effects:** In higher doses, salicylates suppress several antigen–antibody reactions including inhibition of antibody production, Ag–Ab aggregation and antigen-induced release of histamine. These effects might also contribute to the beneficial effects in rheumatic fever.
10. **Uric acid excretion:** Uric acid is excreted by secretion from the distal tubules. In a dose of 1–2 g/day, aspirin increases plasma urate levels by urate retention because it interferes with urate secretion by the distal tubules.

    Large doses of >5 g/day increase urate excretion because it inhibits reabsorption of urate by proximal tubule causing uricosuria. But, its uricosuric effect cannot be used therapeutically because high doses are required and such doses result in prominent adverse effects.
11. **Blood:** Even in small doses, aspirin irreversibly inhibits platelet cyclo-oxygenase (acetylates COX) and thereby TXA_2 synthesis by the platelets (Flowchart 10.1). It, therefore, interferes with platelet aggregation and prolongs the bleeding time. Even a single dose can irreversibly inhibit TXA_2 synthesis which is for the life of the platelets (8–11 days). **Platelets contain only COX-1**. Fresh platelets have to be formed to restore TXA_2 activity, because platelets cannot synthesize proteins as they have no nuclei— which means, COX cannot be regenerated. Moreover, aspirin inhibits platelet COX in the portal circulation itself and, therefore, even small doses (40 mg daily) of aspirin is adequate for its antiplatelet aggregatory effects.

    Other NSAIDs are reversible inhibitors of platelet cyclo-oxygenase.
12. **Local effects:** Salicylic acid when applied locally is a keratolytic. It also has mild antiseptic and fungistatic properties. Salicylic acid is also an irritant for the broken skin.

Pharmacokinetics

Salicylates being acidic are rapidly absorbed from the stomach and the upper small intestine. But aspirin as such is poorly soluble, hence not well-absorbed. When administered as microfine particles, absorption increases. Thus particle size, pH of the gut, solubility of the preparation and presence of food in the stomach influence the absorption.

Flowchart 10.1: Antiplatelet activity of aspirin

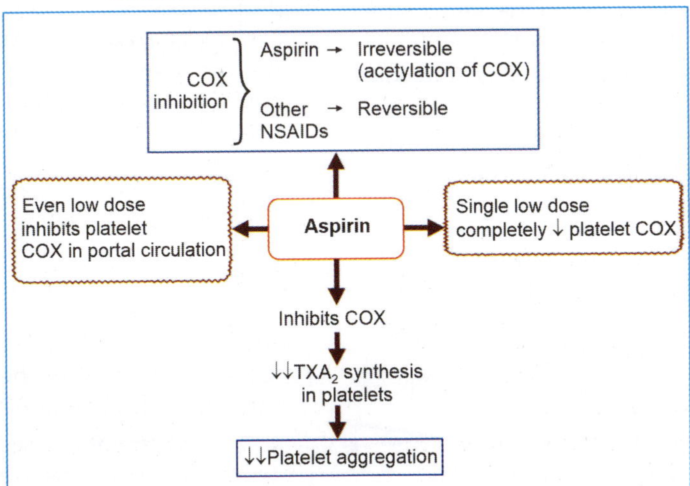

Salicylic acid and methylsalicylate are absorbed from the intact skin. They are extensively bound to plasma proteins. Aspirin is deacetylated in the liver, plasma and other tissues to release salicylic acid which is the active form. Plasma t½ of aspirin is 3–5 hr. Fresh COX is synthesized in the tissues in about 6–12 hr and, therefore, the duration of action. Elimination is dose dependent. It follows first order kinetics in small doses and zero order kinetics in higher doses. Therefore, in anti-inflammatory doses, t½ increases to 12 hr. Salicylates are excreted in the urine. Alkalinization of the urine hastens the excretion of salicylates.

Adverse Effects

Analgesic doses are generally well tolerated but anti-inflammatory doses are usually associated with adverse effects especially when used over a long period.

1. *GI tract:* Nausea, epigastric distress, vomiting, erosive gastritis, peptic ulcer, increased occult blood loss in stools are common.
2. *Nephrotoxicity:* Almost all NSAIDs can cause nephrotoxicity after long-term use **(analgesic nephropathy)** (Flowchart 10.2). Salt and water retention, with hypertension and impaired renal function with acute interstitial nephritis and acute papillary necrosis can occur.
3. *CNS:* Headache, dizziness and confusion.
4. *Allergic reactions* are not common and may be manifested as rashes, urticaria, pruritus, photosensitivity, rhinorrhoea, angioedema, and asthma especially in those with a history of allergies.
5. *Respiratory system:* As aspirin inhibits only cyclo-oxygenase pathway, arachidonic acid is available for conversion by lipoxygenase pathway into leukotrienes. Leukotrienes are powerful bronchoconstrictors. Hence aspirin can precipitate **bronchial asthma** in some individuals. Of the currently available NSAIDs, diclofenac and indomethacin inhibit the synthesis of both PGs and LTs.
6. *Hemolysis:* Salicylates can cause hemolysis in patients with G6PD deficiency. NSAIDs can also rarely cause thrombocytopenia and neutropenia.

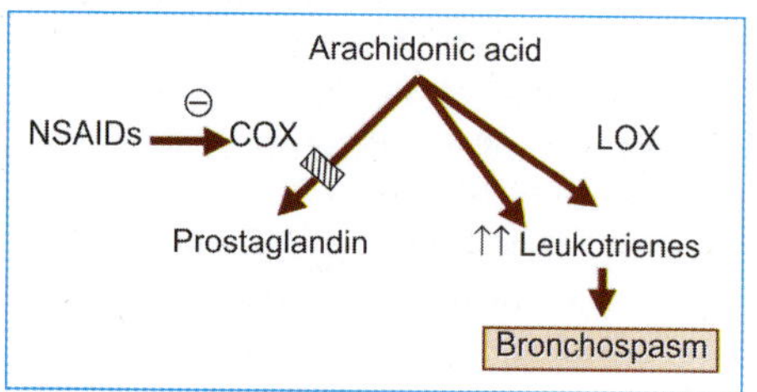

7. *Hepatotoxicity* with heptic necrosis and cholestatic jaundice can also occur when high doses of NSAIDs are used over a long period. Plasma levels of liver enzymes are raised.
8. *Reye's syndrome* seen in children is a form of hepatic encephalopathy which may be fatal. It develops a few days after a viral infection especially influenza and varicella. An increased incidence of this syndrome has been noted when aspirin is used to treat fever. Hence aspirin and other salicylates are contraindicated in children and young subjects <20-year-old with viral fever. Paracetamol may be used to treat fever in such children.
9. *Pregnancy:* Aspirin when taken at term delays the onset of labour due to inhibition of PG synthesis (PGs play an important role in the initiation of labour). Premature closure of ductus arteriosus may occur in the foetus resulting in portal

Flowchart 10.2: Nephropathy by aspirin

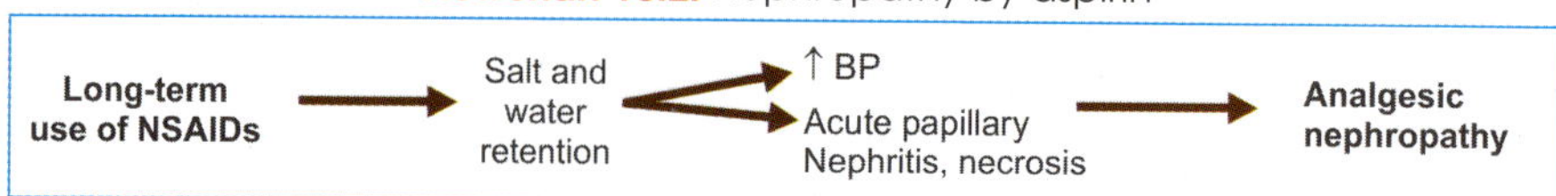

hypertension. It can also increase postpartum bleeding due to inhibition of platelet aggregation.

10. *Salicylism:* Higher doses given for a long time as in treatment of rheumatoid arthritis may cause chronic salicylate intoxication termed 'salicylism'. The syndrome is characterised by headache, vertigo, dizziness, tinnitus, vomiting, mental confusion, diarrhoea, sweating, difficulty in hearing, thirst and dehydration. These symptoms are reversible on withdrawal of salicylates.

Acute salicylate intoxication: Poisoning may be accidental or suicidal. It is more common in children, 15–30 g is the fatal dose of aspirin.

Symptoms and signs: Dehydration, hyperpyrexia, GI irritation, vomiting, sometimes haematemesis, acid–base imbalance, restlessness, delirium, hallucinations, metabolic acidosis, tremors, convulsions, coma and death due to respiratory failure and CV collapse.

Treatment is symptomatic and includes:

1. Gastric lavage to eliminate unabsorbed drugs.
2. IV fluids to correct acid–base imbalance and dehydration.
3. Temperature is brought down by external cooling with alcohol or cold water sponges.
4. If haemorrhagic complications are seen, blood transfusion and vitamin K are needed.
5. The IV fluids should contain Na^+, K^+, HCO_3^- and glucose (to treat hypokalemia and acidosis). Blood pH should be monitored.
6. In severe cases, forced alkaline diuresis with sodium bicarbonate and a diuretic like frusemide is given along with IV fluids. Sodium bicarbonate ionizes salicylates making them water-soluble and enhances their excretion through kidneys.

Precautions and Contraindications

Peptic ulcer, liver diseases, bleeding tendencies and viral fever in children contraindicate the use of aspirin/salicylates

Pregnancy: Aspirin should be avoided in pregnancy because it can cause premature closure of the ductus arteriosus in the foetus. Treatment with NSAIDs should be stopped one week before any surgery because of the risk of bleeding due to antiplatelet effect.

Preparations and dosage of salicylates (Table 10.1).

Uses

1. ***As analgesic:*** For headache, backache, myalgias, arthralgias, neuralgias, toothache and dysmenorrhea. In headache, PGs may be responsible for cerebral vasodilation. NSAIDs inhibit PG synthesis and relieve headache. PG synthesis is

Table 10.1: Transdermal therapeutic system—some examples

Drug	*Preparation*	*Dose*
Aspirin	ASABUF 300, 350 tab; DISPRIN (Aspirin 350 mg and Calcium carbonate 105 mg) ECOSPRIN 75, 150, 325 mg EC- tab	Analgesic—300–600 mg every 6–8 hr Anti-inflammatory—4–6 g/day Antiplatelet effects—75–300 mg/day
Sodium salicylate	325, 650 mg tablets	325–650 mg every 4–8 hr
Salicylic acid	Whitfield's ointment: – Salicylic acid 3% – Benzoic acid 6%	2% ointment; for topical use
Methyl salicylate (oil of wintergreen)	Ointment/liniment for topical use	As counterirritant
Diflunisal	DOLOBID 250, 500 mg tab	250 mg every 8–12 hr

responsible for dysmenorrhea—aspirin effectively relieves pain. The NSAIDs are beneficial in a variety of painful conditions of integumental origin and all these are associated with PG synthesis.

2. ***Fever:*** NSAIDs are useful for the symptomatic relief of fever.
3. ***For inflammatory conditions:*** Aspirin is effective in a number of inflammatory conditions such as arthritis and fibromyositis.
4. ***Acute rheumatic fever:*** In a dose of 4–6 g/day (100 mg/kg/day) in 4–6 divided doses, aspirin brings about a dramatic relief of signs and symptoms in 24–48 hr. The dose is reduced after 4–7 days and maintenance doses of 50 mg/kg/day are given for 2–3 weeks.
5. ***Rheumatoid arthritis:*** Aspirin relieves pain, reduces swelling and redness of joints in rheumatoid arthritis. Joint mobility improves, fever subsides and there is a reduction in morning stiffness. But NSAIDs do not alter the progress of the disease. The relief is only symptomatic.

   Dose: 4–6 g/day in 4–6 divided doses.
6. ***Osteoarthritis:*** NSAIDs provide symptomatic relief in osteoarthritis.
7. ***Postmyocardial infarction and post-stroke:*** Aspirin inhibits platelet aggregation and this may lower the incidence of reinfarction in a low dose of 50 to 300 mg/day. It also decreases the incidence of transient ischemic attacks (TIA) and stroke in such patients.

   Low dose aspirin is also given to patients with angina pectoris with the hope of preventing MI in such patients.

   It is also given in deep vein thrombosis to prevent recurrence.
8. ***Inflammatory bowel disease:*** Mesalamine and sulfasalazine are given orally for local effects in ulcerative colitis. Both are not well absorbed and thereby are available to act on the colon. Mesalamine can be given as rectal suppository or enema. Sulfasalazine is converted to the active metabolite in the colon and acts locally.
9. ***Other uses:***
   i. ***To delay labor:*** Since PGs are involved in the initiation of labour, aspirin delays labour due to PG synthesis inhibition. But such use is associated with the risk of increased bleeding and premature closure of the ductus arteriosus.
   ii. ***Colon cancer prevention:*** Some studies suggest that long-term use of aspirin at low doses is associated with a lower incidence of colon cancer. In familial adenomatous polyposis a hereditary disorder, subjects develop polyps in the colon during younger age and then cancer colon in the older age. Some studies have shown that chemoprophylaxis with aspirin can reduce the risk of colon cancers in such patients.
   iii. ***Patent ductus arteriosus:*** Aspirin may be given to bring about closure of PDA in the newborn.
   iv. ***Bartter's syndrome:*** Excess production of renal PGs is thought to be responsible for Bartter's syndrome characterised by raised plasma renin and aldosterone with hypokalemia. NSAIDs are useful in such patients.
   v. ***Eclampsia:*** Aspirin 60–100 mg daily is recommended in pregnant women with 'high risk' of hypertension. PGs are involved in the genesis of eclampsia and hypertension. Hence, NSAIDs are useful in lowering BP in such patients.
   vi. ***Systemic mastocytosis:*** Excessive proliferation of mast cells in the reticuloendothelial system, bone marrow and other tissues may result in sudden episodes of hypotension. This is due to the release of PGD_2 from the mast cells. Aspirin and other NSAIDs help by PG synthesis inhibition. Histamine blockers to block

the H_1 and H_2 receptors should be given prior to NSAIDs because NSAIDs cause degranulation of mast cells leading to the release of histamine.

vii. ***Niacin flush:*** Niacin used for its hypolipidemic effects often causes intense flushing due to release of PGD_2 from the skin. NSAIDs can be used to prevent flushing as they inhibit PG synthesis.

viii. ***Cataract:*** Aspirin, paracetamol or ibuprofen have been useful to slow the cataract formation. They could act by protecting the lens proteins and preventing changes. However, tolerability may be a problem as higher doses are required.

10. ***Local:*** Salicylic acid is used as a keratolytic, fungistatic and mild antiseptic. Methylsalicylate is a counterirritant used in myalgias. Mesalamine is used in inflammatory bowel disease (*see* page 439).

Drug Interactions

- Salicylates compete for protein binding sites and displace drug molecules resulting in toxicity with warfarin, heparin, naproxen, phenytoin and sulfonylureas. Inhibition of platelet aggregation may increase the risk of bleeding with oral anticoagulants.
- In low doses, salicylates can counter the uricosuric actions of probenecid by decreasing uric acid excretion.
- NSAIDs may blunt the effects of antihypertensives and diuretics by salt and water retention.
- They can potentiate other nephrotoxic drugs because they inhibit PG synthesis in the kidneys.

Diflunisal, a salicylate, has good anti-inflammatory but poor antipyretic activity (poor CNS penetration). It may be used in sprains, rheumatoid and osteoarthritis; available in some countries.

2. PARA-AMINOPHENOL DERIVATIVES

Paracetamol (Acetaminophen)

Phenacetin was the first drug used in this group but, due to severe adverse effects, it was withdrawn. Paracetamol, a metabolite of phenacetin, is found to be safer and effective.

Actions: Paracetamol has analgesic, good antipyretic and **weak anti-inflammatory** properties. The inflammatory sites are rich in peroxides generated by the leukocytes. In the presence of peroxides, paracetamol is a weak inhibitor of COX and thereby PG synthesis. Hence paracetamol has poor anti-inflammatory actions.

Paracetamol is active on cyclo-oxygenase in the brain which accounts for its antipyretic action. In the presence of peroxides which are present at the site of inflammation, paracetamol has a poor ability to inhibit cyclo-oxygenase. It does not stimulate respiration, has no actions on acid–base balance, cellular metabolism, cardiovascular system and platelet function; it is not a uricosuric agent and gastric irritation is mild.

Pharmacokinetics: Paracetamol is well-absorbed orally and 30% protein bound; it is metabolised by the hepatic microsomal enzymes—by glucuronide conjugation (60%) and glutathione conjugation (20%).

Dose: CROCIN 500, 650 mg tab, 120 mg/5 ml suspension, 240 mg/5 ml DS-suspension. DOLO 500, 650 mg tab. 156 mg/ 5 ml, 250 mg/ 5 ml susp.

Adverse effects: In antipyretic doses, paracetamol is safe and well-tolerated. Nausea and rashes may occur. But when large doses are taken, *acute paracetamol poisoning* results. Children are more susceptible because their ability to conjugate by glucuronidation is poor. 10–15 g in adults cause serious toxicity. Symptoms are—nausea, vomiting, anorexia and abdominal pain during first 24 hours. Paracetamol is hepatotoxic and can cause severe hepatic damage. Manifestations are seen within 2–4 days and include increased serum transaminases, jaundice, liver tenderness and prolonged prothrombin time which may progress to liver failure in some patients. Hepatic lesions are reversible when promptly treated.

Nephrotoxicity may result in acute renal failure in some.

Mechanism: A small portion of paracetamol is metabolised to a highly reactive intermediate—**N-acetyl-benzoquinone-imine** which is detoxified generally by conjugation with glutathione. However, when large doses of paracetamol are taken, hepatic glutathione is depleted and the toxic metabolite binds to sulphydryl groups in hepatic proteins resulting in hepatic necrosis.

Chronic alcoholics and infants are more prone to hepatotoxicity.

Treatment: Stomach wash is given. Activated charcoal prevents further absorption. Antidote is—**N-acetylcysteine** (150 mg/kg IV infusion over 15 min repeated as required; oral loading dose—140 mg/kg followed by 70 mg/kg every 4 hr—17 doses)—more effective when given early. N-acetylcysteine partly replenishes the glutathione stores of the liver and prevents binding of toxic metabolites to the cellular constituents.

Uses

- Paracetamol is used as an analgesic in painful conditions like toothache, headache and myalgia
- As an antipyretic.

3. PROPIONIC ACID DERIVATIVES

Ibuprofen is better tolerated than aspirin. Analgesic, antipyretic and anti-inflammatory efficacy is slightly lower than aspirin. It is 99% bound to plasma proteins. Ibuprofen and other propionic acid derivatives are well absorbed, >90% bound to plasma proteins, cross the BBB, also reach the synovial fluid. They are metabolised in the liver and excreted both in bile and through the kidneys.

Ibuprofen is available for oral, parenteral and topical use (gel, cream).

Dose: Ibuprofen: 400–800 mg TDS, BRUFEN 200, 400, 600 FC-tab. IBUGESIC 200, 400, 600 mg FC-tab, 100 mg/5 ml susp, 300 mg SR-cap.

Ketoprofen: KETOPATCH 30 mg patch. OSTOFEN 30 mg cap. RHOFENID 100 mg tab.

Flurbiprofen is used on the eye for its anti-inflammatory properties.

Adverse effects are milder when compared to other NSAIDs and the incidence is low.

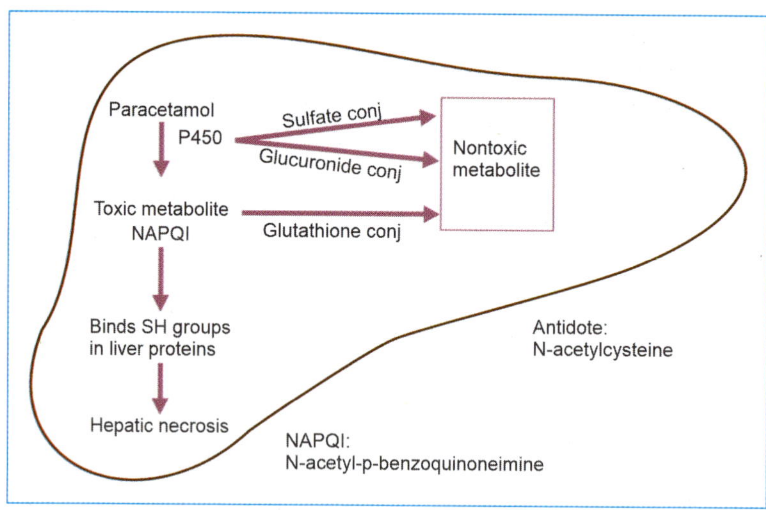

Fig. 10.1: Paracatamol conjugation in liver

Nausea, vomiting, gastric discomfort, CNS effects, hypersensitivity reactions, fluid retention are all similar but **less severe** than phenylbutazone or indomethacin.

Dose: FLUROFEN 100 mg tab. ARFLUR 50, 100 mg tab, 200 mg CR-tab.

Uses

1. As an analgesic in painful conditions.
2. In fever.
3. Soft tissue injuries, fractures, following tooth extraction, to relieve postoperative pain, dysmenorrhea and osteoarthritis.
4. Gout.

Naproxen is longer acting (OD-BD dose) and is a commonly used drug.

Dose: 250–500 mg BD.

4. ACETIC ACID DERIVATIVES

Ketorolac is another PG synthesis inhibitor having good analgesic and anti-inflammatory properties. It is used for its analgesic properties to relieve postoperative pain. It is mostly used parenterally though it can also be given orally.

Indomethacin is a potent anti-inflammatory agent, antipyretic and good analgesic. It is well-absorbed, 90% bound to plasma proteins; t½—4–6 hr. It undergoes enterohepatic circulation.

Dose: 25–50 mg BD-TDS, INDOCID 25 mg cap.

Adverse effects are high—gastrointestinal irritation with nausea, GI bleeding, vomiting, diarrhoea, peptic ulcers and pancreatitis can occur.

CNS effects include headache, dizziness, ataxia, confusion, hallucinations, depression and psychosis.

Hypersensitivity reactions like skin rashes, leukopenia, and asthma in aspirin sensitive individuals. It can also cause bleeding due to decreased platelet aggregation and edema due to salt and water retention.

It should be avoided in patients with renal failure, thrombocytopenia and raised serum bilirubin.

Drug Interactions

- Indomethacin blunts the diuretic action of furosemide and the antihypertensive action of thiazides, furosemide, beta blockers and ACE inhibitors by causing **salt and water retention.** Pancreatic and renal papillary necrosis have been reported occasionally.
- Indomethacin + warfarin—risk of bleeding is higher. Gastric erosions may bleed or the bleeding may not easily stop due to anticoagulant effect.

Uses (Table 10.2)

1. For closure of patent ductus arteriosus (PDA) in premature infants.
2. Though indomethacin is effective in reducing pain and inflammation in RA, ankylosing spondylitis, gout and psoriatic arthritis, wide range of adverse effects have made it the least preferred of the NSAIDs.
3. Epidural indomethacin is tried for pain relief in patients who have undergone laminectomy.
4. Topical
   i. Eye drops in inflammation.
   ii. As mouthrinse—to suppress gingival inflammation.

Dose: 25 –50 mg BD-QID. INDOCAP, MICROCID 25, 75 mg SR-cap.

Sulindac has weaker analgesic, antipyretic and anti-inflammatory actions but is less toxic. Does not antagonize the diuretic and antihypertensive actions of thiazides. It may be used as an alternative drug for inflammatory conditions.

5. FENAMATES (ANTHRANILIC ACID DERIVATIVES)

Fenamates are analgesic, antipyretic, anti-inflammatory drugs with less efficacy, and are more toxic; contraindicated in children. They should not be used for more than one week.

Table 10.2: Topical preparations of NSAIDs

NSAID	Preparation	Brand name
Salicylic acid	6% w/w oint	KERALIN with hydrocortisone acetate and benzoic acid.
	3% oint	MYCODERM with benzoic acid and menthol
	2.2% ear drops	METHAZIL with 6% methanol
Diclofenac diethyl ammonium	1.16% gel	VOVERAN, Relaxyl, Inac gel.
	eye drops	DIFENIC 0.1% w/v, OXALGIN 0.1% w/v
Piroxicam	0.5% gel	DOLONEX gel, PIROX gel.
Ibuprofen	50 mg gel	ACKS gel with mephenisin,methyl salicylate and menthol
Flurbiprofen	0.03% w/v eye drops	OCUFLUR
Indomethacin	1% w/v eye drops	INDOCAP ophthalmic drops.
Naproxen	10% gel	XENOLID gel.
Ketorolac tromethamine	0.5% w/v eye drops	KETANOV eye drops Ketlur
Nimesulide	10 mg gel	NIZU gel with menthol 50 mg and methyl salicylate 100 mg.

They are not preferred. Mephenamic acid is the fenamate in use.

Adverse effects GI side effects are similar to aspirin but GI bleeding is less. Diarrhea is common.

- As an analgesic in myalgias;
- Mefenamic acid is commonly used in dysmenorrhea (250–500 mg TDS).

6. PYRAZOLONE DERIVATIVES

Phenylbutazone has good anti-inflammatory activity, is more potent, but has poorer analgesic and antipyretic effects. It is a uricosuric agent. However, phenylbutazone is more toxic than aspirin and is poorly tolerated; can cause gastrointestinal side effects, salt and water retention hypothyroidism, haematological toxicity including agranulocytosis and CNS adverse effects. Because of its toxicity, phenylbutazone is **withdrawn from the market** in most countries.

Azapropazone is structurally related to phenylbutazone but is less likely to cause agranulocytosis.

Metamizol is a potent analgesic and antipyretic, but poor anti-inflammatory agent and has no uricosuric properties; 500 mg 3–4 times a day. It offers no advantages over aspirin. Not recommended in children up to 6 years.

ANALGIN, NOVALGIN, 500 mg tab.

Propiphenazone is similar to metamizol.

Dose: 300–600 mg 3–4 times a day (SARIDON).

7. OXICAMS (ENOLIC ACID DERIVATIVES)

Piroxicam is an oxicam derivative, has good anti-inflammatory, analgesic and antipyretic activity. No clinically significant drug interactions are seen; better tolerated as it is less ulcerogenic. It is almost completely absorbed, 99% bound to plasma proteins. It has slow onset of action and is **longer acting**—given once daily (20 mg OD).

Piroxicam is used for rheumatoid arthritis, osteoarthritis, ankylosing spondylitis, acute musculoskeletal pain and postoperative pain and painful dental lesions.

Dose: UGESIC 20 mg tab. DOLONEX 20 mg cap, 20 mg/ml inj. BREXIC 10, 20 mg cap.

Tenoxicam is similar to piroxicam.

Many other oxicams are being developed with the idea of obtaining one which is non-ulcerogenic. Most of them are prodrugs of piroxicam and in lower doses some of them are selective COX-2 inhibitors.

PREFERENTIAL COX-2 INHIBITORS

Diclofenac is an analgesic, antipyretic and anti-inflammatory agent. Its tissue penetrability is good and attains good concentration in synovial fluid which is maintained for a long time. Diclofenac almost selectively inhibits COX-2 as a result is more 'gastric-friendly' and also has poor antiplatelet activity (COX-1 mediated). It is well absorbed, quickly attains therapeutic levels but bioavailability is only 50% due to first pass effects; it is extensively protein bound. It is metabolised by microsomal enzymes in the liver. Adverse effects are similar to other NSAIDs but are milder. Extended release preparations are available. Gel is available for topical application. Ophthalmic preparation is used for postoperative pain; rectal suppository and mouthwashes are also available (Table 10.3).

Aceclofenac is more gastric-friendly as it is more COX-2 selective and is also **longer acting.** Hence it is now preferred over diclofenac.

Dose: Diclofenac: 50 mg BD-TDS. VOVERAN 50 mg cap, gel. INAC gel.

Aceclofenac: 100 mg BD, **DOLOWIN** 100 mg tab.

Uses

Diclofenac and aceclofenac are the most commonly used NSAIDs.

1. Treatment of chronic inflammatory conditions like rheumatoid arthritis and osteoarthritis.
2. Acute musculoskeletal pain, painful dental lesions.
3. Postoperatively for relief of pain and inflammation.
4. ***Eye:*** To reduce ocular inflammation.

Nabumetone is an anti-inflammatory agent with significant efficacy in rheumatoid arthritis and osteoarthritis. It shows a relatively low incidence of side effects, and it is comparatively less ulcerogenic. It is a prodrug and also preferentially inhibits COX-2—both account for the low ulcerogenic potential. It is used in rheumatoid and osteoarthritis.

Dose: NABUFLAM 500 mg tab. NILTIS 500, 750 mg tab.

Meloxicam is similar to piroxicam, but in lower doses, it causes less gastric irritation than piroxicam. It **preferentially binds to COX-2** which could be responsible for less ulcerogenic activity. It is, therefore, better tolerated.

Dose: 7.5–15 mg OD, M-CAM, MELFLAM 7.5, 15 mg tab.

Nimesulide, a sulfonamide compound, has a higher affinity for COX-2 than COX-1. It preferentially inhibits COX-2 and in addition has antihistaminic and antiallergic properties. Nimesulide has analgesic, antipyretic and anti-inflammatory actions like other NSAIDs.

Adverse effects are nausea, epigastric pain, rashes, drowsiness, dizziness and nephrotoxicity. Nimesulide can cause **hepatotoxicity** particularly on prolonged use.

Though nimesulide can be used as an analgesic, antipyretic and anti-inflammatory agent, particularly in patients who develop bronchospasm with other NSAIDs, because

What's in a name? — Melflam or Melphalan

A senior orthopedician prescribed MELFLAM (meloxicam) for joints pain to 50-year-old-Krishnan. The pharmacist read it as melphalan, an anticancer drug—the Doctor's handwriting after all! The patient promptly swallowed the tablets and understandably also obtained relief from joints pain (rheumatoid arthritis) as melphalan is also an immunosuppressant. Unfortunately he asked for a refill(!) and continued the medication for almost 2 months when he started experiencing full blown effects of bone marrow depression, which was almost fatal. The cause was detected with great difficulty and was referred to a superspeciality hospital in Mumbai. After several weeks of intensive care, the patient recovered but sued the doctor for his negligence.

Table 10.3: Properties of some commonly used NSAIDs

NSAID	*Properties*	*Adverse effects*	*Uses*
Aspirin	Analgesic, anti-inflammatory, rheumatic fever, rheumatoid, psoriatic and osteoarthritis, closure of PDA; to delay labor or antiplatelet activity in post-stroke and post-MI	Gastritis, nausea, allergic reactions, precipitation of bronchial asthma, nephro-toxicity, hepatotoxicity, Reye's syndrome, delayed onset of labour, salicylism	Antiplatelet activity even in low dose, **good anti-inflammatory,** analgesic, Uricosuric agent. Irreversible inhibitor of COX-1 and COX-2
Paracetamol	Fever, as analgesic in head-ache, backache, dysmenor-rhoea, myalgia and other painful conditions	Less gastric irritant, large doses—hepatotoxicity (toxic metabolite N-acetyl-benzoquinone-imine)	Good analgesic, antipyretic but weak anti-inflammatory (weak PG inhibition in the periphery). Antidote: n-acetylcysteine
Diclofenac	Chronic inflammatory condi-tions, rheumatoid arthritis, osteoarthritis, acute musculo-skeletal pain and post-operative pain	Same as aspirin	Good concentration in **synovial fluid,** adverse effects milder; **aceclo-fenac** is longer acting and more gastric friendly
Ibuprofen, naproxen	Analgesic anti-inflammatory, and antipyretic, all actions milder than aspirin	Same as aspirin, but milder	Good analgesic, anti-inflammatory, antipyretic
Piroxicam	Arthritis, musculoskeletal pain	Same as aspirin, but milder gastric irritant.	Good analgesic, antipyretic anti-inflammatory. **Longer acting—OD dose**
Phenylbutazone	Rheumatoid arthritis, osteoarthritis, ankylosing spondylitis	Same as aspirin, but more salt and water retention, more toxic than aspirin.	Salt and water retention, poor analgesic, antipyretic **Not preferred**
Indomethacin	Rheumatoid, psoriatic arthritis; good anti-inflammatory and antipyretic but toxicity is high	Toxicity high-peptic ulcera-tion, oedema, agranulo-cytosis, hypothyroidism, insomnia, vertigo, optic neuritis, blurred vision, convulsions	Because of toxicity, it is **withdrawn** in many countries
Mephenamic acid	Dysmenorrhoea, myalgias	Gastric irritation, diarrhoea	Efficacy low, more toxic, contraindicated in children, used for short periods
Celecoxib	Good anti-inflammatory, analgesic, antipyretic	Higher risk of CV throm-botic events; Nausea, gastritis—milder, rashes, drowsiness, dizziness, nephrotoxicity, hepatotoxicity	Does not inhibit platelet aggregation, highly selective COX-2 inhibitor

of the risk of hepatotoxicity, nimesulide is **now banned** in most countries including India.

SELECTIVE COX-2 INHIBITORS

Coxibs

Though NSAIDs are extremely useful drugs, they are poorly tolerated particularly when they are used for long periods. Gastric irritation is the common side effect which limits its use. Selective inhibition of COX-2 was found to be advantageous because COX-2 is involved in inflammation and COX-1 which is protective on gastroduodenal mucosa is spared (Fig. 10.2). Some of the older NSAIDs have relative selectivity for selective COX-2 (meloxicam) but

COMPARE AND CONTRAST

Aspirin and Celecoxib (nonselective and selective COX-2 inhibitors)

Features	*Aspirin*	*Celecoxib*
Chemistry	Salicylic acid derivative	Sulfonamide derivative
COX inhibition	Non-selective (COX-1, COX-2)	Selective COX-2 inhibitor
Ulcerogenic effect on gastric mucosa	+++ (Significant)	+ (Mild)
t½	Short (2–3 hours)	Long (6–12 hours)
Effect on platelet function	Inhibits platelet aggregation	Does not
Risk of Reye's syndrome in children	Present	Nil
Risk of thrombosis, atherogenesis	Nil	Present
Cardiovascular toxicity	No significant effect	Risk of MI
Cerebrovascular toxicity	No significant effect	Risk of stroke
Use in post-MI patients	Recommended	Contraindicated
Prominent action	Analgesic, antipyretic, anti-inflammatory	Analgesic, antipyretic, anti-inflammatory
PG synthesis	Inhibited	Inhibited

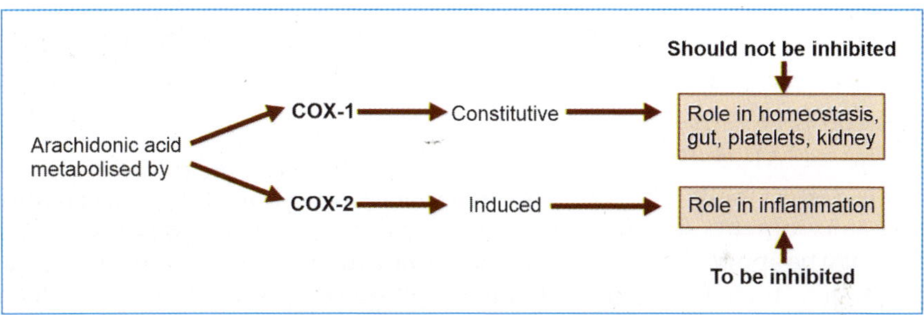

Fig. 10.2: Role of COX-1 amd COX-2

highly selective COX-2 inhibitors with several times greater selectivity for COX-2 have been synthesized—like the coxibs—**celecoxib, parecoxib and etoricoxib.** These drugs have analgesic, anti-inflammatory and antipyretic effects like non-selective NSAIDs but with much less gastric ulcerogenic effects. They also do not inhibit platelet aggregation because COX-1 is involved in platelet function. However, many of the coxibs have been withdrawn due to the adverse effects.

Adverse Effects

Clinical studies have shown that use of selective COX-2 inhibitors increase the risk of cardiovascular and cerebrovascular thrombotic events—**may increase the risk of myocardial infarction and stroke. Hence most of them (like rofecoxib) were withdrawn** from the market and the others are under supervision. They are indicated only in patients who cannot tolerate NSAIDs and are at a high risk of developing peptic ulcer.

Celecoxib

Celecoxib, a diaryl substituted compound is highly selective COX-2 (10–20 times) inhibitor. It has good anti-inflammatory, analgesic and antipyretic properties but does not affect platelet aggregation. In such indications too, they should be used in the minimum effective dose for a short period only.

Celecoxib is better tolerated because of **milder gastric irritation (due to COX-2 selectivity)**. It can cause hypertension and edema which can be troublesome in patients with cardiovascular problems. It can be used in acute painful conditions like postoperative pain, dysmenorrhea and dental pain as well as in osteoarthritis and rheumatoid arthritis in patients who cannot tolerate other NSAIDs.

Dose: Anti-inflammatory—100–200 mg OD- BD. COXIB, CELCOX, ZECOXIB 100, 200 mg cap.

Etoricoxib is highly selective for COX-2 and long acting to be given once daily. It is better tolerated than other selective COX-2 inhibitors.

Dose: ETOXIB, HICOX 60, 90, 120 mg tab.

Parecoxib, a prodrug of valdecoxib, can be given parenterally.

Topical NSAID Preparations

Topical NSAID preparations (Table 10.2). Some of the NSAIDs like diclofenac, ibuprofen and paracetamol are available for topical use as ointments and transdermal patch. They may be applied to the site of pain to avoid systemic toxicity. Some systemic absorption occurs but efficacy of these is low. Many NSAIDs are also available as eye drops.

Drugs that Inhibit Both Cyclo-oxygenase and Lipoxygenase

Diclofenac, ketoprofen and **indomethacin** are drugs that block both cyclo-oxygenase and lipoxygenase. These are less likely to precipitate acute attacks of bronchial asthma because they also inhibit leukotriene synthesis.

Atypical NSAID

Diacerin has been found to have useful activity in osteoarthritis patients. It inhibits interleukin-1β (IL-1β) which is involved in the inflammation as well as destruction of the joint cartilage in patients with osteoarthritis. It is well tolerated with minor adverse effects like mild diarrhea which could subside on continued use. It colors the urine a deep yellow. Diacerin is used for long-term, generally 6–8 months in osteoarthritis.

Clinical Pharmacology

- NSAIDs afford symptomatic relief of pain—are good antipyretic and anti-inflammatory agents.
- Aspirin is mostly used for antiplatelet effects while other better tolerated NSAIDs may be used for inflammatory conditions.
- Diclofenac, aceclofenac, ibuprofen and piroxicam are commonly used. They are also available for topical use as gels, cream and as eye drops.
- All of them cause gastric irritation but the extent varies. Hence should be taken with food.
- Paracetamol is safe and effective for fever, myalgia and conditions of milder pain.
- Diclofenac is particularly useful in joints pain as it attains good concentration in the synovial fluid and remains there for a long period.
- Analgesic nephropathy, salt and water retention are seen with prolonged use of higher doses of NSAIDs.

[1] From Medical Council of India, *Competency based Undergraduate Curriculum for the Indian Medical Graduate*, 2018;1:136–144.

CHAPTER 11

Drugs Used in Rheumatoid Arthritis and Gout

Competency achievement: The student should be able to:

PH 1.16 Describe mechanism/s of action, types, doses, side effects, indications and contraindications of the drugs which act by modulating autacoids, including: Antihistaminics, 5-HT modulating drugs, NSAIDs, drugs for gout, anti-rheumatic drugs, drugs for migraine.[1]

Rheumatoid arthritis (RA) is a chronic, progressive, autoimmune, inflammatory disease, mainly affecting the joints and the periarticular tissues. Antigen–antibody complexes trigger the pathological process. Mediators of inflammation released in the joints initiate the inflammatory process. The earliest lesion is vasculitis, followed by synovial edema and infiltration with inflammatory cells. There is local synthesis of prostaglandins and leukotrienes. Prostaglandins cause vasodilation and pain. The inflammatory cells release lysosomal enzymes which cause damage to bones and cartilage.

Drugs used in the treatment of rheumatoid arthritis are:

I. NSAIDs
II. Glucocorticoids
III. DMARDs
1. ***Immunosuppressants:*** Methotrexate, cyclophosphamide, azathioprine, cyclosporine, leflunomide, chloroquine, hydroxychloroquine
2. ***Biological agents:***
   a. *TNF-alpha blockers:* Etanercept, infliximab, adalimumab, certolizumab, golimumab
   b. *Other biologicals:* Abatacept, anakinra, rituximab, kanakinumab, tocilizumab, lituximab
3. ***Miscellaneous:*** Gold salts, penicillamine, sulphasalazine

NONSTEROIDAL ANTI-INFLAMMATORY DRUGS

Nonsteroidal anti-inflammatory drugs only **provide symptomatic relief** but do not modify the course of the disease. Long-term use of these drugs is associated with significant toxicity; higher doses are required for anti-inflammatory activity. Aspirin, ibuprofen, diclofenac, naproxen, and piroxicam are commonly used. Most of the selective COX-2 inhibitors except 1–2 are now withdrawn due to toxicity.

GLUCOCORTICOIDS

Detailed pharmacology is discussed in Chapter 39. Glucocorticoids have anti-inflammatory and immunosuppressant activity. They produce prompt and dramatic relief of symptoms but do not arrest the progress of the disease. However, long-term use of these drugs leads to several adverse effects. Moreover, on withdrawal of glucocorticoids, there may be an exacerbation of the disease. Therefore, glucocorticoids are used only as adjuvants. They may be used to treat exacerbations. Low dose long-term treatment with prednisolone (5–10 mg/day) or IM depot methylprednisolone 80–160 mg are used in some patients. Intra-articular corticosteroids are helpful to relieve pain in severely inflamed joints.

DISEASE MODIFYING ANTI-RHEUMATIC DRUGS

Disease modifying anti-rheumatic drugs (DMARDs) are also called disease modifying drugs (DMDs). These are reserved for patients with progressive disease who do not obtain satisfactory relief from NSAIDs. They are capable of arresting the progress of the disease and inducing remission in these patients. Recent studies have shown that RA causes significant systemic effects that shorten life expectancy. This has renewed interest in the use of DMDs in RA. The effects of these drugs may take 6 weeks to 6 months to become evident and are, therefore, also called slow-acting anti-rheumatic drugs (SAARDs).

Immunosuppressants

Methotrexate, cyclophosphamide, azathioprine and leflunomide are the immunosuppressants used in RA. They are cytotoxic drugs and are reserved for patients with seriously crippling disease with reversible lesions after conventional therapy has failed. Among the immunosuppressants, methotrexate is the best tolerated.

Methotrexate: In lower doses than that used in cancers (*see* page 671), methotrexate affords significant benefit in patients with rheumatoid arthritis. Mechanism of action of methotrexate in RA is probably that:

- It increases adenosine levels which is a potent inhibitor of inflammation.
- Methotrexate also inhibits cytokines, directly suppresses the cells involved in inflammation and immunological diseases and stimulates apoptosis of these cells.
- Inhibition of DHFR could influence macrophage and lymphocyte function.

Methotrexate is now the **most commonly used drug** in autoimmune disorders. Leucovorin rescue may be given to reduce toxicity. Toxicity includes nausea, mucosal ulcers, bone marrow suppression and hepatotoxicity. Weekly regimens of low oral doses are better tolerated.

Dose: ALLTREX 2.5 mg tab, 5 mg/ml inj. CARDITREX 2.5 mg tab, 25 mg vial.

Azathioprine, a purine analog, is a prodrug converted to 6-thioguanine in the body. It suppresses the cell-mediated immunity and inhibits T and B cell function. It is used as an alternative to methotrexate.

Dose: AZORAN 25 mg tab. AZAP 50 mg tab.

Cyclophosphamide, an alkylating agent, also inhibits T cell and B cell function. It is given orally in RA and other autoimmune disorders.

Dose: CYPHOS, NEOPHOS 200, 500 mg 1 g inj. ONCOMIDE 50 mg tab, 200, 500 mg, 1 g, vial.

Leflunomide is a prodrug. The active metabolite inhibits autoimmune T cell proliferation and production of autoantibodies by B cells. Leflunomide is orally effective, undergoes enterohepatic circulation and has a long t½ of 5–40 days.

Adverse effects include diarrhoea and raised hepatic enzymes. It can also cause weight gain, hypertension and sometimes alopecia.

Leflunomide is used with methotrexate in rheumatoid arthritis patients not responding to methotrexate alone.

Dose: Initially 100 mg daily for 3 days followed by 20 mg OD. CLEFT, LEFRA, RUMALEF 10, 20 mg tab. LEFUMIDE, LISIFEN 10, 20 mg FC-tab.

Cyclosporine is an immunosuppressant that has now been approved for use in RA, SLE, psoriasis and polymyositis. It is given orally 2–5 mg/kg/day and the dose is gradually increased.

Mycophenolate mofetil has been occasionally used in RA but its efficacy is yet to be established.

Hydroxychloroquine and chloroquine: These antimalarial drugs (*see* page 634) are found to be useful in mild non-erosive rheumatoid arthritis. They induce remission in 50% of patients. Mechanism of action is not exactly understood but they are known to depress cell-mediated immunity.

Toxicity: Chloroquine and hydroxychloroquine accumulate in tissues leading to toxicity. The most significant side effect is the **retinal damage** on long-term use. This toxicity is **less common and reversible** with **hydroxychloroquine which is, therefore, preferred over chloroquine in rheumatoid arthritis.** Every 3 months eyes should be tested. Other adverse effects include myopathy, neuropathy and irritable bowel syndrome.

Chloroquine: CADIQUIN 250, 500 mg tab.

Hydroxychloroquine: Dose: 400 mg/day for 4–6 wks; maintenance dose—200 mg/day. HCQS 200, 400 mg tab. ZY-Q 200 mg tab.

Biological Agents

TNF-α Blocking Agents

Cytokines, particularly tumor necrosis factor (TNF-α) plays an important role in the process of inflammation. TNF-α produced by macrophages and activated T cells, acts through TNF-α receptors to stimulate the release of other cytokines. TNF-α blocking drugs infliximab, entanercept and adalimumab, are found to be useful in rheumatoid arthritis.

Infliximab is a monoclonal antibody which specifically binds with high affinity to human TNF-α. When given in combination with methotrexate, it slows the progression of rheumatoid arthritis. It is given intravenously as an infusion 3–5 mg/kg every 8 hr. It has a long t½ of 9–12 days. Adverse effects of the combination include increased susceptibility to upper respiratory infections; dormant tuberculosis may become active. Nausea, headache, cough, sinusitis, skin rashes and allergic reactions can occur. Rarely hepatitis and activation of viral hepatitis have been reported. Antinuclear and anti-DNA antibodies may develop and this can be largely avoided by giving methotrexate along with infliximab.

Dose: 3–5 mg / kg 8 hrly. REMICADE 10 mg vial

Uses: Infliximab can be used in many conditions of autoimmune aetiology like ankylosing spondylitis, Crohn's disease, psoriasis, ulcerative colitis and sarcoidosis. Infliximab is used in RA along with methotrexate or one of the other DMARDs.

Etanercept is a recombinant fusion protein that binds to TNF-α molecules. It is given subcutaneously and is found to slow the progression of the disease in rheumatoid arthritis patients. It is also found to be useful in psoriatic and juvenile arthritis. Etanercept is also given with methotrexate and the combination has a higher efficacy.

Pain, itching and allergic reactions at the site of injection, anti-etanercept antibodies and anti-DNA antibodies have been detected.

Dose: 50 mg weekly SC. ENBREL 25, 50 mg inj.

Adalimumab is an anti-TNF monoclonal antibody which acts similar to infliximab but is less immunogenic. It is given SC 40 mg/week. It is used along with methotrexate for better efficacy.

Certolizumab is an anti-TNF-α antibody which neutralizes TNF-α. It is given subcutaneously every 2–4 weeks in moderate to severe RA as monotherapy with other DMARDs

Golimumab—another anti-TNF-α antibody used SC with methotrexate every 4 weeks in moderate to severe RA.

Other Biologicals

Abatacept inhibits the activation of T cells. It has a long t½ of 13–16 days. Given as IV infusion 800–1000 mg and repeated after 2 and 4 weeks brings about a symptomatic improvement. The infusion is then repeated at monthly intervals. It is well tolerated, may cause hypersensitivity reactions on infusion. Abatacept may increase the risk of upper respiratory infections particularly if combined with TNF alpha blockers and the combination should be avoided.

Anakinra is a recombinant IL-1 receptor antagonist tried in patients not responding to other DMARDs.

Rituximab is an anti-B lymphocyte monoclonal antibody against B cells and is used in lymphomas (*see* page 680). Reduction in B cells suppresses the inflammatory process, inhibits the release of cytokines. It has been approved for use in moderate to severe active RA along with methotrexate.

Tocilizumab—IL-6, a proinflammatory cytokine is produced by most inflammatory cells including T cells and B cells. Tocilizumab is **an IL-6 antagonist** (antibody) which binds to IL-6 receptors and blocks its action. Tocilizumab may be used (IV once in 4 weeks) as monotherapy or with a DMARD in moderate to severe RA who have failed to respond to other DMARDs. Increased susceptibility to infection is a limiting factor. It is also found to be useful in Covid-19 infections.

Miscellaneous Anti-Rheumatic Drugs

Gold salts: Aurothiomalate and auranofin are **no more preferred** because of their toxicity and the availability of safer agents. Gold depresses cell-mediated immunity (CMI). Treatment with gold is associated with several adverse effects. Dermatitis, hepatotoxicity, nephrotoxicity, encephalitis, peripheral neuritis, pulmonary fibrosis and bone marrow suppression can occur.

d-Penicillamine is a metabolite of penicillin, a chelating agent that chelates copper. Its actions and toxicities are similar to gold and hence it is not preferred.

Sulphasalazine is a compound of sulphapyridine and 5-amino salicylic acid. In the colon, sulphasalazine is split by the bacterial action and sulphapyridine gets absorbed. This has anti-inflammatory actions though the mechanism is not known.

Adverse effects include gastrointestinal upset and skin rashes.

Dose: 500–1000 mg BD-TDS. IWATA 500 mg tab.

Immunoadsorption apheresis: Extracorporeal immunoadsorption of plasma for the removal of IgG-containing immunocomplexes has been approved for the treatment of moderate to severe rheumatoid arthritis. The duration of benefit varies from a few months to several years. Adverse effects are mild and tolerable.

Diet and inflammation: Clinical studies have shown that when patients of rheumatoid arthritis are given a diet (such as marine fish) rich in unsaturated fatty acids like omega-3 fatty acids. viz eicosapentaenoic acid and docosahexaenoic acid (*see* page 390), there is a decrease in morning stiffness, pain and swelling of the joints. Unsaturated fatty acids compete with arachidonic acid for uptake and metabolism. Moreover, the metabolic products of unsaturated fatty acids are only weak inflammatory mediators when compared to the products of arachidonic acid metabolism. Adequate consumption of marine fish should be recommended. For people who do not eat fish, eicosapentaenoic acid 1–4 g/day may be given as tablets. It serves as an adjuvant.

Clinical Pharmacology

- In mild RA, NSAIDs are tried. Diclofenac is the first choice but presently aceclofenac is preferred to diclofenac because it is more gastric-friendly, longer acting and better tolerated.
- In patients presenting with pain and swelling, a short course of glucocorticoids is given, followed by methotrexate or hydroxychloroquine.
- Methotrexate (low dose) can be given for long-term suppression but bone marrow and liver functions should be monitored.
- Patients not responding to methotrexate are given second-line drugs—leflunomide, etanercept or infliximab. Etanercept and infliximab are very expensive.
- Physiotherapy is given to prevent joint stiffness and improve mobility.

PHARMACOTHERAPY OF GOUT

Gout is a familial metabolic disorder characterised by recurrent episodes of acute arthritis due to deposits of monosodium urate in the joints and cartilage. There is an inherent abnormality of purine metabolism resulting in over production of uric acid—a major end product of purine metabolism. As uric acid is poorly water-soluble, it gets precipitated—especially at low pH and deposited in the cartilages of joints and ears, subcutaneous tissues, bursae and sometimes in kidneys. An acute attack of gout occurs as an inflammatory reaction to crystals of sodium urate deposited in the joint tissue. There is infiltration of granulocytes which phagocytize the urate crystals and release a glycoprotein that causes joint destruction. The joint becomes red, swollen, tender and extremely painful.

Secondary hyperuricaemia may be drug-induced or may occur in lymphomas, leukaemias and polycythemia. Chemotherapy and radiation could also result in hyperuricaemia due to increased metabolism of nucleic acids and thereby increased production of uric acid. Several drugs can also induce hyperuricaemia. Gout may also be due to decreased excretion of uric acid.

Strategy in the treatment of gout is either to decrease the biosynthesis of uric acid or increase its excretion.

Drugs Used in Gout

In acute gout

- Colchicine, NSAIDs

In chronic gout

1. *Uric acid synthesis inhibitors*
   Allopurinol, febuxostat, rasburicase, pegloticase
2. *Uricosuric drugs*
   Probenecid, sulphinpyrazone, benzbromarone, lesinurad

Colchicine is an alkaloid of *Colchicum autumnale*. It is a unique anti-inflammatory agent effective only against gouty arthritis. It is not an analgesic and also does not alter the production of uric acid.

Actions: In gout, colchicine is highly effective in acute attacks and it dramatically relieves pain within a few hours.

Mechanism of action: Colchicine inhibits the migration of granulocytes into the inflamed area and the release of glycoprotein by them. It binds to the protein tubulin and prevents its polymerization into microtubules and inhibits the migration of leukocytes and also their phagocytosis.

Other actions: Colchicine binds to microtubules and arrests cell division in metaphase. It increases gut motility by neurogenic stimulation.

Pharmacokinetics: Colchicine is rapidly absorbed orally, metabolised in the liver and undergoes enterohepatic circulation.

Dose: COLJOY, ZYCOLCHIN 0.5 mg tab.

Adverse effects are dose related. Nausea, vomiting, diarrhea and abdominal pain are the earliest side effects. Though these may be avoided by giving colchicine intravenously, it can cause serious toxicity and hence IV colchicine should be avoided. Anemia, leukopenia and alopecia may be seen. In high doses, hemorrhagic gastroenteritis, nephrotoxicity, muscular paralysis, acute renal failure, respiratory failure, shock and fatal CNS depression can occur.

Uses

1. *Acute gout:* Colchicine 1 mg orally initially, followed by 0.5 mg every 2–3 hours relieves pain and swelling within 12 hours. But diarrhea limits its use.
2. *Prophylaxis:* Colchicine may also be used for the prophylaxis of recurrent episodes of gouty arthritis 0.6 mg OD-TDS.

NSAIDs afford symptomatic relief in the treatment of gout due to their anti-inflammatory activity. Indomethacin is the most commonly used agent in acute gout. Piroxicam, naproxen, diclofenac and other newer NSAIDs are also used. They relieve an acute attack in 12–24 hours and are better tolerated than colchicine. They can be given in lower doses for 2–4 weeks. But NSAIDs are not recommended for long-term use due to their toxicity.

Allopurinol is an analog of hypoxanthine and inhibits the biosynthesis of uric acid.

Mechanism of action: Purine nucleotides are degraded to hypoxanthine. Uric acid is produced from hypoxanthine as shown in Fig. 11.1. Allopurinol and its metabolite alloxanthine both inhibit the enzyme xanthine oxidase and thereby prevent the synthesis of uric acid. The plasma concentration of uric acid is reduced.

Pharmacokinetics: Allopurinol is 80% absorbed orally; t½ of allopurinol is 2–3 hr; and t½ of alloxanthine, 24 hr.

Adverse effects are mild. Hypersensitivity reactions include fever and rashes. Gastrointestinal irritation, headache, nausea and dizziness may occur.

Attacks of acute gouty arthritis may be seen frequently during the initial months of treatment with allopurinol.

Drug interactions: The anticancer drugs, 6-mercaptopurine and azathioprine, are metabolised by xanthine oxidase. Hence when allopurinol is used concurrently, the dose of these anticancer drugs should be reduced.

Uses: Allopurinol is used in chronic gout and secondary hyperuricaemia. Initial dose is 100 mg/day and may be gradually increased to 300 mg/day depending on the response. Colchicine or an NSAID should be given during the first few weeks of allopurinol therapy to prevent the acute attacks of gouty arthritis. On treatment with allopurinol, tophi are gradually resorbed and the formation of renal stones is prevented. In patients with large tophaceous deposits, both allopurinol and uricosuric drugs can be given.

Dose: 100–300 mg OD. ALORIC, ALURID, CIPLORIC 100, 300 mg tab.

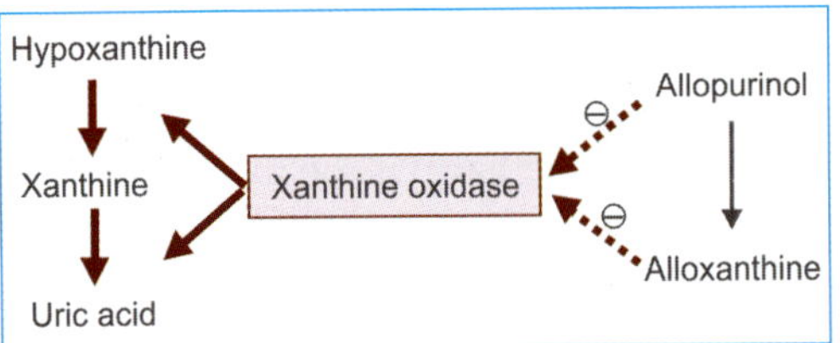

Fig. 11.1: Biosynthesis of uric acid. Both allopurinol and alloxanthine suppress the enzyme xanthine oxidase

Febuxostat is another xanthine oxidase inhibitor but is not a purine. It reduces the formation of xanthine and uric acid. Like allopurinol, treatment with febuxostat can cause gout flares. It can also cause nausea, diarrhea, headache and altered liver function.

Febuxostat is well absorbed and extensively metabolised in the liver. It is used in the dose of 80–120 mg for the treatment of chronic gout.

Uricase Analogs

Rasburicase: Uricase (urate oxidase) is an enzyme present in mammals but absent in human beings. It converts uric acid to allantoin which is a highly soluble product easily excreted by the kidneys. Rasburicase is recombinant uricase and **pegloticase** is pegylated uricase (attached to methoxy-polythylene glycol mPEG). Given intravenously (4–12 mg) it rapidly reduces uric acid levels in 1–3 days, maintaining it up to 21 days.

$$\text{Uric acid} \xrightarrow{\text{Uricase}} \text{Allantoin} \longrightarrow \text{Excreted}$$

Adverse effects include **allergic reactions**, gout flare, nausea, anemia and methaemoglobinaemia. They are to be avoided in G6PD deficiency.

Rasburicase and pegloticase are indicated in **tumor lysis syndrome** and **refractory chronic gout.**

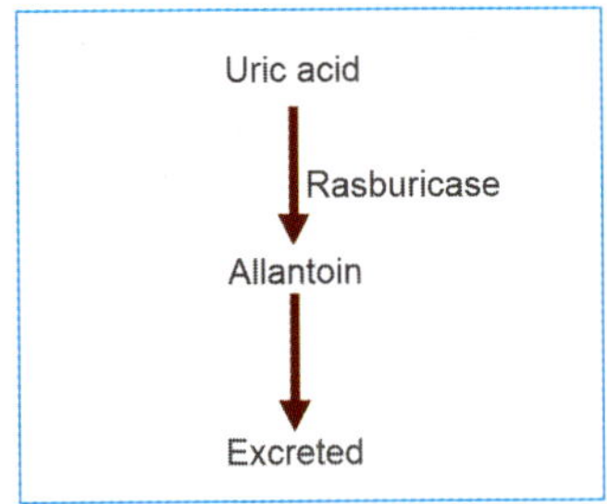

Uricosuric Drugs

Probenecid is an organic acid developed to inhibit the renal tubular secretion of penicillin in order to prolong its action.

Probenecid blocks tubular reabsorption of uric acid and thereby promotes its excretion. Plasma urate pool decreases and tophoceous deposits are gradually reabsorbed. It is ineffective in presence of renal insufficiency as it acts through the kidney. It is well-absorbed and well-tolerated. Adverse effects include gastrointestinal irritation and skin rashes. Large amounts of water should be given to prevent the formation of renal stones.

Probenecid is indicated in chronic gout and secondary hyperuricaemia. It is started with 500 mg once a day and gradually increased to 1 g/day. Probenecid may also precipitate acute attacks of gout due to fluctuating urate levels.

Dose: 0.5–1g OD. BENCID 500 mg tab.

Sulphinpyrazone, a pyrazolone derivative, is another uricosuric drug which has actions and adverse effects similar to probenecid. Duration of action is similar to probenecid—given once or twice daily. It is used in chronic gout in an initial dose of 200 mg/day and gradually increased to 400–800 mg/day.

ANTURAN 100, 200 mg tab.

Benzbromarone is a uricosuric drug which acts by inhibiting renal tubular reabsorption of uric acid. It is a potent uricosuric given 40–80 mg, once daily. It is used as an alternative in patients allergic to other drugs. Benzbromarone can also be used in combination with allopurinol.

Interleukin-1 receptor antagonist anakinra is being studied for a possible role in gout.

Lesinurad is a uric acid transporter 1 (URAT 1) inhibitor to be used along with a xanthine oxidase inhibitor like allopurinol or febuxostat when a single drug is inadequate in gout. It has been approved for use in some countries.

Clinical Pharmacology

- Allopurinol dose should be reduced in renal failure.
- Many drugs like loop diuretics, thiazides, some anticancer drugs and pyrazinamide can precipitate gout and concurrent use requires dose reduction.
- Colchicine is not freely available in India.
- NSAIDs should be avoided in presence of urate nephropathy and nephritis—patient should be screened for these before using NSAIDs.

[1] From Medical Council of India, *Competency based Undergraduate Curriculum for the Indian Medical Graduate*, 2018;1:136–144.

Unit IV

Anaesthetics

CHAPTER 12

Local Anaesthetics

> *Competency achievement:* The student should be able to:
> **PH 1.17** Describe the mechanism/s of action, types, doses, side effects, indications and contraindications of local anesthetics.[1]

INTRODUCTION

Local anaesthetics (LA) are drugs that block nerve conduction when applied locally to nerve tissue in appropriate concentrations. Their action is completely reversible. They act on every type of nerve fibre and can cause both sensory and motor paralysis in the innervated area. They act on axons, cell body, dendrites, synapses and other excitable membranes that utilize sodium channels as the primary means of action potential generation.

Cocaine was the first agent to be isolated by Niemann in 1860. In spite of its addiction potential, cocaine was used for 30 years as a surface anaesthetic. In an effort made to improve the properties of cocaine, procaine was synthesized in 1905. It ruled the field for the next 50 years. In 1943, lignocaine was synthesized by Lofgren and it continues to dominate the field till today.

Classification of local anaesthetics based on the route of administration and duration of action.

Classification

I. Injectable
1. *Short-acting:* Procaine, chloroprocaine
2. *Intermediate-acting:* Lignocaine, prilocaine
3. *Long-acting*: Tetracaine (amethocaine), bupivacaine, dibucaine, ropivacaine, etidocaine.

II. Surface anaesthetics: Lignocaine, cocaine, tetracaine, benzocaine, oxethazaine proparacaine.

CHEMISTRY

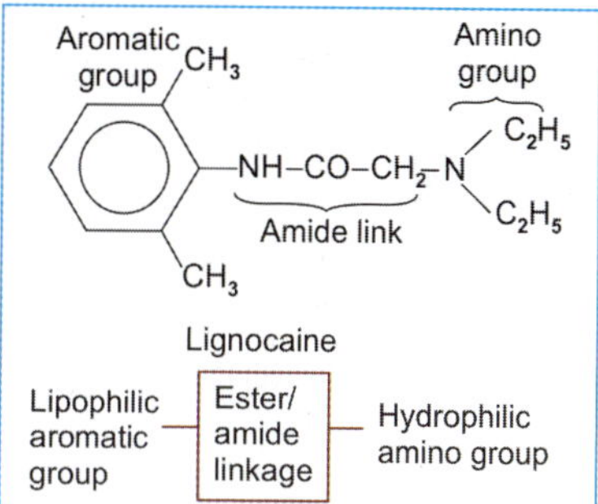

Local anaesthetics are bases and consist of a hydrophilic amino group on one side and a lipophilic aromatic residue on the other, joined by an intermediate chain through an **ester** or **amide** linkage. Since ester links are more prone to hydrolysis than amide links, generally esters have a shorter duration of action.

Since local anaesthetics are weak bases and the infected tissues have a low extracellular pH, LAs ionise in such medium and a very low fraction of non-ionised LA is available for diffusion into the cell. Therefore, LAs are much **less effective in infected tissues.** Depending on the linkage, LAs can be grouped as:

Esters	Amides
Cocaine	Lignocaine (lidocaine)
Procaine	Mepivacaine
Tetracaine	Bupivacaine
Benzocaine	Ropivacaine
Chloroprocaine	Etidocaine
	Prilocaine
	Articaine
Note:	
Esters	*Amides*
Single 'i' in all names	*Double 'i' in all names*

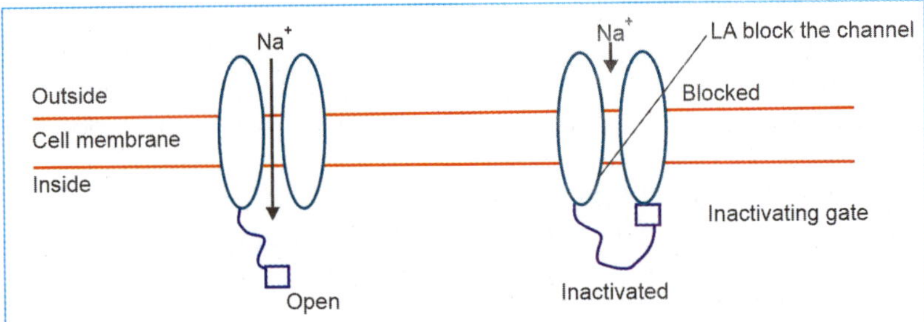

Fig. 12.1: Mechanism of action of local anaesthetics. In the open state the Na^+ moves in and within milliseconds the channel is inactivated due to closure of the inactivating gate. LA block the sodium channels

Mechanism of Action

Local anaesthetics prevent the generation and the conduction of nerve impulses (Fig. 12.1). The primary mechanism of action is blockade of voltage-gated sodium channels.

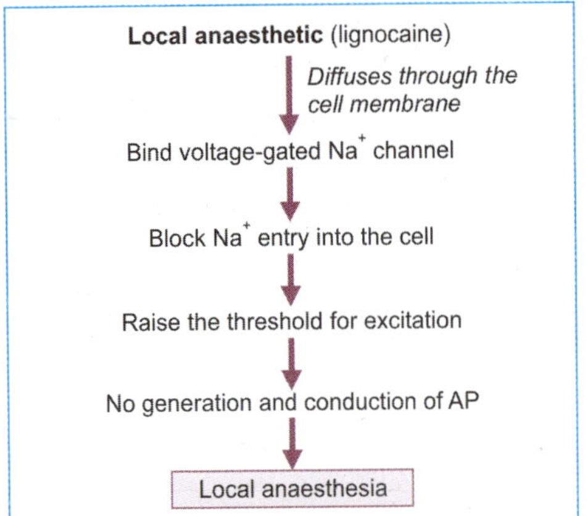

Local anaesthetics diffuse through the cell membrane and bind to the voltage-sensitive sodium channels from the inner side of the cell membrane. They prevent the increase in permeability to Na^+ and gradually raise the threshold for excitation. With increasing concentration, impulse conduction slows, rate of rise of action potential (AP) declines. Threshold for electrical excitability increases. AP amplitude decreases and finally the ability to generate an AP is abolished. These result from binding of LA to more and more sodium channels. Thus it prevents the generation of an AP and its conduction.

- Small nerve fibres are more susceptible as they present a greater surface area per unit volume and such fibres also are shorter. Thus smaller fibres are blocked first—autonomic fibres are blocked first followed by sensory fibres conducting pain, temperature sense, then touch, pressure and vibration sensations in the same order. This is called **differential blockade.**
- Sensory and motor fibres are equally sensitive. Fibres with a high firing rate, like sensory fibres, have a small diameter.
- Small non-myelinated fibres are blocked more readily than the myelinated. However, if the diameter is same, the myelinated nerves are blocked faster than nonmyelinated nerves.

Addition of a **vasoconstrictor like adrenaline** (1:1,00,000 to 1:2,00,000) or **phenylephrine** (1:20,000):

1. Prolongs the **duration of action** of LAs by slowing the rate of absorption from the site of administration.
2. **Reduces systemic toxicity** of LAs because the absorption rate is reduced and as it gets absorbed, it gets metabolised.

ACTIONS

Systemic Actions

Depending on the concentration attained in the plasma, any LA can produce systemic effects. LAs interfere with the functions of all organs in which conduction or transmission of impulses occur. Thus CNS, autonomic ganglia, NMJ and all muscles are affected.

- *CNS:* Local anaesthetics depress the cortical inhibitory pathway thereby allowing unopposed activity of excitatory components. This loss of inhibition is manifested as restlessness, tremors and may proceed to convulsions. The central stimulation is followed by generalised CNS depression and death may result from respiratory failure.
- *CVS:* The primary site of action is the myocardium—lignocaine decreases excitability, conduction rate and force of contraction (quinidine like effects).
- *Blood vessels:* LAs cause hypotension which is due to sympathetic blockade. They also cause arteriolar dilatation. Cocaine, however, causes a rise in BP due to sympathetic stimulation. Since procaine is short-acting, procainamide is used as an antiarrhythmic. Bupivacaine is more cardiotoxic than other LAs.
- *Smooth muscle:* LAs depress contractions in the intact bowel. They also relax vascular and bronchial smooth muscles.
- *Local actions:* On local administration, LAs bring about reversible loss of sensation as already discussed. Depending on the site of administration, the extent of anaesthesia varies (*see* uses).

Pharmacokinetics: Local anaesthetics are rapidly absorbed from the mucous membranes and abraded skin. Rate of absorption is dependent on the vascularity of the area. Thus vasoconstriction decreases the absorption. Toxicity depends on the balance between absorption and metabolism, i.e. if it gets metabolised as it gets absorbed, then toxicity is less. Binding to tissues decreases the concentration in systemic circulation and thereby toxicity. Ester-linked LAs are rapidly hydrolysed by plasma pseudocholinesterase and in the liver. Amide linked LAs are metabolised by the liver microsomes by dealkylation and hydrolysis and are not effective orally (as antiarrhythmics). They undergo extensive first pass metabolism. The metabolism of lignocaine is influenced by hepatic blood flow.

ADVERSE EFFECTS (Table 12.1)

Systemic Effects

1. *Hypersensitivity reactions* including skin rashes, dermatitis, asthma or rarely anaphylaxis are more common with ester type of drugs. Ester type LAs are metabolised to PABA derivatives. These are responsible for allergic reactions while with amides, allergy is rare. Intradermal sensitivity test should be done before using these drugs. Drugs (including adrenaline) to manage such reactions should be kept ready. Moreover, allergy is most often due to the preservative methylparaben. Preparations that do not contain this preservative are now available.
2. *CNS:* Dizziness, sedation, auditory and visual disturbances, mental confusion and disorientation. Higher doses induce anxiety, nystagmus, muscle tremors, convulsions and respiratory failure because LAs depress the cortical inhibitory pathways leading to CNS stimulant effects. Intravenous diazepam controls convulsions. In fact, these can be prevented by preanaesthetic administration of diazepam (1–2 mg/kg), especially if large doses are to be used. In all patients who may need larger doses of an LA including for infiltration, premedication with BZD helps.
3. *CVS:* Blockade of sodium channels in the myocardium by LA results in myocardial depression with decrease in the force of

Table 12.1: Adverse effects of local anaesthetics

CNS	: Dizziness, confusion, anxiety, tremors, occasionally convulsions and respiratory depression
CVS	: Hypotension, bradycardia, arrhythmias
Hypersensitivity reactions	: Rashes, dermatitis, asthma, rarely anaphylaxis

contraction, bradycardia, excitability and conduction velocity; rarely cardiac arrest can occur. Lignocaine is used in arrhythmias. LAs also cause vasodilation resulting in hypotension. In contrast, cocaine causes vasoconstriction and hypertension as it blocks the reuptake of noradrenaline in the adrenergic nerve terminals—**bupivacaine is the most cardiotoxic.** Rarely cardiac arrest can occur.

Lipid rescue: Intravenous infusion of lipid has shown to overcome cardiotoxicity and CNS toxicity due to bupivacaine. The basis for this benefit is not exactly known but may be because the lipophilic compound extracts the lipophilic drug from the tissues and could restore energy to the myocardium. The lipid resuscitation has also been tried to treat the toxicity of other drugs like CNS toxicity due to LA and haloperidol-induced ventricular tachycardia.

4. *Local irritation* can be seen with bupivacaine. Wound healing may be delayed.

INDIVIDUAL COMPOUNDS

A. Injectable (Table 12.2)

1. *Lignocaine* is the most widely used LA. It is fast and long-acting. It is useful for all types of blocks. Maximum anaesthetic effect is seen in 2–5 minutes and lasts for 30–45 minutes. In contrast to other LAs, lignocaine causes drowsiness and mental clouding. Though it is a good corneal anaesthetic, it is not generally preferred because it causes irritation.

XYLOCAINE 4% Topical solution, 2% Jelly, 5% ointment, 1% and 2% inj., 5% for Spinal anaesthesia, 10% Lignocaine spray.

2. *Bupivacaine HCl* is more potent and longer acting than lignocaine—it is widely used. But it can cause more cardiotoxicity than others. 0.25–0.75% inj with or without adrenaline. **Levobupivacaine** HCl is a derivative of bupivacaine that seems to be less neurotoxic and less cardiotoxic than bupivacaine.

BUPIVAN 0.25%, 0.5% inj. MARCAIN 0.5%, 1% inj.

3. *Ropivacaine* is similar to bupivacaine except that it is less cardiotoxic.

2–10% inj, NAROPIN 2 mg/ml, 5 mg/ml 7.5 mg/ml inj, 10 mg/ml (10 ml, 20 ml) inj.

4. *Chloroprocaine HCl* potency is twice that of procaine and its toxicity is lower because of its more rapid metabolism.

5. *Etidocaine HCl:* Its analgesic action lasts 2–3 times longer. It is used for epidural (1%) and all types of infiltration and regional anaesthesia.

6. *Mepivacaine:* Action is more rapid in onset and more prolonged than that of lignocaine.

7. *Prilocaine HCl* has an intermediate onset of action and duration of action is longer. It is less toxic to CNS due to large volume of distribution but can cause methaemoglobinaemia. Because of its toxicity, its use is restricted to dental procedures and IV regional anaesthesia.

8. *Cocaine* produces euphoria and is a drug of dependence and abuse. It is a surface anaes-

Table 12.2: Duration of action and uses of some local anaesthetics

Drug	Duration of anaesthesia (min)		Uses
	Plain	with adrenaline	
Tetracaine	120–240	240–280	Topical, spinal anaesthesia
Lignocaine	30–60	60–120	Topical, infiltration, nerve block, spinal, epidural and IV regional anaesthesia
Mepivacaine	45–90	120–360	Nerve block, epidural anaesthesia
Bupivacaine	120–240	240–480	Infiltration, nerve block, spinal, epidural anaesthesia
Ropivacaine	120–360	240–360	Infiltration, nerve block, spinal, epidural anaesthesia
Benzocaine			Topical anaesthesia
Dibucaine			Topical anaesthesia
Oxethazaine			Topical anaesthesia (used in peptic ulcer)

thetic. It is a protoplasmic poison and hence cannot be injected. Cocaine was used for ocular anaesthesia earlier. But it causes constriction of conjunctival vessels, clouding and sometimes corneal sloughing and is, therefore, not used to produce corneal anaesthesia. Cocaine is used topically for anaesthesia of upper respiratory tract. It has the advantage of being a vasoconstrictor and a local anaesthetic—both in one.

9. *Procaine* was widely used once, but is now replaced by other agents. It is hydrolysed to PABA which interferes with the action of sulfonamides. It is rapidly absorbed following parenteral administration. It is ineffective when applied topically because it is poorly absorbed from the mucous membranes—thus not useful as a surface anaesthetic.

MERICAINE 2% inj, NOVOCAINE 1%, 10%, 2% inj.

10. *Tetracaine (amethocaine)* is a PABA derivative and is 10 times more toxic and more active than procaine. It is used on the eye as 0.5% drops, ointments 0.5% and cream 1% for topical use. 0.25 to 0.5% injection is used for spinal anaesthesia.

PONTOCAINE 0.5% eye drops 1%, 2% inj. AK-T-caine 0.5%, 1%, 2% inj.

B. Local anaesthetics used only on the eye

1. *Benoxinate HCl* within 60 seconds of administration produces corneal anaesthesia enough to perform tonometry. Less irritation, no mydriasis. Used as 0.4% eye drops.

BENDZON 0.4% eye drops.

2. *Proparacaine HCl* produces a little or no initial irritation—0.5% ophthalmic solution is the most commonly used surface anaesthetic on the eye.

PARACAINE 0.5% eye drops.

3. **Tetracaine** is also used on the eye as 0.5% eye drops.

C. Local anaesthetics used on the skin and mucous membranes

LAs used on the skin and mucous membranes are **dibucaine, dyclonine hydrochloride** and **pramoxine hydrochloride**. These drugs are effective when used topically in the symptomatic relief of anal and genital pruritus, poison ivy rashes, acute and chronic dermatoses. Dibucaine is the most potent, most toxic and longest-acting LA. It is available as cream and ointment.

UPERCAINAL cream 1%. NUPERCAINE 0.5% inj.

D. Poorly soluble anaesthetics: These are too slowly absorbed to be toxic. They can be applied to wounds directly and ulcerated surfaces as they produce sustained anaesthetic effect, e.g. benzocaine. **Benzocaine** is a PABA derivative. It is poorly soluble in water because of which it remains at the site for a longer time and toxicity is low as absorption is poor. It is used topically to anaesthetise the skin and mucous membrane. It can also be used as a suppository for anorectal lesions, dusting powder on wounds and as lozenges in stomatitis.

ZOKEN GEL 20% gel.

Butamben is similar to benzocaine.

USES OF LOCAL ANAESTHETICS

Local anaesthesia is the loss of sensation without the loss of consciousness or impairment of the central control of vital functions. Depending on the site and technique of administration, LA can be:

1. **Surface anaesthesia:** Anaesthesia of mucous membrane of the eye, nose, mouth, tracheobronchial tree, oesophagus and genitourinary tract can be produced by direct application of the anaesthetic solution. Tetracaine 2%, lignocaine 2–10%, proparacaine 0.5% and benoxinate 0.4% are most often used. Phenylephrine (but not adrenaline as its penetration is poor) produces vasoconstriction on topical application and prolongs the duration of action.

Anaesthesia is entirely superficial and does not extend to submucosal structures. But LAs are absorbed from mucous membranes and may result in systemic toxicity. Patient should be cautioned to expectorate the excess solution to avoid excess absorption. Local anaesthetics can also be used on abraded skin. Surface anaesthesia is used for the following:

i. *On the eye*
   a. For tonometry, surgery
   b. To remove foreign bodies from the cornea and conjunctiva
   c. For preoperative preparation.
ii. *Others:* Nasal lesions, stomatitis, sore throat, tonsillectomy, endoscopies, intubation, gastric ulcer, burns, proctoscopy, fissure and piles.

An eutectic mixture containing 2.5% each of lignocaine and prilocaine at room temperature has a lower melting point than either of the drugs. This is emulsified and applied as a cream to anaesthetise the intact skin (should not be used on abraded skin). The cream should be applied on the skin under an occlusive dressing and can produce anaesthesia up to a depth of 5 mm. It can be used for procedures like venipuncture and skin graft harvesting.

2. **Infiltration anaesthesia:** Injection of a local anaesthetic solution directly into the tissue can be: (i) Superficial—only into the skin, or (ii) into deeper structures including intra-abdominal organs. Duration can be doubled by adrenaline (1:2,00,000). Adrenaline should not be used:

i. Around end arteries to avoid necrosis, and
ii. Intracutaneously to avoid sloughing.

Drugs used are LIGNOCAINE (0.5–1%), PROCAINE (0.5–1%) and BUPIVACAINE (0.125–0.25%).

Corneal anaesthetics used clinically

Proparacaine	Benoxinate
Tetracaine	Lignocaine

Advantage: By using infiltration anaesthesia, it is possible to provide anaesthesia without disruption of normal bodily functions.

Disadvantage: In major surgeries, systemic toxicity due to local anaesthetic is likely as large amounts of the anaesthetic are required for such procedures.

Uses: For minor procedures like incisions, drainage of an abscess, excision, etc.

3. **Field block:** Subcutaneous injection of a LA solution proximal to the site to be anaesthetised, interrupts nerve transmission in the region distal to the injection. Sites such as forearm, scalp, anterior abdominal wall and lower extremity are used for field block. Knowledge of the relevant neuroanatomy is essential.

Advantage: With a small dose of the drug, anaesthesia could be provided to a greater area.

4. **Nerve block:** Injection of a solution of a LA about/around individual peripheral nerves or nerve plexuses produces larger areas of anaesthesia with a smaller amount of the drug than the above techniques. Anaesthesia starts a few centimetres distal to the injection.

COMPARE AND CONTRAST

Lignocaine and Cocaine

Features	***Lignocaine***	***Cocaine***
Source	Synthetic	Natural—*Erythroxylon coca*
Chemistry	Amide	Ester
Euphoria	Nil	Produces
Abuse potential	Nil	Abused since centuries
CV effects	↓ cardiac contraction →↓ BP	Arrhythmias, vasoconstriction → hypertension
Surface anaesthesia	Yes	Yes (but not used)
IV use	Injected IV	Protoplasmic poison—cannot be injected IV

COMPARE AND CONTRAST

Procaine (Ester type) and Lignocaine (Amide type)

Features	***Procaine***	***Lignocaine***
Chemistry	Ester	Amide
Absorption	Poor	Good
Onset of action	Slow	Rapid
Metabolism	Metabolised by plasma cholinesterases	Metabolised in liver by microsomal enzymes
In liver disease	Can be used	Toxicity likely
Allergic reactions	Ester type—allergy more likely	Amidetype—allergy less common
Penetrability	Poor	Good
Surface anaesthesia	Not a surface anaesthetic	Surface anaesthetic
Use	Not preferred	Widely used

Nerve block anaesthesia is useful for:

1. Blocks of brachial plexus for procedures on the arm (distal to deltoid).
2. Intercostal nerve blocks to anaesthetise anterior abdominal wall.
3. Cervical plexus block for surgery of the neck.
4. Sciatic and femoral nerve blocks for surgeries distal to the knee.
5. Blocks of nerves at wrist and ankle.
6. Radial and ulnar nerve block at the elbow.
7. Sensory cranial nerves block.
8. Facial and lingual nerves block.
9. Inferior alveolar nerve block for extraction of lower jaw teeth.

Onset of action is within 3 minutes with lignocaine. Duration depends on lipid solubility and protein binding. Anaesthesia lasts longer than by field block or infiltration techniques. Nerve blocks are done for tooth extraction, operations on the eye, limbs and in neuralgias.

5. **Spinal anaesthesia** (SA)*:* Local anaesthetic solution is injected into the subarachnoid space between L2–3 or L3–4 below the lower end of the spinal cord. The drug acts on nerve roots. Lower abdomen and lower limbs are anaesthetised and paralysed. The level of anaesthesia can be altered by the volume of injection, specific gravity of the solution and posture of the patient. Generally, a hyperbaric solution (in 10% glucose) is injected. Iso- and hypobaric solutions can also be given. Level of sympathetic block produced is 2 segments higher and motor paralysis 2 segments lower than sensory or cutaneous anaesthesia. Duration depends on the concentration, dose and the drug itself. Lignocaine, tetracaine, bupivacaine and ropivacaine are used for spinal anaesthesia.

Advantages: Safe, affords good analgesia and muscle relaxation and there is no loss of consciousness. In cardiac, pulmonary and renal diseases, SA may be preferred over general anaesthesia whenever possible.

Uses: Surgical procedures on the lower limb, pelvis, lower abdomen, obstetric procedures, caesarean section and other operations are done on spinal anaesthesia.

Complications of SA

i. *Hypotension and bradycardia:* Sympathetic blockade results in relaxation of vascular smooth muscles which causes venous pooling of the blood leading to decreased venous return, decreased cardiac output and hypotension.

Key Box 12.1: Other drugs with local anaesthetic property

- Chlorpromazine
- Propranolol
- Quinine
- H1 antihistamines

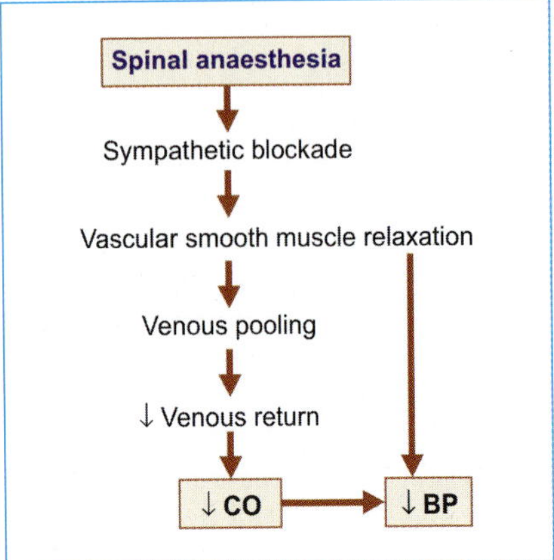

ii. *Respiratory paralysis:* Hypotension and ischaemia of the respiratory centre results in respiratory failure. Due to paralysis of the abdominal muscles, cough reflex is less effective resulting in stasis of respiratory secretions, leading to respiratory infections.

iii. *Headache* due to leakage of CSF can be treated with analgesics.

iv. *Cauda equina syndrome* is uncommon—control over bladder and bowel sphincters is lost because of damage to nerve roots.

v. *Sepsis*—resulting in meningitis

vi. *Nausea and vomiting*—premedication can be given to prevent this.

6. **Epidural anaesthesia:** LA is injected into the spinal extradural space. It acts on nerve roots while small amounts diffuse into subarachnoid space. It is technically more difficult and comparatively larger volumes of the anaesthetic are needed. After repeated injections, tachyphylaxis may develop.

Advantages

1. Sensory blockade is 4–5 segments higher than motor blockade. This difference is useful for obstetric analgesia, as the mother has painless labour and can still cooperate in the process of labour and is conscious throughout.
2. As there is no risk of injecting into SA space, there are no chances of infection.

Epidural opioids may be used to provide analgesia for postoperative pain and terminal cancer pain. Small doses of the opioids are required compared to oral doses (e.g. 0.2–0.5 mg morphine) to provide good analgesia.

7. **Intravenous regional anaesthesia (Bier's block):** This type of anaesthesia is useful for rapid anaesthetization of an extremity (upper or lower). A rubber bandage is used to force the blood out of the limb (veins) and a tourniquet is applied to prevent the re-entry of the blood. A dilute solution of the local anaesthetic is then injected intravenously into a distal vein. It diffuses into extravascular tissues. Onset of anaesthesia is in 2 minutes. Because of the pain produced by the tourniquet, this type of anaesthesia is used for procedures lasting less than one hour. About 25% of the drug enters into the systemic circulation. This type of anaesthesia is more commonly used on the upper limbs though it can also be used on the legs and the thighs.

Clinical Pharmacology

- LAs are less effective in inflamed and infected tissues.
- Intradermal sensitivity tests should be done before using. History of allergy should be taken.
- Allergy is more common with ester type LA.
- Adrenaline may be used to prolong the duration of action of infiltration and nereve block anaesthetics. However, it should bot be added when the anaesthesia is required around structures supplied by end arteries.
- Symptoms of CNS stimulation may be prevented by prior administration of diazepam, if larger dose of LA use is intended.

[1] From Medical Council of India, *Competency based Undergraduate Curriculum for the Indian Medical Graduate*, 2018;1:136–144.

CHAPTER 13

General Anaesthetics

Competency achievement: The student should be able to:

PH 1.18 Describe the mechanism/s of action, types, doses, side effects, indications and contraindications of general anaesthetics, and pre-anesthetic medications.[1]

INTRODUCTION

General anaesthetics (GA) are agents that bring about reversible loss of sensation and consciousness. Before 1846, alcohol, opium, packing a limb with ice and concussion, i.e. making the patient unconscious by a blow on the head were used to relieve surgical pain. Dr Horace Wells, a dentist, tried to demonstrate the effect of nitrous oxide as an anaesthetic in 1844 but was unsuccessful as he removed the gas bag too early. Dr William Morton who was present at the demonstration, worked on it and in 1846 demonstrated ether anaesthesia successfully. Chloroform was introduced by James Y Simpson in 1847. Since then several anaesthetics have been synthesized over the decades. Halothane was introduced into anaesthetic practice by Johnstone in 1956.

STAGES OF GENERAL ANAESTHESIA

Guedel described four stages using ether anaesthesia

1. ***Stage of analgesia*** is from the beginning of inhalation of the anaesthetic up to loss of consciousness. Reflexes and respiration are normal.
2. ***Stage of delirium:*** This stage is from loss of consciousness to beginning of surgical anaesthesia. It may be associated with excitement—shouting, crying and violent behaviour.
3. ***Stage of surgical anaesthesia:*** This stage is of 4 planes. As anaesthesia passes to deeper planes, respiratory depression is seen. There is gradual loss of reflexes and relaxation of skeletal muscles. BP falls and HR increases.
4. ***Stage of medullary paralysis*** is seen only with overdose. It is the stage of medullary depression. Cessation of breathing, circulatory failure and death may follow.

The stages are not clearly demarcated in the actual use of anaesthesia in the present day because of the concomitant use of other drugs to aid anaesthesia.

Ideal anaesthetic: An ideal anaesthetic should be pleasant, non-irritating, provide adequate analgesia, immobility and muscle relaxation; should be non-inflammable and administration should be easy and controllable and have a wide margin of safety. Induction and recovery should be smooth and should not affect cardiovascular functions. It should be inexpensive.

MECHANISM OF ACTION OF GENERAL ANAESTHETICS

The exact mechanism of action of general anaesthetics is not known. The most accepted mechanisms of action are as follows:

1. Inhaled and some intravenous anaesthetics bind to specific sites on GABA receptor chloride channels and activate these receptors. By this they increase the inhibitory neurotransmission and depress the CNS.

2. Inhalational anaesthetics also enhance the sensitivity of glycine-gated chloride channels to glycine. These glycine receptors bring about inhibitory neurotransmission in the brainstem.
3. Some anaesthetics, like ketamine and nitrous oxide, bind to and inhibit the N-methyl-D-aspartate (NMDA) receptors.
4. Inhalational and intravenous agents act at multiple sites in the nervous system and depress the neuronal activity at many sites in the brain.
5. Some GA may activate the potassium channels in the brain leading to hyperpolarization of the membranes and thereby inhibitory effect. This is in addition to their effects on the $GABA_B$ receptors.

General anaesthetics are classified as inhalational and intravenous anaesthetics as given below.

INHALATIONAL ANAESTHETICS

Pharmacokinetics: Inhalational anaesthetics are administered at a specific concentration. Since the brain is a highly perfused organ, steady state can be achieved quickly. When the steady state is reached, the partial pressure of the anaesthetic in the lung and the brain are equal and this makes it possible to monitor the anaesthesia. But, for anaesthetics with high solubility in blood and tissues, rise in alveolar partial pressure (and thereby induction) is slower. Such anaesthetics need to be administered at higher pressures.

Factors which influence the partial pressure (PP) of the anaesthetic attained in the brain are:

1. *Partial pressure of the anaesthetic in the inspired gas:* Higher the partial pressure of the anaesthetic in the inspired air, greater is its quantity moving into the blood.
2. *Pulmonary ventilation:* Delivery of the anaesthetic into the alveoli is directly proportional to pulmonary ventilation.
3. *Alveolar exchange:* When ventilation perfusion is appropriate, volatile anaesthetics freely diffuse across the alveoli.
4. *Solubility of the anaesthetic in the blood:* Lower the solubility of the anaesthetic in the blood, faster is the rise of its PP in the blood and faster is the induction.
5. *Solubility of the anaesthetic in the tissue:* Anaestheics which are more soluble in tissues like the adipose tissue, require a longer time to attain equilibrium.
6. *Cerebral blood flow:* Since the blood flow to the brain is high, GAs reach it rapidly and if other factors are favourable, anaesthesia can be rapidly attained.

Minimum alveolar concentration (MAC) is the lowest concentration of the anaesthetic in the alveoli that immobilizes 50% of subjects in response to a surgical skin incision. MAC

Classification

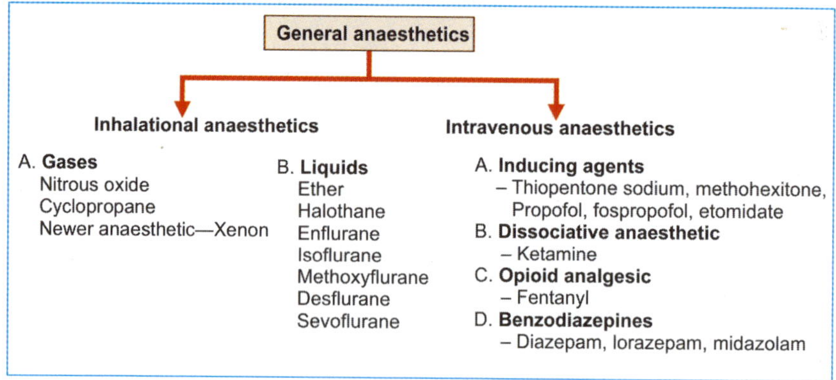

is used to describe the potencies of different volatile anaesthetics.

Second gas effect: When certain anaesthetics like nitrous oxide are administered in high concentrations, the other anaesthetic gases are also pulled in and their alveolar tension rises more rapidly. This is known as second gas effect.

Concentration effect: When an anaesthetic is administered in high concentrations, its alveolar tension rises more rapidly than when the same gas is inhaled in lower concentration. For example, if 75% nitrous oxide is administered, its alveolar tension rises faster than 50% nitrous oxide administration.

Elimination: Once the administration of the anaesthetic is discontinued, recovery from anaesthesia depends on the rate of elimination of anaesthetics from the brain. The same factors which influence induction also influence recovery. Most anaesthetics are eliminated unchanged. Inhalation anaesthetics are eliminated from the lungs. Agents which are soluble in fat and tissues require longer time for elimination and, therefore, recovery is slower.

Actions of Inhaled Anaesthetics

CNS: Inhaled anaesthetics increase cerebral blood flow by decreasing cerebral vascular resistance, they also decrease the metabolic rate of the brain and may increase intracranial pressure.

Kidney and liver: Volatile anaesthetics decrease glomerular filtration rate, renal and hepatic blood flow. Halothane and its derivatives decrease cardiac output and arterial pressure. The effect on heart rate is variable—some cause tachycardia and some bradycardia.

Respiratory system: All inhaled anaesthetics are respiratory depressants—decrease tidal volume, ventilation and also mucociliary function. However, all of them also are bronchodilators.

CVS: Inhaled anaesthetics tend to reduce the myocardial contractility, oxygen requirements, arterial pressure and also produce some coronary vasodilation.

Toxicity of general anaesthetics: Repeated use of halothane may occasionally cause hepatitis. The incidence is lesser with other inhalational agents. A metabolite of enflurane can cause nephrotoxicity on prolonged exposure. Malignant hyperthermia (halothane) and megaloblastic anaemia (N_2O) are other adverse effects.

INDIVIDUAL ANAESTHETICS

Nitrous Oxide

Priestly discovered nitrous oxide in 1776 and was used by Horace Wells in 1944 for its anaesthetic properties. Nitrous oxide is a gas with a slightly sweetish odour. It produces light anaesthesia without significant depression of respiration or vasomotor centre.

Advantages

1. Strong analgesic.
2. Induction is rapid and smooth.
3. Non-irritating and non-inflammable.
4. Recovery is rapid.
5. Postoperative nausea is not significant.
6. Has little effect on respiration and cardiovascular functions, hence ideal for combination.
7. It is non-toxic to liver, kidney and brain and is quickly removed from the lungs.
8. It is inexpensive.

Disadvantages

1. It is less potent and should be used with other agents.
2. Poor muscle relaxant.
3. N_2O displaces nitrogen in the air-filled cavities and while doing so, it enters the cavities faster, i.e. even before nitrogen escapes. This results in expansion of such cavities leading to pneumothorax and air embolus. Hence, N_2O should be avoided in such patients.

4. Repeated use can depress the bone marrow.
5. Long-term exposure (like in staff of operation theatre) to low doses can impair DNA synthesis which may result in foetal abnormalities on conception. May also cause vitamin B_{12} deficiency.

Status in anaesthesia: Nitrous oxide is used as an adjuvant to other anaesthetics. Nitrous oxide (~50%) is used along with oxygen (30%) to provide analgesia and sedation during dental procedures.

Ether

Ether is a colourless volatile liquid. It is highly inflammable; vapours are irritating.

Advantages

1. Potent and reliable anaesthetic.
2. Good analgesic.
3. Effects on cardiovascular and respiratory functions are not significant in therapeutic doses; reflexes are well-maintained.
4. It is a bronchodilator.
5. Provides full muscle relaxation in deep anaesthesia.
6. Does not sensitize the heart to adrenaline.
7. Easy to administer as complicated equipment is not necessary.
8. Inexpensive.

Disadvantages

1. It is inflammable—hence diathermy is contraindicated.
2. Highly soluble in body tissues—induction is slow and unpleasant.
3. Irritating → increases respiratory secretions. Premedication with atropine is essential—laryngeal spasm may occur during induction.
4. Postoperative nausea, vomiting common.
5. Recovery is slow.

Status in anaesthesia: Ether is not preferred now because of its flammability and irritant property. However, it is still used in some centres in developing countries because it is inexpensive, easy to administer (by open drop method) and relatively safe.

Halothane

Halothane is a colourless volatile liquid with a sweet odour. It is non-irritant and non-inflammable.

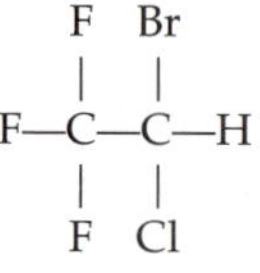

Halothane

Advantages

1. Potent, non-inflammable anaesthetic.
2. Induction is smooth and rapid—in 2–5 min surgical anaesthesia can be produced.
3. Non-irritant—therefore, does not augment salivary or bronchial secretions.
4. Recovery is rapid.
5. Postoperative nausea and vomiting are of low incidence.

Disadvantages

1. Neither a good analgesic nor a muscle relaxant.
2. Direct myocardiac depressant—cardiac output and BP start falling and heart rate may decrease. It sensitizes the heart to the arrhythmogenic action of adrenaline.
3. It also causes some respiratory depression.
4. Severe hepatitis which may be fatal occurs in 1: 50,000 patients. A metabolite may be responsible for this toxicity.
5. **Malignant hyperthermia**—a genetically determined reaction occurs rarely but could be fatal. Succinylcholine accentuates this effect of halothane. It is due to intracellular release of calcium from the sarcoplasmic reticulum which causes muscle contraction and increased heat production. It is treated with dantrolene.
6. Halothane increases cerebral blood flow by cerebral vasodilation which can increase intracranial pressure. This could be troublesome in patients with intra-

COMPARE AND CONTRAST
Nitrous oxide, Ether and Halothane

Features	*Nitrous oxide*	*Ether*	*Halothane*
State	Gas	Liquid	Liquid
Potency	Low	Good	Good
Flammability	No	Inflammable	No
Irritant property	No	Yes	No
Analgesia	Good	Good	Poor
Effect on CV function and respiration	Not significant	Not significant	Significant (depressant)
Muscle relaxation	Poor	Good	Very poor
Risk of hepatitis	No	No	Yes
Induction and recovery	Smooth and rapid	Unpleasant and slow	Smooth and rapid
Use in anaesthesia	Used as adjuvant along with oxygen	Rarely used	Commonly used

cranial tumours and cerebral oedema. Halothane should be avoided in them.

7. Halothane reduces renal blood flow and GFR.

Status in anaesthesia: Halothane was till recently one of the most popular anaesthetics. Analgesics and muscle relaxants are used as adjuvants. Properties such as non-flammability, non-irritancy, bringing about rapid induction and recovery have made it an important anaesthetic but now its use has largely declined as the newer safer derivatives are available. However, in India, it is still extensively used.

Enflurane

Enflurane is similar to halothane except that:

1. It is metabolised to a lesser extent than halothane—therefore, safer regarding the liver toxicity.
2. Does not sensitize the heart to adrenaline.

However, enflurane may precipitate seizures in epileptics and should be avoided in them. For the same reason, isoflurane is preferred to enflurane. A metabolite of enflurane is nephrotoxic and prolonged use has to be avoided.

Isoflurane

Isoflurane is an isomer of enflurane and is similar to halothane. It differs as follows:

1. More potent than halothane.
2. Does not sensitize the heart to adrenaline—safer in patients with myocardial ischaemia.
3. Metabolism is negligible (99% excreted unchanged through the lungs), therefore, safer regarding the liver toxicity.
4. It does not provoke seizures.
5. Preferred anaesthetic in neurosurgical procedures because it causes milder cerebral vasodilation and less increase in intracranial pressure than other anaesthetics.

Isoflurane is extensively used now for maintenance of anaesthesia. However, it can cause hypotension.

Desflurane

Desflurane is a congener of isoflurane. It has all the advantages of isoflurane. In addition, desflurane has low solubility in blood and tissues, because of which it rapidly attains therapeutic concentrations in the alveoli. Therefore, induction and recovery are very rapid and smooth.

Desflurane also has some disadvantages:

- It is pungent—may induce coughing and sometimes laryngospasm. It is, therefore, used for maintenance of anaesthesia and is not preferred for induction.

- Because of low volatility, a special vaporizer is required for administration.
- It can cause transient sympathetic stimulation and tachycardia.

Sevoflurane

Sevoflurane is the latest introduction to inhalation anaesthetics. It has the benefits of desflurane but is not pungent. It has the advantages of rapid and smooth induction and recovery because of low solubility in blood and tissues. It is a good bronchodilator. This also makes it suitable for day-case surgeries and for anaesthesia in children. It is available in India and is used at several centres.

Disadvantages

1. Sevoflurane is chemically unstable and is degraded by carbon dioxide absorbants (sodalime) to a metabolite **(compound A)** that can cause nephrotoxicity. Postoperative restlessness is avoided by premedication with midazolam.
2. Sevoflurane undergoes biotransformation (about 3%) in the liver to release fluoride ions which can cause nephrotoxicity.
3. Can precipitate malignant hyperthermia in genetically susceptible individuals.

If the above disadvantages of sevoflurane are overcome, we would have an ideal anaesthetic.

NEWER ANAESTHETIC

Xenon

Xenon is an inert gas that has properties very close to an *ideal anaesthetic.* It is available in selected centres in some countries.

Advantages

- Rapid induction, insoluble in blood and tissues.
- Rapid recovery.
- Potent anaesthetic.
- No effect on hepatic, renal or pulmonary function.
- No significant CV effects—no effect on CO, HR or BP.
- Not metabolised in the body.

Disadvantage

Currently xenon cannot be manufactured but can only be extracted from air. This makes it very expensive and largely unaffordable to most patients. If this problem is taken care of, xenon could top the list of anaesthetics.

Oxygen in Anaesthesia

Oxygen should be added routinely to inhalational agents to protect against hypoxia (especially when halothane or nitrous oxide is used). When oxygen is not available, ether is the safest agent for maintenance of anaesthesia.

INTRAVENOUS ANAESTHETICS

Intravenous anaesthetics allow an extremely rapid induction because the blood concentration can be raised rapidly—in one arm brain circulation (~11 sec), there is loss of consciousness. But when we administer anaesthetics intravenously, there is no channel for quick elimination like the lungs. Moreover, elimination of inhaled anaesthetics can be hastened by inducing hyperventilation, while this is not possible with intravenous anaesthetics. Hence, IV anaesthetics are used for induction because of the rapid onset of action and anaesthesia is maintained by an inhalational agent (Table 13.1).

A. Inducing Agents

Thiopentone sodium is an ultrashort-acting barbiturate which when administered IV, rapidly induces hypnosis and anaesthesia **without analgesia**. It is highly water-soluble. Extravasation of the solution produces intense pain, necrosis and gangrene. If accidentally injected into an artery, there would be severe vasospasm.

On IV injection (3–5 mg/kg as a 2.5% solution), thiopentone sodium produces unconsciousness in 20–30 sec. Duration of

Table 13.1: Intravenous anaesthetics

Drug	*Main features*	*Uses*
Thiopental	• Fast onset of action • CV and profound respiratory depression	For induction Medicolegal use **'truth serum'**
Propofol	• Fast onset and recovery • Pain at injection site • CV and respiratory depression • Antiemetic property	Short procedures
Etomidate	• Fast onset and recovery • Less CV and respiratory depression • Involuntary movements during induction • Suppresses adrenal steroidogenesis • Pain at injection site	For induction particularly in patients with low cardiovascular reserve
Ketamine	• Slow onset • Good analgesia and amnesia • No respiratory depression, no hypotension • ↑ BP • Hallucinations and involuntary movements during recovery	Short procedures particularly in children
Midazolam	• Slow onset and recovery • Less CV and respiratory depression	Short procedures like endoscopy, fracture reduction
Fentanyl + Droperidol	• Slow onset and recovery • Profound analgesia	Short procedures

CV: Cardiovascular

action is 4–7 minutes. It is highly lipid-soluble, rapidly crosses the BBB and gets rapidly redistributed in the body tissues leading to termination of its action.

Thipentone is metabolised slowly—if administered repeatedly, may accumulate in the body fat leading to prolongation of its effects.

Advantages

Quick onset of action; induction is smooth, rapid and pleasant.

Disadvantages

- Neither a good analgesic nor muscle relaxant.
- It cannot be used alone as the dose required results in delayed recovery, respiratory and circulatory depression.
- A short period of apnoea occurs. Overdosage results in profound **respiratory depression**. Artificial ventilation has to be given.
- Severe hypotension, hiccoughs may occur. Hypotension should be treated with plasma expanders, head low position and pressor agents.
- Should not be mixed with acidic drugs because barbiturates may be precipitated.

Uses

1. Thiopentone sodium is used for induction of anaesthesia before the administration of inhalational anaesthetics.
2. To control convulsions in status epilepticus not responding to antiepileptics.
3. Medicolegal use—**'truth serum'**—thiopentone sodium is used in subanaesthetic doses to produce altered consciousness when the capacity of a person to concoct stories and lie is lost. It is used in interrogation of suspects.

Precautions: Equipment for resuscitation should be ready.

Methohexitone is similar to thiopentone but is more potent. It is not preferred due to toxicity.

Propofol: Propofol is an oily liquid with several advantages making it the most preferred IV anaesthetic.

Advantages

- Quick induction (30 sec) and rapid recovery (4 min) are possible from a single dose.
- Has antiemetic property—an added advantage.
- Because of rapid recovery, it is particularly preferred for 'day cases' when the patient has to be discharged the same day.
- Propofol can be safely used in pregnant women.

Disadvantages

- Propofol causes respiratory depression like thiopental.
- Vasodilation → decreased PVR → fall in BP.
- Direct negative inotropic effect—depression of cardiac contractility.
- Pain on injection (oily liquid) is troublesome but can be prevented by diluting it and combining with lignocaine.
- Prolonged use can occasionally cause propofol infusion syndrome characterised by skeletal muscle necrosis, metabolic acidosis, hyperkalaemia, renal failure, arrhythmias and CV collapse.
- Though rare—can cause histamine release and anaphylactoid reactions.

Uses

1. Propofol is used for **induction** and maintenance of GA for short procedures of up to 1 hour duration. The effect of a single dose is terminated by **redistribution**. It is rapidly metabolised in the liver by conjugation.
2. Propofol can be used for **total IV anaesthesia** as continuous infusion or intermittent injection for short surgical procedures like endoscopies, burns dressing and other such conditions in poor risk patients.
3. Propofol may also be used in subanaesthetic doses to treat **postoperative nausea** and **vomiting**.

The lipid formulation of propofol causes pain. **Fospropofol** is a water-soluble prodrug, converted to propofol and formaldehyde. It does not cause pain at the injection site but the onset of action and recovery are slow because it is a prodrug.

Etomidate is similar to thiopental but it differs in that:

- It is rapidly metabolised—as a result recovery is fast.
- Less cardiovascular and respiratory depression.

Disadvantages

- Involuntary movements and excitatory effects during induction.
- Pain at the injection site.
- Postoperative nausea and vomiting.
- Adrenocortical suppression on long-term use.

Etomidate is preferred for induction in patients with cardiovascular problems.

B. Dissociative Anaesthetic

Ketamine is a phencyclidine derivative. In anaesthetic doses, it produces a trans-like state known as *dissociative anaesthesia* characterised by intense analgesia, immobility, amnesia and a feeling of dissociation from ones own body and surroundings with or without actual loss of consciousness. Thus ketamine produces both **analgesia and anaesthesia.**

Mechanism of action: Ketamine acts by blocking the NMDA receptor which is an excitatory amino acid receptor (*see* Fig. 14.1, page 202).

Ketamine is highly lipid-soluble and gets rapidly distributed into highly perfused organs and then redistributed to less vascular structures. Ketamine hydrochloride 1–2 mg/kg slow IV or 10 mg/kg IM.

Ketamine produces dissociative anaesthesia within 3–5 min which lasts for 10–15 min after a single injection. Amnesia lasts for 1–2 hr. Premedication with atropine is needed. Return to 'consciousness' is gradual. Delirium with vivid dreams and disorientation may be accompanied. If diazepam is administered pre- and postoperatively, delirium can be avoided. Heart rate, CO and BP are increased due to sympathetic stimulation.

Advantages

- Provides profound **analgesia and amnesia**; can be used as the sole agent for minor procedures.
- Respiration is not depressed (or mild), does not induce hypotension.
- Less likely to induce vomiting.
- Pharyngeal and laryngeal reflexes are only slightly affected.
- Convenient to use as it may be given by various routes including epidural IV, IM and rectal.
- It is of particular value in **children** and **poor-risk patients** and also in **asthmatic** patients since it does not induce bronchospasm but may in fact produce bronchodilation.
- Ketamine is also useful in poor-risk cardiogenic shock—as it increases HR, CO and BP.

Disadvantages

- Hallucinations, delirium (psychotomimetic effects), involuntary movements and nystagmus may occur during recovery, if used as a sole agent. Diazepam may be used as preanaesthetic medication to prevent these symptoms.
- Ketamine increases the BP, heart rate and cardiac output—may be dangerous in hypertensives.
- Ketamine increases cerebral blood flow and intracranial pressure.

Uses

1. Ketamine is used for short surgical and diagnostic procedures particularly in poor-risk patients.
2. Ketamine is now available for **topical** use in some countries for joints pain.

Contraindications: Hypertension, CCF, cerebral haemorrhage, increased intracranial tension, psychiatric disorders and pregnancy before term—it is an ecbolic.

Precautions: Pulse and BP should be closely monitored; during recovery patients must remain undisturbed and under observation.

C. Opioid Analgesics

Fentanyl: High potency opioids, fentanyl and sufentanil, have been used as adjuncts to general anaesthetics to provide analgesia. They have also been used (in high doses) with BZDs to attain general anaesthesia. Fentanyl is a short-acting (30–50 min) and potent synthetic opioid analgesic (*see* page 263). Short-acting derivatives of fentanyl-like alfentanil and remifentanil have been used for the induction of anaesthesia along with other IV anaesthetics. They can be used epidurally in low doses to provide postoperative analgesia. However, potent opioids, like fentanyl, in larger doses can induce **thoracic wall rigidity** which interferes with mechanical ventilation.

Neuroleptanalgesia: A combination of a neuroleptic (droperidol) with an analgesic (fentanyl) is used. Droperidol is a rapidly acting, potent neuroleptic related to haloperidol. When the combination is given IV, a state of neuroleptanalgesia is produced. This is characterised by quiescence, psychic indifference and intense analgesia without loss of consciousness. It lasts for 30–40 min. FENTANYL 0.05 mg + DROPERIDOL 2.5 mg/ml- 4 to 6 ml of the solution is infused IV over 10 min. Patient is drowsy but cooperative. It was employed for endoscopies and other diagnostic and minor surgical procedures. However, the combination causes significant respiratory depression, hypotension, bradycardia and EPS (due to droperidol) during recovery. Hence, it is **not commonly used now**.

COMPARE AND CONTRAST
Halothane and Thiopentone Sodium

Features	***Halothane***	***Thiopentone***
Chemistry	Fluorinated compound	Barbiturate
State	Liquid	Liquid
Route of administration	Inhalation	Intravenous
Onset of action	In minutes	In seconds
Recovery	Medium	Fast (8–10 min)
Cardiac effect	Sensitizes heart to the effects of adrenaline	No such effects
Equipment for administration	Special equipment required	Not required
Risk of malignant hyperthermia	Present	Nil
Use in anaesthesia	For maintenance	For induction
Contraindication	Previous halothane hepatitis	Acute intermittent porphyria

Neuroleptanaesthesia: Addition of 65% N_2O + 35% O_2 to the above combination produces neuroleptanaesthesia.

D. Benzodiazepines

Benzodiazepines, like diazepam, lorazepam and midazolam, are used to induce or supplement anaesthesia. They cause sedation, amnesia and reduce anxiety which are beneficial in such patients. BZDs may be employed alone in procedures like endoscopies, reduction of fractures, cardiac catheterisation and cardioversion. IV **midazolam** is particularly preferred as it is faster and shorter-acting (peak effect in two minutes and sedation for 30 minutes), more potent, does not cause significant respiratory and cardiovascular depression and does not cause pain or irritation at the injection sites. BZDs are also used as preanaesthetic medication.

E. Other Drugs

1. **Alpha 2 adrenergic agonists: Dexmedetomidine** is a highly selective alpha 2 adrenergic agonist that produces sedation and analgesia. Advantages are that the respiratory depression and hypotension are mild. It is used intravenously as an adjunct to anaesthesia in minor surgical procedures like endoscopies, burn dressing and other such conditions in poor-risk patients and in ICU for short-term sedation.
2. **Neurosteroids: Eltanolone** does not cause any significant cardiovascular or respiratory depression or cerebrovascular effects. It is undergoing clinical trials for use in anaesthesia.

PREANAESTHETIC MEDICATION

Prior to anaesthesia, certain drugs are administered in order to make anaesthesia safer and more pleasant and is known as preanaesthetic medication. It is given in order to:

1. Decrease anxiety
2. Provide amnesia for the preoperative period
3. Relieve preoperative pain, if present
4. Make anaesthesia safer
5. Reduce side effects of anaesthetics
6. Reduce gastric acidity.

To achieve the above purpose, more than one drug is required. An informative, supportive, preoperative visit by the anaesthesiologist is very much essential.

Sedative hypnotics: Antianxiety agents like benzodiazepines are used extensively as preanaesthetic medication. They reduce anxiety and produce sedation. Diazepam 5–10 mg is given orally. It also produces amnesia. Barbiturates are not preferred due to the disadvantages like respiratory depression.

Antihistamines have sedative, antiemetic and anticholinergic properties and are useful as preanaesthetic medication, e.g. promethazine.

Antiemetics: Metoclopromide, domperidone or ondansetron may be used. Antihistamines with antiemetic properties may also be used.

Anticholinergic drugs: Some irritant anaesthetics, like ether, increase the salivary and respiratory secretions. The secretions from the oral cavity and trachea may creep into the larynx inducing laryngospasm. They may enter into the lungs causing aspiration pneumonia. This indicated the need for drugs that reduce secretions. Fortunately, we now have less irritant anaesthetics and secretions are less of a problem. Atropine 0.6 mg IM or scopolamine 0.6 mg IM or glycopyrrolate 0.2 mg IM can be used. Scopolamine produces more sedation.

Anticholinergics
- Reduce the secretions.
- Prevent bradycardia due to vagal stimulation.
- Prevent laryngospasm which is due to excessive secretions.

Glycopyrrolate: As compared to atropine—
- Glycopyrrolate is longer acting,
- is a better antisialagogue,
- is less likely to cause significant tachycardia,
- also produces less sedation than scopolamine (Flowchart 13.1).

Drugs that reduce acidity: General anaesthetics may induce vomiting. This is associated with an increased risk of aspiration into the respiratory tract because normal protective airway reflexes are blunted by anaesthetics. Aspiration of the acidic gastric contents into the lungs cause damage to the lungs. H_2 blockers like ranitidine decrease gastric acid secretion (*see* page 418) and are given on the night before surgery. Decrease in gastric secretions reduces the damage to lungs, if aspiration occurs while on anaesthesia.

Gastrokinetic agents: Metoclopramide is a dopamine antagonist that promotes gastrointestinal motility and increases the tone of oesophageal end of the stomach. This speeds up gastric emptying. The combination of H_2 blocker + metoclopramide provides best protection against aspiration.

Opioids, like morphine and pethidine, reduce anxiety and apprehension, provide analgesia and reduce the dose of the anaesthetic required. But they depress respiration and may cause hypotension, postoperative constipation, and urinary retention; they precipitate bronchial asthma and delay recovery.

Balanced Anaesthesia

Since it is not possible to achieve ideal anaesthesia with a single drug, multiple drugs are employed (anaesthetic adjuncts) to attain

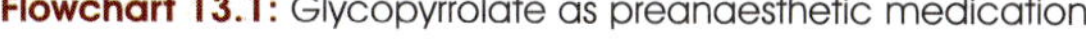

Flowchart 13.1: Glycopyrrolate as preanaesthetic medication

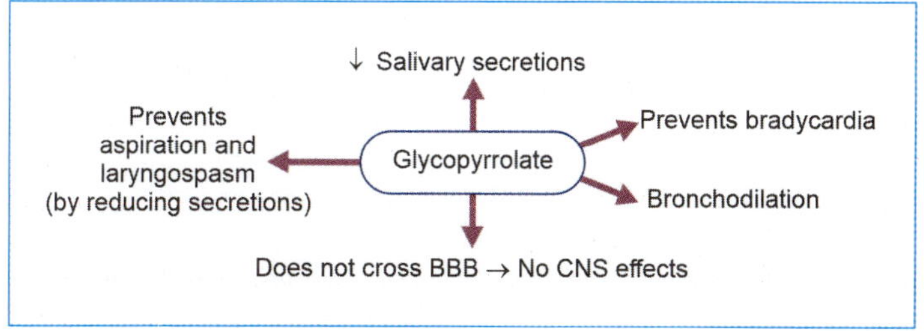

this—preanaesthetic medication, IV anaesthetics for induction, inhalational agents for maintenance, oxygen, skeletal muscle relaxants and analgesics. This is termed balanced anaesthesia.

Conscious Sedation

Conscious sedation is a state when the patient has sedation and amnesia without being unconscious. Such a state is attained by combination of a sedative (midazolam) and an analgesic (fentanyl). The patient responds to commands but is drowsy. For longer action, diazepam may be combined with pethidine. It is reasonably safe as antidotes for both drugs are available (flumazenil and naloxone). Propofol may be used in place of midazolam. Conscious sedation can be employed for minor surgical and diagnostic procedures. In addition, regional block with local anaesthetics may be used for short surgical procedures. It should, however, be avoided in COPD or psychotic patients and in pregnancy.

Clinical Pharmacology

- Hypotension can occur during anaesthesia—BP should be constantly monitored.
- Respiratory depression—anaesthetics abolish ventilatory reflexes. Ventilation should be assisted.
- Hypothermia is common due to cool OT temperature, cold IV fluids, vasodilation leading to heat loss, and low metabolic activity.
- Laryngospasm, aspiration of gastric contents and delirium during recovery are the common problems to be avoided in GA.
- Post-anaesthetic nausea and vomiting should be prevented by antiemetics.
- Pneumonia—postoperatively is rare but should be borne in mind.

[1] From Medical Council of India, *Competency based Undergraduate Curriculum for the Indian Medical Graduate*, 2018;1:136–144.

Unit V

Central Nervous System

14. Sedative Hypnotics
15. Antiepileptic Drugs
16. Drugs used in Neurodegenerative Disorders—Parkinsonism and Alzheimer's Disease
17. Drugs used in Psychiatric Disorders: Antipsychotics and Antianxiety Agents
18. Antidepressants and Mood Stabilizers
19. Opioid Analgesics and Antagonists
20. Alcohols
21. CNS Stimulants and Drugs of Abuse

CHAPTER 14

Sedative Hypnotics

INTRODUCTION

The central nervous system is the most complex of all the systems in the body. Several drugs act on the CNS including drugs used therapeutically and those used for pleasurable effects. Drugs may stimulate or depress the CNS. To understand the effects of drugs, a basic idea of the important neurotransmitters acting on the CNS (Table 14.1) and their receptors is very much essential.

The central neurotransmitters include:

- **Excitatory transmitters**
  Glutamate, aspartate

Table 14.1: Central neurotransmitters and their receptors

Transmitter	*Receptor*
Excitatory	
Glutamate	NMDA
	AMPA
	Kainate
	Metabotropic
Inhibitory	
GABA	$GABA_A$
	$GABA_B$
Glycine	Glycine
Others	
Noradrenaline	α_1, α_2, β_1, β_2 β_3,
Dopamine	$D_{1\text{-}5}$
Acetylcholine	Muscarinic (M_{1-5})
5-Hydroxytryptamine	5-$HT_{1A, 2A, 3, 4}$
Histamine	$H_{1\text{-}4}$
Tachykinins	$NK_{1,2,3}$
Opioid peptides	*K*, μ, δ
Endocannabinoids	CB_1
Orexins	OX_1,OX_2

- **Inhibitory transmitters**
  GABA, glycine
- **Other transmitters** (mediate both excitatory and inhibitory effects)
  Noradrenaline, dopamine, 5-HT, acetylcholine, histamine, adenosine, tachykinins, opioid peptides, endocannabinoids.

EXCITATORY NEUROTRANSMITTERS

Glutamate is the chief excitatory neurotransmitter present throughout the CNS. It is stored in synaptic vesicles and is released into the synapse by exocytosis. It acts on specific glutamate receptors for excitatory amino acid receptors. Aspartate also acts like glutamate in certain regions of the brain.

Excitatory amino acid (EAA) receptors are of 4 subtypes:

- NMDA } Ionotropic receptor
- AMPA } Ionotropic receptor
- Kainate } Ionotropic receptor
- Metabotropic receptor—GPCR

B & C is a ligand-gated ion channel, a pentamer and activated by glycine and glutamate (Fig. 14.1).

The NMDA receptors mediate slow excitatory responses and also play a role in the long-term adaptive changes in the brain. Drugs like ketamine, phencyclidine, memantine and magnesium block the NMDA receptor channels. Ketamine produces dissociative anaesthesia.

AMPA and kainate receptors are involved in fast excitatory transmission and are both activated by glutamate. Symptoms of CNS

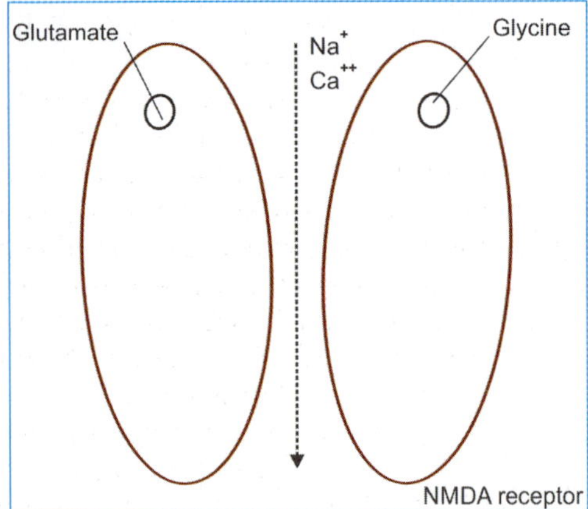

Fig. 14.1: NMDA receptor is a ligand-gated ion channel. Binding of glutamate and glycine opens the channel resulting in entry of Ca^{++} and some Na^{+}

depression include drowsiness, sedation, hypnosis, disorientation, unconsciousness, coma and death.

Metabotropic receptors are involved in long-term adaptive changes in the brain.

Symptoms of CNS stimulation: Excitement, insomnia, tremors, convulsions, coma and death.

INHIBITORY NEUROTRANSMITTERS

GABA is the principal inhibitory neurotransmitter in the brain. Agonists may bind to different sites on the GABA receptor. There are two subtypes of GABA receptors. $GABA_A$ and $GABA_B$ receptors. A third type—$GABA_c$ is now known to exist. $GABA_A$ receptor is a ligand-gated chloride channel while $GABA_B$ receptors are G-protein-coupled receptors.

Drugs like benzodiazepines and barbiturates bring about their effects by acting on the $GABA_A$ receptors. Flumazenil is a $GABA_A$ antagonist. Baclofen is a $GABA_B$ receptor agonist which brings about skeletal muscle relaxation.

	$GABA_A$ receptor	*$GABA_B$ receptor*
Location	Brain	Spinal cord
Receptor	Cl^- channel	GPCR
Effect	Hypnosis	Muscle relaxation
	Anticonvulsant	–
Agonist	Diazepam	Baclofen

Excitatory postsynaptic potential (EPSP): When an excitatory neurotransmitter activates specific receptors on the postsynaptic membrane, the permeability of the membrane to cations (Na^+, Ca^{++}) increases — this is excitatory postsynaptic potential.

Inhibitory postsynaptic potential (IPSP): Binding of an inhibitory neurotransmitter to the specific receptors on the postsynaptic membrane results in increased permeability of the postsynaptic membrane to K^+ and Cl^- and is known as IPSP.

Glycine is an inhibitory transmitter in the brainstem and spinal cord. It acts on glycine receptor which is a ligand-gated chloride channel. Tetanus toxin inhibits the release of glycine in the spinal cord resulting in powerful muscle spasms.

Other transmitters in the CNS include noradrenaline, dopamine, acetylcholine, serotonin, histamine, purines, nitric oxide, tachykinins, endogenous opioid peptides (enkephalins, endorphins and dynorphins) and endocannabinoids.

SEDATIVE HYPNOTICS

Competency achievement: The student should be able to:

PH 1.19 Describe the mechanism/s of action, types, doses, side effects, indications and contraindications of the drugs which act on CNS (including anxiolytics, **sedatives and hypnotics,** antipsychotic, anti-depressant drugs, anti-manics, opioid agonists and antagonists, drugs used for neurodegenerative disorders, antiepileptics drugs).[1]

Sedative is a drug that produces a calming or quietening effect and reduces excitement. It may induce drowsiness. **Hypnotic** is a drug that induces sleep resembling natural sleep. Both sedation and hypnosis may be considered as different grades of CNS depression.

All human beings need sleep. Approximately 1/3rd of our life is spent in sleep.

Sleep can be classified into two types depending on the physiological characteristics:

1. NREM (non-rapid eye movement) sleep
2. REM (rapid eye movement) sleep.

NREM sleep is of 0 to 4 levels of depth.

Stages or Levels of NREM Sleep

Stage 0 : From lying down to falling asleep.

Stage 1 : Eye movements are less and the body muscles begin to relax—lightest stage of sleep—5 to 10% of total sleep time.

Stage 2 : Eye movements are further reduced but the person is still easily arousable—involves 50% of total sleep time.

Stage 3 : Deeper sleep with minimum eye movements and not easily arousable. Stages 3 and 4 together are called delta or slow wave sleep; it is refreshing and a decrease in delta sleep is poor quality sleep.

Stage 4 : It is the deepest level of sleep. In this stage, the metabolic rate is the lowest and growth hormone secretion is highest. There are no eye movements and muscles are fully relaxed—if awakened, there is disorientation for 1–2 minutes. Makes up 20% of total sleep time.

These stages of NREM alternate with REM sleep throughout the night for brief periods.

REM sleep is associated with dreaming, enhanced heart rate, breathing and brain activity and relaxation of voluntary muscles; dreams can be recollected; REM sleep makes up 20–25% of total sleep time.

Insomnia is sleeplessness. It is insufficient or poor quality sleep which could lead to undesirable day time consequences. Insomnia may be primary or secondary. **Primary** insomnia is sleeplessness that is not attributable to medical, psychiatric or environmental causes. This is uncommon. Insomnia may be **secondary** to a variety of clinical conditions including medical and psychiatric illness, stress, drug induced or simply due to lack of adequate physical activity.

Since centuries, man has sought the help of drugs and other remedies for insomnia.

Classification

1. Benzodiazepines

Long-acting (24–48 hr)

Diazepam, chlordiazepoxide
Clonazepam, flurazepam
Chlorazepate, clobazam

Short-acting (12–24 hr)

Temazepam, lorazepam
Oxazepam, nitrazepam
Alprazolam, halazepam.

Ultra short acting (<6 hr)

Triazolam, Midazolam

2. Newer agents

Melatonin and congeners

Melatonin, ramelteon, tasimelteon

Z hypnotics

Zolpidem, zopiclone, eszopiclone, zaleplon

Orexin receptor antagonists

Suvorexant, almorexant, filorexant

3. Barbiturates

Phenobarbitone, mephobarbitone, pentobarbitone, secobarbitone, thiopentone, hexobarbitone

4. Miscellaneous

Paraldehyde, chloral hydrate, glutethimide, meprobamate

BENZODIAZEPINES (BZDs)

Chlordiazepoxide was the first BZDs to be introduced into clinical medicine in 1961 and since then about 2000 BZDs have been synthesized, of which 35 are now in clinical use.

Pharmacological Actions

The most important actions of BZDs are on the CNS and include:

1. Sedation and hypnosis
2. Reduction in anxiety
3. Anaesthesia
4. Muscle relaxation
5. Anticonvulsant effects
6. Amnesia.

Hypnosis: BZDs hasten the onset of sleep. At slightly higher doses, they induce sleep (hypnosis) and increase the duration of sleep. The stage 2 NREM sleep is prolonged while the duration of REM sleep and stage 4 NREM is decreased. The suppression of REM sleep is very little with BZD. The quality of sleep resembles natural sleep more closely when compared to other older hypnotics. Tolerance develops to this effect gradually after about 1–2 weeks of use.

Sedation or anxiolytic effects: BZDs reduce anxiety and aggression and produce a calming effect. Alprazolam has additional antidepresant properties. Psychomotor and cognitive functions are also depressed.

Anaesthesia: BZDs produce CNS depression in a dose-dependent manner. Sedation, hypnosis, stupor, anaesthesia and coma are the different grades of CNS depression. BZDs in higher doses than that used for sedation produce general anaesthesia which can reach up to stage III of anaesthesia. Midazolam is used as an IV anaesthetic. BZDs including diazepam, lorazepam and midazolam can be used as adjuvants to general anaesthetics, but they carry the risk of prolonging respiratory depression which could be due to their longer half-lives. These effects can be reversed by flumazenil.

Muscle relaxant action: BZDs reduce muscle tone by a central action. They depress the spinal polysynaptic reflexes which maintain the muscle tone. Generally, anxiety is associated with an increased muscle tone and may be responsible for aches and pains in these patients. The muscle relaxation by BZDs adds to their beneficial effects in such patients. High doses also depress transmission at the NMJ.

Anticonvulsant effects: BZDs increase the seizure threshold and act as anticonvulsants. They suppress the development and spread of seizures. Several BZDs have somewhat selective anticonvulsant effects which is seen at doses that do not produce profound CNS depression. Diazepam is used intravenously for the treatment of status epilepticus and rectally in febrile convulsions. Other BZDs, like clonazepam, are used in the treatment of absence seizures and myoclonic seizures in children. Nitrazepam and lorazepam also have useful antiepileptic activity.

Amnesia: BZDs produce anterograde amnesia, i.e. loss of memory for the events happening after the administration of BZDs. This property is an advantage when BZDs are used in surgical procedures as the patient does not remember the unpleasant events. However, this may be a disadvantage when used for other indications particularly over a long time.

Other Actions

- *Cardiovascular functions:* In higher doses, BZDs decrease BP, increase heart rate and also depress respiration. In patients with impaired cardiac function, regular therapeutic doses of BZDs can cause significant CV depression especially on parenteral administration. Toxic doses result in depressed myocardial contractility and vascular tone leading to cardiovascular collapse.
- *Respiration:* BZDs in higher doses can cause respiratory depression. It can be profound in patients with pre-existing respiratory disease.
- Diazepam decreases nocturnal gastric acid secretion.

Mechanism of Action

GABA is the principle inhibitory neurotransmitter of the central nervous system and it acts through GABA receptors. BZDs bring about their effects through GABA, i.e. they modulate the response to GABA by acting on $GABA_A$ receptors. Benzodiazepines bind to the $GABA_A$ receptor present in the neurons of the CNS. They bind (Fig. 14.2) at a site which is different from the GABA-binding site and enhance the affinity of GABA for the receptor. GABA enhances chloride ion conductance through this receptor and this effect is potentiated or intensified by BZDs. BZDs bind

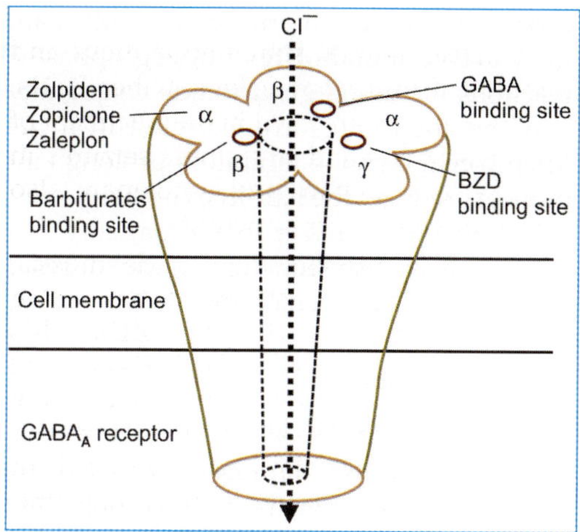

Fig. 14.2: GABA$_A$ receptor is a pentamer made of 5 subunits (2α, 2β and 1γ). BZDs, GABA, barbiturates and newer non-BZD hypnotics bind to different sites on the GABA$_A$ receptor to facilitate the opening of the Cl^- channel. Binding of agonists opens the Cl^- ion channels. β carbolines bind to the BZD receptors and produce opposite effects (inverse agonists)

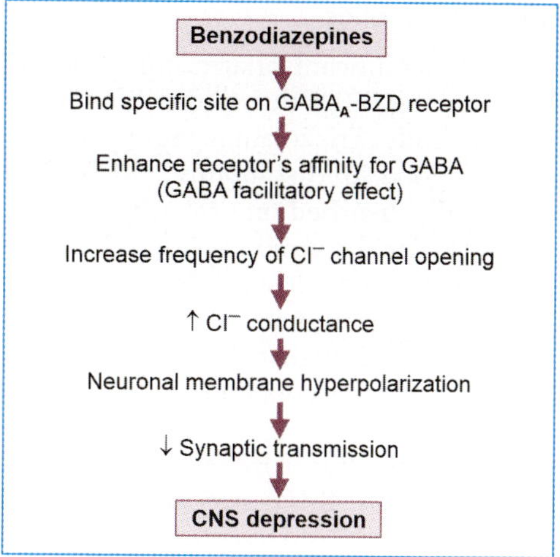

to the receptor (BZ$_1$ subtype) and increase the **frequency** of chloride channel opening in response to GABA. This in turn leads to an increased flow of chloride ions into the neurons, resulting in hyperpolarization of these neuronal membranes which in turn, results in decreased synaptic transmission (Table 14.2).

BZDs as Hypnotics

When compared to barbiturates:

1. *Sleep quality:* BZDs induce better quality sleep which more closely resembles natural sleep and has less hangover. The suppression of REM sleep is lesser when compared to barbiturates. On discontinuation of BZDs, the rebound REM is less intense.
2. *Cardiorespiratory function:* In hypnotic doses, they do not affect respiration or cardiovascular functions.
3. *Safety:* BZDs have a higher safety margin and are safer than barbiturates even in overdoses. The respiratory depression in overdoses is milder and unlikely to be fatal.
4. *Overdose:* In BZD overdosage, a specific BZD antagonist—**flumazenil** is available to reverse the symptoms.
5. *Enzyme induction:* BZDs do not cause microsomal enzyme induction and, therefore, do not alter the blood levels of other drugs.
6. *Dependence:* BZDs have lower abuse liability—dependence and withdrawal symptoms are mild.
7. Also, other disadvantages like 'drug automatism' is less likely and increased porphyrin levels caused by barbiturates is not seen with BZDs.

Because of the above advantages, BZDs are the preferred sedative hypnotics over barbiturates.

Table 14.2: Effects of ligands on GABA$_A$ receptor BZD binding site (BZD receptor)

	Agonist	*Antagonist*	*Inverse agonist*
• *Ligand*	BZD	Flumazenil	Beta carbolines
• *Principle effects*	Sedation, hypnosis, antianxiety, anticonvulsant, muscle relaxation	Blocks and reverses the BZS effects	Arousal, anxiety, increased muscle tone, convulsions

Pharmacokinetics

There are significant pharmacokinetic differences among BZDs due to the differences in lipid solubility. Triazolam is rapidly absorbed as it has good lipid solubility. All BZDs are **completely absorbed** on oral administration. Intramuscular absorption is slow—hence **oral route is preferred.** Most BZDs are extensively bound to plasma proteins (e.g. diazepam 99%).

BZDs are widely distributed in the tissues. They cross the placenta and are also excreted in the milk.

Duration of action of BZDs varies depending on metabolism. BZDs are metabolized by oxidation and hydroxylation reactions catalysed by the microsomal enzymes of the cytochrome P450 family, mostly CYP3A4. The metabolites of some of the BZDs particularly long-acting ones like chlorazepate are also active, thereby prolonging the duration of action. Nordiazepam, a metabolite of diazepam, has a t½ of 40 hr. On repeated administration, cumulative effects may be seen with some of the long-acting agents in a few days. The duration of action gets prolonged and may result in drowsiness which gets carried to the next morning also. BZDs and their **active metabolites** undergo phase II reactions including glucuronide conjugation and the conjugates are excreted in urine. Microsomal enzyme inhibitors prolong (and inducers reduce) the half-lives of many of the BZDs including diazepam. In patients with serious hepatic dysfunction, lower doses of BZDs should be given (Table 14.3).

Drug Interactions

CNS depressants + BZD → increased sedation

1. All other CNS depressants add to the effects of sedative hypnotics (Table 14.4). For example: Alcohol, opioid analgesics, antipsychotics, antiepileptics, antidepressants and sedative antihistamines given concurrently can cause significant CNS depression.
2. Microsomal enzyme inhibitors like ketoconazole, omeprazole, erythromycin and others prolong the t½ of BZDs.
3. Though BZDs are extensively bound to plasma proteins, displacement interactions are **not** clinically significant.

Table 14.3: Dose and duration of action of some commonly used hypnotics

Hypnotic	*Hypnotic dose (mg)*	*Duration of action (hrs)*	*Trade names*
Long-acting (24-48 hr)			
Diazepam	5–10	24–48	CALMPOSE 5, 10 mg tab, 5 mg/ml inj.
Chlordiazepoxide	10–20	24–48	CLOXIDE, LIBRIUM 10, 25 mg tab,
Intermediate to short acting (upto 24 hrs)			
Nitrazepam	5–10	24	BARONITE, DORMIN, NIPAM, NITRAVET 5, 10 mg tab.
Alprazolam	0.25–0.5	24	ALPRAX .025, 0.5, 1, 1.5 mg. ALPAM 0.25 mg tab
Triazolam	0.125–0.25	<6	HYPAM 0.25, 0.125, 0.5 mg tab.
Midazolam	7.5–10	<6	MIDAZ, MIDZOL, SEDEVEN 5 mg/ml, 1 mg/ml inj.
Lorazepam	1–2	12–18	L-ZEPAM, ATIVAN 1,2 mg tab. LORA 2 mg inj.
Temazepam	10–20	12–18	RESTORIL 7.5 mg tab.
Newer agents			
Zolpidem	5–10	<4	ZOLDEM, ZLEEP 5, 10 mg tab.
Zaleplon	5–20	<4	ZAPLON 5, 10 mg tab
Zopiclone	7.5–10	<4	ZICLONE 7.5 mg tab.
Melatonin	2–10	4–6	MELOSET, 3 mg tab
Ramelteon	4–16	4–6	ROZEREM, 8 mg tab

Table 14.4: Other drugs that can produce sedation

• Most antipsychotics	• Alcohol
• Most antidepressants	• Reserpine
• Some antihistamines	• Opioids
• Clonidine	• Methyldopa
• Most antiepileptics	• Tizanidine

Adverse Effects

BZDs are generally well tolerated and are fairly safe drugs. The common side effects include drowsiness, confusion, dizziness, amnesia, lethargy, weakness, headache, blurred vision, ataxia, disorientation, daytime sedation, worsening of sleep apnoea and **impaired motor coordination** as well as judgement such as driving skills, therefore, while on BZDs **driving should be avoided**. Some patients may experience nightmares. BZDs can impair learning ability due to **depressed cognitive functions**. When given to a pregnant mother during labour, BZDs cause hypotonia and respiratory depression in the neonate.

In some patients, BZDs may cause paradoxical irritability and anxiety.

Tolerance and Dependence

Both tolerance and dependence liability are less with BZDs as compared to barbiturates. Patients develop some tolerance to the sedative effects after 1–2 weeks of continued use and higher doses are required. Partial cross-tolerance between different sedative hypnotics and alcohol is noted.

Both physiologic and psychological dependence develop on repeated long-term administration of BZDs. BZDs now come under **'Schedule H'** drugs. The withdrawal symptoms are mild and slow in onset because of the longer plasma half-lives of most BZDs, but they may be abrupt and more intensive with short-acting agents. Severity of withdrawal symptoms also depends on the dose and duration of use. Withdrawal symptoms include anxiety, nervousness, tremors, anorexia, dizziness, insomnia, restlessness, bad dreams and may rarely cause convulsions.

Acute Overdosage

Overdosage of BZDs is quite common due to the extensive use and relatively easy availability of this group of drugs. They induce sleep but the respiratory depression is mild and hence are fairly safe drugs. The availability of a specific antagonist—**flumazenil** makes it safer to use BZDs because poisoning can be treated. Cardiovascular depression can be quite significant. BP and ventilation have to be maintained. Ventilatory support may be needed. Flumazenil reverses all the effects of BZDs. However, constant monitoring is required as flumazenil is short acting. Renal function should be watched for. Haemodialysis or haemoperfusion may be needed in some cases.

Uses of BZDs

1. **Insomnia** is a common problem in the present days with rising stress and anxiety. Various factors could contribute to insomnia including lifestyle, unsuitable sleep environment like extremes of temperature, noisy or too bright room and the type of bed.

Several **nonpharmacological measures** can help to overcome insomnia like following a regular bedtime, avoiding naps during daytime, avoiding stimulants like coffee and sentimental discussions at bedtime, adequate exercise or physical activity through the day, proper food habits and following relaxation or meditation techniques before sleeping. When such measures fail, drugs may be needed to induce sleep.

An ideal hypnotic should be fast acting, produce adequate duration of sleep resembling natural sleep with minimum or no hangover. Benzodiazepines (or one of the newer drugs) may be considered. Long-acting BZDs can produce sedation and cause daytime drowsiness. Among the BZDs, lorazepam, oxazepam, nitrazepam, temazepam or triazolam may be used. After some days of use, tolerance develops to the sedative effects.

Insomnia has been divided into three categories (by the National Institute of Mental Health Consensus Development Conference) as follows:

i. ***Transient insomnia:*** May be due to acute stress or air travel to a new time zone, sudden change in place, jet lag, etc. It could last for a few days usually <3 days. A low dose of a short-acting hypnotic may be given for 2–3 days or as required. Observing good sleep hygiene and reassuring the patient that a few days of lack of sleep is not harmful could often solve the problem.

ii. ***Short-term insomnia:*** Insomnia of more than 3 days may last for 2–3 weeks and is due to stressful situations in the work and family life or medical illness. A short-acting hypnotic may be required for a maximum of 2–3 weeks and is gradually withdrawn with good sleep hygiene, exercises and other measures.

iii. ***Long-term insomnia:*** Insomnia of >3 weeks. Needs proper evaluation to find the cause. It could be secondary to a variety of causes including chronic alcoholism, drug dependence, sleep apnoea, drugs (Table 14.4) noctural hyperacidity or psychiatric illnesses. Nonpharmacological measures should be given adequate importance. If required, a hypnotic may be given intermittently—once in 2–3 days. Since sleep apnoea is aggravated by BZDs and other hypnotics, they are contraindicated in these patients.

2. **In anxiety states:** BZDs are the most commonly used anxiolytics for the treatment of anxiety states and anxiety neuroses (*see* page 272). Any of the BZDs except the ultrashort-acting ones may be used. They are also useful in panic attacks. Alprazolam has demonstrated good efficacy in panic attacks and in agoraphobia (*Agora* = market place *phobs* = fear of being suddenly incapacitated in the public—an irrational fear of leaving the familiar setting of home and entering into the open external life situations because one might feel trapped or unable to escape and is often associated with panic attacks).

3. **As anticonvulsants:** IV diazepam is the drug of choice in the treatment of status epilepticus. Rectal administration of diazepam is used in febrile convulsions. Clonazepam or clobazam is used as adjuncts with other antiepileptic drugs.

4. **Muscle relaxation:** BZDs are centrally acting muscle relaxants used in chronic muscle spasm and spasticity.

5. **As preanaesthetic medication:** For their sedation, amnestic and anxiolytic effects, BZDs are useful.

6. **General anaesthesia:** IV midazolam or diazepam is used as an intravenous anaesthetic. BZDs are also used to supplement anaesthesia.

7. **Minor procedures:** Like endoscopies, fracture reduction, cardiac catheterization, prior to ECT and in other minor procedures intravenous diazepam is used.

8. **During alcohol withdrawal:** BZDs are useful in patients during withdrawal of alcohol or other sedative-hypnotics and opioids.

9. **In psychiatry:** For the initial control of mania, diazepam is used as an adjuvant.

Benzodiazepine Antagonist

Flumazenil is a competitive antagonist at the BZD receptor. It competes for the same binding site as BZDs on the GABA receptor and blocks the effects of BZDs, zolpidem, zopiclone, eszopiclone and zaleplon as well as the inverse agonists (beta carbolines).

Flumazenil is given IV as (oral bioavailability is very low) to overcome the effects of BZDs. It is rapid and short acting. The disadvantage with flumazenil is its short action and the symptoms of BZD overdosage recur in 3–4 hr as most BZDs are longer acting due to the active metabolites. Hence, dose needs to be repeated and constant monitoring is needed. Adverse effects include nausea, confusion and dizziness. It may rarely induce seizures.

Uses

1. To reverse BZD sedation/anaesthesia
2. In BZD overdosage.

NEWER AGENTS

Melatonin and its Congeners

Melatonin, the hormone secreted by the pineal gland, is known to regulate sleep. It is secreted at night and plays an important role in the circadian rhythm (chronobiotic). Its levels rise and fall accordingly with increasing levels seen in the evening and decreasing towards the dawn.

It acts on two types of **melatonin receptors**—melatonin 1 (MT_1) and melatonin 2 (MT_2) which are GPCRs. It does not depress the CNS; MT_1 receptors mediate sleep while MT_2 receptors are involved in circadian rhythm. Melatonin improves the quality of sleep and helps in withdrawing benzodiazepines after long-term use. However, its role in the maintenance of sleep is not proved.

Administered orally 30–60 min before bedtime in the dose of 2–10 mg, melatonin is considered a natural remedy for insomnia and is free from the disadvantages of BZDs.

Uses

1. **Insomnia:** Hypnotic for short periods and also for chronic insomnia.
2. To help **withdraw** hypnotics like BZDs in elderly dependents.
3. **Jet lag:** Melatonin may be used to overcome jet lag and other conditions of disturbed biorhythm.
4. **Ageing:** The secretion of melatonin decreases with age and, therefore, it is supplemented with the hope that it retards ageing.

Ramelteon, an agonist of the melatonin receptors (both MT_1 and MT_2), is a novel hypnotic drug. Ramelteon reduces the latency of persistent sleep. Advantages are that it does not modify the sleep architecture, there is no rebound insomnia or other major withdrawal symptoms, is well tolerated and is also useful in chronic insomnia with no known abuse liability. Since it is metabolised by microsomal enzymes, the duration of action is prolonged by microsomal enzyme inhibitors and in liver failure (contraindicated).

Dose: 4–16 mg 30 min before going to bed.

Adverse effects include dizziness and fatigue. There could be an increase in prolactin levels and decrease in testosterone.

Tasimelteon: Tasimelteon is another melatonin agonist similar to ramelteon.

Z Hypnotics

The newer agents **zolpidem, zopiclone, eszopiclone and zaleplon** are sedative hypnotics.

- They are not BZDs but produce their effects by binding to the $GABA_A$ receptors and facilitate the inhibitory actions of GABA (Fig. 14.1).
- They are specific hypnotics. They lack antianxiety, anticonvulsant and muscle relaxant properties unlike BZDs.
- The modification of sleep pattern is negligible in therapeutic doses.
- The risks of dependence and tolerance are lower than with BZDs and withdrawal symptoms are milder.
- These newer agents are used for short periods to treat insomnia.
- They are all rapid- and short-acting agents and produce minimum hangover.
- Their actions are blocked by flumazenil.

Zolpidem

Zolpidem is a good hypnotic but has weak anticonvulsant, anxiolytic and muscle relaxant effects.

Zolpidem does not suppress deep sleep (stages 3 and 4 NREM sleep) and the suppression of REM sleep is negligible. It is short acting (t½—2 hr) but the effects on sleep continue for a longer time even after stopping zolpidem. The duration of sleep is 8 hr after a single dose (Table 14.2).

It is well absorbed from the gut and metabolized in the liver by microsomal enzymes—cytochrome P450 (CYP3A4). Dose should be reduced in hepatic dysfunction.

Adverse effects include dizziness and diarrhoea.

Zaleplon

Zaleplon was introduced for clinical use in 1999. It is rapidly absorbed when given on an empty stomach, has a fast onset but short duration of action (t½—1 hr)—hence patients fall asleep quite fast but the nocturnal awakenings and total sleep time are not much affected. It is metabolised in the liver both by microsomal and non-microsomal enzymes. Microsomal enzyme inhibitors prolong the duration of action of zaleplon. No significant adverse effects are reported in therapeutic doses—well tolerated—may occasionally cause headache, dizziness and nausea. Zaleplon is to be avoided in pregnancy and lactating mothers.

Zaleplon has the following advantages:

i. In therapeutic doses, there is no risk of daytime hangover.
ii. Withdrawal symptoms are very mild after stopping it.
iii. Has rapid onset but short duration of action—hence should be taken just before going to sleep.
iv. No significant tolerance develops.
v. No significant abuse potential.
vi. No significant side effects in therapeutic doses.

Uses: Because zaleplon has a rapid onset of action, it is useful in patients who require a long time to fall asleep (long sleep latency). Duration of sleep is not much prolonged with zaleplon.

Zopiclone

Zopiclone is another new hypnotic. Its actions resemble those of BZDs. Zopiclone binds to the $GABA_A$ receptor (Fig. 23.1) and potentiates the effects of GABA. It does not suppress REM sleep but prolongs deep sleep (stages 3 and 4 NREM).

Eszopiclone

Eszopiclone is the S enantiomer of zopiclone—it prolongs the total sleep time. It is metabolized by hepatic microsomal enzymes (cytochrome p450—CYP3A4), has a half-life of 6 hr which is altered by microsomal enzyme inducers and inhibitors.

Mild tolerance to the hypnotic effects of eszopiclone develops after long-term use of 4–6 months.

Adverse effects include dryness of mouth, metallic taste; higher doses can cause impaired psychomotor performance.

Uses of Z Hypnotics

The newer drugs have similar efficacy as BZDs in the treatment of insomnia with the advantages of rapid action and minimum day-after drowsiness and less amnesia. They are recommended for short periods as their long-term safety is yet to be established.

Orexin Receptor Antagonists

Orexins are peptide neurotransmitters in the CNS which control wakefulness. Orexin levels are high in the day and low at night. Orexins act on the receptors OX_1 and OX_2. Orexin receptor antagonists **suvorexant** (10 mg at bedtime), **almorexant** and **filorexant** are new class of drugs useful in insomnia. They block the binding of wake-promoting neuropeptides orexin A and orexin B to the orexin receptors.

BARBITURATES

Barbiturates are derivatives of barbituric acid and were the largest group of hypnotics in clinical use until the 1960s.

Classification

Based on the duration of action:

Long-acting
- Phenobarbitone, mephobarbitone

Short-acting
- Pentobarbitone, butobarbitone

Ultrashort-acting
- Thiopentone, hexobarbitone, methohexitone

Mechanism of Action

Barbiturates bind to a specific site on the GABA receptor Cl^- channel complex (which is different from the BZD binding site). They facilitate inhibitory neurotransmission by **prolonging the duration of opening** of the chloride ion channels by GABA and they hyperpolarise the neural membrane. At high concentrations, barbiturates directly enhance the chloride conductance, i.e. by a GABA-mimetic effect.

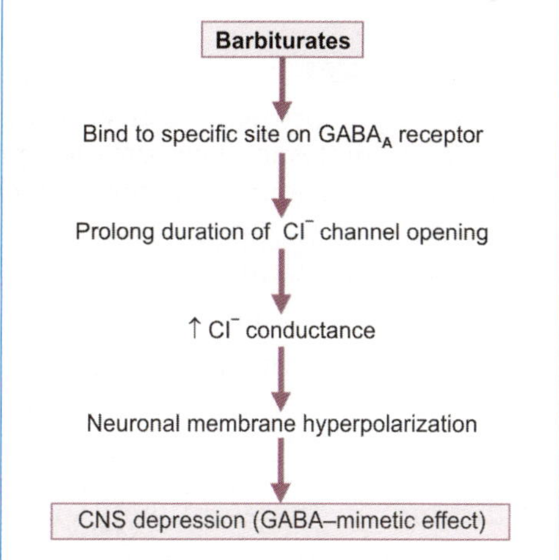

Pharmacological Actions

CNS

Barbiturates cause depression of all excitable tissues of which CNS is the most sensitive.

Sedation and hypnosis: In hypnotic doses, barbiturates induce sleep and prolong the duration of sleep. The REM–NREM sleep cycle is altered with decreased duration of REM and prolonged NREM sleep. On waking up, there is some hangover with headache and residual sedation.

Barbiturates reduce anxiety, impair short-term memory and judgement. They can produce euphoria and are drugs of addiction while some people may experience dysphoria. Barbiturates produce hyperalgesia (increased sensitivity to pain). Therefore, barbiturates, when given as hypnotics for a patient in pain may be more troublesome than being of any benefit.

Anaesthesia: In higher doses, barbiturates produce general anaesthesia. The ultrashort-acting barbiturates like thiopentone are used intravenously for this effect.

Anticonvulsant effects: All barbiturates have anticonvulsant action. **Phenobarbitone** and mephobarbitone have specific anticonvulsant activity in subhypnotic doses and are used in the treatment of epilepsy.

Respiratory System

Barbiturates cause significant depression of respiration. High doses cause profound respiratory depression and also bring about a direct paralysis of the medullary respiratory centre. BZDs in higher doses can cause respiratory depression. It can be profound in patients with pre-existing respiratory disease.

Cardiovascular System

Hypnotic doses of barbiturates produce a slight reduction in blood pressure and heart rate as seen during natural sleep. Toxic doses of barbiturates produce a significant fall in BP due to direct decrease in myocardial contractility and vasomotor centre depression.

Skeletal Muscles

Higher doses of barbiturates depress the excitability of the neuromuscular junction.

Pharmacokinetics

Barbiturates are well-absorbed and widely distributed in the body. The highly lipid-soluble barbiturates, like thiopentone, have a fast onset of action while duration of action is short due to **redistribution** into adipose tissues. Barbiturates are metabolised in the liver. They are hepatic **microsomal enzyme inducers.** The metabolites are excreted in the urine.

Adverse Reactions

Hangover due to residual depression of the CNS may be accompanied by nausea, vomiting, vertigo and diarrhoea. Distortions of mood, impaired judgement and fine motor skills may be evident. Barbiturates may cause excitement and irritability in some patients particularly children.

Barbiturates cause **respiratory depression** and in the presence of respiratory disorders even the hypnotic doses of barbiturates can cause serious respiratory depression. **Hypersensitivity reactions** like skin rashes, swelling of the eyelids and lips and rarely exfoliative dermatitis may be seen.

Drug automatism: As barbiturates cause confusion, disorientation and amnesia, patient may repeatedly take the tablets resulting in overdosage. This phenomenon is 'drug automatism'. It is seen to some extent with BZDs also.

Barbiturates are contraindicated in porphyrias because they increase porphyrin synthesis.

Tolerance and Dependence

On repeated administration, tolerance develops to the effects of barbiturates.

Development of both psychological and physical dependence to barbiturates make them one of the drugs with abuse liability. Withdrawal symptoms include anxiety, restlessness, abdominal cramps, hallucinations, delirium and convulsions.

Acute Barbiturate Poisoning

The fatal dose of phenobarbitone is 6–10 g. Manifestations include respiratory depression with slow and shallow breathing, hypotension, skin eruptions, cardiovascular collapse and renal failure.

Treatment: There is no specific antidote. The measures include:

1. **Gastric lavage** followed by administration of activated charcoal to prevent further absorption of barbiturates.
2. **Artificial ventilation** and oxygen administration.
3. **General supportive measures** like maintenance of BP, patent airway, adequate ventilation and oxygen administration.
4. **Forced alkaline diuresis** with sodium bicarbonate, a diuretic and IV fluids will hasten the excretion of long-acting barbiturates through the kidneys since they are acidic drugs.
5. **Haemodialysis** should be done, especially if there is renal failure.

Uses of Barbiturates

Because of respiratory depression and abuse liability, barbiturates are generally not preferred.

1. *Anaesthesia:* Thiopentone sodium is used IV for the induction of general anaesthesia.
2. *Neonatal jaundice:* Phenobarbitone is a microsomal enzyme inducer because of which it enhances the production of glucuronyl transferase—the enzyme required for metabolism and excretion of bilirubin. It, therefore, helps in the clearance of jaundice in the neonates.
3. *Antiepileptic:* Phenobarbitone is used as an antiepileptic (*see* page 219).
4. *Sedation and hypnosis:* Not preferred.
5. *Preanesthetic medication:* Not preferred.

MISCELLANEOUS

Chloral hydrate is used as an alternative to BZD. It has a bad taste and is an irritant—

Table 14.5: Drugs that can cause insomnia

• Ephedrine	• Levodopa
• Amphetamine	• Amantadine
• Caffiene	• SSRIs
• Chloroquine	• Anorexiants
• Metronidazole	• Nicotine

causes nausea and vomiting. It produces hypnosis without affecting respiratory and cardiovascular functions.

Meprobamate has sedative and antianxiety properties but is now **not recommended.** It produces respiratory depression, ataxia and is a drug of abuse—not preferred.

Paraldehyde is a colourless, transparent, pungent, inflammable liquid. It is an irritant and can dissolve plastic—cannot be given by a plastic syringe. It is a good hypnotic causing little hangover. Paraldehyde also has anticonvulsant properties. It can be given rectally, intramuscularly or orally.

Uses

1. As anticonvulsant in status epilepticus (particularly in children), tetanus and eclampsia.
2. Hypnotic—rarely used.

Clinical Pharmacology

- For patients with sleep onset problems, zolpidem, zopiclone, zaleplon or ramelteon are the first-line agents.
- For patients with sleep onset as well as sleep maintenance problems, controlled release zolpidem or eszopiclone is the preferred choices and BZDs are the second line drugs in these patients.
- Optimizing sleep hygiene, cognitive behavioural therapy and enhancement of slow wave sleep (with sodium oxybate, gabapentin, trazodone or tiagabine) may also be useful.
- BZDs, like alprazolam, acting for almost 24 hours, produce day- time drowsiness and long-term use should be avoided.
- Cognitive impairment with prolonged use of BZDs can also be a problem.

[1] From Medical Council of India, *Competency based Undergraduate Curriculum for the Indian Medical Graduate*, 2018;1:136–144.

CHAPTER 15

Antiepileptic Drugs

Competency achievement: The student should be able to:

PH 1.19 Describe the mechanism/s of action, types, doses, side effects, indications and contraindications of the drugs which act on CNS (including anxiolytics, sedatives and hypnotics, antipsychotic, anti-depressant drugs, anti-manics, opioid agonists and antagonists, drugs used for neurodegenerative disorders, **antiepileptics drugs**).[1]

Epilepsy is a common neurological abnormality that affects about 0.5–1% of the population worldwide. **Epilepsy** is a chronic disorder of brain function characterised by recurrent seizures often accompanied by episodes of unconsciousness and/or amnesia.

Seizure indicates a transient alteration in behaviour because of disordered firing of groups of brain neurons (Key Box 15.1). Such discharges may spread to other parts of the brain to different extents. In most of the cases, the cause is not known. It may be due to various reasons including trauma during birth process, head injury, childhood fevers, brain tumours, meningitis or drug induced. Genetic inheritance of single gene defects accounts for epilepsy in a small percentage of patients.

TYPES OF EPILEPSY

Seizures have been classified into partial and generalised seizures.

Focal onset Seizures

Partial seizures account for about 60% of all epilepsies and begin focally in the cortex, i.e. they involve focal brain regions. They are classified as simple partial in which there is no impairment of consciousness and complex partial seizures with impairment of consciousness. When reticular formation is affected unconsciousness results.

1. **Focal aware seizures:** There is no impairment of consciousness. The manifestations depend on the site in the cortex that is activated by the seizure, e.g. if the motor cortex representing the right thumb is involved, there is recurrent contractions of the right thumb. If the sensory area representing the left palm is involved, there

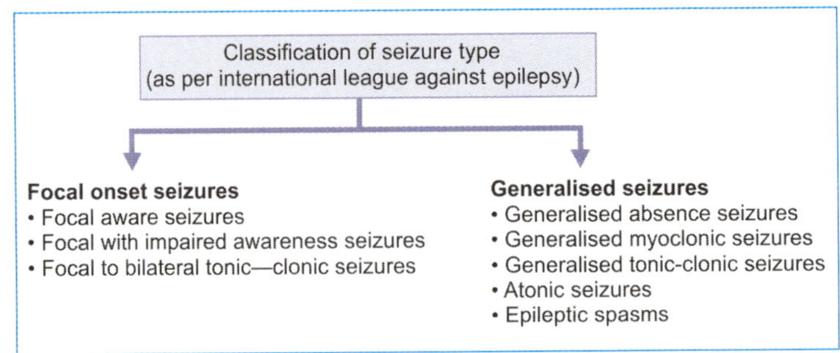

Key Box 15.1: Seizure, convulsions and epilepsy

- Seizure is an episode of brain dysfunction due to abnormal discharge of cerebral neurons.
- Convulsions are involuntary, violent and spasmodic/ prolonged contraction of the skeletal muscle.
- Epilepsy is a disease due to disorder of brain function characterized by episodes of seizures.

is numbness or paresthesia of the left palm. This type of seizures lasts for 20–60 seconds.

2. **Focal with impaired awareness seizure** is the most common type of epilepsy. This is characterised by purposeless movements like lip-smacking, hand wringing or swallowing that lasts for 30 sec to 2 minutes. Consciousness is impaired and may be preceded by an *aura.*
3. **Focal to bilateral tonic-clonic seizures:** Simple or complex partial seizure may evolve into a generalised seizure.

Generalised Seizures

Generalised seizures account for 40% of all epilepsies and are usually of genetic aetiology. Generalised seizures affect the whole brain. They may be:

1. *Generalised absence seizures (earlier petit mal):* In this, there is a sudden onset of impaired consciousness associated with staring. The person stops all on-going activities and the episode lasts for a brief period usually less than 30 seconds.
2. *Generalised myoclonic seizures* involve a sudden, brief, shock-like contraction of the muscles. It may be limited to a part of the body or may affect the whole body.
3. *Generalised atonic seizures (drop attacks)* are characterised by sudden loss of postural tone and the head may drop for a few seconds or the person may drop to the ground for no obvious reasons.
4. *Generalised tonic-clonic seizures (earlier grand mal epilepsy)* are characterised by sudden loss of consciousness followed by sustained contraction of muscles throughout the body (known as tonic phase), lasting for 1 minute and then, a series of jerks, i.e. periods of muscle contraction alternating with periods of relaxation (clonic phase) lasting for 2–4 minutes follow. CNS depression then occurs and the person goes into sleep. Injury may occur during the convulsive episode.

Status Epilepticus

Status epilepticus is continuous or recurrent seizures of any variety without recovery of consciousness between the attacks.

ANTIEPILEPTICS

Antiepileptics can be classified as follows:

Classification

1. ***H**ydantoins*	Phenytoin, mephenytoin
2. ***B**arbiturates*	Phenobarbitone, mephobarbitone
3. ***D**eoxybarbiturate*	Primidone
4. ***I**minostilbene*	Carbamazepine
5. ***S**uccinimide*	Ethosuximide
6. ***G**ABA transaminase inhibitors*	Valproic acid, vigabatrin
7. ***B**enzodiazepines*	Diazepam, clonazepam, lorazepam, clorazepate
8. ***M**iscellaneous*	Magnesium sulphate Acetazolamide
Newer agents	
9. ***M**ost commonly used*	Levetiracetam, lacosamide, lamotrigine, topiramate.
10. Drugs influencing **G**ABA	Gabapentin, pregabalin, vigabatrin, tiagabine, stiripentol
11. ***O**thers*	Felbamate, zonisamide, rufinamide, retigabine, parempanel

Mnemonic: This **H**appy **B**irth **D**ay **IS** **G**oing to **B**e **M**y **M**ost **G**ala **O**ne

Mechanism of Action of Antiepileptics

The strategies to treat epilepsy include enhancing GABA-mediated inhibition, reducing excitatory transmission or modifying the ionic conductances. Thus, antiepileptics act by one or more of the following mechanisms (Fig. 15.1, Flowchart 15.1)

- **Na^+ channel blockers** cause Na^+ channel blockade and prolongation of their inactive state and delaying their recovery, e.g. phenytoin, carbamazepine, lamotrigine.
- **Ca^{++} channel blockers** (thalamic-T type) block low threshold Ca^{++} current in the thalamic neurons—control absence seizures, e.g. ethosuximide.
- Increasing GABA-mediated inhibition by:
  - acting on GABA receptors, e.g. benzodiazepines, pregabalin, gabapentin
  - inhibiting GABA metabolism—valproate
  - potentiating GABA—- topiramate
- Blocking excitatory glutamate receptors—felbamate

PHENYTOIN

Phenytoin (diphenylhydantoin) was synthesized in 1908, but its anticonvulsant property was discovered only in 1938.

Phenytoin

Pharmacological Actions

CNS Phenytoin has good antiseizure activity and is one of the most effective drugs against generalised tonic-clonic seizures and partial seizures. It brings about its effects without causing general depression of the CNS.

Mechanism of Action

Phenytoin causes blockade of the voltage-dependent sodium channels and **stabilizes the neuronal membrane.** It inhibits the generation of repetitive action potentials (Fig. 15.1).

Voltage-dependent Na^+ channels enter an inactive stage after each action potential. Phenytoin blocks the Na^+ channels which are in an inactivated state and delay the recovery of these channels from inactivation. It decreases the number of channels which are available for the generation of action potentials and inhibits excitability of these voltage-dependent Na^+ channels. Phenytoin preferentially blocks high frequency firing (neurons in normal state have low frequency firing while in seizures, high-frequency firing occurs) (Flowchart 15.2 and Key Box 15.2).

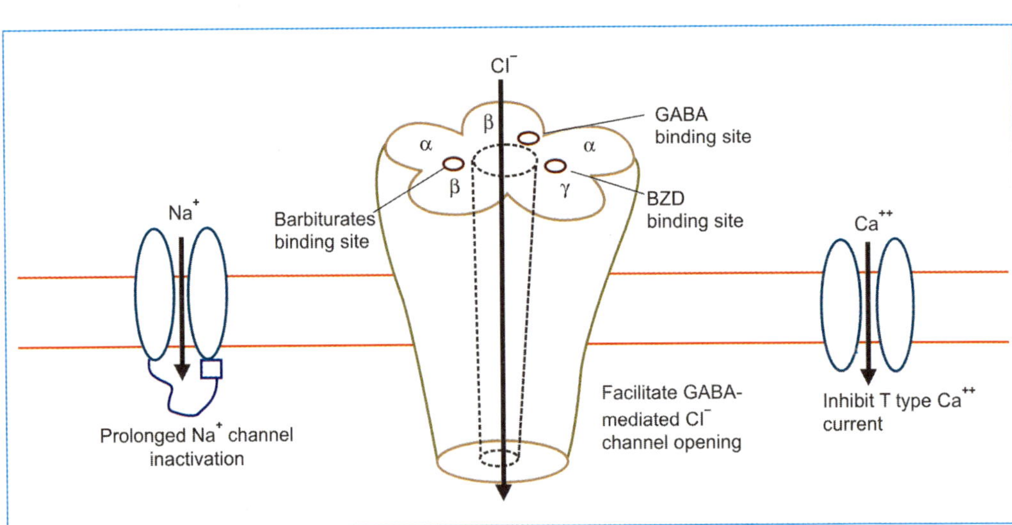

Fig. 15.1: Mechanisms of action of antiepileptics. Antiepileptics may act by blockade of Na^+ channels, by facilitating GABA activity or by blockade of Ca^{++} current

Flowchart 15.1: Clinical correlation of mechanism of action and uses of antiepileptics

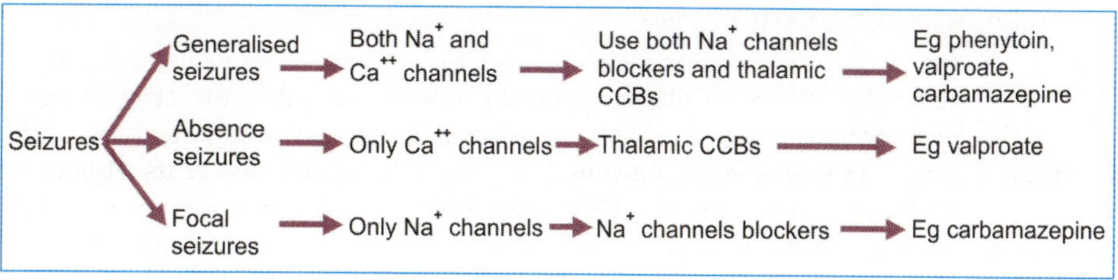

Pharmacokinetics

Phenytoin is poorly water-soluble—hence absorption is slow but is almost complete on oral administration. Phenytoin **should not be** given IM because absorption is unpredictable and a fraction of the drug may also precipitate in the muscle. **Fosphenytoin** can be given IM (*see* below). Phenytoin is 90% bound to plasma proteins. The t½ of phenytoin ranges from 12–36 hr with longer t½ at higher concentrations. Valproic acid competes with phenytoin for plasma protein binding sites and may result in phenytoin toxicity. It is metabolised in the liver initially by first order and later by zero order kinetics as the dose increases. Therefore, monitoring of plasma concentration is useful. Phenytoin is an enzyme inducer. Glucose containing fluids are not suitable for infusion of phenytoin.

Dose: 100 mg BD. Children 5–8 mg/kg/day. EPTOIN 50, 100 mg tab, 30 mg/ml susp, 50 g/ml amp. FENTOIN-ER 100 mg ER-Cap. EPICENT 100 mg tab.

Adverse Effects

Adverse effects depend on the dose, duration and route of administration (Table 15.1).

1. *Nausea*, vomiting, epigastric pain, anorexia.
2. *Nystagmus*, diplopia, ataxia are common.
3. *Gingival hyperplasia* is more common in children on prolonged use. It could be because phenytoin inhibits the enzyme collaginase and alters collagen metabolism. It also promotes angiogenesis in the gingival tissue through increased activity of growth factors. It is more common in children and good oral hygiene should be followed.

Flowchart 15.2: Mechanism of action of phenytoin

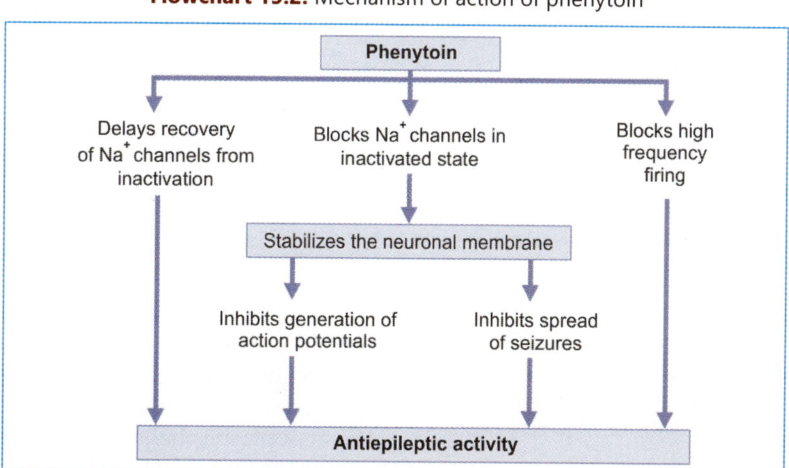

Table 15.1: Prominent adverse reactions and therapeutic uses of some antiepileptic drugs

Drug	*Important adverse reactions*	*Indication*
Phenytoin	Ataxia, gingival hyperplasia, diplopia, cardiac conduction blocks, hirsutism, neuropathy, megaloblastic anaemia	GTCS and focal onset seizures
Carbamazepine	Ataxia, diplopia, vertigo, drowsiness, antidiuretic effects, cardiac conduction blocks	GTCS and focal onset seizures
Phenobarbitone	Sedation, ataxia, nystagmine, megaloblastic anaemia, osteomalacia	GTCS, focal onset and gen myoclonic seizures, SE
Ethosuximide	Gastritis, drowsiness, dizziness, headache	Gen absence seizures
Valproic acid	Gastritis, hepatotoxicity, sedation, alopecia, weight gain	GTCS, focal onset seizures, gen myoclonic, absence seizures
Clonazepam and clobazam	Sedation	Gen absence seizures, gen myoclonic seizures, infantile spasms
Levetiracetam	Drowsiness, dizziness, ataxia, weakness	Refractory focal, gene tonic—clonic and gen myoclonic seizures
Lamotrigine	Diplopia, drowsiness, ataxia, dizziness	GTCS, focal onset, gen absence seizures
Gabapentin	Drowsiness, dizziness, ataxia	GTCS, focal onset seizures
Topiramate	Drowsiness, confusion, paraesthesias, renal stones, weight loss, migraine	GTCS, focal onset seizures, gen absence seizures
Zonisamide	Drowsiness, confusion, cognitive impairment	GTCS, focal onset and gen myoclonic seizures

GTCS: Generalised tonic-clonic seizures; SE: Status epilepticus, gen: Generalised

4. *Peripheral neuropathy*—on long-term use with diminished deep tendon reflexes.
5. *Endocrine*
   - Hirsutism, acne due to increased secretion of androgens and coarsening of facial features.
   - Hyperglycaemia—as phenytoin inhibits insulin release.
   - ↓ release of ADH.

Key Box 15.2: Phenytoin

- Blocks Na^+ channels.
- Blocks high frequency firing seen in seizures.
- Blocks Na^+ channels in an inactivated state and delays their recovery.
- Main adverse effects—vestibular effects, GI disturbances; long-term use—gum hyperplasia, hirsutism and megaloblastic anaemia.
- Teratogenic.
- May worsen myoclonic and atonic seizures.
- Use: Focal onset and GTCS, SE, trigeminal neuralgia, cardiac arrhythmias

   - Osteomalacia, hypocalcaemia—due to altered metabolism of vitamin D and inhibition of intestinal absorption of calcium.
   - Phenytoin also reduces target tissue sensitivity to vitamin D.
6. *Hypersensitivity*—rashes, SLE, hepatic necrosis, lymphadenopathy and neutropenia. Idiosyncratic reactions including hepatic necrosis, **Stevens-Johnson syndrome** and SLE have been reported.
7. *Megaloblastic anaemia*—as phenytoin decreases absorption and increases excretion of folates.
8. *Cardiotoxicity*—phenytoin can cause cardiac conduction blocks.
9. *Teratogenicity*—when taken by the pregnant lady, phenytoin produces **foetal hydantoin syndrome** characterised by hypoplastic phalanges, cleft palate, harelip and microcephaly in the offspring.

Toxic doses: Intravenous administration of phenytoin in higher doses results in cardiac arrhythmias, hypotension and CNS depression. When high doses are given orally, cerebellar and vestibular effects are prominent; vestibular effects include nystagmus, vertigo, diplopia and ataxia. Drowsiness, delirium, confusion, hallucinations, disorientation, altered behaviour and coma follow.

Uses

1. Generalised tonic-clonic seizures (GTCS) and focal onset seizures (not useful in absence seizures).
2. Status epilepticus—phenytoin is used by slow IV injection.
3. Trigeminal neuralgia—as an alternative to carbamazepine.
4. Cardiac arrhythmias—phenytoin is useful in digitalis-induced arrhythmias (*see* page 378).

Drug Interactions

- Phenytoin is an enzyme inducer. Given with phenobarbitone, both increase each other's metabolism. Also phenobarbitone competitively inhibits phenytoin metabolism.
- Carbamazepine and phenytoin enhance each other's metabolism.
- Valproate displaces protein bound phenytoin and may result in phenytoin toxicity.
- Cimetidine and chloramphenicol inhibit the metabolism of phenytoin resulting in toxicity.
- Antacids $\downarrow$ absorption of phenytoin.

Fosphenytoin is a prodrug of phenytoin that has certain advantages over phenytoin for parenteral use:

- It is quickly converted to phenytoin in the body.
- More potent.
- Less cardiotoxic.
- Safer on the intestine.
- It can be injected into a glucose drip unlike phenytoin.
- Drip rate can be faster than phenytoin.
- Can be given IM.
- Damage to the vessel wall is milder than with phenytoin.

Because of the above advantages, fosphenytoin is preferred over phenytoin in status epilepticus.

Dose: 20 mg/kg IV FOSOLIN 75 mg/ml inj.

Mephenytoin, ethotoin and phenacemide are congeners of phenytoin. Ethotoin can be used as an alternative in patients allergic to phenytoin. Adverse effects of ethotoin are milder. Phenacemide is used in patients with refractory partial seizures when other drugs fail. It is a highly toxic drug.

PHENOBARBITONE

Phenobarbitone (*see* page 211) was the first effective antiepileptic drug to be introduced in 1912. It still remains one of the widely used drugs.

Antiepileptic actions: Phenobarbitone has specific antiepileptic activity and raises the seizure threshold. Primidone which is rarely used now is metabolised to phenobarbitone. Phenobarbitone is effective in tonic-clonic seizures and is ineffective in absence seizures. Though other barbiturates also have anticonvulsant effects, the dose required produces significant sedation.

Mechanism of action: Barbiturates enhance the inhibitory neurotransmission in the CNS by enhancing the activation of $GABA_A$ receptors and thus facilitating the GABA-mediated opening of chloride ion channels (Fig. 15.1). Barbiturates also reduce glutamate-mediated excitation.

Pharmacokinetics: Oral absorption of phenobarbitone is slow but complete. About 50% is bound to plasma proteins. It is a microsomal enzyme inducer and can result in many drug interactions.

Dose: 60 mg OD-TDS. GARDENAL 60, 30 mg tab. 20 mg/5 ml syrup. PHENETONT, BARBEE 30, 60 mg tab.

Adverse effects: Sedation is the most common side effect. Tolerance develops to some extent to sedation after prolonged use. Phenobarbitone, like phenytoin, can also cause nystagmus, ataxia, megaloblastic anaemia and osteomalacia. Skin rashes and other hypersensitivity reactions can occur.

Uses: Phenobarbitone is still one of the widely used antiepileptics because of its efficacy and low cost.

It is used in:

1. Generalised tonic-clonic seizures.
2. Focal onset seizures.

Primidone is metabolized to phenobarbitone in the body. The mechanism of action, however, seems to resemble phenytoin. It is effective in partial and generalised tonic-clonic seizures. Absorption of primidone is complete and is gradually converted to phenobarbitone. Primidone is started at low doses and gradually increased to attain steady state. Adverse effects are that of phenobarbitone.

Dose: 250–500 mg BD MYSOLINE 250 mg tab.

CARBAMAZEPINE

Carbamazepine is a tricyclic compound closely related to imipramine. It is one of the most commonly used antiepileptic drugs.

Antiseizure activity: Carbamazepine has good antiseizure activity. Its mechanism of action and antiepileptic actions are similar to phenytoin, i.e. it blocks sodium channels. It is effective in generalised tonic-clonic seizures and focal onset seizures.

Carbamazepine is also useful in the treatment of trigeminal neuralgia (severe pain along the distribution of the trigeminal nerve) and glossopharyngeal neuralgia. It is also found to be beneficial in mood disorders. Carbamazepine has mild antidiuretic effects.

Pharmacokinetics: Absorption is slow and erratic; has a t½ of 30–36 hours. It is a powerful microsomal enzyme inducer and after repeated administration, its t½ reduces to 8–12 hr due to **'autoinduction'** (enhances its own metabolism). Therefore, patients on carbamazepine need therapeutic drug monitoring.

Dose: 200–400 mg TDS. Extended release preparation given twice daily. TEGRETOL, VERSITOL, ZEPTOL 100, 200, 400 mg, 100 mg/5 ml syrup.

Adverse effects: Drowsiness, vertigo, ataxia, diplopia, blurring of vision, nausea, vomiting and dizziness are common. Driving is dangerous for patients on carbamazepine. It also causes water retention due to antidiuretic effects. Hypersensitivity reactions, like skin rashes, may occur. Haematological toxicity includes leukopenia, thrombocytopenia and rarely agranulocytosis and aplastic anaemia. It is a teratogen.

Drug interactions: Carbamazepine is an enzyme inducer—can increase **its own metabolism** and that of other drugs like phenytoin, valproic acid and clonazepam.

Mnemonic for salient features of carbamazepine

A to H of hot antiepileptic carbamazepine not to forget Neuralgias

A—Autoinduction
B—Bipolar mood disorder
C—Chronic neuropathic pain
D—anti-Diuretic
E—Enzyme inducer
F—Focal onset seizures
G—Generalised tonic-clonic seizures
H—Hemifacial spasm
Neuralgias—trigeminal and glossopharyngeal

Uses

1. Generalised tonic clonic seizures (grand mal epilepsy)—commonly used drug.
2. Focal onset seizures—especially temporal lobe epilepsy.
3. Trigeminal neuralgia and glossopharyngeal neuralgia—carbamazepine is the

drug of choice for these neuralgias and has to be given for several months.
4. It is also effective in hemifacial spasm following facial palsy.
5. Useful in chronic neuropathic pain and in tabetic pain.
6. Bipolar mood disorder—carbamazepine is used as an alternative to lithium as a mood stabilizer (*see* page 253).

Oxcarbazepine and **eslicarbazine** are prodrugs and the active metabolites act similar to carbamazepine in actions and uses.

Advantages over carbamazepine:
- Fewer hypersensitivity reactions,
- Milder induction of microsomal enzymes—hence fewer drug interactions.
- Eslicarbazine is longer acting, hence once daily dosing.

Oxcarbazepine has been tried as an alternative to carbamazepine in focal onset seizures. Enzyme induction due to these drugs can result in oral contraceptive failure.

Dose: 900–1800 mg/day. OXEP, OXEPTAL, CARBOX 150, 300, 600 mg tab.

ETHOSUXIMIDE

Ethosuximide is a succinimide. It raises the seizure threshold.

Mechanism of action: Ethosuximide reduces the low threshold calcium currents (T-currents) in the thalamic neurons. These T-calcium currents are thought to be responsible for absence seizures.

Pharmacokinetics: Absorption is complete on administration of oral dosage forms. It is metabolised in the liver. It has a t½ of about 40 hr, but is given twice daily to avoid gastrointestinal adverse effects.

Adverse effects: The most common adverse effects are nausea, vomiting, epigastric pain, gastric irritation and anorexia. These can be avoided by starting with a low dose and gradually increasing it. CNS effects like drowsiness, fatigue, lethargy, euphoria, dizziness, headache and hiccough are dose-related effects. Hypersensitivity reactions like rashes, urticaria, leukopenia, thrombocytopenia or pancytopenia have been reported.

Uses: Ethosuximide is the drug of choice for generalised absence seizures but currently valproate is preferred by most clinicians.

VALPROIC ACID

Valproic acid (salt-sodium valproate) is a very effective antiepileptic drug useful in many types of epilepsies including absence seizures, focal onset and generalised tonic-clonic seizures.

Divalproex sodium is a combination of valproic acid and sodium valproate. The combination is said to have a better bioavailability and is better tolerated.

Mechanism of action: Valproic acid acts by multiple mechanisms.
1. It enhances the levels of GABA by:
   - Increasing the synthesis of GABA—by increased activity of GABA synthetase enzyme.
   - Decreasing the metabolism of GABA—by inhibiting GABA transaminase enzyme.
2. Like phenytoin, valproic acid blocks the sodium channels.
3. Like ethosuximide valproate decreases low threshold Ca^{++} current (T-currents) in the thalamus.

Pharmacokinetics: Valproate is well absorbed when given orally, but food may delay its absorption, 90% bound to plasma proteins and is metabolised in the liver. Clearance is dose-dependent with half-life varying from 9 to 18 hr.

Adverse effects: Gastrointestinal symptoms, like nausea, vomiting, epigastric distress, occur initially. Weight gain is common. Tremors, sedation, ataxia, rashes and alopecia are rare. Sodium valproate can cause hepatotoxicity in children below 2 years of age which can be fatal. Hepatotoxicity is thought to be an idiosyncratic response. Though it is more likely to occur in children below 2 years of age who are also on other antiepileptics, hepatotoxicity can occur in patients of all age groups. Hence, careful monitoring of liver functions is mandatory. Valporic acid should be avoided in patients with hepatic dysfunction. Idiosyncratic thrombocytopenia has also been reported.

Valproic acid is teratogenic, it can cause neural tube defects including spina bifida.

Drug interactions: Valproate increases plasma phenytoin levels by displacing it from plasma protein binding and also inhibiting its metabolism. Valproate inhibits the metabolism of carbamazepine and phenobarbitone. Valproate inhibits the clearance of lamotrigine.

Uses

1. Used in focal onset and generalised seizures. Valproic acid is particularly useful in absence seizures and myoclonic seizures. In patients with both absence seizures and generalised tonic-clonic attacks, valproate is the drug of choice. It is also effective in juvenile myoclonic seizures.
2. Valproate is useful as a mood stabilizer in bipolar mood disorder (*see* page 253).
3. It has been tried in the prophylaxis of migraine.

BENZODIAZEPINES

Benzodiazepines have useful anticonvulsant properties. **Diazepam** is the drug of choice in status epilepticus and febrile convulsions. Diazepam may also be given rectally and is the preferred route in febrile convulsions. **Lorazepam** may be used in place of diazepam (0.1 mg/kg IV) as it is effective and longer acting. **Clonazepam** is a potent antiepileptic useful in absence and myoclonic seizures. It has the advantage of being long-acting but causes significant sedation—should be started with low doses and gradually increased. Tolerance develops both to sedation and antiepileptic effects. **Nitrazepam** has also been used in myoclonic seizures and infantile spasms. **Clorazepate** is used as an add-on drug in complex partial seizures. **Clobazam** causes less sedation and is effective in most types of epilepsies—used as an adjuvant (0.1 mg/kg/day) to other antiepileptic drugs.

MISCELLANEOUS DRUGS

Magnesium sulphate given intravenously, has anticonvulsant properties. It is used to prevent and treat convulsions in eclampsia in pregnant women. In addition, magnesium sulphate relaxes the uterus and also reduces the BP which may be beneficial in such patients.

Acetazolamide, a carbonic anhydrase inhibitor, has antiseizure activity particularly in absence seizures. Because of the rapid development of tolerance and several adverse effects with its use, acetazolamide is not a preferred antiepileptic.

NEWER ANTIEPILEPTICS

Most commonly used:

1. **Levetiracetam,** an analog of piracetam, is effective against partial and secondarily generalized seizures. Mechanism of action is not exactly known, but it binds to a protein (synaptic vesicular protein) in the synapse and modifies the release of glutamate and GABA.

Advantages: It is not an enzyme inducer—no related drug interactions; almost **completely absorbed** and can be given both oral and IV.

Adverse effects include drowsiness, dizziness, weakness, ataxia and in some patients psychotic symptoms.

Uses: Levetiracetam can be used as an add-on drug in refractory partial seizures, generalised tonic-clonic seizures and myoclonic seizures.

It is also being prescribed as the antiepileptic in pregnancy.

Dose: 250–1000 mg BD. EPICTAL. LEVTAM 250, 500, 700 mg tab.

Brivaracetam and **seletracetam** are analogs similar to levetiracetam.

2. **Lamotrigine** has a broad-spectrum of antiepileptic activity. It prolongs the inactivation of sodium channels and also inhibits the release of the excitatory amino acids like glutamate. Lamotrigine is completely absorbed on oral administration and is metabolized by glucuronidation. Lamotrigine may cause skin rashes, drowsiness, nausea, ataxia, blurred vision and dizziness. It is used either alone or with other drugs in focal onset and generalized seizures. Absence and myoclonic seizures also respond.

Drug interactions: Phenytoin, phenobarbitone and carbamazepine reduce the t½ of lamotrigine by 6–8 hours, whereas valproic acid increases the t½ of lamotrigine by inhibition of glucuronidation—lamotrigine dose should be reduced by 50%.

Dose: 50–300 mg/day. LAMEPIL, LAMOIG 25, 50, 100 mg tab.

3. **Topiramate,** a monosaccharide, acts by multiple mechanisms:

- It blocks the sodium channels.
- Enhances $GABA_A$ receptor currents and thereby potentiates the effects of GABA.
- Also blocks AMPA receptors (glutamate receptor).

It is effective in focal onset and generalized seizures.

Dose: Started with 50 mg/day—gradually increased to 200–600 mg/day. EPITOP 25, 50, 100 mg tab. TOPEX, TOPIVA 25, 50, 100 mg tab.

Adverse effects include fatigue, drowsiness, dizziness and nervousness. It can promote the formation of **renal calculi** because it inhibits the enzyme carbonic anhydrase; dysguisia and cognitive dysfunction have been reported. It is teratogenic.

Uses: Topiramate can be used as add-on therapy in **refractory epilepsy** and in **Lennox-Gastaut syndrome**. It has also been used as monotherapy or add-on therapy in **focal onset**, **generalised** and in **absence seizures** and infantile spasms. Topiramate is also effective in **migraine** headache.

4. **Lacosamide (LCM)** is a functionalised amino acid that demonstrates efficacy in epilepsy and in neuropathic and chronic pain. Lacosamide selectively enhances sodium channel slow inactivation but has no effects of fast inactivation. In the clinical trials, LCM was well tolerated. Nausea, dizziness, sedation, headache and diplopia were reported. LCM is orally effective, completely absorbed and has a t½ of 13 hr.

LCM is approved for use in the treatment of partial seizures as an adjuvant and as monotherapy in diabetic neuropathic pain.

Dose: 50–100 mg BD.

Drugs influencing GABA

5. **Gabapentin** and 6. **pregabalin** called "gabapentinoids" are analogs of GABA, designed to cross the BBB. However, they do not act directly on GABA receptors. Their exact mechanism of action is not known. They bind to α-2 δ-1 subunit of voltage gated calcium channels and may decrease glutamate release at the excitatory synapses.

Both are absorbed well—gabapentin is highly lipid soluble. Absorption depends on a carrier protein and does not increase with an increase in dose because it gets saturated, hence, both are safe. Both gabapentinoids are not bound to plasma proteins and do not influence the plasma concentration of other drugs—no significant drug interactions known.

Adverse effects: Both are well tolerated. Common adverse effects include ataxia, fatigue, drowsiness and dizziness. Tolerance develops to these effects in 1–2 weeks. Weight gain due to water retention and peripheral oedema may be seen in a small percentage of patients.

Dose: Gabapentin 300 mg OD-TDS. GABA 200 mg cap; GABACENT 100, 300 mg tab

Pregabalin 75–150 mg BD. GABAWIN, PREGABIN 75, 150 mg tab.

Uses

1. *Focal onset seizures:* Gabapentin and pregabalin are used as add-on drugs particularly in refractory focal seizures, started with a low dose and gradually increased to therapeutic levels.
2. *Neuropathic pain:* Both gabapentinoids are effective in neuropathic pain including post-herpetic neuralgia, diabetic neuropathy and chronic pain associated with spinal cord injury.
3. *Fibromyalgia:* Pregabalin relieves symptoms of fibromyalgia.
4. *Migraine:* Pregabalin is also tried in migraine.
5. Bipolar mood disorders and other anxiety disorders could respond to pregabalin.

7. **Vigabatrin** is a GABA analogue which acts by irreversibly inhibiting the enzyme GABA transaminase, thereby raising brain GABA levels. It can cause depression in some patients. Vigabatrin is useful in patients not responding to other antiepileptics.

8. **Tiagabine,** a GABA analogue, inhibits the reuptake of GABA into neurons and thereby enhances extracellular GABA levels. It may cause tremors, drowsiness, dizziness and confusion. Tiagabine can be used as add-on drug for refractory partial seizures. It has also been tried as monotherapy.

9. **Stiripentol** enhances GABA release and improves GABAergic transmission in the brain. It is a microsomal enzyme inhibitor and enhances the levels of other antiepileptics given concurrently. It is used as an add on drug with clobazam and valproate in refractory generalized seizures in children.

Others

10. **Felbamate,** an analogue of meprobamate is found to have good antiepileptic action. It blocks the NMDA receptors in addition to its weak sodium channel blocking effect. However, felbamate can sometimes cause serious adverse effects like aplastic anaemia and hepatitis because of which it is employed only in refractory epilepsy.

11. **Zonisamide,** a sulfonamide derivative, acts by inhibiting T type Ca^{++} currents and also by blocking Na^{+} channels. It is well tolerated and is indicated in refractory partial and generalised tonic-clonic and myoclonic seizures as well as infantile spasms.

Advantages: No drug interactions with other antiepileptic drugs are known. Almost completely absorbed, has a long t½ of 1–3 days.

Dose: 100–600 mg/day. ZONEGRAN 100 mg FC-tab. ZONISEP 25, 50, 100 mg tab.

12. **Parempanel,** an AMPA receptor antagonist, blocks the AMPA receptor and prevents repetitive discharge. Effective in a single daily dose in partial seizures and is well tolerated in most patients. However, it can cause serious behaviour disturbances in some patients particularly those with pre-existing psychiatric illness.

Since parampanel is metabolized by the microsomal enzymes, risk of related drug interactions with inducers and inhibitors should be considered while prescribing. Parempanel may be used in **refractory partial seizures**.

13. **Retigabine:** It is a potassium channel facilitator approved as an add-on drug in refractory partial seizures. Adverse effects include sedation, weight gain, confusion, disturbed bladder function, QT prolongation and ocular toxicity. A unique adverse effect is the bluish discolouration of the skin on prolonged use.

14. **Rufinamide,** a triazole derivative, acts on the sodium channels and is useful in Lennox-Gastaut syndrome and may also be effective in partial seizures.

CLINICAL PHARMACOLOGY

- In all patients of epilepsy, an attempt should be made to detect the cause. The

Table 15.2: Choice of antiseizure drugs

Types of seizures	*Preferred drugs*	*Alternative drugs*
1. Focal aware seizures 2. Focal with impaired awareness seizures 3. Focal to bilateral tonic-clonic seizures	Carbamazepine, phenytoin, valproic acid	Gabapentin, lamotrigine, topiramate
4. Generalised absence seizures	Ethosuximide, valproate	Clonazepam, lamotrigine
5. Generalised tonic-clonic seizures	Carbamazepine, phenytoin, valproic acid	Lamotrigine, topiramate, phenobarbitone, levetiracetam
6. Generalised tonic-clonic + generalised absence seizures	Valproic acid	
7. Generalised myoclonic seizures	Valproic acid	Clonazepam, levetiracetam
8. Status epilepticus	Diazepam, lorazepam, fosphenytoin, general anaesthesia	Clonazepam, lamotrigine, phenobarbitone
9. Febrile convulsions	Diazepam (rectal)	Lorazepam

goal of therapy is to keep the patient free of seizures (Table 15.2) without interfering with normal daily activity. Treatment should be started with a single drug at a low dose; dosage is increased gradually, preferably by monitoring the drug levels in plasma. If a single drug is not effective, another drug should be tried.

- Good compliance is very important for success. Regarding the duration—decision should be made on an individual basis and dose should be very gradually reduced over months to avoid status epilepticus.
- Almost all antiepileptics produce side effects related to the CNS. Drowsiness is the most common side effect of most of them.

  The ratio of ED_{50} (neurological impairment) to ED_{50} (seizure protection) is called **protective index.** Higher the protective index, safer is the drug.
- Most antiepileptics are sedatives—patients should be warned about this and adjust the time of intake.
- Alcohol potentiates CNS depression of antiepileptics.
- Most antiepileptics are teratogenic.
- Carbamazepine needs TDM.
- Monitor liver function of patients on sodium valproate.
- Patient's attendants should be taught how to protect the patient in case of a convulsion like protection of tongue and airway.
- Drug interactions may occur among different antiepileptics and should be kept in mind.
- Antiepileptics should always be tapered. If stopped suddenly, risk of status epilepticus.
- Single daily dose ensures better compliance.

Febrile convulsions: Two to four per cent of children experience convulsions during fever; of them 2–3% become epileptics. Treatment is controversial. Children <18 months developing febrile convulsions, those with neurological abnormalities and those with seizures lasting for >15 minutes, complex seizures—all these have greater risk of recurrence. Diazepam (0.5 mg/kg) given orally or rectally at the onset of fever prevents convulsions. Timely use of paracetamol and tepid sponging prevent high fever. If convulsions occur, diazepam (rectally or intravenously) can be used.

Status epilepticus is a neurological emergency which may be fatal. **Lorazepam** 0.1 mg/kg IV is the drug of choice in status epilepticus. **Diazepam** IV 5–10 mg every 10–15 minutes up to 30 mg is an alternative. **Fosphenytoin** is now preferred to phenytoin in status epilepticus. Earlier phenytoin (IV) was given. A loading dose 500–1000 mg phenytoin (max 1000 mg in 24 hr) takes 15–20 min to act. Some prefer to combine diazepam and phenytoin (60 mg/min). Patient could require **ventilatory support**. Patients who do not respond to phenytoin, phenobarbitone may be given in higher doses 100–200 mg (total 400–800 mg). Respiratory depression is expected. If seizures continue, **general anaesthesia** with propofol or thiopental is the last resort. Thiopentone sodium/propofol 3–5 mg/kg followed by 30–100 mg/min—dose adjusted to suppress seizures guided by EEG. Airway maintenance is important. After the control of seizures, long-term antiepileptic therapy is needed.

Absence status (absence seizures going into status epilepticus) **IV diazepam/lorazepam** is the drug of choice.

Treatment of Epilepsy in Pregnancy

In pregnancy, antiepileptics should be continued because abrupt discontinuation increases the risk of status epilepticus which is hazardous to the foetus. Children of mothers receiving antiepileptic drugs in pregnancy have a 2–3 times increased risk of developing congenital defects. Most antiepileptics are teratogenic—phenytoin can cause 'fetal hydantoin syndrome' and sodium valproate can cause neural tube defects. Though **carbamazepine** use was associated with major malformations like microcephaly and growth retardation, the incidence and the defects were the same as that seen in mothers who did not receive antiepileptics. **Levetiracetam** has been found to be a good choice in pregnancy. Lamotrigine has also been used though it could increase the risk of cleft lip. However, seizures in a pregnant lady are harmful to the foetus. Thus it has been agreed upon that epilepsy should be well controlled before pregnancy.

Lowest possible doses of antiepileptics should be continued in pregnancy. Treatment should be restricted to a single drug as far as possible. Folic acid supplementation (500 μg daily) should be given during 2nd and 3rd trimester to avoid neural tube defects. Vitamin K_1 10 mg/day is given for last 2–4 weeks to avoid vitamin K deficiency and bleeding disorders.

[1] From Medical Council of India, *Competency based Undergraduate Curriculum for the Indian Medical Graduate*, 2018;1:136–144.

CHAPTER 16

Drugs used in Neurodegenerative Disorders—Parkinsonism and Alzheimer's Disease

Competency achievement: The student should be able to:

PH 1.19 Describe the mechanism/s of action, types, doses, side effects, indications and contraindications of the drugs which act on CNS, (including anxiolytics, sedatives and hypnotics, antipsychotic, antidepressant drugs, antimanics, opioid agonists and antagonists, **drugs used for neurodegenerative disorders,** antiepileptics drugs).[1]

ANTIPARKINSONIAN DRUGS

Parkinsonism is a chronic, progressive, motor disorder characterised by rigidity, tremors and bradykinesia. Other symptoms include excessive salivation, abnormalities of posture and gait, seborrhoea and mood changes. It was described by James Parkinson in 1817 and is, therefore, named after him.

The incidence is about 1% of population above 65 years of age. It is usually idiopathic in origin but can also be drug induced. In idiopathic parkinsonism, there is degeneration of nigrostriatal neurons in the basal ganglia resulting in dopamine deficiency (Fig. 16.1). The balance between inhibitory dopaminergic neurons and excitatory cholinergic neurons is disturbed. Dopamine synthesized in the dopaminergic nerve terminals acts on dopamine receptors. Of the 5 subtypes (D_1–D_5) of the DA receptors, all types are present in different parts of the brain, but striatum is rich in D_1 and D_2 subtypes and are important in the pathophysiology of parkinsonism.

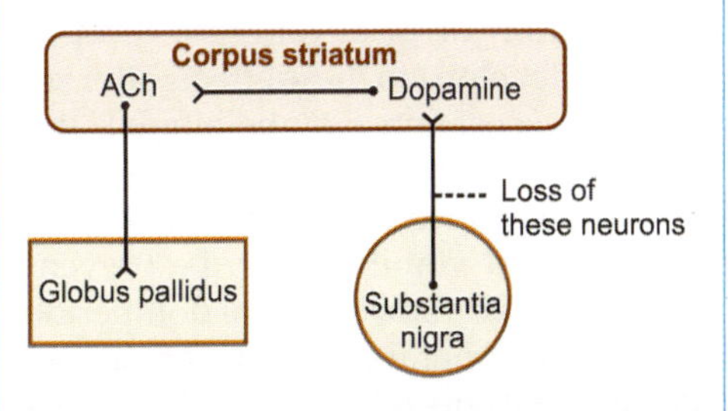

Fig. 16.1: Pathophysiology of parkinsonism: Nigrostriatal neurons degenerate resulting in ↓DA content in these neurons

Antiparkinsonian drugs can only help to alleviate the symptoms and improve the quality of life. The two strategies in the treatment are:

i. To enhance dopamine activity
ii. To depress cholinergic overactivity.

Often combination of drugs are used to influence both functions. Drugs used in Parkinson's disease (PD) can be classified as:

Classification

1. **Drugs that increase dopamine influence**
   i. **DA precursor**
   Levodopa
   ii. **Dopaminergic agonists**
   Bromocriptine, pergolide
   Lisuride, ropinirole, pramipexole
   Rotigotine, apomorphine
   iii **Dopamine metabolism inhibitors**
   - ***MAO_B inhibitors:*** Selegiline, rasagiline, safinamide
   - ***COMT inhibitors:*** Tolcapone, entacapone

   iv. **DA releaser**
   Amantadine
   v. **Peripheral dopa decarboxylase inhibitors**
   Carbidopa, benserazide
2. **Drugs influencing cholinergic system**
   i. **Central anticholinergics**
   Benzhexol (trihexyphenidyl), benztropine, biperidien
   ii. **Antihistamines**
   Diphenhydramine
   Orphenadrine, promethazine

DOPAMINE PRECURSOR

Levodopa

Though parkinsonism is due to dopamine deficiency, dopamine is of no therapeutic value because it does not cross the blood–brain barrier. Levodopa is a prodrug which is converted to dopamine in the body. Levodopa crosses the BBB and is taken up by the surviving nigrostriatal neurons. It is converted to DA in the dopaminergic neurons of the striatum.

HO, HO, CH_2–CH–COOH, NH_2

Levodopa

$$\text{Levodopa} \xrightarrow{\textit{Dopa decarboxylase}} \text{Dopamine}$$

Antiparkinsonian effect: On administration of levodopa, there is an overall improvement in the patient as all the symptoms subside.

Bradykinesia, rigidity and tremors respond. There is an improvement in sialorrhoea, seborrhoea, mood changes and general motor performance. The patient shows more interest in the surroundings.

However, some studies have shown that levodopa may generate oxidative stress damaging the dopaminergic neurons on long-term use.

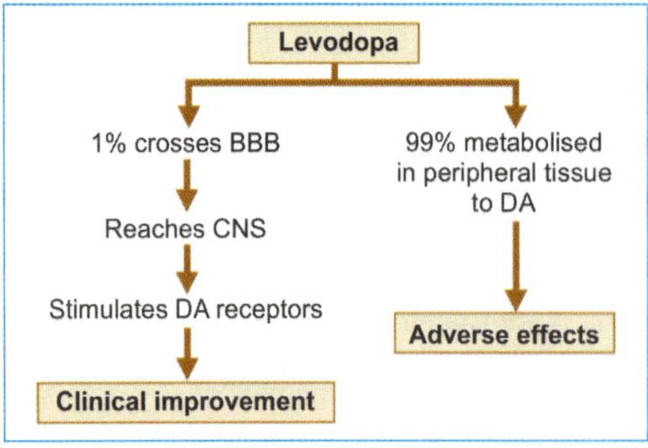

Other Actions

Large amounts of levodopa are converted to dopamine in the periphery which brings about other actions.

- *CTZ:* Dopamine stimulates the CTZ to induce vomiting.
- *CVS:* It causes postural hypotension, tachycardia and arrhythmias. Dopamine is a catecholamine.
- *Endocrine:* Dopamine suppresses the prolactin secretion.

Pharmacokinetics

Levodopa is rapidly absorbed from the small intestine. An active transport process that is meant for amino acids is responsible for absorption and transport of levodopa into the brain across the BBB. Therefore, some amino acids in food compete with levodopa for both absorption and transport into the brain. Presence of food delays its absorption. If gastric emptying is delayed, bioavailabilty is reduced due to higher first pass metabolism. It undergoes first pass metabolism in the gut and the liver. Its t½ is 1–2 hours. 1–2% of an oral dose reaches the brain.

Adverse Reactions

As nearly 99% of levodopa is converted to dopamine in the periphery, several adverse effects are expected. Nausea, vomiting, anorexia, postural hypotension, palpitation and occasionally arrhythmias can occur due to stimulation of β_1 adrenergic receptors. Tolerance develops to these effects after some time. Taste sensation may be altered. It can cause mydriasis and may raise IOP → should be avoided in glaucoma. The peripheral effects viz nausea and vomiting may be prevented by concurrent administration of domperidone which is a peripheral dopamine antagonist.

Behavioural effects like anxiety, depression, hallucinations, mania, trauma, confusion and sometimes psychosis can occur. Dopaminergic drugs including levodopa should not be withdrawn abruptly—may precipitate neuroleptic malignant syndrome with confusion, rigidity and hyperthermia. Excessive dopaminergic activity (due to levodopa) in the limbic system could be responsible for these effects.

Abnormal involuntary movements, like facial tics, grimacing and choreoathetoid movements of the limbs, may develop after a few months of use and require reduction in the dose of levodopa.

Fluctuation in response to levodopa can occur after 2–5 years of use—known as 'on-off' phenomenon—where the patient swings alternately from periods of good response to severe disabling disease. The reduced response or 'wearing off' of effect may increase over time.

Uses

Levodopa is the most effective drug in idiopathic parkinsonism but is not useful in drug-induced parkinsonism. However, on long-term use, there is 'wearing-off' of therapeutic effects. Sustained release formulations are now tried so that the therapeutic levels can be constantly maintained. It has recently come to light that in the process of metabolism of levodopa, free radicals are generated, which may produce oxidative damage and death of nigrostriatal fibres. This has been a concern for use of levodopa to initiate therapy.

Drug Interactions

1. Pyridoxine enhances peripheral decarboxylation of levodopa and thus reduces its availability to the CNS.
2. Phenothiazines and metoclopramide are DA antagonists. They reverse the effects of levodopa.
3. Non-selective MAO inhibitors prolong the action of levodopa and may result in hypertensive crisis.

Precautions and Contraindications

- Levodopa should be avoided in patients with psychosis and narrow angle glaucoma.
- Levodopa should be used with caution in patients with IHD, hepatic and renal disorders.
- Peptic ulcer—risk of gastrointestinal bleeding.
- Malignant melanoma and its premalignant skin lesions—careful monitoring required because levodopa is the precursor of melanin and may stimulate the growth of melanoma.

Carbidopa and Benserazide

These are peripheral dopa decarboxylase inhibitors. When carbidopa and benserazide are given with levodopa, they prevent the formation of dopamine in the periphery. They do not cross the BBB and hence allow levodopa to be converted to DA in the CNS. The combination is synergistic and, therefore, levodopa is always given with carbidopa/ benserazide.

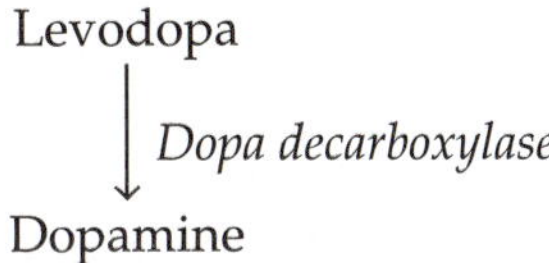

Advantages of the Combination

1. Dose of L-dopa can be reduced by 75%.
2. Response to L-dopa appears earlier.
3. Side effects like vomiting and tachycardia are largely reduced.
4. Pyridoxine does not interfere with the treatment.

Preparations and Dose

Fixed dose combination of 1:10 or 1:4, i.e. 10 mg carbidopa with 100 mg levodopa or 25 mg carbidopa with 100/250 mg levodopa is available. LEVOPA-C, TIDOMET forte levodopa 250 mg + carbidopa 25 mg tab. SYNDOPA carbidopa—25, 50 mg, Levodopa—100, 200 mg. BENSPAR levodopa 100 mg + Benserazide 25 mg.

DOPAMINE RECEPTOR AGONISTS

Dopaminergic agonists have the advantages of **directly stimulating the DA receptors** and do not depend on the enzymes for convertion to active metabolites (unlike levodopa). They are less likely to generate free radicals which could damage the dopaminergic neurons. They are longer acting than levodopa and are the first-line drugs in Parkinson's disease.

Bromocriptine and pergolide, the older agents, are ergot derivatives. Bromocriptine is an agonist at D_2 and a partial agonist at D_1 while pergolide is an agonist at both D_1 and D_2 receptors. The newer agents **ropinirole** and **pramipexole** are non-ergot derivatives, are selective D_2 and D_3 agonists, are better tolerated than older agents and quickly attain therapeutic levels (hence dose titration can be done faster). Their adverse effects are milder except that they may cause some sleep disorders. Being longer-acting, they are less likely to cause dyskinesia and 'on-off' phenomenon.

DA agonists are well absorbed given orally. Dopamine agonists are all longer acting because of which they are useful in the treatment of 'on-off' phenomenon.

Adverse effects include nausea, vomiting, anorexia, dyspepsia and skin eruptions. Ergot derivatives can cause postural hypotension or hypertension initially and first dose phenomenon → sudden cardiovascular collapse. Cardiac arrhythmias can occur.

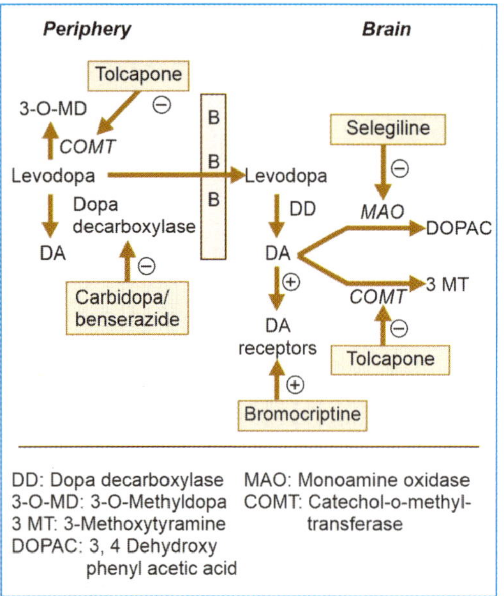

Fig. 16.2: Sites of action of drugs in parkinsonism

Psychiatric disturbances like hallucinations, confusion, impulsive behaviour (betting, gambling, sexual overactivity due to loss of impulse control) are reported but are reversible. Sleep disorders with uncontrolled sleep may require withdrawal of DA agonists. Patients should be warned to avoid driving. These drugs should be started with a low dose and gradually increased. **Pergolide has been withdrawn** due to cardiovascular toxicity.

Uses: Newer agents are preferred-ropinirole and pramipexole are used for:

1. Initiation of therapy in PD as first-line drugs.
2. In the treatment of on-off phenomena.
3. Restless leg syndrome-ropinirole or pramipexole is taken 2–3 hours before sleep.

Pramipexole 0.125–1.5 mg TDS, PARPEX 0.5, 1, 1.5 mg.

Ropinirole 0.25–4–8 mg TDS, ROPIN, ROPITOR 0.25, 0.5, 1, 2 mg tab

Rotigotine another DA agonist, has been used as a **transdermal** patch so that constant dopaminergic stimulation is possible. In addition to the side effects of other DA agonists, local reaction to the patch can also occur. **Lisuride** is similar to bromocriptine but is also a serotonin receptor agonist and not commonly used.

Apomorphine is used subcutaneously (2–6 mg) for short periods as 'rescue' medication to tide over akinesia in patients receiving regular dopaminergic medication. Since apomorphine is an emetic, suitable antiemetic (domperidone) should be given.

DRUGS THAT INHIBIT DA METABOLISM

MAO_B Inhibitor

Of the two types of monoamine oxidases MAO_B selectively metabolises dopamine. Selegiline is a selective MAO_B inhibitor in therapeutic doses but in higher doses it also inhibits MAO_A. MAO_B is present in DA containing regions of the CNS. Selegiline prolongs the action of levodopa by preventing its degradation. Some studies suggest that selegiline may delay the progression of parkinsonism.

Adverse effects include nausea, postural hypotension, confusion and hallucinations.

Uses

Mild cases of parkinsonism are started on selegiline. It is also used as an adjunct to levodopa as it prolongs the action of levodopa and the dose of levodopa can be reduced.

Dose: 5 mg each at breakfast and lunch; should be avoided at night as it causes insomnia. SELERIN, JVMAX 5 mg tab.

Rasagiline is more potent than selegiline. It may also slow the course and progression of disease by a neuroprotective effect like selegiline.

The risk of drug interactions—serotonin syndrome (*see* page 250), if taken with TCA or SSRIs, should be borne in mind.

Safinamide is a newer drug under develoment which inhibits MAO-B as well as DA reuptake.

COMT Inhibitors

Tolcapone and entacapone inhibit the peripheral metabolism of levodopa by inhibiting the enzyme COMT—thereby they increase the bioavailability of levodopa. Tolcapone crosses the BBB and enhances the availability of levodopa in the brain. The duration of action of levodopa is prolonged and the response is smoother with reduced on-off periods.

Both are rapidly absorbed; entacapone has peripheral effects, whereas tolcapone has both central and peripheral effects.

Adverse effects: Adverse effects are nausea, diarrhoea orthostatic hypotension, dyskinesias, sleep disturbances, confusion and hallucinations mostly due to increased effects of L-dopa. Dose of levodopa should be reduced by 30%. Tolcapone can also cause hepatotoxicity, raised hepatic enzymes and rarely acute hepatic failure which may be fatal. Liver function needs to be monitored every 2 weeks and this makes entacapone more preferred.

Uses: COMT inhibitors are used as add-on drugs in parkinsonism. A fixed dose combination of levodopa and carbidopa with entacapone is available in some countries.

ENTACAPONE Dose: 200 mg 1 tab with every dose of LEVODOPA. COMTAN, EMTACOM 200, 400 mg tab.

DRUGS THAT RELEASE DOPAMINE

Amantadine is an antiviral drug but was found to be effective in parkisonism. It enhances the release of DA in the brain and also diminishes the re-uptake of DA. Amantadine is also an adenosine receptor antagonist and adenosine receptors are found to inhibit the D_2 receptors. Thus this action may also help patients with parkinsonism. The response starts early and its adverse effects are minor. Large doses produce insomnia, irritability, excitement, headache, constipation, dizziness, vomiting, postural hypotension, hallucinations, ankle oedema and livido reticularis.

Amantadine is used in mild cases of parkinsonism. It can also be used along with levodopa as an adjunct. Amantadine is used for short periods as the response may be blunted after a few weeks. Dyskinesias may also subside.

Dose: 100 mg BD-TDS. AMANTREL, COMANTREL 100 mg tab.

ANTICHOLINERGICS

The cholinergic overactivity is overcome by anticholinergics. They block the muscarinic receptors in the striatum. Tremors, seborrhoea and sialorrhoea are reduced more than rigidity and bradykinesia. Atropine derivatives like benzhexol (trihexyphenidyl), biperiden, procyclidine and benztropine are used.

Clinical Pharmacology

- Parkinsonism should be treated only when symptoms are bad enough to initiate therapy.
- Treatment is mostly symptomatic.
- Selegiline and rasagiline have been shown in some studies to delay the progress of PD.
- Treatment is initiated with selegiline or DA agonists like ropinirole/pramipexole.
- Levodopa is always given with carbidopa and is still the mainstay of treatment in PD. However, generation of free radicals causing oxidative stress and thereby damaging nigrostriatal fibre is a cause of concern.
- All drugs are started with a low dose and gradually titrated.
- After about 2–3 years of use, disease progression, decreased response and on-off phenomena may complicate treatment.
- To smoothen the on-off phenomenon, ropinirole/pramipexole and entacapone may be used as adjuvants.
- Drug holidays: When adverse effects become seriously troublesome or when the response to drugs is inadequate, a drug holiday for a short period (3–21 days) may be tried. Some of the adverse effects may subside and the response after restarting may be better. However, there are certain disadvantages like increased risk of venous thrombosis, pulmonary embolism and depression, hence it is no more recommended.

Antihistamines, like orphenadrine, owe their beneficial effects in parkinsonism to their anticholinergic properties. Atropine-like side effects such as dry mouth, constipation, urinary retention and blurred vision may be encountered.

Uses

Anticholinergics are used as: (i) Adjuncts to levodopa, (ii) drugs of choice in drug-induced parkinsonism.

Benzhexol Dose: 2–10 mg/day PARKIN, PACITANE 2 mg tab.

Orphenadine: Dose: 100–300 mg/day. ORPHIDAL 50 mg tab. **Peribedil:** Dose: 50–100 mg/day. TRIVASTAL-LA 50 mg tab.

DRUG-INDUCED EXTRAPYRAMIDAL REACTIONS

Drugs like reserpine, metoclopramide and phenothiazines can induce extrapyramidal reactions. Reserpine depletes dopamine (catecholamines) stores, while metoclopramide and phenothiazines are dopamine antagonists. Several types of extrapyrimidal reactions may be induced—symptoms of **drug induced parkinsonism** are almost similar to idiopathic parkinsonism.

Treatment: Whenever possible the drug responsible for it should be withdrawn—this usually reverses the symptoms. Low doses of benzhexol (or other anticholinergics) are given along with antipsychotics to prevent and treat EPS.

Dystonias which are painless, spasmodic contractions of muscles (e.g. torticollis, trismus) may be seen following metoclopramide or phenothiazines. Promethazine inj 25 mg may be followed by 1–2 oral doses.

Levodopa or other dopamine agonists are **not effective in drug-induced parkinsonism because DA receptors are blocked** by drugs like metoclopramide and phenothiazines.

DRUGS USED IN ALZHEIMERíS DISEASE

Alzheimer's disease (AD) is a neurodegenerative disorder, characterized by progressive impairment of memory and cognitive functions. Other symptoms like depression, anxiety and disturbed sleep may also be seen. Pathological features include atrophy of the cerebral cortex and loss of neurons—mainly cholinergic neurons with multiple senile (amyloid) plaques and neurofibrillary tangles in the brain. Since there is loss of cholinergic neurons, drugs that enhance cholinergic function have been tried. Many other drugs have also been used to improve cognitive functions with variable results.

Tacrine is a centrally acting cholinesterase inhibitor. It enhances cholinergic transmission

Drugs used in Alzheimer's disease

Cholinesterase inhibitors
Tacrine, rivastigmine, donepezil, galantamine
Nootropic agents (cognition enhancers)
Piracetam, aniracetam, cerebrolysin
NMDA receptor antagonist
Memantine
Others
Piribedil, ginkgo biloba

in the brain. But it is short acting and also causes various side effects including nausea, vomiting, abdominal cramps, diarrhoea and hepatotoxicity. The newer agents ***rivastigmine, donepezil*** and ***galantamine*** are better tolerated with fewer side effects. They are selective central anticholinesterases—hence do not cause the GI side effects which are due to peripheral cholinergic activity. They increase acetylcholine levels in the surviving neurons and have produced good response—cognitive function improves and the symptom score shows benefit. They are not hepatotoxic and are longer acting. All are started at low doses which are gradually increased. Donepezil has the advantage of longer action and once a day administration.

Preparations

Rivastigmine 1.5–6 mg BD. RIVAMER 1.5, 3, 4.5 and 6 mg cap.

Donepezil: 5 mg HS. DONECEPT 5, 10 mg cap.
Galantamine: 4 mg BD. GALAMER 4, 8, 12 mg tab.

Nootropic agents have not shown consistent results in Alzheimer's disease.

Memantine is an NMDA receptor antagonist found to be useful in patients with moderate to severe AD. The benefit is thought to be due to blockade of glutamate-induced excitotoxicity. Memantine is well tolerated as the adverse effects are mild and reversible—may cause dizziness and headache. It is used in moderate to severe AD. Started with 5 mg OD and increased to 10 mg BD.

NSAIDs: Small doses of aspirin (and other NSAIDs) have been shown to delay the onset of AD. However, further studies are needed to prove their benefit.

Amyotropic Lateral Sclerosis

Amyotropic lateral sclerosis is a rapidly progressive motor neuron disorder that is characterised by damage to motor neurons of the ventral horn of the spinal cord that control the voluntary muscles. Manifestations include progressive muscle weakness, atrophy, fasciculations and spasticity. Both upper and lower motor neurons are affected. Till now it was treated symptomatically—for example, muscle relaxants, like baclofen, are used for spasticity. The only drug that was recently made available for the treatment of ALS in riluzole.

Riluzole blocks the sodium channels and calcium channels. It is an NMDA/glutamate receptor antagonist. It increases survival. It is orally effective, highly protein bound and given 50 mg BD. It is well tolerated. Nausea, diarrhoea and rarely hepatotoxicity are noted.

Ginkgo biloba: An extract of the chinese plant contains ginkgoflavon glycosides. It is thought to act as a PAF antagonist and decreases the production of TXA_2 and inhibits platelet aggregation. It has been used as a cognition enhancer—but the benefits have yet to be proved.

GINKOCER, GINKOBA 40 mg tab.

[1] From Medical Council of India, *Competency based Undergraduate Curriculum for the Indian Medical Graduate*, 2018;1:136–144.

CHAPTER 17

Drugs used in Psychiatric Disorders: Antipsychotics and Antianxiety Agents

Competency achievement: The student should be able to:

PH 1.19 Describe the mechanism/s of action, types, doses, side effects, indications and contraindications of the drugs which act on CNS, (including anxiolytics, sedatives and hypnotics, **antipsychotic**, antidepressant drugs, anti-manics, opioid agonists and antagonists, drugs used for neurodegenerative disorders, antiepileptics drugs).[1]

Since ages, man has sought the help of drugs to modify behaviour, mood and emotion.

Psychoactive drugs were used both for recreational purposes and for the treatment of mental illnesses (*Psyche* = mind).

In 1931, Sen and Bose showed that *Rauwolfia serpentina* is useful in the treatment of insanity. ECT was introduced in 1937 for the treatment of depression. In 1950, chlorpromazine was synthesized in France and its usefulness in psychiatric patients was demonstrated in 1952. Since the second half of the twentieth century, extensive research has been carried out in psychopharmacology and we now have several useful drugs in this branch of pharmacology.

Psychiatric conditions are broadly divided into:

- Organic mental disorders
- Psychoses
- Neuroses
- Personality disorders.

1. Organic Mental Disorders

An organic cause is present in these disorders, i.e. a definable toxic, metabolic or pathological change—e.g. head injury.

2. Psychoses

Of the psychiatric disorders, psychoses are the most severe forms and involve a marked impairment of behaviour, inability to think coherently, and to comprehend reality. Patients have no 'insight' into these abnormalities and have hallucinations and delusions. These include functional disorders where there is no organic cause like in schizophrenia, delusional disorders (paranoia) and affective (mood) disorders.

Schizophrenia: Schizophrenia affects about 1% of population, starts at an early age and is highly incapacitating. It has a strong hereditary tendency and is a **disorder of thinking**—earlier called split mind. Schizophrenia is characterised by delusions, hallucinations, irrational conclusions, interpretations and withdrawal from social contacts. Symptoms are grouped as positive and negative. ***Positive symptoms*** include delusions, hallucinations and disorders of thought while ***negative symptoms*** include poor concentration, social withdrawal, poverty of speech and lack of initiative and energy. Negative symptoms generally indicate poor prognosis and these symptoms do not respond to antipsychotic drugs. Patients with chronic schizophrenia have progressive shrinkage of the brain.

The pathology is not exactly understood but available evidence suggest overactivity of the neurotransmitters mainly dopamine and probably others including glutamate (NMDA receptors), 5-HT and noradrenaline in the brain. The **dopamine theory** was proposed by Carlson which is based on indirect evidences. Drugs that increase DA activity in the brain (amphetamine—increases DA release, bromocriptine—DA agonist) produce psychotic episodes akin to schizophrenia. Drugs that reduce dopaminergic activity (DA antagonists like chlorpromazine, DA storage depletor—reserpine) control symptoms of schizophrenia and also prevent amphetamine-induced behavioural changes.

Glutamate theory: NMDA receptor antagonists like ketamine and phencyclidine produce symptoms of psychosis. There is decrease in glutamate concentration and glutamate receptor density in the brain of schizophrenic patients—a postmortem finding. Glutamate has excitatory and DA has inhibitory effects on the striatal neurons. Decrease in glutamate or excess of DA would result in uninhibited sensory inputs to reach the cortex. It is also proposed that DA overactivity is responsible for positive symptoms while deficient NMDA-receptor activity is the cause for negative symptoms.

Other transmitters: Hallucinogens like LSD are serotonin agonists and also influence NMDA receptors—modulate 5-HT and DA release at many sites. Most atypical antipsychotics act by blocking the 5-HT_{2A} receptors or influencing NA receptors and some by stimulating 5-HT_{2C} receptors. The whole area is complex and much needs to be understood.

3. Neuroses

Neuroses are the milder forms of psychiatric disorders and include anxiety, panic disorders, obsessions, irrational fears and reactive depression as seen following tragedies.

4. Personality Disorders

Personality disorders include paranoid, schizoid, histrionic, avoidant, antisocial and obsessive compulsive personality types.

Drugs used in psychiatric illnesses may be grouped as:

1. *Antipsychotics:* Used in psychoses.
2. *Antidepressants:* Used in affective disorders.
3. *Mood stabilizers:* Used in bipolar mood disorders.
4. *Antianxiety drugs:* Used in anxiety related disorders.

Psychotropic drugs are drugs used in mental illnesses—they are drugs capable of affecting the mind, emotions and behaviour.

Neuroleptic is a drug that reduces initiative, brings about emotional quietening and induces drowsiness.

Tranquilizer is a drug that brings about tranquillity by calming, soothing and quietening effects. This is the older terminology. Neuroleptics or antipsychotics were called 'major tranquilizers' and antianxiety drugs were called 'minor tranquilizers'. These terminologies are no longer used.

ANTIPSYCHOTICS (NEUROLEPTICS)

Classification

1. *Classical/typical/First generation neuroleptics*

A. *Phenothiazines*

Aliphatic side chain:	Chlorpromazine Triflupromazine
Piperidine side chain:	Thioridazine
Piperazine side chain:	Trifluoperazine Fluphenazine

B. *Butyrophenones*

Haloperidol	Droperidol
Trifluperidol	Penfluridol

C. *Thioxanthenes* — Thiothixene, Flupenthixol

2. *Atypical/Second generation neuroleptics*

Clozapine	Olanzapine
Risperidone	Quetiapine
Paliperidone	Ziprasidone
Amisulpride	Sertindole
Zotepine	Aripiprazole
Asenapine	

3. *Newer drugs* — Cariprazine, brexpiprazole

4. *Miscellaneous*

Reserpine	Loxapine Pimozide

CHLORPROMAZINE (CPZ)

Delay and Deniker demonstrated the antipsychotic effect of chlorpromazine. It has a wide variety of actions (hence the brand name Largactil) because it blocks the actions of several neurotransmitters including adrenaline, dopamine, histamine, acetylcholine and serotonin.

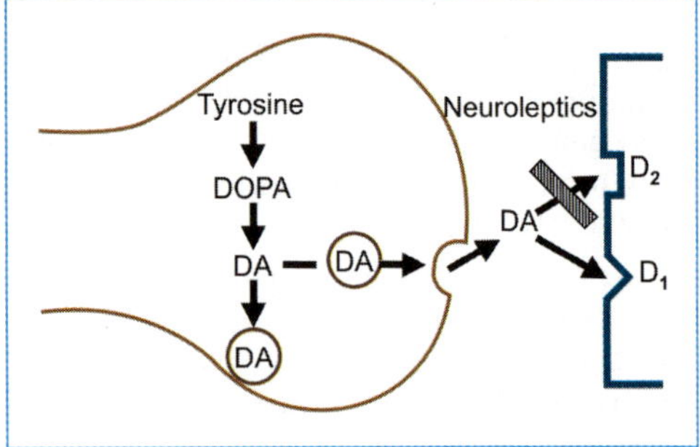

Fig. 17.1: Mechanism of action of neuroleptics. Neuroleptics block the dopamine D_2 receptors and act as antipsychotics

Mechanism of Action

Typical or first generation neuroleptics act by blocking the dopamine D_2 receptors in the CNS (Fig. 17.1). There are 5 subtypes of dopamine receptors—D_1 to D_5. They are all G-protein-coupled receptors. As proposed in DA hypothesis, dopaminergic overactivity mainly in the limbic area is thought to be responsible for schizophrenia, and typical antipsychotics block dopamine D_2 receptors in the CNS particularly in the limbic and mesolimbic area.

Some drugs like phenothiazines also block D_1, D_3 and D_4 receptors. However, antipsychotic efficacy correlates with D_2 blocking ability. Dopamine receptor blockade also is responsible for the classical side effects (Fig. 17.2) of these agents including extrapyramidal effects.

Pharmacological Actions

CNS: Behavioural effects—in normal subjects, CPZ reduces motor activity, produces drowsiness and indifference to surroundings. In psychotic agitated patients, it induces neuroleptic syndrome, reduces aggression, initiative, impulsiveness and motor activity, relieves anxiety and brings about emotional quietening and drowsiness. Hallucinations, delusions and disordered thought gradually subside. In animal studies, neuroleptics selectively inhibit conditioned avoidance response. They induce sedation and normalise the sleep disturbances characteristic of psychoses.

Other CNS Actions

1. *Cortex:* CPZ lowers seizure threshold and can precipitate convulsions in untreated epileptics.
2. *Hypothalamus:* CPZ decreases gonadotrophin secretion and may result in amenorrhoea in women. It increases the secretion of prolactin resulting in galactorrhoea and gynaecomastia.

COMPARE AND CONTRAST

Typical and atypical antipsychotics/First and second generation antipsychotics

Features	***Chlorpromazine***	***Clozapine***
Group	Typical antipsychotic	Atypical antipsychotic
Mechanism of action	D_2 receptor blocker	D_4 blocker, weak D_2 blocker, 5-HT_{2A} blocker
Absorption	Poor: Bioavailability ~30%	Good: 45–65%
Potency	High	Low
Extrapyramidal adverse effects	High	Very low
Sedation	High	Low
Hypotension	+++	+
Galactrorrhoea, gynaecomastia	Yes	No
Risk of angranulocytosis	No	Yes

Seradase—do not put me to sleep

Rudresh, a diabetic, was an in-patient for drainage of an abscess. He was prescribed Seradase 10 mg (serratiopeptidase) tablets. The patient was found to be unusually drowsy the whole day and had extrapyramidal symptoms. On investigating the cause, it was found that the patient was given Seranase 10 mg (haloperidol) in place of seradase. Such medication errors can put both the patient and the doctor including the nurse into trouble.

3. *Basal ganglia:* CPZ acts as a dopamine antagonist and, therefore, results in extrapyramidal motor symptoms (drug-induced parkinsonism).
4. *Brainstem:* Vasomotor reflexes are depressed leading to a fall in BP.
5. *CTZ:* Neuroleptics block the dopamine (DA) receptors in the CTZ and thereby act as antiemetics.

Autonomic nervous system: The actions on the ANS are complex. CPZ is an alpha blocker. The alpha blocking potency varies with each neuroleptic. CPZ also has anticholinergic properties which leads to side effects. The degree of anticholinergic activity also varies with each drug.

CVS: Neuroleptics produce orthostatic hypotension due to alpha receptor blockade action and reflex tachycardia. CPZ also has a direct myocardiac depressant effect like quinidine.

Local anaesthetic: CPZ has local anaesthetic properties—but is not used for the purpose since it is an irritant.

Kidney: CPZ depresses ADH secretion and has weak diuretic effects.

Tolerance develops to the sedative and hypotensive actions while no tolerance is seen to the antipsychotic actions.

Pharmacokinetics

CPZ is incompletely absorbed following oral administration and also undergoes significant

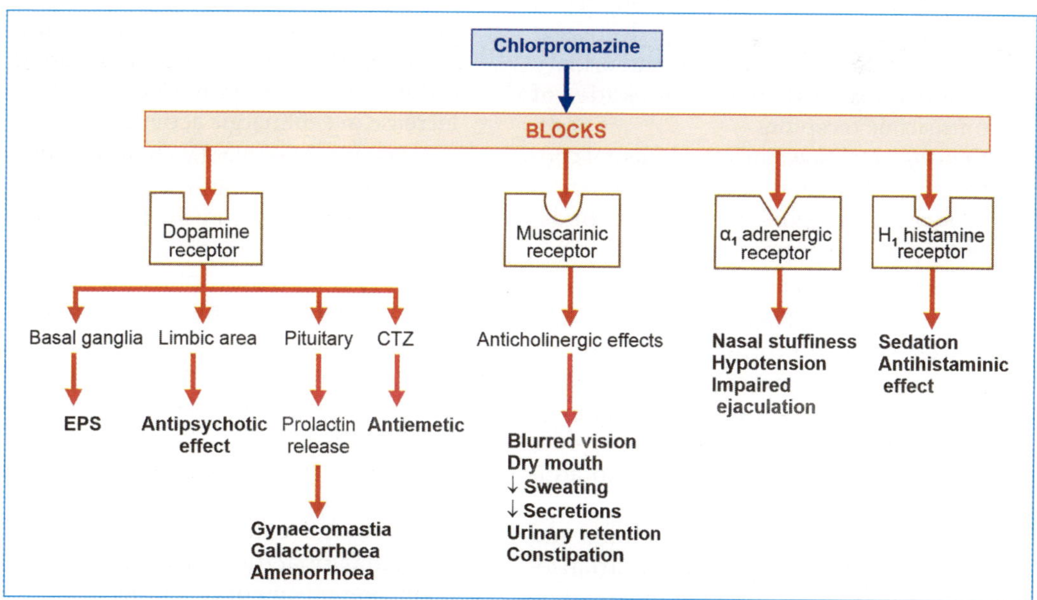

Fig. 17.2: Chlorpromazine and other neuroleptics block dopamine, muscarinic, α_1 adrenergic and H_1 histamine receptors which is responsible for their wide range of actions and adverse effects.

first pass metabolism (bioavailability is 30%). It is highly protein bound; has a t½ of 20 to 24 hr and is, therefore, given once a day.

Dose: 100–800 mg daily. LARGACTIL 10, 25, 50, 100 mg tab; 25 mg/5 ml syr; 50 mg/2 ml inj.

Adverse Reactions

Antipsychotics have a high therapeutic index and are fairly safe drugs (Fig 17.2).

1. ***Cardiovascular and autonomic effects:*** Antipsychotics can cause postural hypotension and palpitation both due to **alpha receptor blockade** and central effects. Parenteral administration may cause more prominent **hypotensive** effect.
   Some of the antipsychotics like CPZ, haloperidol, ziprasidone and pimozide in higher doses can cause prolongation of QT interval—may lead to arrhythmias in overdosage. Caution is required for concurrent use with other drugs that also prolong QTc like mefloquine, halofantrine, quinine and some antiarrhythmics.
   Nasal stuffiness and inhibition of ejaculation is due to α blockade; blurred vision, dry mouth, reduced sweating, decreased gastric motility, constipation and urinary retention result from blockade of muscarinic receptors.
2. ***CNS effects:*** Drowsiness and mental confusion are common, several neurological syndromes involving the extrapyramidal system are the prominent side effects.

Extrapyramidal symptoms

i. *Acute dystonias:* Facial grimacing, tics, muscle spasms, protruding tongue and similar involuntary movements can occur in the first **few days** of starting antipsychotics especially the high potency ones like haloperidol. They respond to anticholinergics.

ii. *Parkinsonism:* Bradykinesia, tremors and rigidity including the typical 'parkinsonian face' may be noticed in the first **few weeks.** It responds to anticholinergic antiparkinsonian drugs.

iii. *Perioral tremors:* Also called 'rabbit syndrome' may occur **after several months** of antipsychotic therapy—anticholinergics are useful.

iv. *Akathesia:* It is a feeling of intense discomfort which compels the person to be continuously moving, like constant walking. It necessitates a reduction in antipsychotic dosage and treatment with propranolol or other antianxiety drugs.

v. *Tardive dyskinesia:* Appears after months or **years of therapy** and is characterised by involuntary movements of the face, tongue, eyelids, trunk and limbs. It can be disabling. Atypical antipsychotics like clozapine may be used in such patients because of the lower incidence of EPS.

vi. *Malignant neuroleptic syndrome:* It is characterised by immobility, rigidity, tremors, fever, dysphagia, stupor or coma with autonomic effects like fluctuating blood pressure and heart rate. It is associated particularly with parenteral use of high potency neuroleptic. Though it is rare, it can be fatal and could be due to sudden reduction of dopaminergic activity or increase in cholinergic activity.

   Treatment: Neuroleptic should be stopped immediately. Tepid water sponging to reduce the high body temperature, skeletal muscle relaxants like dantrolene or diazepam; bromocriptine may help to increase central dopaminergic activity.

3. ***Endocrine disturbances:*** Gynaecomastia, amenorrhoea and galactorrhoea due to DA receptor blockade on pituitary lactotrophs.
4. ***Ocular toxicity:*** Long-term use of high doses of some antipsychotics particularly thioridazine can cause corneal and lenticular opacities as well as retinal pigmentation and degeneration.
5. ***Hypersensitivity reactions:*** Jaundice, agranulocytosis and skin rashes.

Drug Interactions

Neuroleptics enhance the sedative effects of CNS depressants, alpha blockers and of anticholinergic drugs. When combined with these groups of drugs, the effects may be additive.

Neuroleptics inhibit the actions of dopamine agonists and L-dopa.

Uses

Neuroleptics are given orally (chlorpromazine 100–800 mg). In acute psychosis, they may be given intramuscularly and the response is seen in 24 hr while in chronic psychosis it takes 2–3 weeks of treatment to demonstrate the beginning of obvious response.

1. *Psychiatric conditions:* Psychoses including **schizophrenia** and organic brain syndromes like delirium and dementia all respond to antipsychotics.The manic phase of bipolar mood disorder responds to antipsychotics and generally atypical antipsychotics are used.
2. *Other neuropsychiatric syndromes:* Neuroleptics are useful in the treatment of several syndromes with psychiatric features like psychoses associated with chronic alcoholism, Huntington's disease and Gilles de La Tourette's syndrome.
3. *Hiccough:* CPZ can control intractable hiccough though the mechanism of action is not known.
4. *Nausea, vomiting:* Prochlorperazine is a good antiemetic as it blocks the DA receptors in the CTZ and in the stomach. It is used in vomiting due to radiation sickness and drug-induced vomiting.
5. *Pruritus:* Promethazine also blocks—H_1 receptors and is useful in pruritus.
6. *Neuroleptanalgesia:* Droperidol is used with fentanyl for neuroleptanalgesia.

INDIVIDUAL ANTIPSYCHOTICS

The antipsychotics differ in their potency, sedative, autonomic and extrapyramidal effects and to some extent in pharmacokinetic parameters.

Phenothiazines

The aliphatic and piperidine derivatives are less potent but produce more sedation and weight gain. Piperazine derivatives are more potent and pharmacologically more selective compared to others. **Triflupromazine,** a neuroleptic with aliphatic side chain, is mostly used as an antiemetic. **Thioridazine** has prominent anticholinergic properties—EPS are less but hypotension, arrhythmias and anticholinergic effects are common. Thioridazine can cause ocular side effects like lenticular opacities and retinal degeneration and is therefore not preferred for long-term use. **Trifluoperazine, fluphenazine** with piperazine side chain have high potency with less prominent side effects but EPS do occur.

Trifluoperazine: Dose 5–10 mg/day NEOCALM 5, 10 mg tab, Arkazine 1, 5 mg tab.

Thioridazine: Dose: 100–400 mg/day. RIDAZINE, THIOZINE-10, 25, 50 and 100 mg tab.

Triflupromazine: Dose: 10–30 mg/day. SIQUIL 10 mg tab, 10 mg/ml inj.

Fluphenazine: Dose: 1–10 mg/day. ANATENSOL 1 mg tab, 25 mg/ml inj. FLUDECAN 25 mg/ml inj.

Butyrophenones

The butyrophenones have higher potency and fewer autonomic side effects.

Haloperidol, a butyrophenone, is a potent antipsychotic with actions similar to chlorpromazine. It differs from chlorpromazine in that it has lesser incidence of autonomic side effects and is, therefore, preferred in older patients. Also epileptogenic property is relatively less and has a long t½ of 24 hr. It does not cause weight gain.

Haloperidol is useful in acute schizophrenia and is the drug of choice in Gilles de la Tourette's syndrome and Huntington's disease.

Dose: 2–20 mg SERENASE 0.5, 1.5, 2 mg tab

Trifluperidol is more potent than haloperidol. Dose: 1–8 mg/day, TRIPERIDOL 0.5 mg tab, 2.5 mg/ml inj.

Penfluridol structurally related to haloperidol is a long-acting neuroleptic—can be given once a week in the dose of 20–60 mg orally. FLUMAP 4, 10, 20 mg tab.

Thioxanthines

Thioxanthines are chemically related to phenothiazines and are similar to them. **Flupenthixol** has additional antidepressant properties. It is available as depot preparation for injection and is suitable for maintenance therapy of schizophrenia.

Dose: 3–5 mg daily FLUANXOL 0.5, 1, 3 mg tab.

Atypical or Second Generation Antipsychotics

The newer atypical antipsychotics are second generation agents with weak D_2 blocking properties but prominent 5-HT_2 antagonistic actions. They have the following advantages over first generation agents:

1. Extrapyramidal side effects are absent or of much lower intensity.
2. Low endocrine side effects—particularly no raised prolactin levels, hence no galactorrhoea and no gynaecomastia.
3. Effective in suppressing both positive and negative symptoms of schizophrenia
4. Effective in resistant cases of psychosis.

Atypical antipsychotics are used as **first-line** drugs in newly diagnosed patients (because of lower incidence of EPS) and in patients having troublesome EPS with conventional antipsychotics. However, their efficacy is not superior to conventional antipsychotics.

Clozapine is an effective antipsychotic. It blocks the dopamine D_1 and D_4 receptors but has low affinity for D_2 receptors, hence very low incidence of EPS. Clozapine also blocks 5-HT_{2A}, alpha adrenergic, muscarinic and H_1 histamine receptors. Clozapine is metabolised by microsomal enzymes mainly CYP 3A4 in the liver.

Adverse effects: The most important disadvantage with clozapine is that it may cause agranulocytosis in some patients, which can be fatal. Hence it is not preferred.

Clozapine can also cause sedation, weight gain, hyperglycaemia, urinary incontinence, hypotension and tachycardia. Clozapine is epileptogenic (Table 17.1).

Olanzapine is similar to clozapine in actions and has the added advantage that it does not cause agranulocytosis. It blocks D_2, 5-HT_2, alpha adrenergic, muscarinic and H_1 histamine receptors. It is well absorbed on oral administration. It has a t½ of 24–30 hr—given once daily; effective against both positive and negative symptoms of schizophrenia. The incidence of EPS is negligible. No rise in prolactin levels and sexual dysfunction. However, **anticholinergic side effects, weight gain, hyperglycaemia** and hypertriglyceridaemia can occur. These side effects are particularly of concern in diabetics. It is used in mania, schizoaffective disorders and in Tourette's syndrome.

Dose: 2.5–10 mg daily. OLANDUS 2.5, 5, 7.5, 10 mg tab. OLZAP 5, 10 mg tab.

Quetiapine is an effective antipsychotic, similar in actions to clozapine. Blocks 5-HT_{1A}, 5-HT_2, D_2, alpha 1, alpha 2, M_1 and H_1 receptors. Since it is a weak D_2 blocker, EPS and hyperprolactinaemia are less marked; weight gain, hypotension and drowsiness are moderate. Quetiapine is completely absorbed on oral use, has a short t½ of 6 hr—hence given twice daily. The initial dose is 25 mg BD gradually increased over 4–6 days to 300–400 mg per day.

SEROQUIN, SOCALM 25, 100, 200 mg tab. QUITIPIN 25, 50, 100, 200, 300 mg tab.

Risperidone blocks serotonin (5-HT_{2A}) and dopamine (D_2) receptors which is responsible for its antipsychotic activity. Risperidone also blocks alpha adrenergic and H_1 histamine receptors. It is effective against both positive and negative symptoms of schizophrenia. Risperidone is one of the most commonly used atypical antipsychotics. Adverse effects

Table 17.1: Salient features of antipsychotics

Drug	*Salient features*
Chlorpromazine	Prototype drug
Triflupromazine	Used as antiemetic
Thioridazine	Anticholinergic effects, less EPS; causes lenticular opacities, retinal degeneration
Trifluoperazine	High potency less prominent side effects
Fluphenazine,	Potent, low autonomic side effects but high EPS
Haloperidol	Potent, low autonomic side effects, preferred in elderly, DOC in Tourette's, Huntington's disease
Trifluperidol	High potency
Flupenthixol	Additional antidepressant preparation.
Loxapine	Fast onset, short action—similar to phenothiazines
Clozapine	D_1, D_4, 5-HT_{2A} blocker, weak D_2 blocker, low EPS, low sedation, no galactorrhoea, gynaecomastia; but risk of agranulocytosis.
Olanzapine	Long t½—once daily; suppresses both positive and negative symptoms of schizophrenia
Risperidone	Less EPS, less sedation, most commonly used.
Pimozide	Weak alpha, M_1 blocker → low autonomic side effects; long action, Use: Tourette's syndrome, psychoses.

DOC: *Drug of choice*

include nausea, anorexia, agitation and drowsiness. EPS, tardive dyskinesia and raised prolactin levels do occur but are of low incidence. Increased incidence of cerebrovascular disease is reported.

Risperidone is generally used in the dose of 1–3 mg twice daily. Doses higher than this cause higher incidence of side effects. Risperidone is used in schizophrenia and other psychotic conditions. It is also available as long acting injection.

RISPOND, RISPERDAL 1, 2, 3, 5 mg tab, 1 mg/ml liquid.

Paliperidone is the active metabolite of risperidone. **Iloperidone** is an antagonist at D_2 and 5-HT_2 receptors.

Ziprasidone is an effective antipsychotic with actions and mechanism of action similar to risperidone. It acts by blocking the **5-HT_{2A}**, **5-HT_{2C}** and **5-HT_{2D}** receptors and has agonistic activity at 5-HT_{1A} receptors. It also inhibits the reuptake of 5-HT and NA due to which it has additional antidepressant and anxiolytic effects. Ziprasidone also blocks D_2, H_1 and alpha receptors; causes some sedation, hypotension but incidence of EPS is low. It prolongs QT interval and may cause arrhythmias particularly if other arrhythmogenic drugs are coadministered. Ziprasidone is given twice daily as it has a t½ of 8 hr. It is used in mania.

Dose: 40–160 mg/day. ZIPSYDON, 20, 40, 80 mg tab.

Amisulpride: Some newer agents like amisulpride and **remoxipride** have a high affinity for D_2 receptors. Amisulpride is also a potent D_3 antagonist. Its actions and advantages are similar to risperidone. It is useful in schizophrenia.

Aripiprazole is a partial agonist at the dopamine D_2 and 5-HT_{1A} receptors and an antagonist at **5-HT_{2A}** receptors. The antipsychotic activity may be attributed to actions at all these three receptors. Side effects include tachycardia, nausea, dyspepsia and hypothyroidism. Weight gain and hyperlipidemia are also minimum. EPS, gynaecomastia and galactorrhoea are much milder. Aripiprazole has a long t½ of ~3 days. It is metabolised by microsomal enzymes. It is approved for use in schizophrenia, mania and bipolar mood disorders.

Dose: 5–30 mg/day. ARIPRA, ARILAN-10, 15 mg tab.

NEWER DRUGS

Brexpiprazole is an atypical antipsychotic. It is similar to aripiprazole with lower risk of agitation and restlessness compared to aripiprazole.

Cariprazine is a new class of antipsychotic. It acts at multiple receptors:

i. It is selective D_3 partial agonist—may have beneficial effects in negative symptoms
ii. D_2 antagonist
iii. 5-HT_2 antagonist

Cariprazine is indicated in schizophrenia and bipolar disorder.

OTHER ANTIPSYCHOTICS

Loxapine has a fast onset and short duration of action. Actions are similar to phenothiazines. It is used in psychotic disorders including schizophrenia.

Dose: Initially 10–50 mg increased over 7–10 days to 100 mg/day. LOXAPAC 10, 25, 50 mg caps.

Pimozide is a DA blocker with weak blocking actions on α-adrenergic and cholinergic receptors—hence, low autonomic side effects. It also has a long duration of action. It is used in Tourette's syndrome (1–2 mg/day) and in psychoses (2–4 mg/day).

PIMODAC, NEURAP 2, 4 mg tab.

Reserpine acts by depleting monoamines, i.e. NA and DA. Since it causes serious side effects including depression, it is not used.

ANTIANXIETY DRUGS (ANXIOLYTICS)

Anxiety is tension or apprehension which is a normal response to certain situations in life. It is a universal human emotion. However, when it becomes excessive and disproportionate to the situation, it becomes disabling and needs treatment.

Benzodiazepines (*see* page 203) have good antianxiety actions and are the most commonly used drugs for anxiety. They are CNS depressants. Alprazolam, in addition, has antidepressant properties.

Classification

Benzodiazepines
Diazepam, chlordiazepoxide
lorazepam, alprazolam

5-HT agonist–antagonists
Buspirone, gepirone, ipsapirone

Beta-blockers
Propranolol

Sedative antihistamine
Hydroxyzine

Buspirone

Buspirone is an azapirone with good anxiolytic properties. It differs from BZDs in many aspects. It is a selective 5-HT_{1A} partial agonist. 5-HT_{1A} receptors are inhibitory autoreceptors and binding of buspirone inhibits the release of 5-HT. Buspirone is also a weak D_2 antagonist. It is useful in mild to moderate anxiety. Antianxiety effect develops slowly over 2 weeks. Unlike diazepam, it is not a muscle relaxant, not an anticonvulsant, does not produce significant sedation, tolerance or dependence and is not much useful in panic attacks.

Buspirone is rapidly absorbed and metabolised in the liver, undergoes extensive first pass metabolism. Microsomal enzyme inducers like rifampicin shorten the t½ while enzyme inhibitors like erythromycin prolong its t½.

Dose: 5–15 mg OD or TDS. BUSPIN, BUSCALM 5, 10 mg tab

Adverse effects are mild including headache, dizziness, nausea, tachycardia, nervousness, paraesthesias and rarely, restlessness.

Uses

Buspirone is used in mild to moderate anxiety and is particularly beneficial when sedation is to be avoided. **Ipsapirone** and **gepirone** are similar to buspirone.

COMPARE AND CONTRAST
Diazepam and Buspirone

Features	*Diazepam*	*Buspirone*
Chemistry	Benzodiazepine	Azapirone
Receptor involved	$GABA_A$	$5\text{-}HT_{1A}$, D_2
Sedation	Yes	Not significant
Muscle relaxant effect	Yes	No
Anticonvulsant effect	Yes	No
Tolerance	Can develop	Unlikely
Dependence	Can develop	Unlikely
In panic attacks	Effective	Not very effective
Onset of anxiolytic effect	Quick	Delayed

Beta-Blockers

In patients with prominent autonomic symptoms of anxiety like tremors, palpitation and hypertension, propranolol (*see* page 99) may be useful. β-blockers are also useful in anxiety inducing states like public speaking and stage performance. They can be used as adjuvants to benzodiazepines.

Sedative Antihistamine

Hydroxyzine is an antihistaminic with anxiolytic actions—but due to high sedation, it is not used.

Clinical Pharmacology

- Atypical antipsychotics like risperidone and olanzapine are the most commonly used antipsychotics.
- Conventional antipsychotics cause troublesome side effects like EPS. However, these agents have a lower cardiometabolic risk, are less expensive and are used as sedating, short-term agents for management of acute psychosis.
- The choice of atypical antipsychotic agent depends mainly on target symptoms to be treated like positive/negative symptoms or aggression and side effects.
- All atypical antipsychotics carry the risk of cardiometabolic disorders and weight gain.
- Agents least likely to induce sedation include ziprasidone and aripiprazole. Risperidone and paliperidone may or may not cause sedation. In cases where sedation would be beneficial, options include quetiapine, clozapine, olanzapine or augmentation with a benzodiazepine.

[1] From Medical Council of India, *Competency based Undergraduate Curriculum for the Indian Medical Graduate*, 2018;1:136–144.

CHAPTER 18

Antidepressants and Mood Stabilizers

Competency achievement: The student should be able to:

PH 1.19 Describe the mechanism/s of action, types, doses, side effects, indications and contraindications of the drugs which act on CNS, (including anxiolytics, sedatives and hypnotics, antipsychotic, **anti-depressant drugs**, anti-manics, opioid agonists and antagonists, drugs used for neurodegenerative disorders, antiepileptics drugs).[1]

Mood disorders, also called affective disorders, are a group of psychoses associated with changes of mood, i.e. depression and mania.

Depression is a common psychiatric disorder but the aetiology of it is not clear.

Depression could be:

1. Unipolar
   - Reactive depression
   - Endogenous depression
2. Bipolar mood disorder or manic depressive illness.

Unipolar Depression

Reactive depression is due to stressful and distressing circumstances in life.

Endogenous depression is major depression and results from a biochemical abnormality in the brain. Deficiency of monoamine (NA, 5-HT) activity in the CNS is thought to be responsible for endogenous depression. Symptoms are:

- Emotional symptoms—sadness, misery, hopelessness, low self-esteem, loss of interest and suicidal thoughts.
- Biological symptoms—fatigue, apathy, loss of libido, loss of appetite, lack of concentration and sleep disturbances.

Bipolar Depression

Bipolar depression is characterised by alternate episodes or periods of mania and depression. It was earlier called manic depressive psychosis (MDP) or manic depressive illness (MDI). The patient has cyclical mood swings. It is less common and is associated with a hereditary tendency. Mania can be considered opposite of depression with elation, over-enthusiasm, over-confidence, often associated with irritation and aggression.

Pathophysiology of endogenous depression: Endogenous depression has been thought to be due to a deficiency of the monoamines in the cortical and limbic systems—called the '**monoamine hypothesis'** (serotonin, norepinephrine and dopamine). The pathophysiology of depression is also explained by a newer 'neurotrophic hypothesis'. It suggests that certain nerve growth factors, like **brain-derived neurotrophic factor (BDNF),** control neurogenesis. Loss of the neurotrophic effects leads to atrophic changes in certain parts of the brain and is associated with depression.

Drugs used in Affective Disorders

Antidepressants act by enhancing the monoamine levels in the brain either by inhibiting their reuptake or preventing their degradation.

Classification

1. ***Selective serotonin reuptake inhibitors (SSRIs)***
   Fluoxetine, fluvoxamine, paroxetine, citalopram, escitalopram, sertraline
2. ***Tricyclic antidepressants (TCAs)***
   Imipramine, desipramine, clomipramine, amitriptyline, nortriptyline, doxepin
3. ***Serotonin norepinephrine reuptake inhibitors (SNRIs)***
   Venlafaxine, desvenlafaxine, duloxetin, milnacipran
4. ***Atypical antidepressants***
   Mianserine, amineptine, tianeptine, bupropion, reboxetine, mirtazapine, amoxapine, atomoxetine maprotiline, trazodone, nefazodone, vortioxetine
5. ***Monoamine oxidase (MAO) inhibitors***
   Phenelzine, tranylcypromine, moclobemide.

SELECTIVE SEROTONIN REUPTAKE INHIBITORS (SSRIs)

SSRIs include fluoxetine, fluvoxamine, paroxetine, citalopram, sertraline and escitalopram. They are now considered the first-line drugs in depression.

Mechanism of Action

SSRIs block the reuptake of serotonin from the synapse into the serotonergic nerve endings by inhibiting the **serotonin transporter** (SERT). About 80% reuptake is inhibited and more serotonin is available at the synapse which in turn results in transcription of certain proteins leading to the production of related proteins like BDNF responsible for the effects of SSRIs. Hence, they enhance serotonin levels in these synapses (Fig. 18.1).

TCAs were the first-line drugs and were widely used till the advent of SSRIs. Presently, SSRIs have taken over the place to a large extent because of several advantages over TCAs (*see* Compare and Contrast).

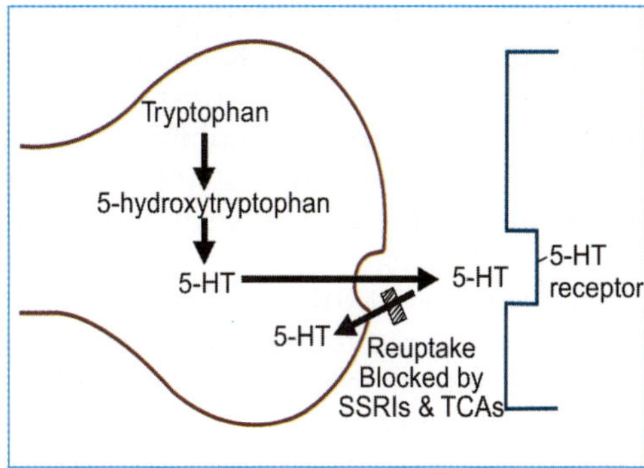

Fig. 18.1: Mechanism of action of SSRIs. They block the reuptake of serotonin and improve serotonergic transmission

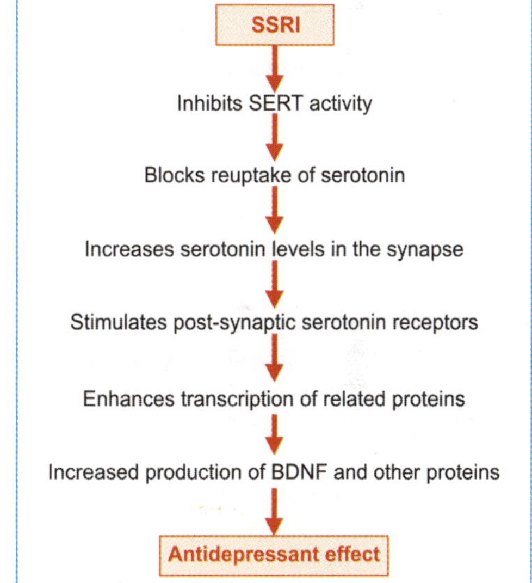

Advantages of SSRIs over TCAs

- Low cardiovascular side effects.
- Anticholinergic side effects are negligible.
- Less sedation.
- Preferred in elderly because of lower anticholinergic effects (anticholinergic effects like constipation and urinary retention may be troublesome in the elderly).
- Safer in overdose (this is particularly advantageous in patients with depression who may have suicidal tendencies).
- Due to low side effect profile, SSRIs are generally well tolerated and accepted by patients.

Pharmacokinetics: SSRIs are well absorbed when given orally, most are bound to plasma proteins. SSRIs are microsomal enzyme inhibitors—though each of them inhibit different isoforms. Fluoxetine is converted to an active metabolite norfluoxetine—prolonging the action to 7–10 days.

Escitalopram is 1000 times more potent than citalopram. Moreover, unlike with other SSRIs, drug interactions are uncommon with escitalopram (Table 18.1).

Adverse effects: Adverse effects to SSRIs include nausea, vomiting, insomnia, headache, restlessness, anxiety and **sexual dysfunction**—may interfere with ejaculation. Inhibition of platelet function may result in ecchymosis. **Serotonin syndrome**—*see* page 250.

TRICYCLIC ANTIDEPRESSANTS

Tricyclic antidepressants (TCAs) like imipramine have been extensively used in the treatment of depression for a few decades (Fig. 18.2). TCAs are less expensive than SSRIs and are, therefore, still in use.

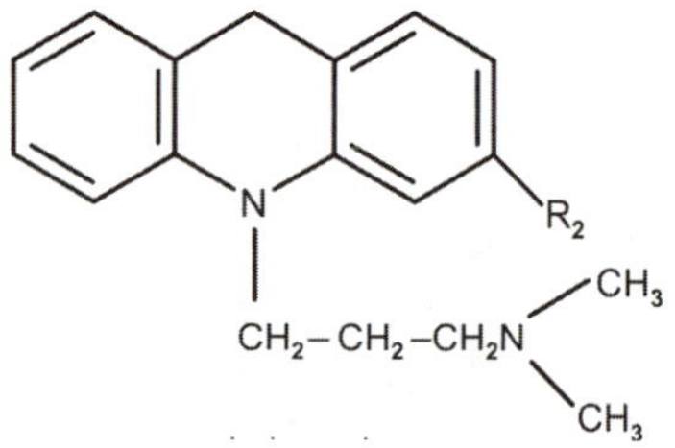

Pharmacological Actions

1. *CNS:* In normal subjects, TCAs cause dizziness, drowsiness, confusion and difficulty in thinking. In depressed patients, after 2–3 weeks of treatment, elevation of mood occurs; the patient shows more interest in the surroundings and the sleep pattern becomes normal.

   Mechanism of action (Fig. 18.3)*:* TCAs block the reuptake of both NA and serotonin into the presynaptic terminals by binding to the transporters, viz. serotonin transporter (SERT) and norepinephrine transporter (NET). The synaptic levels of these monoamines increase and thereby prolong their action on the receptors. Thus TCAs potentiate amine neurotransmission in the CNS. The extent of binding and selectivity for SERT and NET varies with each TCA.

2. *CVS:* Postural hypotension and tachycardia (due to blockade of α_1-adrenergic

N
R2
CH3
$CH_2-CH_2-CH_2N$
CH3

Fig. 18.2: Imipramine

Table 18.1: Therapeutic dose, preparations and unique features of SSRIs

Drug	*Dose (mg/day)*	*Preparation*	*Unique features*
Fluoxetine	20–50	FLUZE 20 mg cap.	Longest acting due to active metabolites; duration 7–10 days; 4 wks withdrawal for washout; more agitation.
Fluvoxamine	50–200	FLUATOR 50 mg tab. REVILIFE, 50, 100 mg tab.	Less agitation, shorter acting, inhibits microsomal enzymes → DI.
Paroxetine	20–50	DEPROX 10 mg tab. PAROTIN, 10, 20, 40 mg tab.	Weight gain, GI side effects significant
Sertraline	50–200	SERTA 25, 50, 100 mg tab. SERTIMA, 50, 100 mg tab.	Milder enzyme inhibition—DI lower. Long acting metabolite; bioavailability low—45%.
Citalopram	20–40	C-PRAM, C-TALO 10, 20 40 mg tab.	Lesser DI, avoid in patients with suicidal tendencies.
Escitalopram	10–20	TALO, ESCITA 10, 20 mg tab.	Enantiomer of citalopram, more potent and safer than it. DI uncommon

DI: Drug interactions

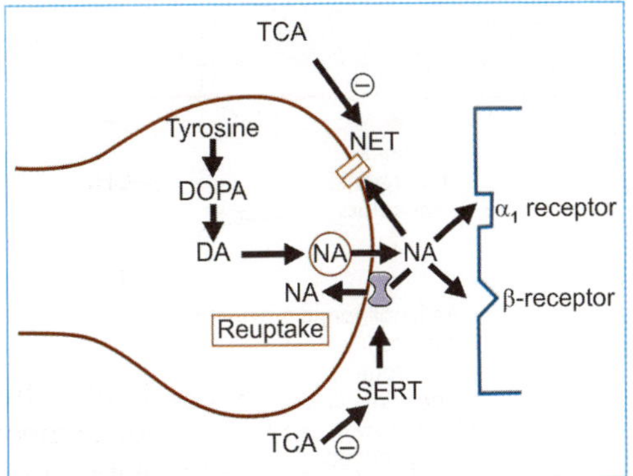

Fig. 18.3: Mechanism of action of tricyclic antidepressants. 80% of noradrenaline and serotonin released into the synaptic cleft enters into the synaptic neuron by reuptake through SERT and NET. This reuptake is blocked by TCA

and muscarinic receptors) can be severe in overdosage.

3. *ANS:* TCAs have anticholinergic properties and cause dry mouth, blurred vision, constipation and urinary retention.

Pharmacokinetics

TCAs are rapidly absorbed, extensively protein bound and metabolised in the liver. Microsomal enzymes are involved in the metabolism of TCAs and can result in drug interactions. TCAs are converted to active metabolites and thereby have a longer action. They have a long t½ and can be given once daily—at night to avoid daytime sedation. On prolonged administration, accumulation can occur resulting in cumulative toxicity.

Adverse Effects

- Sedation, confusion, postural hypotension, tachycardia and sweating.
- Anticholinergic side effects like dry mouth, constipation, blurred vision and urinary retention are also relatively common.
- TCAs may precipitate **convulsions** in epileptics—they lower the seizure threshold; may cause hallucinations and mania in some patients.
- Many TCAs may also cause **weight gain** due to increased appetite.
- TCAs can also cause cardiac **arrhythmias**.
- *Acute toxicity* is manifested by (mimic symptoms of atropine poisoning) delirium, excitement, hypotension, convulsions, fever, arrhythmias, respiratory depression and coma.

Treatment: Physostigmine may be given to overcome atropine like effects; sodium bicarbonate for acidosis, diazepam or phenytoin for seizures and lignocaine/propranolol for arrhythmias—with other supportive measures. Gastric lavage, IV fluids and respiratory support are needed.

COMPARE AND CONTRAST

Imipramine (TCA) and Fluoxetine (SSRIs)

Features	*Imipramine*	*Fluoxetine*
Chemistry	Tricyclic compound	Bicyclic compound
MOA	Inhibits reuptake of serotonin and NE	Inhibits reuptake of serotonin
Antiholinergic effects	Present	Absent
Hypotension	Yes	Nil
Cardiac arrhythmias	Possible	Nil
Sedation	Significant	Mild
Safety margin	Relatively low	Good
Tolerability	Poor	Good
Onset of action	Slow	Faster
Plasma half life	9–24 hr	48–72 hr
Cost	Less expensive	More expensive

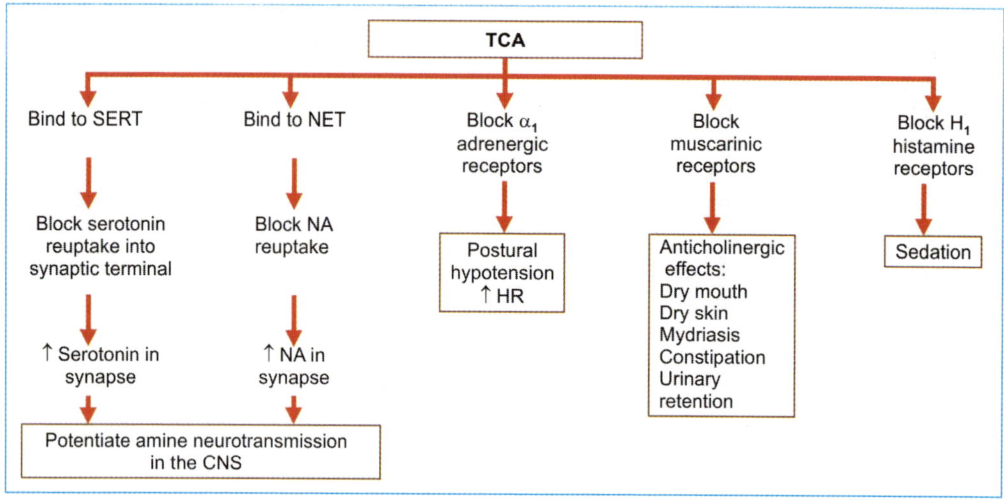

Fig. 18.4: Mechanism of action, actions and adverse effects of TCAs

Tolerance and Dependence

Tolerance develops gradually to the sedative and anticholinergic effects over 2–3 weeks. Starting with a low dose and gradually increasing the dose minimizes the side effects.

Following long-term treatment, TCAs should be gradually withdrawn, as withdrawal symptoms like headache, anxiety and chills can occur due to physical dependence.

Drug Interactions

1. Tricyclics potentiate sympathomimetics—even small amounts of adrenaline used with local anaesthetics can cause serious hypertension.
2. Highly protein bound drugs like phenytoin, aspirin and phenylbutazone displace TCAs from binding sites resulting in toxicity.
3. TCAs potentiate the effects of alcohol and other CNS depressants.
4. TCAs have anticholinergic effects and this effect gets added up with other drugs.

SEROTONIN NOREPINEPHRINE REUPTAKE INHIBITORS (SNRIs)

Venlafaxine, desvenlafaxine, duloxetine, milnacipran inhibit the reuptake of both serotonin and norepinephrine at the presynaptic neurons by binding to SERT and NET like TCA. Unlike TCA, they do not have anticholinergic, α-blocking or antihistaminic effects—hence fewer side effects. SNRIs are also useful in chronic pain.

Venlafaxine is thought to be faster acting and may be useful in patients not responding to other antidepressants. Venlafaxine has a short t½ (~5 hr) and needs to be given twice daily; it is safe in overdosage. If abruptly stopped or if doses are missed, withdrawal symptoms are common. Venlafaxine is better tolerated than the TCAs because it does not block alpha adrenergic, muscarinic and histamine H_1 receptors and, therefore, is devoid of the related adverse effects.

Dose: 75–150 mg/day. VENLA, VENAXIN 25, 37.5, 75 mg tab, 150 mg SR- cap.

Desvenlafaxine is a metabolite of venlafaxine. **Milnacipran** is similar to other SNRIs.

Duloxetine is similar to venlafaxine, is well absorbed and metabolised by microsomal enzymes.

Dose: 30–80 mg/day. DULIFE, DELOK 20, 30 mg cap.

ATYPICAL ANTIDEPRESSANTS

Atypical antidepressants include bupropion, mianserin, mirtazapine, amoxapine, maprotiline, trazodone and nefazodone. Atypical antidepressants act by enhancing the monoamine levels in the brain either by inhibitng their reuptake or preventing their degradation.

Mirtazapine blocks 5-HT_2, 5-HT_3 and α_2 receptors and enhances the release of NA and 5-HT. It is faster acting—action starts by one week of treatment. It causes sedation but other side effects are negligible.

Dose: 15–45 mg/day. MIRAZ 7.5, 10 mg tab. RISTRA 15, 30 mg tab.

Bupropion is a weak DA reuptake inhibitor and has CNS stimulant effects. It is well absorbed orally and is used in depression with anxiety. Bupropion is also used to help cessation of smoking (along with nicotine patch). It can cause insomnia, agitation but does not cause sexual side effects.

Dose: 150–300 mg/day. BUPDEP 150 mg SR- tab. BUPISURE 150 mg ER-tab.

Amoxapine is a derivative of the antipsychotic loxapine. It has side effect profile like the TCAs and hence are not preferred.

Mianserin acts by blocking presynaptic α_2 receptors but toxicity including blood dyscrasias, seizures and liver dysfunction has limited its use.

Dose: 30–100 mg/day. DEPNON, SERIAAC 10, 30 mg tab. TETRADEP 10, 20, 30 mg tab.

Trazodone and **nefazodone** are now known to act as serotonin antagonists and are also weak serotonin reuptake inhibitors. Trazodone is short acting (t½ 6 hr). It can cause postural hypotension and priapism due to its α_1-blocking effects. Nefazodone causes sedation and mild postural hypotension. Both lack anticholinergic activity and were once extensively used but they cause profound **sedation** and nefazodone causes **hepatotoxicity**. Hence both are not preferred now.

Dose: 50–200 mg/day. SERTIMA, SETEX 50, 100 mg tab.

Vortioxetine: It is a newly introduced antidepressant with complex actions on sertonin receptors. It is an antagonist at 5-HT_3, 5-HT_7 and 5-HT_{1D} receptors, agonist at 5-HT_{IA} receptors and partial agonist at 5-HT_{IB} receptors. Like SSRIs, it also inhibits SERT but to a smaller extent. It may also improve cognition. Gastrointestinal side effects and serotonergic effects (like SSRIs) including sexual dysfunction are reported.

Dose 10–20 mg OD.

MAO INHIBITORS

Monoamine oxidase (MAO) is an enzyme which metabolizes NA, 5-HT and DA. Drugs which inhibit this enzyme, enhance the neuronal levels of monoamines like NA, DA and 5-HT. MAO exists as two isozymes—MAO_A and MAO_B. MAO_A is selective for 5-HT.

MAO inhibitors include:

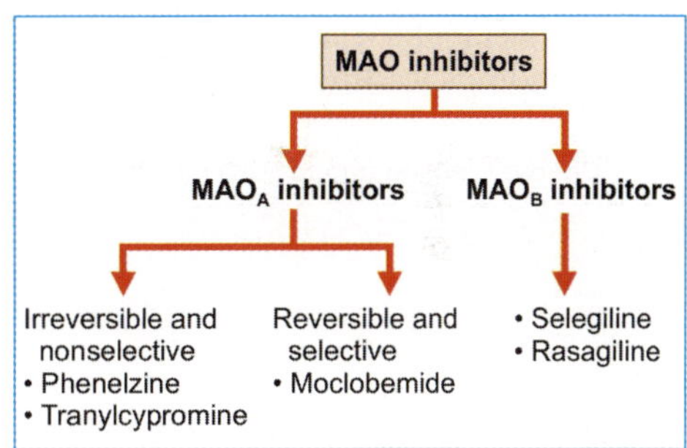

Nonselective and irreversible MAO inhibitors have the following features:

- Irreversibly inhibit the enzyme MAO and enhance neuronal levels of noradrenaline, dopamine and 5-HT.
- Antidepressant actions develop slowly over weeks of treatment and MAO activity recovers over 1–2 weeks on stopping the drug.
- Side effects are orthostatic hypotension, weight gain, restlessness, insomnia (due to CNS stimulation), anticholinergic effects and, rarely, liver dysfunction.

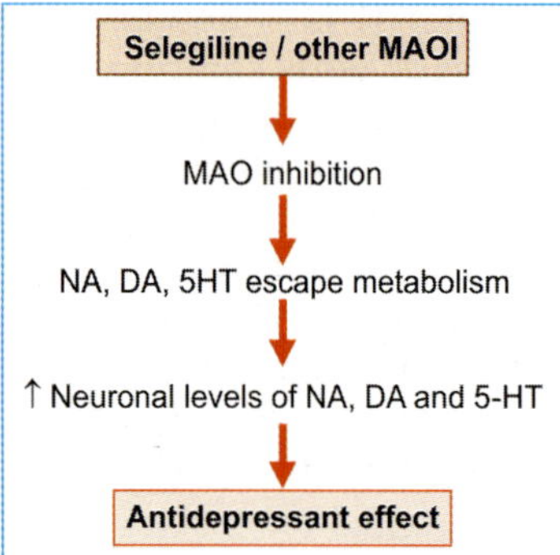

- Abrupt stopping can result in **withdrawal syndrome** with confusion, excitement and even psychosis.
- They interact with many drugs and food. Patients on MAO inhibitors taking tyramine containing food like cheese, beer, wines, yeast, buttermilk and fish—develop severe hypertension and is known as ***'cheese reaction.'*** Tyramine is normally metabolised by MAO in the gut wall. On inhibition of MAO by drugs, tyramine escapes metabolism and displaces NA from nerve endings leading to hypertension.

Cheese reaction due to MAO inhibitors

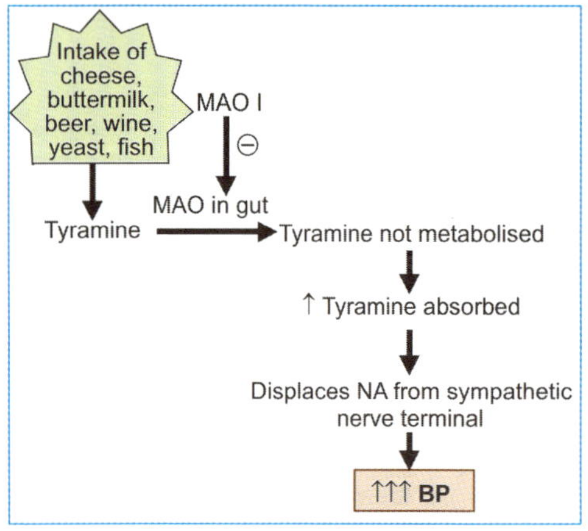

- ***Serotonin syndrome:*** When an SSRI and an MAO inhibitor are administered concurrently, there could be a significant increase in serotonin levels in the synapses—this is because of both reduced reuptake and inhibition of metabolism. Raised serotonin levels can result in hyperthermia, restlessness, sweating, muscle rigidity, aggressive behaviour, tremors, seizures and coma. It can be fatal. This pharmacodynamic interaction can also occur when there is a potentiation of serotonergic activity with drugs like amphetamines, cocaine (5-HT release) tryptophan (5-HT synthesis), buspirone, and sumatriptan (5-HTagonist). Hence such combinations should be avoided.

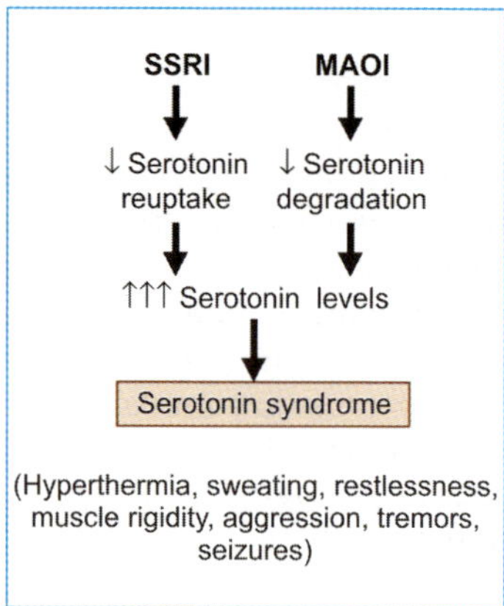

- Because of the side effects and drug interactions, MAO inhibitors are not the preferred antidepressants.

Reversible inhibitor of MAO_A (RIMA)—Moclobemide is a reversible, competitive, selective MAO_A inhibitor. It is short-acting and MAO activity recovers within 1–2 days after stopping the drug. It is found to be an effective antidepressant and has the advantages that it is not a sedative, does not produce cardiovascular and anticholinergic side effects. Hence, it is well tolerated. No significant drug interactions are seen. Adverse effects include nausea, insomnia, headache, dizziness and liver dysfunction.

Moclobemide is used in mild to moderate depression as an alternative to TCA. It is also useful in anxiety related mood disorders.

Dose: 150 mg BD-TDS. RIMAREX, TRINA 150, 300 mg tab.

Uses of Antidepressants

1. **Endogenous depression:** Antidepressants are used over a long period. The response appears after 2–3 weeks of treatment. The choice of drug depends on the side effects and patient factors like age. SSRIs are the most commonly used antidepressants. In severe depression with suicidal tendencies, electroconvulsive therapy (ECT) is given.
2. **Panic attacks:** Acute, recurrent, brief episodes of anxiety are known as panic attacks. Post-traumatic stress disorders, panic attacks and other anxiety disorders—all respond to antidepressants.
3. **Obsessive compulsive disorders (OCDs):** OCDs are characterised by repeated anxiety—provoking thoughts and compulsive behaviour to overcome such anxiety. OCDs respond to SSRIs/ clomipramine along with counselling.
4. **Other anxiety disorders:** SSRIs are effective in several anxiety states like post-traumatic stress disorders, phobias and social anxiety. They may be preferred over BZDs in many of these conditions.
5. **Disorders of pain:** Antidepressants that inhibit the uptake of both serotonin and norepinephrine (SNRIs) are found to influence ascending pain pathway and are effective in chronic pain, including diabetic neuropathy, backache, post-herpetic neuralgia and fibromyalgia.
6. **Psychosomatic disorders:** Newer anti-depressants are tried in irritable bowel syndrome, chronic fatigue, tics and sleep apnoea.
7. **Bulimia nervosa:** It is an eating disorder associated with episodic excessive eating and responds to SSRIs.
8. **Premenstrual syndrome:** It may be prominent in some women with dysphoria when SSRIs may be given for 2 weeks prior to menstruation and the cycles may be repeated. Flushing and other vasomotor symptoms seen in perimenopausal women also respond to SSRIs.
9. **Smoking withdrawal:** Bupropion has been shown to reduce the urge in people who need to quit smoking.
10. **Nocturnal enuresis** in children may be treated with antidepressants only when other measures fail and drugs are indicated.
11. **Other indications:** Migraine, attention deficit hyperactivity disorder, chronic fatigue, urinary stress incontinence and chronic alcoholism—may result in depression—antidepressants are tried.

MOOD STABILIZERS

Mood stabilizers control the mood swings that are seen in bipolar mood disorders. They are also called ***antimanic drugs***. Lithium salts (lithium carbonate and lithium citrate) have been used for several decades but several antiepileptics like carbamazepine, valproic acid and gabapentin and antipsychotics like aripiprazole, olanzapine and risperidone are now approved for use. Antipsychotics like chlorpromazine and haloperidol are used in acute episodes of mania.

Mood stabilizers include: Lithium, valproic acid, carbamazepine.

Others: Lamotrigine, topiramate

Lithium

Lithium is a monovalent cation. Cade, in 1949, discovered the beneficial effects of lithium in bipolar mood disorder. Since then, it has been widely used. On prophylactic use in bipolar mood disorder (manic-depressive illness), lithium acts as a mood stabilizer. It prevents swings of mood and thus reduces both the depressive and manic phases of the illness. Given in acute mania, it gradually suppresses the episode over weeks.

Mechanism of Action

Mechanism of action of lithium is **complex** and not fully understood. It is thought that lithium acts by the following mechanisms.

1. **Inositol pathway:** Lithium interferes with the regeneration of inositol (Fig. 18.5). It

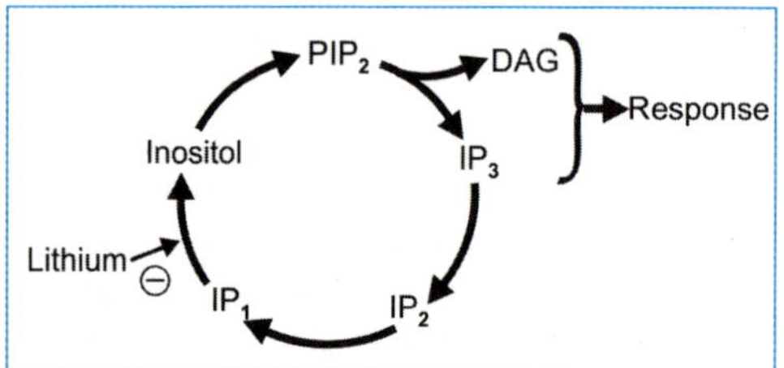

Fig. 18.5: Mechanism of action of lithium. Lithium inhibits monophosphatases that convert IP to inositol

inhibits inositol monophosphatase and other enzymes and thereby inhibits the conversion of IP_3 to inositol, leading to a depletion of phosphatidyl inositol biphosphate (PIP_2). This results in a reduction in the formation of the second messengers IP_3 and DAG leading to a reduction in the receptor activity. Lithium selectively inhibits signal transduction in the hyperfunctioning neurons as seen in mania. Lithium inhibits monophosphatases that convert IP to inositol.

2. **Effect on electrolytes:** Lithium can compete with and replace sodium at many sites including neurons. It may alter neuronal functions resulting in its mood stabilizing effects.
3. **G-proteins:** Lithium inhibits the receptor-mediated activation of G-proteins in the CNS, i.e. they could uncouple receptors from their G-proteins. This action could also contribute to its mood stabilizing action.
4. **Neurotransmitters:** Lithium inhibits the release of noradrenaline and dopamine from the nerve terminals. Lithium also prevents the supersensitivity of the receptors induced by dopamine antagonists (antipsychotics).

Pharmacokinetics

Lithium is a small ion and mimics the role of sodium in excitable tissues. Given orally it is well-absorbed. It is filtered at the glomerulus but reabsorbed like sodium. Steady state concentration is reached in 5–6 days. Lithium is secreted in sweat, saliva and breast milk. Since safety margin is narrow, **plasma lithium concentration needs to be monitored** (0.5–1 mEq is the therapeutic plasma concentration) 3–5 mEq can cause fatal toxicity.

Adverse Effects

Lithium is a drug of low therapeutic index and side effects are common.

- Nausea, vomiting, mild diarrhoea, oedema, thirst and polyuria occur initially in most patients.
- Tremors are common with therapeutic doses and it responds to propranolol.
- Hypothyroidism is due to reversible inhibition of thyroid function. TSH may be monitored once in 6 months.
- On long-term use, lithium can cause nephrogenic diabetes insipidus—should avoid dehydration while on lithium.
- Weight gain can also occur. As the plasma concentration rises, CNS effects like coarse tremors, drowsiness, giddiness, confusion, ataxia, blurred vision and nystagmus are seen. In severe overdosage, delirium, muscle twitchings, convulsions, arrhythmias and renal failure develop.

Precautions

1. Minimum effective dose should be used.
2. Patients should always use the same formulation.
3. Patients should be made aware of the first symptom of toxicity.
4. Lithium is contraindicated in pregnancy.

Drug Interactions

1. Diuretics enhance Na^+ loss and lithium absorption from the kidney. This increases plasma lithium levels resulting in toxicity.
   Lithium + Diuretics
   Diuretic → ↑ Na^+ loss → ↑ Li^+ reabsorption (in place of Na^+)
   ↓
   Toxicity ← ↑ plasma Li^+
2. NSAIDs decrease lithium elimination and increase toxicity.

Uses

1. **Prophylaxis of bipolar mood disorder:** Episodes of mania and depression and their severity are reduced.
2. **Acute mania:** Since the response to lithium is slow, neuroleptics are preferred.
3. **Depression:** Lithium is tried along with other antidepressants as an add-on drug in the treatment of severe recurrent depression.
4. **Leucopenia:** Lithium increases leukocyte count and has been used in leukopenia following cancer chemotherapy.
5. **Other uses:** Lithium is tried in recurrent neuropsychiatric disorders, childhood mood disorders, hyperthyroidism and inappropriate ADH secretion syndrome.

Other Mood Stabilizers

Because of difficulty in using lithium like, need for monitoring plasma levels, risk of toxicity in renal dysfunction and potential for drug interactions, other drugs are being tried. The antiepileptics ***carbamazepine, sodium valproate and lamotrigine*** are found to be useful, less toxic alternatives (*see* Chapter 15).

Carbamazepine is found to be effective in preventing the relapses of bipolor mood disorder and in the treatment of acute mania. It can be combined with lithium for better therapeutic effects but lithium can enhance the toxicity of carbamazepine.

Mechanism of action is not understood. Carbamazepine may be used alone in mild cases as a mood stabilizer.

Dose: Started with 200 mg twice daily and may be increased if required.

Sodium valproate can be tried alone in mild to moderate cases or along with lithium in refractory cases. It is now known that sodium valproate has antimanic effects and is presently the first-line mood stabilizer. It has several advantages.

- It is almost as effective as lithium.
- It may be effective in patients not responding to lithium.
- Safer
- Better tolerated
- Dose can be rapidly titrated upwards.
- It is well tolerated and adverse effects are milder as compared to lithium. Nausea may be experienced in some patients.
- It can be combined with other antipsychotics and the combination is well tolerated.
- Valproic acid is now considered the first-line drug in the initial treatment of mania.

Dose: Started with 750 mg/day—may be increased to 1500–2000 mg/day.

Other antiepileptics: Lamotrigine, gabapentin topiramate and other newer antiepileptics are being tried in the prophylaxis of bipolar mood disorder as alternatives to lithium.

Other drugs: Antipsychotics like risperidone, olanzapine, quetiapine and aripiprazole are also being tried.

Riluzole, a neuroprotective agent used in amyotrophic lateral sclerosis, is also being tried in mood disorders.

Clinical Pharmacology

- SSRIs are the most commonly used. They are long-acting (once daily). Fluoxetine is the longest acting (7–10 days) hence, stop 4 weeks for 'washout' before using MAO inhibitor.
- Fluoxamine inhibits microsomal enzymes leading to drug interactions–needs caution.
- TCAs and MAO inhibitors are now second-line drugs tried in patients who do not respond to SSRIs. Their dose is titrated over several weeks.
- TCAs are cheaper than SSRIs making them still widely prescribed in developing countries.
- MAO inhibitors are not commonly used now.
- Bupropion and nortriptyline are used for cessation of smoking.
- Valproate and carbamazepine are the most commonly used drugs in bipolar disorder. Oxcarbazepine has been prescribed 'Off label' by many psychiatrists because it is less sedating, less bone marrow toxic and has fewer drug interactions than carbamazepine.

[1–5] From Medical Council of India, *Competency based Undergraduate Curriculum for the Indian Medical Graduate*, 2018;1:136–144.

CHAPTER 19

Opioid Analgesics and Antagonists

Competency achievement: The student should be able to:

PH 1.19 Describe the mechanism/s of action, types, doses, side effects, indications and contraindications of the drugs which act on CNS, (including anxiolytics, sedatives and hypnotics, antipsychotic, antidepressant drugs, antimanics, **opioid agonists and antagonists**, drugs used for neurodegenerative disorders, antiepileptics drugs).[1]

Pain or algesia is an unpleasant subjective sensation. It cannot be easily defined. Pain is a warning signal and indicates that there is an impairment of structural and functional integrity of the body. It is the most important symptom that brings the patient to the doctor and demands immediate relief. Prompt relief of pain instills enormous confidence in the patient regarding the doctor's treating ability.

Types of Pain

Pain arising from the skin and integumental structures, muscles, bones and joints is known as **somatic pain.** It is usually caused by inflammation and is well-defined or sharp pain.

Pain arising from the viscera is vague, dull-aching type, difficult to pinpoint to a site and is known as **visceral pain.** It may be accompanied by autonomic responses like sweating, nausea and hypotension. It may be due to spasm, ischaemia or inflammation.

When pain is referred to a cutaneous area which receives nerve supply from the same spinal segment as that of the affected viscera, it is known as **referred pain**, e.g. cardiac pain referred to the left arm.

Pain consists of two components—the original 'sensation' and the 'reaction' to it. The original sensation is carried by the afferent nerve fibres and is the same in all. The reaction component differs widely from one person to another. Perception of pain is enhanced in presence of anxiety. A person who is already in stress can poorly tolerate pain.

Pain may be acute or chronic. Acute pain may result from wounds, irritants, burns or from ischaemia. The cause is usually well defined. In chronic pain, the origin may not be well defined. Example: Pain due to arthritis, cancers and neuroplasmic pain.

ANALGESICS

Analgesic is a drug which relieves pain without loss of consciousness. Analgesics only afford symptomatic relief from pain without affecting the cause.

Analgesics are of 3 classes:

1. Opioid or morphine type of analgesics
2. Non-opioid or aspirin type of analgesics.
3. *Adjuvant analgesics:*
   a. Antiepileptics—pregabalin, gabapentin, carbamazepine, lamotrigine
   b. Antidepressants—amitriptyline, venlafaxine, duloxetine, citalopram, escitalopram

OPIOID ANALGESICS

Opium is the dark brown gummy exudate obtained from the poppy capsule *(Papaver somniferum).* On incising the unripe seed capsule, a milky juice emerges which turns brown on drying and this is crude opium. The word opium is derived from Greek in which

Table 19.1: Location of opioid receptors

Receptor	Location	Function
μ	Thalamus, periaqueductal gray area, nucleus tractus solitarius, area postrema, dorsal horn	Analgesia, respiratory depression, euphoria, sedation, miosis, constipation
K	Cerebral cortex, hippocampus, striatum, midbrain dorsal horn, medulla	Analgesia, respiratory depression, dysphoria, sedation, miosis, constipation
δ	Same as above + myenteric plexus trigeminal nucleus	Analgesia, respiratory depression, constipation

'opos' means juice. Opium has been in use since 4000 BC. It was used both for medicinal and recreational purposes. By 18th century, opium smoking was popular in Europe. It was Serturner who isolated a pure opium alkaloid in 1806. He named it **Morphine** after *Morpheus,* the Greek God of dreams. As the research progressed, opium was found to contain 20 alkaloids. By around 19th century, the pure opium alkaloids were available for therapeutic use—but because they were equally abused, efforts were made to isolate the analgesic property, i.e. to obtain an opioid that is only an analgesic and has no euphoric effects. In the process, various agonists, antagonists and partial agonists were synthesized. **'Opioid'** is the term used for drugs with morphine-like actions. They were earlier called narcotic analgesics.

Endogenous Opioid Peptides and Opioid Receptors

There are three families of endogenous opioid peptides released in the body in response to pain *viz.* ***enkephalins, endorphins*** **and** ***dynorphins***. Endorphins are good analgesics. We now also know of endomorphins. This indicate that we have a natural system in the body that releases various opioid peptides in response to pain. These opioid peptides act on the opioid receptors *mu* (μ), *kappa* (κ), *delta* (δ) and N/OFQ, to relieve pain (Table 19.1). Most pharmacological effects of opioids are mediated through μ receptors.

They are abundant in the spinal cord, periaqueductal grey area and in the affective areas, *viz* limbic system and cortex. They are also present in the peripheral tissues.

Dynorphins are endogenous ligands for κ receptors.

'**Endomorphins**' are endogenous ligands for μ receptors with a high affinity. Endomorphin-1 and endomorphin-2 are known.

Nociceptin/orphanin FQ is another type of endogenous opioid peptide recently identified. It acts on the **nociceptin N/OFQ receptor** which is widely distributed in the CNS and periphery.

All of the opioid receptors have been cloned. Subtypes have been suggested for each of them, viz μ_1 μ_2, δ_1, δ_2 and κ_1, κ_2 and κ_3. μ_1 mediates analgesia, euphoria and dependence while μ_2 receptors may be involved in respiratory depression and constipation. However, more information on these is yet to be available.

Classification

1. **Agonists**
   Morphine, codeine
   Pethidine, methadone, oxycodone, oxymorphone, fentanyl, diphenoxylate, loperamide, dextropro poxyphene, tramadol, tapentadol
2. **Mixed agonist–antagonists**
   Pentazocine, nalbuphine, butorphanol, buprenorphine, nalorphine
3. **Antagonists**
   Naloxone, naltrexone, nalmephene, naloxegol

Opioids can also be classified depending on their source as:

1. **Natural opium alkaloids:**
   Morphine, codeine, noscapine
2. **Semisynthetic derivatives:**
   Heroin, oxymorphone, pholcodeine
3. **Synthetic opioids:**
   Pethidine, methadone, fentanyl, oxycodone, dextromethorphan, diphenoxylate, loperamide, dextropropoxyphene, tramadol, tapentadol

MORPHINE

Morphine is the most important alkaloid of opium. Though many new opioids with actions similar to morphine have been synthesized, none of them are superior to morphine as an analgesic. Morphine is discussed as the prototype of the group.

Mechanism of Action

1. Morphine and other opioids produce their effects by acting on specific **opioid receptors** (Fig. 19.1). These receptors are abundant in the CNS and other tissues. The opioid receptors are *mu* (μ), *kappa* (κ) and *delta* (δ) receptors.

   All opioid receptors are G-protein-coupled receptors. Stimulation of these receptors inhibits adenylate cyclase resulting in decreased intracellular cAMP formation.
2. They also facilitate the opening of K^+ channels leading to hyperpolarisation.
3. In addition to this, they inhibit the opening of calcium channels.

All these result in a decrease in the intracellular calcium which, in turn, decrease the release of neurotransmitters. Various neurotransmitters including dopamine, glutamate, GABA, NA, 5-HT and substance P are involved in the transmission of pain impulses.

Opioids also directly inhibit the transmission in the dorsal horn ascending pathway. Opioids stimulate the descending pain control pathway—from the midbrain and brainstem to the dorsal horn of the spinal cord. Opioid receptors are abundant in these areas including the periaqueductal grey (PAG) area, substantia gelatinosa and the spinal cord.

Pharmacological Actions

I. Central Nervous System

1. ***Analgesia:*** Morphine is a potent analgesic and relieves pain without loss of consciousness. Dull aching visceral pain is relieved better than sharp pricking pain. In higher doses, it relieves even the severe pain as that of biliary colic. Morphine alters both the perception and reaction to pain. It raises the pain threshold and thus increases the capacity to tolerate pain. Further, it alters the emotional reaction to pain.

   Euphoria and sedation also contribute to its analgesic effects.
2. ***Euphoria, sedation and hypnosis:*** Morphine produces a feeling of well-being termed *euphoria*. It is this effect which makes it an important drug of abuse. Rapid intravenous injection of morphine produces a warm flushing of the skin and

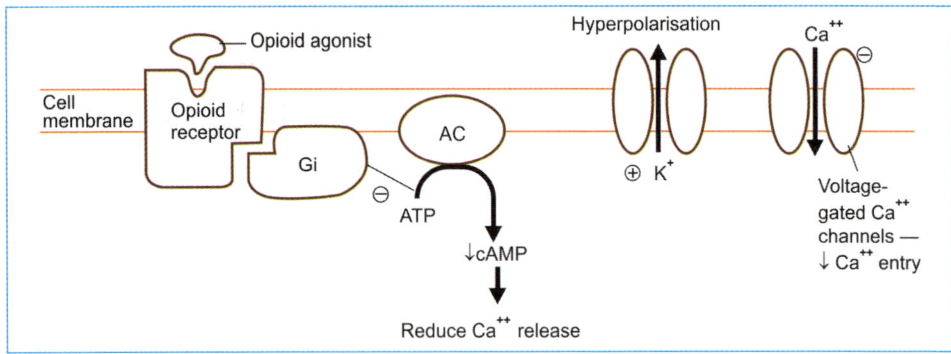

Fig. 19.1: Mechanisms of action of opioids. Opioid receptors are G-protein-coupled receptors. Stimulation of these receptors ↓cAMP formation, ↑K^+ efflux causing hyperpolarisation and also inhibit Ca^{++} entry through voltage-gated Ca^{++} channels. AC=Adenylyl cyclase; cAMP=cyclic-AMP

an immensely pleasurable sensation in the lower abdomen lasting for about 45 seconds which is known as 'high', 'rush' or 'kick'. The person loses rational thinking and is lost in colourful day dreams. It also produces drowsiness, a calming effect, inability to concentrate, feeling of detachment and indifference to surroundings.

The effects of morphine may not be pleasurable in all. A person has to learn to perceive its pleasurable effects. It may produce dysphoria in some.

3. ***Respiration:*** Morphine produces significant respiratory depression. It directly depresses the respiratory centre in the brainstem. This action is dose dependent. It depresses all phases of respiratory activity—rate and tidal volume. It may also alter the rhythm to produce irregular and periodic breathing. Death from morphine poisoning is almost always due to respiratory arrest.

   Morphine suppresses neurogenic (originating in RAS), chemical (hypercapnoeic) and hypoxic drive in the order. The respiratory centre is insensitive to increased plasma CO_2 concentration. With toxic doses, breathing is maintained by hypoxic drive.

   Sedation and indifference to surroundings add to the depression.

4. ***Cough centre:*** Morphine directly depresses the cough centre and thereby suppresses cough. Opioids should be used as antitussives only in presence of dry cough because in presence of respiratory secretions suppression of cough results in accumulation of the secretions and its consequences.

5. ***Nausea and emesis:*** Morphine directly stimulates the CTZ in the medulla causing nausea and vomiting. In higher doses, it depresses the vomiting centre and hence there is no vomiting in poisoning. Therefore, emetics should not even be tried in morphine poisoning.

6. ***Pupils:*** Morphine produces miosis resulting in a characteristic pinpoint pupil in high doses. This is due to stimulation of (EW) nucleus of the third cranial nerve. Thus, by a central effect, it produces miosis. Hence, morphine used as eye drops does not produce miosis.

7. ***Vagus:*** Morphine stimulates vagal centre causing bradycardia.

8. ***Heat regulation:*** Opioids shift the equilibrium point of heat-regulating centre so that body temperature falls slightly.

9. ***Truncal rigidity:*** Higher doses of highly lipid-soluble opioids like fentanyl have been found to enhance the tone of the large trunk muscles by acting at the supraspinal levels–**Wooden chest syndrome**. Truncal rigidity results in a decrease in the thoracic compliance and thereby interferes with breathing. A neuromuscular blocker or opioid antagonist may be used to overcome truncal rigidity.

10. ***Excitatory effect:*** In high doses, opioids produce convulsions. They may increase the excitability of the spinal cord.

II. Peripheral Actions

1. ***Cardiovascular system:*** In therapeutic doses, morphine produces hypotension by:
   - Direct peripheral vasodilatation
   - Inhibition of baroreceptor reflexes

In higher doses, it causes depression of the vasomotor centre and provokes histamine release—both contributing to a fall in BP. Postural hypotension and fainting may occur.

2. ***GIT:*** Opioids decrease the motility of the gut.
   - *Stomach:* Gastric motility is decreased resulting in increased gastric emptying time. Oesophageal reflux may increase. Gastric acid secretion is reduced. Opioids increase the tone of the antrum and first part of the duodenum which

also contribute to delayed emptying by almost 12 hr and this can retard the absorption of orally given drugs.

- *Intestines:* Morphine diminishes all intestinal secretions, delays digestion of food in the small intestine; resting tone is increased. There can be spasms of the intestine. The tone of the sphincters is increased leading to spasm. The intestinal motility (propulsive) is markedly diminished. The resulting delay in the passage of the intestinal contents in the large intestine, together with reduced secretions and inattention to the sensory stimuli for defaecation reflex—all contribute to produce marked constipation. The effects of morphine on the gut are by stimulation of the μ and δ receptors in the gut.

3. ***Other smooth muscles:***
   - *Biliary tract:* Morphine causes spasm of the sphincter of Oddi. Intrabiliary pressure rises and may cause biliary colic. Atropine partly antagonises this while opioid antagonists relieve it.
   - *Urinary bladder and ureter:* Tone and amplitude of contractions of the ureter is increased; tone of external sphincter and volume of the bladder are increased. Hence, if opioids are used to relieve colic, they may worsen the pain due to increase in the tone of the ureters. Opioids inhibit urinary voiding reflex. All these result in urinary retention especially in the elderly male with prostatic hypertrophy.
   - *Uterus:* No significant effect—may prolong labour in high doses.
   - *Bronchi:* Morphine causes release of histamine from the mast cells leading to bronchoconstriction. This together with respiratory depression, can be dangerous in asthmatics.
4. ***Renal function:*** Opioids decrease renal plasma flow and thereby depress renal function. They also have an antidiuretic effect.
5. ***Neuroendocrine effects:*** Morphine acts in the hypothalamus to inhibit the release of gonadotrophin-releasing hormone and CRF, thus decreasing blood levels of FSH, LH, ACTH and beta endorphins. Tolerance develops after long-term use. These effects are reversible on cessation of therapy.
6. ***Miscellaneous***
   - *Pruritus:* Administration of opioids particularly parenteral can induce flushing of the skin, itching and sometimes urticaria. These effects may be attributed both to histamine release and to its central effects.
   - *Immune system:* Opioids also have complex immunomodulatory properties by effects on lymphocyte proliferation, antibody production and chemotaxis.

Pharmacokinetics

Given orally, absorption of morphine is slow and incomplete. Morphine undergoes extensive first pass metabolism. Bioavailability is 20 to 40%.

Given subcutaneously, onset of action is in 15–20 min, peak effect in 1 hr, t½ 2–3 hr and duration of action is 3–5 hr. Morphine is metabolised in the liver by glucuronide conjugation. The active metabolite morphine-6-glucuronide is more potent than morphine and is excreted through the kidneys. Morphine undergoes enterohepatic circulation.

Dose: 10–50 mg oral, 10–15 mg SC/IM inj, 2–6 mg IV; 2–3 mg epidural. MORCONTIN CONTINUS—10, 30, 40, 100 mg continuous release tablets.

Some opioids are also given as rectal suppositories while highly lipid-soluble opioids are available as transdermal preparations.

Dose: Table 19.2.

Adverse Effects

Morphine can produce a wide range of adverse effects like nausea, vomiting, drowsiness, dizziness, sedation, mental clouding, respiratory depression, constipation, dysphoria, urinary retention and hypotension.

Apnoea: Administration of morphine to the mother in labour can cause apnoea in the newborn because morphine crosses the placenta, reaches the foetal brain, attaining high levels and causes apnoea.

Naloxone injection to the umbilical cord reverses this effect.

Allergic reactions including skin rashes, pruritus and wheal at the site of injection of morphine may be seen. Morphine is a histamine liberator and this action is responsible for the allergic effects. Rarely intravenous injection can cause anaphylaxis due to the same reason. It is a drug of dependence.

Tolerance

Repeated administration of morphine results in the development of tolerance to some of its effects including respiratory depression, analgesia, sedation and euphoriant effects and other CNS depressant effects. Constipation and miosis show no tolerance. Though lethal dose of morphine is about 250 mg, addicts can tolerate morphine in grams. Patients in pain can also tolerate a higher dose of morphine. Cross-tolerance is seen among different opioids.

Tolerance is mainly pharmacodynamic, where the cells adapt to the effects of the drug—at the receptor level, though pharmacokinetic mechanisms like increased metabolism also contribute. An addict needs progressively higher doses to get his 'kick' or 'rush'.

Dependence

Opium has been a drug of addiction for many centuries. Its ability to produce euphoria makes it a drug of addiction. Opioids produce both psychological and physical dependence. Sudden cessation of opioids or administration of opioid antagonists produce significant withdrawal symptoms in such dependent individuals. Manifestations are lacrimation, sweating, yawning, anxiety, apprehension, restlessness, rhinorrhoea and tremors—seen 8–12 hr after the last dose. The person craves for the drug. As the syndrome progresses, fever, insomnia, abdominal colic, severe sneezing, violent yawning, diarrhoea, blurring of vision due to mydriasis, hypertension, severe dehydration, gooseflesh, palpitation, prostration and cardiovascular collapse can occur. There is profound weakness, depression and irritability. Gooseflesh is due to pilomotor activity; skin resembles that of a plucked turkey. Hence, the word 'cold turkey' is used for symptoms of abrupt withdrawal. Abdominal cramps, pain in the bones and muscles of the back and limbs are also characteristic.

In spite of all these disturbing symptoms, withdrawal symptoms are generally not life-threatening. Administration of a suitable opioid, dramatically and completely reverses the symptoms of withdrawal. Without treatment, symptoms disappear in 7–10 days.

Withdrawal in the Newborn

Babies born to mothers who were addicts prior to delivery will also be dependent. Withdrawal symptoms may be irritability, excessive crying, tremors, frantic suckling of fists, diarrhoea, sneezing, yawning, vomiting and fever. Tincture of opium 0.2 ml/kg/3–4 hr is started at birth and gradually withdrawn.

Opioid Deaddiction

Morphine is slowly withdrawn over several days and substituted by **oral methadone.**

Advantages of methadone administration are:

1. Methadone is effective orally and by this route no 'kick' is experienced.
2. It is more potent, long-acting and prevents withdrawal symptoms because it is slowly released from the tissues.

The dose is adjusted as per the degree of dependence—1 mg methadone for every 4 mg of morphine (once a day). Methadone is then gradually withdrawn.

Clonidine a central α_2 agonist can suppress some of the autonomic withdrawal symptoms like anxiety, nausea, vomiting and diarrhoea. It is given for 7–10 days and withdrawn over 3–4 days. Night-time sedation with a hypnotic like **diazepam** is helpful.

Most addicts can be completely withdrawn from opioids in about 10 days though mild tolerable withdrawal symptoms persist. Symptoms like insomnia, malaise, restlessness, irritability, fatigue and GI hyperactivity may last up to several months.

Precautions and Contraindications

1. Avoid opioids in patients with respiratory insufficiency, COPD.
2. Acute bronchospasm may be precipitated by morphine in patients with bronchial asthma.
3. In extremes of age—more susceptible to respiratory depression.
4. Head injury—morphine is contraindicated because (Flowchart 19.1):
   i. CO_2 retention due to respiratory depression—increased CSF pressure thereby increasing the intracranial tension.
   ii. Causes marked respiratory depression.
   iii. Vomiting, miosis and mental clouding seen with morphine interfere with the diagnosis and assessment of progress in head injuries.
5. In hypovolaemic shock, morphine further decreases the BP.
6. Opioids potentiate CNS depressants.
7. Undiagnosed acute abdomen—morphine relieves pain and may interfere with the diagnosis. It induces vomiting and its spasmogenic effect may add to its drawbacks. Hence, it can be administered only after the diagnosis is established, if necessary.
8. Pregnancy—opioids should be avoided.
9. Renal and hepatic dysfunction—opioids should be avoided or dose reduced.
10. Partial agonists like pentazocine should not be mixed with pure agonists (like morphine) → reduced analgesic effect.

Flowchart 19.1: Morphine is contraindicated in head injury

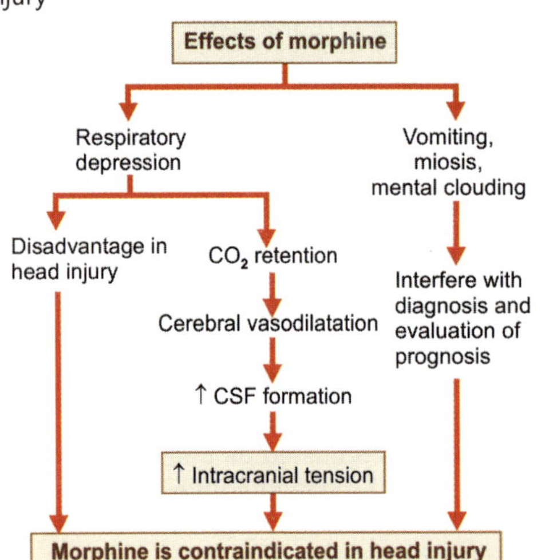

Acute Morphine Poisoning

Poisoning may be accidental, suicidal or homicidal. Lethal dose in non-addicts is about 250 mg but addicts can tolerate grams of morphine. Signs and symptoms include respiratory depression with shallow breathing, pin-point pupils, hypotension, shock, cyanosis, flaccidity, stupor, hypothermia, coma and death due to respiratory failure and pulmonary oedema.

Treatment

1. Positive pressure respiration.
2. Maintenance of BP.
3. Gastric lavage with potassium permanganate to remove unabsorbed drug.
4. Specific antidote is naloxone—0.4–0.8 mg IV repeated every 10–15 min.

Drug Interactions

1. Opioids potentiate CNS depressants and enhance the effects of drugs like sedative hypnotics, alcohol and antipsychotics—respiratory depression may be dangerous.

COMPARE AND CONTRAST
Morphine and Pethidine

	Morphine	**Pethidine**
Source	Natural opium alkaloid	Synthetic
Potency	More potent	Less potent (1/10th of mophine)
Corneal anaesthesia	No effect	Corneal anaesthetic
Higher doses	Profound CNS depression	CNS stimulation (due to norpethidine)
Antitussive property	Good	Poor or nil
Constipation effect	Marked	Less
Analgesic dose	10 mg	100 mg
Anticholinergic effect	Absent	Present
Use during labour	Significant respiratory depression in the neonate	Less neonatal respiratory depression—hence preferred over morphine
Tendency to produce seizures	No	Significant in higher doses

2. Concurrent use of opioids with MAO inhibitors can result in hyperpyrexia, coma and hypertension.

Other Opioids

Heroin or **diamorphine** or **diacetyl morphine** is converted to morphine in the body. It has higher lipid solubility because of which euphoric effects are faster and greater resulting in higher abuse potential. It has a strong smell of vinegar. Though it can be used as an analgesic, it is banned in most countries.

Apomorphine is modified morphine molecule and is a potent emetic. It induces emesis by stimulating the dopamine receptors in the CTZ. It is used as an emetic (*see* page 424).

Levorphanol is similar to morphine but it is longer acting.

Codeine is a naturally occurring opium alkaloid. It is less potent (one-sixth) than morphine as an analgesic (60 mg codeine = 10 mg morphine). Codeine depresses the cough centre in **subanalgesic doses**. It is effective orally and is well-absorbed. It produces less respiratory depression and is less constipating. Codeine has less addiction liability and tolerance is uncommon. Hence, is used as an antitussive. Duration of action is 4–6 hr. About 10% of codeine is converted to morphine. Constipation is the most common side effect.

Uses: Codeine is a commonly used antitussive. It is also available in combination with paracetamol for analgesia. It is to be given at bedtime.

Dose: 10–30 mg antitussive dose; 30–60 mg analgesic dose CODEINE LINCTUS 30 mg/ 5 ml; (CODOPLUS-Codeine 30 mg + Paracetamol 500 mg).

Oxycodone is available as a controlled release formulation for moderate to severe pain.

Papaverine is devoid of opioid and analgesic activity.

Noscapine is a naturally occurring opium alkaloid. In therapeutic doses, it has no significant actions on the CNS except for antitussive effects. Hence, it has no disadvantages of opioids. In large doses, it may cause bronchoconstriction due to the release of histamine. Noscapine is highly effective and safe. The only adverse effect is nausea. It is used as a cough suppressant.

Dose: 15–30 mg, 3–4 times a day, TUXYNE syr, COSCOPIN linctus, Noscapine 15 mg with Aspirin, Caffeine, Chlorpheniramine and Pseudoephedrine.

Several other centrally acting antitussives have been synthesized including, pholcodeine, and dextromethorphan.

Pholcodeine is as effective as codeine as an antitussive; has a long half-life and, therefore, can be given once a day.

Dextromethorphan Methorphan is a codeine analog. Its l-isomer and d-isomers have different properties. Dextromethorphan has no analgesic or addictive properties. It acts centrally to elevate the threshold for coughing for which it is as effective as codeine. Toxicity is very low; extremely high doses cause CNS depression. Antitussive dose: 10–30 mg, 3–4 times a day.

Tramadol is a synthetic codeine analog. It is an effective analgesic but its mechanism of action is not clear. It is a weak opioid agonist. In addition, it **blocks the reuptake of serotonin in the CNS** and inhibits the function of noradrenaline transporter.

Nausea is a common side effect. Other adverse effects include drowsiness, dryness of mouth and sedation. Respiratory depression is mild. It is a drug of dependence. It may precipitate seizures. Intravenous administration of tramadol can cause **truncal rigidity**. It should be avoided in patients on MAO inhibitors because tramadol inhibits serotonin uptake.

Tramadol is used in acute and chronic pain, like postoperative pain and neuralgias.

Dose: 50–100 mg oral/IM/IV infusion. URGENDOL, CONTRAMOL 50 mg cap, 100 mg SR tab 50 mg/ml. TRAMAZAC 50 mg caps.

Tapentadol is similar to tramadol in structure, actions and adverse effects. It may be used for treatment of moderate to severe pain. Dose 50, 75 and 100 mg. Sustained release and immediate release tablets are also available.

PETHIDINE AND ITS DERIVATIVES

Pethidine (Meperidine)

Pethidine is a phenylpiperidine derivative of morphine. Though chemically it is very much different from morphine, many of its actions resemble that of morphine. It was accidentally found to have opioid effects when efforts were made to obtain anticholinergic drugs. When compared to morphine (Table 19.2):

- Pethidine is 1/10th as potent as morphine (100 mg pethidine = 10 mg morphine). However, efficacy as an analgesic is equal to morphine.
- The onset of action is more rapid and duration of action is shorter.
- It produces corneal anaesthesia.
- It is not a good antitussive.
- It is less constipating, causes less urinary retention
- In some patients, it may cause dysphoria.
- It also has anticholinergic effects which can cause dry mouth, tachycardia and blurring of vision.
- Release of histamine is milder.
- May produce a negative inotropic effect.
- In toxic doses, pethidine sometimes produces CNS stimulation with tremors, restlessness and convulsions instead of sedation. This is because of the toxic metabolite—norpethidine.

Adverse effects are similar to morphine except that constipation and urinary retention are less common. Anticholinergic side effects like blurred vision, dry mouth and tachycardia are common. If tachycardia is to be avoided in some patients, pethidine should not be given. Pethidine may also produce a negative inotropic effect.

Preparations dose: 25–100 mg IM/SC, PETHIDINE HCl 100 mg/2 ml inj 50, 100 mg tab.

Uses

1. **In pain:** Pethidine is used as an **analgesic** in visceral pain and also for other indications of morphine. Because of its better oral efficacy and less spasmogenic effect, pethidine is preferred to morphine.
2. **During labour:** Given during labour, pethidine produces less respiratory depression in the newborn when compared to morphine. Moreover, it does not interfere with uterine contractions and

Table 19.2: Salient features of opioid analgesics

Name	*Dose (mg)*	*Duration of analgesia (hrs)*	*Salient features*
Morphine	20–40	4–5	Prototype; poor BAB
Ethylmorphine	16–32	6–8	Better BAB, oral use
Methadone	10	4–6	Orally effective, long-acting, bound to tissues, Use: Analgesic, opioid deaddiction.
Pethidine	50–100	2–4	Anticholinergic, corneal anaesthetic, norpethidine in toxicity; use: Preanaesthetic and obstetric analgesia
Fentanyl	0.05–0.2	1–2	High potency, highly lipid-soluble, fast-acting, does not increase intracranial pressure, not a histamine liberator
Codeine	30–60	3–5	Antitussive in subanalgesic doses.
Dextropropoxyphene	60	4–6	Longer acting, good BAB, irritant—not used parenterally Large doses—respiratory arrest, death.
Pentazocine	30–60	3–4	κ agonist, weak μ agonist; dysphoria; hypertension, tachycardia, CI in myocardial infarction.
Nalbuphine	10–15	3–6	Ceiling effect for respiratory depression; high doses → dysphoria
Buprenorphine	0.3–0.6	4–8	Potent, highly lipid-soluble, long-acting; SL administration similar to pentazocine
Tramadol	50–100	4–6	5-HT and NA reuptake blocker, weak μ agonist; avoid with MAO inhibitors.

labour and is, therefore, preferred to morphine for obstetric analgesia.

3. **Preanaesthetic medication:** Pethidine can also be used as preanaesthetic medication.

Derivatives of Pethidine

Derivatives of pethidine include fentanyl and its congeners (sufentanil, alfentanil, remifentanil) alphaprodine, diphenoxylate and loperamide.

Fentanyl

Advantages

- It is about 100 times more potent than morphine as an analgesic.
- Fentanyl is highly lipid-soluble and fast-acting (maximum effect within 5 minutes).
- Fentanyl has mild effects on the cardiovascular system. It slightly reduces HR and BP. Hence, it is found to be safer than other opioids in cardiovascular surgeries.

Flowchart 19.2: WHO analgesic ladder

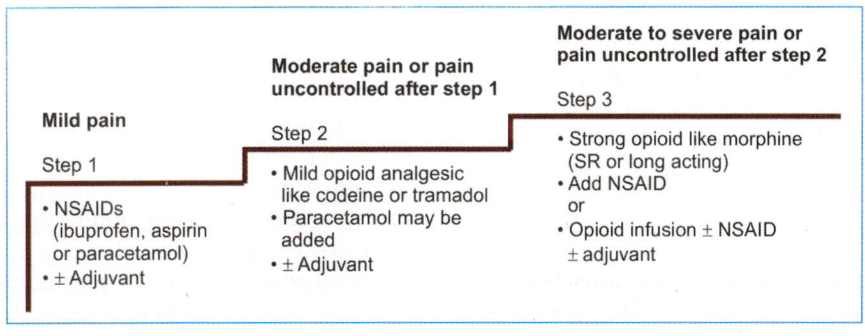

- **Transdermal patches** of fentanyl are available which act for 48 hours.
- Unlike morphine, fentanyl does not increase the intracranial pressure.
- Fentanyl is not a histamine liberator.
- It can be used in combination with droperidol, a neuroleptic agent to produce neuroleptanalgesia.

Because of the above advantages, fentanyl is a commonly used opioid analgesic.

Dose: 0.05–2 mg inj DUROGESIC Transdermal patches—deliver 25, 50 or 75 μg/hr for 2–3 days. SUBLIMAZE, TROFENTYL 50 μg/ml inj.

For **neuroleptanalgesia** the combination is given IV to produce sedation and intense analgesia without loss of consciousness. This state is maintained for 30–40 minutes as both have rapid- and short-action (*see* page 195). Patient is drowsy but responds to commands. A fixed dose combination is available with 0.05 mg fentanyl + 2.5 mg droperidol per ml. 5 ml is the dose used IV over 10 minutes.

Uses

1. Neuroleptanalgesia is used for short surgical procedures especially in 'poor-risk' patients.
2. Epidural fentanyl is used for post-operative and obstetric analgesia. For this, morphine/fentanyl may be combined with local anaesthetics so that lower doses of both drugs are sufficient.
3. Fentanyl can also be used in chronic pain where opioid use is permissible. Transdermal fentanyl patch delivers fentanyl constantly to relieve pain and may be used in severe painful conditions like terminal cancer pain. Constant watch for respiratory depression is needed. Fentanyl is also available as a lozenge and as a **'lollipop'** for transmucosal drug delivery.

Adverse Effects

Bolus doses of fentanyl cause **muscle rigidity**. This can be reduced by avoiding bolus doses. Other adverse effects include nausea, vomiting and respiratory depression.

Congeners of fentanyl: Alfentanil and remifentanil are faster acting (act within one minute) and recovery is rapid. Remifentanil is rapidly metabolised by tissue esterase. They are used for short surgical procedures. Sufentanil is 5 times more potent than fentanyl. **Diphenoxylate** and its metabolite difenoxin reduce gastrointestinal motility and are used orally in the treatment of diarrhoea (*see* page 437). They are used in combination with atropine to reduce the risk of abuse.

Loperamide is also an antidiarrhoeal drug with no other significant opioid effects (*see* page 437).

Methadone

Methadone, a synthetic opioid, has actions similar to morphine. Its outstanding features are:

- It is an effective analgesic.
- It is effective by many routes including oral, rectal, SC, IV and spinal routes.
- It is effective in certain types of neuropathic and cancer pain which are not relieved by morphine. Methadone is therefore, now a preferred analgesic.
- It has a long duration of action (t½ 24–36 hours) and, therefore, effectively suppresses withdrawal symptoms in addicts.

Mechanism of Action

1. Methadone is a μ receptor agonist.
2. Methadone also blocks NMDA receptors.
3. Blocks monoaminergic receptor uptake transporters.

The latter two actions may be responsible for its better efficacy as an analgesic in certain types of pain.

Methadone is about 90% bound to plasma proteins; it is also firmly bound to proteins in various tissues, including brain. After repeated administration, it gradually accumulates in tissues. When administration is discontinued, the drug is slowly released from the binding sites. Methadone is metabolised by microsomal enzymes like CYP3A4 in the liver. Hence, microsomal enzyme inhibition by drugs and hepatic failure can enhance blood levels of methadone. This probably accounts for its milder withdrawal symptoms. As euphoric effects are less intense, abuse potential is less. Tolerance develops more slowly. In addicts, withdrawal symptoms are gradual in onset, less intense, but prolonged.

Dose: 10 mg oral or IM PHYSEPTONE 10 mg inj, 2 mg/5 ml Linctus.

Uses

1. *Substitution therapy:* In opioid dependence 1 mg oral methadone is given for every 4 mg morphine in 2–3 divided doses for 2–3 days. When methadone is stopped, withdrawal symptoms appear but are mild and tolerable.
2. *Opioid maintenance:* Gradually increasing doses of methadone are given orally to produce a high degree of tolerance. 50–100 mg/day. Such subjects do not experience the pleasurable effects of IV morphine and other opioids and they give up the habit.
3. *Methadone* can also be used as an *analgesic.*

LAAM (L-alpha-acetyl-methadol) is a derivative of methadone with longer duration of action than methadone so that it can be given three times a week. It is used to prevent withdrawal symptoms in addicts.

Dextropropoxyphene: Propoxyphene is a congener of methadone and dextro and levo isomers are available. Dextropropoxyphene binds to the opioid receptors and produces effects similar to morphine. It is less constipating, longer acting and has good oral bioavailability—but it is an irritant when given parenterally. Large doses cause CNS stimulation. Several deaths have been reported with its use as it gets rapidly absorbed and causes respiratory arrest and hypotension. It also has abuse potential and efficacy is low.

Used in mild to moderate pain and is marketed in combination with aspirin but is not preferred now. **Dextropropoxyphene 32 mg + aspirin 600 mg**

PARVODEX 60 mg cap. SUDHINOL 65 mg + Paracetamol 650 mg.

Levopropoxyphene is a weak opioid agonist devoid of other effects but is a good antitussive used in the dose of 50–100 mg 4–6 times a day.

Ethoheptazine: Ethoheptazine is related to pethidine and has mild analgesic effects with low addiction potential. It is used orally in combination with NSAIDs for relief of pain.

EQUAGESIC Aspirin 325 mg + Ethoheptazine Citrate 75 mg tab—1 tab TDS.

Uses of Morphine and its Congeners

Dose: Morphine 10 to 20 mg IM/SC; 20 mg tablet of ethylmorphine.

1. *Analgesic:* Morphine is one of the most effective analgesics available. It affords **symptomatic relief of pain** without affecting the underlying disease. It is an excellent analgesic for severely painful conditions such as acute myocardial infarction, fractures, burns, pulmonary embolism, terminal stages of cancer, acute pericarditis, spontaneous pneumothorax and postoperative pain. In excruciating pain, morphine can be given IV.

   In **myocardial infarction,** morphine relieves pain and thereby apprehension. As a result, reflex sympathetic stimulation is reduced and shock is minimized—it can be life saving.

   - Morphine is given with atropine to relieve **renal and biliary colic.** Atropine relieves spasm of the sphincter of Oddi. Morphine relieves pain but may cause spasm of the sphincter of Oddi which in turn raises intrabiliary pressure. Hence along with morphine, atropine is given which relieves spasm of the sphincter of Oddi.
   - Since opiate receptors are present in the spinal cord, epidural morphine can be

used to produce **epidural analgesia.** Such analgesia is segmental in distribution and there is no interference with motor function or autonomic changes and no systemic adverse effects. Small doses of morphine can produce profound analgesia for 12–24 hours.

- *Obstetric analgesia:* Pethidine is preferred to morphine for this condition as it causes milder respiratory depression in the newborn.
- Opioids can be liberally given to control the pain of **terminal illness** like cancers.
- Opioids should ***not*** *be* freely used in case of other chronic pain due to their addiction liability.

Various **alternative routes** of administration are tried for opioids—in order to reduce their systemic effects and provide longer duration of analgesia particularly for patients with chronic pain. Morphine and other opioids are being tried as intraspinal infusion, rectal, transmucosal, transdermal administration and by inhalation. In patient-controlled analgesia (PCA) with opioids, the patients decide their own need for the analgesic. A specific dose of the opioids is pushed through an intravenous device; careful monitoring is needed to avoid overdosage.

2. *Acute left ventricular failure/acute pulmonary oedema:* Intravenous morphine is used to alleviate the dyspnoea of LVF and pulmonary oedema in which the response may be dramatic. The mechanism is not clear. The relief may be due to:
   i. Alteration in the patient's reaction to impaired respiratory function.
   ii. Reduction in the workload of the heart due to decreased fear and apprehension because reduced anxiety decreases sympathetic stimulation which in turn decreases cardiac work done.
   iii. Cardiovascular effects like decreased PVR leading to shifting of blood from pulmonary to peripheral circulation, thereby reducing cardiac workload.

   Morphine is contraindicated in bronchial asthma and pulmonary oedema due to respiratory irritants.

3. *In anaesthesia*
   i. *Preanaesthetic medication:* Morphine and pethidine are commonly used as preanaesthetic medication. They reduce anxiety, provide analgesia, allow smoother induction and reduce the dose of the anaesthetic required. But they have certain disadvantages:
      - Opioids depress respiration.
      - Morphine precipitates bronchospasm and is dangerous in patients with poor respiratory reserve.
      - They cause vasomotor depression.
      - They may induce vomiting.
      - They may interfere with pupillary response to anaesthesia because they cause miosis.
      - Postoperative urinary retention and constipation may be troublesome.
   ii. *Special anaesthesia:* High doses of morphine can be used IV to produce general anaesthesia
   iii. *Neuroleptanalgesia:* Fentanyl with droperidol can be used to produce neuroleptanalgesia.
   iv. *Epidural analgesia:* Morphine can be used epidurally for the relief of postoperative and chronic pain.

4. *Diarrhoea:* Opioids are effective for the symptomatic treatment of diarrhoea. Synthetic opioids—diphenoxylate and loperamide, are preferred as antidiarrhoeals. **Eluxadoline** is an agonist at μ and κ receptors with prominent effects on the gut. It is used to overcome abdominal pain and diarrhoea associated with inflammatory bowel disease. It does not induce constipation. It can rarely cause pancre-

atitis and is reversible on withdrawal of the drug.

5. *Cough:* Though morphine is an effective antitussive, codeine is the preferred opioid for this purpose. Now many nonaddictive antitussives are available (*see* page 406).
6. *Shivering:* Pethidine reduces shivering and this property could be by its action on α_2 adrenoceptors. Other opioids also have this property but are weaker than pethidine.
7. *Sedative:* Morphine relieves anxiety in threatened abortion without affecting uterine motility. It is an useful sedative in the presence of pain.

MIXED AGONISTS AND ANTAGONISTS

They include—pentazocine, cyclazocine, nalbuphine, buprenorphine, butorphanol and nalorphine.

Pentazocine: In an attempt to develop an analgesic with less addiction liability and low adverse effects, pentazocine was developed. Pentazocine is a κ receptor agonist.

- CNS effects of pentazocine are similar to morphine. 20 mg pentazocine = 10 mg morphine. Euphoria is seen only in low doses. With higher doses—above 60 mg, dysphoria can occur due to k receptor stimulation.
- Sedation and respiratory depression are less marked.
- It has weak antagonistic properties at μ receptors.
- Tolerance and dependence develop on repeated use.
- CVS: In contrast to morphine, pentazocine increases BP and heart rate and thereby increases cardiac work. It is, therefore, **not suitable in myocardial infarction.**
- Biliary spasm and constipation are less severe.

Preparations: Pentazocine can be given both orally and parenterally. It undergoes first pass metabolism.

Dose: 50–100 mg oral; 30–60 mg IM, SC, IV inj FORTWIN, PENTAWIN 30 mg inj SC IV.

Adverse effects: Sedation, sweating, dizziness, nausea, dysphoria with anxiety, nightmares and hallucinations which are unpleasant are seen above 60 mg. As it is an irritant, IM injection can be painful and cause sterile abscesses.

Uses

Pentazocine is a commonly used opioid analgesic especially in postoperative and chronic pain—abuse liability is less than morphine.

Cyclazocine is similar to pentazocine.

Nalbuphine is an agonist–antagonist—more potent than pentazocine. It is a good analgesic. Though it produces respiratory depression like morphine, it has a ceiling effect for respiratory depression at 30 mg, i.e. an increase in dose beyond 30 mg does not increase respiratory depression further. Higher doses produce dysphoria. Used as an analgesic 10–20 mg IM.

Buprenorphine is a highly lipid-soluble synthetic thebaine congener. It is a partial μ agonist, 25 times as potent as morphine. Though onset of action is slow, duration of analgesia is long. Other CNS effects are similar to morphine while respiratory depression is less marked. Patients exhibit lower degree of tolerance and dependence liability. Withdrawal syndrome appears late and is mild.

Dose: 0.3–0.6 mg SC, IM or sublingual (oral not available), TIDIGESIC, 0.2 mg SL tab, 0.3 mg/ml inj. BUPRIGESIC, PENTOREL 0.3 mg/ml inj.

Uses

Chronic pain like in terminal cancer patients. Buprenorphine can also be used as a maintenance drug in opioid addicts as the withdrawal symptoms are mild.

Butorphanol is similar to pentazocine but is more potent than it. It causes tachycardia similar to it but does not increase the BP and dysphoria may be milder. Indication and contraindications are similar to pentazocine. Butorphanol is available for **intranasal administration.**

Dose: 1–2 mg IM/IV, BUTRUM 1, 2 mg/ml inj.

Nalorphine is also an agonist–antagonist. At low doses, it is a good analgesic but, with increase in dose, there is no increase in analgesia. It causes dysphoria (κ agonist) and respiratory depression even in low doses. Hence, it cannot be used as an analgesic. At high doses, it acts as an antagonist and counters all the actions of opioids.

Uses

Nalorphine may be used in acute opioid poisoning. It can also be used for the diagnosis of opioid addiction.

Newer Agonistñantagonists

Meptazinol is a short-acting agonist–antagonist with additional anticholinergic effects. It produces short duration analgesia with less respiratory depression and is, therefore, suitable for obstetric analgesia.

Dezocine is a partial agonist at μ receptors. Its analgesic actions are similar to morphine but respiratory depression does not increase with an increase in dose (ceiling effect).

OPIOID ANTAGONISTS

Naloxone acts as a competitive antagonist to all types of opioid receptors. It is a pure antagonist. In normal individuals, it does not produce any significant actions. But in opium addicts, given IV, it promptly antagonises all the actions of morphine including respiratory depression and sedation and precipitates withdrawal syndrome. It also blocks the action of endogenous opioid peptides—endorphins, enkephalins and dynorphins. It blocks the analgesia produced by placebo and acupuncture. This suggests that endogenous opioid peptides are responsible for analgesia by these techniques.

Given orally it undergoes high first pass metabolism and is metabolised by the liver. Hence, it is given intravenously. Duration of action is 1–2 hours . It is metabolised by glucuronide conjugation.

Dose: 0.4 mg IV. NARCOTAN 0.4 mg/ml and 0.04 mg/ml Ampoules.

Uses

1. Naloxone is the drug of choice for morphine overdosage. 0.1–0.4 mg is injected intravenously. The dose should be repeated after every 1–2 hr as naloxone is short acting and respiratory depression may recur again. Constant monitoring is, therefore, required till the patient fully recovers from opioid overdosage.
2. It is also used to reverse neonatal asphyxia due to opioids used in labour.

   Dose: 5–10 μg/kg repeated, if required.
3. Naloxone can also be used for the diagnosis of opioid dependence—it precipitates withdrawal symptoms.
4. Hypotension seen during shock could be due to endogenous opioids released during such stress. Naloxone has been found to be beneficial in reversing hypotension.

Naltrexone is another pure opioid antagonist. It is:

- More potent than naloxone
- Orally effective
- Has a longer duration of action of 1–2 days.
- Naltrexone is well absorbed when given orally but undergoes first pass metabolism.

Dose 50–100 mg/day. NALTIMA 50 mg tab.

Uses

1. Naltrexone is used for 'opioid blockade' therapy in post-addicts is found to be effective (50–100 mg/day orally single dose or on alternate days) so that even if the addicts take an opioid, they do not

experience the pleasurable effects and, therefore, lose the craving.

2. Alcohol craving is also reduced by naltrexone and is used to prevent relapse of heavy drinking (*see* page 273).

Nalmefene

Nalmefene is a derivative of naltrexone. It is orally effective (but only an IV preparation is available) and longer acting. It has better bioavailability and is not hepatotoxic. It is used in opioid overdosage.

Peripheral Opioid Antagonists

1. **Methylnaltrexone and Naloxegol** are mu opioid antagonists acting peripherally and they reverse the opioid-induced constipation in patients receiving long-term treatment with opioids for chronic cancer pain (0.25 mg in the morning).
2. **Alvimopan** blocks the μ receptors in the gut and does not significantly penetrate CNS. It is used in the treatment of postoperative ileus following bowel resection.
3. **Diprenorphine, naloxonazine, naltrindole and naloxone benzoyl-hydrazone** are other opioid antagonists.

Clinical Pharmacology

- Opioids are schedule H drugs and should not be casually prescribed. Because of the risk of abuse, even when prescribed, it should be for a short period except in terminally ill patients.
- Terminally ill cancer patients can be given adequate opioids to relieve pain and reduce suffering.
- Tramadol, tapentadol, pethidine and pentazocine are commonly used opioids.
- Nausea is common with tramadol. IV tramadol in addition can cause truncal rigidity and should be used carefully.
- Postoperative pain (or other painful conditions associated with significant inflammation) require additional NSAIDs. Opioid monotherapy is generally insufficient for adequate pain control in such patients.

[1] From Medical Council of India, *Competency based Undergraduate Curriculum for the Indian Medical Graduate*, 2018;1:136–144.

CHAPTER **20**

Alcohols

Competency achievement: The student should be able to:

PH 1.20 Describe the effects of acute and chronic ethanol intake.[1]

PH 1.21 Describe the symptoms and management of methanol and ethanol poisonings.[2]

ETHYL ALCOHOL (ETHANOL)

Ethyl alcohol is a monohydroxy alcohol manufactured by fermentation of sugars. It is a colourless, volatile, inflammable liquid. The ethanol content of various alcoholic beverages ranges from 4 to 55%. For commercial use, alcohol is largely produced from mollases which is a by-product when sugar is manufactured from sugarcane.

Actions

1. ***Local:*** On topical application, ethanol evaporates quickly and has a cooling effect. It is an astringent—precipitates surface proteins and hardens the skin. 40–50% alcohol is a rubefacient and counterirritant. Alcohol is also an antiseptic. **At 70%, it has maximum antiseptic properties,** which decreases above that. It could be because presence of some water allows the alcohol to enter the bacterial cell and kill the bacteria. It is not effective against spores.
2. ***CNS:*** Alcohol is a CNS depressant. Small doses cause euphoria, relief of anxiety and loss of social inhibitions. Moderate doses, blunt the reflexes and impair muscular coordination and visual acuity making driving dangerous. With higher doses, mental clouding, impaired judgement, fine and precise movement, drowsiness and loss of self-control result. High doses cause stupor and coma. Death is due to respiratory depression.

   Alcohol may precipitate convulsions in epileptics. Tolerance develops on long-term use.
3. ***CVS:*** The actions are dose dependent. Small doses cause cutaneous vasodilation resulting in flushing and feeling of warmth. Large doses cause hypotension due to depression of myocardium and vasomotor centre. Arrhythmias may also be seen in heavy drinking or 'binge drinking'. Chronic heavy drinking is associated with hypertension.

   Chronic moderate drinking, however, has shown to prevent coronary heart disease and stroke. It could be because of raised HDL, raised tissue plasminogen activator and because it could also inhibit inflammatory processes in atherosclerosis.
4. ***GIT and liver:*** Alcohol is an irritant—increases gastric secretion and produces vasodilation and warmth. It is an appetizer. Chronic alcoholism results in chronic gastritis.

   Chronic consumption of moderate amounts of alcohol results in accumulation of fat in the liver, liver enlargement, followed by fatty degeneration and cirrhosis.

   Alcohol induces hepatic microsomal enzymes.

Heavy drinking is associated with both acute and chronic pancreatitis.

5. *Other effects*
   - Though alcohol is called an aphrodisiac, this effect could just be due to loss of inhibition.
   - Low doses taken over a long time increases HDL and lowers LDL cholesterol.
   - Alcohol is a diuretic (↓ADH secretion).
   - It interferes with folate metabolism and may cause megaloblastic anaemia.
   - Chronic alcoholics also develop nutritional deficiencies including vitamin deficiencies.
   - Chronic alcoholism is often associated with osteoporosis though the exact cause is not known.
   - Though alcohol causes a feeling of warmth, heat loss is increased due to vasodilation and should not be used for 'warming up' in cold surroundings. Food value is 7 calories/gram.

Mechanism of Action

Ethanol acts by:

1. Inhibiting central neuronal nicotinic cholinergic receptors
2. Inhibiting excitatory NMDA and kainate receptor functions.
3. Promoting the function of 5-HT_3 receptors.
4. Ethanol also influences many ion channels including K^+ channels.

Pharmacokinetics

Alcohol is rapidly absorbed from the stomach and is metabolised in the liver by dehydrogenases (Fig. 20.1).

Metabolism follows zero order kinetics—a constant amount is metabolised per unit time, i.e. about 10 ml absolute alcohol is metabolised per hour. Hence, when higher doses are taken blood alcohol rises significantly resulting in toxicity. It is excreted through kidneys and lungs.

Drug Interactions

1. Alcohol potentiates other CNS depressants including hypnotics, opioids and antipsychotics.
2. Sulfonylureas, metronidazole and griseofulvin have disulfiram like effects on alcohol consumption—should be avoided.
3. Alcohol is an enzyme inducer and can hasten the metabolism of other drugs.
4. Alcohol increases gastric acidity which gets added up, if patients also receive NSAIDs and other gastric irritants.

Uses

1. *Antiseptic:* 70% alcohol is applied topically.
2. *Bedsores:* When rubbed on to the skin, alcohol hardens the skin and prevents bedsores—it is an astringent.
3. *Fever:* Alcoholic sponges are used for reduction of body temperature in fevers.
4. *Appetite stimulant:* About 50 ml of 6–10% alcohol given before meals is an appetite stimulant.
5. *Neuralgias:* In severe neuralgias like trigeminal neuralgia, injection of alcohol around the nerve causes permanent loss of transmission and relieves pain.
6. *In methanol poisoning* (*see* page 273).

Acute Alcoholic Intoxication

Acute alcoholic intoxication causes severe gastritis, hypotension, hypoglycaemia, respiratory depression, coma and death. Fatal blood alcohol concentration is >400 mg/dl but

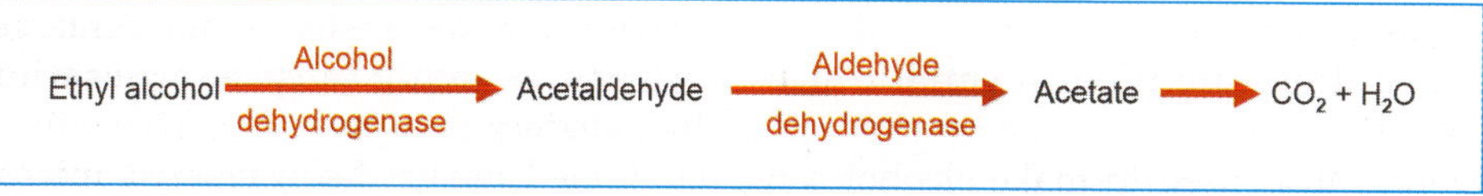

Fig. 20.1: Metabolism of ethanol

varies due to tolerance in chronic alcoholics. Treatment measures include gastric lavage, airway maintenance, positive pressure ventilation and maintenance of fluid and electrolyte balance. Haemodialysis is needed in severe intoxication. Hypoglycemia needs glucose; thiamine should be administered to prevent Wernicke's encephalopathy. Blood potassium and phosphate should be checked and corrected, if required.

Chronic Alcoholism

Chronic alcoholism causes dependence. Wernicke's encephalopathy, Korsakoff's psychosis, tremors, cirrhosis of liver, hypertension and cardiomyopathy can occur. In addition, nutritional deficiencies such as polyneuritis, anaemia and pellagra can occur. Chronic alcoholism is also associated with increased risk of cancer of the oropharynx, larynx, oesophagus and liver. In pregnant women, alcohol is teratogenic. Even moderate drinking during pregnancy can produce **fetal alcohol syndrome** with manifestations like low IQ, microcephaly, growth retardation and facial anomalies. It can also cause stillbirths and abortions.

Drugs used in Alcohol Dependence

Alcohol dependence is a common social evil which is difficult to treat.

Abrupt withdrawal: Sudden cessation of alcohol in chronic alcoholics results in withdrawal symptoms including anxiety, tremors, insomnia, increased motor activity and reduced threshold for seizures which are prominent for 1–2 days but may persist in milder form for many months. Diazepam helps overcome most withdrawal symptoms. Other measures include correcting electrolyte imbalance, thiamine replacement, watching for seizures and treatment of seizures, if any, and reassurance.

Several drugs are tried in **chronic alcoholism**

1. **Disulfiram** is used to make alcohol consumption an unpleasant experience so that the person gives up drinking. Disulfiram inhibits the enzyme aldehyde dehydrogenase. If alcohol is consumed after taking disulfiram, acetaldehyde accumulates and within a few minutes it can produce flushing, throbbing headache, nausea, vomiting, sweating, hypotension and confusion—called **the antabuse reaction,** due to accumulation of acetaldehyde. The effect lasts for 7–14 days after stopping disulfiram. Therefore, the person develops aversion to alcohol and often gives up the habit.

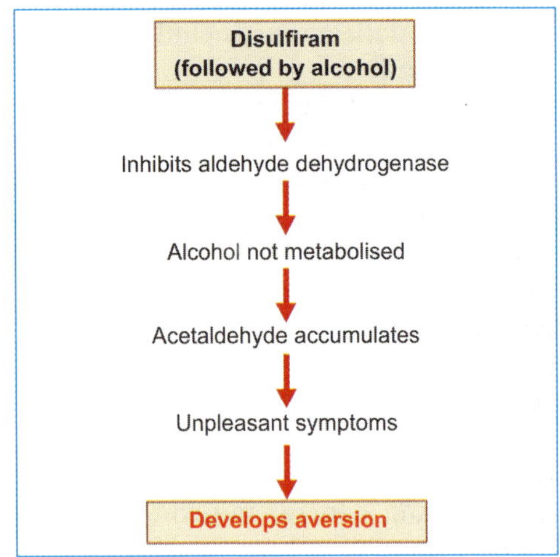

However, willingness on the part of the person to give up the habit goes a long way in the success of this aversion therapy. The reactions can sometimes be very severe and, therefore, treatment should be given in a hospital.

Other drugs that cause antabuse reaction—Key Box 20.1

Contraindications: Patients with liver disease, patients physically dependent on alcohol.

2. **Benzodiazepines:** Long-acting BZDs like diazepam to reduce the symptoms of alcohol withdrawal—benzodiazepines relieve symptoms like anxiety and insomnia. They should be continued and gradually tapered over several months.

Key Box 20.1: Some drugs that can precipitate disulfiram-like reaction

Metronidazole	Some cephalosporins
Sulfonylureas	Phenylbutazone
Griseofulvin	Nitrofurantoin

3. **Clonidine,** an α_2-receptor agonist, reduces the release of sympathetic neurotransmitters while propranolol blocks the effects of sympathetic overactivity like tremors and tachycardia.

4. **Naltrexone** is an orally effective opioid antagonist which has been thought to be useful in alcohol withdrawal. It is given in the dose of 50 mg once daily. A long-acting IM preparation to be given once a month is also available. Several studies have shown naltrexone to reduce alcohol craving and 'relapse' of heavy drinking. Naltrexone can cause nausea. Naltrexone and disulfiram should not be given concurrently as both can cause hepatotoxicity. Moreover, chronic alcoholics are likely to have an already damaged liver. **Nalmefene** can also be used in place of naltrexone.

5. **Acamprosate,** an NMDA receptor antagonist, has been found to be useful in preventing relapse of heavy drinking and in achieving alcohol abstinance.

6. **Ondansetron,** a 5-HT_3 antagonist antiemetic, has been shown to reduce alcohol consumption and is being evaluated for use in alcohol withdrawal.

7. **Other drugs:** Baclofen, a $GABA_B$ receptor antagonist (*see* page 133), and topiramate (*see* page 223), an antiepileptic drug, are tried. **Rimonabant,** a CB_1 cannabinoid receptor antagonist, has also been found to be useful in alcohol withdrawal.

8. **Psychosocial therapy** and counselling by a psychologist also help.

METHYL ALCOHOL (METHANOL, WOOD ALCOHOL)

Methanol is used to denature ethyl alcohol. It has no therapeutic value. Ingestion results in methanol poisoning. Methanol can also be absorbed through the skin. Methanol is converted to formaldehyde—catalysed by alcohol dehydrogenase; formaldehyde is converted to formic acid by the action of aldehyde dehydrogenase (Fig. 20.2). Toxic effects are due to formic acid.

Manifestations of toxicity may take about 30 hr to appear as they are due to the metabolites and include vomiting, headache, visual distrubances, vertigo, severe abdominal pain, hypotension, delirium, acidosis and coma. Formic acid has affinity for optic nerve and causes retinal damage resulting in blindness. There are reports of even 15 ml of methanol causing blindness. Death is due to respiratory failure.

Treatment

1. *Correction of acidosis:* As acidosis hastens retinal damage, immediate correction of acidosis with IV sodium bicarbonate infusion helps in preventing blindness.
2. *Protect eyes:* Patient should be kept in a dark room to protect the eyes.
3. *Gastric lavage:* Should be given.
4. *BP and ventilation:* Must be maintained.
5. *Ethyl alcohol:* Should be given immediately. It competes with methanol for

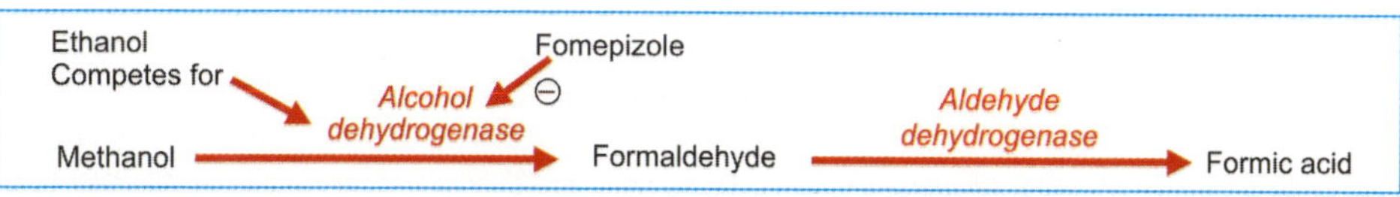

Fig. 20.2: Metabolism of methanol

alcohol dehydrogenase because of its higher affinity for alcohol dehydrogenase. It thus slows the metabolism of methanol and prevents the formation of toxic metabolites. A loading dose of 0.6 g/kg is followed by an infusion of 10 g/hour.

6. *Antidote:* **Fomepizole** specifically inhibits the enzyme alcohol dehydrogenase and thereby prevents the formation of toxic metabolites—formaldehyde and formic acid. Fomepizole is considered the antidote in methanol poisoning. It has the advantage over alcohol that it does not cause any intoxication by itself. Fomepizole is also effective in ethylene glycol poisoning.
7. *Haemodialysis:* Should be started at the earliest possible to enhance the removal of methanol.

Clinical Pharmacology

- Metabolised by zero order kinetics—blood alcohol levels rise disproportionately with higher doses.
- Microsomal enzyme inducer—related drug interactions are likely in chronic alcoholics.
- Therapeutic uses are limited; topically in bedsores—for astringent, antiseptic effects systemically in methanol poisoning.
- CNS depression additive with other drugs like sedative antihistamines, sedative hypnotics.
- Long-term use of 3–4 drinks per day can cause serious hepatotoxicity.
- Thiamine (vitamin B_1) should be administered to people consuming alcohol regularly to avoid Wernicke's and Korsakoff syndrome.
- Disulfiram, naltrexone may help in overcoming chronic alcohol dependence; metronidazole, sulfonylureas, griseofulvin, some cephalosporins, phenylbutazone and nitrofurantoin—also have disulfiram like effects.

[1–2] From Medical Council of India, *Competency based Undergraduate Curriculum for the Indian Medical Graduate*, 2018;1:136–144.

CHAPTER 21

CNS Stimulants and Drugs of Abuse

Competency achievement: The student should be able to:

PH 1.22 Describe drugs of abuse (dependence, addiction, stimulants, depressants, psychedelics, drugs used for criminal offences).[1]

PH 1.23 Describe the process and mechanism of drug deaddiction.[2]

Drugs that have a predominantly stimulant effect on the CNS may be broadly divided into:

1. **Respiratory stimulants**
   Doxapram, nikethamide
2. **Psychomotor stimulants**
   Amphetamine, cocaine, methylxanthines
3. **Convulsants**
   Leptazol, strychnine.

RESPIRATORY STIMULANTS

Respiratory stimulants are also called ***analeptics***. These drugs stimulate respiration and are sometimes used to treat respiratory failure. Though they may bring about temporary improvement in respiration, the mortality is not reduced. They have a low safety margin and may produce convulsions. The availability of ventilators has reduced the need for analeptics.

Doxapram appears to act mainly on the brainstem and spinal cord and increase the activity of medullary respiratory and vasomotor centres. Doxapram in low doses can selectively stimulate respiration. Given intravenously as an infusion.

1–2 mg/kg/hr or 40–80 mg IM.

Adverse effects are nausea, cough, restlessness, muscle twitching, hypertension, tachycardia, arrhythmias and convulsions.

Uses

1. Doxapram is occasionally used IV as an analeptic in acute respiratory failure.
2. Apnoea in premature infants not responding to theophylline.

Nikethamide is not used because of the risk of convulsions.

PSYCHOMOTOR STIMULANTS

Amphetamine and **dextroamphetamine** are sympathomimetic drugs (*see* page 91).

Cocaine is a CNS stimulant, produces euphoria and is a drug of abuse (*see* page 182).

Methylxanthines

Caffeine, theophylline and theobromine are the naturally occurring xanthine alkaloids. The beverages—coffee contains caffeine; tea contains theophylline and caffeine; cocoa has caffeine and theobromine.

Actions

CNS: Caffeine and theophylline are CNS stimulants. They bring about an increase in mental alertness, a reduction of fatigue, produce a sense of well-being and improve motor activity and performance with a clearer flow of thought. Caffeine stimulates the respiratory centre. Higher doses produce irritability, nervousness, restlessness, insomnia, excitement and headache. High doses can result in convulsions.

CVS: Methylxanthines increase the force of contraction of the myocardium and increase the heart rate and, therefore, increase the cardiac output. But, they also produce peripheral vasodilatation which tends to decrease the BP. The changes in BP are, therefore, not consistent. Caffeine causes vasoconstriction of cerebral blood vessels.

Kidneys: The xanthines have a diuretic effect and thereby increase the urine output.

Smooth muscle: Xanthines cause relaxation of smooth muscles especially the bronchial smooth muscle (*see* page 399).

Skeletal muscle: Xanthines enhance the power of muscle contraction and thereby increase the capacity to do muscular work by both a central stimulant effect and the peripheral actions.

GI tract: Xanthines increase the secretion of acid and pepsin in the stomach and are gastric irritants.

Pharmacokinetics

Methylxanthines are well absorbed orally, widely distributed and are extensively metabolised in the liver; t½ 7–12 hr. In higher doses t½ may be prolonged due to saturation of metabolizing enzymes. Premature infants have a longer t½ of 24–36 hr.

Adverse Effects

Adverse effects include nervousness, insomnia, tremors, tachycardia, hypotension, arrhythmias, headache, gastritis, nausea, vomiting, epigastric pain and diuresis. High doses produce convulsions. Tolerance develops after sometime. Habituation to caffeine is common.

Uses

i *Headache:* Because of the effect of caffeine on cerebral blood vessels, it is combined with ergotamine for the relief of migraine headache. Caffeine is also combined with aspirin/paracetamol for the treatment of headache.

ii. *Bronchial asthma:* Theophylline is used in the treatment of bronchial asthma.

iii. *Apnoea in premature infants:* Episodes of prolonged apnoea (>15–20 sec) may be seen in premature infants which if too frequent may result in neurologic and other tissue damage due to hypoxia. When no primary cause can be detected, methylxanthines may be used orally or IV. Theophylline or caffeine may be used for 1–3 weeks to reduce the duration of episodes of apnoea which may be seen in premature babies.

CONVULSANTS

Strychnine is an alkaloid obtained from the seeds of *Nux vomica.* On administration, it produces tonic convulsions—opisthotonus followed by coma and death. It acts as a competitive antagonist of the inhibitory neurotransmitter glycine—mainly stimulates the spinal cord and in higher doses the entire nervous system. **Strychnine is of no therapeutic value.** Poisoning can be treated by IV diazepam or clonazepam. Ventilatory support may be needed. 1:1000 potassium permanganate solution or tannic acid 2% solution can be used to adsorb the alkaloid and prevent its absorption. All sensory stimuli produce exaggerated reflexes and should, therefore, be avoided.

Leptazol or pentylene tetrazol is a CNS stimulant. By a direct effect on the central neurons, it produces convulsions. It is mostly used as an experimental drug to induce convulsions. Poisoning with leptazol is treated with diazepam.

NOOTROPICS

Nootropics are drugs that improve memory and cognition. They are also called cognition enhancers.

Piracetam described as a 'nootropic agent' is thought to protect cerebral cortex from hypoxia and improve learning and memory. In higher doses, it also inhibits platelet aggregation. Adverse effects include insomnia, weight-gain, nervousness, depression and gastrointestinal disturbances.

Piracetam and **aniracetam** have been tried in dementia, myoclonus, stroke and other cerebrovascular accidents; alcoholism, Alzheimer's disease, behavioural disorders and learning problems in children and in vertigo. The beneficial effects in all these are not proved.

DRUGS OF ABUSE AND ADDICTION

Several drugs have been used for recreational purposes—for their pleasurable effects. Drug abuse is often closely associated with drug dependence. Dependence may by physical or psychological (*see* page 63). Sudden withdrawal of such drugs of dependence can result in withdrawal symptoms which are difficult to tolerate. The word drug **addiction** is generally used to mean drug dependence.

Drug habituation is milder involvement with the drug and withdrawal causes only mild discomfort.

Mechanisms of Addiction

All drugs of abuse are known to increase dopamine levels at different sites of the mesolimbic projections. Selective activation of DA neurons leads to behavioural changes as in addiction.

Based on the molecular targets—the drugs of addiction bind to—GPCRs, ion channels and DA transporter.

Repeated drug use can result in **'reinforcement'**. Reinforcement is the tendency of a pleasure-producing drug to lead to repeated self administration. This leads to drug-seeking behaviour and plays a major role in the neuroadaptation process. Reinforcement can be positive reinforcement, i.e. pleasurable effects or negative reinforcement, i.e. withdrawal symptoms.

During acute withdrawal, dopaminergic and opioidergic functions are significantly compromised with decreased DA release and decreased D2 receptor number.

Drugs of dependence include (some examples):

1. **CNS stimulants**
   Amphetamines, methylphenidate, cocaine, caffeine, nicotine, bath salts (designer drugs)
2. **CNS depressants**
   Opioids—morphine, heroin, pethidine
   Ethyl alcohol
   Barbiturates
   Benzodiazepines
   Methaqualone
3. **Hallucinogens**
   LSD, mescaline, phencyclidine (PCP)
   Psilocybine, psilocin
   Dimethyltryptamine (DMT)
   Diethyltryptamine (DET)
   Cannabinoids
   Gama-hydroxybutyric acid (GHB)

Drugs which are not discussed in the respective chapters have been dealt here.

CNS Stimulants

Cocaine, amphetamines and their **analogs** including **methamphetamine, methylphenidate and 3,4 methylene dioxymethamphetamine** (MDMA, 'ecstasy') are CNS stimulants. MDMA inhibits monoamine transporters and also releases 5-HT, NA and DA—leading to euphoria and psychotomimetic effects. It is often called a **'party drug'** as it causes euphoria, loss of inhibitions and a feeling of being energised. Long-term abuse of these stimulants can result in changes in the personality, paranoid behaviour, depression, irritability and even psychosis. Withdrawal can result in depression, drowsiness, dysphoria, fatigue and bradycardia.

Caffeine: Long-term intake of caffeine can cause dependence. Withdrawal symptoms like headache and lethargy can occur.

Nicotine is an alkaloid present in tobacco and is a commonly used drug of dependence—is highly addicting. Tobacco is used for smoking (as cigarettes) as well as by other routes (like nasal insufflation of snuff) and by chewing.

Methylphenidate is structurally related to amphetamine and is a mild CNS stimulant. It brings about the release of catecholamines from intracellular stores and may also directly stimulate the adrenergic receptors. It improves alertness, increases attention span, reduces fatigue and irritability. Methylphenidate is also an anorexient and like other CNS stimulants cause insomnia and in higher doses produce convulsions.

CNS Depressants

Sedative hypnotics like barbiturates, benzodiazepenes and meprobamate are abused for their pleasurable effects and anxiolytic properties. Barbiturate over dosage can often be fatal.

Ethanol is the most common and oldest agent of abuse. Chronic drinkers develop withdrawal symptoms on suddenly stopping alcohol and develop a craving for the drug (*see* page 272).

Hallucinogens

Hallucinogens or psychotogenic drugs are drugs that can produce psychosis. They are also called **psychotomimetics, psychedelics or psychodysleptics.**

Hallucinogens include:

Lysergic acid diethylamide (LSD) is a semi-synthetic derivative related to the ergot alkaloid ergometrine. Like ergometrine, it is also an uterine stimulant. It was synthesized by Hoffmann in 1938.

Pharmacological effects: LSD is very potent and a dose of 20–30 µg can bring about its effects. It produces euphoria, emotional out bursts, visual illusions, altered perception, terror, impairment of judgement, mood and thinking ability. Mood swings and a feeling of disintegration of the person can be highly frightening. LSD also produces sympathetic stimulation, anxiety-tremors and nausea. The symptoms last from 8 to 12 hours. LSD is effective both orally and parenterally—but is usually taken orally.

Phencyclidine (PCP) causes CNS stimulation, hallucinations (mainly auditory), psychotic behaviour and dissociative anaesthesia (ketamine, a PCP derivative is used for dissociative anaesthesia), sweating, tachycardia, hypertension and nystagmus. Overdosage with PCP and ketamine can be fatal.

Mescaline is obtained from a cactus and has hallucinogenic effects like LSD.

Cannabinoids

Cannabis obtained from the hemp plant (*Cannabis sativa*) has been used for its pleasurable effects since several centuries. ***Marijuana*** is the name given for dried leaves and flowering heads of the plant, while ***hashish*** or ***charas*** is the dried solid, black resinous substance obtained from the leaves of the plant. ***Ganja*** is the dried female inflorescence. All these forms are used for smoking while ***Bhang*** is taken orally and consists of dried leaves of cannabis.

Actions

CNS: Δ^9 tetrahydrocannabinol (THC) is the principal constituent of cannabis that is responsible for psychopharmacological effects. On smoking, THC is absorbed and the effects start within minutes. It has a t½ of ~4 hours. It produces euphoria, uncontrolled laughing, a feeling of relaxation, altered time sense, visual distortions, a dream-like state followed by drowsiness and poor motor co-ordination. These effects may vary from person to person based on the personality of the individual. **Prolonged use up to 1 year can result in schizophrenia.**

Mechanism of action: Cannabinoids act on the cannabinoid receptors CB1 and CB2. CB1 receptors are widely distributed in the CNS including cerebral cortex, hypothalamus, limbic system, cerebellum and basal ganglia; CB1 is also present in the gut and adipocytes. CB2 is present in the periphery. ***Anandamide*** is an endogenous substance that binds the cannabinoid receptors. Its physiological role is not clear.

Other actions: Cannabinoids also produce:

- Tachycardia, vasodilation and hypotension
- Conjunctivae are red because of vasodilation
- Bronchodilation
- Reduce intraocular pressure.
- Increased appetite.

They also have analgesic and antiemetic properties (dronabinol, *see* page 428). Due to the pain relief seen in chronic pain, medicinal use of cannabis in pain has been studied. However, risk of schizophrenia on long-term use particularly in genetically predisposed people, discourages such use. Chronic heavy marijuana smokers may experience bronchitis, airway obstruction, precancerous changes in the lung and worsening of angina.

Rimonabant, an inverse agonist at the CB_1 receptor, is useful in smoking cessation and also prevents weight gain in smokers after they quit smoking but is a banned drug in India.

Tolerance and dependence: The development of tolerance to the effects of hallucinogens is rapid—even after 3–4 doses tolerance can be evident but is also overcome rapidly. Long-term use results in some dependence. Withdrawal symptoms are mild and remain for a short period—with irritability, restlessness, insomnia, nausea and muscle cramps.

Date rape drugs and club drugs

GHB is known as **'date rape'** drug while amphetamines, GHB and MDMA are known as 'club drugs'. MDMA is also called 'party drug'.

γ-hydroxybutyrate (GHB), sodium oxybate or γ-hydroxybutyric acid is a $GABA_B$ agonist. It is formed endogenously from GABA but its functions are not known. Though GHB was used as a general anaesthetic, it is not preferred due to its low safety margin. It is largely abused for its effects including euphoria, improved sensory perceptions and anterograde amnesia—it particularly prevents memory retention. Because of these effects and also being tasteless and odourless, it can be mixed with drinks; it also has a quick action (acts in about 30 minutes). GHB is popularly known or misused as 'date rape drug'. The victim is unable to recollect the events. In high doses, GHB may inhibit DA release and also blocks its activation by other drugs of abuse. Hence it may be useful to prevent craving of some drugs of abuse.

Treatment of Dependence

Addiction is a social evil. Treatment of dependence is a great challenge as it involves motivation and absolute determination on the part of the addict along with dedicated efforts of the family and the deaddiction team. Measures for deaddiction include:

1. Detoxification—involves complete but gradual stoppage of the addicting drug.

2. Pharmacotherapy—Administration of suitable drugs to reduce the severity of withdrawal symptoms. For example, insomnia is most common with drugs like opioids, alcohol and cannabis. Diazepam or clonidine given at night helps to overcome insomnia and reduce anxiety. Also for drugs like opioids, replacement with a suitable alternative like methadone (*see* page 259), reduces the severity of withdrawal symptoms. To quit tobacco smoking, replacement with nicotine chewing gum or transdermal patches are used to prevent withdrawal.

3. Prevention of relapse—following the deaddiction program, many may crave for the drug or may have a tendency to go back to addiction. This should be prevented to successfully achieve complete deaddiction. For prevention of alcohol relapse (*see* page 272), drugs like naltrexone and for nicotine deaddiction varenicline has been used.

4. Cognitive behavioural therapy—help from a psychologist in counselling and CBT go a long way in preventing relapse and also aid in rehabilitation.

Drugs used for Criminal Offences

Almost all of the drugs of abuse have played a major role in criminal offences. Drugs influencing the CNS including alcohol, cannabis, cocaine, amphetamine have been used either to facilitate criminal offences by the offender or as stupifying agents to 'knock off' the victim. Drug addicts also take to crimes for financial gains either to avoid the withdrawal symptoms or for pleasurable effects. Hence getting rid of drug addiction can help in the overall development of the country.

Drugs used in Tobacco Smoking Withdrawal

Nicotine: Administered by different routes as nicotine transdermal patches, nasal spray, inhaler or nicotine chewing gum, nicotine containing lozenges.

Bupropion: A weak DA reuptake inhibitor with CNS stimulant effects is used along with nicotine.

Rimonabant: Cannabinoid CB1 receptor antagonist and inverse agonist has been tried. It has also been used as an anorexiant.

Varenicline: A nicotinic receptor (N_n) partial agonist has been useful in some patients to quit smoking.

[1–5] From Medical Council of India, *Competency based Undergraduate Curriculum for the Indian Medical Graduate*, 2018;1:136–144.

Unit VI

Drugs Acting on the Kidney

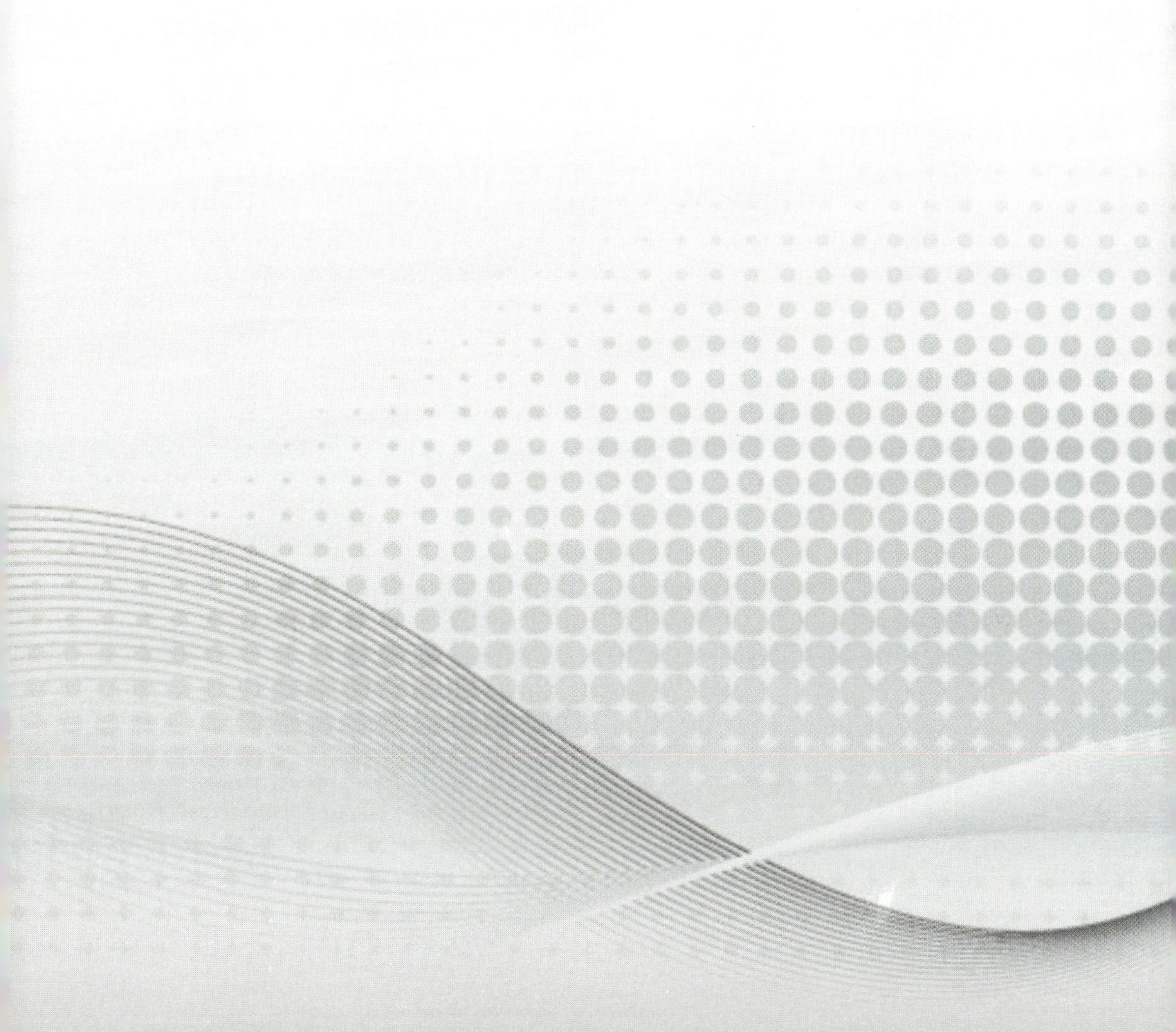

CHAPTER 22

Diuretics and Antidiuretics

Competency achievement: The student should be able to:

PH 1.24 Describe the mechanism/s of action, types, doses, side effects, indications and contraindications of the drugs affecting renal systems including diuretics, antidiuretics–vasopressin and analogues.[1]

Kidney, the excretory organ of our body, serves the important functions of excretion of waste products and regulation of fluid volume and electrolyte content of the extracellular fluid.

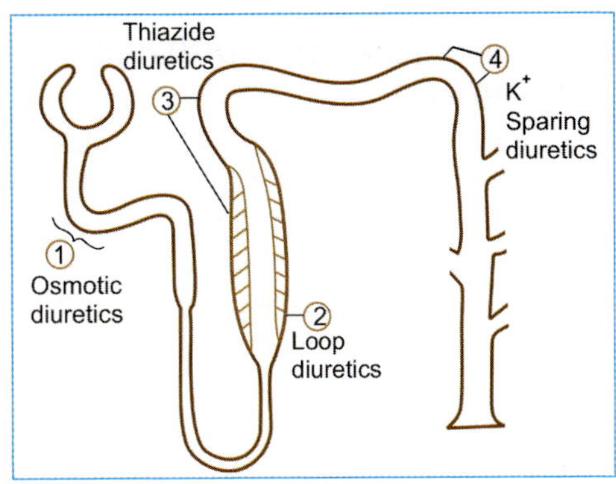

Fig. 22.1: Simplified diagram of a nephron showing sites of action of diuretics: (1) Proximal tubule—osmotic diuretics, mannitol, adenosine antagonists; (2) Ascending limb of Henle's loop—loop diuretics; (3) Early distal tubule— thiazides; (4) Distal tubule and collecting duct—K^+ sparing diuretics

PHYSIOLOGY OF URINE FORMATION

Normally about 180 litres of fluid is filtered by the glomerulus everyday, of which 99% gets reabsorbed and about 1.5 litres of urine is formed. The nephron is the functional unit of the kidney. The three basic processes involved in the formation of urine are glomerular filtration, tubular reabsorption and active tubular secretion. For simplification, the nephron can be divided into four sites (Fig. 22.1).

Proximal Tubule

Nearly 85% of sodium bicarbonate, 65% of sodium, potassium, calcium and magnesium and almost 100% of filtered glucose, and other organic solutes including amino acids are absorbed in the proximal tubule (PT). Water is reabsorbed passively to maintain the osmolality proportionate to the salt absorption.

Sodium transport in the proximal tubule takes place by four mechanisms, *viz* (i) through Na^+/H^+ exchanger, (ii) by direct entry of Na^+, (iii) transport of Na^+ and K^+ along with glucose, amino acids and phosphates and (iv) the specific symporters. The reabsorption of large bicarbonate ion and other organic solutes including amino acids in the PT create a passive force for the transfer of chloride ions in between the tubular cells.

Osmotic diuretics act at the PT. Adenosine A1 receptor antagonists, a new class of drugs, also act on the proximal tubule and the collecting duct.

Henle's Loop

In the thin descending limb of the loop of Henle, water is reabsorbed by osmotic forces. Hence, osmotic diuretics are acting here too. The thick ascending limb actively reabsorbs sodium chloride (25% of filtered sodium) from the lumen (but is impermeable to water) by Na^+, K^+, $2Cl^-$ cotransporter. 'Loop diuretics' selectively block this Na^+, K^+, $2Cl^-$ cotransport in the loop of Henle and selectively inhibit NaCl reabsorption. Na^+, K^+, $2Cl^-$ cotransporter is a glycoprotein with 12 domains. Frusemide, a loop diuretic, binds to the Cl^- binding site of the transporter and inhibits it. Loop diuretics are the most efficacious of all diuretics.

Distal Convoluted Tubule (DCT) and Collecting Duct

In the early distal tubule, sodium chloride (about 10%) is reabsorbed by an electrically neutral Na^+ and Cl^- transporter. This transporter is blocked by thiazide diuretics. This segment is also relatively impermeable to water. Calcium is reabsorbed by an apical calcium channel in the DCT epithelial cells and by basolateral Na^+/Ca^{++} exchanger. Potassium is secreted in exchange for Na^+ in the DCT and the collecting duct (CD) and is largely under the influence of aldosterone. All diuretics that modify the K^+ secretion act at these sites.

The final composition and concentration of urine is determined at the collecting duct. In the CD, absorption of water is under the control of antidiuretic hormone (ADH, arginine vasopressin). ADH acts by controlling the number of water channels called aquaporins. ADH increases the expression of aquaporins—inserted into the apical membrane of the cells in the collecting tubule. ADH also regulates the transfer of urea by stimulating the insertion of urea transporter UT1 molecules into the cells of collecting tubule in the renal medulla. The concentration of urea in the medulla is responsible for high osmolarity of the medulla.

The secretion of ADH is controlled by the plasma volume and serum osmolality. The renal function is also influenced by atrial natriuretic peptide which enhances sodium excretion in presence of sodium overload. Renin–angiotensin–aldosterone system and the prostaglandins released locally in the kidneys also influence the renal function.

Renal autacoids: Adenosine, prostaglandins and natriuteric peptides are produced in the kidney and exert physiological effects on the kidney. Adenosine has significant influence on GFR and the sodium transport. Though prostaglandins are produced in the kidney, their role in renal physiology is yet to be understood. PGE_2 has significant role in Na^+ and water transport. Natriuretic peptides including urodilatin produced in the distal tubule influence the sodium reabsorption. Several drugs influence these and thereby modify renal physiology.

DIURETICS

Diuretic is an agent which increases urine and solute excretion. A **natriuretic** is an agent which increases sodium excretion from the kidney while an **aquaretic** is a drug that increases the excretion of water.

Diuretics may be classified as follows:

Classification

1. **High efficacy diuretics**
   - Furosemide, bumetanide, piretanide, ethacrynic acid, torsemide, azosemide
2. **Moderate efficacy diuretics**
   - ***Thiazides***
     Benzothiadiazines—chlorothiazide, hydrochlorothiazide, polythiazide, bendroflumethiazide, benzthiazide
   - ***Thiazide-related agents***
     Chlorthalidone, clopamide, indapamide, metolazone, xipamide
3. **Low efficacy diuretics**
   - ***Potassium sparing diuretics***
     Triamterene, amiloride, spironolactone, eplerenone.
   - ***Carbonic anhydrase inhibitors***
     Acetazolamide, methazolamide, dorzolamide
   - ***Osmotic diuretics***
     Mannitol, urea, glycerol
   - ***Methylxanthines***
     Theophylline

Contd...

Contd...

4. Newer agents
- ***Vasopressin antagonists***
  Conivaptan, tolvaptan, lixivaptan
- ***Adenosine A1 receptor antagonist***
  Rolophylline
- ***SGLT2-inhibitors***
  Dapagliflazin, canagliflazin

HIGH EFFICACY, HIGH CEILING OR LOOP DIURETICS

Frusemide (Furosemide)

Frusemide a sulfonamide derivative, is the most popular loop diuretic. It is a powerful diuretic.

Actions and Mechanism of Action

Frusemide acts by inhibiting $NaCl^-$ reabsorption in the thick ascending limb of the Henle's loop (Fig. 22.2). It blocks the Na^+, K^+, $2Cl^-$ symporter in the thick ascending limb of the Henle's loop because of which it is called a loop diuretic. It greatly increases the excretion of Na^+ and Cl^- in the urine (Flowchart 22.1). Because a large amount of $NaCl^-$ is absorbed in this segment, loop diuretics are highly efficacious. Diuretic response increases with dose and over-enthusiastic treatment can cause dehydration as several litres of urine may be produced in a single day (high ceiling of effect).

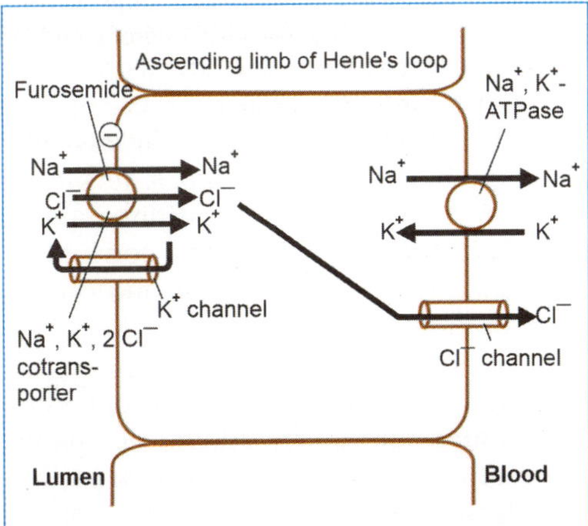

Fig. 22.2: Mechanism of action of loop diuretics

Other Actions

- Loop diuretics also enhance the excretion of K^+, Ca^{++} and Mg^{++} (but Ca^{++} is reabsorbed in the distal tubule—hence generally no hypocalcaemia). K^+ excretion is increased because it is exchanged with higher amounts of Na^+ that reaches the distal tubule. Prolonged use can cause hypomagnesemia.
- They increase reabsorption of uric acid in the proximal tubule.
- High ceiling diuretics cause **vasodilation in renal vasculature** and increase renal blood flow. On long-term use, they alter renal haemodynamics to reduce fluid and electrolyte reabsorption in the proximal tubule.
- Loop diuretics enhance renin release.
- Frusemide is also a weak carbonic anhydrase inhibitor, hence it increases the excretion of HCO_3^- and phosphate.
- Intravenous frusemide causes **venodilatation and reduces left ventricular filling pressure**. It thus relieves pulmonary congestion in acute congestive heart failure and in pulmonary edema even before the onset of diuresis. This effect may be PG-mediated (induction of PG synthesis in the kidneys).
- Loop diuretics also **induce the synthesis of PGE_2** (through COX-2) which inhibits reabsorption of salt in the loop of Henle, thereby contributing to their diuretic action.
- Frusemide is also secreted in the proximal tubule where it blocks the free water clearance. This contributes to a small extent to its diuretic effects.

Pharmacokinetics

Frusemide and other loop diuretics are rapidly and almost **completely absorbed** orally. Given intravenously frusemide acts in 2–5 minutes, while following oral use, it takes 20–40 minutes. Plasma t½ is 1½ hours and duration of action is 2 to 4 hours. They are

Flowchart 22.1: Actions of frusemide (loop diuretics)

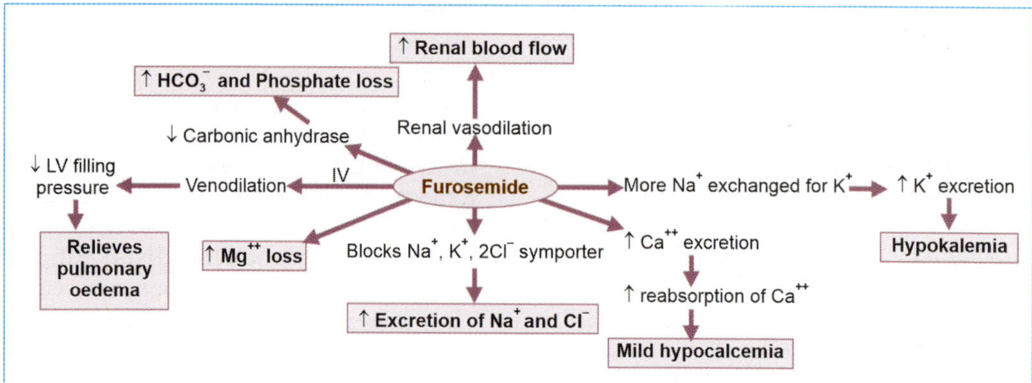

extensively and firmly bound to plasma proteins and, therefore, cannot enter the glomerular filtrate. Loop diuretics reach the ascending limb of Henle's loop by being secreted in the proximal tubule by organic acid transport system. They are partly metabolized in the liver and the metabolites are excreted by the kidneys by glomerular filtration and tubular secretion.

Dose: 20–80 mg OD in the morning. LASIX 40 mg tab, 20 mg/ml; inj, FROSENSEX 40, 100 mg tab.

Bumetanide is a sulfonamide like frusemide but is 40 times more potent (1 mg bumetanide = 40 mg frusemide). Bioavailability is 80% and the onset of action is faster than frusemide. It is better tolerated because the adverse effects like hypokalemia, ototoxicity, hyperglycaemia and hyperuricaemia are milder but may cause myopathy. Bumetanide may be effective in some patients not responding to frusemide.

Dose: 1–5 mg orally OD in the morning. 2–4 mg IM/IV. BUMET 1 mg tab, 0.25 mg/ml inj.

Ethacrynic acid is more likely to cause adverse effects particularly ototoxicity and hence is not commonly used.

Torsemide is a recently introduced loop diuretic. It is longer acting and, therefore, can be given once a day. It is rapidly and almost completely absorbed. It is mostly metabolized in the liver and, therefore, the dose needs to be reduced in liver failure.

Adverse Effects of Loop Diuretics

1. *Hypokalaemia and metabolic alkalosis:* Because loop diuretics inhibit reabsorption of sodium in the loop of Henle, a high sodium fluid is delivered to the collecting duct. In the collecting duct, K^+ and H^+ are secreted in large amounts in exchange for sodium leading to hypokalaemia and metabolic alkalosis. **Hypokalaemia** is dose dependent and can be quite troublesome in higher doses on prolonged diuretic use especially in patients who also have low dietary intake of potassium or in patients with cardiac failure and cirrhosis.

   Symptoms of hypokalaemia are seen with serum potassium levels less than 2.5 mEq/L (normal serum K levels are 4.5–5 mEq/L). Manifestations include irritability, drowsiness, confusion, dizziness, muscle weakness and cardiac arrhythmias.

   Hypokalaemia can be prevented and corrected by high dietary intake of K^+, oral KCl supplements or by adding a K^+ sparing diuretic. Hypokalaemia should be particularly prevented in post-MI patients and in patients who are also receiving digitalis.

2. *Hyponatraemia, dehydration, hypovolaemia and hypotension:* All these are due to diuresis and natriuresis—should be treated with saline infusion. Dilutional hyponatraemia may follow brisk diuresis. When salt and water are lost due to rapid diuresis, body tries to compensate by increasing retention of water and salt. However, salt retention is not possible because of the diuretics and only water gets retained. This results in dilution of ECF and hyponatraemia leading to electrolyte imbalance and oedema remains despite diuretic therapy. Diuretics should be withheld temporarily and fluid restricted. Electrolyte disturbances may be corrected.
3. *Hyperuricaemia:* Hypovolaemia leads to increased uric acid absorption in the proximal tubule. Hence, loop diuretics can cause hyperuricaemia and may precipitate acute gout particularly on long-term use. Allopurinol may be needed.
4. *Hypocalcaemia:* After prolonged use, loop diuretics may cause hypocalcaemia—this may result in osteoporosis on long-term use.
5. *Hypomagnesaemia:* It develops after prolonged use of loop diuretics and is more pronounced in patients with dietary magnesium deficiency. Oral magnesium supplements may be needed.
6. *Ototoxicity:* Na^+, K^+, $2Cl^-$ cotransport is important in the inner ear. Loop diuretics cause hearing loss by a toxic effect on the hair cells in the internal ear. Associated tinnitus and vertigo may also occur. Ototoxicity is more common with **ethacrynic acid.** It is dose-related; seen in higher doses, more common on IV administration and in the patients with renal dysfunction and is generally reversible except with ethacrynic acid. Concurrent use of other ototoxic drugs like aminoglycosides should be avoided.
7. *Hyperglycaemia and hyperlipidaemia* are mild in therapeutic doses.
8. *GIT disturbances* like nausea, vomiting and diarrhoea are common with ethacrynic acid.
9. *Allergic reactions* like skin rashes are more common with sulfonamide derivatives, since all loop diuretics except ethacrynic acid are sulphonamides, allergic reactions like skin rashes and eosinophilia can occur.
10. Weakness, fatigue, hypotension, dizziness and muscle cramps are mostly due to hypokalaemia.
11. In cirrhosis patients, rapid diuresis may lead to undesirable consequences.

Uses

1. *Oedema:* Loop diuretics are highly effective for the relief of oedema of all origins like cardiac, hepatic or renal oedema. In chronic congestive cardiac failure, loop diuretics reduce venous and pulmonary congestion.
2. *Acute renal failure or acute kidney injury (AKI):* Loop diuretics increase the urine output and K^+ excretion. They are also useful in impending acute renal failure. In chronic renal failure, large doses are needed.
3. *Cerebral oedema:* Frusemide is used as an alternative to or in combination with osmotic diuretics.
4. *Acute pulmonary oedema and acute LVF:* It is quickly relieved by IV frusemide (Flowchart 22.2) due to its immediate vasodilator effect and then by diuretic action.
5. *Forced diuresis*
   - In poisoning due to drugs like barbiturates and salicylates, frusemide is used with IV fluids.
   - Anion overdosage—poisoning due to fluoride, iodide and bromide respond to furosemide along with saline infusion (to avoid hyponatraemia and dehydration).

Flowchart 22.2: Frusemide in pulmonary oedema

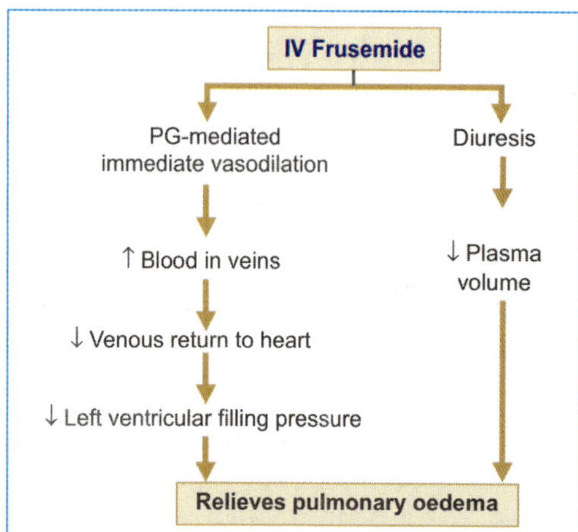

6. *Hypertension*—with renal impairment may be treated with loop diuretics. Thiazides are the preferred diuretics in primary hypertension.
7. *Acute hypercalcaemia and hyperkalaemia:* Loop diuretics enhance excretion of Ca^{++} and K^+ and are useful in acute hypercalcaemia and hyperkalaemia but Na^+ and Cl^- should be replaced to avoid hyponatraemia and hypochloraemia.

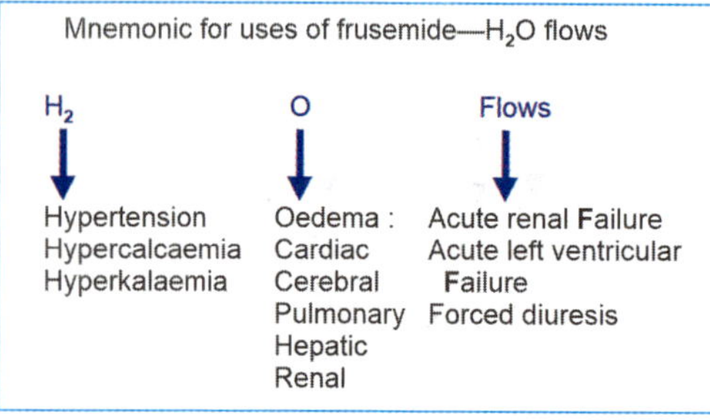

THIAZIDES AND THIAZIDE-LIKE DIURETICS

Chlorothiazide was the first thiazide to be synthesized. In contrast to loop diuretics, all thiazides have a sulfonamide group (Fig. 22.3).

Actions and Mechanism of Action

Thiazides have a moderate efficacy as diuretics because 90% of the filtered sodium

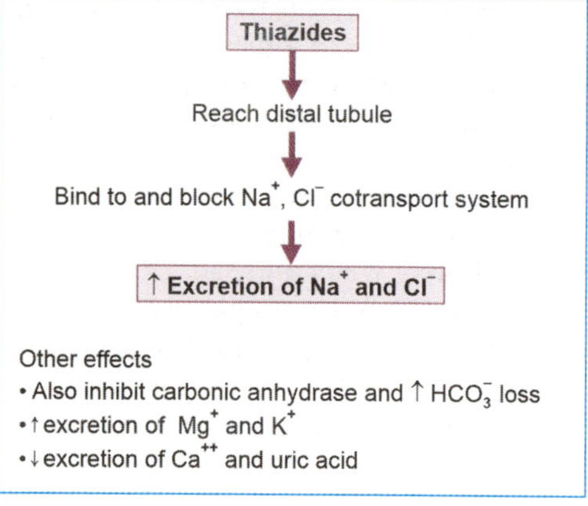

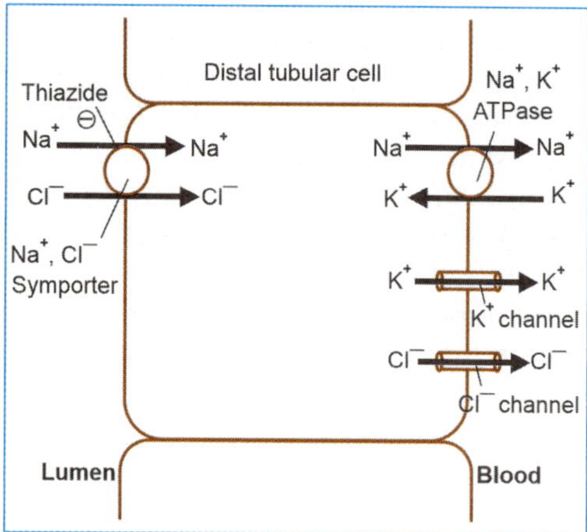

Fig. 22.3: Mechanism of action of thiazide diuretics

is already reabsorbed before reaching the distal tubule. This group of drugs **bind to the Cl^- site of Na^+, Cl^- cotransport system and block the system**. They thus enhance the excretion of Na^+ and Cl^- in the early distal tubule. The primary site of action of thiazides is the early distal tubule. Since the Na^+, Cl^- cotransport takes place on the luminal side of the distal tubular cells, thiazides should reach the luminal fluid to block this transport. Like frusemide, thiazides are also largely bound to plasma proteins and reach the tubular fluid by being secreted by the proximal tubular organic acid secretory system. From there, they move along the nephron to the distal tubule which is their site of action. Thiazides also inhibit carbonic anhydrase activity and increase bicarbonate loss. They enhance the excretion of Mg^+ and K^+ (in distal segments, Na^+ in the lumen is exchanged for K^+ which is then excreted). In contrast to loop diuretics, thiazides inhibit urinary excretion of Ca^{++} and uric acid resulting in **hypercalcaemia** and **hyperuricaemia**.

Concurrent administration of a thiazide and loop diuretics have a **synergistic effect** because loop diuretics deliver a larger amount of sodium to the distal tubule where thiazides act.

Thiazides may cause hyperglycaemia and may precipitate diabetes in borderline hyperglycaemic patients. This could be due to inhibition of insulin release (which may be secondary to hypokalaemia).

Another peculiar paradoxical action of thiazides is that they reduce glomerular filtration and reduce the urine output in patients with diabetes insipidus. Such patients do not respond to the ADH and excrete large volumes of dilute urine. Thiazides help by reducing GFR and positive free water clearance.

Pharmacokinetics

Thiazides are well-absorbed orally and are rapid acting—act within 60 minutes. Duration varies from 6 to 48 hr (Table 22.1). They are excreted by the kidney. Since thiazides are organic acids, they are secreted into the proximal tubules. They are also partly excreted by the hepatobiliary acid secretory system. The more lipid-soluble agents have longer action because of larger volume of distribution and tubular reabsorption.

Table 22.1: Dose and duration of action of commonly used diuretics

Diuretic	*Daily dose (mg)*	*Duration (hr)*
Furosemide	20–80 mg	3–6
Bumetanide	0.5–2 mg	3–6
Indapamide	2.5–5 mg	18–24
Hydrochlorothiazide	25–100	8–12
Polythiazide	1–3	24–48
Chlorthalidone	50–100	48–72
Xipamide	20–60	24–36
Metolazone	5–10	18–24
Spironolactone	50–100	6–12
Triamterene	50–100	4–6
Amiloride	5–10	20–24

Adverse Effects

- **Hypokalaemia** is the most important side effect of thiazide use. For more information *see* page 286.
- **Metabolic alkalosis,** hyperuricaemia, hypovolaemia, hypotension, dehydration, hyponatraemia, hypomagnesaemia, hypochloremia, hypercalcaemia, and hyperlipidaemia are similar to that seen with loop diuretics.
- **Hyperglycaemia** induced by thiazides may precipitate diabetes mellitus probably by inhibition of insulin secretion. The exact mechanism is not known but correction of hypokalaemia also reduces hyperglycaemia. It is more common when long-acting thiazides are used for a long time.
- Thiazides can cause impotence in men.
- Weakness, fatigue, anorexia, gastrointestinal disturbances and allergic reactions like rashes and photosensitivity can also be seen.

Uses

1. *Hypertension:* Thiazides are the first-line drugs (*see* page 336).
2. *Congestive heart failure:* Thiazides are useful in the management of oedema due to mild to moderate CHF.
3. *Oedema:* Thiazides may be tried in hepatic (cirrhosis) or renal oedema. Renal oedema may be due to nephrotic syndrome, acute glomerulonephritis or chronic renal failure. Metolazone may be combined with loop diuretics in severe refractory oedema.
4. *Renal stones and hypercalciuria:* Hypercalciuria with renal stones can be treated with thiazides which reduce calcium excretion.

5. *Diabetes insipidus:* Thiazides benefit such patients by reducing plasma volume and GFR—a paradoxical effect.

Indapamide

Indapamide is particularly suitable in hypertension because it is claimed to lower blood pressure in subdiuretic doses and in such doses adverse effects are milder. It is well absorbed orally and has a long duration of action to permit once a day dosing.

Dose: 2.5–5 mg OD, LORVAS 2.5 mg tab.

POTASSIUM SPARING DIURETICS

Potassium sparing diuretics may act by two ways. They may be aldosterone antagonists (spironolactone) or directly inhibit ion channels in distal tubule and collecting duct (triamterene, amiloride) (Fig. 22.4).

Spironolactone

Aldosterone regulates the sodium absorption and potassium secretion in the collecting tubule and ducts. It enhances the Na^+ reabsorption through Na^+ channels in the collecting tubule and enhances K^+ secretion. Aldosterone enters the cells of the collecting duct and binds to the mineralocorticoid receptor in the cell. The agonist-receptor complex moves to the nucleus and directs the synthesis of aldosterone-induced proteins (AIP) which are responsible for the actions of aldosterone.

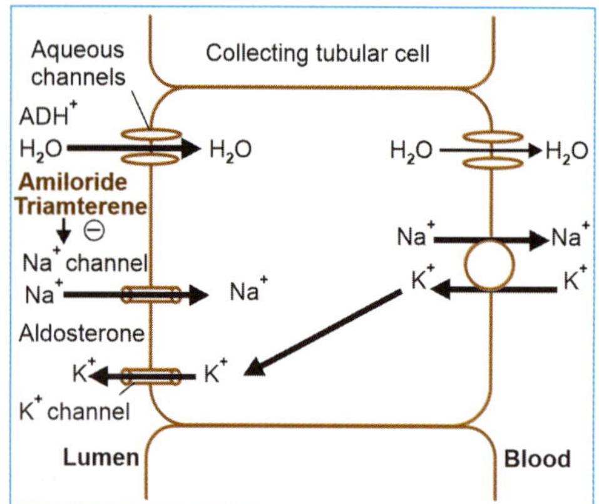

Fig. 22.4: Mechanism of action of potassium sparing diuretics. Spironolactone antagonises the action of aldosterone while amiloride and triamterene directly inhibit the Na^+ channels (ADH promotes reabsorption of water through aqueous channels—it also increases the number of these channels)

Spironolactone is a synthetic steroid which is structurally similar to aldosterone. It is an **aldosterone antagonist**. Spironolactone binds to the mineralocorticoid receptors on the distal tubule and collecting duct and competitively inhibits the action of aldosterone. As major amount of Na^+ is already reabsorbed in the proximal parts, spironolactone has low efficacy. It also reduces K^+ loss due to other diuretics. It enhances the excretion of calcium by a direct action on the renal tubules.

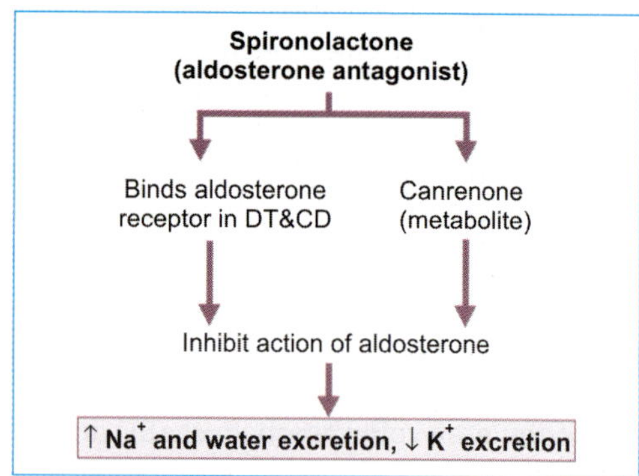

Spironolactone is given as microfined powder to enhance bioavailability (75%). It is highly bound to plasma proteins and has a slow onset of action. It is metabolized in the liver. The metabolites formed are active. A metabolite **canrenone** has a long t½ of almost 18 hr while that of spironolactone is 1–2 hr.

Preparations

Dose: 25–50 mg, ALDACTONE 25, 100 mg tabs, SPIROMIDE SPIRONOLACTONE 50 mg + FUROSEMIDE 20 mg tab.

Adverse Effects

Endocrine side effects including gynaecomastia, impotence in men, hirsutism and

COMPARE AND CONTRAST

Hydrochlorothiazide and Frusemide

Features	*Hydrochlorothiazide*	*Frusemide*
Efficacy	Low	High
Site of action	Early distal tubule	Ascending limb of loop of Henle
Mechanism of action	Inhibits Na^+, Cl^- symport	Inhibits Na^+, K^+, $2Cl^-$ cotransport
Onset of action	1 hour	In minutes (20–40)
Duration of action	Long (8–12 hr)	Short (36 hr)
Response to increasing dose	No significant increase	Increases (dose dependent)
Hyperuricaemia	Higher incidence	Low
Blood glucose	May incarease—contraindicated in diabetics	No significant effect—not contraindicated
Ototoxicity	Not known to cause	Can cause
Primary use	Hypertension	Oedema

menstrual irregularities in women are seen with large doses of spironolactone. It binds to the androgen and progesterone receptors and also interferes with steroidogenesis.

Hyperkalaemia: Spironolactone can cause mild to significant hyperkalaemia particularly in patients with renal insufficiency or when other hyperkalaemic drugs are given.

Drowsiness, metabolic acidosis GI disturbances, and skin rashes can occur.

Amiloride and triamterene are directly acting agents which enhance Na^+ excretion and reduce K^+ loss by acting on ion channels in the distal tubule and collecting duct. They block the Na^+ transport through the sodium-channels in the luminal membrane. Since K^+ secretion is dependent on Na^+ entry, these drugs reduce K^+ excretion. Amiloride is the drug of choice in lithium-induced diabetes insipidus.

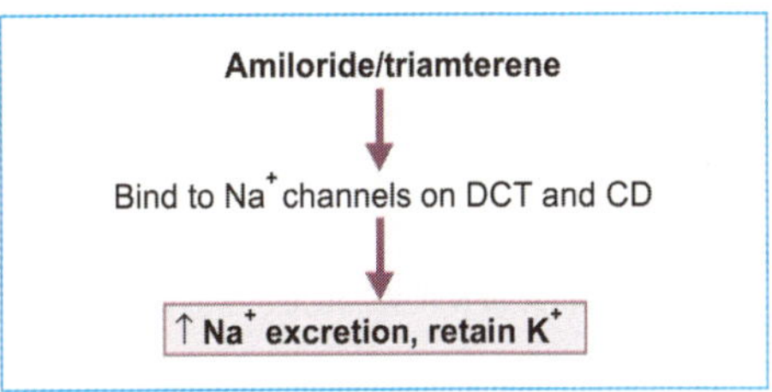

Preparations

Amiloride: Dose: 5-10 mg/day, AMINIDE-Amiloride 5 mg + Furosemide 40 mg tab

KSPAR-Amiloride 5 mg + Hydrochlorothiazide 50 mg tab.

Triamterene: Dose 50-100 mg/day, DITIDE Triamt 50 mg + Benzthiazide 25 mg tab, FRUSEMENE TRIAMT 50 mg + Furosemide 20 mg tab

Potassium canrenoate is a prodrug that gets converted in the body to canrenone, the active metabolite of spironolactone. It has actions similar to spironolactone and has the advantage that it can be given parenterally. The hormonal side effects are much less intense.

Eplerenone is an analog of spironolactone having greater selectivity for mineralocorticoid receptors and blocks them. Stimulation of androgen and progesterone receptor by eplerenone is very much less compared to spironolactone. Thus the hormonal adverse effects are much less but can cause hyperkalaemia. It is orally effective; t½ 4–6 hr and is metabolized in the liver by microsomal enzymes.

Eplerenone is used in the treatment of hypertension. Started with 50 mg once daily the dose may be raised, if required to a maximum of 100 mg. It may be used as monotherapy or with other drugs. Eplerenone may also be used in heart failure in place of spironolactone but is expensive.

Preparations

Dose: 50-100 mg, EPLERAN 25 mg, 50 mg tab.

COMPARE AND CONTRAST
Frusemide and Spironolactone

Features	Frusemide	Spironolactone
Chemistry	Sulfonamide	Synthetic steroid
Sites of action	Ascending limb of loop of Henle	Distal tubule and collecting duct
Mechanism of action	Blocks $Na^+/K^+/2Cl^-$ cotransport	Aldosterone antagonist
Efficacy	High	Low
Onset of action	Quick—2–5 minutes	Slow—may take several days
Effect on K^+	↑Excretion–hypokalaemia	↓Excretion–hyperkalaemia
Unique adverse effect	Ototoxicity	Gynaecomastia, hirsutism
Primary use	• CCF, oedema, ascites • Pulmonary oedema	• Hyperaldosteronism • As adjuvant to other diuretics to reduce K^+ loss
Contraindications	Allergy to sulfonamides	Peptic ulcer

Drug Interactions

- Aspirin causes salt and water retention and counters the action of spironolactone.
- Oral potassium supplements should be avoided while on K^+ sparing diuretics.
- Hyperkalaemia gets added up with ACE inhibitors and ARBs.

Uses of Potassium Sparing Diuretics

1. *With thiazides and loop diuretics* to prevent potassium loss.
2. *Oedema:* In cirrhosis and renal oedema where aldosterone levels may be high.
3. *Hypertension:* Along with thiazides to avoid hypokalaemia and for additive effect.
4. *Primary or secondary aldosteronism:* Spironolactone is used.
5. Lithium-induced diabetes insipidus—amiloride is drug of choice

CARBONIC ANHYDRASE INHIBITORS

Carbonic anhydrase is an enzyme that catalyses the formation of carbonic acid which spontaneously ionises to H^+ and HCO_3^-. This HCO_3^- combines with Na^+ and is reabsorbed.

$$H_2O + CO_2 \rightleftharpoons H_2CO_3$$
$$H^+ + HCO_3^- \rightleftharpoons HCO_3^-$$

By inhibiting the enzyme, carbonic anhydrase inhibitors block sodium bicarbonate reabsorption and cause HCO_3^- diuresis. Carbonic anhydrase is present in the nephron, ciliary body of the eyes, gastric mucosa, pancreas and other sites.

Acetazolamide, a sulfonamide derivative, is a carbonic anhydrase inhibitor and enhances the excretion of sodium, potassium, bicarbonate and water. The loss of bicarbonate leads to metabolic acidosis. There is some increase in chloride clearance. Other actions include:

1. *Eye:* The ciliary body of the eye secretes bicarbonate into the aqueous humour. Carbonic anhydrase inhibition results in decreased formation of aqueous humour and thereby reduces intraocular pressure.
2. *Brain:* Bicarbonate is secreted into CSF and carbonic anhydrase inhibition reduces the formation of CSF.

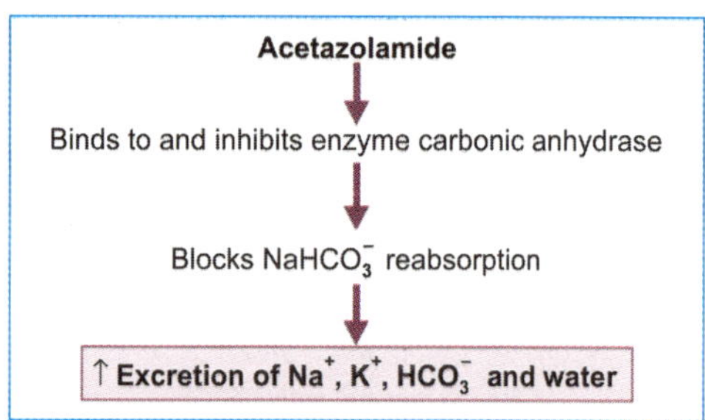

Pharmacokinetics: Acetazolamide is well absorbed orally, onset of action is within 60–90 minutes and duration of action is 8–12 hr. It is excreted unchanged by the kidney.

Preparations

DIAMOX, SYNOMOX 250 mg tab. Dose: 250 mg OD-BD.

Adverse Effects

1. Metabolic acidosis due to HCO_3^- loss.
2. Renal stones—Ca^{++} is lost with HCO_3^- resulting in hypercalciuria. This excess Ca^{++} may precipitate resulting in the formation of renal stones.
3. Hypokalaemia, drowsiness and allergic reactions can occur.

Uses

1. *Glaucoma:* Intraocular pressure is decreased by acetazolamide; it is given orally. Methazolamide (50–100 mg 8 hrly) and dichlorphenamide (50 mg OD-TDS) are also used orally in glaucoma. Newer ones like brinzolamide and dorzolamide are better tolerated and are available as eye drops.
2. *Alkalinization of urine:* It is required in overdosage of acidic drugs. Also, uric acid and cysteine excretion can be enhanced by HCO_3^- use as these are soluble in alkaline urine.
3. *Metabolic alkalosis:* Acetazolamide enhances HCO_3^- excretion. Alkalosis due to excess diuretics in patients with heart failure responds to acetazolamide.
4. *Mountain sickness:* In mountain climbers who rapidly ascend great heights, severe pulmonary oedema and/or cerebral oedema may occur particularly in unacclimatized persons. Initial symptoms of mountain sickness include headache, dizziness, nausea and weakness. Acetazolamide may relieve symptoms by reducing the formation as well as the pH of CSF—it can also be used for prophylaxis.
5. *Epilepsy:* Acetazolamide is used as an adjuvant as it increases the seizure threshold.
6. *Hyperphosphataemia:* When hyperphosphataemia is severe, it can be treated with acetazolamide to increase the urinary phosphate excretion.

> ***Mnemonic for uses***
>
> **MEGHA Mountain**
>
> **M:** Metabolic alkalosis
> **E:** Epilepsy
> **G:** Glaucoma
> **H:** Hyperphosphatesia
> **A:** Alkalinization
> **Mountain:** Mountain sickness

OSMOTIC DIURETICS

Mannitol is a pharmacologically inert substance not absorbed orally and causes osmotic diarrhoea. When given IV, mannitol gets filtered by the glomerulus but is not reabsorbed. It causes water to be retained in the proximal tubule and descending limb of Henle's loop by osmotic effect resulting in water diuresis, hence also called **aquaretic**. Mannitol also opposes the action of ADH in the collecting tubule. There is also some loss of sodium.

Adverse effects are dehydration, ECF volume expansion (water is extracted from cell due to osmotic effect), hyponatraemia (due to volume expansion), headache, nausea, vomiting and allergic reactions. Mannitol and other osmotic diuretics are contraindicated in pulmonary oedema as they could worsen it by expansion of plasma volume.

Uses

1. To maintain urine volume and prevent oliguria in conditions like massive haemolysis, rhabdomyolysis, shock and severe trauma. In such situations, mannitol prevents renal failure. It is given as a slow infusion of 500–1000 ml over 24 hr, after a test dose of 12.5 g IV because all patients with oliguria may not respond to mannitol. In patients who have already gone into renal failure, mannitol **can be dangerous** since it can cause pulmonary

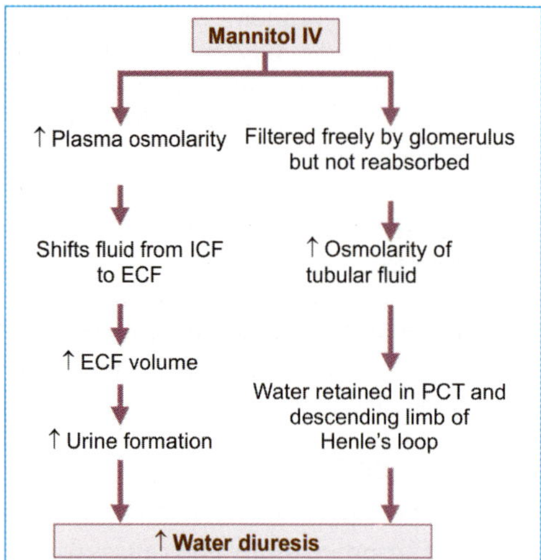

oedema and may precipitate heart failure due to volume expansion.

2. To reduce intracranial and intraocular pressure—following head injury and glaucoma, respectively. Fluid from the oedematous cells in the brain gets mobilized due to higher osmolarity (in about 60–90 minutes) and the intracellular volume shrinks. Similarly intraocular pressure too drops.

Preparations

Dose: 1–2 g/kg IV infusion. MANNITOL 10%, 20% in 100 and 500 ml bottles.

Glycerol (glycerine) is effective orally—reduces intraocular and intracranial pressure. It can be used topically to relieve oedema including corneal oedema.

Methylxanthines, like theophylline have mild diuretic effect.

Urea: Because of its unpleasant taste and availability of more efficient osmotic agents, urea is not generally used as a diuretic now.

NEWER AGENTS

Vasopressin Antagonists

A new class of drugs called arginine vasopressin (AVP) receptor antagonists have been found to induce diuresis. Three drugs have been introduced in this group, viz **conivaptan, tolvaptan and lixivaptan** (the vaptans). They inhibit the effects of ADH in the collecting tubule and cause free water diuresis. Conivaptan is an antagonist of V_{1a} and V_2 receptors while lixivaptan, tolvaptan and satavaptan are V_2 antagonists. Conivaptan is given parenterally while tolvaptan and lixivaptan are effective orally.

Uses

Patients with syndrome of inappropriate ADH secretion (SIADH), should be treated with restriction of water intake. If response is inadequate, the vaptans enhance free water excretion and correct hyponatraemia. Clinical studies have shown them to be useful in these patients. Serum sodium levels should be monitored to avoid hypernatraemia and nephrogenic diabetes insipidus. Conivaptan has been approved for use in euvolemic hyponatraemia.

Adenosine A1 Receptor Antagonists

Adenosine A1 receptor antagonists are a recently introduced class of drugs which decrease NaCl reabsorption in the proximal tubule and the collecting duct.

Rolophylline belongs to this group and is undergoing clinical trials for use in cardiac failure.

Sodium Glucose Cotransporter 2 (SGLT 2) Inhibitors

Most of the glucose (90%) is reabsorbed through SGLT2 and inhibition of this transporter can lower the reabsorption and thereby enhance the renal excretion of glucose. Dapagliflozin and canagliflazine, the SGLT2 inhibitors, are used in the treatment of diabetes mellitus (*see* page 517).

Diuretic Resistance

Inability to reduce plasma sodium levels despite using full therapeutic dose of diuretics is diuretic resistance. Resistance to diuretics could be due to multiple reasons like higher sodium intake, reduced absorption of the diuretic, inadequate renal blood flow as in CCF leading to lower amounts of it reaching the kidney. Chronic renal failure and nephrotic syndrome patients may also be refractory to diuretics. Diuretic resistance may be managed with:

- Upgradation from a lower to a higher efficacy diuretic.
- Using a suitable combination.
- Reduced salt intake helps.
- Timing the diuretic intake 30 to 60 minutes before food also works because renal diuretic levels would be high enough to avoid slat retention.
- NSAIDs can cause salt and water retention and are a common cause of diuretic resistance—hence they should be avoided.

Drug Interactions with Diuretics

1. Frusemide and ethacrynic acid are highly protein bound and may compete with drugs like warfarin and clofibrate for protein binding sites.
2. Other ototoxic drugs like aminoglycosides should not be used with loop diuretics to avoid enhanced toxicity.
3. Hypokalaemia induced by diuretics enhance digitalis toxicity.
4. NSAIDs blunt the effect of diuretics as they cause salt and water retention to avoid enhanced toxicity. It could be because of inhibition of PG synthesis in the kidneys.
5. Diuretics enhance lithium toxicity by reducing renal excretion of lithium.
6. Other drugs that cause hyperkalaemia (ACE inhibitors) and oral K^+ supplements should be avoided with K^+ sparing diuretics because, given together they can cause severe hyperkalaemia.
7. Diuretics potentiate the antihypertensive effects of drugs used in hypertension.
8. Probenecid competes with furosemide and thiazides for tubular secretion and counter their diuretic effect as smaller amounts of these diuretics reach the tubular fluid. Diuretics also counter the uricosuric effects of probenecid as they cause hyperuricaemia.

Contraindications for Diuretics

1. *Toxaemia of pregnancy:* Diuresis induced in pregnancy results in reduced foetal circulation which may result in foetal death. Hence diuretics are contraindicated in pregnancy-induced hypertension.
2. *Hepatic cirrhosis:* Diuretics can cause mental disturbances and hepatic coma in cirrhosis patients. The combined effect of raised NH_3 levels, alkalosis and hypokalaemia may be responsible for this. Hence diuretics should be used carefully in them.

Combination of Diuretics

- When diuresis produced by a single diuretic is inadequate or in refractory patients, a combination of them may be used. Drugs acting at different sites should be combined. A thiazide with a loop diuretic provides good diuresis—a synergistic combination. However, they could result in profound dehydration and electrolyte disturbances and should be used for short periods in preferably hospitalized patients.
- A potassium sparing diuretic may, however, be added to a thiazide or loop diuretic for long-term use.

ANTIDIURETICS

Antidiuretics are drugs that reduce urine volume. These include:

1. Antidiuretic hormone (vasopressin)
2. Vasopressin analogs
   - Desmopressin
   - Terlipressin
   - Lypressin
   - Felypressin
3. Thiazide diuretics
4. Miscellaneous
   - Chlorpropamide
   - Carbamazepine

Antidiuretic Hormone (ADH)

Antidiuretic hormone is secreted by the posterior pituitary along with oxytocin. It is synthesized in the supraoptic and paraventricular nuclei of the hypothalamus, transported along the hypothalamohypophyseal tract to the posterior pituitary and is stored there. ADH is released in response to two stimuli—dehydration and rise in plasma osmolarity.

Vasopressin Receptors

ADH acts on vasopressin receptors—V_1 and V_2. V_1 receptors mediate vasoconstriction while V_2 receptors mediate water retention in the collecting duct (Flowchart 22.3). Both are G-protein-coupled receptors. V_1 receptors are of two subtypes—V_{1a}—present on vascular and other smooth muscles, urinary bladder, platelets, liver and CNS. V_{1b} receptors are present on the anterior pituitary.

V_2 receptors are present in the renal collecting ducts where they enhance reabsorption of water. The stimulation of V_2 receptors activates adenylyl cyclase leading to ↑cAMP synthesis resulting in phosphorylation of the specific proteins. This in turn increases the number of aqueous channels inserted in the collecting duct.

Actions

ADH enhances water reabsorption by acting on the collecting duct. ADH activates the V_2 receptors present on the cell membrane of the collecting duct and increases the water permeability of these cells. ADH causes vasoconstriction and raises BP-mediated by V_1 receptors. All vasculature including cutaneous, mesenteric, coeliac and coronary are constricted. It also acts on other smooth muscles to increase constriction and peristalsis in the gut (can cause cramps). Vasopressin contracts the uterus.

Vasopressin is given parenterally SC/IM/IV injection.

Flowchart 22.3

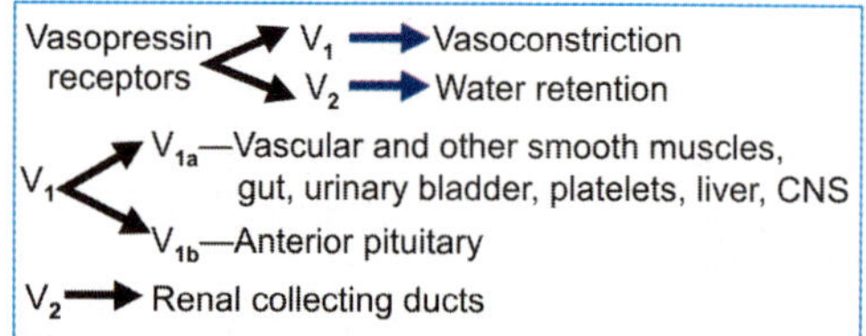

Adverse effects: When used intranasally ADH can cause nasal irritation, allergy, rhinitis and atrophy of the nasal mucosa. Other effects include nausea, abdominal cramps (due to contractions of the uterus) and backache.

Uses

Mediated through V_1 Receptors

1. Bleeding oesophageal varices—ADH constricts mesenteric blood vessels and may help. Analogs like desmopressin, terlipressin and lypressin can be used.
2. Before abdominal radiography—ADH promotes expulsion of gases from the bowel.
3. Cardiac arrest—IV vasopressin has been found to be useful in reverting the asystolic cardiac arrest.

Mediated through V_2 Receptors

1. Diabetes insipidus (DI) of pituitary origin also known as central DI or neurogenic DI—is treated with desmopressin. It requires life long treatment in most cases (Flowchart 22.4).
2. *Nocturnal enuresis:* Desmopressin given at bedtime either orally or intranasally along with restriction of fluid intake at bed time largely controls bed wetting. It should be given only for short periods. Blood pressure should be monitored.
3. *Bleeding disorder:* Haemophilia and von Willebrand's disease—ADH may release factor VIII and prevent bleeding.
4. *Renal concentration test:* A small dose of desmopressin (2 µg) can enhance the urine concentration to a great extent, if the kidneys are normal.

Flowchart 22.4: Treatment of diabetes insipidus

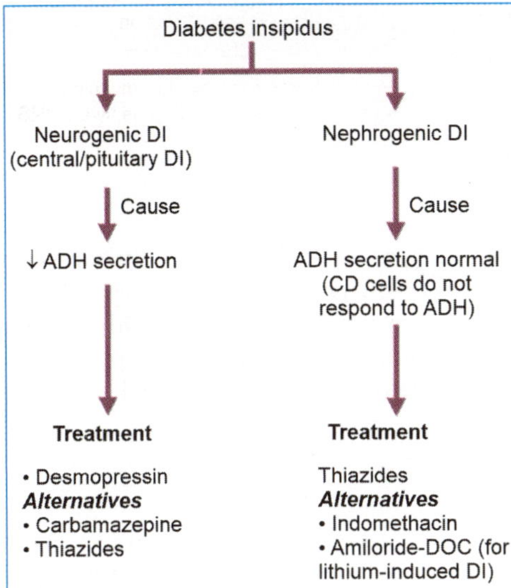

Vasopressin Analogs

Desmopressin is selective for V_2 receptors and is longer acting and more potent than vasopressin. Given orally, bioavailability is 1–2% and intranasally bioavailability is 10–20%. Hence requirement of oral dose is 10–15 times higher than intranasal dose. Desmopressin is used for conditions where V_2 agonist is required.

Dose: INTRANASAL: 10–40 μg/day in 2–3 divided doses. Oral: 100–200 μg TDS.

Terlipressin is a prodrug of vasopressin and is longer acting while felypressin is short acting. It is used for bleeding oesophageal varices. **Felypressin** is used with local anaesthetics to prolong the duration of action because of its vasoconstrictor properties. **Lypressin** is another analog used in place of ADH.

Miscellaneous

Thiazides: Paradoxically thiazides reduce urine volume in diabetes insipidus of both pituitary and renal origin by an unknown mechanism.

Chlorpropamide, an oral hypoglycaemic, sensitizes the kidney to ADH action.

Carbamazepine, an antiepileptic, stimulates ADH secretion.

Vasopressin Antagonists

Drugs that block the vasopressin receptors, viz. conivaptan, tolvaptan and lixivaptan are now available for the treatment of inappropriate or elevated ADH secretion. **Demeclocycline and lithium** also have anti-ADH effects but are not used for this purpose as they cause many adverse effects.

Clinical Pharmacology

- All diuretics can cause electrolyte disturbances.
- Hyponatraemia can be dangerous particularly in patients with cardiac diseases.
- In CHF, the dose of the diuretic used is adjusted to reduce 1 kg body weight per day.
- Diuretics are often administered on alternate days.
- The risk of hypokalaemia is higher in cirrhosis patients.
- In severe cirrhosis with ascites, vigorous diuresis should be avoided as it may precipitate hepatic coma and azotemia which can be fatal.
- Diuretic resistance/tolerance may develop; avoiding dehydration may prevent the development of resistance.
- If required for a long term, it is preferable to use a combination of K^+ sparing diuretic with loop/thiazide diuretics.

[1] From Medical Council of India, *Competency based Undergraduate Curriculum for the Indian Medical Graduate*, 2018;1:136–144.

Unit VII

Blood

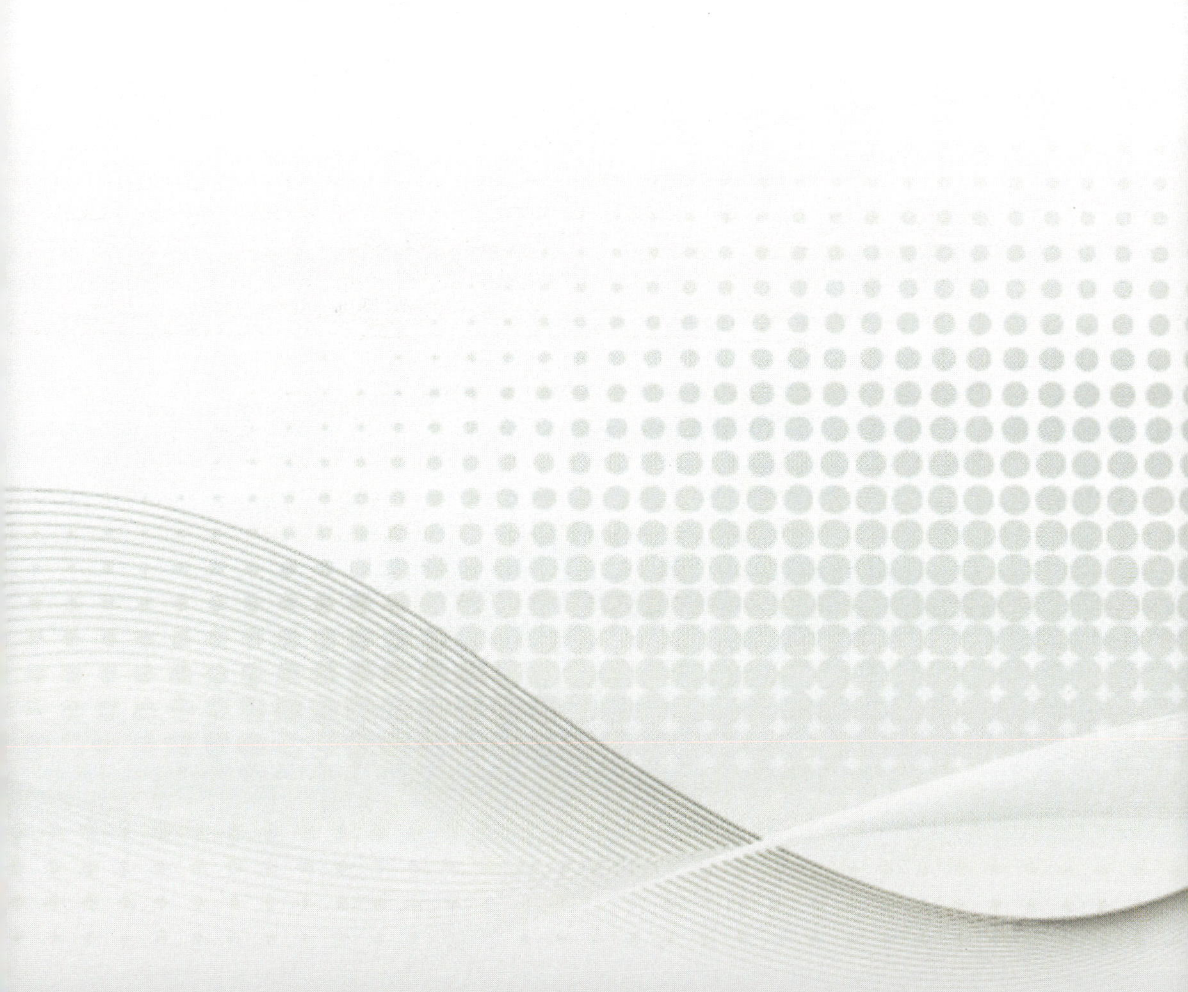

CHAPTER 23

Drugs used in the Disorders of Coagulation

Competency achievement: The student should be able to:

PH 1.25 Describe the mechanism/s of action, types, doses, side effects, indications and contraindications of the drugs acting on blood, like anticoagulants, antiplatelets, fibrinolytics, plasma expanders.[1]

Haemostasis is the spontaneous arrest of bleeding from the damaged blood vessels. In the process, complex interactions take place between the injured vessel wall, platelets and clotting factors.

Following injury, there is local vasoconstriction and platelet adhesion—forming a plug which temporarily stops bleeding. This is reinforced by fibrin for long-term haemostasis.

Clotting factors are proteins synthesized by the liver. Two systems—the extrinsic and the intrinsic system are involved in the process of coagulation. Several proteins interact in a cascading series to form the clot (Fig. 23.1).

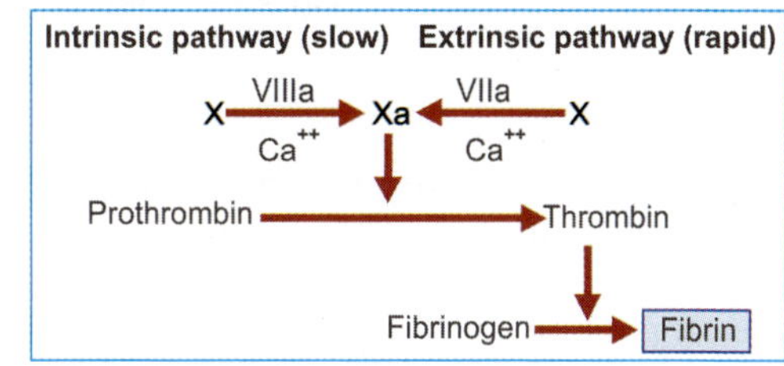

Fig. 23.1: Major reactions of blood coagulation

Anticoagulants are drugs that reduce the coagulability of the blood (Fig. 23.2).

Classification

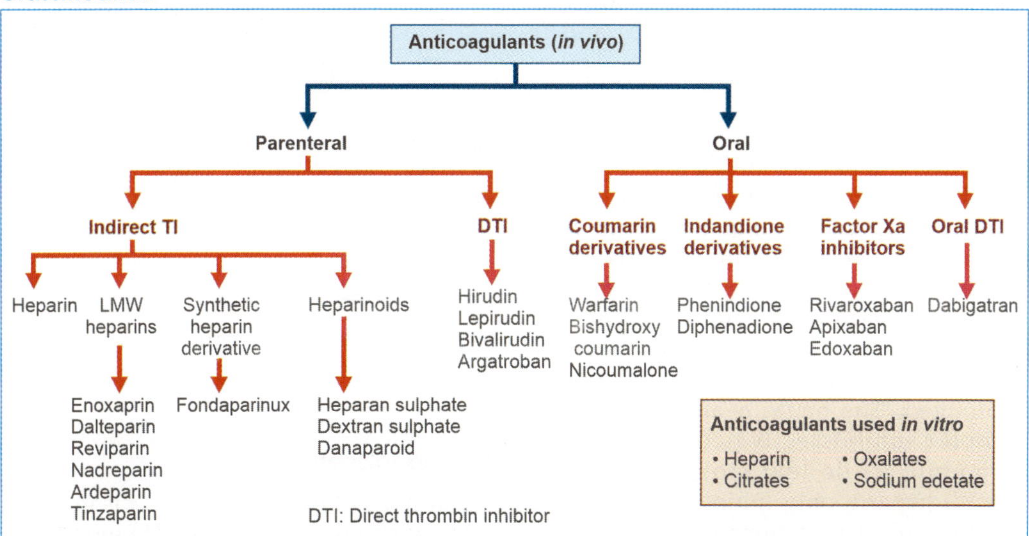

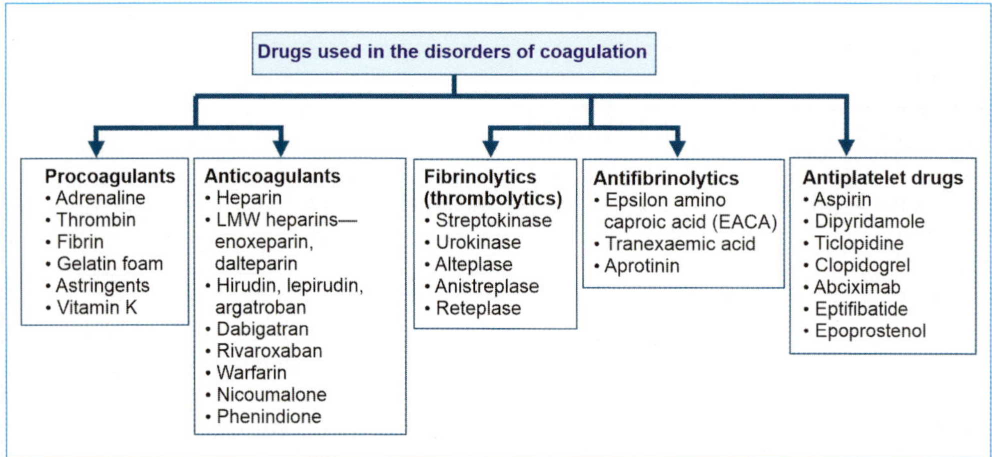

Fig. 23.2: Drugs used in coagulation disorders

HEPARIN

Heparin was discovered by McLean, a medical student in 1916. It was named 'heparin' as it was first extracted from the liver. It is a mucopolysaccharide found in the mast cells of the liver, lungs and intestinal mucosa. Heparin is the strongest acid in the body. It is a glycosaminoglycan.

Actions

Heparin is a powerful anticoagulant that acts instantaneously both *in vivo* and *in vitro.*

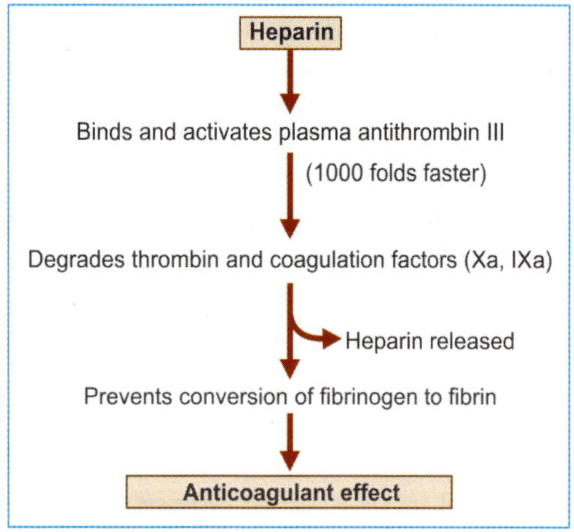

Mechanism of Action

Antithrombin III is a peptide that is synthesized in the liver and circulates in the plasma. Heparin activates plasma antithrombin III. Antithrombin III binds to and inhibits the activated thrombin and coagulation factors (Xa and IXa). This is a physiological reaction, but heparin accelerates it by 1000 times. Clotting time is prolonged. The heparin–antithrombin III complex inhibits activated factor X and thrombin, while low molecular weight (LMW) heparin only inhibits factor X and not thrombin. Unfractionated heparin (UFH standard heparin) has a molecular weight of 10,000–30,000 while LMW heparins have short chains with molecular weight 4,000–7,000.

Other Actions

Heparin activates lipoprotein lipase which hydrolyses triglycerides present in the plasma and thus clears the plasma of lipids.

Pharmacokinetics

Heparin is not effective orally. It is given IV or SC. **It should not be given IM because—**

- It may cause haematomas at the site of injection due to local bleeding which also results in erratic absorption
- It causes irritation.

Given intravenously the onset of action is immediate, reaches peak in 5–10 minutes and clotting time returns to normal in 2–4 hours. Treatment is monitored by the aPTT (preferable) or clotting time. Heparin is metabolised by heparinase in the liver.

Because of its large molecular size, heparin does not cross the placental barrier. Therefore, **heparin can be used in pregnancy,** if an anticoagulant is needed.

Heparin administration and dose: Heparin is given as an IV infusion of 5000 units bolus dose followed by 1000–1500 units per hour infusion with the help of an infusion pump. aPTT is maintained 1.5 to 2 times the control. Clotting time is maintained at 1.8 to 2.5 times the normal mean aPTT value. Anti-Xa activity may also be used to assess heparin concentration. During cardiopulmonary bypass, high doses of heparin is used to prevent coagulation. Intermittent heparin administration may be done by an IV bolus injection of 10,000 units followed by 5000 units every 4–6 hr.

For prophylaxis, low dose heparin is given subcutaneously—5000 units every 8–12 hours. However, this regimen has now been shown to be less efficacious but the advantage is that it does not require constant monitoring.

Preparations

BEPARINE, HEPARIN SODIUM, NUPARIN, HEPLOCK inj 1000 IU/ml and 5000 IU/ml in 5 ml vials for injection, No-Clot 5000 IU inj THROMBOPHOB Ointment, HEPGEL—for topical use.

Adverse Reactions

1. **Bleeding** is the most common, major adverse effect of heparin. Careful monitoring and dose control will prevent this to a great extent.
2. **Hypersensitivity reactions:** For commercial use, heparin is obtained from bovine lung or porcine intestine. Because of its animal origin, allergic reactions are quite common.
3. **Heparin-induced thrombocytopenia (HIT):** Heparin-induced platelet aggregation and formation of antiplatelet antibodies—both result in thrombocytopenia and a systemic hypercoagulable state. Platelet count is reduced to less than 1.5 l/dl. The antigen–antibody complexes may damage the vessel wall triggering thrombosis leading to occlusion of peripheral arteries and disseminated intravascular coagulation. Though both venous and arterial thrombosis can occur, venous thrombosis is common. The incidence is higher in surgical patients. Confirmatory test is by heparin-independent platelet activation assay. This paradoxical complication of heparin therapy can occur in 1–4% of patients treated with standard heparin for atleast a week, but can be serious. It is less common with LMW heparins. Heparin should be stopped immediately at the first sign of thrombocytopenia. HIT can occur faster, if patients have received heparin within the previous 3–4 months as the patients may have circulating antibodies to heparin.
4. **Alopecia** is reversible. Occurs in 0.5% of patients after about 5–10 days of starting heparin therapy.
5. **Osteoporosis** can occur on long-term use of heparin—the cause is unknown.
6. **Hypoaldosteronism:** Heparin can inhibit the synthesis of aldosterone and may result in hyperkalaemia.

Precautions

- Platelet count should be frequently monitored.
- If there is formation of a new clot in heparin treated patients—HIT should be considered.
- If HIT develops, a direct thrombin inhibitor should be given.

Heparin Resistance

Resistance to heparin could be due to both pharmacokinetic and pharmacodynamic reasons. Higher concentration of heparin binding proteins in plasma competitively inhibit the binding of heparin to antithrombin. Heparin clearance may be accelerated in some patients leading to resistance. Resistance to heparin is detected when the dose of heparin needed to maintain the therapeutic aPTT is increased.

Contraindications to Heparin Therapy

Bleeding disorders, heparin-induced thrombocytopenia, thrombocytopenic purpura, infective endocarditis, threatened abortion, haemophilia, severe hypertension, intracranial haemorrhage, cirrhosis, ulcers in the gut, renal failure and neurosurgery are contraindications for heparin use.

Low molecular weight (LMW) heparins include enoxaparin, dalteparin, reviparin, nadreparin, etc. LMW heparins are obtained by chemical/enzymatic treatment of standard heparin (UFH). Apart from being equally efficacious, LMW heparins have a favourable pharmacokinetic profile. They have a shorter chain and lower molecular weights when compared to UFH. Since LMW heparins inhibit factor Xa only and have just a weak effect on thrombin, aPTT or clotting time are not prolonged. Plasma low molecular weight heparin levels can be determined by assay of anti-Xa units and therapeutic levels should be maintained at 0.5–1.5 units/ml. Anticoagulant dose is calculated based on the body weight. LMW heparins should be used carefully in patients with renal dysfunction. Anti-Xa assay may be used to monitor the dose in patients with renal failure.

LMW heparins have the following advantages over standard heparins:

1. Better bioavailability following SC injection.
2. Longer action once or twice daily administration.
3. Predictable pharmacokinetics and plasma levels. Frequent aPTT monitoring is not required.
4. Lower risk of bleeding
5. Lower risk of osteoporosis
6. Lower incidence of thrombocytopenia and thrombosis.

Uses

LMW heparins are used in the prevention and treatment of venous thrombosis and pulmonary embolism; they are also useful in unstable angina and to maintain the patency of tubes in dialysis patients.

Several LMW heparins are available for therapeutic use:

1. Enoxaparin 1 mg/ kg. SC twice daily
   Prophylaxis 40 mg once daily
2. Reviparin 0.25 ml SC once daily
3. Dalteparin 200 IU/kg SC once daily
   Prophylaxis 2500 to 5000 IU, SC once daily
4. Ardeparin 2500–5000 IU SC once daily
5. Nadroparin: 4000 IU/0.4 ml 6000 IU/0.6 ml inj
6. Tinzaparin 3500 IU SC once daily

Heparin Antagonist

Mild heparin overdosage can be treated by just stopping heparin because heparin is short acting. In severe heparin overdose, an antagonist may be needed to arrest its anticoagulant effects. **Protamine sulphate** is a protein obtained from the sperm of certain fish. Given intravenously, it neutralises heparin (1 mg for every 100 units of heparin). In the absence of heparin, protamine sulphate can itself act as a weak anticoagulant. Hence, overdose should be avoided. Protamine sulphate is a strongly basic protein which binds with the strongly acidic groups of heparin forming a stable complex which is devoid of anticoagulant activity. Whole blood transfusion may be needed.

Strongly basic Protamine sulfate —Binds→ Strongly acidic heparin → Inactive complex

Synthetic heparin derivatives: Fondaparinux a factor Xa inhibitor, is a synthetic pentasaccharide, binds to antithrombin and mediates inhibition of factor Xa. It is given by SC inj 2.5 mg once daily, has a rapid onset of action, the response is predictable, t½ 17–21 hr and is excreted in the urine. It is given once a day and does not require frequent coagulation monitoring. The risk of HIT is lower than with even LMW heparins. However, it should not be given in patients with renal dysfunction.

Uses: Fondaparinux is used for the prevention and treatment of deep vein thrombosis and pulmonary embolism and for the thromboprophylaxis in patients undergoing hip or knee surgery.

Idraparinux, a longer acting derivative of fondaparinux, has a t½ of 5–6 days.

Heparinoids

Heparan sulfate present in some tissues is similar to heparin. It is believed to be responsible for thrombolytic activity on the vascular endothelium

Danaparoid is a mixture of heparinoids and acts by inhibiting factor Xa. It does not prolong aPTT and is longer acting. It is used subcutaneously in the treatment of deep vein thrombosis and in other conditions as an alternative to heparin.

DIRECT THROMBIN INHIBITORS (DTI)

Most DTIs are given parenterally but recently some oral DTIs have been developed.

Parenteral DTIs

Hirudin present in the saliva of leech has been synthesized by recombinant DNA technology for clinical use. **Lepirudin** and **bivalirudin** are hirudin analogs—irreversibly bind thrombin on both the fibrin binding site and the catalytic site and inhibit its protease activity. They can inactivate fibrin-bound thrombin in the clots since their activity is independent of antithrombin III. The action is monitored by aPTT; there is no specific antidote unlike heparin.

Lepirudin is excreted by the kidneys and, therefore, should be used carefully in renal impairment. Bivalirudin is only 20% excreted through the kidneys and is safer.

Antibodies develop to lepirudin and on reexposure, risk of anaphylaxis exists. Lepirudin has been approved for use in patients with heparin-induced thrombocytopenia. Bivalirudin may be used in patients undergoing coronary angioplasty.

Argatroban, a direct thrombin inhibitor, binds thrombin and has a quick but short action. Given as an IV infusion, it may be used in HIT and treatment monitored with aPTT.

ORAL ANTICOAGULANTS

Cattle that were fed on spoiled sweet clover hay, developed a haemorrhagic disease in North America in 1924. This turned out to be due to bishydroxycoumarin, an anticoagulant in the spoiled sweet clover. Many related compounds were then developed and are also being used as rat poison. Warfarin is a commonly used anticoagulant (Table 23.1).

Mechanism of Action

Warfarin and its congeners act as anticoagulants only *in vivo* because they act by interfering with the synthesis of vitamin K dependent clotting factors in the liver. They block the gamma-carboxylation of glutamate residues in prothrombin, factors VII, IX and X. Gamma-carboxylation is necessary for these factors to participate in coagulation (Fig. 23.3).

The onset of action is slow; it develops over 1–3 days because oral anticoagulants do not destroy the already circulating clotting factors. Prothrombin time (PT) is measured to

Table 23.1: Pharmacokinetics and preparations of oral anticoagulants used clinically

Drug	*t½ (hr)*	*Duration of action*	*Dose (mg) LD*	*MD*	*Trade name, preparations*	
Warfarin sodium	36–48	4–7 days	10–15	2–10	UNIWARFIN	5 mg tab
Dicumarol	24–100	4–7 days	200 × 2 days	50–100	DICUMORAL	50 mg tab
Nicoumalone	18–24	2–3 days	8–12	2–8	ACTIROM	1,2,4 mg tab

LD—Loading dose MD—Maintenance dose

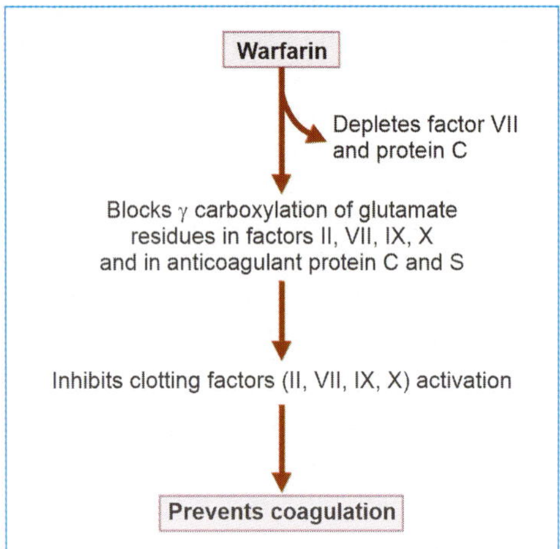

Fig. 23.3: Mechanism of action of warfarin

monitor the treatment. It takes 5–7 days for PT to return to normal after stopping oral anticoagulants.

Pharmacokinetics

Warfarin is completely absorbed orally (100% bioavailability) and is 99% bound to plasma proteins. Warfarin is available as a mixture of levo- and dextrorotatory forms, levorotatory form being more potent. They are metabolized by glucuronide conjugation and are excreted in the urine. Warfarin is also metabolized by microsomal enzymes CYP2C9. People inheriting a genetic variant of CYP2C9 metabolise warfarin at a slow rate and, therefore, the risk of bleeding is higher in such people. Pharmacokinetic profile (Table 23.1).

Bishydroxycoumarin (dicumarol) is poorly tolerated because of the GIT distrubances. Absorption is slow and unpredictable.

Nicoumalone can cause ulcers in the mouth apart form the gastrointestinal disturbances and dermatitis (Table 23.2).

Phenindione and ethyl biscoumacetate are not used therapeutically due to toxicity. Diphenadione is used as a rodenticide.

Adverse Effects

Haemorrhage is the main side effect. Bleeding in the intestines or brain can be troublesome. Minor episodes of epistaxis and bleeding gums are common. Purple toe syndrome—a painful blue tinged discoloration of plantar surfaces and sides of toes but is reversible. It is due to release of cholesterol emboli from athermatous plaque. Treatment depends on the severity.

- Stop the anticoagulant.
- Fresh blood transfusion is given to supply clotting factors.
- **Antidote** The specific antidote is **vitamin K_1 oxide.** It allows the synthesis of clotting factors. But even on IV administration, the response to vitamin K_1 oxide needs several hours. Hence in emergency, **fresh frozen plasma** is necessary to counter the effects of oral anticoagulants.

Table 23.2: Factors influencing oral anticoagulant activity

Factors increasing activity	*Factors reducing activity*
Poor diet, bowel disease, liver disease and chronic alcoholism—result in vitamin K deficiency	Pregnancy—there is increased synthesis of clotting factors Hypothyroidism—there is reduced degradation of clotting factors.

COMPARE AND CONTRAST
Standard Heparin and LMW Heparin

Features	***Standard Heparin***	***LMW Heparin***
Mol. weight	10,000–20,000	4,000–7,000
Source	Natural	Semisynthetic (chemical treatment of std. heparin)
Thrombin activity in therapeutic doses	Inhibited	Not inhibited
Effect on tests of clotting	Significant	Not significant
Lab. monitoring	Required	Not required
SC bioavailability	Low (20–30%)	Good (70–90%)
Duration of action	Short (2–4 hr)	Long (18–24 hr)
Frequency of administration	Every 4–6 hr	Once a day
Dose dependent clearance	Yes	No
Risk of bleeding	Present	Low
HIT	Likely (++++)	Less likely (++)

HIT: Heparin-induced thrombocytopenia

Other adverse effects include allergic reactions, gastrointestinal disturbances and teratogenicity.

Orally Acting DTIs

Oral DTIs have a rapid onset of action, predictable absorption and plasma levels. Routine frequent monitoring of anticoagulant therapy is not essential. Hence they are preferred in several conditions.

Dabigatran is an orally effective DTI administered orally as dabigatran etexilate which is a prodrug converted to dabigatran. In patients with renal impairment, dose should be reduced. Adverse effects include GI disturbances and bleeding. PTT and thrombin time will be prolonged.

It is long acting—given once daily.

Advantages

- **Frequent monitoring is not required** and there is no risk of significant drug interactions unlike heparin.
- **Idarucizumab**, an antidote to dabigatran, has been very recently developed. It binds to dabigatran with high affinity and completely reverses the actions of dabigatran in 5 minutes.

Because of the above advantages, these orally acting DTIs may soon replace warfarin for long-term anticoagulation therapy.

Dabigatran is currently approved for the prevention of venous thromboembolism in patients who have undergone surgeries for hip or knee replacement.

Factor Xa Inhibitors

Rivaroxaban and apixaban are the orally effective direct inhibitors of factor Xa. Rivaroxaban has a good oral bioavailability, fast onset of action and is extensively protein bound. Apixaban is gradually absorbed and has a long t½. Both are metabolised by CYP450 enzymes. Rivaroxaban is approved for the prevention and treatment of deep vein thrombosis and prevention of venous thrombosis in hip and knee surgery. Apixaban is approved for prevention of stroke in atrial fibrillation (without valvular heart diaease). Edoxaban is under clinical trials for use in deep vein thrombosis and pulmonary embolism. Efforts have been made to develop oral anticoagulants that do not require monitoring.

COMPARE AND CONTRAST

Heparin and Dicoumarol/Warfarin

Features	***Heparin***	***Dicoumarol/Warfarin***
Source	Natural	Synthetic
Chemistry	Mucopolysaccharide	Coumarin derivative
Route of administration	Parenteral	Oral
Site of action	*In vivo* and *in vitro*	*In vivo only*
Onset of action	Immediate	Slow (1–3 days)
Duration of action	Short (2–4 hr)	Long (4–7 days)
Mechanism of action	Activates antithrombin III which inhibits thrombin, factors Xa and IXa	Inhibits synthesis of clotting factors (II, VII, IX, X)
Antagonist	Protamine sulfate	Vitamin K_1 oxide
Monitoring with	aPTT/clotting time	Prothrombin time/INR
Safety in pregnancy	Yes	No
Used for	Initiation of therapy	Maintenance therapy

INR: International normalized ratio

Drug Interactions

Many drugs **potentiate** warfarin action

1. Drugs that inhibit platelet function - NSAIDs, like aspirin, increase the risk of bleeding.

   NSAIDs + Warfarin → ↑ Bleeding

2. Drugs that inhibit hepatic drug metabolism like cimetidine, chloramphenicol and metronidazole enhance plasma levels of warfarin.

   Enzyme inhibitors (Chloramphenicol, cimetidine) → ↓ Warfarin metabolism → ↑ Warfarin levels

Some drugs reduce the effect of oral anticoagulants

1. Drugs that enhance the metabolism of oral anticoagulants—microsomal enzyme inducers, like barbiturates, rifampicin, griseofulvin, enhance the metabolism of oral anticoagulants. When these drugs are suddenly withdrawn, excess anticoagulant activity may result in haemorrhages.
2. Drugs that increase the synthesis of clotting factors, like oral contraceptives, counter the effect of oral anticoagulants.

Uses of Anticoagulants

Anticoagulants can prevent the extension of thrombus but cannot destroy the existing clots. Heparin has rapid and short action which makes it suitable for initiating treatment while warfarin is suitable for long-term maintenance due to its slow and prolonged action and convenience of oral use.

1. **Venous thrombosis and pulmonary embolism**—anticoagulants prevent extension of thrombus and recurrence of embolism.
2. **Postoperative, post-stroke patients; bedridden patients** due to leg fractures and other causes—who cannot be ambulant for several months—anticoagulants prevent venous thrombosis and pulmonary embolism in such patients.
3. **Rheumatic valvular disease:** Anticoagulants prevent embolism.
4. **Unstable angina:** Heparin reduces the risk of myocardial infarction in patients with unstable angina.
5. **Vascular surgery, artificial heart valves and haemodialysis** anticoagulants prevent thromboembolism.
6. **Covid-19:** As thromboembolism has been found to be associated with deaths in covid, anticoagulants are started in moderate to severe cases. Heparin or a LMW heparin may be given and continued on oral anticoagulants after the patient gets discharged.

Contraindications to Anticoagulant Therapy

- Bleeding disorders including thrombocytopenia.
- Severe hypertension
- Malignancies
- Bacterial endocarditis
- Liver and kidney diseases.

THROMBOLYTICS (FIBRINOLYTICS)

Thrombolytics lyse the clot or thrombi by activating the natural fibrinolytic system.

Plasminogen circulates in the plasma and also some of it is bound to fibrin. Tissue plasminogen activator (tPA) activates plasminogen which is converted to plasmin. Plasmin degrades fibrin—thereby dissolving the clot. Thrombolytic agents are:

- First generation agents
  Streptokinase, urokinase
- Second generation agents
  Alteplase, duteplase, tenecteplase, reteplase, anistreplase.

Streptokinase obtained from β-haemolytic streptococci activates plasminogen. Antistreptococcal antibodies present in the blood due to previous streptococcal infections inactivate a large amount of streptokinase.

Streptokinase is antigenic and can cause allergy. The antibodies formed may persist for five years. Hence, if thrombolytics are required during that period, others like tPa or urokinase should be used. Streptokinase also causes hypotension (Table 23.3).

Anistreplase (anisoylated plasminogen streptokinase activator complex, APSAC) is a form of streptokinase which is long acting and can be injected in a single IV bolus of 30 units over 3–5 minutes. Hence it is more convenient to use. Coronary reperfusion is better than with streptokinase—has greater activity on clot than on free plasminogen, and also has thrombolytic activity. But it also causes fibrinogenolysis and allergic reactions.

Urokinase is an enzyme prepared from cultures of human kidney cells (it was first isolated from human urine—hence the name). It activates plasminogen and converts it to plasmin.

Tissue plasminogen activator (tPA) preferentially activates plasminogen that is bound to fibrin which means circulating plasminogen is largely spared. Chances of reocclusion may be reduced by use of heparin and antiplatelet drugs.

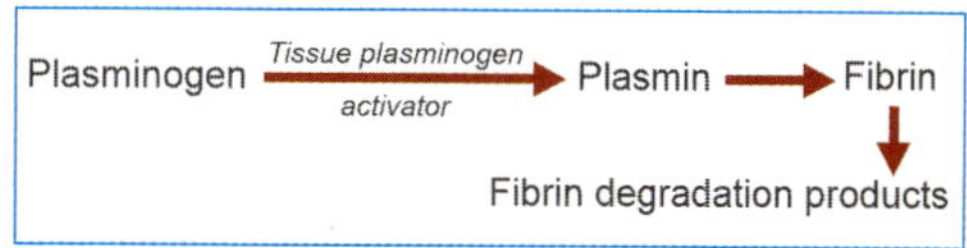

Alteplase and duteplase are tPA produced by recombinant DNA technology. They are very expensive.

Reteplase is modified human tPA obtained by genetic engineering. It is claimed to have the following advantages over tPA:

- Faster reperfusion
- Bleeding tendency is negligible.

Tenecteplase is longer acting and can be given as an IV bolus injection. Its ability to bind fibrin is better than that of alteplase.

Table 23.3: Dose of fibrinolytics

Drug	*Loading dose*	*Maintenance dose*	*Brand name*
Streptokinase	2.5 lakh units	1 lakh unit/hr for 24–72 hr	STREPTASE
Urokinase	3 lakh units over 10 min	3 lakh units/hr for 12 hr	UROKEN
Alteplase	60 mg over 60 min	20 mg/hr for 2 hr	ACTILYSE
Reteplase	10 units	10 units after 30 minutes	RETAVASE
Tenecteplase	0.5 mg/kg single inj		ELAXIM
Anistreplase	30 mg over 3–5 min single inj.		EMINASE

Sclerosing agent IV !

Rajan, a 45-year-old man, suffering from oesophageal varices was prescribed a sclerosing agent for local injection. The drug was injected intravenously in the arm instead of local injection. Sclerosing agents are irritants. Therefore, IV injection resulted in severe thrombophlebitis and the patient was in great pain. Though it is the nurse who gave the injection in this case, it is the responsibility of the doctor to ensure proper administration of the medicine.

Adverse Effects of Thrombolytics

Bleeding is the major toxicity of all thrombolytics. Hypotension and fever can occur. Allergic reactions are common with streptokinase.

Uses

Several studies have confirmed the efficacy of fibrinolytic therapy in patients with myocardial infarction. All of them have the same therapeutic value.

1. *Acute myocardial infarction:* Intravenous thrombolytics given immediately reduce the mortality rate in acute MI. They should be given within 6 hr but preferrably immediately because early treatment largely reduces mortality.
2. *Severe deep vein thrombosis* and large pulmonary emboli, ascending thrombophlebitis are also treated with fibrinolytics.
3. *Peripheral vascular diseases:* Intra-arterial, thrombolytics have been tried.

Contraindications to Thrombolytic Therapy

- Recent surgery, injury, gastrointestinal bleeding, stroke.
- Severe hypertension.
- Bleeding disorders.

ANTIFIBRINOLYTICS

Antifibrinolytics are drugs that inhibit fibrinolysis—they block the binding of plasminogen to fibrin and inhibit the dissolution of clot.

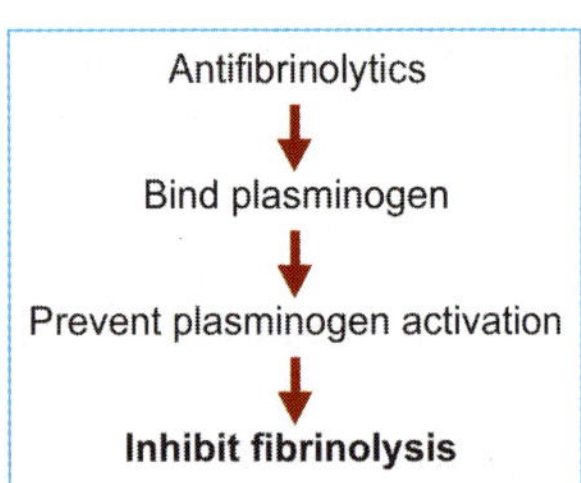

Epsilon aminocaproic acid (EACA): It is an analog of the amino acid lysine interacts with the lysine binding sites on plasminogen and plasmin and blocks them—thus plasminogen activation and at higher doses proteolytic activity of the plasmin is inhibited and the clot is stabilized. Given orally it is rapidly absorbed.

Adverse effects include nausea, abdominal discomfort, dyspepsia, conjunctival erythema, skin rashes and rarely intravascular thrombosis. If injected rapidly intravenously, it can cause hypotension and bradycardia.

Preparations and Dose: 100 mg/kg loading dose (max 10 g) followed by 50 mg/kg (max 5 g) four times a day for 2–3 days, AMICAR, HEMOCID, HEMOSTAT 500 mg tab, 5 g. 20 ml inj.

Therapeutic uses of EACA are:

a. As an antidote in overdose of thrombolytic therapy.
b. Dental surgery, tooth extraction in haemophiliacs.
c. To reduce bleeding in some cases of trauma, surgical procedures, cardiac surgeries, prostatic surgery.
d. To prevent recurrence of upper gastrointestinal haemorrhage.
e. PPH and some cases of primary menorrhagia.
f. Bleeding in patients with thrombocytopenia.

COMPARE AND CONTRAST

Anticoagulants and thrombolytics

Features	*Anticoagulants*	*Thrombolytics*
Examples	**Heparin, warfarin**	**Streptokinase, urokinase**
Route of administration	Oral and parenteral	Only parenteral
Action	Prevent clot formation	Dissolve clot
Mode of action	Activate anticoagulant mechanism or inhibit clotting factors	Activate natural fibrinolytic system
Primary side effects	Bleeding	Bleeding
Primary use	Deep vein thrombosis, pulmonary and other embolism	MI, severe deep vein thrombosis, large pulmonary emboli
Use in MI	During and after angioplasty	Prior to angioplasty or as alternative to it
Cost	Most (like warfarin) are inexpensive	All are expensive
Duration of use	May be long-term	Short-term only

Contraindications

1. Haematuria—risk of ureteric obstruction, colic due to the unlysed clot (called clot colic)
2. Intravascular coagulation

Tranexaemic acid (TA) is an analog of EACA and a derivative of lysine—like EACA it binds competitively to plasminogen, inhibits conversion of plasminogen to plasmin and thus inhibits fibrinolysis. It is more potent and longer acting than EACA.

TA is given by oral, topical and by IV routes t½ after IV inj is 1½ hr.

Preparations: Dose: 1–1.5 g 6 to 8 hourly TRANOSTAT 500 mg tab, 100 mg/ml inj.

Uses

To arrest bleeding in hyperplasminaemic states which result from damage to tissues that are rich in plasminogen activator as in the following conditions:

a. Overdosage of fibrinolytics
b. Menorrhagia, postpartum haemorrhage
c. After cardiac surgeries including cardiopulmonary bypass
d. Bleeding peptic ulcer
e. Following dental procedures to prevent bleeding in patients with haemophilia as a mouthwash
f. After prostate surgery, tonsillectomy
g. Epistaxis, bleeding from eye injury
h. Hereditary angioedema—in this rare condition, plasmin-induced uncontrolled activation of the complement system takes place.

Adverse effects include nausea, diarrhoea, headache, giddiness and hypertension.

Aprotinin, a naturally occurring polypeptide, is a protease inhibitor—it inhibits kallikrein, plasmin, trypsin and chymotrypsin. It also protects platelets from mechanical injury—thus aprotinin inhibits the initiation of clot formation and fibrinolysis.

Aprotinin has been used in patients with cardiac surgeries like cardiopulmonary bypass surgery and heart valve replacement to reduce blood loss. It can also be used in fibrinolytic overdosage.

Aprotinin is obtained from bovine lung and can, therefore, cause allergic reactions. It can also cause thrombosis and renal toxicity.

Aprotinin is used intravenously but can also be used topically.

Dose: Started with 5 lakh units, followed by 2 lakh units every 4 hr as slow IV infusion. Units for aprotinin is KIU, i.e. kallikrein inactivator units. TRASYLOL (5 lakh units in 50 ml inj) APROGEN 1 lakh and 5 lakh units inj.

ANTIPLATELET DRUGS

Platelets form the initial haemostatic plug at the site of vascular injury and are also involved in the formation of atherosclerosis. By inhibiting the platelet function, thrombosis and atherosclerotic vascular disease can be largely prevented.

Antiplatelet drugs or drugs interfering with platelet function (Fig. 23.4) include:

1. *PG synthesis inhibitors*: Aspirin
2. *Phosphodiesterase inhibitor:* Dipyridamole
3. *ADP antagonists:*
   Ticlopidine, clopidogrel, prasugrel
   Newer drugs—cangrelor, ticagrelor
4. *Glycoprotein IIb/IIIa receptor antagonists:*
   Abciximab, eptifibatide, tirofiban
5. *Others:* PGI_2, cilostazol, ridogrel.

Aspirin

The prostaglandin thromboxane A_2 promotes platelet aggregation. Aspirin inactivates cyclooxygenase (COX) by irreversible acetylation of the enzyme and thereby inhibits the synthesis of thromboxane A_2 even in low doses (75 mg/day). The COX inhibition is irreversible and the effect lasts for 7 to 10 days—till fresh platelets are formed. Aspirin inhibits the synthesis of both TXA_2 which promotes platelet aggregation and PGI_2 which inhibits it. However, in low doses given once daily, it is found to inhibit only TXA_2 production without significant effect on PGI_2 production. Hence aspirin is used in low doses for thromboprophylaxis—such doses also reduce the risk of gastrointestinal adverse effects of aspirin since these are dose related. Several studies have shown that aspirin (and other antiplatelet drugs) effectively reduces the incidence of stroke and MI in the susceptible individuals.

Dose: 50–300 mg/day ECOSPRIN 75, 150, 325 mg tab LOPRIN 75 mg tab.

Aspirin resistance: When thrombosis occurs inspite of aspirin prophylaxis, it can be considered as aspirin resistance. The incidence of resistance is about 30%. The significance of resistance to antiplatelet drugs, the cause for it and the methods for testing resistance are being studied.

Dipyridamole: Dipyridamole is a phosphodiesterase inhibitor which interferes with platelet function by increasing platelet cyclic-

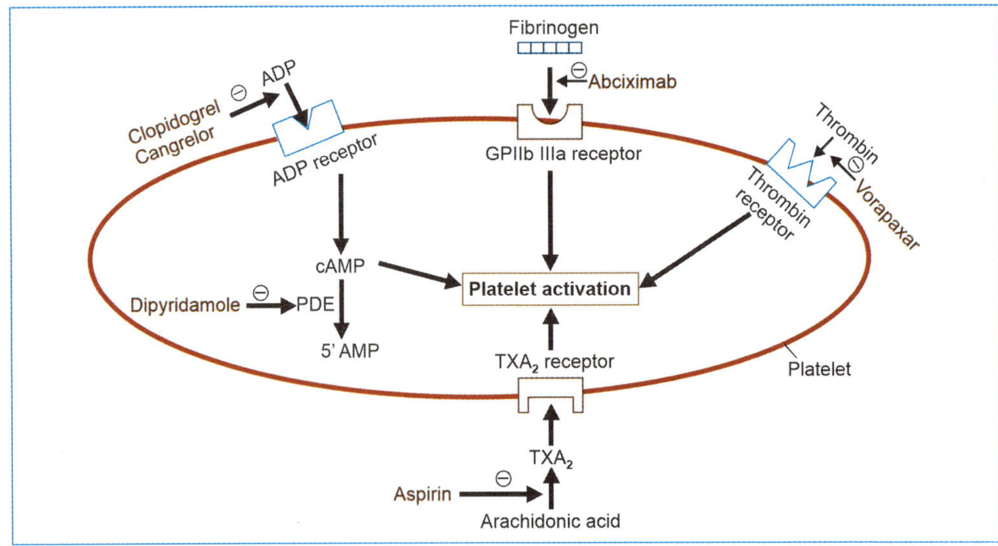

Fig. 23.4: Sites of action of antiplatelet drugs

AMP levels. It is used along with aspirin or warfarin for the prophylaxis of thromboemboli in patients with prosthetic heart valves. A study (The European Stroke Prevention Study-2) has shown that a modified release form of dipyridamole used in patients with transient ischaemic attacks or stroke, reduced the risk of stroke similar to aspirin and the effects were additive with aspirin. It does not increase the risk of bleeding. Headache has been reported. Dipyridamole is extensively bound to plasma proteins and has a t½ of 12 h.

Preparations: Dose: 25–100 mg TDS, PERSANTIN, CARDIWELL: 25, 75, 100 mg tabs.

ADP Antagonists

Clopidogrel, prasugrel and **ticlopidine,** the theinopyridines, are ADP antagonists. ADP binds to the receptors on platelets to bring about platelet aggregation. ADP antagonists are all prodrugs and the active metabolites bind to and **irreversibly block the ADP receptors** and thereby prevent activation of platelets—thus inhibit platelet aggregation. The effects are additive with aspirin because the mechanisms of action are different. However, clopidogrel is more expensive than aspirin and the combination is much more expensive. Hence the combination should be used only in conditions like acute coronary syndrome, MI and in coronary angioplasty.

Ticlopidine is well absorbed orally, and after repeated administration cumulative effect is seen. Clopidogrel has about 50% bioavailability. Though onset of action is slow (3–7 days), it is dose dependent and an oral loading dose of 300 mg of clopidogrel can attain antithrombotic effects within about 5 hours. The antiplatelet effects remain for 7–10 days even after stopping the drug.

Preparations and dose

Clopidogrel 75 mg OD (300 mg loading dose), CLOPID, CLODREL, CLOPILET 75 mg tab.

Ticlopidine 250 mg OD TICLOP, 250 mg tab.
Prasugrel 5–10 mg OD. PRASUREL 5, 10 mg tab.

Adverse effects: Clopidogrel is generally preferred to ticlopidine because of its side effect profile—safer and better tolerated.

They can cause rash, diarrhoea, epigastric pain, neutropenia and rarely bleeding.

Ticlopidine can also cause nausea, diarrhoea, and idiosyncratic blood dyscrasias including leucopenia, and thrombocytopenia.

Uses: Clinical trials have shown ADP antagonists to be effective in preventing vascular events in patients with angina and transient ischaemic attacks. They are also used for thromboprophylaxis in patients undergoing insertion of coronary stents and in coronary angioplasty. Ticlopidine is generally not preferred. **Prasugrel** is approved for patients with acute coronary syndrome. Compared to clopidogrel, prasugrel has a more rapid onset of action and more efficient platelet inhibition but the risk of bleeding exists.

Ticagrelor and **cangrelor** block ADP receptors P2Y12 and thereby inhibit platelet aggregation.They are approved for use in acute coronary syndrome but bleeding should be watched for.

Glycoprotein IIb/IIIa Receptor Antagonists

Fibrinogen, vitronectin, fibronectin and von Willebrand factor bind to glycoprotein IIb/IIIa receptor complex on the platelets and mediate platelet aggregation by platelet agonists like thrombin, collagen and TXA_2. Thus their receptor complex acts as final common pathway for platelet aggregation. Drugs that block these receptors inhibit platelet aggregation induced by all platelet agonists.

Abciximab is a monoclonal antibody which binds GP IIb/IIIa receptor complex and inhibits platelet aggregation. It can cause bleeding and rarely—allergic reactions. It is used parenterally in patients undergoing coronary angioplasty and other percutaneous coronary intervention and in acute coronary syndromes. Abciximab is given along with aspirin and heparin, it reduces the incidence of restenosis and its consequences. Abciximab is expensive.

Eptifibatide and **tirofiban** are peptides given as IV infusion. They bind to the IIb/IIIa receptors and block them. Orally effective IIb/IIIa inhibitors are being developed. They are short acting and are tried in unstable angina and myocardial infarction as alternatives to abciximab.

Others

- *Epoprostenol* (PGI_2) can be used during haemodialysis to prevent platelet aggregation and platelet loss, as an alternative to heparin in patients in whom heparin is contraindicated. It is directly injected into the dialysis circuit. Epoprostenol has a short t½ of 2 of 3 minutes and is, therefore, given as infusion but can also be given SC. The other indications are severe pulmonary hypertension and circulatory shock since PGI_2 is also a potent vasodilator.
- *Cilostazol* is a phosphodiesterase III inhibitor. It has vasodilator and antiplatelet aggregatory properties. It is used in intermittent claudication as it increases pain-free walking distance.
- *Ridogrel:* Drugs like ridogrel that have dual actions of blocking thromboxane A_2 receptor and also inhibiting the synthesis of TXA_2, are found to be useful in selectively inhibiting thromboxane synthesis and enhancing PGI_2 synthesis. They are in different stages of development.

Uses of Antiplatelet Drugs

1. **Ischaemic heart diseases:** Thromboprophylaxis helps in preventing the formation of clot and thereby prevent MI.
   a. *Myocardial infarction:* 300 mg aspirin is given immediately after MI to reduce the risk of reinfarction, improve survival and reduce mortality. Clopidogrel or abciximab may be used along with aspirin or as alternatives to it. In post- MI patients, long-term low-dose aspirin (75–150 mg daily) is continued to prevent reinfarction after thrombolytic therapy.
   b. *Unstable angina:* Aspirin reduces the risk of acute MI. Aspirin 150 mg daily is given with heparin and then later with warfarin.
   c. *Stable angina pectoris:* All patients with coronary artery disease including angina would require prophylaxis with 75 to 150 mg aspirin daily to prevent MI.
2. **Cardiac procedures:** Following coronary artery angioplasty, stenting and coronary bypass grafting, aspirin is used either alone or in combination with clopidogrel or abciximab to reduce the risk of reocclusion. Heparin is used along with antiplatelet drugs in coronary angioplasty.
3. **Atrial fibrillation:** If oral anticoagulants cannot be used, antiplatelet drugs may be given.
4. **Prosthetic heart valves:** Formation of microthrombi on the artificial heart valves is an expected risk—emboli can also develop. In order to prevent these complications, aspirin or dipyridamole may be combined with warfarin.
5. **Cerebrovascular disease:** Transient cerebral ischaemic attacks called 'mini-strokes' require thromboprophylaxis. Aspirin reduces the incidence of stroke in them. In cerebral thrombosis patients, long-term use of antiplatelet drugs prevents recurrence. Aspirin may be combined with dipyridamole for a synergistic effect. Clopidogrel is also effective.
6. **Vascular grafts:** To prevent occlusion and maintain patency of the vascular grafts, antiplatelet drugs are used.
7. **Peripheral vascular disease:** Antiplatelet drugs are used for thromboprophylaxis in intermittent claudication.
8. **Haemodialysis:** Epoprostenol (PGI_2) is injected into the blood entering the

dialysis unit in order to prevent platelet aggregation and thereby thrombus formation during haemodialysis and in haemofiltration.

9. **Pulmonary hypertension:** Epoprostenol is used in both primary and secondary pulmonary hypertension.

COAGULANTS

Coagulants are drugs that promote coagulation (procoagulants) and control bleeding. They are also called **haemostatics.** They may be used locally or systemically. Local haemostatics are called **styptics.** Physical methods like application of pressure, tourniquet or ice can control bleeding.

Styptics are local haemostatics that are used on bleeding sites like tooth socket and wounds. They are:

1. **Adrenaline:** Sterile cotton soaked in 1:10,000 solution of adrenaline is commonly used in tooth sockets and as nasal packs for epistaxis. Adrenaline arrests bleeding by vasoconstriction.
2. **Thrombin** powder is dusted over the bleeding surface following skin grafting. It is obtained from bovine plasma.
3. **Fibrin** obtained from human plasma is available as sheets. It is used for covering or packing bleeding surfaces.
4. **Gelatin foam** is porous spongy gelatin used with thrombin to control bleeding from wounds. It gets completely absorbed in 4 to 6 weeks and can be left in place after suturing of the wound.
5. **Thromboplastin powder** is used in surgery as a styptic.
6. **Astringents,** like tannic acid, are used on bleeding gums.

Coagulants used Systemically

Vitamin K

Vitamin K is a fat-soluble vitamin essential for the biosynthesis of clotting factors. There are three compounds: Vitamin K_1—present in food from plant source, vitamin K_2—produced in the gut by bacteria and vitamin K_3—a synthetic compound used therapeutically.

Actions: Vitamin K is essential for the biosynthesis of clotting factors—prothrombin and factors VII, IX and X by the liver.

Vitamin K deficiency results from liver diseases, malabsorption, long-term antibiotic therapy and rarely by dietary deficiency. It is manifested as bleeding tendencies.

Adverse reactions are seen on parenteral administration—allergic reactions and jaundice can occur.

Uses

1. Vitamin K deficiency—may result from various causes. Dietary deficiency is uncommon. Prolonged use of antibacterials destroy the intestinal flora leading to vitamin K deficiency. Malabsorption syndrome, prolonged parenteral nutrition, obstructive jaundice and liver disease all result in vitamin K deficiency and require adequate vitamin K supplementation—5–10 mg/day orally or parenterally till the dificiency is corrected. INJEK 1 mg inj (phytomenadione)
2. *Newborn babies* lack intestinal flora and have low levels of prothrombin and other clotting factors. Routine administration of vitamin K (1 mg IM) prevents haemorrhagic disease of the newborn.
3. Oral anticoagulant toxicity.

Other Coagulants

Fresh plasma or whole blood are useful in most coagulation disorders as they contain all the clotting factors. Other concentrated plasma fractions like fibrinogen, factors II, VII, VIII, IX and X are available for the treatment of specific deficiencies.

Fibrinogen obtained from pooled human plasma is used to control bleeding in haemophilia, antihaemophilic globulin (AHG) deficiency and acute afibrinogenemic states.

Antihaemophilic factor obtained from pooled human plasma or from recombinant DNA technology is used in haemophiliacs and in AHG deficiency to control bleeding episodes.

Desmopressin: An analog of vasopressin increases factor VIII and von Willebrand factor levels by 3–5 folds in patients with mild haemophilia A and in von Willebrand's disease. It normalizes the bleeding time in patients with congenital defects of platelet function and is also useful in bleeding secondary to other conditions like uremia and NSAID-induced bleeding. Adverse effects include flushing, headache, tachycardia, water retension, mild hypertension and hyponatraemia.

Ethamsylate reduces capillary bleeding probably by increasing capillary wall stability by an anti-hyaluronidase activity. It may correct abnormal platelet adhesion and promote platelet aggregation by inhibition of PGI_2 synthesis. Ethamsylate is used to arrest or prevent bleeding in PPH, menorrhagia, epistaxis, after tooth extraction and in similar indications as tranexamic acid. It does not stabilize fibrin and, therefore, has no antifibrinolytic activity. Ethamsylate may be given orally and by IV inj.

Preparations and dose: 250–500 mg tab TDS

Pause, Ethamsyl 250, 500 mg tab; 250 mg/2 ml inj.

Snake venom: Some snake venom like Russell's viper venom stimulate thrombokinase and promote coagulation.

SCLEROSING AGENTS

Sclerosing agents are irritant substances. They are injected locally to the varicose veins, oesophageal varices and into piles. They cause local inflammation and obliterate these veins. The compounds used are:

- *Sodium tetradecyl sulfate* is a detergent used as 3% solution for sclerotherapy SETROL 3% Inj.
- *Phenol 5%* in vegetable oil—2–5 ml is injected into the vein.
- *Ethanolamineoleate* 5%: 1–5 ml.
- *Polydocanol* 3% is a detergent—2 ml injection
- *Sodium linoleate:* 2–5 ml injection.

PLASMA EXPANDERS

When there is sudden loss of blood or plasma as seen in conditions like extensive bleeding, the gross reduction in blood volume results in underperfusion of tissues and can be rapidly fatal.

To restore the intravascular volume, the component that is lost should ideally be replaced like plasma in burns and blood after haemorrhage. However, in emergency, immediate volume replacement is important to maintain the blood pressure and tissue perfusion. In such situations, plasma expanders are used. These are high molecular weight substances which when infused IV exert osmotic pressure and remain in the body for a long time to increase the volume of circulating fluid. An ideal plasma expander should exert oncotic pressure comparable to plasma, be long-acting, non-antigenic and pharmacologically inert.

Plasma expanders include:

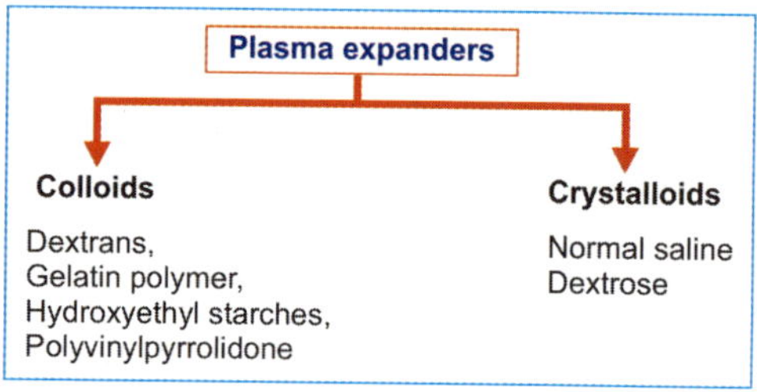

Colloids and crystalloids: Colloids are large molecules which on infusion, remain in the vascular system (unlike crystalloids) and are effective as plasma expanders. Colloids are more potent than crystalloids and are superior to them in maintaining plasma volume for longer periods. However, they are more expensive than crystalloids. **Crystalloids** are solutions that can pass through a semi-permeable membrane as against colloids which cannot do so. Normal saline and dextrose are some crystalloids (*see* page 348).

Dextrans (Dextran 70 mol wt 70,000 and dextran 40 mol wt 40,000) are polysaccharides obtained from sugar beet. Their osmotic pressure is similar to that of plasma proteins. Dextran 70 effectively expands the plasma volume which remains so for almost 24 hours. It interferes with coagulation, blood grouping and cross-matching. It is slowly excreted by glomerular filtration and partly metabolised over weeks by oxidation.

Dextran 40 is faster but shorter acting. It can improve microcirculation in shock by **preventing rouleax formation** of RBCs and have an **anti-sludging effect**. It can clog renal tubules resulting in renal failure—though rare should be watched for. Allergic reactions are common as dextrans are antigenic.

Dextrans have a long shelf-life (10 years) and can be easily sterilized. Dextrans are the commonly used plasma expanders and of the two, dextran 70 is more commonly used.

Dextran—70: LOMODEX 70, 500 ml in normal saline or 5% DEXTROSE.

Gelatin products like degraded gelatin polymer (polygeline) have a mol wt of 30,000 and a duration of action of 12 hours. Gelatin polymers can remain stable for almost 3 years at a pH of 7.2–7.3. They do not interfere with coagulation, blood grouping and cross-matching. They are not antigenic and can rarely cause urticaria, allergic reactions and bronchospasm. Degraded gelatin polymer is a polypeptide. It has a long shelf life and is excreted gradually by the kidneys. It is used for priming the heart-lung and dialysis machines.

HAEMACCEL, SERACCEL 500 ml; 100 ml contains gelatin Polymer 3.5 g along with electrolytes.

Hydroxyethyl starch (hetastarch) starch maintains blood volume for a long period. Hetastarch is a mixture of 90% amylopectin of different molecular sizes with an average molecular weight of 4.5 lakhs. Used as 6% solution for infusion, it expands blood volume and stabilizes it for almost 24 hr. Smaller molecules are excreted faster than the larger ones and the larger ones may have a longer t½ of up to 17 days. Hetastarch accelerates erythrocyte sedimentation. It does not interfere with coagulation.

Adverse effects are fever, chills (flu-like symptoms) vomiting, anaphylactoid reactions with urticaria and bronchospasm; other allergic reactions are rare.

EXPAN 6% inj in 100 ml, 500 ml.

Hetastarch may be used in shock to expand the plasma volume, in burns and other conditions associated with extensive fluid loss.

Polyvinylpyrrolidone (PVP): It is a synthetic, water-soluble polymer used as a 3.5% solution. It is partly excreted through the kidneys and part of it is stored in reticuloendothelial cells, Kupfer cells in liver, skeletal muscles and skin for a long period. PVP binds penicillin and insulin in the plasma. It is not preferred due to various disadvantages like—it provokes histamine release and interferes with blood grouping.

OSMOPLASMA 3.5% solution in normal saline.

Human albumin is obtained from pooled human plasma. It is given as 5% or 20% solution. 100 ml of the 20% solution is osmotically equivalent to 800 ml of whole blood. It is nonantigenic, does not interfere with coagulation, blood grouping or cross-matching. It also does not carry the risk of transmitting serum hepatitis as the preparation is heat treated. It is expensive.

Human albumin is used in oedema, burns, hypovolaemic shock, hypoproteinaemia, acute liver failure and in dialysis. Allergic reactions and fever can occur though rarely.

ALBUMED 5%, 20% inj, ALBUPAN 50, 100 ml inj.

Uses of Plasma Expanders

These are used as plasma substitutes in hypovolaemic shock, burns and in extensive fluid loss—as an emergency measure to restore plasma volume.

Contraindications

Plasma expanders are contraindicated in cardiac failure, pulmonary oedema, renal failure and severe anaemia.

Clinical Pharmacology

- LMW heparins are superior to standard heparin as anticoagulants. Though they are expensive, in practice cost works out to be only slightly more than heparin because of the repeated aPTT monitoring required for standard heparin.
- Low dose aspirin (75–150 mg) is the most commonly used antiplatelet drug.
- The only conditions where a combination of clopidogrel + aspirin is required are acute coronary syndrome, post-MI and coronary angioplasty.
- In presence of acid peptic disease, clopidogrel is better tolerated than aspirin.
- Ticlopidine is not preferred due to adverse effects—it is presently out of market.
- In using anticoagulants, drug interactions should be taken care of as they are very common clinically, particularly warfarin + NSAIDs → haematemesis.
- Streptokinase is the fibrinolytic used in India due to its low cost while in developed countries, tenecteplase is used because of better efficacy but is more expensive.

[1] From Medical Council of India, *Competency based Undergraduate Curriculum for the Indian Medical Graduate*, 2018;1:136–144.

Unit VIII

Cardiovascular System

CHAPTER 24

Renin-Angiotensin-Aldosterone System and other Vasoactive Peptides

Competency achievement: The student should be able to:

PH 1.26 Describe mechanisms of action, types, doses, side effects, indications and contraindications of the drugs modulating the renin-angiotensin and aldosterone system.[1]

ANGIOTENSIN

Angiotensins are peptides synthesized from the precursor angiotensinogen. Angiotensinogen, a circulating protein synthesized in the liver is converted sequentially to angiotensin I (Ang I), angiotensin II (Ang II) and angiotensin III (Fig. 24.1). The enzymes involved are also depicted in Fig. 24.1.

Angiotensin-converting enzyme (ACE) which catalyses the conversion of Ang I to Ang II is widely distributed in the body. It is present in blood vessels, kidneys, heart, brain, lungs, adrenals and other tissues. Angiotensin II, the most potent angiotensin acts through angiotensin receptors (AT_1 and AT_2) present on the tissues. The plasma renin levels (t½–5 min) determine the generation of Angiotensin II. Angiotensin I is rapidly converted to angiotensin II. Angiotensin II has a short t½ of 1 min and is converted to angiotensin III which is much less potent than angiotensin II, but has similar biological actions. Angiotensin II (AngII) and angiotensin III act as stimuli for secretion of aldosterone from the adrenal cortex. Angiotensin IV is the smallest biological peptide which produces its effects on the CNS and periphery and the effects are different from angiotensin II. There are

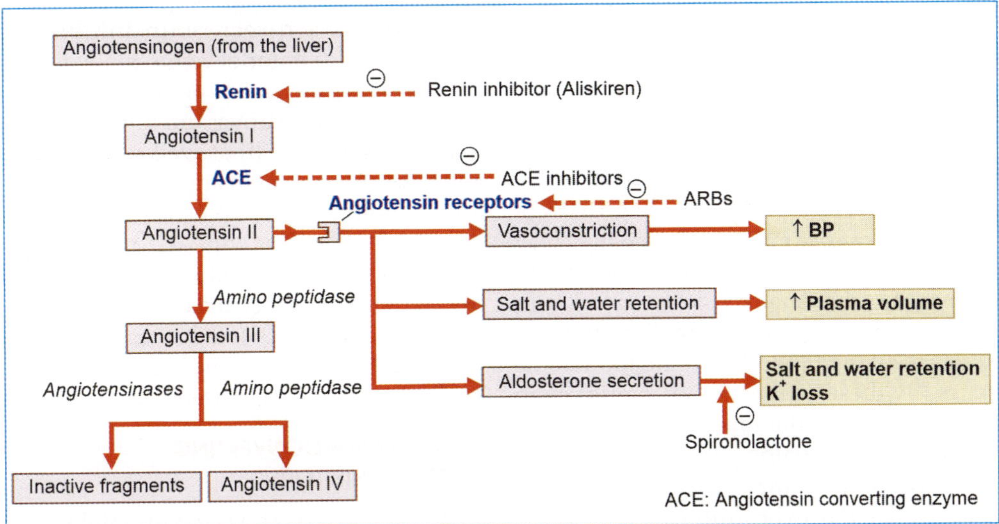

Fig. 24.1: Synthesis and metabolism of angiotensins and drugs acting at various sites

additional local renin-angiotensin systems in tissues like the heart, brain, and kidneys which generate Ang-II.

Angiotensin receptors: Ang-II brings about its effects by acting on angiotensin receptors which are G-protein-coupled receptors. There are of two types—AT_1 and AT_2.

AT_1 receptors are present in the vascular and myocardial tissue, brain, kidney and adrenal glomerular cells, mediate their effects through different transducer mechanisms in different tissues. In the vascular and other smooth muscle cells, it is the phospholipase C, IP_3/DAG pathway which mediates the effects of AT_1 receptors. Activation of AT_1 receptors mediates vasoconstriction, growth and hypertrophy of the myocardium. AT_2 receptors mediate the effects almost opposite to that of AT_1 receptors—they inhibit cell growth and hypertrophy, promote vasodilation and myocardial fibrosis.

AT_2 receptors are present in the brain, vascular endothelium, kidney and in the foetal tissue. However, the significance of AT_2 receptors is not clearly known and all the major actions of angiotensin are mediated through the AT_1 receptors.

Actions

Angiotensin II causes vasoconstriction resulting in increased blood pressure. It stimulates the synthesis of aldosterone by the adrenal cortex, increases sodium reabsorption by the kidneys and increases the secretion of vasopressin. Angiotensin II also promotes the growth of vascular and cardiac muscle cells and may play a role in the development of cardiac hypertrophy as in hypertension. Angiotensin II also enhances the permeability of the endothelium in large arteries resulting in fluid accumulation in the tissues. By these actions, renin–angiotensin system regulates the fluid and electrolyte balance as well as blood pressure.

Angiotensin II increases the force of contraction of the myocardium by promoting the influx of calcium. Angiotensin II can also stimulate the sympathetic system and increase myocardial contractility. It promotes the growth of cardiac muscle cells and is involved in the enhancement of vascular intimal thickness. These actions over a long period play an important role in the development of myocardial hypertrophy and remodelling in long-standing hypertension. The ventricular remodelling that follows myocardial infarction is also brought about by Angiotensin II.

Other Actions

Angiotensin II contracts many other smooth muscle cells, enhances the synthesis and release of aldosterone from the adrenal cortex. Promotes Na^+/H^+ exchange resulting in sodium and water retension and acting centrally, it induces ADH release.

Drugs that Interfere with Renin–Angiotensin–Aldosterone System

Drugs that interfere with renin–angiotensin–aldosterone system (RAAS) include:

- Direct renin inhibitors
- Angiotensin-converting enzyme inhibitors
- Angiotensin receptor blockers.

DIRECT RENIN INHIBITORS

Aliskiren is a direct renin inhibitor—a competitive inhibitor of renin, binds to renin and prevents the action of angiotensinogen. Ang I and its derivatives are not formed and Ang I, Ang II, Ang III as well as aldosterone levels fall. Hence renin angiotensin system is inhibited at a higher level. Some natriuresis occurs and BP falls as with ACE inhibitors and ARBs. Aliskiren also reduces left ventricular hypertrophy. It is approved for use in hypertension (*see* page 338). Other uses are under evaluated. It is contraindicated in diabetic nephropathy, pregnancy and renal failure.

ANGIOTENSIN-CONVERTING ENZYME INHIBITORS

Angiotensin-converting enzyme inhibitors are drugs that prevent the convertion of Ang-I to

Ang-II by inhibiting the ACE. Captopril was introduced in 1977 and was followed by several of them including **enalapril**, **lisinopril**, **ramipril**, **benazepril**, **fosinopril** and **quinapril**.

Pharmacological Actions

Administration of ACE inhibitors reduces the blood pressure due to a reduction in peripheral arterial resistance. The fall in BP is due to inhibition of Ang II formation and to raised bradykinin levels. Bradykinin is a potent vasodilator metabolized by kininase II which we now know is the same as ACE. Thus inhibition of ACE will prevent the degradation of bradykinin and contributes to the fall in BP. The reduction in BP is associated with a fall in plasma angiotensin II and aldosterone levels and an increase in plasma renin activity. The left ventricular hypertrophy is reversed. In patients with congestive heart failure, ACE inhibitors enhance cardiac output by a reduction in ventricular afterload.

Pharmacokinetics

ACE inhibitors are generally well-absorbed. **Except captopril and lisinopril** all others are prodrugs. They differ in their potency and pharmacokinetic properties like bioavailability, distribution, plasma t½ and excretion. Most ACE inhibitors are excreted through the kidney. Hence their dose should be reduced in renal dysfunction.

Adverse Effects

ACE inhibitors are well-tolerated by most patients. Adverse effects include:

1. ***Persistent dry cough:*** Due to increased bradykinin levels (20% incidence) is more common in women. It may require withdrawal of the ACE inhibitors. An angiotension II receptor antagonist may be used in such patients (see below).
2. ***Hypotension:*** On initiation of therapy, ACE inhibitors may cause significant hypotension—'first dose phenomenon'. Hence, treatment should be started with small doses and if patients are already on diuretics—temporarily diuretics should be stopped.
3. ***Hyperkalaemia:*** ACE inhibitors may cause hyperkalaemia particularly in patients on K^+ sparing diuretics, NSAIDs, beta blockers or with K^+ supplements. In other patients, hyperkalaemia is not very significant.
4. ***Dysgeusia:*** An altered taste sensation is more common with captopril—it is, however, reversible.
5. ***Angioneurotic oedema:*** ACE inhibitors can rarely cause (0.1% incidence) angio-oedema with swelling in the lips, nose, larynx and airway obstruction. It may be due to increased bradykinin levels and can be fatal. ACE inhibitors should be immediately withdrawn at the first sign of angio-oedema. Severe cases may need adrenaline and glucocorticoids.
6. ***Skin rashes:*** ACE inhibitors can occasionally cause skin rashes which are self-limiting.
7. ***Teratogenicity:*** Given during second and third trimesters of pregnancy, ACE inhibitors can cause various foetal malformations including foetal growth retardation, malformed lungs and even death. ACE inhibitors are, therefore contraindicated in pregnancy.

Mnemonic for ADR

Captopril **HAD SHOT A N**aughty **P**ig

Captopril: Cough
H: Hypotension
A: Angioedema
D: Dysgeusia
S: Skin rashes
H: Hyperkalemia
O: Others—nausea
T: Teratogenicity
A: Abdominal pain
N: Neutropenia
P: Proteinuria

8. ***Other effects:*** They can cause headache, nausea, abdominal pain, proteinuria and rarely, neutropenia. **Neutropenia** is more common in patients with collagen diseases and should be watched for. ACE inhibitors can precipitate acute renal failure in patients with renal artery stenosis.

Uses

1. *Hypertension:* ACE inhibitors are presently the first-line antihypertensives and are useful in the treatment of hypertension of all grades due to all causes (*see* page 337).
2. *Congestive cardiac failure:* ACE inhibitors are now considered the first-line drugs in chronic heart failure (*see* page 353)
3. *Myocardial infarction:* ACE inhibitors started within 24 hr and given for several weeks prevent the development of CCF and reduce mortality. In post-MI patients, ACE inhibitors are used to reduce the long-term mortality and prevent ventricular remodelling and development of cardiac failure.
4. *Prophylaxis in coronary artery disease:* In patients who are at a high risk of ischaemic cardiovascular conditions like MI and stroke, ACE inhibitors are protective and afford significant benefit by reducing the risk of MI, stroke, heart failure, diabetes and sudden death. They are useful to prevent reinfarction in post-myocardial infarction.
5. *Diabetic nephropathy:* Studies have shown that in patients with diabetic nephropathy, long-term treatment with an ACE inhibitor prevents the progression of renal disease and retards the worsening of renal function. They reduce albuminuria, intraglomerular pressure and check hyperfiltration.
6. *Chronic renal failure:* CRF—due to causes other than diabetes also responds to ACE inhibitors which delay the progression of the failure.
7. *Scleroderma renal crisis:* ACE inhibitors may be life saving in these patients. They prevent an increase in BP and deterioration of renal function.

Precautions and Contraindications

- Started with a low dose and gradually increased every 1–2 weeks to the required dose.
- ACE inhibitors are contraindicated in **pregnancy.**
- Should not be combined with K^+ sparing diuretics → cause hyperkalemia.
- At the first sign of angio-oedema, ACE inhibitors should be stopped.
- ACE inhibitors are contraindicated in patients with renal artery stenosis as they can cause renal failure in them.
- ACE inhibitors may increase the plasma levels of digoxin.

Individual ACE Inhibitors

After the introduction of captopril in 1977, several ACE inhibitors have been introduced. Their actions are similar but have minor pharmacokinetic differences and are as follows:

Captopril is absorbed rapidly from the gut, bioavailability 70%; food interferes with its absorption—hence should be given 1 hr before meals. It is largely excreted through the kidneys. Pharmacokinetic properties (Table 24.1).

Enalapril is a prodrug converted to enalaprilat in the liver. It is devoid of the sulfhydryl group. Enalapril is more potent and longer acting; food does not interfere with its absorption and first dose phenomenon is milder (since it is a prodrug). For the same reason, the onset of action is also slower. It is largely excreted through the kidneys and dose reduction is required in renal dysfunction. Dysguisea and leukopenia are less frequent (*see* Compare and Contrast—Captopril and Enalapril).

Lisinopril does not require activation in the body (not a prodrug). Absorption is slow and duration of action is >24 hr. It is excreted unchanged by the kidneys.

Table 24.1: Pharmacological features of some ACE inhibitors

Drug	*Active/metabolite*	*Bioavailability*	*Duration of action (hr)*	*Daily dose*
Catropril	Active	65–70%	6–12	25–50 mg BD-TDS
Enalapril	Enalaprilat	45–50%	22–24	2.5–20 mg OD
Lisinopril	Active	20–25%	>24	5–40 mgOD
Ramipril	Ramiprilat	55–50%	>24	1.25–10 mg OD
Fosinopril	Fosiniprilat	25–30%	12–24	10–60 mg OD
Perindopril	Perindoprilat	15–20%	>24	2–8 mg OD

Perindopril is converted (20% of the dose) to the active compound perindoprilat in the body.

Ramipril is a long-acting ACE inhibitor which is widely distributed in the tissues because of its high lipophilicity. Since it is bound to the tissues and is slowly released from them, the active compound ramiprilat has a long t½.

Trandolapril is converted to trandolaprilat and has a long duration of action. Other ACE inhibitors like **fosinopril, imidapril, cilazepril, quinapril and zofenopril** share similar properties.

ANGIOTENSIN RECEPTOR BLOCKERS (ARBs)

Drugs that block the angiotensin receptors antagonise the effects of angiotensin II.

Losartan was the first orally effective AT_1 receptor antagonist to be developed. Of the two subtypes of angiotensin II receptors, AT_1 receptors are present in vascular and myocardial tissue, brain, kidney and adrenal glomerular cells. Losartan has a high affinity for AT_1 receptors when compared to AT_2 receptors, and blocks the effects of angiotensin II. It, therefore, relaxes vascular smooth muscles, promotes salt and water excretion and reduces plasma volume. Losartan is thus a selective competitive blocker of AT_1 angiotensin receptors, binds firmly to the receptor and dissociates slowly from it.

The affinity of Losartan is 1000 times and valsartan 20,000 times more for AT_1 receptors than AT_2. By blocking the effects of angiotensin II, ARBs relax the vascular smooth muscles, promote salt and water excretion and reduce plasma volume. Thus there is a decrease in peripheral vascular resistance, and reduced cardiac output (due to reduced venous return). On long-term administration of ARBs, plasma renin activity increases.

COMPARE AND CONTRAST

Captopril and Enalapril

Features	***Captopril***	***Enalapril***
Chemistry	Contains sulfhydryl group	Contains carboxyl group
Drug status	Active	Prodrug (enalaprilat)
Potency	Less	More
Bioavailability	65–70%	45–50%
Peak effect in	1 hr	4–6 hr
Duration of action	6–12 hr	22–24 hr
Absorption	Food interferes	Food does not interfere
Dysguisea	Fairly common	Uncommon

Advantages of ARBs over ACE Inhibitors

1. The main advantage of ARBs over ACE inhibitors is that there is **no increase in bradykinin levels** and its associated adverse effects like dry cough and angio-oedema.
2. Losartan is also a competitive antagonist of thromboxane A_2 and **inhibits platelet aggregation**. A metabolite of losartan reduces cyclooxygenase dependent PG synthesis.
3. In addition to reducing BP, ARBs also **reduce the proliferation** of arteriolar intima.
4. Reduction in Ang II synthesis by ACE inhibitors may stimulate the formation of **Ang II by alternative pathways** (e.g. by chymase) leading to blunting of their efficacy. ARBs do not have this disadvantage since they block the receptors. However, the significance of this in a clinical setting is not yet known.

Pharmacokinetics

Several ARBs have been synthesized with minor pharmacokinetic variations apart from differences in their affinity for the AT_1 receptors. They are candesartan, irbesartan, valsartan, telmisartan, eprosartan and olmesartan **(sartans)**.

ARBs are all given orally. Their bioavailability is generally <50%. Losartan is partly converted in the liver to a metabolite which is 10–20 times more potent and longer acting than losartan. They are all extensively protein bound; excretion is mostly through the gut and to a minor extent by the kidneys.

Losartan Dose: 25–50 mg OD. LOSAR 2, 50, 100 mg tab. NUSAR 25, 50 mg tab

Candesartan Dose: 8 mg OD CANDELONG 4, 8, 16 mg tab. CANDESAR 4, 8 mg tab.

Telmisartan Dose: 20–80 mg OD. TELISTA 20, 40 mg tab. TELSOR 20, 40, 80 mg tab.

Valsartan Dose: 80–160 mg OD. VALZAAR 20, 40, 80 mg tab

Adverse Effects

ARBs are well tolerated. They can cause hypotension and hyperkalaemia like ACE inhibitors. Angio-oedema is rare. Weakness, headache, dizziness and epigastric distress are reported occasionally but are mild.

ARBs are contraindicated in pregnancy because of their teratogenic potential.

Uses of ARBs

1. *Hypertension:* ARBs are used in the treatment of hypertension in similar indications as that of ACE inhibitors—as alternatives to ACE inhibitors. They can be considered as first-line drugs in hypertension. Losartan, candesartan and irbesartan are available in India. ARBs can be usefully combined with diuretics.
2. *Cardiac failure:* ARBs may be used as alternatives to ACE inhibitors in cardiac failure, i.e. in patients who poorly tolerate ACE inhibitors. The therapeutic benefits are comparable to enalapril. Some studies show captopril to be more effective in reducing mortality in heart failure patients. However, another trial using valsartan showed it to be as effective as captropril in patients with MI complicated by heart failure. With the available data, ACE inhibitors are now the first-line drugs in cardiac failure and ARBs are reserved for patients who are unable to tolerate an ACE inhibitor.
3. *Diabetes mellitus with renal dysfunction:* ARBs are considered to be '**reno-protective**' in patients with type 2 diabetes mellitus. They prevent or delay the development of renal failure in such patients and ARBs are now considered the drugs of choice in them.
4. *Prevention of stroke:* Clinical trials have shown that in hypertensive patients with LV hypertrophy, ARBs have reduced the risk of stroke.
5. *Atrial fibrillation:* Irbesartan has been shown to maintain cardiac rhythm in patients with chronic atrial fibrillation.

6. *Portal hypertension:* Losartan has been found to be safe and effective in patients with portal hypertension and cirrhosis. Hence, it is now recommended in these patients.

OTHER VASOACTIVE SUBSTANCES

Several vasoactive peptides are released in the body which influence the vascular tone under different circumstances. Many of them have been identified and their role in the maintenance of homeostasis is being explored. Several agonists and antagonists are being developed. Vasoactive peptides include:

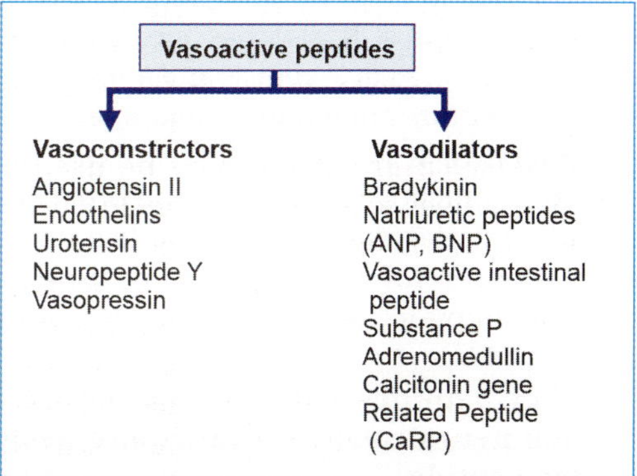

Some of them which are likely to be of pharmacological importance are discussed below.

Vasoconstrictors

Endothelins (ET) secreted by the vascular endothelial cells are the most **powerful vasoconstrictors.** Three isoforms of the peptide are ET-1, ET-2 and ET-3. ET-1 present mostly in the vascular endothelium, ET-2 in the intestines and kidneys while ET-3 is present in the brain.

Synthesis and release of endothelins occurs in response to various vasoconstrictor substances released during injury and inflammation—like cytokines, thrombin, angiotensin II and growth factors. There are 2 types of **endothelin receptors**—ET_A and ET_B. Responses mediated through ET_A receptors include vasoconstriction, bronchoconstriction and aldosterone secretion while ET_B is mostly present in the brain and to some extent in other organs.

Pathophysiological Role

Endothelins are involved in the:

- Control of the **vascular** tone and peripheral vascular resistance.
- Release of various hormones like aldosterone, adrenaline, atrial natriuretic peptide, hypothalamic and pituitary hormones and in thyroglobulin synthesis.
- Maintaining uteroplacental blood flow.
- Genesis of several cardiovascular diseases, bronchial asthma and pulmonary hypertension.
- They may have a role in cerebral, coronary and renal vasospasm.
- An endothelin antagonist **Bosentan** has been found to be useful in the treatment of pulmonary hypertension but may cause hepatotoxicity and is teratogenic.
- **Sitasextan** and **ambisextan** are analogs of bosentan with similar properties. Other endothelin receptor antagonists are being developed for use in pulmonary hypertension, hypertension and other cardiovascular disorders.

Urotensin II is a powerful vasoconstrictor, acts on urotensin (UT) receptors present on the vascular smooth muscles, heart, brain and spinal cord. Antagonists of UT receptors have been found to be of value in cardiac failure, diabetes and renal diseases and are under development.

Vasodilators

Kinins are vasodilator peptides formed from the precursor kininogen by the action of the enzymes called kallikreins. Kallikreins are present in the plasma, kidneys, pancreas, intestines, salivary glands and other tissues. (*Kallikreas* = Pancreas in Greek). Kinins include **bradykinin and kallidin**. They bring about their effects by acting on B_1 and B_2 receptors and both are G-protein-coupled receptors. Kinins are rapidly degraded by kininase II which is same as ACE (Fig. 24.1).

Actions: Kinins are potent vasodilators and cause a brief fall in BP. They stimulate contraction of other smooth muscles—thus they induce bronchospasm in asthmatics, slow contraction of intestines (Brady = slow) and uterus. Kinins mediate inflammation, and stimulate the pain nerve endings. They enhance vascular permeability and induce oedema. **Aprotinin** inhibits kallikrein and has been tried in acute pancreatitis. Bradykinin B_2 receptor antagonist **icatibant** is effective in hereditary angio-oedema. It has also been under evaluation for use in airway disease, ascites, drug-induced angio-oedema and pancreatitis.

Antagonists of B_1 receptors are under development.

Natriuretic Peptides

Atrial natriuretic peptide (ANP), brain natriuretic peptide (BNP) and C-type natriuretic peptide (CNP) are the endogenous natriuretic peptides. ANP is synthesized, stored and released mostly in the atrium, BNP in the brain and ventricles and CNP in the brain, kidneys and blood vessels. Mechanical stretch of the heart (as due to volume overload), exercise, sympathetic stimulation, glucocorticoids and vasopressin are some of the factors which trigger the ANP release.

The major effects of natriuretic peptides are: (i) to increase the excretion of sodium and water, (ii) relax the vascular smooth muscles leading to a fall in blood pressure and (iii) to inhibit the release of renin, aldosterone, ADH and endothelins. Natriuretic peptides antagonize the effects of the renin angiotensin system. The natriuretic peptides act on specific ANP receptors.

Nesiritide is recombinant human BNP which is a vasodilator and a diuretic. It has been tried in acute decompensated heart failure.

The peptides have a short half-life and are metabolized by neutral endopeptidases like neprilysin. **Sacubitril** is a **neprilysin inhibitor** which enhances natriuretic peptide levels and is useful in heart failure (*see* page 357).

Other Peptides

Vasoactive intestinal peptide produces vasodilation in most vascular beds including coronary arteries. It also has inotropic and chronotropic effects. Agonists and antagonists of VIP receptors are under development.

Substance P is an arteriolar dilator but causes contraction of intestinal and bronchial smooth muscles. **Aprepitant,** an antagonist at the receptor for substance P, is used in chemotherapy-induced nausea and vomiting (*see* page 427).

Other peptides with **role in the CNS** include **neurotensin** and **calcitonin gene-related peptides**.

Clinical Pharmacology

- ACE inhibitors and ARBs are preferred drugs in diabetes with hypertension.
- ACE inhibitors have better efficacy than ARBs.
- Dry cough (20% incidence) is the commonest side effect of ACE inhibitors.
- To avoid first dose effect, all ACE inhibitors are started with low dose at night.
- They have been shown to postpone the onset of diabetes mellitus.

[1] From Medical Council of India, *Competency based Undergraduate Curriculum for the Indian Medical Graduate*, 2018;1:136–144.

CHAPTER 25

Calcium Channel Blockers

The discovery of the calcium channels in the cardiac myocyte helped in understanding the mechanisms involved in smooth muscle contraction. Calcium influx occurs during the contraction of cardiac and smooth muscle cells. Verapamil (synthesized in 1962) was the first agent found to have calcium channel blocking properties and many more drugs soon followed.

CALCIUM CHANNELS

There are four types of calcium channels.

1. **Voltage-gated calcium channels**—operated by membrane potential.
2. **Receptor-operated channels**—activated by agonists like adrenaline, noradrenaline, angiotensin II and some hormones which enhance calcium influx into the cells. The agonists also promote the release of Ca^{++} from the sarcoplasmic reticulum.
3. **Stretch-operated channels**—present in the blood vessels are sensitive to stretch and promote calcium influx when stretched. These are also called leak channels as small amounts of Ca^{+} leak into the resting cells, but it is pumped out by Ca^{++}ATPase.
4. A fourth type of channel, i.e. **Na^{+}-Ca^{++} exchange channel** which can operate in both directions, i.e. for influx and extrusion is also known.

Voltage-gated calcium channels are activated when the membrane potential drops to –40 mV or lower. There are 3 major subtypes of voltage-sensitive channels, viz. L, T and N type.

- *L type:* Long-lasting current/slow channels are present in **cardiac, smooth muscle** and endocrine cells as well as neurons.
- *T type:* Transient current/fast channel present in neurons and endocrine cells are blocked by drugs like ethosuximide and flunarizine.
- *N type:* Neural channel found in neurons is involved in neurotransmitter release.
- Two other subtypes P/Q and R are now known—present in nerve terminals and involved in the release of neurotransmitters.

The **L type** is the most common type and the rate of activation and inactivation of this channel is slow. It consists of the main α_1 subunit which encloses the calcium channel along with other subunits namely α_2, β, γ and δ.

Calcium channel blockers bind to the α_1 subunit and block the L type calcium channels. Dihydropyridines, verapamil and diltiazem bind to different sites on the α_1 subunit.

Calcium Channel Blockers (CCB)

Dihydropyridines (DHP)

Nifedipine	Nitrendipine
Nimodipine	Felodipine
Nisoldipine	Isradipine
Amlodipine	Lacidipine
Benidipine	Clevidipine
Nicardipine	

Others

Verapamil	Diltiazem

Mechanism of Action

The depolarisation of the cardiac and most smooth muscle cells depends on the entry of extracellular calcium into the cell through the calcium channels. Intracellular calcium is also increased by receptor-mediated action, i.e. agonist-induced calcium release—mediated by the second messenger IP_3. This calcium triggers the release of intracellular calcium from the sarcoplasmic reticulum. All these calcium ions are responsible for bringing about contraction of the cardiac and smooth muscle cells including the vascular smooth muscles.

Calcium channel antagonists inhibit the entry of calcium by blocking the L-type of calcium channels. The CCBs bind to both the open and inactivated state of Ca^{++} channels resulting in a decreased frequency of opening of the channels in response to depolarization. This decreases Ca^{++} current and Ca^{++} entry into the cardiac and vascular smooth muscle cells leading to relaxation. In the cardiac myocyte, the reduced Ca^{++} results in decreased cardiac contractility, heart rate and conduction velocity.

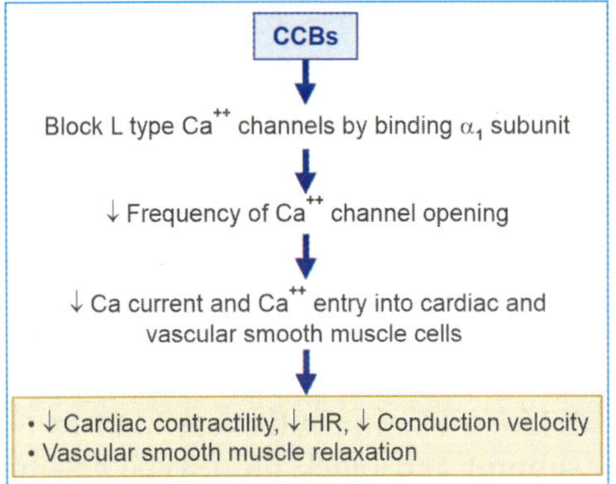

The CCBs also to some extent reduce the Ca^{++} influx through receptor-operated channels while other types of calcium channels poorly respond.

Actions

CCBs bring about the following effects:

1. *Smooth muscle:* The smooth muscle cells including vascular smooth muscles are relaxed by CCBs (Fig. 25.1).
   - *Vascular smooth muscle:* Vascular smooth muscles are very sensitive to the effects of CCBs. Relaxation of the arteriolar smooth muscles results in reduced peripheral vascular resistance and blood pressure. The effect on venous beds is not significant. Reflex tachycardia may occur with some CCBs like nifedipine. Dihydropyridine CCBs have prominent effects on the blood vessels compared to heart, i.e. they are vascular selective.

   Coronary circulation: CCBs dilate the coronary vessels, increasing the coro-

Table 25.1: Bioavailability, dose, route of administration and indications of CCBs

CCB	*Bioavailability*	*Dose and route*	*Indications*
Nifedipine	50–70%	5–20 mg TDS 10 mg SL	Angina, hypertension, Raynaud's phenomenon
Amlodipine	60–70%	5–10 mg OD	Hypertension, angina, coronary vasospasm
Felodipine	15–25%	5–10 mg OD	Hypertension, angina, Raynaud's phenomenon
Nicardipine	30–35%	20–40 mg TDS	Hypertension, angina, Raynaud's phenomenon
Isradipine	15–25%	2.5–10 mg BD	Hypertension, angina, Raynaud's phenomenon
Nitrendipine	10–30%	5–20 mg OD	Hypertension, angina, Raynaud's phenomenon
Nisoldipine	7–10%	20–40 mg OD	Hypertension
Nimodipine	12–35%	30–60 mg 4 hrly	Subarachnoid haemorrhage
Verapamil	20–35%	40–120 mg TDS 2.5–10 mg slow IV	Angina, coronary spasm, hypertension, migraine
Diltiazem	40–60%	30–60 mg QID 20 mg slow IV	Angina, coronary spasm, hypertension, Raynaud's phenomenon

Isoptin—what are you doing? 

Leela, a 40-year-old lady, was admitted for cardiac arrhythmias. She was prescribed isoptin (verapamil). The intern reported to the doctor that the patient's heart rate was not coming down and instead had severe tachycardia. When the medication was checked, it was found that the patient was receiving isoprin (isoprenaline) and not isoptin. This medication error was the reason for her tachycardia which was, however, brought to light before any mishap.

nary blood flow. Hence, they are useful in variant angina.

- *Other smooth muscles:* Gastrointestinal and bronchial smooth muscles are relaxed. CCBs relax the uterus for which they may be useful in premature labour.

2. *Heart:* Calcium influx plays a major role in contraction of the cardiac myocyte. CCBs interfere with the Ca^{++} influx through the Ca^{++} channels. They also delay the recovery of the channels. Thus they have a negative inotropic effect. They depress the myocardial contractility, reduce heart rate and in higher doses slow AV conduction. CCBs also decrease cardiac output particularly verapamil and diltiazem; the effects are dose dependent. They reduce cardiac work done and along with decreased PVR there is a decrease in myocardial oxygen consumption. Verapamil depresses the SA node. Verapamil, diltiazem and bepridil have more prominent cardiac effects than vascular effects when compared to DHPs.
3. *Skeletal muscles:* Because the skeletal muscle uses intracellular calcium for contraction and does not depend on calcium influx during depolarization, there is no skeletal muscle relaxation with CCBs.
4. *Other effects:*
   - Verapamil in high doses inhibits insulin release.
   - CCBs may interfere with platelet aggregation and prevent atheroma formation in animals but these effects have not been proved in humans.
   - Verapamil blocks the P-glycoprotein which is involved in the efflux of drugs out of cancer cells. Thus it may reverse the resistance of cancer cells to chemotherapy. Its clinical significance is yet to be established. Similarly, it may also have a role in reversing the resistance of malarial parasite to chloroquine.

Pharmacokinetics: CCBs are well absorbed but undergo extensive first pass metabolism, hence most have lower bioavailability. They are all

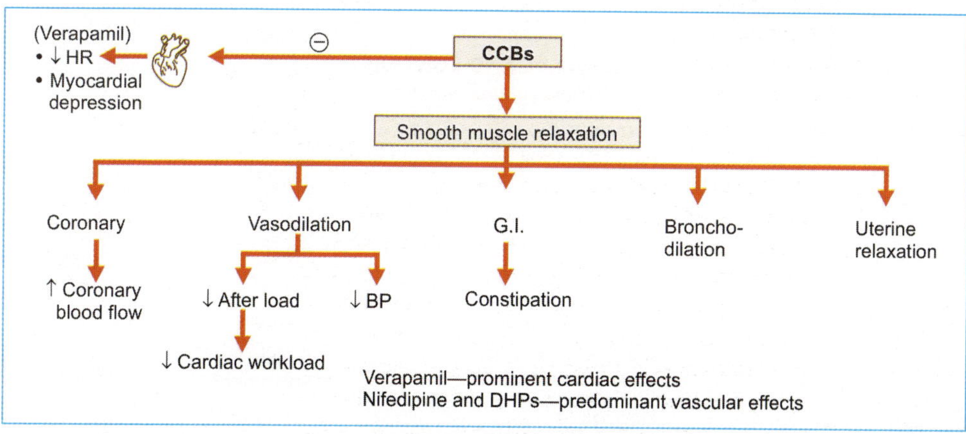

Fig. 25.1: Actions of CCBs

highly plasma protein bound (70–99%) and are metabolised in the liver. Onset of action is in 30–60 minutes after oral administration while on IV use the action is quick, e.g. verapamil peak effects are seen in 15 minutes.

Therapeutic Uses

1. *Ischaemic heart disease:*
   i. *Angina pectoris:* In chronic stable angina, verapamil and diltiazem are used for the prophylaxis. They decrease myocardial oxygen demand by a mild negative inotropic effect and decreased after load. They also inhibit exercise-induced tachycardia and cause coronary vasodilatation. Among the DHPs, amlodipine may be combined with beta blockers like atenolol because DHPs have a tendency to produce tachycardia and thereby worsen angina.
   ii. *Vasospastic angina:* Since CCBs are coronary vasodilators and relieve pain, they are considered the drugs of choice in variant angina. Though many DHPs have been tried, verapamil and amlodipine are the most commonly used CCBs in vasospastic angina.
   iii. *Unstable angina:* Verapamil may be used to reduce cardiac work load along with other lines of treatment in unstable angina (DHPs are contraindicated for the risk of reflex tachycardia).
2. *Hypertension:* Long-acting CCBs or sustained release preparations may be used in chronic hypertension. In hypertensive crisis, nifedipine is used sublingually or the capsule is bitten and swallowed. Amlodipine is the preferred agent because of its long half-life, good patient compliance and tolerability. CCBs are preferred in hypertension with low renin levels. Several studies have shown short-acting DHPs to have increased mortality due to fluctuating BP. Hence long-acting DHPs are to be used. CCBs are also suitable for combination with most other antihypertensives. However, verapamil should not be combined with β-blockers for the risk of significant cardiac depression.
3. *Arrhythmias:* Verapamil, diltiazem and bepridil have antiarrhythmic properties. Verapamil is used in PSVT and to control ventricular rate in atrial flutter or fibrillation. Verapamil, diltiazem and bepridil depress the SA and AV nodes, AV conduction and prolong the recovery of the Ca^{++} channels. They are employed to protect the ventricles from atrial tachyarrhythmias (because they depress AV conduction). IV verapamil and diltiazem

COMPARE AND CONTRAST

Verapamil and Nifedipine

Features	***Verapamil***	***Nifedipine***
Bioavailability	Poor (20–35%)	Good (50–70%)
Sublingual form	Not available	Available
t½	6 hr	4 hr
Effects on heart	Prominent	Weak
AV conduction	Depressed	No effect
Cardiac output	May be decreased	Increased
Cardiac contractility	May be decreased	Increased
Effects on vasculature	Mild	Prominent
Reflex tachycardia	Negligible	Prominent
Use in arrhythmias	Used	Not used

are also used in supraventricular tachyarrhythmias.

4. *Peripheral vascular diseases:* Nifedipine, felodipine and diltiazem can be used in Raynaud's disease for their vasodilator effects. Verapamil can increase the maximum walking ability in intermittent claudication (*see* page 371).
5. *Other uses*
   i. **Hypertrophic cardiomyopathy:** Verapamil produces beneficial effects. Verapamil improves diastolic function and exercise performance and relieves symptoms.
   ii. **Migraine:** Verapamil is useful for the prophylaxis of migraine.
   iii. **Subarachnoid haemorrhage:** Vasospasm that follows subarachnoid haemorrhage is believed to be responsible for neurological defects. As nimodipine brings about cerebral vasodilatation, it is used to treat neurological deficits in patients with cerebral vasospasm.

      Dose: 40–60 mg orally every 4–6 hr for 3 weeks.
   iv. **Atherosclerosis:** There are claims that dihydropyridines slow the progress of atherosclerosis. In postmyocardial infarction patients, verapamil reduces mortality and the risk of reinfarction.
   v. **Preterm labour:** Nifedipine inhibits uterine contractions and is found to be useful in delaying labour in premature uterine contractions.
   vi. **Cardiac transplantation:** Studies have shown that diltiazem suppresses the formation of post-transplant coronary atheroma.
   vii. **Diabetic nephropathy:** In type II diabetes patients, verapamil may be used as an alternative to an ACE inhibitor to slow the development of diabetic nephropathy because verapamil has a protective effect on the renal function and inhibits the development of harmful vascular changes.
   viii. **Smooth muscle hyperactivity:** CCBs are also found to be beneficial in conditions of smooth muscle hyperactivity as in achalasia. Verapamil is used in nocturnal leg cramps.

Individual CCBs

Verapamil has prominent myocardiac depressant action (negative inotropic effects), AV conduction is depressed. It does not cause reflex tachycardia. As it is a myocardiac depressant, usually, bradycardia is seen. Hence, it should not be combined with β-blockers. Fall in BP is mild as the vasodilator effect of verapamil is less potent.

Verapamil is almost completely absorbed on oral use but undergoes significant first pass metabolism; bioavailability is 20–35%.

Diltiazem has less potent vasodilator effects but is a myocardiac depressant though weaker than verapamil.

Adverse Effects

Verapamil and diltiazem produce constipation, bradycardia, heart block, hypotension and skin rashes. They may precipitate CCF in patients with diseased heart. Long-term use of CCBs can cause gum hyperplasia.

Dihydropyridine CCBs

Nifedipine is a potent vasodilator and causes a significant fall in BP and evokes reflex tachycardia.

Dihydropyridine CCBs block the Ca^{++} channels in the vascular smooth muscles at lower concentration than that needed to depress the heart. Hence they have weak myocardiac depressant effects. Nifedipine inhibits platelet aggregation. Smooth muscles of the bronchi, ureter and uterus are relaxed. Nifedipine can be given sublingually, orally and parenterally.

Adverse effects of nifedipine are headache, flushing, palpitation, dizziness, fatigue, hypotension, leg cramps and ankle oedema.

Other Dihydropyridines

Amlodipine

Advantages

- Amlodipine has a favourable pharmacokinetic profile.
- Completely absorbed
- First pass metabolism is milder and bioavailability is better (60–70%).
- Absorption is slow and steady hence plasma drug levels rise gradually without sudden alterations. Hence side effects like flushing, headache, dizziness and palpitation are much less compared to other DHPs.
- Has a **long t½** and is **suitable for once daily use**.

Because of above advantages amlodipine is a commonly used CCB.

Dose: 5–10 mg OD.

Nimodipine is highly lipid-soluble, crosses the BBB and selectively relaxes the cerebral blood vessels. Hence, it may be useful in patients with subarachnoid haemorrhage and haemorrhagic stroke.

Dose: 30–60 mg 4 hourly.

Nicardipine is highly vascular selective and brings about cerebral vasodilation, like nimodipine. It is a better coronary vasodilator compared to nifedipine and has been used by intravenous and intracerebral arterial infusion to prevent cerebral vasospasm in patients with stroke. It has a short t½ of 4 hr. Intra-arterial verapamil has also been used for this purpose.

Felodipine, nitrendipine and isradipine are similar to nifedipine with some pharmacokinetic variations. They have:

- Higher vascular selectivity,
- Longer acting → can be given once daily.

Lacidipine: It is highly lipid-soluble and has a high degree of vascular selectivity because it attains a higher concentration in the vascular smooth muscle. It is long acting and can be given once daily. It is used in the treatment of hypertension.

Benidipine: Dissociates slowly from the binding site on smooth muscle cell and is, therefore, longer acting. It is used in hypertension and angina.

Lercanidipine: It is a long-acting DHP given once daily in hypertension.

Clevidipine is a recently introduced CCB for IV infusion.

Drug Interactions

Verapamil + β blocker → ↑ Myocardial depression

1. Verapamil and diltiazem should be avoided in patients receiving beta-adrenergic blockers or other myocardiac depressants because the myocardiac depressant effects get added up.
2. Verapamil can precipitate digoxin toxicity by increasing digoxin levels (verapamil reduces digoxin excretion) by inhibiting digoxin transporter p-glycoprotein.

Verapamil → ↓ digoxin excretion → digoxin toxicity

3. Verapamil inhibits the microsomal enzyme CYP3A4 because of which it enhances the blood levels of statins, cyclosporin, theophylline, carbamazepine, sildenafil and ketoconazole.

Clinical Pharmacology

- All CCBs are generally well tolerated.
- Pedal oedema is the commonest side effect of all CCBs.
- Amlodipine is the commonly used CCB in hypertension.
- Diltiazem and verapamil are the commonly used CCBs in arrhythmias.
- In presence of depressed AV conduction, verapamil and diltiazem should be avoided, whereas nifedipine may be used safely.

CHAPTER 26

Antihypertensive Drugs and Drugs used in Shock

Competency achievement: The student should be able to:
PH 1.27 Describe the mechanisms of action, types, doses, side effects, indications and contraindications of antihypertensive drugs and drugs used in shock.[1]

Hypertension is an elevation of systolic and/or diastolic BP above 140/90 mm Hg. It is a common cardiovascular entity. Hypertension may be *primary* (essential) hypertension, where the cause is not known or *secondary*, when it is secondary to other conditions like renal, endocrine or vascular disorders.

As per Joint National Committee (JNC) guidelines on hypertension, blood pressure is graded as:

Category	*SBP mm Hg*		*DBP mm Hg*
Normal	<120	and	<80
Prehypertension	120–139	or	80–89
Hypertension, Stage 1	140–159	or	90–99
Hypertension, Stage 2	≥ 160	or	≥100

Key: SBP = systolic blood pressure; DBP = diastolic blood pressure

Blood pressure is determined by cardiac output (CO) and total peripheral vascular resistance (PVR). Blood pressure is controlled by baroreceptor reflexes acting through the autonomic nervous system along with renin-angiotensin-aldosterone system.

Prolonged hypertension damages the blood vessels of the heart, brain and the kidneys and may result in several complications like stroke, coronary artery disease or renal failure. Hence hypertension needs to be treated even though as such it does not generally produce obvious troublesome symptoms.

Antihypertensives act by influencing the BP regulatory systems, *viz.* the autonomic nervous system, renin-angiotensin system, calcium channels or sodium and water balance (plasma volume).

CLASSIFICATION

Antihypertensives may be classified as given below.

1. DIURETICS

Diuretics have been in use for the treatment of hypertension since several decades. The anti-hypertensive effects of diuretics are mild—

Antihypertensives may be classified as

Classification	
1. Diuretics	
• *Thiazides*	Hydrochlorothiazide, chlorthalidone, indapamide
• *Loop diuretics*	Frusemide, bumetanide, torsemide
• *K^+ sparing diuretics*	Spironolactone, amiloride, triamterene
2. Drugs acting on renin-angiotensin system	
• Angiotensin Converting Enzyme Inhibitors	Captopril, enalapril, lisinopril, ramipril, perindopril, fosinopril, trandolapril, quinapril, benazepril

Contd...

• Angiotensin II Receptor Blockers	Losartan, candesartan, valsartan, eprosartan, irbesartan, olmesartan
• Renin Inhibitor	Aliskiren
3. Sympatholytics	
• *Centrally acting drugs*	Clonidine, methyldopa, guanabenz, guanfacine
• *Ganglion blockers*	Trimethaphan
• *Adrenergic neuron blockers*	Guanethidine, reserpine
• *Adrenergic receptor blockers:*	
α-blockers	Prazosin, terazosin, doxazosin, phenoxybenzamine, phentolamine
β-blockers	Propranolol, atenolol, esmolol, metoprolol
Mixed α- and β-blockers	Labetalol, carvedilol
4. Ca^{++} channel blockers	Nifedipine, nicardipine, nimodipine, amlodipine, verapamil
5. Vasodilators	
• *Arteriolar dilators*	Hydralazine, minoxidil, diazoxide
• *Arteriolar and venular dilators*	Sodium nitroprusside

BP falls by 15–20 mm Hg over 2–4 weeks. Diuretics act as antihypertensives as follows:

Diuretics enhance the excretion of sodium and water resulting in reduced plasma volume → ↓ **CO**→ ↓ **BP.**

Though initially the fall in BP is due to reduced plasma volume and cardiac output, after continued treatment, by about 6–8 weeks, CO returns to normal due to **compensatory mechanisms.** It is then that the PVR declines. Reduction in body sodium stores results in low intracellular sodium levels. Such low sodium in vascular smooth muscle cells leads to relaxation of vasculature and decreased peripheral vascular resistance.

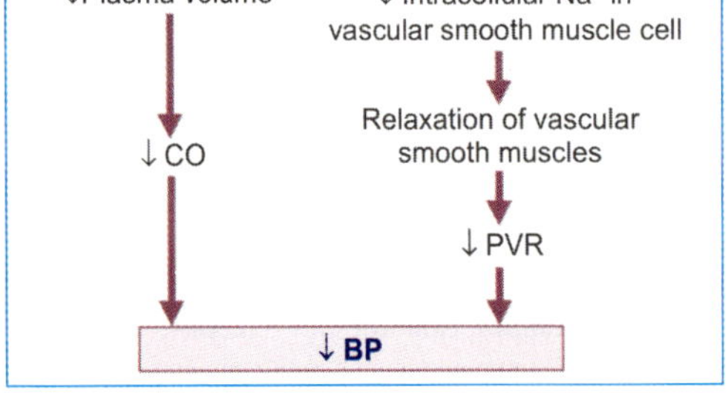

Diuretics in hypertension

Diuresis

Immediate effect: ↑ Na^+ and water excretion → ↓Plasma volume → ↓ CO → ↓ BP

Long-term use (6–8 weeks): ↓ Body sodium → ↓ Intracellular Na^+ in vascular smooth muscle cell → Relaxation of vascular smooth muscles → ↓ PVR → ↓ BP

Restriction of dietary salt intake will reduce the dose of the diuretic needed. On long-term treatment with diuretics, PVR is reduced but CO and heart rate are not altered.

Thiazides are the first-line antihypertensives and are inexpensive. An initial dose of 12.5 mg daily hydrochlorothiazide/ chlorthalidone is given. If the response is not adequate, the dose may be increased to a maximum of 25 mg daily. They may be combined with a K^+ sparing diuretic which is the best way to avoid hypokalaemia—1.25 mg amiloride with 12.5 mg hydrochlorothiazide (in the ratio 1:10). Thiazides may be used in combination with other antihypertensives particularly with those that cause salt and water retention as a side effect and the antihypertensive action is synergistic.

Indapamide is related to thiazides and is particularly useful in hypertension because it:

- **Lowers BP in subdiuretic doses.**
- May also have **additional vasodilator properties.**
- Can be administered **once daily**—long acting.
- Causes milder electrolyte disturbances.

Loop diuretics: Although loop diuretics, like frusemide, are powerful diuretics, their antihypertensive efficacy is low (weaker than thiazides). Frusemide is short acting and the loss of salt and water are compensated quickly by an increased reabsorption of Na^+ and water. Hence uniform reduction in vascular resistance cannot be achieved. Side effects like electrolyte disturbances are more profound with loop diuretics. They are used only in hypertension with chronic renal failure or congestive heart failure and in hypertensive crisis to rapidly lower the BP.

2. DRUGS ACTING ON RENIN ANGIOTENSIN ALDOSTERONE SYSTEM

Angiotensin-Converting Enzyme (ACE) Inhibitors

Angiotensin II is a powerful vasoconstrictor. Aldosterone also raises the BP by increasing the plasma volume (Fig. 26.1). ACE inhibitors prevent the formation of angiotensin II and (indirectly) aldosterone. There is vasodilation and decrease in PVR resulting in a fall in BP. ACE also degrades bradykinin and ACE inhibitors raise the bradykinin levels which is a potent vasodilator. This also contributes to the fall in BP.

The blood flow to the kidneys, brain and heart increases due to selective vasodilation and thus maintains adequate blood supply to these vital organs. For more detailed pharmacology of ACE inhibitors, *see* Chapter 24.

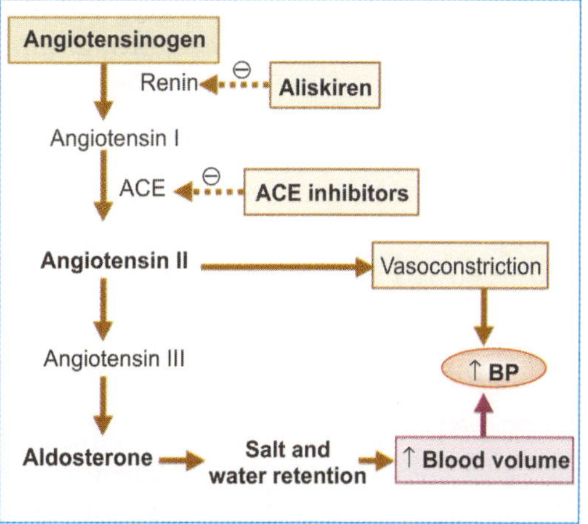

Fig. 26.1: Renin–angiotensin system

Status in Hypertension

- ACE inhibitors are presently the first-line antihypertensives.
- ACE inhibitors are useful in the treatment of hypertension of all grades due to all causes.
- Addition of a diuretic potentiates their antihypertensive efficacy. They are generally combined with thiazides without a K^+ sparing diuretic because there can be significant hyperkalaemia, when an ACE-I is combined, with a K^+ sparing diuretic.
- ACE inhibitors are well tolerated.
- They are specially indicated as antihypertensives in:
  a. Hypertension with left ventricular hypertrophy because hypertrophy is gradually reversed by ACE inhibitors.
  b. Patients with diabetes mellitus because ACE-I slow the development of nephropathy.
  c. Renal diseases with hypertension—ACE inhibitors slow the progression of chronic renal diseases like glomerulosclerosis.
  d. Patients with co-existing IHD including post-MI patients.
  e. In severe hypertension, they may be combined with other antihypertensives like β-blockers, CCBs or diuretics.

Angiotensin II Receptor Blockers (ARBs)

Losartan, candesartan, irbesartan, valsartan and telmisartan are some AT_1 receptor antagonists in clinical use (*see* page 325). There are 2 subtypes of angiotensin II receptors—AT_1 and AT_2. AT_1 receptors are present in vascular and myocardial tissue, brain, kidney and adrenal glomerular cells. ARBs have high affinity for AT_1 receptors when compared to AT_2 receptors. By blocking AT_1 receptors, ARBs block the effects of angiotensin II. They thus relax vascular smooth muscles, promote salt and water excretion and reduce the plasma volume.

The main advantage of ARBs over ACE inhibitors is that there is no increase in bradykinin levels and its associated adverse effects like dry cough and angio-oedema. ARBs are all given orally (Dose: Refer to Table 26.1).

Adverse effects: ARBs are well tolerated. They can cause hypotension and hyperkalaemia like ACE inhibitors. Angio-oedema is rare. ARBs are contraindicated in pregnancy because of their teratogenic potential.

Status in hypertension: ARBs are used in the treatment of hypertension in similar indications as that of ACE inhibitors as alternatives to ACE inhibitors. They can be considered as the first-line drugs in hypertension. Losartan, candesartan, irbesartan and olmesartan are available in India. ARBs can be usefully combined with diuretics.

Renin Inhibitor

Aliskiren is a direct renin inhibitor or renin antagonist that blocks the effects of renin, thereby reducing the blood pressure. Use of several drugs, like ACE inhibitors, ARBs and diuretics, tends to bring about a compensatory rise in the plasma renin levels. Because aliskiren blocks the effects of renin, its action is synergistic with these drugs. It can also be used as monotherapy and is orally effective. Aliskiren is contraindicated in pregnancy.

Adverse effects include hyperkalaemia, angio-oedema, hypotension, dizziness and rashes.

Dose: 150–300 mg OD, TEKTURNA ENALKIREN 100 mg.

3. SYMPATHOLYTICS

Sympatholytic drugs may be used to interfere with sympathetic activity at different levels including centrally, at the ganglia, neurons and receptors (Fig. 26.2).

Drugs Acting Centrally

Clonidine, an imidazoline derivative, is a selective α_2-agonist. Stimulation of α_2 autoreceptors in the CNS (in the vasomotor centre and hypothalamus) decreases central sympathetic outflow, blocks the release of noradrenaline from the nerve terminals leading to a fall in BP and bradycardia. There is a reduction in heart rate, cardiac output and a decrease in PVR but an increase in renal blood flow.

Clonidine is lipid-soluble and attains peak effect in 3–5 hr after oral administration. Dose is 100–300 micrograms twice daily. It is

Table 26.1: Dose and route of administration of some commonly used antihypertensives

Antihypertensives	*Daily dose*	*Routes*
Hydrochlorothiazide + amiloride	12.5–25 mg + 1.25–2.5 mg OD	Oral
Losartan	50 mg OD	Oral
Clonidine	100–300 μg	Oral
Methyldopa	250–500 mg BD-TDS	Oral
Atenolol	25–100 mg OD	Oral
Prazosin	2–20 mg OD	Oral
Hydralazine	25–50 mg q OD-TDS	Oral
Diazoxide	50–100 mg every 5–10 min	IV
Sodium nitroprusside	0.2–0.3 mg/min	IV
Nifedipine	10 mg 5–20 mg BD-TDS	SL Oral

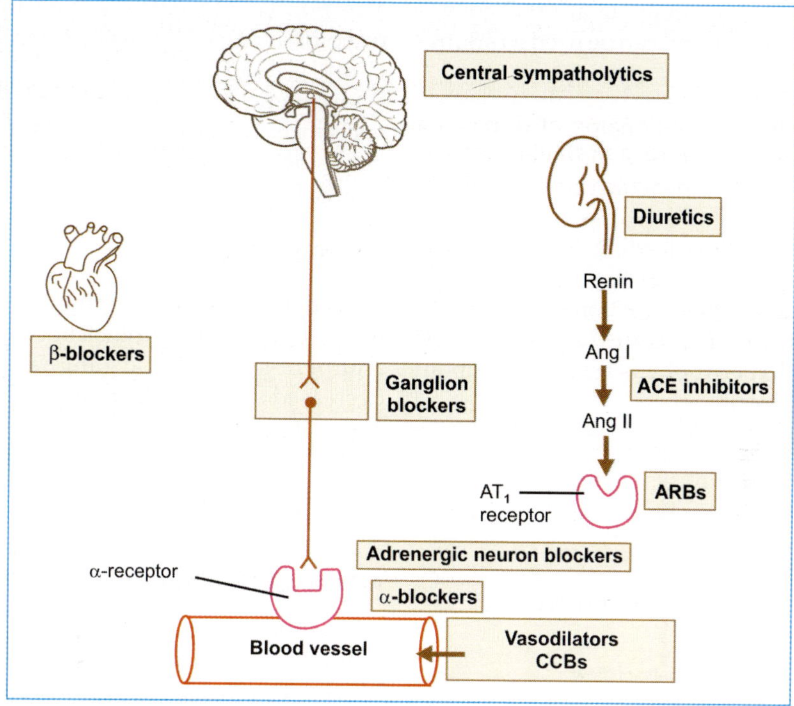

Fig. 26.2: Sites of action of antihypertensive drugs

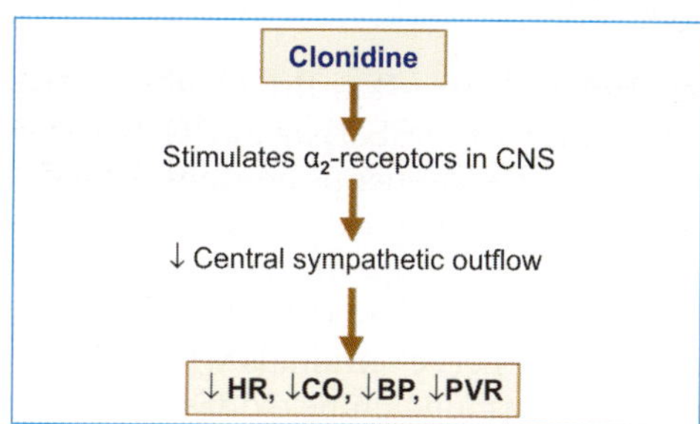

available as a transdermal patch which is effective for 7 days and is to be applied over the arm once a week. Adverse effects are milder with the transdermal preparation.

Adverse effects include drowsiness, dryness of mouth, nose and eyes; parotid gland swelling and pain, fluid retention, constipation and impotence. Sudden withdrawal of clonidine will lead to rebound hypertension, headache, tremors, sweating and tachycardia. Hence the dose should be tapered.

Uses

Mild to moderate hypertension: Clonidine was commonly used earlier but now other drugs are preferred because of the side effect profile of clonidine. However, as it is inexpensive, it is still used for the purpose in developing countries.

Other Uses

1. *In opioid withdrawal:* Most withdrawal symptoms in opioid addicts are of sympathetic overactivity and can be benefited by treatment with clonidine.
2. *Diabetic neuropathy:* Clonidine controls diarrhoea by improving absorption of NaCl and water in the gut by stimulation of α_2 receptors in the intestines.
3. *With anaesthetics:* Clonidine given preoperatively reduces the dose of the general anaesthetic needed due to its analgesic effects.

Guanfacine and **guanabenz** are α_2 agonists similar to clonidine and can be used as antihypertensives.

Alpha methyldopa, an analog of dopa, is a prodrug. It is metabolised in the body to α-methyl norepinephrine which is an α_2-agonist and acts like clonidine. It reduces central sympathetic outflow leading to a fall in BP. Renin levels also fall but renal blood flow is well maintained. Onset of action is about 4–6 hr and duration of action 12–24 hr. Left ventricular hypertrophy is reversed in about 12 weeks of treatment.

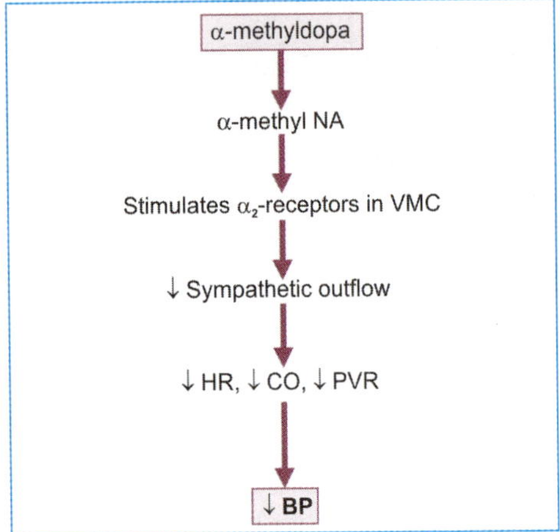

Adverse effects are sedation, dryness of mouth and nose, nightmares, depression, vertigo, extrapyramidal signs, raised prolactin levels, headache, postural hypotension and impotence.

On prolonged use, salt and water retention may blunt the antihypertensive effect (called pseudotolerance) and needs a diuretic to be added.

Uses

Methyldopa is used in mild to moderate hypertension along with a diuretic. It is safe in hypertension during pregnancy and is the preferred antihypertensive in such patients. Started with 250 mg twice daily, the dose may be increased to a maximum of 750 mg BD.

Moxonidine: Moxonidine is an imidazole I_1 receptor agonist, stimulates I_1 receptor in the medulla leading to reduction in central sympathetic drive and peripheral vascular resistance. The efficacy is similar to clonidine but is better tolerated with fewer adverse effects. Dose: 0.2 to 0.6 mg

Ganglion Blockers

Trimethaphan is the only ganglion blocker that is in use. These drugs block both sympathetic and para-sympathetic ganglia resulting in decreased sympathetic tone and a fall in BP. Trimethaphan is given intravenously to produce controlled hypotension during certain surgical procedures due to its rapid and short action (15 minutes) *see* page 125.

Adrenergic Neuron Blockers

Guanethidine depletes the stores of noradrenaline in the adrenergic neurons and also blocks its release. Because of the adverse effects like postural hypotension, diarrhoea and sexual dysfunction, guanethidine is not used.

Reserpine is an alkaloid obtained from *Rauwolfia serpentina* (Sarpagandhi) that grows in India. In the adrenergic neurons, it binds to the vesicles that store monoamines like noradrenaline, dopamine and 5-HT and destroys these vesicles. The monoamines then leak into the nerve terminals where they are destroyed by monoamine oxidase. Reserpine thus depletes the stores of these monoamines and reduces BP. Depletion of monoamines particularly dopamine is thought to be responsible for the antipsychotic effects of reserpine (*see* page 242).

Reserpine depletes monoamines throughout the body, in both central and peripheral neurons. Reserpine thus causes various side effects like drowsiness, depression, nightmares, parkinsonism, postural hypotension, oedema, weight gain, gynaecomastia and sexual dysfunction. Though it is generally not preferred, it has the advantages of being inexpensive, effective, long acting (once daily dose) and generally well tolerated when given with a diuretic.

Adrenergic Receptor Blockers

α-blockers

Nonselective α-blockers like phenoxybenzamine and phentolamine are used in the treatment of hypertension due to pheochromocytoma. Selective α_1-blockers like prazosin, terazosin and doxazosin block the α_1-receptors in arterioles and venules and thereby dilate both arterioles and venules. Peripheral vascular resistance is decreased leading to a fall in BP with only mild tachycardia.

30–60 minutes after the first dose of prazosin, the patient could experience postural hypotension which may lead to fainting particularly if the patient suddenly gets up from lying down position. This **'First dose phenomenon'** can be avoided by starting with a low dose (prazosin 0.5 mg) given at bedtime and the dose is gradually increased. α_1-blockers can also cause dizziness, headache and palpitation. α_1-blockers are used in mild to moderate hypertension; when used as monotherapy, salt and water retention can occur—hence they may be combined with diuretics and β-blockers.

α_1-blockers are particularly suitable in hypertensive men who also have BPH because of the benefit these afford in both.

β-blockers

β-blockers are mild anti-hypertensives. Blockade of cardiac β_1 receptors results in decreased myocardial contractility and cardiac output. Thus they reduce the BP due to a fall in the cardiac output. They also lower plasma renin activity and have an additional central antihypertensive action.

β-blockers are effective and well-tolerated and are of special value in patients who also have arrhythmias or angina. They may be used alone but are also suitable for combination with other antihypertensives, particularly with drugs that cause tachycardia as their side effect (*e.g.* vasodilators). They are useful in mild to moderate hypertension.

Atenolol is the preferred β-blocker because of the advantages like once a day dosing, absence of CNS side effects and β_1 selectivity. β-blockers should always be tapered while withdrawing.

Metoprolol may be given as a sustained release preparation for twice daily use. It is particularly preferred in patients with concurrent hypertension and heart failure.

Esmolol is a short-acting β_1-blocker with a half life of about 10 min. It is given intravenously as a loading dose of 0.5–1 μg/kg followed by an infusion (50–300 μg/kg/min). Esmolol is suited for use in intraoperative and postoperative hypertension and in hypertensive emergencies.

Third generation β blockers with β1 blocking effects which also stimulate β2 receptors and increase NO production like nebivolol are found to have clinical benefits but higher cost may be a limiting factor particularly for long term use.

α- and β-blockers

Labetalol and carvedilol block α_1- and β-receptors. They are used IV in the treatment of hypertension in pheochromocytoma and in hypertensive emergencies.

4. CALCIUM CHANNEL BLOCKERS

Calcium channel blockers (CCBs, *see* Chapter 25) are another important group of antihypertensives. They dilate the arterioles resulting in reduced peripheral vascular resistance. Nifedipine produces some reflex tachycardia while this is not seen with verapamil and diltiazem as they are cardiac depressants. Fluid retention is negligible unlike other arteriolar dilators. CCBs were earlier considered first-line antihypertensives and were extensively used. But several recent large scale studies have shown them to have many disadvantages. They are not preferred in patients who also have left ventricular hypertrophy and previous myocardial infarction. Short-acting dihydropyridines produce frequent changes in BP and sympathetic activity and hence should be avoided in hypertension.

Use in Hypertension

- CCBs are well-tolerated and effective.
- CCBs are particularly effective in elderly patients.
- CCBs may be used as monotherapy or in moderate to severe HT along with other antihypertensives.
- It has now been shown that sublingual nifedipine does not actually achieve therapeutic plasma concentrations quicker than oral formulations. Thus in HT emergencies, short-acting DHPs can be used parenterally.
- There is a growing concern that use of CCBs, especially short-acting ones, is associated with increased mortality and risk of sudden death.
- Sustained release preparations or long-acting dihydropyridine CCBs may be used for smoother control of BP.
- IV clevidipine can be used when parenteral CCB is needed for quick reduction of BP.

5. VASODILATORS

Vasodilators relax the vascular smooth muscles thus reducing BP due to decreased peripheral vascular resistance. Salt and water retention and reflex tachycardia are common with vasodilators.

Hydralazine

Hydralazine is a **directly acting arteriolar dilator.** The fall in BP is associated with tachycardia, renin release and fluid retention. Coronary, cerebral and renal blood flow are increased.

Given orally, hydralazine is well absorbed but first pass metabolism is extensive (25% bioavailability). Hydralazine is metabolised by **acetylation** in the liver (like INH) and the rate of acetylation is genetically determined—people may be fast or slow acetylators. Fast acetylators have lower bioavailability and, therefore, poorer antihypertensive effects.

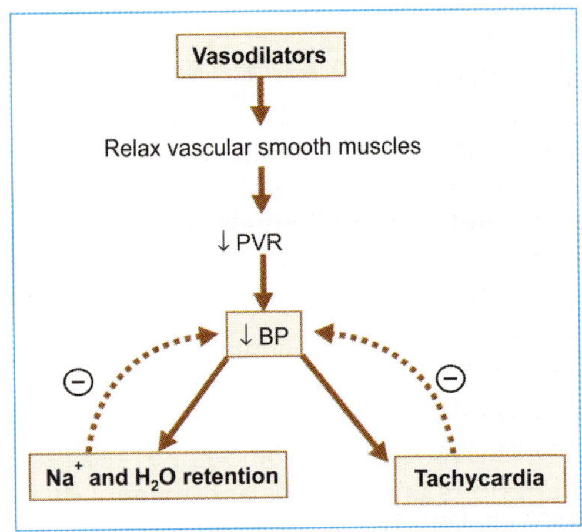

Dose: 25–50 mg OD-TDS, NEPRESOL 25 mg tab.

Adverse effects are headache, dizziness, flushing, palpitation, nausea, anorexia, hypotension and salt and water retention. It may precipitate angina and arrhythmias because of increased O_2 demand due to reflex tachycardia and decreased myocardial blood supply due to peripheral vasodilatation.

Hydralazine can cause hypersensitivity reactions with drug fever, peripheral neuropathy, **serum sickness** and **Sweet's syndrome** (febrile neutrophilic dermatosis). A syndrome resembling lupus erythematosus (arthralgia, fever, myalgia, pleuritis, pericarditis) may occur with high doses of hydralazine, and is more common in **slow acetylators.** It is reversible on withdrawal of hydralazine.

Fast acetylators → ↓ drug levels → less drug effect

Slow acetylators → ↑ drug levels → ADR: SLE

Uses: Hydralazine is used with a β-blocker and/or a diuretic in moderate to severe hypertension not controlled by the first-line drugs. Hydralazine may be combined with nitrates in hypertensives with cardiac failure. It can be given in hypertension during pregnancy (2nd and 3rd trimesters).

Minoxidil

Minoxidil is a directly acting arteriolar dilator used in severe hypertension not responding to other drugs. Minoxidil is a prodrug—converted to minoxidil sulfate which **opens up the potassium channels** in the smooth muscles. Opening of the K^+ channels causes efflux of K^+ resulting in hyperpolarisation and smooth muscle relaxation. It is an effective antihypertensive.

Minoxidil can cause sodium and water retention leading to oedema, it can also cause palpitations, anginal episodes, headache and sweating. Hence minoxidil must be combined with a diuretic and a β-blocker. **Hypertrichosis** on the face, arms, legs and back make it unacceptable in women.

Uses

1. *Hypertension:* Minoxidil is used with a diuretic—as a reserve drug—in patients with severe hypertension who do not respond to other drugs. Minoxidil is started with a low dose of 5 mg daily and is gradually increased to 40–50 mg. Loniten 2.5, 10 mg tab.
2. *Baldness:* Minoxidil directly stimulates the growth of hair on prolonged use (hypertrichosis). It appears to activate the gene that controls the protein of hair shaft—by this it stimulates the maturation and growth of cells of the hair shaft. Hence it is used topically (2% solution) for the correction of *alopecia.* Young men with relative alopecia are more likely to respond. Continued use of minoxidil is needed in patients who respond because cessation of treatment may result in hair fall. On topical use, minoxidil can rarely cause dermatitis.

   MINTOP, COVERIT 2% solution for topical use.

Diazoxide

Diazoxide is related to thiazide diuretics and is a potent **arteriolar dilator.** Its mechanism of action is like that of minoxidil. Diazoxide can cause **hyperglycaemia** because it inhibits the insulin secretion from pancreas. Other side effects include salt and water retention, palpitation and myocardial ischaemia. It is used intravenously in **hypertensive emergencies** where monitoring of infusion is not possible. Diazoxide has a long duration of action (24 hours) and is suitable in such situations.

Sodium Nitroprusside

It is a **rapidly acting** vasodilator and it relaxes both **arterioles and venules**. Both peripheral resistance and cardiac output are reduced resulting in lower myocardial oxygen consumption.

Nitroprusside acts through the release of nitric oxide which activates guanylyl cyclase, resulting in the formation of cGMP which relaxes the vascular smooth muscles. On IV administration, it is rapid (<30 seconds) and short-acting (3 minutes) allowing rapid titration of the dose. This makes it suitable for use in **hypertensive emergencies** with close monitoring and in severe heart failure.

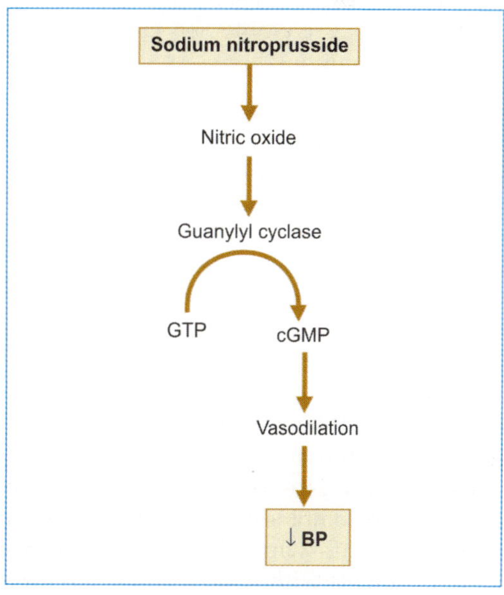

Sodium nitroprusside is taken up into the RBCs and **cyanide** is released. The cyanide is metabolized by the mitochondrial enzyme and a sulfur group is added to get thiocyanate which is gradually excreted by the kidneys.

The following points are to be noted in using sodium nitroprusside.

1. Sodium nitroprusside acts within seconds. Hence, BP should be monitored constantly.
2. The drug should be dissolved in 2 ml of 5% dextrose solution and then diluted in IV fluids.
3. Sodium nitroprusside is light sensitive. The infusion bottle and the tubing must be protected from light by an opaque wraping. Fresh solution should be made before each use.
4. If the colour changes, the infusion should be discarded.
5. If infusion is prolonged, blood levels of cyanide and thiocyanate levels should be checked.
6. Sodium nitroprusside is used for emergency control of BP and in severe heart failure. Use should not be prolonged for more than 2–3 days.
7. It should preferably be used with an infusion pump.

Adverse reactions are palpitation, sweating, weakness, nausea, vomiting and hypotension.

In higher doses, nitroprusside gets converted to cyanide and thiocyanate which can result in toxicity. Accumulation of **thiocyanide** can result in symptoms of toxicity like nausea, anorexia, weakness, disorientation, psychosis, muscle spasm and convulsions. Higher doses can result in severe hypotension, metabolic acidosis, arrhythmias and death. Administration of **sodium thiosulphate** along with nitroprusside prevents the accumulation of cyanide.

Alternatively, hydroxocobalamin may be given which combines with cyanide to form cyanocobalamin which is a nontoxic compound. Patients with renal dysfunction may fail to excrete thiocyanate efficiently, resulting in its gradual accumulation over days. Methaemoglobinaemia is also known following infusion of nitroprusside. It should be avoided in pregnancy.

Uses

1. ***Hypertensive emergencies:*** Nitroprusside is the drug of choice. Started with 0.5 μg/kg/min infusion and may be gradually increased up to 10 μg/kg/min. The BP should be constantly monitored.
2. ***Myocardial infarction***—used in situations where short-term reduction of myocardial workload is required as in severe heart failure and MI.

Fenoldopam is a D_1 dopamine receptor agonist, brings about dilation of peripheral arteries and also loss of sodium. It has a short t½ of 10 minutes and is given as an IV infusion. Fenoldopam is found to be useful in hypertensive emergencies and postoperative hypertension, particularly when there is impaired renal function. Started with a low dose of 0.1 μg/kg/min, it is gradually increased every 20 minutes till adequate response is attained (maximum dose 1.6 μg/kg/min).

Adverse effects include flushing, headache, palpitation and hypotension. It should be avoided in patients with glaucoma since it can raise the intraocular pressure. Fenoldopam has efficacy similar to sodium nitroprusside but is devoid of thiocyanate-related complications.

Drug Interactions of Antihypertensives

1. Sympathomimetics and tricyclic antidepressants can antagonise the effects of sympatholytics.
2. First generation antihistamines add to sedation produced by clonidine and methyldopa.

   Clonidine/methyldopa + Ist generation antihistamines → ↑ sedation
3. NSAIDs tend to cause salt and water retention and may reduce the effect of antihypertensives.

TREATMENT OF HYPERTENSION

Since hypertension *per se* does not produce troublesome symptoms but requires life long treatment in most patients, it is necessary to educate the patient regarding the need for treatment and the importance of good patient compliance. Several of the antihypertensive drugs can cause unacceptable side effects and this may further complicate treatment. Hence in every patient diagnosed to be a hypertensive, decision has to be made whether pharmacotherapy is needed or BP can be controlled with nonpharmacological measures. Prehypertension can be managed with diet, weight reduction, adequate exercises and moderation of alcohol intake. Once the decision to use drugs is made, the choice of drugs needs consideration of several factors including patient's age, severity of the disease, presence of other diseases and risk factors for coronary artery diseases.

Joint National Committee (JNC 8) recommendations for treatment of hypertension were released in 2014.

Stage 1 hypertension is to be treated with a thiazide diuretic or an ACE inhibitor/ARB/CCB. Commonly used are telmisartan and amlodipine. If uncontrolled by adequate doses of one drug, a second drug may be added.

Stage 2 hypertension would require a combination of 2 drugs—a thiazide with ARB/ACEI/CCB. In patients with chronic kidney disease, treatment should be initiated with an ACE inhibitor/ARB with or without other antihypertensives.

Hypertensive crises: Hypertensive crises include hypertensive emergencies and urgencies. Though these terminologies are no more in use in many countries, several clinicians find it useful to manage such situations.

Hypertensive emergencies are situations with very high BP (210/120 mm Hg) associated with **target organ damage.** They may be life-threatening. Conditions like malignant hypertension, hypertensive encephalopathy, acute myocardial infarction, dissecting aneurysm of aorta, acute LVF with pulmonary oedema, eclampsia and hypertensive crisis in pheochromocytoma are some hypertensive emergencies. ***Malignant hypertension*** is severe hypertension associated with vascular damage due to arteriolopathy. It is a medical emergency manifested by papilloedema, retinal haemorrhages and hypertensive encephalopathy.

Hypertensive urgencies are conditions with highly elevated BP but no target organ damage.

Hypertensive crises require treatment in an ICU with **constant monitoring** of BP. Blood pressure should be **lowered gradually**. This is because, in patients with chronic hypertension, autoregulatory changes would have taken place in the blood vessels of vital organs. Sudden reduction in BP may cause hypoxia of vital organs.

Pareneral drugs are preferred and **IV sodium nitroprusside** under close monitoring is the drug of choice (Table 26.2). **IV esmolol, diazoxide, fenoldopam, nitroglycerine, labetalol, hydralazine, CCBs like nicardipine and sublingual nifedipine** are alternatives. BP should be constantly monitored because drugs like sodium nitroprusside can bring down BP suddenly which results in hypoperfusion of vital organs. Diuretics like furosemide reduce volume overload. As soon as possible switching over to oral drugs is desirable because the control of BP is smoother with oral antihypertensives.

Hypertension in Pregnancy

The antihypertensives found to be safe in pregnancy are **methyldopa** orally for maintenance and **hydralazine** parenterally for reduction of BP in emergencies. However, they should be used only after the first trimester. Dihydropyridine CCBs like

Table 26.2: Drugs in hypertensive emergencies

Drug	*Dose*	*Duration of action*
Sodium nitroprusside	0.5 to 10 μg/kg/min IV infusion	1–2 min
Nifedipine	10 mg sublingual	2–3 hours
Nitroglycerin	5 to 100 μg/min IV infusion	3–5 min
Fenoldopam	0.1 to 1.6 μg/kg/min IV infusion	15–30 min
Hydralazine	10 to 20 mg IV bolus or 10–50 mg IM	4–8 hours
Esmolol	50 to 300 μg/kg/min IV infusion	10–15 min
Labetalol	20 to 80 mg IV every 10 min (Max 300 mg)	3–6 hours

nifedipine may be used but should be withdrawn during labour as they may inhibit uterine contractions. Other drugs like **prazosin** and **clonidine** can also be used. **Cardioselective β-blockers** like **atenolol** and **acebutolol** may be used in pregnancy but nonselective β-blockers should be avoided as they may reduce blood supply to the placenta leading to reduced size of the placenta and low birth weight.

Failure of treatment: Control of BP achieved may not be satisfactory in some patients. Reason could be many. Poor patient compliance, excessive salt intake, drugs that counter effects of antihypertensives or progression of the disease itself. Patients should be adequately educated regarding the importance of low sodium diet, exercises, body weight reduction in the obese and good patient compliance.

Combination of Antihypertensives

When it is not possible to achieve adequate control of BP with a single drug, a combination of drugs may be used. Antihypertensives may also be combined to overcome the side effects of one another. This also allows use of lower doses of each drug. Sympatholytics and vasodilators cause fluid retention which can be overcome by adding a diuretic.

Vasodilators like nifedipine and hydralazine evoke reflex tachycardia. This can be countered by β-blockers, while propranolol may cause initial rise in peripheral vascular resistance which is countered by vasodilators. Combination of ACE inhibitors and diuretics is synergistic.

Resistant hypertension: It includes:

- BP uncontrolled even on 3 drugs of different classes one of which is a diuretic.
- BP controlled but requiring 4 or more drugs of different classes.

Lifestyle modifications: Dietary approaches to stop hypertension (DASH) includes diet comprising of grain and grain products, fruits, vegetables, low fat diary products, nuts, seeds and legumes, i.e. diet less in sodium salt.

Non-pharmacological measures: Low salt diet (<2.4 g/day), moderate exercises, weight reduction, and *transcendental* meditation—all go a long way in controlling the blood pressure. Smoking and alcohol should be given up. These measures also help in reducing the dose of the antihypertensive needed.

Drugs used in pulmonary hypertension

- Prostaglandin analogs—iloprost, epoprostenol
- Sildenafil
- Calcium channel blockers
- Diuretics
- Oral anticoagulants
- Oxygen administration
- Endothelin receptor antagonists like bosentan
- For severe pulmonary hypertension—inhaled nitric oxide

Clinical Pharmacology

- The BP reading in a doctor's clinic/hospital tends to be higher due to anxiety. Multiple readings preferably in the domestic set up in supine and standing posture should be considered before starting antihypertensive therapy.
- Salt restriction is equal to one antihypertensive tablet; patient should be convinced so that they reduce the excess salt intake by avoiding pickles, papad, dry fish and preserved food. The practice of salt taken on the plate must be avoided by all and salt restriction reduces BP in all including nonhypertensives.
- Alcohol, smoking, hyperlipidaemia, obesity, diabetes mellitus should all be controlled.
- Systolic hypertensives should preferably be started with low doses of antihypertensives and gradually increased.
- In Western population, average salt intake is 4–6 g/day while in India it is 12–14 g/day.
- In South America, a race exists which does not consume salt whatsoever and none of them have hypertension.
- While using sodium nitroprusside, monitoring treatment is very important because if unmonitored, BP drops rapidly and can even be fatal.
- IV enalapril, labetalol, sodium nitroprusside and NTG are available for hypertensive emergencies.

PHARMACOTHERAPY OF SHOCK

Competency achievement: The student should be able to:
PH 1.27 Describe the mechanisms of action, types, doses, side effects, indications and contraindications of antihypertensive drugs and **drugs used in shock.**[1]

Shock is acute circulatory failure with underperfusion of tissues. It needs immediate treatment and can be rapidly fatal, if not appropriately taken care of.

Clinical features: In shock, symptoms of sympathetic overactivity are generally seen—like pallor, sweating, cold extremities and tachycardia.

Shock may be of different types and causes.

1. **Hypovolaemic shock:** Decreased blood volume due to sudden loss of plasma or blood as in haemorrhage, burns or dehydration can result in hypovolaemia and under perfusion of all tissues including vital organs. This stimulates a complex compensatory response which also includes sympathetic stimulation. There is vasodilation in the vital organs and peripheral vasoconstriction. These help to maintain the cardiac output for a short period.

Depending on the severity of hypovolaemia, shock ensues in more severe cases and the compensatory changes themselves would result in inappropriate vasodilation, loss of fluid from the capillaries into the tissues and excessive peripheral vasoconstriction, all leading to extensive tissue hypoxia, acidosis, hypotension, pulmonary oedema and finally multiorgan failure resulting in death.

Treatment of hypovolaemic shock is by prompt replacement of fluids and electrolytes (*see* below). Blood pressure should be monitored.

2. **Septic shock:** Septic shock is precipitated by severe bacterial infection. It may be due to release of bacterial toxins—which could be exotoxins or endotoxins. These trigger the release of cytotoxic mediators including interleukins, PGs, TNF-α, PAF, cytokines and others, resulting in vasodilation.

It is called **warm shock** since the skin is warm (not cold as in other types of shock) due to peripheral vasodilation. The peripheral vascular resistance falls and cardiac output increases for some time. Inflammatory mediators are responsible for vascular injury with an increased permeability and other pathological changes in shock. Though there is an increase in cardiac output initially, it is maldistributed and there is formation of microthrombi with abnormal microcirculation and is, therefore, also called distributive shock.

Treatment: Immediate treatment of shock is as important as controlling the infection. General measures include correction of acidosis, blood volume, maintenance of BP and appropriate antibiotics in adequate doses. Ventilatory support may be given, if required.

3. **Cardiogenic shock:** Cardiogenic shock is due to failure of pumping of the blood by the heart as is in myocardial infarction or acute myocarditis. IV morphine is the drug of choice to relieve pain and anxiety (*see* page 266).

4. **Anaphylactic shock:** Anaphylactic shock is a Type I hypersensitivity reaction. Antigen–antibody reaction on the surface of mast cells and basophils triggers the release of massive amounts of histamine and other mediators of inflammation.

The important clinical features are hypotension, bronchospasm and laryngeal oedema. It can be rapidly fatal and, therefore, needs to be treated immediately.

Treatment

i. **Adrenaline** 0.3–0.5 ml of 1:1000 solution is injected intramuscularly; it promptly reverses the symptoms because it is the physiological antagonist of histamine and can be life saving. If needed, another dose may be repeated after 15–20 minutes. In very severe shock, adrenaline 1:10,000 solution may be injected intravenously slowly in the dose of 500 µg over 5–10 minutes.
ii. **Airway** should be maintained. **Salbutamol** nebulization may be given to relieve bronchospasm.
iii. **Foot end of the bed** should be elevated to improve BP. Suitable **plasma expanders** and vasopressors, like norepinephrine or dopamine, may be needed.
iv. **Hydrocortisone hemisuccinate** 100 mg may be given intravenously. Once the patient recovers, a short course of oral prednisolone may be given. Antihistamines **chlorpheniramine** 20 mg may be injected by slow IV injection. It may take care of some of the manifestations of allergy. However, it is not the primary drug as many other mediators of inflammation other than histamine are also released in anaphylaxis.

5. **Neurogenic shock:** Neurogenic shock is due to venous pooling as following spinal anaesthesia, severe head injury, spinal cord injury, abdominal or testicular trauma (vagal inhibition).

Treatment: Blood volume replacement should be done. A vasopressor, like noradrenaline, may be given intravenously to improve the vascular tone.

General guidelines for the treatment of shock

- The cause should be identified and treated.
- BP and plasma volume should be maintained with appropriate intravenous fluids.
- The foot end of the bed should be elevated. This increases venous return which raises the BP to some extent based on the requirement. Vasopressors, like dopamine, may be given intravenously when the BP cannot be brought up by IV fluids. Plasma expanders may help in maintaining the plasma volume when there is severe hypovolaemia.
- Acid–base and electrolyte disturbances should be corrected.
- Adequate urine output should be ensured.
- Ventilatory support and oxygen administration may be given, if required.

INTRAVENOUS FLUIDS

Intravenous fluids are sterile solutions meant for intravenous administration. The content and quantity of solute varies. Intravenous fluids are used for replacement of fluid, electrolytes and nutrition.

Types of IV Solutions

Intravenous solutions are of 3 types depending on osmolality—*isotonic, hypotonic and hypertonic* (Flowchart 26.1).

Plasma osmolality is nearly equal to 300 mmol/l. Osmolality of 10% dextrose is 505 mmol/l.

Intravenous fluids may also be grouped as:

1. ***Maintenance fluids***—5% dextrose in half normal saline
2. ***Replacement fluids***—normal saline, dextrose saline (DNS), Ringer lactate, Isolyte—M, P, G and E

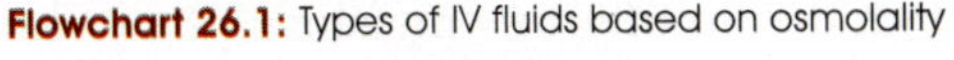

Flowchart 26.1: Types of IV fluids based on osmolality

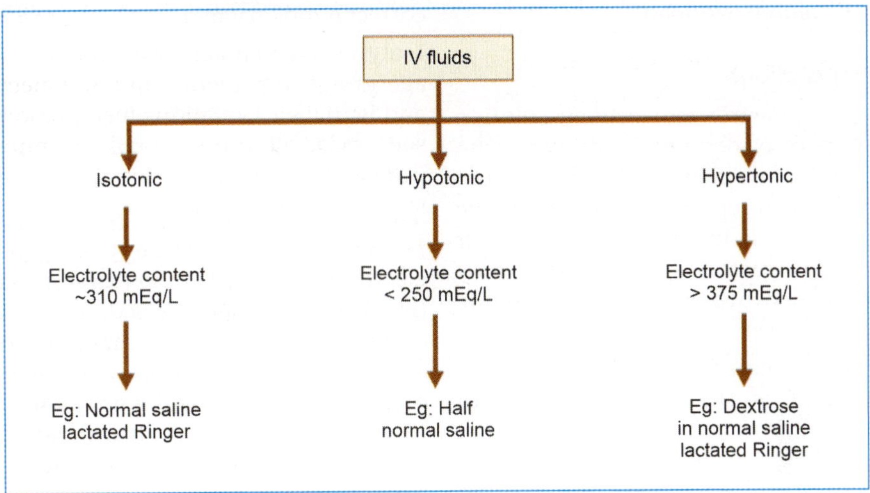

3. ***Special fluids*** (for special indications)—25% dextrose, sodium bicarbonate, potassium chloride.

Isotonic fluids: As isotonic fluids have an osmolality nearly equal to that of ECF, they do not alter the size of RBCs (neither shrink not swell). One litre of isotonic solution expands ECF by 1 litre, but it quickly diffuses into the ECF compartment and, therefore, the plasma volume is increased only by ¼ litre (250 ml). Hence **around 3 litres of isotonic fluid is needed to replenish volume of one litre of lost blood.** However, patients with hypertension and cardiac failure need careful monitoring to avoid fluid overload.

Normal saline solution: 0.9% sodium chloride—remains in the ECF because the electrolytes make up its osmolality. It is used in hyponatraemia. It should be avoided in heart failure, pulmonary oedema and renal impairment.

Lactated Ringer solution: It contains potassium, calcium and sodium chloride. It is used to correct dehydration, hyponatraemia and to replace gastrointestinal fluids. Many other similar solutions are available with minor changes in the electrolyte content.

Hypotonic fluids: These replace cellular fluid because they are hypotonic as compared to plasma. Half normal saline (0.45% sodium chloride solution) is the commonly used hypotonic solution but other electrolyte solutions are also available. Hypotonic sodium solution is used in hypernatraemia and other hyperosmolar conditions. Overdosage can result in intravascular fluid depletion, hypotension, cellular oedema and later cell damage.

Hypertonic fluids: Dextrose is used as a 5% solution. The plasma volume expansion is minimum because dextrose gets metabolised and water gets distributed in all compartments in the body. Infusion of 1 litre of dextrose can raise the plasma volume by just 100 ml but it contains 50 grams of glucose and, therefore supplies nutrition (170 kcal/l).

Dextrose 5% in normal saline or lactated Ringer's solution or in hypotonic solution has osmolality more than ECF. 50% dextrose solution may be administered in hypoglycaemia or to supplement calories. Since these solutions are strongly hypertonic, they should be injected into central veins for rapid dilution. Hypertonic saline solutions draw water from the cells and the cells shrink. They should be injected slowly and carefully to avoid ECF volume overload.

Isolyte Preparations

Isolyte-G is a **gastric** replacement solution containing glucose, sodium chloride, potassium chloride, ammonium chloride and sodium metabisulphate. It replaces electrolytes in the gastric juice that is lost during vomiting or continuous nasogastric aspiration which may lead to hypochloraemic, hypokalaemic metabolic alkalosis.

Isolyte-M is a **maintenance** fliud with 5% dextrose and is the richest source of potassium. It contains glucose, sodium chloride, sodium acetate, potassium chloride, dibasic potassium phosphate and sodium metabisulphate. Isolyte-M is also useful to correct hypokalaemia.

Isolyte-P is a maintenance fluid for paediatric age group to provide fluid and electrolytes and in diabetes insipidus It contains glucose, sodium lactate, dibasic potassium phosphate, potassium and magnesium chloride and sodium metabisulphite.

Isolyte-E is replacement solution with electrolytes matching the **extracellular** fluid (ECF). It contains glucose, sodium chloride and acetate, sodium citrate, potassium chloride, magnesium chloride and sodium metabisulphate. **Isolyte is the only fluid which replaces magnesium.** It thus provides all ECF electrolytes, corrects metabolic acidosis, supplies energy and replaces the lost water.

[1] From Medical Council of India, *Competency based Undergraduate Curriculum for the Indian Medical Graduate*, 2018;1:136–144.

CHAPTER 27

Treatment of Cardiac Failure and Pharmacology of Cardiac Glycosides

Competency achievement: The student should be able to:

PH 1.29 Describe the mechanisms of action, types, doses, side effects, indications and contraindications of the drugs used in congestive heart failure.[1]

PHYSIOLOGICAL CONSIDERATIONS

The cardiac muscle is a specialised tissue with unique properties like excitability, contractility and automaticity. The myocardium has two types of cells—the contracting cells and the conducting cells. The contracting cells participate in the pumping action of the heart. SA node, AV node and His-Purkinje system comprise the conducting tissue of the heart. Parts of the conducting tissue have the characteristic property of automaticity. **Automaticity** is the ability of the cell to generate electrical impulses spontaneously. Normally, the SA node acts as the pacemaker. **Excitability** is the ability of the cell to undergo depolarization in response to a stimulus. **Contractility** is the ability of the myocardium to contract adequately and pump the blood out of the heart.

Cardiac Action Potential

When a stimulus reaches the cardiac cell, specific ions move into and out of the cell eliciting an action potential. Such movement of ions across the cardiac cell may be divided into five phases (Fig. 27.1).

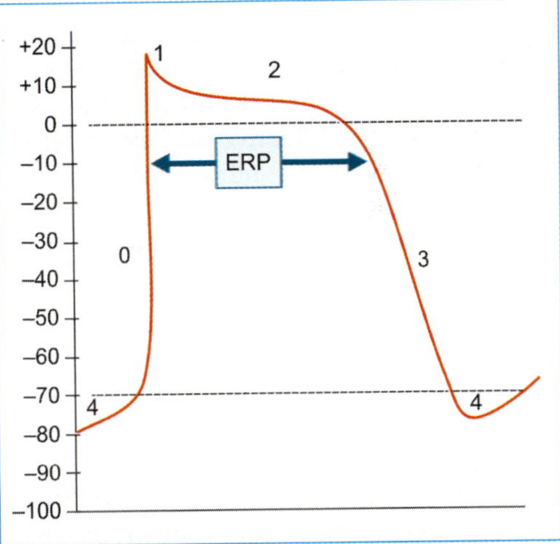

Fig. 27.1: Cardiac action potential phases 0–4: Phase 0 indicates rapid depolarisation; Phases 1–3 indicate repolarisation; Phase 4—gradual depolarisation during diastole

Phase 0 is rapid depolarisation of the cell membrane during which there is opening of the voltage-gated sodium channels and fast entry of sodium ions into the cell through the sodium channels. The channels close in 1–2 milliseconds when they enter an inactivated state. This is followed by repolarisation.

Phase 1 is a short, initial, rapid repolarisation due to efflux of potassium ions and the membrane potential returns towards 0 mV.

Phase 2 is a prolonged plateau phase due to slow entry of calcium ions into the cell through the calcium channels. Cardiac cell differs from other cells in having this phase of action potential.

Phase 3 is a second period of rapid repolarisation with potassium ions moving out of the cell through the potassium channels (Ikr).

Drugs that interfere with K^+ channels prolong the action potential by delaying this phase of repolarisation.

Phase 4 is the resting phase during which potassium ions return into the cell while sodium and calcium ions move out of it and the resting membrane potential is restored and the sodium channels recover from inactivation.

During phases 1 and 2, the cell does not depolarise in response to another impulse, i.e. it is in **absolute refractory period.** During phases 3 and 4, the cell is in **relative refractory period** and may depolarise in response to a powerful impulse. Effective refractory period (ERP) begins with the action potential and includes the absolute refractory period.

Cardiac conduction: The cardiac impulse originates in the SA node and spreads throughout the atrium, enters the AV node and is then carried through the right and left bundle branches to the right and left ventricles. Conduction velocity of an impulse is reflected by the slope of the action potential. If the conduction is depressed, the slope is reduced.

The cardiac output is determined by heart rate and stroke volume. The stroke volume in turn depends on the preload, afterload and contractility. **Preload** is the load on the heart due to the volume of blood reaching the left ventricle. It depends on the venous return. **Afterload** is the resistance to the left ventricular ejection, i.e. the total peripheral vascular resistance.

Congestive Cardiac Failure (CCF)

Congestive cardiac failure is one of the common causes of morbidity and mortality with almost 50% mortality at 5 years. In congestive cardiac failure, the heart is unable to provide adequate blood supply to meet the body's oxygen demand. The pumping ability of the heart is reduced and the cardiac output decreases. Thus ventricles are not completely emptied resulting in increased venous pressure in the pulmonary and systemic circulation. The ejection fraction (EF) decreases—the normal EF of the left ventricle is 55–65% while in chronic heart failure it falls to less than 40%.

All these result in tachycardia, pulmonary and peripheral oedema, dyspnoea, reduced exercise tolerance, with liver and heart enlargement. As a compensatory mechanism, there is stimulation of the **sympathetic system**, **renin–angiotensin system** and **release of atrial natriuretic peptides** which help in maintaining the cardiac output.

Atria, ventricles and vascular endothelium store natriuretic peptides and release them in volume overload. These peptides increase renal excretion of salt and water and dilate vascular smooth muscles. The endothelins are also released. The myocardium undergoes structural alterations like **ventricular hypertrophy** and **remodelling** to adapt itself to the stressful situation. These compensatory changes maintain the cardiac output for sometime.

Low output failure could result from ischaemic heart disease, hypertension, valvular and congenital heart diseases. It generally responds to treatment.

High output failure results from anaemia, thyrotoxicosis, beriberi and certain congenital heart diseases causing AV shunts. This type of failure responds poorly to drugs and the cause needs to be corrected.

Cardiac failure may also be categorised as systolic failure or diastolic failure.

Systolic failure (systolic dysfunction) or ejection failure is the inability of the ventricles to pump and empty adequately. Contractility and ejection fraction are reduced as in ischaemic heart diseases and myocarditis. The ventricles are dilated and, therefore, need to develop higher tension in its walls to eject the blood efficiently.

Laplace's Law

Wall tension = Intraventricular pressure × Ventricular radius

Diastolic failure is filling failure and occurs when the ventricles are not filled adequately during diastole because of both stiffening and inadequate relaxation during diastole. As the filling is reduced, cardiac output is reduced. However, ejection fraction may be normal. In patients with ventricular hypertrophy as in prolonged hypertension, aortic stenosis, hypertrophic cardiomyopathy and congenital heart diseases, diastolic failure is seen.

Some patients may have both systolic as well as diastolic dysfunction.

DRUGS USED IN CONGESTIVE CARDIAC FAILURE

The aim of treatment in congestive cardiac failure is to reduce morbidity and mortality by restoring cardiac output and relieving congestion.

The drugs used (Flowchart 27.1) in CCF include:

The drugs used in CCF include:

1. ***Diuretics:*** Frusemide, bumetanide, spironolactone, eplerenone
2. ***Vasodilators***
   a. Arteriolar dilators—hydralazine
   b. Venodilators—organic nitrates
   c. Arteriolar and venular dilators—ACE inhibitors, ARBs, sodium nitroprusside, prazosin, CCBs.
3. ***Positive inotropic drugs*** (inotropes)
   a. Cardiac glycosides—digoxin, digitoxin
   b. β adrenergic agonists—dobutamine, dopamine, dopexamine
   c. Phosphodiesterase (PDE) inhibitors—amrinone, milrinone
   d. Newer inotropes—levosimendan, istaroxime
4. ***Others:*** Beta-adrenergic blockers.
5. ***Newer drugs:*** Ivabradine, sacubitril, serelaxin, ularitide.

1. ***Diuretics:*** Loop diuretics like **frusemide** are the first-line drugs in CCF. They increase salt and water excretion and reduce blood volume. By this, they *reduce preload* and venous pressure, improve cardiac performance and relieve oedema and afford rapid symptomatic relief. However, they have some disadvantages.

- Long-term diuretic therapy may cause hypokalaemia (hence should be combined with potassium sparing diuretics).
- They activate renin–angiotensin system leading to deleterious effects on the cardiovascular system.
- Resistance develops on prolonged use.
- Diuretics do not stop the progression of the heart failure and only suppress the symptoms.

Hence the current recommendation in mild heart failure is **diuretics for short periods** as and when required. IV frusemide along with an ACE inhibitor is particularly useful in acute heart failure. Long-term frusemide therapy may be needed in more severe disease.

Spironolactone and eplerenone, the K^+ sparing diuretics are aldosterone antagonists. The role of aldosterone in the pathophysiology of cardiac failure is now clearly established. Spironolactone, though a weak diuretic, can benefit the patients with heart failure because it antagonises the effects of aldosterone including raised plasma volume and preload. They have been shown to reduce morbidity and mortality when given along with ACE inhibitors in patients with severe heart failure.

2. ***Vasodilators:*** Vasodilators reduce the mortality in patients with cardiac failure. Vasodilators may be arteriolar or venular dilators or both.

a. **Arteriolar dilators** (e.g. hydralazine) relax arterial smooth muscles, thus reducing peripheral vascular resistance and thereby the **after load**. As a result, the workload on the heart is reduced and the ventricles can pump out more blood.

   Hydralazine being an arteriolar dilator improves renal function as it causes good renal vasodilation. It may be given in combination with a nitrate in patients who have some contraindication for ACE inhibitors/ARBs. The combination improves long-term survival though less than with ACE inhibitors.

b. **Venodilators** (e.g. nitrates) reduce the venous return to the heart (**preload**) thus reducing the stretching of the ventricular

Flowchart 27.1: Algorithm for treatment of congestive heart failure

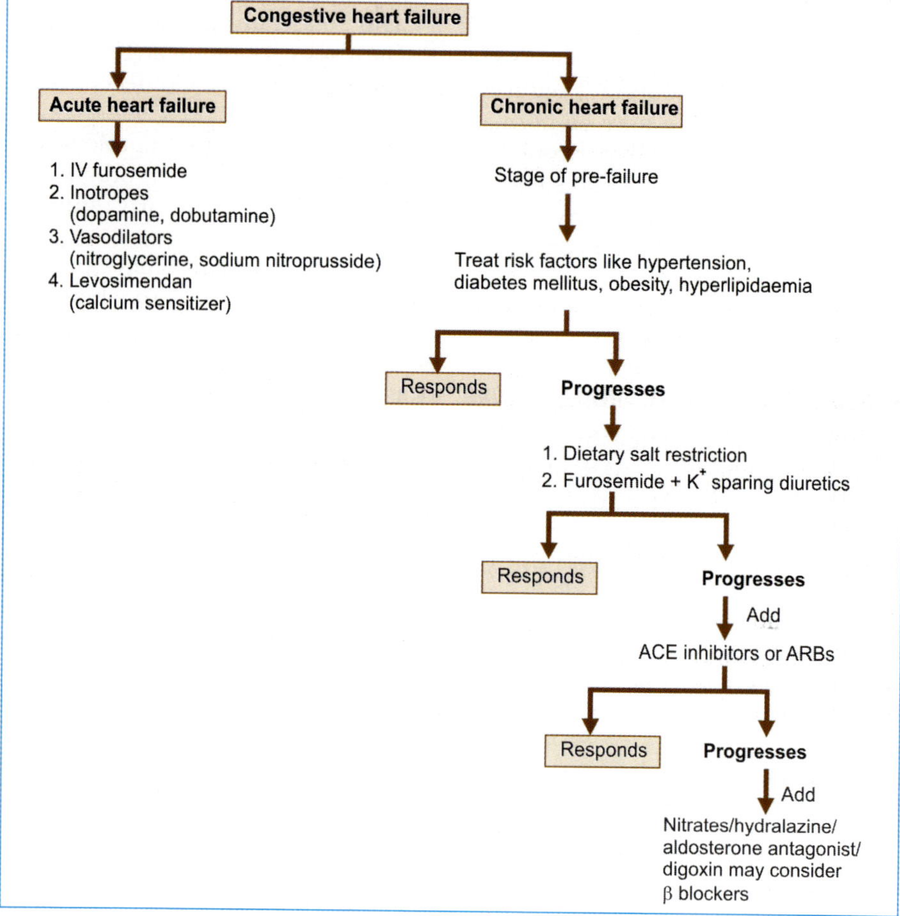

walls and myocardial oxygen requirements. *Organic nitrates:* Nitroglycerine and isosorbide dinitrate are good vasodilators with a rapid and short action. They can be used for short periods to decrease the ventricular filling pressure in acute heart failure.

Nitroglycerine can be used IV in acute CCF. Nitrates may also be given in combination with hydralazine.

c. **Arteriolar and venular dilators** (e.g. ACE inhibitors, sodium nitroprusside, prazosin) reduce both preload and afterload.
   i. *Angiotensin-converting enzyme inhibitors (ACE-I) like captopril, enalapril act by:*

- ***Reduction of afterload:*** Angiotensin II is a powerful vasoconstrictor present in the plasma in high concentrations in cardiac failure. ACE inhibitors prevent the conversion of angiotensin I to angiotensin II and thereby cause vasodilatation and reduce the afterload. Reduced afterload helps to increase cardiac output (Flowchart 27.2).
- ***Reduction of preload:*** Aldosterone causes salt and water retention and increases plasma volume. ACE-I prevent the formation of aldosterone (by reducing Ang-II) and thereby

Flowchart 27.2: Rationale for use of ACE inhibitors in CCF

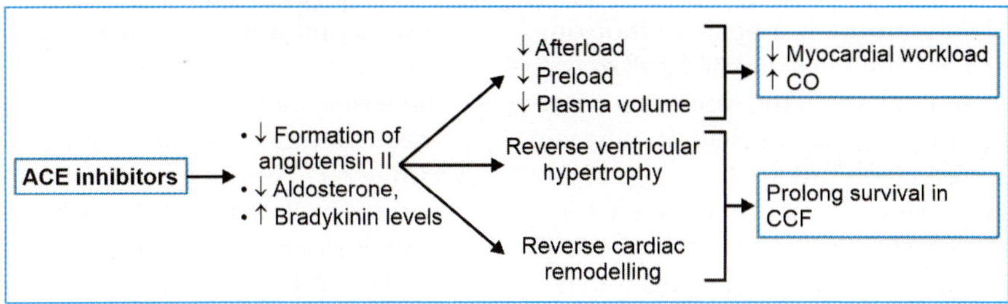

reduce the preload. They also prevent bradykinin degradation and **increase bradykinin levels** which also causes vasodilatation.

- ***Reversing compensatory changes***: Angiotensin II formed locally in the myocardium is responsible for various undesirable compensatory changes like ventricular hypertrophy and ventricular remodelling seen in CCF. ACE-I reverse these changes.

ACE inhibitors are thus the ***most preferred*** drugs in chronic congestive cardiac failure. Several studies have shown them to **prolong survival.** They produce beneficial effects even in resistant heart failure. They are useful in patients who have hypertension. ACE-I and ARBs have disease modifying effects—they reverse or prevent ventricular hypertrophy and remodelling in all grades of heart failure including asymptomatic LV dysfunction. Therefore, **ACE inhibitors are recommended in all patients with heart failure**. ARBs may be used as alternatives. Direct renin inhibitor aliskiren is being studied for its efficacy in CCF.

ii. *Sodium nitroprusside:* Sodium nitroprusside is a powerful vasodilator. Since it dilates both arterioles and venules, it reduces both ventricular filling pressure and peripheral arterial resistance. It is given IV, has a rapid (30–60 sec) and short action (3 minutes). Hence it is useful in acute severe heart failure.

iii. *Prazosin:* Prazosin, an α_1 antagonist, is a vasodilator. It can be used in acute heart failure for longer periods than nitrates.

iv. *Calcium channel blockers (CCBs):* These are not routinely used in heart failure because of their myocardiac depressant effect. Amlodipine may be tried when other vasodilators are contraindicated.

3. *Positive inotropic agents:*

   a. *Cardiac glycosides:* When the patients do not respond to diuretics and ACE inhibitors, digoxin may be given. Digoxin improves cardiac performance in the dilated, failing heart. If there is associated atrial fibrillation, digoxin is the preferred drug. Pharmacology of cardiac glycosides is discussed later.

Mechanism of action of some drugs in CCF

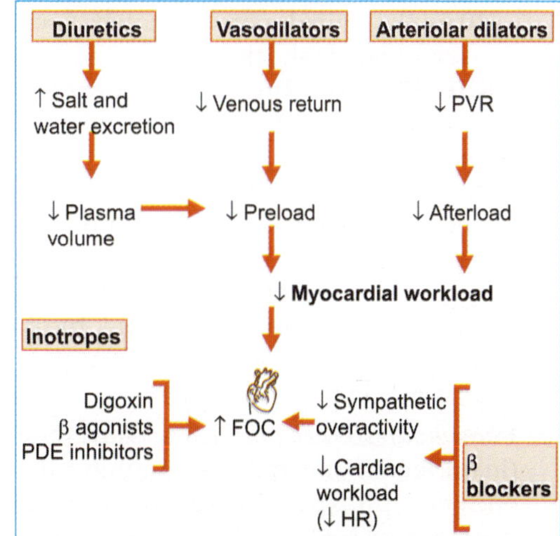

b. ***β*-adrenergic agonists**

(i) Dobutamine is a positive inotropic agent. It stimulates the cardiac β_1 receptors and enhances the force of contraction of the cardiac muscle. It increases the cardiac output without significant tachycardia. It also produces some vasodilation by stimulating the β_2 receptors. The mild tachycardia that is produced may itself be troublesome in patients with IHD, where it may also cause arrhythmias. Dobutamine may be used for short periods in some patients with chronic heart failure. It may be given as intermittent infusion which relieves the symptoms and the benefit may persist for several weeks. Dobutamine is useful in patients with acute heart failure that may be seen in cardiac surgeries or MI as an infusion in the dose of 2–8 µg/kg/min as temporary support to the failing heart. Development of tachyphylaxis is another reason that limits its longer use.

INOJECT, CARDIFORCE 12.5 mg/ml inj.

(ii) Dopamine may be used in patients with associated renal impairment because dopamine increases renal perfusion in addition to increased cardiac output. Infused at a rate of 3–10 µg/kg/min dopamine may be used in cardiogenic shock.

(iii) Dopexamine is an agonist at dopamine D_1, D_2 and β_2 adrenergic receptors because of which it has vasodilator properties—reduces peripheral vascular resistance and improves renal blood flow. Thus cardiac workload reduces due to reduced afterload. It also has mild inotropic properties by β_1 receptor stimulation. Dopexamine may be useful in heart failure.

c. ***Phosphodiesterase inhibitors:* Amrinone** (inamrinone) and **milrinone** inhibit the enzyme phosphodiesterase (which degrades cAMP) resulting in increased cAMP levels. They increase the force of contraction and also cause vasodilation. Because of the adverse effects and increased mortality seen with the use of these drugs, they are not preferred. However, they may be used for short periods in severe heart failure. Milirinone has shorter t½ and fewer side effects.

Sildenafil inhibits PDE5 which is abundant in the lungs. It has been found to be useful in patients with pulmonary hypertension and CHF. Sildenafil improves cardiac function, haemodynamics of the heart and overcomes ventricular hypertrophy and enhances exercise capacity.

d. *Newer inotropes:* **Levosimendan:** In addition to PDE inhibition, levosimendan sensitizes the troponin system to calcium and thereby has positive inotropic effects—**'calcium sensitizer'**. It also has vasodilator properties including coronary vasodilation and has been approved for use in heart failure. It is not an arrhythmogenic drug. Levosimendan may be used in acute decompensated heart failure as an alternative to dopexamine. It is used intravenously in a loading dose of 6–24 µg/kg followed by 0.05–0.2 µg/kg/minute.

Istaroxime is undergoing clinical trials for use in heart failure. It acts as an inotropic agent in two ways—inhibits Na^+, K^+-ATPase like digoxin and also facilitates the sequestration of calcium in the sarcoplasmic reticulum. It has some advantages over digoxin like being less arrhythmogenic.

Other newer drugs like **nesiritide** (a recombinant natriuretic peptide), vasopressin receptor antagonists like **conivaptan** and **tolvaptan** are under clinical trials for use in heart failure.

4. *Others*

β-adrenergic blockers: Though β-blockers are negative inotropic agents, several recent studies have shown that when used carefully along with other drugs, β-blockers can improve long-term survival (*see* page 103).

The strongest **disadvantage** of beta adrenergic blockers is their **negative inotropic effect.** However, several recent studies have shown that when used appropriately as an add-on drug, some of the beta blockers like **bisoprolol, metoprolol** and **carvedilol** reduce mortality and improve long-term survival in stable and severe heart failure. Beta blockers should be started with a low dose and gradually titrated upwards. The reduced ejection fraction due to reduced contractility that may be seen initially, gradually improves after 8–10 weeks of treatment. Though the exact reason for the beneficial effect is not understood, it could be because of (i) the reduction of the negative effects of sympathetic overactivity including apoptosis and remodelling effects, (ii) up-regulation of beta receptors and (iii) decreased heart rate.

Beta blockers are useful in mild to moderate heart failure with dilated cardiomyopathy and systolic dysfunction. A long-acting preparation, like sustained release metoprolol, is preferred.

5. *Newer drugs*
   a. **Ivabradine** selectively blocks the I_f current in the SA node, i.e. it inhibits cardiac pacemaker channels thereby reducing heart rate without depressing myocardial contractility (*see* page 368). Useful in chronic heart failure in patients who do not tolerate β blockers.
   b. **Sacubitril:** Neprilysin is an enzyme that degrades natriuretic peptides. Sacubitril inhibits **neprilysin**, thereby increasing the levels of natriuretic peptides. It is found to be useful in heart failure with or without valsartan (an ARB).
   c. **Serelaxin** is human relaxin-2, a peptide which activates VEGF, vascular endothelin B receptor and also enhances nitric oxide (NO) production, leading to renal and systemic vasodilatation. It is found to be useful in acute heart failure.
   d. **Ularitide** is synthetic urodilatin, a natriuretic peptide which regulates renal sodium and water excretion and has been shown to be beneficial in acute heart failure.

PHARMACOLOGY OF CARDIAC GLYCOSIDES

Cardiac glycosides are obtained from the plants of the foxglove family. Though these plants were known to Egyptians 3000 years ago, they were irrationally used. William Withering, an English physician, first described the clinical effects of digitalis in CCF in 1785.

Source: Digitoxin is obtained from the leaves of *Digitalis purpurea*. From the leaves of *Digitalis lanata*, digitoxin and digoxin are derived and the seeds of *Strophanthus gratus* contain ouabain. They are all called cardiac glycosides but digoxin is the glycoside used clinically because of its favourable pharmacokinetic properties. The word digitalis is used to mean cardiac glycosides.

Chemistry: The glycosides consist of an aglycon attached to sugars. The aglycone consists of a steroid ring with an unsaturated lactone ring attached to it. The aglycon has pharmacodynamic activity while sugars influence pharmacokinetic properties.

Pharmacological Actions

1. *Cardiac actions:* The primary effects of digitalis on the heart are:
   - Positive inotropic effects
   - Cardiotonic effects
   - Reduction in heart rate.

   a. *Positive inotropic effects:* Cardiac glycosides increase the force of contraction of the heart—the stroke volume increases and thereby the cardiac output. These effects are dose dependent. The systole is shortened and the diastole is prolonged which allows more rest to the heart and better filling of the coronaries. The ventricles are more completely emptied because of more forceful contractions. The inotropic effects are more pronounced on the failing heart.

b. *Tone:* Cardiac glycosides are cardiotonic drugs. The resting tension in the myocardial fibre increases.

c. *Heart rate:* Reduced by cardiac glycosides and this reduces workload.

Bradycardia is due to:

- Increased vagal tone
- Decreased sympathetic overactivity due to improved circulation
- By a direct action on SA and AV nodes.

d. *Coronary circulation:* Coronary circulation improves due to increased cardiac output and prolonged diastole during which the coronaries get filled better.

e. *Blood pressure:* No significant effects on BP in CCF patients. Pulse pressure may increase.

f. *Electrophysiological effects:* The effects on *electrophysiological properties* of the heart vary with dose and in different parts of the heart. These effects are a result of both direct and autonomic effects of digitalis. The action potential duration is reduced which may be due to increased potassium conductance following increased intracellular calcium. Digitalis shortens the refractory period of the purkinje fibres, the atria and the ventricular muscles. The automaticity of the ventricles and the Purkinje cells are enhanced but more pronounced effect is on AV conduction. Cardiac glycosides **depress AV conduction** and increase the AV nodal refractory period.

Digitalis also produces the characteristic ECG changes like T wave inversion, changes in P wave, increased PR interval (in AV node), shortened QT interval and ST segment depression.

2. ***Extracardiac actions***
   - *Kidney:* Diuresis occurs which relieves oedema in CCF patients.
   - *CNS:* High doses stimulate CTZ resulting in nausea and vomiting.

Mechanism of action: Cardiac glycosides inhibit the enzyme Na^+, K^+-ATPase—also called ***'sodium pump'*** present on the cardiac myocytes (Fig. 27.2). This results in an increase in the intracellular Na^+ and Ca^{++}. Thus more calcium is available for contraction, resulting in increased force and velocity of contraction. Inhibition of the 'sodium pump' increases intracellular sodium. This prevents Ca^{++} extrusion and also drives more calcium into the cell during depolarisation through voltage-sensitive calcium channels. Excess calcium is stored in the sarcoplasmic reticulum and thus cardiac glycosides increase the amount of calcium released during each action potential.

Pharmacokinetics: Digoxin is well-absorbed (Table 27.1). Presence of food in the stomach delays absorption. Bioavailability varies with different manufacturers and because the safety margin is low, in any given patient, the preparations from the same manufacturer should be used. Glycosides are cumulative drugs. Therapeutic concentration is 0.5 to 1.4 ng/ml.

Digoxin: Dose 0.125–0.5 mg daily is the slow loading and maintenance dose.
Digitran, Digox, Lanoxin 0.25 mg tab.

Digitalization: Response to digoxin develops over 5–7 days with the maintenance dose as given in mild to moderate cases of CCF. However, when rapid response is required, rapid digitalization can be done by more frequent dosing with constant monitoring 0.5–0.75 mg every 8 hours.

Adverse effects: Cardiac glycosides have a low safety margin and adverse effects are common. They inhibit Na^+, K^+-ATPase in all excitable tissues—including neurons and smooth muscle cells where spontaneous activity is increased and this action is

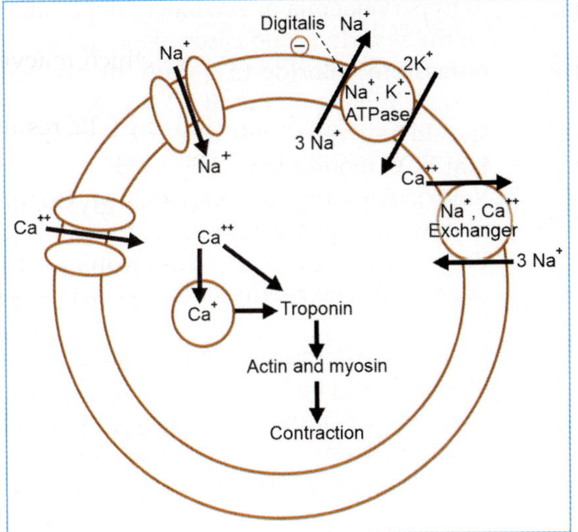

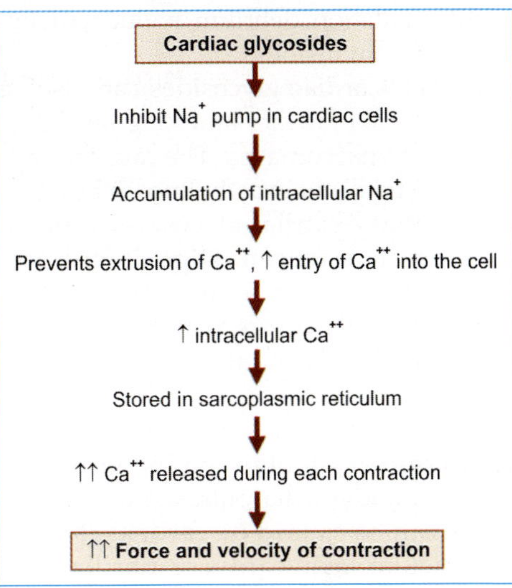

Fig. 27.2: Mechanism of action of cardiac glycosides. Cardiac glycosides inhibit the Na^+, K^+-ATPase pump and increases intracellular Na^+ which in turn prevents Ca^{++} extrusion. Thus more calcium is available for contraction

Table 27.1: Comparison between digoxin and digitoxin

Feature	*Digoxin*	*Digitoxin*
Source	*Digitalis lanata*	*Digitalis purpurea and lanata*
Pharmacokinetics		
• Route of administration	Oral, IV	Oral, IV
• Bioavailability	40–60%	90–100%
• Plasma protein binding	25%	95%
• Onset of action	15–30 min	30–120 min
• t½	40–48 hr	5–7 hr
• Time for digitalization (without loading dose)	5–7 days	25–30 days
Route of elimination	Renal excretion	Hepatic metabolism
Therapeutic utility	Most used among cardiac glycosides	Rarely used
Use	Used for initiation and maintenance therapy	Was used earlier for maintenance therapy

responsible for toxicity. Despite its toxicity, digitalis continues to be used. Toxicity can be cardiac and extracardiac.

1. *Extracardiac*

- Gastrointestinal toxicity—anorexia, nausea, vomiting and diarrhoea are the first symptoms to appear. Cardiac glycosides directly stimulate the CTZ which is responsible for nausea and vomiting.

  It is important to recognise these first symptoms of toxicity while at the same time vomiting may also be due to CCF itself.
- Neurotoxicity—digitalis can cause vertigo, blurred vision, disturbances of colour vision, headache, confusion, neuralgia,

disorientation, delirium, hallucinations and rarely convulsions.

- *Others:* Cardiac glycosides can also cause allergic skin rashes and long-term use can cause gynaecomastia. The cause for gynaecomastia is not exactly known but it could be because cardiac glycosides structurally resemble estrogen. Digoxin crosses the placental barrier to an extent that foetal blood levels of digoxin are higher than maternal and can cause toxicity.

2. Cardiac Toxicity

Arrhythmias of any type including extrasystoles, bradycardia, pulses bigeminy and AV block can be caused by cardiac glycosides. Ventricular tachycardia or fibrillation and paroxysmal atrial tachycardia can also occur but rare. Factors that influence digitalis-induced cardiotoxicity are:

- **Hypokalaemia** enhances digoxin toxicity. This is because potassium and digitalis inhibit each other's binding to the sodium pump which means hyperkalaemia reduces the effects of cardiac glycosides while hypokalaemia enhances their effects and thereby toxicity. Moreover, excess of potassium can suppress abnormal cardiac automaticity and thereby overcome digoxin toxicity to some extent. Unfortunately, plasma K^+ is not an indicator of myocardial K^+ status. Vomiting, diarrhoea and diuretic therapy may all result in hypokalaemia and potentiate digoxin toxicity.
- **Hypercalcaemia** can enhance cardiac toxicity particularly arrhythmias due to digitalis as it can hasten the filling up of intracellular Ca^{++} stores.
- Rapid digitalization and IV administration are likely to precipitate toxicity.
- Patients with poor cardiac status especially elderly are more prone to digoxin toxicity.

Treatment of Toxicity

1. Stop digitalis
2. Oral or parenteral K^+ supplements are given (but K^+ is contraindicated in presence of hyperkalaemia or AV block) depending on the severity. Mild cases respond to oral potassium chloride (5 g daily in divided doses). When parenteral K^+ is required, it should be given slowly as a drip with constant ECG monitoring.
3. Ventricular arrhythmias are treated with IV phenytoin/lignocaine.
4. Bradycardia is treated with atropine and supraventricular arrhythmias with propranolol.
5. In severe toxicity, temporary cardiac pacemaker should be inserted.
6. Antidigoxin immunotherapy (Digibind obtained from sheep) is now available. **Antidigoxin antibodies** bind cardiac glycosides and reverse their effects. These antibodies are life saving in severe toxicity due to cardiac glycosides.

Precautions and Contraindications to Digitalis Therapy

- Hypokalaemia—enhances toxicity
- MI, thyrotoxicosis patients—more prone to arrhythmias
- Patients with acid–base imbalance—more prone to toxicity
- Avoid in myocarditis, elderly, AV block and in renal failure.

Drug interactions—Table 27.2.

Uses

1. *Heart failure:* Digoxin increases the force of contraction, ejection fraction and thereby improves tissue perfusion. The sympathetic overactivity and the compensatory increase

Table 27.2: Drug interactions

Drugs that enhance digoxin toxicity
• Diuretics (due to hypokalaemia), calcium
• Quinidine, verapamil, methyldopa—↑ digoxin levels
Drugs that reduce digoxin levels
• Antacids, neomycin, metoclopramide—↓ absorption
• Rifampicin, phenobarbitone—hasten metabolism due to enzyme induction

in salt and water retention are both countered. Hence the peripheral resistance is reduced and thereby the afterload. All these effects further improve the cardiac output, performance in the failing heart and relieve the symptoms. Mild to moderate cases of low output failure are treated with diuretics and vasodilators (ACE inhibitors preferred). When the patients do not respond to these, digoxin may be given. Digoxin improves cardiac performance in the dilated, failing heart. If there is associated atrial fibrillation, digoxin is the preferred drug. Once the patient is stabilized, digitalis may be gradually withdrawn. However, if the patient deteriorates, digoxin has to be restarted.

2. *Cardiac arrhythmias:*
   a. *Atrial fibrillation:* Digitalis reduces ventricular rate in atrial fibrillation depressing the velocity of AV conduction. It enhances the ERP of the AV node. Thus the number of impulses reaching the ventricles from the atrium are reduced which means ventricular rate is reduced. The vagal tone is also increased. The effect is dose dependent and, therefore, the dose should be adjusted to get the required ventricular rate (70–80/min). A beta blocker or verapamil may be added which also help to reduce the dose of digoxin needed.
   b. *Atrial flutter:* Atrial rate of 200–350/min is atrial flutter. Digoxin slows the AV conduction and produces a degree of AV block by increasing the ERP of the AV node. It thus reduces the ventricular rate as in atrial fibrillation. Cardioversion and radiofrequency ablation may also be employed to abolish atrial flutter but prevention of recurrence can be done with digoxin.
   c. *Paroxysmal supraventricular* tachycardia (PSVT): Reentry in the SA and AV nodes is responsible for supraventricular tachyarrhythmia. Digoxin can be used IV to terminate these arrhythmias and in AV nodal tachycardia. Because of its vagomimetic effects and depression of AV conduction, digitalis is useful in these arrhythmias. However, adenosine, verapamil and diltiazem are the preferred drugs in PSVT.

Phosphodiesterase Enzymes and Inhibitors

Phosphodiesterases (PDEs) are enzymes that hydrolyse cyclic nucleotides—cAMP and cGMP. There are 11 subtypes of PDEs of which some hydrolyse cAMP while some have affinity for cGMP. Some of the PDEs inhibit both cAMP and cGMP. Inhibition of PDEs can enhance the levels of cAMP and cGMP leading to several therapeutically useful effects. Some of them are in clinical use and others are being studied for possible therapeutic applications.

Therapeutic Applications of PDE Inhibitors

Non-selective PDE inhibitors

Methylaxanthines
- Theophylline—bronchodilator
- Pentoxyphylline—vasodilator

Selective PDE inhibitors

1. PDE III inhibitors
   - Dipyridamole, cilastazol—vasodilation and antiplatelet aggregation
   - Amrinone, milrinone—inotropes
   - Levosimendan
2. PDE IV inhibitors—roflumilast (antiinflammatory and immunomodulatory)
3. PDE V inhibitors—sildenafil, verdenafil, tadalafil (used in erectile dysfunction)

Clinical Pharmacology

- Spironolactone, eplerenone reduce mortality as well as morbidity in CCF.
- β-blockers should be started only when the patient is in compensated heart failure. Carvedilol is now the preferred β-blocker in CCF.
- ACE inhibitors should be used in all patients with CCF unless contraindicated.
- ACE inhibitors have better efficacy than ARBs due to raised bradykinin levels. ARB is an alternative.
- Salt, water and physical activity restriction are important lifestyle modifications in CCF.

[1] From Medical Council of India, *Competency based Undergraduate Curriculum for the Indian Medical Graduate*, 2018;1:136–144.

CHAPTER 28

Drugs used in Ischaemic Heart Disease

Competency achievement: The student should be able to:

PH 1.28 Describe the mechanisms of action, types, doses, side effects, indications and contraindications of the drugs used in ischaemic heart disease (stable, unstable angina and myocardial infarction), peripheral vascular disease.[1]

Ischaemic heart disease is a common cause of death across the world. It may manifest as angina pectoris, unstable angina and in more severe cases as myocardial infarction.

ANGINA PECTORIS

Angina pectoris is the chief symptom of ischaemic heart disease (IHD) characterised by sudden, severe, substernal discomfort or pain which may radiate to the left shoulder and along the flexor surface of the left arm. The heart receives 4% of the cardiac output. However, coronary circulation has two disadvantages—(i) the coronary arteries are end arteries, (ii) the oxygen extraction capacity of the myocardium is high even at rest. Hence, in presence of increased demand, extraction cannot be further improved unlike the skeletal muscles. Moreover, the coronaries get filled only during the diastole. Myocardial oxygen consumption is mainly determined by **preload** (venous return and stretching of the heart), **afterload** (peripheral arterial resistance) and **heart rate**. When the oxygen supply to the myocardium is insufficient for its needs, myocardial ischaemia develops. Pain is due to accumulation of metabolites in the cardiac muscle.

William Heberden first described angina as a separate disease entity (*angere* = to strangulate, *pectus*-chest). A large percentage of patients may not experience pain as such but may have substernal discomfort or suffocation/uneasiness.

Three forms of angina are:

1. *Classical angina* (stable angina, angina of effort, exertional angina). Pain is induced by exercise or emotion, both of which increase myocardial oxygen demand (even a heavy meal can precipitate angina). In such patients, there is narrowing of the coronary arteries due to atherosclerosis and, therefore, the coronaries cannot dilate to increase the blood supply during exercise. Hence, there is an imbalance between oxygen supply and demand.
2. *Variant or Prinzmetal angina* (described by Myran Prinzmetal) occurs at rest and is caused by spasm of the coronary artery.
3. *Unstable angina:* A combination of factors like increased myocardial O_2 demand, coronary vasospasm and platelet aggregation may result in angina called unstable angina which requires immediate treatment.

Acute coronary syndrome is anginal pain occurring at rest due to rupture of the atherosclerotic plaque leading to coronary thrombosis and includes unstable angina and myocardial infarction.

ANTIANGINAL DRUGS

Drugs are used to improve the balance between oxygen supply and demand either by increasing oxygen supply to the myocardium (coronary dilation) or by reducing the oxygen demand (reducing preload/afterload/heart rate or all of these).

Classification

1. *Nitrates:* Nitroglycerin, isosorbide dinitrate, isosorbide mononitrate, pentaerythritol tetranitrate
2. *Calcium channel blockers:* Verapamil, diltiazem, amlodipine, nifedipine
3. *β-blockers:* Propranolol, atenolol, etc.
4. *Potassium channel openers:* Nicorandil, pinacidil
5. *Miscellaneous:* Dipyridamole, Ivabradine
   Antiplatelet drugs: Aspirin, clopidogrel
   Cytoprotective drugs: Trimetazidine ranolazine.

NITRATES

Nitroglycerin was introduced for the treatment of angina in 1879.

Mechanism of Action

Nitrates are vasodilators (Fig. 28.1). They are converted to **nitric oxide** by the enzymes mitochondrial glutathione-S-transferase and aldehyde reductase. NO activates vascular guanylyl cyclase which in turn increases the synthesis of cGMP. This cGMP brings about dephosphorylation of protein kinases (prevents interaction of actin with myosin). It also reduces free cytosolic calcium by preventing calcium release from the sarcoplasmic reticulum or by increasing Ca^{++} efflux. These effects result in relaxation of smooth muscles including vascular smooth muscles. Thus it causes vasodilation and also relaxation of other smooth muscles.

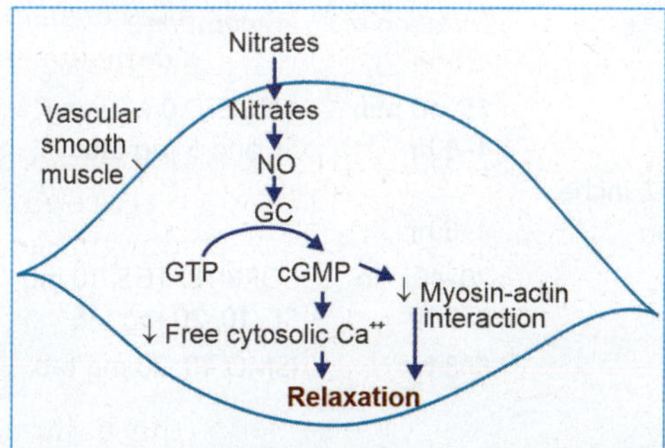

Fig. 28.1: Mechanism of action of nitrates

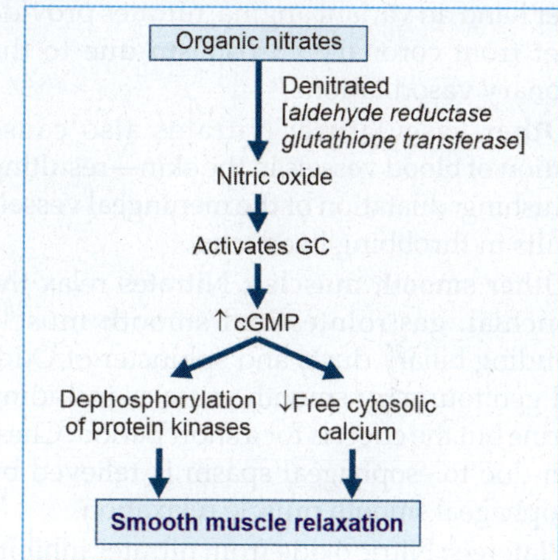

Pharmacological Actions

Reduction in preload: Nitrates are predominantly **venodilators**—thus, with dilation of capacitance vessels, there is pooling of blood in the veins leading to less venous return. When the blood reaching the heart is reduced, the preload and thereby the **myocardial workload** are **reduced.**

As per the Laplace's law, a decrease in ventricular pressure and heart size as due to reduced venus return, results in a reduction in the myocardial wall tension that needs to be developed and, therefore, reduces the oxygen requirement.

Reduction in afterload: Nitrates also cause some arteriolar dilation which is significant in higher doses. Thus they reduce the vascular resistance leading to a reduction in afterload.

Coronary dilation: Nitrates also bring about some coronary vasodilation. There is a significant increase in coronary blood flow in a normal person but in the presence of atherosclerotic coronary artery disease, the increase is not much.

In angina: The beneficial effects of nitrates in stable angina are due to their vasodilator properties. The **reduction in preload and afterload** leads to a decrease in the myocardial workload which in turn results in a **decrease in the myocardial oxygen demand.** On the other hand, in variant angina, nitrates provide relief from coronary vasospasm due to the coronary vasodilation.

Other vasculature: Nitrates also cause dilation of blood vessels in the skin—resulting in flushing; dilatation of the meningeal vessels results in throbbing headache.

Other smooth muscles: Nitrates relax the bronchial, gastrointestinal smooth muscle including biliary ducts and sphincter of Oddi and genitourinary smooth muscles including uterine but the effect is for a short period. Chest pain due to esophageal spasm is relieved by oesophageal smooth muscle relaxation.

Platelets: Nitric oxide from nitrates inhibits platelet aggregation by activating guanylyl cyclase leading to an increase in cGMP. Though the actual extent of the beneficial effect of nitrates in a clinical setting is not known, it may be particularly of help in patients with unstable angina.

Pharmacokinetics

Nitrates are well absorbed orally but they undergo extensive first pass metabolism. All nitrates have good lipid solubility.

Nitroglycerin, isosorbide dinitrate, isosorbide mononitrate and pentaerythritol tetranitrate are the nitrates used in angina. Isosorbide mononitrate is longer acting (needs to be given twice daily) and has 100% bioavailability. Amyl nitrite is used in cyanide poisoning.

Preparations

Nitrates are available for oral, sublingual, parenteral use and as ointment and trans dermal patches for topical use. Topical preparations are used for the prevention of nocturnal episodes of angina. However, there is an increased risk of development of tole rance with topical and slow release preparations (Table 28.1).

Adverse Effects

Headache is common; flushing, sweating, palpitation, weakness, postural hypotension and rashes can occur. Rashes are more common with pentaerythritol tetranitrate. **Tolerance** to vascular effects of nitrates develops on repeated long-term use particularly when continuous high plasma nitrate levels are present. Activation of **compensatory responses,** like tachycardia, salt and water retention, may contribute to the development of tolerance. By adopting proper dosing schedule, tolerance can be avoided. The patient must be **free of nitrates for at least 8 hours** of the day to prevent the development

Table 28.1: Some nitrates used in angina pectoris

Drug	*Dose and route*	*Duration of action*	*Preparation*
Nitroglycerin (NTG)	0.5 mg SL	15–40 min	ANGISED 0.3, 0.5 mg
	5 mg oral	4–8 hr	SL and 5 mg tab.
	2% Skin oint applied 1–2 inches on the precardial region	4–6 hr	
Isosorbide dinitrate	5–10 mg SL	20–40 min	SORBITRATE 5, 10 mg
	10–20 mg oral	2–3 hr	SL, 10, 20 mg tab
Isosorbide mononitrate	10–20 mg oral	6–8 hr	ISMO 10, 20 mg tab

of tolerance. Tolerance can also be minimized by twice/thrice daily dosing schedule.

Monday morning disease: Nitrates are used in factories where explosives are manufactured. Workers joining duty initially experience headache, flushing and palpitations but soon develop tolerance. When they are away at weekends and join back on Monday morning, the symptoms recur, called 'Monday morning disease/sickness'.

Nitrates should not be abruptly withdrawn after long-term use because they can precipitate acute angina and spasm of the vascular and other smooth muscles. Thus nitrates are said to cause a sort of dependence.

Drug Interactions

Nitrates and sildenafil: Cyclic-GMP is metabolised by phosphodiesterase. Sildenafil (Viagra), a drug used in erectile dysfunction, is a phosphodiesterase inhibitor. It thus increases cGMP activity resulting in relaxation of the cavernosal as well as vascular smooth muscles. Vasodilation results in hypotension. Sildenafil potentiates the action of nitrates and together they can cause severe hypotension with reflex tachycardia resulting in MI. Sudden deaths have been reported due to myocardial infarction.

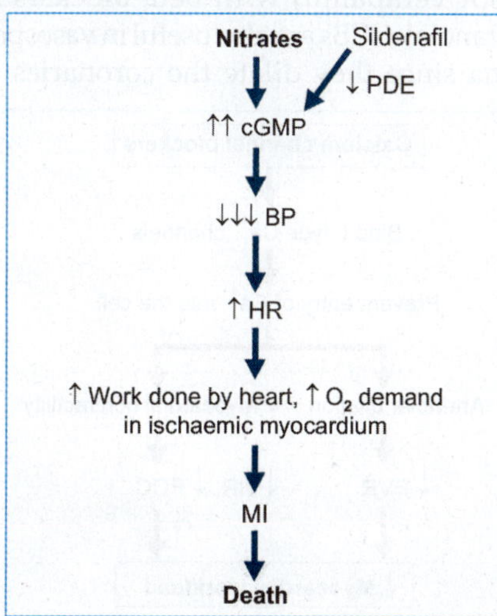

Uses

1. *Exertional angina*
   - *Acute episode:* Sublingual nitroglycerin is the drug of choice for acute anginal attacks. It relieves pain in 2 to 5 minutes. If the pain is not relieved, the dose may be repeated—up to 3 tablets in 15 minutes. Isosorbide dinitrate may also be used though it is slower acting than sublingual NTG. The patient should be advised to take the tablet in a sitting position since the sudden reduction in BP can result in fall due to syncope.
   - *Prophylaxis:* NTG can be used for acute as well as chronic prophylaxis. When patient is expected to have a known exertion like walking uphill, a tablet of sublingual NTG can be used for prevention of angina (acute prophylaxis). Nitrates are also used orally for the prophylaxis of angina. Longer acting nitrates are preferred for this but patients can develop tolerance to nitrates. Nitroglycerin ointment may be applied over the chest specially to control angina at night. Transdermal patch delivers nitroglycerin constantly for 24 hours.
2. *Vasospastic angina:* Nitroglycerin relieves pain by relieving coronary vasospasm.
3. *Unstable angina:* Intravenous nitroglycerin helps to relieve pain but the exact reason for the benefit is not understood. Both a reduction in cardiac workload and coronary vasodilation may be of value in such patients. NTG is started in the dose of 5–10 μg/min and gradually titrated up to 20 μg/min depending on the requirement.
4. *Cardiac failure:* Nitrates are useful due to their vasodilator property. Nitroglycerin given SL or IV helps patients with acute LVF by reducing the preload which in turn reduces the cardiac workload. Constant monitoring is required.
5. *Myocardial infarction:* IV nitroglycerin is used by many physicians to reduce

Unstable angina not gastritis! ☹

A 53-year-old obese but otherwise healthy man at the peak of his career complained of discomfort in the retrosternal region. It was passed off as gastritis and self-treated with antacids. The discomfort recurred on and off and on the third day the patient died a sudden death while he was travelling in his car. The patient had a massive MI and the discomfort he had earlier was retrospectively diagnosed as unstable angina.

cardiac workload. The dose should be carefully adjusted to avoid tachycardia and hypotension.

6. *Cyanide poisoning* (Fig. 28.2): Cyanide rapidly binds to cytochrome oxidase and other vital enzymes resulting in inhibition of cellular respiration and blocks the utilization of oxygen. It requires immediate treatment. Amylnitrite is given by inhalation and sodium nitrite by IV injection (10 ml of 3% solution). Sodium thiosulphate is given IV (50 ml of 25% solution). Nitrites convert haemoglobin to methaemoglobin which has a high affinity for cyanide and binds to cyanide forming cyanmethaemoglobin. Sodium thiosulphate reacts with cyanmethaemoglobin to form thiocyanate which is easily excreted by the kidneys. It thus protects the important enzymes from binding to cyanide. Early treatment is very important.

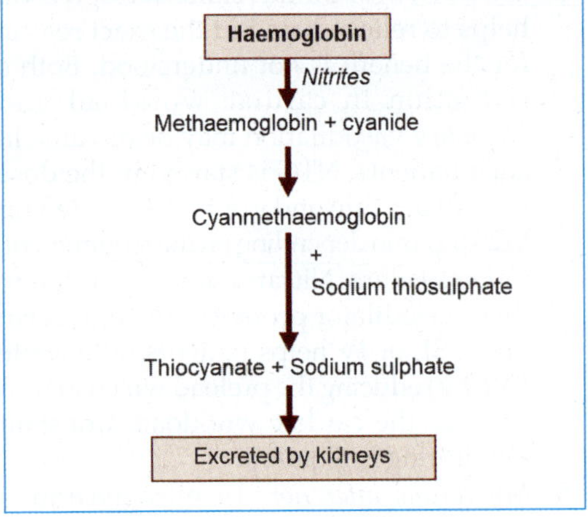

Fig. 28.2: Treatment of cyanide poisoning

7. *Other uses*
   - **To relieve oesophageal spasm.** Sublingual NTG is taken just before meals to counter the spasm.
   - Sublingual nitroglycerin is also useful as a **spasmolytic** to relieve biliary colic.

CALCIUM CHANNEL BLOCKERS

Calcium channel blockers (*see* chapter 25) relax the arterioles leading to a decrease in the peripheral vascular resistance and a reduction in the afterload. Some reflex tachycardia can occur particularly with dihydropyridines. However, some CCBs, particularly verapamil and diltiazem, also depress the myocardial contractility thereby reducing the heart rate and force of contraction. This results in reduced cardiac workload and oxygen consumption. CCBs also dilate the coronaries thereby increasing the coronary blood flow.

CCBs are used for the prophylaxis of exertional angina. They can be combined (except verapamil) with beta blockers like propranolol. CCBs are also useful in vasospastic angina since they dilate the coronaries and

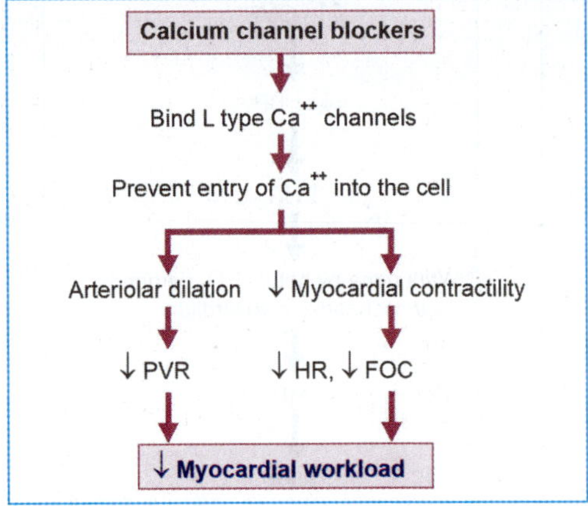

relieve vasospasm. In fact they are preferred over nitrates in vasospastic angina.

β-BLOCKERS

β-blockers reduce the frequency and severity of attacks of exertional angina and are useful in the prevention of angina. Exercise, emotion and similar situations increase sympathetic activity leading to increased heart rate, force of contraction and BP, thereby increasing O_2 consumption by the heart. β-blockers **prevent angina** by blocking all these actions and thereby prevent an increase in the myocardial workload and oxygen demand (Fig. 28.3). β-blockers improve exercise tolerance. They are used for the long-term prophylaxis of classical angina and may be combined with nitrates. β-blockers are also useful in unstable angina when judiciously used. β-blockers should always be tapered after prolonged use. β-blockers are **not** useful in variant angina.

POTASSIUM CHANNEL OPENERS

Like the calcium channels, there are several types of potassium channels, viz:

- Voltage dependent,
- ATP sensitive,
- Receptor operated and
- Ca^{++} and Na^+ activated potassium channels.

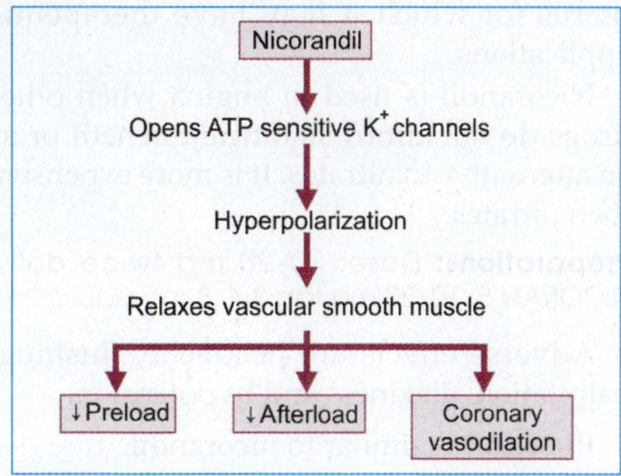

Nicorandil, *pinacidil* and *cromakalim* are potassium channel openers. **Minoxidil** and **diazoxide** also open up K^+ channels and are used in hypertension. Sulfonylureas block the K^+ channels in the pancreatic β-cells, thereby enhancing insulin release. Amiodarone blocks K^+ channels in the heart and prolongs APD—used in arrhythmias.

Nicorandil is an arterial and venous dilator. Opening of the ATP-sensitive K^+ channels results in the efflux of K^+ leading to hyperpolarization and, therefore, relaxation of the vascular smooth muscles. In addition like nitrates it also acts through nitric oxide and reduces the preload and afterload. It causes coronary vasodilation. Nicorandil also relaxes other smooth muscles like the bronchi and

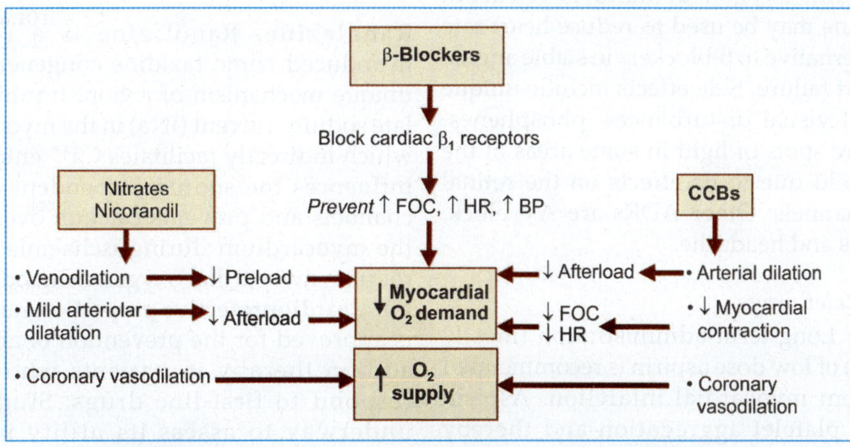

Fig. 28.3: Mode of action and cardiovascular effects of antianginal drugs

uterus for which it may have therapeutic applications.

Nicorandil is used in angina when other drugs do not afford significant benefit or as an alternative to nitrates. It is more expensive than nitrates.

Preparations: Dose: 10–20 mg twice daily. NICORAN 5, 10, 20 mg tab 2,4, 8 mg vial.

Adverse effects are headache, flushing, palpitation, dizziness and hypotension.

Pinacidil is similar to nicorandil.

Other Drugs used in Angina

Dipyridamole: It is a coronary vasodilator (*see* page 312) but it diverts the blood from ischaemic zone **'coronary steal sydrome'** and is, therefore, not beneficial. It inhibits platelet aggregation for which it is used in post-MI and post-stroke patients for prevention of coronary and cerebral thrombosis.

Ivabradine blocks the sodium channels in the SA node and decreases the heart rate **(direct bradycardiac).** It selectively blocks the HCN ion channels which are cardiac pacemaker channels in the SA node. The pacemaker I_f curent is reduced (I_f is funny cation channel) thereby reducing heart rate. Hence diastole is longer, coronaries are filled better and myocardial oxygen demand is reduced. Ivabradine may be used to reduce heart rate as an alternative to β-blockers in stable angina and heart failure. Side effects include unique transient visual disturbances 'phosphenes' which are spots of light in some areas of the visual field due to its effects on the retinal HCN channels. Other ADRs are AV block, dizziness and headache.

Antiplatelet drugs

Aspirin: Long-term administration (mostly life long) of low dose aspirin is recommended to prevent myocardial infarction. Aspirin inhibits platelet aggregation and thereby prevents MI in patients with angina.

Clopidogrel is an ADP antagonist (*see* page 313) which blocks the ADP receptors on platelets and prevent their activation. The antiplatelet effects are additive with aspirin and is used with aspirin in acute coronary syndrome.

Cytoprotective drugs

Trimetazidine: It is claimed to have a protective effect on the ischaemic myocardium and to maintain left ventricular function. Trimetazidine belongs to a new class of drugs that modulate the metabolism in the myocardium. It is a pFOX inhibitor (**P**artial inhibitor of fatty acid **o**xidation), i.e. trimetazidine inhibits the enzyme involved in fatty acid oxidation pathway in the myocardium. It also inhibits the superoxide-induced cytotoxicity to the myocardial cells. Trimetazidine thus protects the myocardium from ischaemic damage. It is also a calcium channel blocker.

It is orally effective and is well tolerated with occasional gastric irritation, fatigue and muscle cramps.

Trimetazidine is used as an add-on drug along with other antianginal drugs in the treatment of angina pectoris.

Preparations: Dose: 20 mg TDS or 35 mg sustained release BD with food. FLAVEDON 20 mg Tab, 35 mg modified release tab. CARVIDON 20 mg tab.

Ranolazine: Ranolazine is a recently introduced trime tazidine congener with a unique mechanism of action. It inhibits the late sodium current (INa) in the myocardium which indirectly facilitates Ca^{++} entry, i.e. it influences the sodium-dependent calcium channels and prevents calcium overload in the myocardium during ischaemia. It thus reduces myocardial oxygen demand. Due to these **cardioprotective properties,** ranolazine is approved for the prevention of angina as add-on therapy in patients who do not respond to first-line drugs. Studies are underway to assess its utility in acute coronary syndrome.

Ranolazine is orally effective with a bioavailability of 30–50%. It prolongs QT interval and, therefore, should be avoided with other drugs that prolong QT interval. It can also cause weakness, postural hypotension, dizziness, headache and constipation.

Dose: 500 mg sustained release tablets BD. RANEXA 100, 500 mg tab.

Oxyphedrine acts by improving myocardial metabolism in hypoxia. However, its efficacy is yet to be proved.

PHARMACOTHERAPY OF ANGINA

Exertional Angina

Coronary angioplasty with insertion of a stent is the preferred treatment in presence of significant narrowing of the coronary arteries. Coronary artery surgery is done when there is severe narrowing. Pharmacotherapy may be an alternative in some patients.

Acute attack: Sublingual nitroglycerin is the drug of choice. If the pain does not subside in 5 minutes, repeat the dose. After the relief of pain, the tablet should be discarded.

Acute prophylaxis: Sublingual nitroglycerin given 15 minutes before an exertion (e.g. walking uphill) can prevent the attack. The prophylactic effect lasts for 30 minutes.

Chronic prophylaxis: Long-acting nitrates or β-blockers (preferred) or calcium channel blockers can be used. All are given orally. If one drug is not effective, a combination of drugs may be used.

Combination of Drugs in Angina

1. *Nitrates + β-blockers:* Very effective in exertional angina. Reflex tachycardia due to nitrates is countered by β-blockers. Ventricular dilatation due to β-blockers is opposed by nitrates.
2. *Nifedipine + β-blockers:* The antianginal effects are additive. Reflex tachycardia due to nifedipine is countered by β-blockers.
3. *Nitrates + CCBs:* Nitrates decrease preload, CCBs reduce afterload and the combination reduces cardiac workload.
4. *CCBs + β-blockers + nitrates:* If the angina is not controlled by 2 drug combinations, 3 drugs can be used. Nitrates reduce preload, CCBs reduce afterload while β-blockers decrease heart rate. This combination is useful in severe angina.

Vasospastic Angina

Nitroglycerin and nifedipine given sublingually and amlodipine are effective in preventing and treating vasospastic episodes.

Unstable Angina

Unstable angina includes:

- Patients with exertional angina developing angina **at rest.**
- Severe, prolonged anginal attacks without ECG evidence of MI.
- Angina developing after myocardial infarction.

Such patients with unstable angina are at a high risk of developing MI or sudden death and need hospitalisation and rigorous treatment for its prevention. The primary goal of treatment is to increase myocardial blood flow.

Drugs used in Unstable Angina

1. *Aspirin:* Platelet aggregation can occlude narrowed coronary arteries and can also release potent vasoconstrictors. Aspirin (75–300 mg daily) prevents platelet aggregation and thereby could prevent myocardial infarction.
2. *Heparin:* In high-risk patients, IV/SC heparin reduces pain.
3. *Nitrates:* Intravenous nitroglycerin reduces the cardiac workload and relieves pain.
4. *Other drugs:* β-adrenergic blockers like atenolol (50–100 mg daily) and; if they are contraindicated, calcium channel blockers like diltiazem and verapamil may be given. Glycoprotein receptor antagonists (abciximab, epitifibatide and tirofiban) inhibit the final steps of platelet aggregation and are being tried in unstable angina.

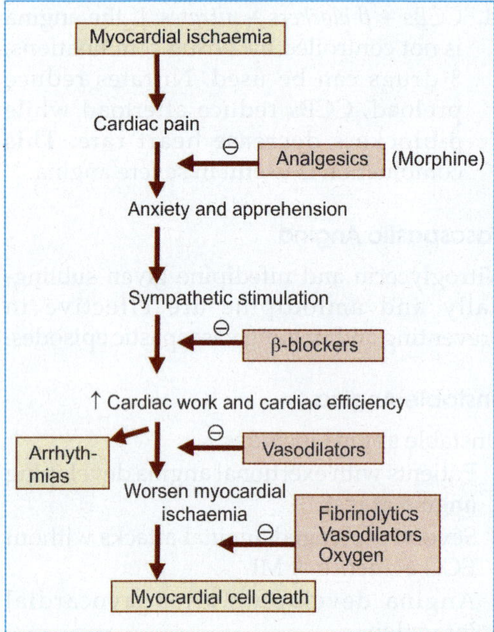

Fig. 28.4: Pathophysiology and sites of drug action in myocardial infarction

DRUGS USED IN MYOCARDIAL INFARCTION

Coronary heart disease is the most important cause of premature death, particularly in the developed countries.

Rupture of an atheromatous plaque in the coronary artery (Fig. 28.4) results in an occlusive thrombus leading to acute myocardial infarction. Symptoms include severe substernal pain radiating to the left shoulder, medial aspect of the left arm with nausea, vomiting, sweating, palpitation and shortness of breath. Patients appear pale and apprehensive. The process of infarction gradually develops (unless it is severe) over 6–8 hours after which there is cell death in the infarcted area. Timely intervention can reduce the extent of damage. Coronary angioplasty with a stent inserted to recanalise the coronary artery is the preferred option. The immediate objective of treatment is to limit the myocardial ischaemia and the consequent cell death. Drugs used are given below.

Immediate Treatment

1. *Analgesics and antianxiety drugs:* Pain due to myocardial ischaemia evokes anxiety and apprehension which result in sympathetic overactivity. This itself could prove deleterious to the heart. Hence a good analgesic, like morphine 10 mg or pethidine 50 mg, is given intravenously through an IV cannula. They relieve pain and thereby reduce anxiety. Hence the demerits of sympathetic overactivity are reduced. Diazepam may also be given to reduce anxiety and produce sedation.
2. *Thrombolytics:* Can limit the extent of damage and reduce mortality, if started at the onset of symptoms. They should be started at the earliest possible (within 6–12 hr). Streptokinase 1.5 million units infusion is given over 1 hour. Urokinase or alteplase may be given as alternatives as 15 mg bolus and 0.5 mg/kg over the next 90 minutes.

   Anistreplase is a form of streptokinase which is convenient to use because it is long acting and, therefore, can be used as a single IV injection. Alteplase is expensive and hence is mostly reserved for patients in whom streptokinase cannot be used (*see* page 309).

   Thrombolytics should be **started at the earliest possible** (within 6–12 hours) because they can limit the extent of damage and reduce mortality.
3. *Antiplatelet drugs:* 300 mg of soluble aspirin should be given orally immediately at the onset of symptoms. It reduces mortality and improves the effect of thrombolysis. Aspirin should be continued for long term (75–150 mg/day) even after the patient recovers from MI. Patients allergic to aspirin may be given oral clopidogrel.
4. *Anticoagulants:* Heparin may be given to prevent the extension of thrombus and also to prevent deep vein thrombosis.
5. *Oxygen:* High flow oxygen should be given by inhalation.

6. *Vasodilators:* Nitroglycerine or sodium nitroprusside may be used as IV infusion to reduce the cardiac workload and decrease mortality. Care should be taken to avoid reflex tachycardia.
7. *Other drugs:*
   i. *β-adrenergic antagonists:* IV atenolol 5–10 mg over 5 minutes or metoprolol 5 mg over 2 minutes should be given at the earliest possible unless contra-indicated as in asthma, heart block or heart failure. β-blockers limit the infarct size, reduce the incidence of arrhythmias and decrease mortality. Later oral β-blockers should be continued.
   ii. *ACE inhibitors:* It should be started within 24 hr. Several studies have shown them to provide long-term survival benefits. They prevent ventricular remodelling and reduce the progression of heart failure. They are continued for long periods after recovery.

Clinical Pharmacology

- Patients with angina should be assessed for coronary artery disease by angiography and suitable intervention like angioplasty/coronary by pass surgery should be considered.
- Associated conditions which increase myocardial workload like anaemia and hyperthyroidism should be looked for.
- Alcohol addicts should gradually withdraw alcohol to avoid withdrawal symptoms. Patient may tend to ignore the pain in angina under the influence of alcohol.
- Antiplatelet drugs like aspirin given lifelong.
- β-blockers/CCBs are the mainstay of treatment.
- Nitrates are only indicated in exertional and unstable angina.
- Diltiazem is the drug of choice in Prinzmetal's angina as nitrates are weaker arteriolar dilators.
- Patients with cardiac problems tend to be depressed psychologically. Adequate counselling and measures to overcome depression including meditation and yoga thearpy are necessary.

   iii. *Inotropic drugs:* Dobutamine or dopamine may be given to support the cardiac function.
   iv. *Antiemetics:* An antiemetic may be given intravenously, if required (pheniramine 25 mg)
   v. *Antiarrhythmics:* Arrhythmias are common in patients in acute MI; suitable antiarrhythmics should be used depending on the arrhythmia.

Long-term Treatment

Once the patient is stabilized, certain drugs are recommended for prevention of further ischaemic events. A stool softener may be given to avoid straining at stools. Long-term administration of low dose aspirin, a β-adrenergic blocker and an ACE inhibitor are useful in reducing long-term mortality.

Risk Factor Management

- Smoking should be stopped.
- Hyperlipidaemia, if any, should be controlled.
- Body weight should be reduced.
- Regular moderate exercises should be advised.
- Adequate control of diabetes and hypertension, if any.

TREATMENT OF PERIPHERAL VASCULAR DISEASES

Peripheral vascular diseases (PVDs) result from reduced blood supply to the lower limbs which may be due to organic occlusion (e.g. thrombus) or vasospasm. Obstruction to the blood flow in the peripheral circulation due to any cause can result in ischaemia of the area distal to it with its related consequences. Drugs are not of much help in organic obstruction. **Vasospastic PVDs** include thromboangitis obliterans (TAO, Buerger's disease), Raynaud's phenomenon, frost bite, vascular complications of diabetes mellitus like gangrene, leg and foot ulcers.

Drugs used in PVD include:

1. *Vasodilators*
   a. CCBs—nifedipine, verapamil
   b. Adrenergic blockers—prazosin, tolazoline
   c. β-adrenergic agonists—isoxsuprine
2. *Anticoagulants* and *antiplatelet drugs*—heparin, warfarin
3. *Other drugs:* Hypolipidaemics (statins), pentoxiphylline, naftidofuryl oxalate, cilostazol, cyclandelate, xanthinol nicotinate.

Vasodilators are of **no significant value** in obstructive PVD because they do not increase the blood flow to the ischaemic areas. Infact they may even harm such an area because general vasodilation may shift the blood to other nonischaemic areas described as **'steal' syndrome**. However, vasodilators may be used in vasospastic diseases like Raynaud's phenomenon. The strategy is to bring about dilation of the arterioles to allow better blood flow to the limbs with minimum hypotension.

- Calcium channel blockers, like nifedipine (5–20 mg thrice daily), are good vasodilators and are beneficial in patients with PVD.
- Alpha adrenergic blockers, like prazosin (0.5 mg twice daily) may be used.
- Beta adrenergic agonists, like isoxsuprine also help to relieve symptoms.

Anticoagulants and antiplatelet drugs: Like heparin and warfarin prevent the formation of clot. They are of value particularly in obstructive peripheral vascular disease. Aspirin 75–150 mg once a day or clopidogrel 10 mg twice daily may be used for this purpose.

OTHER DRUGS

Pentoxiphylline, an analog of xanthine is a phosphodiesterase inhibitor. It reduces the viscosity of the blood and enhances blood flow to the ischaemic areas. It is also claimed to improve the flexibility of the RBCs (called haemorrheological action)—resulting in an improvement of microcirculation and is devoid of steal phenomenon. It potentiates the action of anticoagulants.

Uses: Pentoxiphylline is used in transient ischaemic attacks, non-haemorrhagic stroke, chronic cerebrovascular insufficiency, trophic leg ulcers, gangrene, intermittent claudication (which could be due to diabetes, atherosclerosis or inflammatory vascular disease). Pentoxiphylline is also used in AIDS patients with increased TNF (because pentoxiphylline can inhibits the production of TNF-α) and to improve sperm motility.

Dose: 400 mg 2–3 times a day with food.

Naftidofuryl oxalate is found to be useful in PVD like TAO and in cerebrovascular disorders. Though not a vasodilator, it is said to improve the supply of ATP to the skeletal muscles and reduce their lactate levels—it is called a **'metabolic enhancer'**—thus it improves performance in patients with TAO or intermittent claudication where it increases the walking distance. Naftidofuryl oxalate also blocks 5-HT_2 receptors and inhibits 5HT induced vasoconstriction and platelet aggregation. *Dose:* 100 mg BD to be taken 30 minutes before breakfast and dinner. However, it is found to increase the blood flow to the skin rather than the muscles. It is used in venous leg ulcers.

Dose: 100 mg BD-TDS oral.

Xanthinol nicotinate: Both xanthine and nicotinic acid are vasodilators and xanthinol nicotinate increases blood flow in several vascular beds. Therefore, it has been tried in cerebrovascular insufficiency and PVD. However, clinically, it is not proved to be useful.

Dose: 300–600 mg TDS oral/300 mg IM/slow IV inj. COMPLAMINA.

Cilostazol is a phosphodiestrase III inhibitor. It has vasodilator and antiplatelet effects—improves pain-free walking and maximum walking distance. It can cause headache, diarrhoea, dizziness and tachycardia and is contraindicated in heart failure.

Thromboangiitis Obliterans

Atheroma of the peripheral arteries results in reduced blood supply to the concerned part—usually lower limbs. Histologically, localized inflammatory changes can be seen in the walls of the arteries and veins leading to thrombosis. Initially, there is pain in the legs on walking (intermittent claudication) but later pain even at rest, while in severe cases there could be gangrene of the feet and legs.

The goal is to prevent pain, arrest progression of the disease and decrease the risk of cardiovascular and cerebrovascular events. Patients should first stop smoking. Hyperlipidaemia, if any, should be corrected. **Vasodilators** may be tried. **Quinine** has been tried in a low dose of 200 mg at night to relieve **night cramps**. Surgical treatment is the preferred option. **Angioplasty** of iliac or superficial femoral arteries (with stent placement) is often effective. Other options include arterial bypass grafting or endarterectomy and lastly amputation of the leg in severe cases.

Raynaud's phenomenon: It is a vasospastic disorder. A vasodilator like nifedipine, topical nitroglycerine, indoramin, prazosin or slow infusion of prostacyclin (epoprostenol) help to relieve symptoms. Regular exercises to improve blood supply to the muscles may help. Because **β-blockers can worsen PVD** including Raynaud's phenomenon (due to reduced cardiac output), they should be avoided in these patients. Patients should also be advised to avoid exposure to cold.

[1] From Medical Council of India, *Competency based Undergraduate Curriculum for the Indian Medical Graduate*, 2018;1:136–144.

CHAPTER 29

Antiarrhythmic Drugs

> *Competency achievement:* The student should be able to:
>
> **PH 1.30** Describe the mechanisms of action, types, doses, side effects, indications and contraindications of the antiarrhythmics.[1]

An arrhythmia is an abnormality of the rate, rhythm or site of origin of the cardiac impulse or an abnormality in the impulse conduction. The word dysrhythmia is also used often. The five phases of action potential as shown in Fig. 29.1 in a cardiac myocyte is described on page 351. The normal heart rate in an adult ranges from 60 to 100 beats/min. Factors like myocardial hypoxia, myocardial ischaemia, electrolyte disturbances, trauma, drugs and autonomic influences can cause arrhythmias.

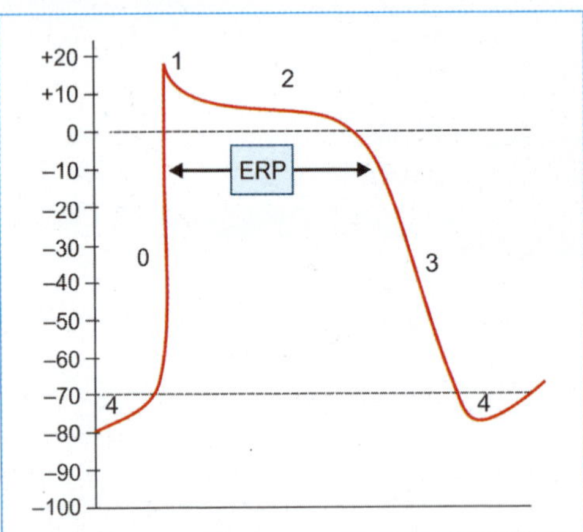

Fig. 29.1: Cardiac action potential: **Phase 0**—rapid depolarisation, **phase 1**—initial rapid repolarisation, **phase 2**—prolonged plateau phase, **phase 3**—second rapid repolarisation, **phase 4**—resting phase. ERP: Effective refractory period

Clinical features include palpitation, syncope, fatigue, breathlessness, cardiac failure and in more severe cases—cardiac arrest.

Mechanisms of Arrhythmogenesis

Cardiac arrhythmias may be due to:

i. Abnormal generation of impulses
ii. Abnormal conduction of impulses.

Disturbances of impulse generation may be due to altered normal and abnormal automaticity or after depolarisations. Disturbances of impulse conduction may be due to repeated activation (re-entry) or conduction blocks.

Thus arrhythmias may originate by one of the following mechanisms:

> ***Mechanisms of Arrhythmogenesis***
>
> *Abnormal impulse generation*
> - Altered normal automaticity
> - Abnormal automaticity
> - After depolarizations — early / delayed
>
> *Abnormal impulse conduction*
> - Re-entry
> - Conduction block—I, II or III degree

1. *After depolarizations* are secondary depolarizations that accompany an action potential. They may be early after depolarizations or delayed after depolarizations. Early after depolarizations occur before achieving full repolarization, i.e. during phase 3 of the action potential. They may develop in hypokalaemia,

hypoxia, acidosis or due to certain drugs. Delayed after depolarizations occur after full repolarization of the membrane, i.e. a premature beat is initiated. Delayed after depolarizations occur in hypocalcaemia, hypokalaemia, due to digitalis or catecholamines.

2. *Abnormal or enhanced automaticity:* An ectopic focus may generate an impulse resulting in arrhythmias. Enhanced automaticity may be due to activation of beta adrenergic receptors, stretching of the cardiac myocytes or hypokalaemia.
3. *Triggered activity:* When an after depolarization leads to an additional action potential, it is called triggered activity.
4. *Reentry* (Fig. 29.2): When there is a conduction block, an impulse may recirculate in the heart and cause repeated reactivation leading to reentry arrhythmias. For reentry to occur, there must be an unidirectional block and slow conduction in a region of the myocardium. Most of the arrhythmias seen clinically (80–90%) are thought to have a reentry mechanism. Drugs help such arrhythmias by either converting the unidirectional block to bidirectional block or prevent reentry by increasing the effective refractory period of the cardiac fibres during reentry.

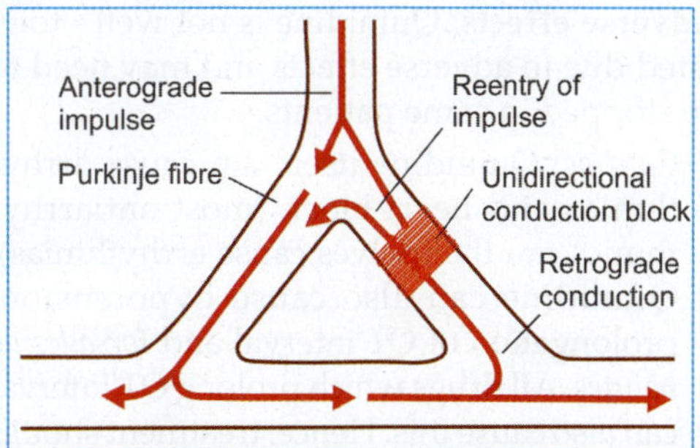

Fig. 29.2: Reentry circuit in the ventricle. The impulse from the SA node generally passes to the AV node, Purkinje fibres and then to the ventricle. When there is a conduction block, an impulse may recirculate in the heart and cause reentry arrhythmias

Types of Arrhythmias

Arrhythmias may be tachyarrhythmias and bradyarrhythmias. **Tachyarrhythmias** may be due to abnormal automaticity, triggered activity or reentry. **Bradyarrhythmias** are generally due to failure of impulse generation in the SA node or failure of impulse conduction in the AV node. In general, tachyarrhythmias can be largely controlled with drugs while bradyarrhythmias poorly respond to pharmacotherapy and may require the placement of a pacemaker.

Based on the site of impulse origin, they may be supraventricular (originating in SA node, AV node and atria) or ventricular arrhythmias (in ventricles) and include:

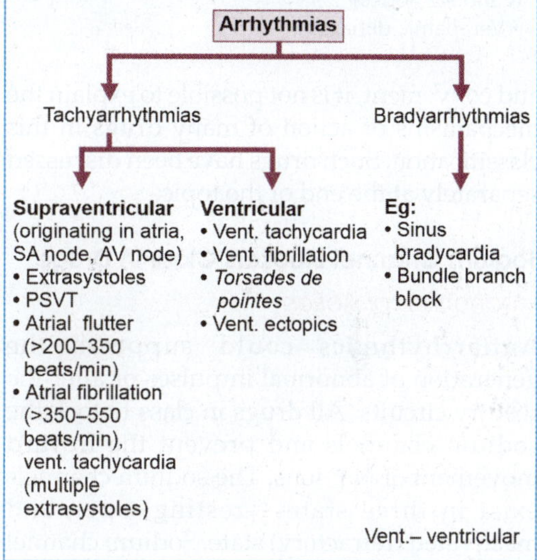

Ventricular arrhythmias are a common cause of death, particularly sudden death. *Torsades de pointes* is a type of ventricular tachycardia with prolonged QT interval. It is so called because of the pattern of ECG changes. In French it means 'twisting of points' and can be fatal. Atrioventricular block is due to depressed conduction in the AV node and bundle of His.

Classification

Based on the cardiac cycle, **Vaughan Williams** classified anti-arrhythmics. Though it is simple

Classification

Class I. Sodium channel blockers

1A. *Prolong repolarization*
- Quinidine, procainamide, disopyramide

1B. *Shorten repolarization*
- Lignocaine, mexiletine, phenytoin

1C. *Little effect on repolarization*
- Encainide, flecainide, propafenone, moricizine

Class II. β-adrenergic blockers

(reduce sympathetic tone)
- Propranolol, acebutolol, esmolol, etc.

Class III. K^+ channel blockers

(Prolong repolarization)
- Amiodarone, dronedarone, vernakalant, bretylium, sotalol, dofetilide, ibutilide.

Class IV. Ca^{++} channel blockers

(Prolong conduction and refractoriness specially in SA and AV nodes)
- Verapamil, diltiazem.

and convenient, it is not possible to explain the mechanisms of action of many drugs in this classification. Such drugs have been discussed separately at the end of the topic.

Sodium Channel Blockers Class IA Drugs

Mechanism of Action

Antiarrhythmics could suppress the generation of abnormal impulses or alter the reentry circuits. All drugs in class I block the sodium channels and prevent the inward movement of Na^+ ions. The sodium channels exist in three states—resting, open and inactivated (refractory) state. Sodium channel blockers preferentially bind Na^+ channels in the open and inactivated state.

Class IA drugs block sodium channels resulting in:

i. Depression of phase 0 depolarization
ii. Prolonged ERP and APD
iii. Slowing of conduction velocity
iv. Suppression of abnormal automaticity (rapid firing channels).

Class IA drugs decrease slope of phase 4 depolarization in pacemaker cells particularly when it is from an ectopic focus. They also prolong repolarization by blocking the K^+ channels.

Quinidine

Quinidine is the D-isomer of quinine obtained from the cinchona bark.

Pharmacological actions: By blocking Na^+ channels, it **depresses all cardiac properties**—automaticity, excitability, conduction velocity and prolongs repolarization—quinidine thus has membrane-stabilizing activity, i.e. it inhibits the propagation of the action potential. By reducing automaticity in the Purkinje fibres and ectopic foci, quinidine overcomes extrasystoles.

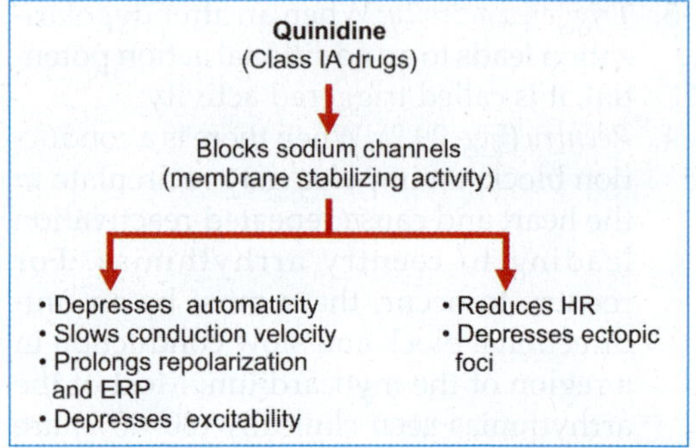

Quinidine has vagolytic (atropine-like) and α-blocking properties. It is also a skeletal muscle relaxant.

Pharmacokinetics: Given orally quinidine is rapidly absorbed, 90% bound to plasma proteins, metabolised in the liver and excreted in the urine. Dose: 100–200 mg TDS

Adverse effects: Quinidine is not well - tolerated due to adverse effects and may need to be stopped in some patients.

- *Cardiac:* Quinidine itself can cause arrhythmias and heart block (most antiarrhythmics can themselves cause arrhythmias). Quinidine can also cause hypotension, prolongation of QT interval and *torsades de pointes*. All drugs which prolong QT interval can also cause this. Hence, treatment should be monitored (Table 29.1).
- *Non-cardiac:* Diarrhoea, nausea, vomiting and hypersensitivity reactions including thrombocytopenia and rarely bone marrow depression, hepatitis and idiosyncratic

Table 29.1: Causes and choice of drugs in cardiac arrhythmias

Arrhythmia	*Cause*	*Treatment*
Sinus tachycardia	↑ sympathetic tone, fever, thyrotoxicosis	• Treat the cause • If severe → propranolol
Atrial extrasystoles	Excess caffeine, nicotine, alcohol	• Treat the cause • Reassurance • If severe → propranolol/disopyramide
Atrial flutter/fibrillation	Rheumatic heart disease, cardiomyopathy, hypertension	• Cardioversion • Propranolol/quinidine/disopyramide/ digoxin/class IC drugs
PSVT	MI, myocarditis, cardiomyopathy, rheumatic heart disease, nicotine, amphetamine	• Vagal manouvers like carotid massage • Verapamil/adenosine • β-blockers
Ventricular ectopics	Normal heart—benign; also in cardiomyopathy, ischaemia, digitalis induced	• β-blockers • Lignocaine
Ventricular tachycardia	Organic heart disease, ventricular dysfunction, drug induced	• Cardioversion • Lignocaine/amiodarone
Ventricular fibrillation	Acute MI, organic heart disease, surgical trauma, drug induced	• Cardioversion • Lignocaine /amiodarone • Class IA drugs for prevention
Digitalis-induced tachyarrhythmias	Digitalis toxicity	• Phenytoin • Potassium • Lignocaine
Sinus bradycardia	Hypothyroidism, ↑ intracranial pressure	• Atropine
AV block	Sick sinus syndrome, IHD, hyperkalemia, myocarditis, congenital heart diseases, drugs (digoxin, verapamil, β-blockers)	• Atropine • Pacemaker

reactions can occur. Higher doses can cause cinchonism like quinine.

Drug Interactions

- Quinidine is a **microsomal enzyme inhibitor**. It raises the plasma levels of propafenone and reduces the conversion of codeine to morphine thereby decreasing its analgesic efficacy.
- Microsomal enzyme inducers, like phenytoin and phenobarbitone, enhance the metabolism of quinidine resulting in therapeutic failure.
- Quinidine reduces the clearance of **digoxin** thereby precipitating digoxin toxicity.
- Quinidine may **potentiate** the effects of SMRs.
- It adds to the myocardiac depressant effects of β blockers, verapamil and potassium → could result in cardiac arrest.

Procainamide, an amide derivative of the local anaesthetic procaine, has the following advantages over quinidine:

- It has weak vagolytic properties.
- It is not an α-blocker.
- It is better tolerated than quinidine.

Procainamide is partly metabolized by acetylation and people can be fast or slow acetylators. Since the t½ is 3–4 hours, it needs to be administered more frequently than quinidine. Procainamide can cause nausea, vomiting and hypersensitivity reactions including systemic lupus syndrome which is more common in slow acetylators. Higher doses can cause hypotension, flushing, heart block and *Torsades de pointes.* Pleuritis and pericarditis are also noted.

Dose: 0.5–1 g oral followed by 0.25–0.5 g every 2 hr. Maintenance dose—0.5 g every 4–6 hr.

Disopyramide is better tolerated than quinidine but has prominent anticholinergic actions. It is used as a second-line drug to prevent recurrences of ventricular arrhythmias and after cardioversion in atrial fibrillation patients.

The significant anticholinergic properties are responsible for adverse effects like dry mouth, blurred vision, constipation and urinary retention. Disopyramide can cause significant myocardiac depression. It can also cause *torsades de pointes.*

Dose: 100–150 mg oral TDS,

Uses of Class IA Drugs

Class IA drugs are useful in almost all types of arrhythmias to prevent recurrences. They are used in **atrial fibrillation** and **atrial flutter** and in **ventricular arrhythmias** to prevent recurrence. Because of the adverse effects, quinidine and procainamide are not preferred by most practitioners in arrhythmias but quinidine can be used in malaria in place of quinine. Procainamide may be used to terminate ventricular tachycardia but is not suitable for long-term use.

Class IB Drugs

Class IB drugs block the sodium channels and also shorten repolarization. They decrease APD and ERP of Purkinje fibres. They have a higher affinity for the ischemic sites. Class IB drugs exhibit least cardiotoxic effects but are neurotoxic.

Lignocaine: Lignocaine, the local anaesthetic, **blocks the sodium channels in the open and inactivated state**. It raises the threshold for action potential and reduces automaticity in the ectopic foci. Lignocaine suppresses the electrical activity of the arrhythmogenic tissues while the normal tissues are not much affected. Lignocaine decreases the action potential duration in ventricles and the Purkinje fibres (but not in the atria). It suppresses the reentry in the ventricular muscle by converting the one way block to two way block or by abolishing the one way block. Given orally lignocaine undergoes high first pass metabolism and has a short t½—hence used parenterally.

It may cause drowsiness, hypotension, blurred vision, confusion and convulsions.

Uses: ***Ventricular arrhythmias:*** Lignocaine is a popular antiarrhythmic and is commonly used. It is used in the treatment of ventricular arrhythmias, especially that caused by acute myocardial infarction or open heart surgery and in digitalis-induced arrhythmias. The ischemic ventricular cells have a long APD and therefore the Na^+ channels remain in an inactivated state for a longer time. **Lignocaine is not useful in atrial arrhythmias because atrial action potentials are so short that sodium channel is in the inactivated state only for a very short period.** Hence, lignocaine does not modify the refractory period or action potential duration of the atria.

Phenytoin: Phenytoin is an antiepileptic also useful in ventricular arrhythmias (not preferred due to toxicity) and digitalis-induced arrhythmias.

Mexiletine: Congener of lignocaine which is orally effective causes dose-related neurologic adverse effects including tremors and blurred vision. Nausea is common. It is used as an alternative to lignocaine in ventricular arrhythmias. It has also been tried in chronic neuropathic pain like diabetic neuropathy.

Class IC Drugs

Class IC drugs including **flecainide, propafenone** and **moricizine** are the most potent sodium channel blockers. Because of the risk of cardiac arrest, sudden death and other adverse effects, they are not commonly used. They are effective in supraventricular arrhythmias including WPW syndrome and to maintain sinus rhythm in atrial fibrillation.

Class II Drugs

β-blockers: β-blockers like propranolol exert antiarrhythmic effects due to the blockade of cardiac β receptors.

- They depress myocardial contractility, automaticity and conduction velocity.
- They decrease the slope of phase 4 depolarization and automaticity in the SA node and Purkinje fibres.
- They also depress AV conduction by prolonging the refractory period of the AV node.
- β-blockers reduce the membrane responsiveness and amplitude of the action potential. The extrasystoles due to catecholamines are suppressed.
- In higher doses, they also have membrane stabilising activity like class I drugs.

Propranolol and cardioselective β-blockers like **atenolol** and **metoprolol** are used in the treatment and prevention of **supraventricular arrhythmias** especially those associated with exercise, emotion or hyperthyroidism. Propranolol is an useful antiarrhythmic in several arrhythmias that are associated with adrenergic stimulation. Propranolol is used **to suppress sinus tachycardia, atrial and nodal extrasystoles and digitalis-induced arrhythmias**. Propranolol is useful in suppressing halothane-induced arrhythmias and in catecholamine-induced arrhythmias in pheochromocytoma. Propranolol is the **drug of choice** in patients with **congenital long QT syndrome.**

Esmolol given intravenously is rapid acting, short-acting and cardioselective. It can be used to treat arrhythmias during surgeries, due to anaesthesia, following myocardial infarction and to control the ventricular rate in atrial fibrillation and flutter (either alone or with digitalis). It is also useful in acute PSVT.

Sotalol: Though a beta blocker, has prominent actions of class III drugs.

Class III Drugs

Potassium Channel Blockers

These drugs prolong the action potential duration and refractory period and delay the repolarization by blocking the potassium channels.

Amiodarone: Amidarone an analog of the thyroid hormone is an iodine-containing compound. It is a powerful antiarrhythmic and acts by multiple mechanisms as follows:

- Blocks the K^+ channels and prolongs APD
- Blocks the sodium and calcium channels
- Blocks the β-adrenergic receptors (nonselective)
- Prolongs ERP—prolongs repolarisation and refractoriness—both absolute and relative refractory period in all cardiac tissues.
- Depresses SA node pacemaker activity (due to inhibition of calcium current)
- Prolongs APD in atrial and ventricular muscles (but shortens the APD in the Purkinje fibres)

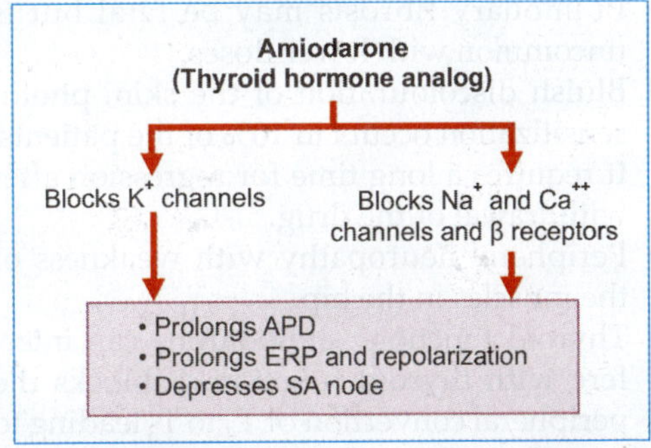

Vasculature: Amiodarone relaxes vascular smooth muscles including coronaries and improves blood flow to the myocardium. Vasodilation in peripheral vasculature results in a decrease in the preload, myocardial workload and thereby oxygen consumption (antianginal effects). Intravenous amiodarone can cause significant hypotension.

Pharmacokinetics: Amiodarone has complex pharmacokinetic properties. Following oral administration, bioavailability is variable (35–65%), onset of action is slow—may vary from 2–3 days to several weeks, duration of action and t½ may range from weeks to months. It is metabolised in the liver by microsomal enzymes. Hence drugs that induce or inhibit microsomal enzymes can alter the plasma levels of amiodarone resulting in many drug interactions. Amiodarone itself inhibits certain microsomal enzymes thereby increasing plasma levels of drugs like digoxin and warfarin. The primary route of excretion is the biliary route.

Adverse effects: Amiodarone can cause various adverse effects including cardiac and extracardiac effects.

Cardiac Effects

Heart block, cardiac failure, QT prolongation, hypotension particularly on IV injection, bradycardia and myocardiac depression.

Extracardiac Effects

- Nausea, gastrointestinal disturbances and hepatitis.
- Pulmonary fibrosis may be fatal but is uncommon with lower doses.
- Bluish discolouration of the skin, photosensitization occurs in 10% of the patients. It requires a long time for regression after withdrawal of the drug.
- Peripheral neuropathy with weakness of the muscles in the hip.
- Thyroid function—amiodarone can interfere with thyroid function. It blocks the peripheral convertion of T_4 to T_3 leading to hypothyroidism. It can also cause hyperthyroidism because it is an iodine-containing compound.
- Corneal microdeposits may develop but are reversible on stopping the drug. Some patients may have visual blurring and halos.

Uses: Amiodarone is useful in a variety of arrhythmias **(broad-spectrum antiarrhythmic)** and is the most efficacious antiarrhythmic drug. However, it is a toxic drug and requires constant monitoring.

- Intravenous amiodarone is used for the treatment and prophylaxis of recurrent and resistant ventricular fibrillation and **ventricular tachycardia** which could be life-threatening.
- Amiodarone may be used to maintain sinus rhythm in paroxysmal atrial fibrillation and in other atrial tachyarrhythmias
- Postoperative junctional ectopic tachycardia.

Dronedarone: Dronedarone, an analog of amiodarone, is devoid of iodine atoms and thereby lacks the resultant adverse effects on thyroid function. Dronedarone, a multi-ion channel blocker like amiodarone, is longer acting—t½ 24 hr. It is useful in patients with atrial flutter and atrial fibrillation.

Celivarone is another derivative under clinical trial.

Vernakalant: It is another multi-ion channel blocker useful in atrial fibrillation. Vernakalant prolongs the atrial effective refractory period and slows AV conduction. It blocks the potassium currents which have an important role in atrial repolarization and thus prolongs atrial ERP. Vernakalant also blocks the sodium channels. It has a short t½ (2 hr) on IV administration but t½ is 12 hr on oral administration. Adverse effects include dysgeusia, hypotension, cough, sneezing and paraesthesias.

In atrial fibrillation, vernakalant is used intravenously to convert to normal sinus rhythm. It is contraindicated in recent MI and heart failure.

Bretylium is an adrenergic neuron blocker used in resistant ventricular arrhythmias.

Sotalol is a nonselective beta blocker and also a blocker of the potassium channels. It prolongs the action potential duration (therefore classified under class III antiarrhythmic drugs) and ERP in the atria, ventricles and the Purkinje tissue. By its beta blocking effects, sotalol depresses the SA and AV nodes.

Adverse effects of sotalol include bradycardia, ventricular fibrillation, torsades de pointes, fatigue, headache, nausea and vomiting.

Uses: Sotalol is useful in ventricular and supraventricular arrhythmias and for maintaining sinus rhythm in atrial fibrillation and atrial flutter. It is often preferred when a beta blocker is needed.

Ibutilide: Ibutilide an analog of sotalol, is a K^+ channel blocker, acts by blocking the potassium currents and prolongs the repolarization.

Ibutilide is not given orally as it undergoes extensive first pass metabolism. It can cause *torsades de pointes* like dofetilide. Ibutilide is used as an IV infusion to quickly convert atrial flutter and fibrillation to sinus rhythm.

Dofetilide: Dofetilide, a selective K^+ channel blocker, selectively blocks the potassium current (IKr) in the myocardial tissues **(pure K^+ channel blocker)** and prolongs APD as well as refractory period. Hyperkalaemia blunts the effects of dofetilide and hence care should be taken to avoid it. Diuretics that cause hypokalaemia potentiate the antiarrhythmic effects of dofetilide. It is effective orally, has a good bioavailability (~100%) though food delays its absorption. Dofetilide is **well tolerated**, the only major adverse effect being *torsades de pointes* (3% incidence) due to prolongation of the QT interval. Clinical trials have shown that other effects like hypotension, hypertension, bradycardia and AV block are similar in incidence as placebo.

It is used orally in atrial fibrillation to convert and to maintain sinus rhythm.

Azimilide: It is a **K^+ channel blocker,** a new class III drug that prolongs cardiac repolarization. It is being studied for its efficacy in supraventricular arrhythmias and for prevention of arrhythmias in post-myocardial infarction patients.

Class IV Drugs

Calcium channel blockers inhibit the inward movement of calcium resulting in reduced contractility, automaticity and AV nodal conduction. Verapamil markedly depresses AV conduction. CCBs block the L type of calcium channels in the myocardium leading to a decrease in the rate of phase 4 depolarization in the SA node and Purkinje fibres. This results in bradycardia and abolishes extrasystoles and after depolarizations. Verapamil, diltiazem, and bepridil have prominent cardiac effects because they block the Ca^{++}channels in the cardiac cells in therapeutic doses.

Verapamil is used to terminate **paroxysmal supraventricular tachycardia** (PSVT). It is given IV 5 mg slowly over 2–3 minutes. It can also be given 80–120 mg TDS orally.

It is also used to control ventricular rate in **atrial flutter or fibrillation** because it depresses the AV nodal conduction.

Diltiazem can be used in place of verapamil. The effects of diltiazem are smilar to verapamil though milder. It is useful in controlling the ventricular rate in atrial flutter and atrial fibrillation for which it is given IV in the dose of 0.25 mg/kg over 10 minutes followed by 5 mg/hr. It may also be used as an alternative to verapamil in the treatment of PSVT.

Drug interactions: Verapamil displaces digoxin from tissue binding sites and also reduces its renal clearance resulting in digoxin toxicity—dose of digoxin should be reduced.

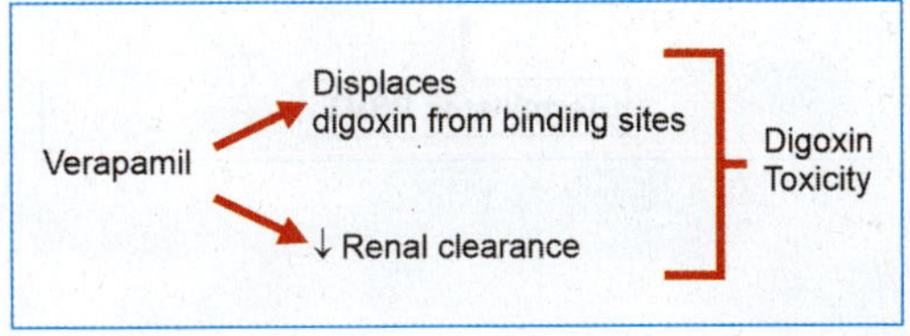

OTHER ANTIARRHYTHMICS

These are not included in Vaughan William's classification.

Adenosine is a purine nucleotide having rapid and short antiarrhythmic action. It is an endogenous substance formed in the metabolism of adenosine triphosphate. Given IV it suppresses automaticity, AV conduction and dilates the coronaries. It shortens the APD and may cause AV block within 10–20 seconds of an IV dose.

Theophylline blocks adenosine receptors and inhibits the action of adenosine. The mechanism of action is not exactly known. Adenosine could act as a potassium channel opener by binding to specific adenosine receptors which are present on the atria, SA and AV nodes. These are G-protein-coupled receptors and activation of them opens the outward potassium currents leading to hyperpolarization.

The action of adenosine is specific for the atria and has **no effect on the ventricles** because there are no adenosine-stimulated potassium channels in the ventricles.

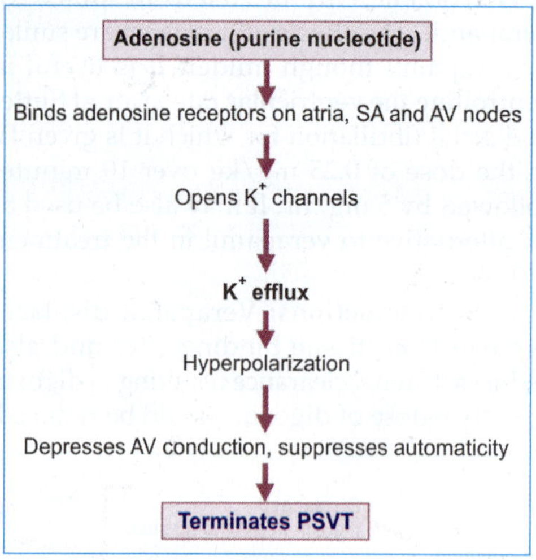

Adenosine (purine nucleotide)
↓
Binds adenosine receptors on atria, SA and AV nodes
↓
Opens K^+ channels
↓
K^+ efflux
↓
Hyperpolarization
↓
Depresses AV conduction, suppresses automaticity
↓
Terminates PSVT

Adenosine has a very short t½ of about 10 seconds and is given as a bolus injection. The duration of action is just 10–20 seconds.

Dose: 6–20 mg ADICAR 6 mg amp.

Adverse effects: Bronchospasm and dyspnoea can be quite profound in asthmatic patients and may take about 30 minutes to subside. Other adverse effects are nausea, flushing, dizziness, chest pain, dyspnoea and headache but are of short duration.

Uses: Adenosine is the drug of choice for acute termination of PSVT including AV nodal reentrant tachycardia. The action of adenosine is so specific to the atria that it can be used for the diagnosis of atrial flutter/arrhythmias. Its brief duration of action is an added advantage for this purpose.

Ivabradine: Selectively blocks the I_f current in the SA node thereby reducing heart rate without depressing myocardial contractility. It is useful in sinus tachycardia as an alternative to beta blockers (0.6 mg IM).

Atropine is used in sinus bradycardia. It acts by blocking M_2 muscarinic receptors.

Digitalis depresses AV conduction, reduces heart rate and increases the force of contraction of the myocardium. Digoxin is used in atrial fibrillation to control the ventricular rate.

Magnesium sulphate 1–2 g is used IV to treat digitalis-induced arrhythmias and *torsades de pointes*. It blocks Ca^{++}, Na^+ and K^+ channels though a weak K^+ blocker.

Potassium is a myocardiac depressant. It brings about a decrease in conduction velocity, automaticity and prolongs the refractory period. Higher doses produce defects in AV conduction. Thus both hypo- and hyperkalemia are arrhythmogenic (digitalis toxicity is potentiated by hypokalaemia). Potassium is used in the treatment of digitalis-induced arrhythmias and in arrhythmias associated with hypokalaemia.

Clinical Pharmacology

Clinical Classification of Antiarrhythmics

Antiarrhythmics used in
- Supraventricular arrhythmias—adenosine, CCBs
- Ventricular arrhythmias—lignocaine
- Both supraventricular and ventricular arrhythmias Amiodarone, β-blockers, procainamide

- All antiarrhythmics are also arrhythmogenic drugs.
- Class IA drugs tend to prolong QT interval.
- Use of drugs for prophylaxis of arrhythmias is now not practiced.
- Amiodarone has good safety margin and broad spectrum of action among antiarrhythmics
- Drug interactions are common with amiodarone
- Adenosine should be given into the central or brachial vein due to its short action and immediately about 10 ml fluid should be pushed into the same vein to flush it.
- Adenosine should **not** be refrigerated—efficacy is lost.
- Adenosine should be avoided in patients on deriphylline because it is an adenosine receptor antagonist.

[1] From Medical Council of India, *Competency based Undergraduate Curriculum for the Indian Medical Graduate*, 2018;1:136–144.

CHAPTER 30

Hypolipidaemic Drugs

Competency achievement: The student should be able to:

PH 1.31 Describe the mechanisms of action, types, doses, side effects, indications and contraindications of the drugs used in the management of dyslipidemias.[1]

Hyperlipoproteinaemias (HPL) are conditions in which the concentration of cholesterol or triglyceride (TG) carrying lipoproteins in the plasma is elevated above normal (Table 30.1). Increase in lipoproteins can hasten the development of atherosclerosis and is a risk factor for myocardial infarction.

Lipids and proteins form complexes called lipoproteins and circulate in the blood vessels. There are four types of lipoproteins:

- Low density lipoproteins (LDL)
- High density lipoproteins (HDL)
- Very low density lipoproteins (VLDL)
- Chylomicrons.

LDL is the primary carrier of cholesterol while VLDL is of triglycerides. There are different pathways for the transport of endogenous and exogenous lipids (Fig. 30.1). In the exogenous pathway, cholesterol and triglycerides absorbed from the gut are transported as chylomicrons. They are hydrolysed to chylomicron remnants by the action of lipoprotein lipase (LPL) and free fatty acids are released which are taken up by muscle and adipose tissue. The chylomicron remnants are transported to the liver.

In the endogenous pathway, cholesterol and triglycerides from the liver are carried as VLDL to the muscle and adipose tissue. Here the triglycerides in VLDL are hydrolysed and free fatty acids released. Thus intermediate density lipoprotein (IDL) and then LDL are formed by the action of lipoprotein lipase. Cells have LDL receptors and LDL is taken up into the cell. When the LDL plasma levels rise, LDL is taken up by the scavenger macrophages. In this process, they are oxidised and such LDL is atherogenic.

Excess cholesterol from the cells is transported to the liver for excretion by reverse cholesterol transport. High density lipoproteins (HDL) take part in this process. They also antagonise atherogenesis by other mechanisms including antiplatelet—aggregatory effect, anticoagulant and other effects. High density lipoproteins decrease the risk of coronary heart disease, are called protective lipoproteins and higher plasma levels of HDL are thus desirable.

Types of Hyperlipoproteinaemias

Based on the lipoprotein fraction that is elevated, lipoprotein disorders may be

Table 30.1: Plasma lipid levels (mg/dl)

	Total CH	*LDL – CH*	*HDL – CH*	*TGs*
Desirable	<200	<100	>40 (men), >50 (women)	<150
Borderline	200–239	130–159	–	150–199
High	>240	>160	>60	>200

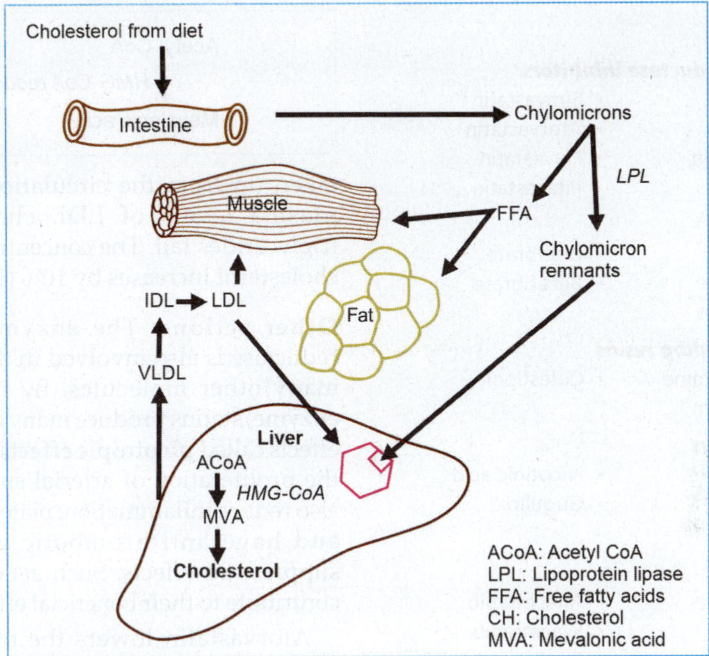

Fig. 30.1: Endogenous and exogenous pathways of lipid transport

broadly grouped into primary and secondary hyperlipidaemias (Table 30.2). Secondary hyperlipidaemias may be secondary to an underlying disorder.

HYPOLIPIDAEMICS

Elevated plasma levels of LDL cholesterol and low levels of HDL cholesterol enhance the risk of CHD along with the other risk factors, viz. smoking, family history of coronary artery disease, male sex, metabolic syndrome, diabetes mellitus and hypertension. Hence hypercholesterolaemia needs to be controlled.

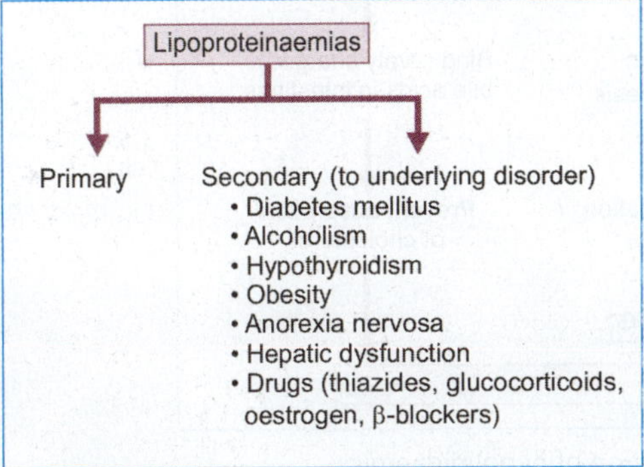

Table 30.2: Types of primary hyperlipoproteinaemias

Type	*Disorder*	*Plasma lipids raised*
I.	Familial LPL deficiency	C, TG
IIa.	Familial hypercholesterolaemia	C
IIb.	Polygenic hypercholesterolaemia	C
III.	Familial dysbetalipoproteinaemia	C, TG
IV.	Hypertriglyceridaemia	TG
V.	Familial combined hyperlipidaemia	C, TG

C: Cholesterol, TG: Triglycerides, LPL: Lipoprotein lipase

Hypolipidaemics are drugs that lower plasma lipid levels in the body.

HMG-CoA Reductase Inhibitors (Statins)

Hydroxymethylglutaryl-CoA (HMG-CoA) is the rate-controlling enzyme in the biosynthesis of cholesterol.

Classification

1. ***HMG-CoA reductase inhibitors***
   - Lovastatin
   - Simvastatin
   - Pravastatin
   - Atorvastatin
   - Rosuvastatin
   - Fluvastatin
   - Pitavastatin
2. ***Fibric acids***
   - Gemfibrozil
   - Clofibrate
   - Fenofibrate
   - Bezafibrate
   - Ciprofibrate
3. ***Bile acid binding resins***
   - Cholestyramine
   - Colestipol
   - Colesevelam
4. ***Miscellaneous***
   - Ezetimibe
   - Nicotinic acid
   - Probucol
   - Gugulipid
   - Neomycin
5. ***Newer drugs***
   CETP inhibitors
   - Anacetrapib
   - Evacetrapib

   DGAT1 inhibitor
   - Pradigastat

   MTP inhibitor
   - Lomitapide

Lovastatin and its congeners are structurally similar to HMG, CoA and are, therefore competitive inhibitors of the enzyme HMG-CoA reductase—**'Reductase inhibitors'.** The synthesis of cholesterol in the liver is reduced. There is an increase in the expression of hepatic LDL receptors so that more of LDL is

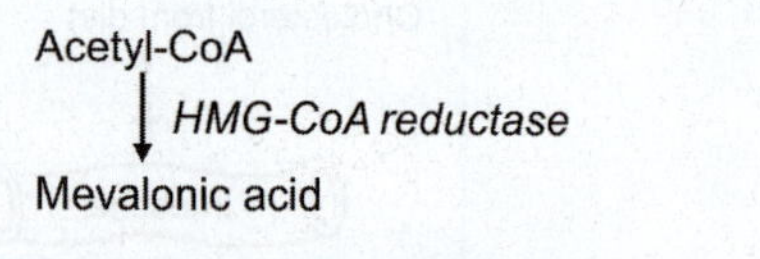

taken up from the circulation. As a result plasma levels of LDL cholesterol and triglycerides fall. The concentration of HDL–cholesterol increases by 10% (Fig. 30.2).

Other actions: The enzyme HMG-CoA reductase is also involved in the synthesis of many other molecules. By inhibiting this enzyme, statins produce many other beneficial effects called **pleotropic effects**. Statins inhibit the proliferation of arterial smooth muscles, also reduce inflammation, platelet aggregation and have antithrombotic and immunosuppressant effects. Such actions could also contribute to their beneficial effects (Fig. 30.3).

Atorvastatin lowers the triglycerides in addition to cholesterol.

Pharmacokinetics: Statins are well absorbed when given orally and food enhances their absorption but may undergo extensive first pass metabolism in the liver. Simvastatin is a prodrug converted to its active metabolite in the liver. Statins are metabolised by the enzyme cytochrome P450. Drugs that induce or inhibit these microsomal enzymes can alter the plasma levels of statins resulting in drug interactions.

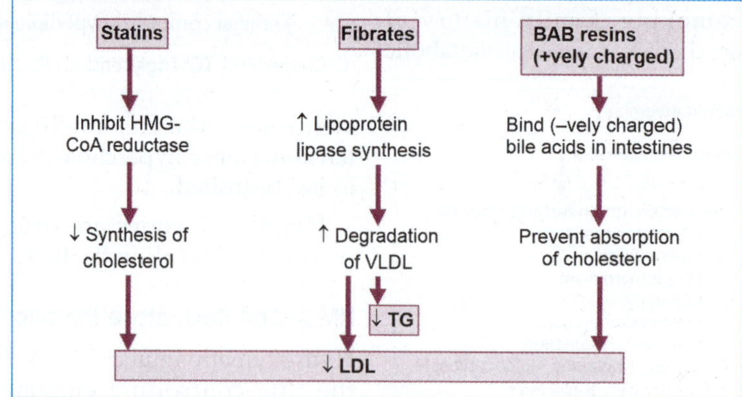

Fig. 30.2: Mechanism of action of hypolipidaemics

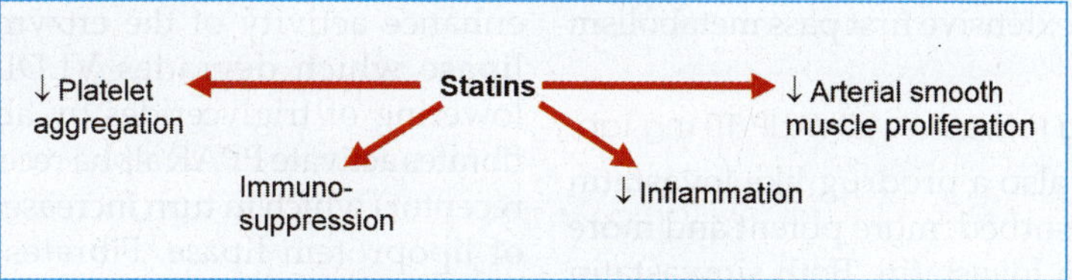

Fig. 30.3: Pleotropic effects of statins

Adverse effects: Include gastrointestinal disturbances, muscle pain, headache, insomnia, rashes, rarely myopathy and angio-oedema.

Treatment with statins can cause hepatotoxicity though not very common. Serum transaminases may be elevated on prolonged therapy. Patients should be watched for hepatotoxicity while on statins, particularly if also on other hepatotoxic drugs or are chronic alcoholics.

All statins can cause **myopathy**, myositis (with myalgia and weakness) and rhabdomyolysis though the incidence is low (<0.1–0.1%). Creatine kinase activity may be raised. In patients with an inherited genetic variation, statins can induce severe myopathy and rhabdomyolysis. Concurrent use of other drugs that also cause myopathy including fibrates, niacin, amiodarone and verapamil should be avoided.

Statins are contraindicated in pregnancy and lactation as they are not proved to be safe in them.

Drug interactions, *see* page 390.

Uses

1. HMG-CoA reductase inhibitors are the first-line drugs (Table 30.2) both for familial and secondary hyperlipidaemias as in diabetes mellitus.
2. Several large scale studies have shown statins to be useful in lowering morbidity and mortality in patients with coronary heart disease. Hence, they are used in patients with MI, angina, stroke and transient ischaemic attacks to lower cholesterol levels.

> Adverse effects of **HMG-CoA R**eductase **I**nhibitors
> **H**—**H**epatotoxicity
> **M**—**M**yositis, **M**yopathy
> **G**—**G**I disturbance
> **Co**—↑**C**reatin kinase
> **A**—**A**llergic reaction, **A**ngio-edema
> **R**—**R**ashes, **R**habdomyolysis
> **I**—**I**nsomnia

Individual Statins

Lovastatin is a prodrug converted to the active drug in the gut. It is incompletely absorbed

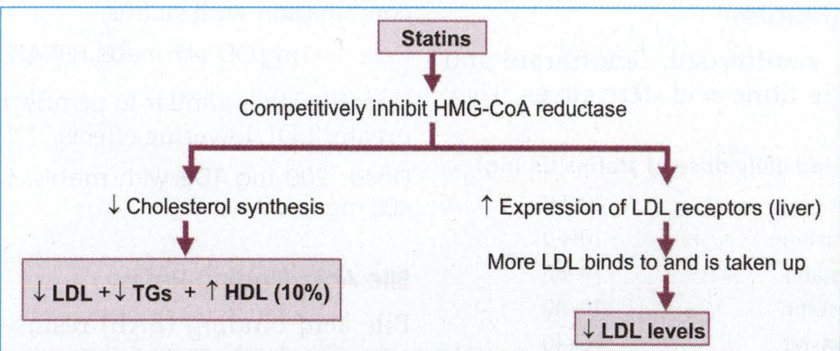

Fig. 30.4: Mechanism of action of statins

and undergoes extensive first pass metabolism by CYP3A4.

LOVADAC 20 mg tab, LOVA, LOVALIP 10 mg tab.

Simvastatin is also a prodrug like lovastatin and is better absorbed, more potent and more efficacious than lovastatin. Both simvastatin and atorvastatin raise HDL levels and may also lower triglycerides.

SIMSTAT, SIMVAS, 5, 10, 20 mg tab.

Fluvastatin is almost completely absorbed; it is metabolized by microsomal enzymes (CYP2C9). Microsomal enzyme inhibitors prolong the action of fluvastatin.

Atorvastatin has good potency and efficacy and a longer duration of action. It effectively lowers LDL-CH and to some extent triglycerides. It is a popular hypolipidaemic and is a commonly used drug.

ATORVA 10, 20, 40, 80 mg tab.

Pravastatin has relatively low efficacy. It also lowers plasma fibrinogen levels.

PRASTATIN, PRAVATOR 10, 20 mg tab.

Rosuvastatin is a fluorinated compound, most potent and longer acting and has good efficacy. It raises HDL-cholesterol in patients who also have raised triglyceride levels. It is metabolized by microsomal enzymes in the liver.

ROSUVAS, NOVASTAT 5, 10, 20 mg tab.

Pitavastatin is a recently introduced statin which binds with high affinity to HMG-CoA reductase. Its actions are similar to atorvastatin.

Fibric Acids (Fibrates)

The fibrates gemfibrozil, fenofibrate and bezafibrate are fibric acid derivatives. They enhance activity of the enzyme lipoprotein lipase which degrades VLDL resulting in lowering of triglycerides by about 40%. The fibrates activate PPAR alpha receptor (a nuclear receptor) which in turn increases the synthesis of lipoprotein lipase. Fibrates also increase HDL levels by 10–15%. Oxidation of fatty acids in the liver and muscle is increased while the lipolysis within the adipocytes is decreased.

In addition to the above actions, fibrates inhibit coagulation and promote thrombolysis which also account for their benefical effects in coronary heart diseases.

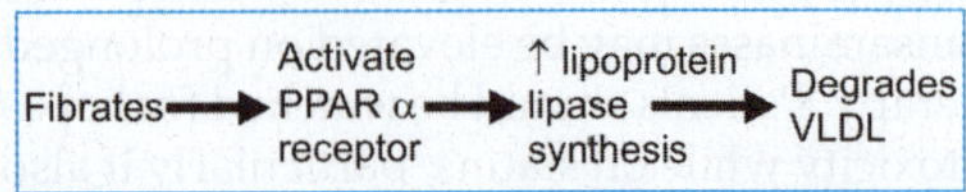

Recommended daily dose of statins (in mg)

Lovastatin	–	10–80
Atorvastatin	–	10–80
Fluvastatin	–	10–80
Pravastatin	–	10–80
Rosuvastatin	–	5–40
Simvastatin	–	5–80

Adverse effects to fibrates include gastrointestinal upset, skin rashes, headache, myositis, muscle cramps and blurred vision. Fibrates can cause rhabdomyolysis particularly in patients with renal failure and when concurrently used with statins, risk of myopathy gets added up. Fibrates should be avoided in patients with renal and hepatic dysfunction.

Gemfibrozil is the drug of choice in patients with increased TG levels and in type III, type IV and type V hyperlipoproteinaemias.

Dose: GEMFIBROZIL 600 mg BD.

Fenofibrate: In addition to lowering TGs, it also lowers LDL-CH and raises HDL-CH. It may be used in place of gemfibrozil or in combination with statins.

Dose: 200 mg OD with meals. FIBRATE 200 mg cap.

Bezafibrate is similar to gemfibrozil and has greater LDL lowering effects.

Dose: 200 mg TDS with meals. BEZALIP 200, 400 mg tab.

Bile Acid Binding Resins

Bile acid binding (BAB) resins—cholestyramine and colestipol (bile acid sequestrants) are not absorbed but they bind bile acids in the intestine and increase their excretion. These resins are highly positively charged and, therefore, bind bile acids which are negatively charged. Bile acids are required for the intestinal absorption of cholesterol. On using bile acid sequestrant, plasma cholesterol and LDL levels fall. The reduction in bile acids stimulates their synthesis but this is also associated with an elevated triglyceride production. Hence bile acid sequestrants should be avoided in patients with increased TG levels. Some studies have shown that colesevelam does not increase TG production to a large extent. However, this needs to be proved. The resins are safe since they are not absorbed.

Colesevelam is a recently developed bile acid sequestrant. It is found to have the following advantages:

1. It is claimed that it does not significantly elevate TG levels.
2. It is available as a tablet which is convenient to take while cholestyramine and colestipol are taken as powders.

Uses

Bile acid binding resins cholestyramine and colestipol can be used in patients with raised LDL levels; they can be used along with lovastatin or nicotinic acid.

Miscellaneous

Ezetimibe is a recently developed drug which selectively inhibits the absorption of cholesterol and other phytosterols by enterocytes. Ezetimibe and its metabolite concentrate in the brush border of the small intestine and interfere with the absorption of cholesterol by inhibiting a specific transport protein NPC1L1 which takes up cholesterol from the intestinal lumen. As a result, there is a decrease in hepatic cholesterol leading to increased clearance of cholesterol from the plasma. The plasma LDL cholesterol decreases by 15–20% with a marginal increase in HDL-CH.

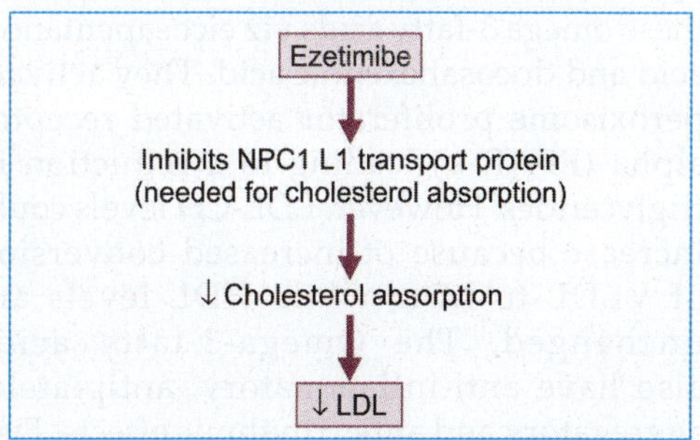

Ezetimibe also blocks the reabsorption of cholesterol that is excreted in the bile. The effects are synergisitc with statins and the combination can bring about a significant (up to 60%) decrease in LDL-CH levels.

Ezetimibe undergoes glucuronide conjugation, enterohepatic circulation and is largely excreted through the gut. It is well tolerated and with available data, can occasionally cause reversible hepatic dysfunction and myositis. It has a long half-life—given 10 mg once daily.

Ezetimibe may be used as monotherapy in patients with mild hypercholesterolaemia or in combination with a low dose of statins in patients who have not had adequate response with statins alone. It may also be used in patients with phytosterolaemia. However, it is not preferred now.

Nicotinic acid, a B group vitamin, in large doses inhibits triglyceride synthesis in the liver and VLDL production resulting in a decrease in LDL, and increase in HDL-cholesterol. The most common adverse effect is flushing, cutaneous vasodilation and a feeling of warmth which are mediated by PGs. This can be avoided by taking niacin after food or 300 mg aspirin taken 30 minutes before niacin. Tolerance develops to this effect in a few days. Other adverse effects include dyspepsia, dryness and pigmentation of the skin.

Dose: Started with 100 mg—gradually increased to 2–6 g/day. NIACIN ER 375 mg tab.

Niacin is used in hypertriglyceridaemia with low HDL levels.

Probucol lowers LDL- and HDL-cholesterol and has antioxidant properties. It is generally not preferred.

Gugulipid obtained from 'gum guggul' lowers plasma cholesterol and triglycerides. It is well tolerated but can cause diarrhoea.

Newer Drugs

Some new drugs that have been introduced are:

1. *PCSK9 inhibitors:* Proprotein convertase subtilisin/kexin type 9 (PCSK9) binds to LDL receptors and degrades them. Inhibition of PCSK9 results in an increase in LDL receptors and thereby LDL levels fall. The monoclonal antibodies **alirocumab** and **evolocumab** are PSCK9 inhibitors with good efficacy (50% reduction) in lowering LDL. However increase in blood glucose levels was noted
2. MTP (microsomal triglyceride transferase protein) inhibitor—lomitapide.
3. CETP (cholesteryl ester transfer protein) inhibitors like anacetrapib which prevent exchange of cholesteryl esters and triglycerides between HDL and lipoproteins.
4. **DAGT1 (diacylglycerol transferase) inhibitor**—pradigastat.
5. Antisense oligonucleotide against apo B100 for familial hypercholesterolaemia—mipomersen.

Drug Interactions with Hypolipidaemics

1. ***With enzyme inducers/inhibitors:*** Most statins are metabolized by the cytochrome P450 enzyme system. Hence grapefruit juice and drugs that inhibit microsomal enzymes (erythromycin, amiodarone, metronidazole, ketoconazole) can raise the plasma levels of statins. Drugs that induce microsomal enzymes like rifampicin, barbiturates, phenytoin, can speed up the metabolism and thereby lower plasma levels of statins.
2. ***Statins + fibrates→↑myositis:*** Concurrent use of statins with fibrates should be avoided because such use can increase the risk of toxicity to the muscle including myositis and rhabdomyolysis.
3. ***BAB resins bind drugs:*** Bile acid sequestrants can bind many drugs like warfarin, digoxin, phenobarbitone, chlorothiazide in the intestines and thereby prevent their absorption. To avoid this, other drugs should be taken 1 hr before or 4 hr after the resins.
4. ***With hepatotoxic drugs →↑ hepatotoxicity:*** Hepatotoxic drugs including alcohol can increase the risk of hepatotoxicity and more frequent monitoring of liver enzymes is needed.
5. ***Fibrates + warfarin:*** Fibrates potentiate the action of warfarin and other coumarin anticoagulants. Hence the dose of anticoagulants should be reduced.

Risk factors for coronary heart disease

1. Age (male >45 years, female >55 years)
2. Family H/o premature CHD
3. Hypertension
4. Low HDL-cholesterol, high LDL-cholesterol
5. Diabetes mellitus
6. Metabolic syndrome

Diet in Dyslipidaemia

Total fat content in the food should be cut so that fat accounts for not more than 20–25% of the total caloric intake and saturated fats to <8%. Alcohol accounts for a large percentage of cases of hypertriglyceridaemia as it increases the hepatic secretion of VLDL. Therefore, cut down on calories, along with exercises and weight reduction and avoiding alcohol are recommended for all patients with hypercholesterolaemia including hypertriglyceridaemia.

Omega 3-fatty acids are known to reduce triglycerides by reducing VLDL triglyceride synthesis in the liver. Fish oils are rich in these omega 3-fatty acids viz eicosapentanoic acid and docosahexenoic acid. They activate peroxisome proliferator activated receptor alpha (PPAR-α) leading to a reduction in triglycerides. However, LDL-CH levels could increase because of increased conversion of VLDL to LDL, while HDL levels are unchanged. The Omega-3-fatty acids also have anti-inflammatory, antiplatelet aggregatory and antiarrhythmic effects. Fish oil may be given as supplement which is available in the form of capsules. It may be used in patients with hypertriglyceridaemia in combination with fibrates. They are also indicated in rheumatoid arthritis (*see* page 172).

Treatment of Dyslipidemia

All patients with hypercholesterolaemia (HCL) first need to modify the diet so that the intake of cholesterol and saturated fat is checked. Lifestyle modification with physical exercises, weight reduction, high fibre diet, restriction of alcohol and cessation of smoking can control hyperlipidaemia to a large extent and it may be all that is needed in patients with mild hypercholesterolaemia. However, in high primary HCL and in familial HCL, drug therapy is required.

Raised LDL: Drug therapy and the goal for LDL levels are guided by the presence of other risk factors in a given patient. In patients with raised LDL-CH and total-CH, statins are the first-line drugs. Monitoring is carried out every 6 weeks. Dose may be increased every 6 weeks if needed till the maximum therapeutic dose. If the control is not adequate despite the optimum dose, ezetimibe may be added. In more severe cases, other drugs may be added (Table 30.3). Several clinical trials have been concluded and we now have clearer guidelines for the treatment of hyperlipidaemias. The US National Cholesterol Education Program (NCEP) ATP III revised guidelines have listed the risk factors for coronary artery disease. According to this, in patients with coronary artery disease, the goal for LDL-CH is 70 mg/dl.

Raised TG Levels: Lifestyle modification, treatment of the cause like diabetes, renal failure, high carbohydrate diet, glucocorticoids and β blockers can reduce triglyceride levels. Reducing LDL and VLDL levels with a statin may also lower TGs. If response is not satisfactory, a fibrate or nicotinic acid may be added. Presence of very high TG levels, i.e. >500 mg/dl, is associated with a risk of pancreatitis and needs drastic measures including lifestyle changes and drugs. Alcohol should be totally stopped.

Low HDL-CH Level: HDL-CH levels <40 mg/dl is considered low. The ratio of total CH:HDL-CH should be ideally <3.5. If it raises above 4.5, the risk is high and most such subjects also have metabolic syndrome. Lifestyle changes largely correct the HDL deficiency. Nicotinic acid and fibrates raise HDL levels but drugs are not indicated only to raise HDL unless other components also need treatment.

Combination of Hypolipidaemics

When adequate control of dyslipidaemia is not achieved with a single agent or when more than one lipid fraction needs to be corrected (as when both LDL and VLDL levels are high), combination of drugs needs to be given. Drugs from two different groups are generally combined. Various combinations are given in Table 30.3.

Table 30.3: Combinations of hypolipidaemics

Hypolipidaemics	*Indications*	*Note*
Statin + BAB resin	Familial hypercholesterolaemia	Administer with a gap of 4 hr
Statin + fenofibrate	Familial hypercholesterolaemia	Higher risk of myopathy
Statin + ezetimibe	Primary HCL, familial HCL	Good synergism
Statin + Niacin	Familial combined HCL	Effective
Fibrate + BAB resin	Familial combined HCL	↑ risk of cholelithiasis
BAB + niacin	Familial combined HCL	—
Statin + resin + niacin and ezetimibe	Severe HCL	Lower dose of each drug is needed

BAB—Bile acid binding, HCL—Hypercholesterolemia

DRUGS USED IN THE TREATMENT OF OBESITY

Obesity is a common problem in the developed countries but is now also increasing in developing countries. It is largely due to sedentary lifestyle and excessive or high calorie food intake. Obesity is recognised as a risk factor for several diseases include cardiac diseases and metabolic syndrome. In treating obesity, emphasis should be on low calorie diet and adequate physical activity. If these fail to control the body weight, drugs may be used but the drugs can be used only for a short period as none of them is proved to be safe for long-term use.

Orlistat: Orlistat acts by irreversibly inhibiting the enzymes gastric and pancreatic lipases—because of which it prevents the breakdown of dietary fat to fatty acids and glycerol. Therefore, it decreases the absorption of lipids. On prolonged administration, orlistat brings about a significant reduction in the body weight. The patient should also receive a low calorie diet and an exercise programme. Orlistat is poorly absorbed from the gut and is mostly excreted unchanged.

Adverse effects are limited to the gut with abdominal cramps, faecal urgency, faecal incontinence, oily faeces and flatulence. It interferes with the absorption of vitamins—hence supplementation is needed. There is also a decreased absorption of oral contraceptives and ciclosporin.

Uses: Orlistat is approved for use in obese individuals. It is also found to be useful in patients with type II diabetes mellitus. In a study where orlistat was given for 4 years in insulin resistant obese diabetics—a 37% reduction in the progression of diabetes was noted.

Drugs in obesity

- Orlistat
- Metformin
- Rimonabant
- Dietary fibre

Sibutramine the uptake of NA and serotonin (5-HT), reduces food intake and also enhances the expenditure of energy by an increase in the metabolic rate.

However, sibutramine can cause, hypertension and an increased incidence of **death due to cardiovascular diseases. Sibutramine is, therefore, withdrawn from the market.**

Amphetamine, dexfenfluramine and fenfluramine have anorexiant effects but are banned due to toxicity and potential for abuse (*see* page 95).

Rimonabant: Rimonabant, a cannabinoid CB_1 receptor antagonist, inhibits lipogenesis, promotes satiety and reduces food intake. Because it can cause depression and other neuropsychiatric side effects, it is **not approved** for use in obesity.

Lifestyle Drugs

Drugs used for non-health-related indications or for indications other than illness to meet the 'lifestyle' requirements are termed 'lifestyle' drugs. Examples include cosmetics, antiobesity drugs, food supplements, anabolic steroids, drugs for erectile dysfunction and oral contraceptives.

Clinical Pharmacology

- Dyslipidaemia is a metabolic disorder and requires almost lifelong medication.
- Atrovastatin and rosuvastatin are the most preferred and safe for long-term treatment as they have **pleiotropic effects,** i.e. antiplatelet, antioxidant, antismooth muscle proliferation and atheromatous plaque stabilization effects.
- Only lipid lowering drugs with pleiotropic effects can bring about a reduction in mortality and morbidity.
- Ezetimibe—no pleiotropic action → hence not preferred.
- Cholesterols are more atherogenic while triglycerides have more thrombogenic effects. 1% reduction in LDL levels approximately reduces mortality and morbidity by 1% over 5 yr.

[1] From Medical Council of India, *Competency based Undergraduate Curriculum for the Indian Medical Graduate*, 2018;1:136–144.

Unit IX

Respiratory System

31. Drugs used in the Treatment of Bronchial Asthma, COPD and Cough

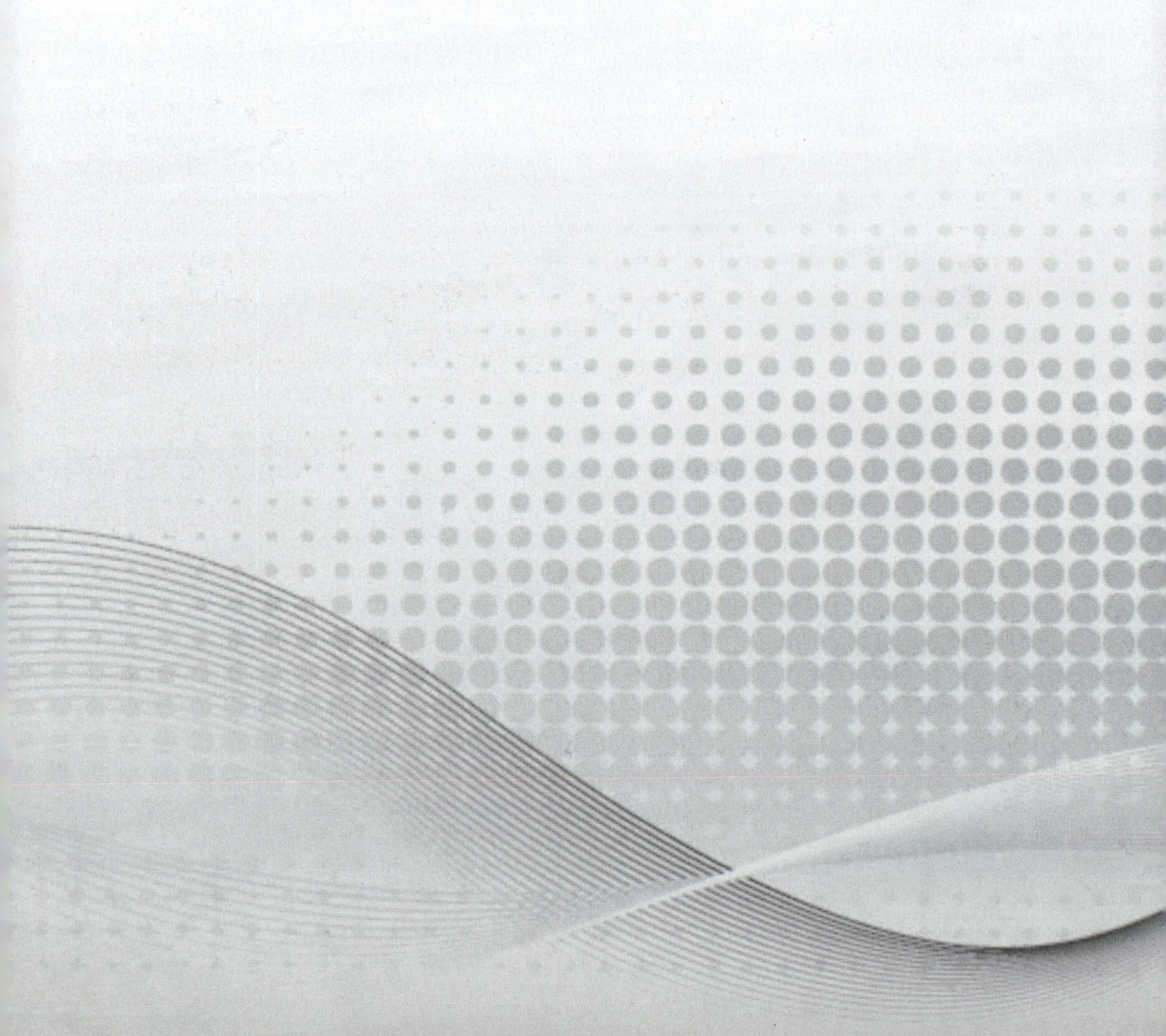

CHAPTER 31

Drugs used in the Treatment of Bronchial Asthma, COPD and Cough

Competency achievement: The student should be able to:

PH 1.32 Describe the mechanism/s of action, types, doses, side effects, indications and contraindications of drugs used in bronchial asthma and COPD.[1]

BRONCHIAL ASTHMA

Bronchial asthma is characterised by dyspnoea and wheeze due to increased resistance to the flow of air through the bronchi. Bronchospasm, mucosal congestion and oedema result in narrowing of airways leading to increased resistance. The tracheobronchial smooth muscle is hyperresponsive to various stimuli like dust, allergens, cold air, infection and drugs. These trigger factors trigger an acute attack.

Antigen–antibody interaction on the surface of mast cells results in (Fig. 31.1):

i. Degranulation of mast cells releasing stored mediators of inflammation
ii. Synthesis of other inflammatory mediators which are responsible for bronchospasm, mucosal congestion and oedema.

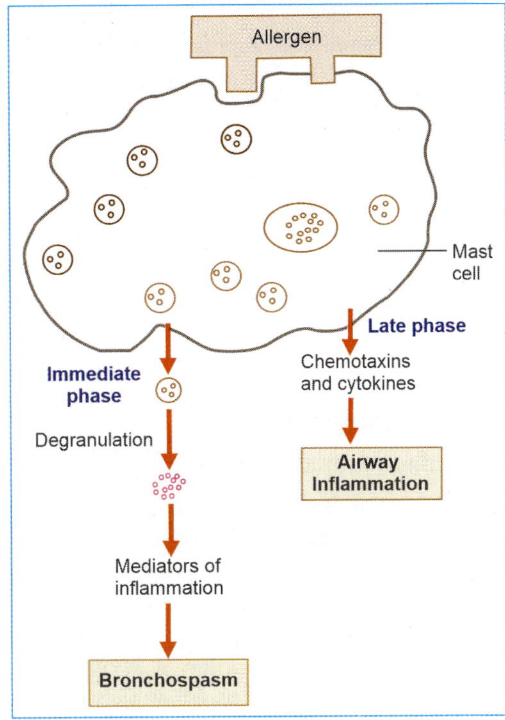

Fig. 31.1: Immediate and late responses of mast cell activation by antigen or allergen

Inflammation is the primary pathology.

Clinically, two types of asthma are identified.

1. *Extrinsic asthma:* Starts at an early age, occurs in episodes; the patient has a family history of allergies.
2. *Intrinsic asthma:* Starts in the middle age and assumes chronic form. There is no family history of allergies.

The clinical symptoms include episodes of wheezing, shortness of breath often associated with cough.

In acute episodes of bronchospasm, the immediate aim is to reverse it with a bronchodilator. In chronic asthmatics, the aim is to prevent bronchospasm. Bronchodilators and anti-inflammatory drugs are the two main classes of drugs used in asthma. Both prevention of inflammatory response and bronchial hyperactivity are important for the long-term control of asthma.

Drugs used in bronchial asthma may be classified as follows:

Classification

1. **Bronchodilators**
   a. *Sympathomimetics*
      i. Selective β_2-agonists
         Short acting – Salbutamol, terbutaline.
         Longer acting – Salmeterol, fenoterol, formoterol, pirbuterol, indacaterol
      ii. Nonselective agents – Adrenaline, isoprenaline, ephedrine.
   b. *Methylxanthines* – Theophylline, aminophylline.
   c. *Anticholinergics* – Ipratropium bromide, tiotropium, atropine.
2. **Anti-inflammatory agents**
   a. Glucocorticoids
      - *Systemic* – Hydrocortisone, prednisolone
      - *Inhalational* – Beclomethasone, budesonide, fluticasone, triamcinolone, mometasone, ciclesonide
   b. Mast cell stabilizers – Disodium cromoglycate, nedocromil, ketotifen.
   c. LT receptor antagonists – Montelukast, zafirlukast.
   d. PDE4 inhibitor – Roflumilast
3. **Anti-IgE antibody** – Omalizumab

BRONCHODILATORS

Sympathomimetics

Sympathomimetics (*see* Chapter 6) are potent bronchodilators and are the most useful drugs to relieve bronchospasm.

Mechanism of Action

Adrenergic agonists stimulate β_2 receptors in the bronchial smooth muscles which in turn cause activation of adenylyl cyclase resulting in increased cAMP levels (Fig. 31.2). This increased cAMP leads to bronchodilatation. The increased cAMP in mast cells inhibit the release of inflammatory mediators. They also reduce bronchial secretions and congestion (by acting on α receptors).

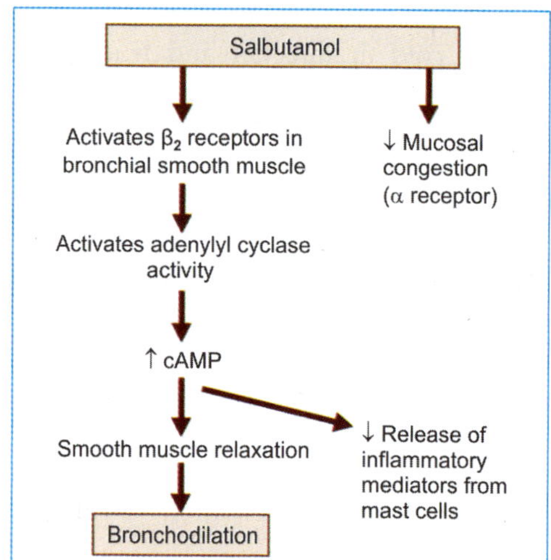

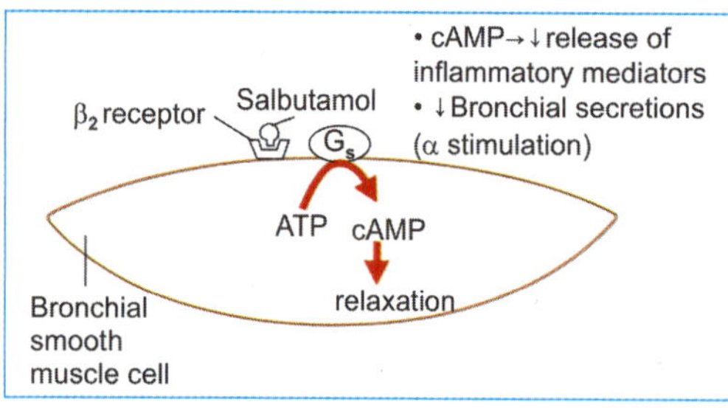

Fig. 31.2: Mechanism of action of β_2 agonists in bronchial asthma

Short-acting β_2 Agonists (SABAs)

Salbutamol (albuterol) and terbutaline are short-acting and selective β_2 agonists. Given by inhalation, they are fastest-acting bronchodilators with peak effect in 10 minutes. The action after inhalation lasts for 3–4 hours.

Adverse effects to β_2 agonists include skeletal muscle tremors, palpitation and nervousness but are mild with aerosols.

Selective β_2 agonists are the most commonly used bronchodilators as they are the most effective, fast-acting, convenient and relatively safe bronchodilators. They are available as metered dose inhalers (Table 31.1), nebulizer solutions, injections and also tablets for oral use (Key Box 31.1). The proper technique in using the inhaler should be taught (Key box 31.2). 'Spacers' (Fig. 31.3) can be used in children and adults who cannot follow the right technique of inhalation. The drug solution is diluted in saline for nebulization. On activation, the nebulizer generates drug particles for inhalation. The particles so generated are of very small size in a metered dose inhaler and the drug needed is of microgram doses (100–200 µg of salbutamol) while a nebulizer forms bigger size particles and, therefore, a higher dose is needed (salbutamol 3–5 mg). β_2 agonists may also be given subcutaneously in patients who cannot reliably take inhalation and require quick action.

On oral administration, salbutamol undergoes high first pass metabolism in the gut with about 50% bioavailability. The duration of action is longer than by inhalation route 4–6 hr.

Dose: Salbutamol 100–200 µg inhalation, 1-4 mg oral. ASTHALIN 100 µg/puff MDI; 2, 4 mg tab. 2 mg/5 ml syrup. AC-HALER, MDI 100 µg/puff

Terbutaline 250 µg inhalation, 2.5-5 mg oral. BRICANYL 2.5, 5 mg tab. 1.5 mg/ml syr. 0.5 mg/ml amp. 250 µg/puff MDI. 10 mg/ml Nebulization solution.

Longer Acting β_2 Agonists (LABAs)

LABAs, like salmeterol, are highly lipid-soluble and, therefore, long acting. That is, they reach the bronchial smooth muscle and dissolve in their cell membrane in high enough concentrations to be long acting (>12 hr). The newer ones including indacaterol, oladaterol and vilanterol are ultralong acting to permit once daily dosing.

Table 31.1: Aerosols in bronchial asthma

Drug	Preparation	Dose
1. Salbutamol	MDI–100 µg/m.d.	1–2 puffs 3–4 times a day
	DPI – 200 µg	3–4 times a day
	Neb soln – 5 mg/ml	2.5 mg 3–4 times a day
2. Salmeterol	MDI – 25 µg/m.d.	50 µg twice daily
	DPI – 50 µg	
3. Terbutaline	MDI – 250 µg/m.d.	1–2 puffs 3–4 times a day
	Neb soln – 10 µg/ml	5 mg 2–4 times a day
4. Ipratropium bromide	MDI – 20, 40 µg/m.d.	1–2 puffs 3–4 times a day
	DPI – 40 µg	
5. Cromolyn sodium	MDI – 1, 2, 5 µg/m.d.	1–2 puffs 3–4 times a day
6. Beclomethasone	MDI – 50, 100, 200 µg/m.d.	400–800 µg/day in 2–3
	DPI – 100, 200, 400 µg	divided doses
7. Budesonide	MDI – 100, 200 µg/m.d.	100–200 µg twice a day
8. Fluticasone	MDI – 25, 50, 125 µg/m.d.	100–250 µg twice a day
	DPI – 50, 100, 250 µg	

MDI—metered dose inhaler md—metered dose Neb soln—Nebulizer solution DPI–Dry powder inhaler

Key Box 31.1: Aerosols in asthma

- β_2 agonists, ipratropium bromide, cromolyn sodium and some glucocorticoids are available for inhalation.
- Use of aerosols largely reduces systemic effects.
- A good aerosol should deliver particles of uniform size in the range of 2–5 micro meters.
- Inhalation can be given by—metered dose inhalers, dry powder inhalers and nebulizers.
- **Metered dose inhalers** are pressurized aerosols which deliver a particular dose of the drug on activation. Advantages—cheaper and portable, but require breathing coordination. Technique—see Key Box 36.2. Chlorofluorocarbon (CFC) propellants used in inhalers are now replaced by a safer hydrofluoroalkane propellant.
- Factors like particle size, breath holding period and rate of breathing all influence effectiveness of inhalers. Even when all these are optimal, only about 2–10% of the drug reaches the bronchioles.
- Use of spacers reduces the need for breathing coordination and increases the amount of drug reaching the lungs.
- **Dry powder inhalers**—rotacaps—have the disadvantages of requiring deep and forceful inspiration which is not possible in children. The powder can cause irritation and cough.
- **Nebulizers** are used in severe bronchospasm. Air or oxygen is passed through a solution of the drug to generate a mist which is inhaled through a mask.

  Advantages

  i. Do not require breathing coordination—a larger dose reaches the bronchioles.
  ii. No use of CFC propellants which are not environment friendly.
  iii. Use is monitored—prevents overdose and inhaler abuse.

  Disadvantages

  i. The device is expensive
  ii. Bigger size → not easily portable.
  iii. A higher dose of the drug is required because the nebulizer generates larger particles.

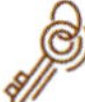

Key Box 31.2: Technique of inhalation

1. Remove the cap from the mouthpiece and shake the inhaler.
2. Breathe out slowly and gently.
3. Place the mouthpiece in the mouth and close the lips around.
4. While breathing in slowly, press the inhaler plunger to release the drug.
5. Hold the breath for at least 10 seconds or longer, if possible.
6. If a second inhalation is required, wait for 1 minute.

Salmeterol is a long-acting selective β_2 agonist. The onset of action is slow (hence not useful in acute attacks) but the effect remains for 12 hours. This is because it is highly lipid-soluble, easily dissolves in the smooth muscle membrane and attains high concentration in these cells. It is used for long-term maintenance and for the prevention of nocturnal asthmatic attacks along with a glucocorticoid.

Dose: 50–100 μg BD. SALMETER, SEROBID 25 μg/ puff MDI. ROTACAP 50 mcg/puff TR-cap, 25 μg MDI.

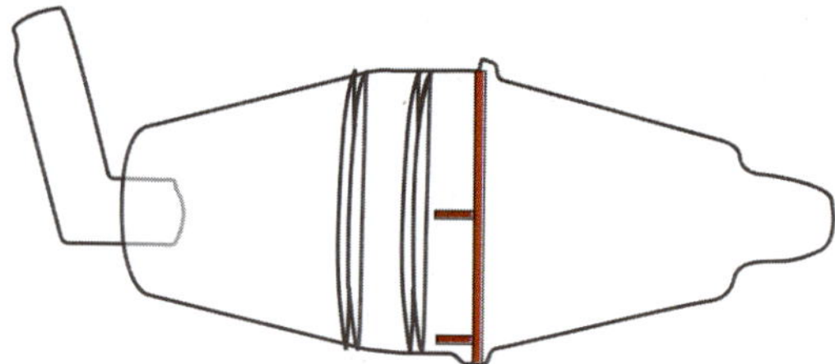

Fig. 31.3: Spacer

Other longer acting agents are also available for use as metered dose inhalers—they are **formoterol, fenoterol, bambuterol and pirbuterol.** Bambuterol is a prodrug of terbutaline which is effective for 24 hours. It is given orally in chronic asthma. Formoterol is fast acting as well as long acting for 12 hr, it is given by inhalation twice daily.

Formoterol: DERIFORM FORATEC 1 puff MDI.
Bambuterol: BAMBUDIL, ASTHAFREE 10, 20 mg tab.

Fenoterol: BEROTEC 100 μg/ puff MDI.

Bitolterol: TORNALATE 0.8% (0.37 mg/puff MDI).

COMPARE AND CONTRAST

	Salbutamol	**Salmeterol**
1. Receptor activated	β_2	β_2
2. Onset of action	Quick	Slow
3. Duration of action	Short (SABA)	Long (LABA)
4. Frequency of use	QID	OD
5. Use in asthma	In acute bronchospasm	Long-term maintenance (not useful in acute attack)
6. Dose	100–200 μg	50–100 μg

Oral β_2 agonists have higher adverse effects than inhaled ones. Muscle tremors, palpitation and nervousness can be significant and are used only in small children who cannot use inhalers and have occasional wheezing (1–4 mg 6 hrly).

Others: Adrenaline and isoprenaline produce prompt bronchodilation. They may be given subcutaneously or by inhalation and the effect lasts for 60–90 min but they are not preferred due to the risk of adverse effects like palpitation, anxiety, restlessness and tremors and in higher doses—cardiac arrhythmias.

Ephedrine produces bronchodilation which is longer lasting but is slow in onset. Because of low efficacy, side effects and availability of better drugs, ephedrine is not preferred.

Status of Sympathomimetics in Bronchial Asthma

β_2 agonists are the first-line drugs for the reversal of bronchospasm. However, the long-term use of β_2 agonists may result in reduced response due to development of tolerance. The β_2 receptors undergo downregulation on continued stimulation by the agonist. Hence management of acute bronchospasm becomes a problem in such patients.

Methylxanthines

Theophylline and its derivatives, like aminophylline, are good bronchodilators.

Mechanism of Action

Methylxanthines act by the following mechanisms:

i. Phosphodiesterase (PDE) is the enzyme that degrades cyclic-AMP. Methylxanthines inhibit PDE (PDE3, PDE5) and thereby enhance cAMP levels. cAMP brings about bronchodilation, and also inhibits the release of mediators of inflammation like cytokines and chemokines.

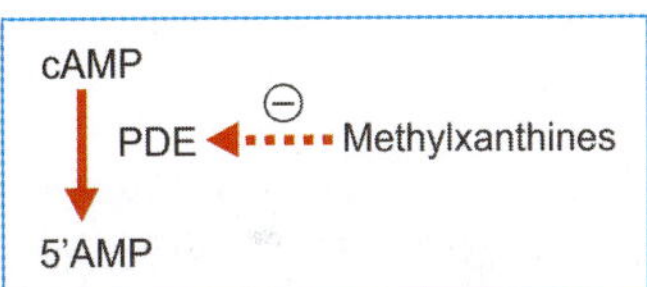

ii. Methylxanthines are **antagonists at adenosine receptors**. It is now known that adenosine induces contraction of smooth muscle cells in the airways and stimulates

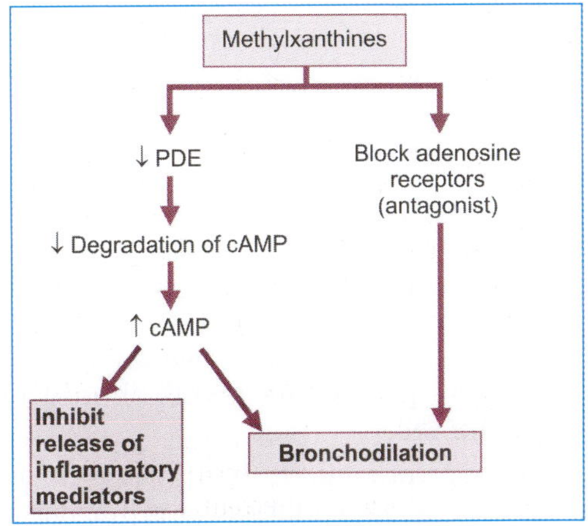

histamine release from airway mast cells. Hence antagonists of the adenosine receptors cause bronchodilation.

iii. Acetylation of histones is involved in the activation of inflammation. Methylxanthines enhance deacetylation of histones and have been also shown to enhance or restore the responsiveness to glucocorticoids in asthmatics and COPD patients.

Pharmacokinetics

Theophylline is well absorbed from the gut, well distributed in the tissues and is metabolised in the liver. Plasma t½ is 7–12 hr in adult. Clearance of theophylline is faster in children. However, neonates and premature babies need a long time to clear theophylline.

Preparations Dose: 200–400 mg TDS. THEOPHYLLINE 400 mg tab. TR-PHYLLINE 125, 250 mg CAP. 80 mg/ 5 ml syrup. 2 ml inj. TSR 200, 400 mg tab.

Aminophylline: Dose-250 mg slow IV over 20 min. MINOPHYL 100 mg tab, 25 mg/ml inj.

Adverse Effects

Theophylline is a drug of **low therapeutic index.** Gastric irritation, vomiting, insomnia, tremors, diuresis, palpitation and hypotension are quite common. Higher doses cause restlessness, delirium, convulsions and arrhythmias. Children may develop behavioural abnormalities on prolonged use—should be avoided.

Status in Bronchial Asthma

Theophylline is a second-line drug in bronchial asthma.

1. *Chronic asthma:* Oral theophylline can be used to control mild to moderate asthma. Etophylline + 80% theophylline (deriphylline) injections (IM) are used to relieve acute attacks. When used over a long term, plasma levels should be monitored.
2. *Acute bronchospasm,* deriphylline IM inj may be used as an alternative to β_2 agonists.
3. *Acute severe asthma* (status asthmaticus): **Aminophylline** is found to be less effective and less safe compared to β_2 agonists. In acute attacks of asthma not responding to β_2 agonists, aminophylline is given intravenously, slowly. In an acute attack, drugs given by inhalation may sometimes fail to reach the bronchioles because of severe bronchospasm. Intravenous aminophylline may then be tried. 250 mg aminophylline should be injected slow IV over 15–20 minutes. Rapid IV injection may cause collapse and death due to hypotension and arrhythmias. Convulsions can also occur and should be carefully watched for.
4. *Other uses—apnoea in premature infants:* Theophylline or caffiene may be used for 1–3 weeks to reduce the duration of episodes of apnoea which may be seen in premature babies.

Anticholinergics

Antimuscarinic drugs relax bronchial smooth muscles but response is slower than to sympathomimetics. Though atropine is a bronchodilator, it is not preferred because of the side effects. Atropine derivatives, **ipratropium bromide and tiotropium bromide** are given by inhalation and their actions are largely confined to the respiratory tract.They block M_1 and M_3 receptors and are poorly absorbed from the gut (if swallowed) and do not cross the BBB. They are more effective in chronic bronchitis including chronic obstructive pulmonary disease (COPD) and are safe and well-tolerated. Unlike atropine, they do not dry up the secretions and hence do not inhibit mucociliary motility. In fact they may increase mucociliary clearance. As a bronchodilator, the efficacy of ipratropium bromide is lower than β_2 agonists but adds to the bronchodilator effects of β_2 agonists. They may also be used as alternatives to β_2 agonists.

Dose: 20–40 μg 3–4 times a day. IPRATOP 20 μg/puff MDI. IPRANASE AQ 40 μg/spray.

Tiotropium bromide is another atropine derivative similar to ipratropium bromide. It is longer acting—a single inhalation can have effect lasting for 24 hrs. It is used in COPD for which tiotropium is particularly suitable due to its longer action. It reduces the frequency and severity of episodes. Tiotropium is also used in bronchial asthma.

Dose: 18 μg 1 ROTACAP OD.

Uses

1. As an adjunct to β_2 agonists particularly in severe bronchospasm and in acute severe episodes. Ipratropium 20–40 μg/puff—2–4 puffs 3–4 times a day or tiotropium 18 μg 1 rotacap OD (They are also available in combination with salbutamol DUOLIN).
2. As a bronchodilator in some cases of chronic bronchitis and COPD.

ANTI-INFLAMMATORY DRUGS

Glucocorticoids

Since inflammation is the primary pathology in bronchial asthma, anti-inflammatory agents afford significant benefit (*see* Chapter 38). Glucocorticoids have been employed in the treatment of bronchial asthma since several decades.

Mechanism of Action

Steroids are not bronchodilators (Fig. 31.4). They suppress the inflammatory response to antigen–antibody reaction, reduce bronchial hyperactivity and thereby reduce mucosal oedema and hyperirritability. Glucocorticoids bind to steroid receptors in the cytoplasm, drug-receptor complex moves to the nucleus, binds to DNA and induces the synthesis of specific mRNA, to bring about the following effects:

1. They decrease the formation of cytokines. These cytokines activate eosinophils and also promote the IgE antibody production.

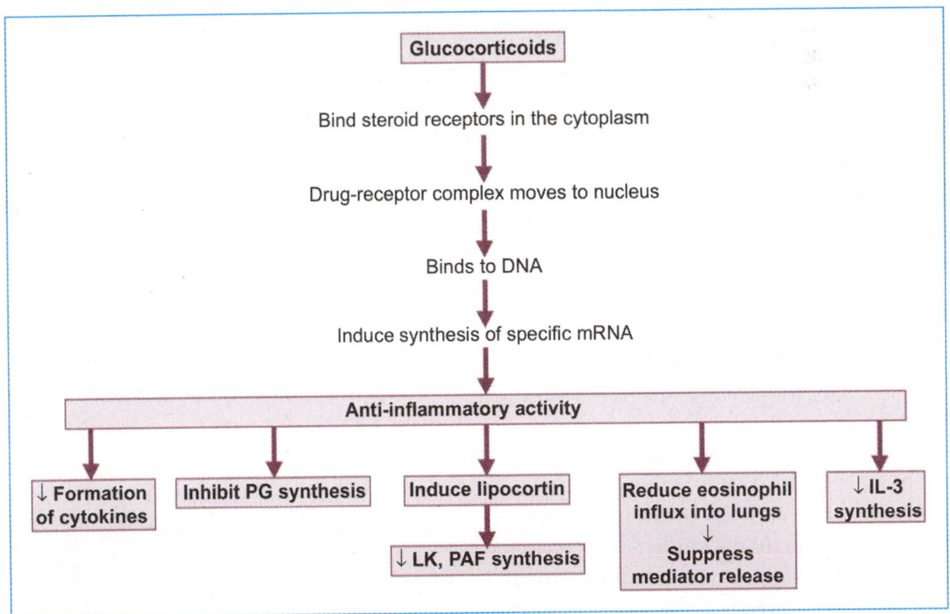

Fig. 31.4: Mechanism of action of glucocorticoids in bronchial asthma

2. Inhibit PG synthesis by inhibiting induction of COX-2.
3. Induce lipocortin and thereby inhibit the production of leukotrienes and PAF.
4. Reduce the influx of eosinophils into the lungs and thus suppress the release of mediators from them. They also inhibit the infiltration of the respiratory passages by mast cells and lymphocytes. After the introduction of inhaled steroids, the concern of adverse effects to glucocorticoids has been largely taken care of. Hence, glucocorticoids have now been extensively used in the prevention and treatment of bronchial asthma. They reduce the frequency and severity of episodes and have also played an important role in improving the quality of life and reducing mortality in asthmatics.
5. Decrease IL-3 synthesis.
6. Restore response to β_2 agonists, if tolerance has developed—by upregulating the β_2 receptors.

Glucocorticoids may be given systemically in acute episodes, if the severity is not controlled by bronchodilators. Oral prednisolone is commonly used (dose 30–60 mg/day). The onset of response requires about 12 hours. In status asthmaticus, glucocorticoids may be given IV. Use of systemic steroids should be restricted for short periods only. Chronic asthma requires prophylaxis with inhaled steroids.

Steroids for Inhalation

The use of inhalational corticosteroids (ICS) largely minimizes the adverse effects of steroids because of the small dose required, but they are not effective in acute attacks and are only of prophylactic value. They prevent episodes of acute asthma, reduce bronchial hyperreactivity and effectively control symptoms. The effect develops after one week of treatment.

Side effects of inhaled steroids include hoarseness of voice (by a direct effect on the vocal cords), sore throat and oropharyngeal candidiasis. Rinsing the mouth and throat with water after each use can reduce the incidence of candidiasis and sore throat. HPA axis suppression is generally not seen in the recommended doses—no clinically significant HPA axis suppression up to 1600 μg/day. But, the drug that is swallowed may be systemically absorbed. Large doses given for a long time may occasionally result in systemic effects of steroids particularly in children. The use of a **'spacer'** reduces this risk and the adverse effects are also less common because the spacer reduces the deposition of the drug in the oropharynx and increases the delivery of the drug to the lungs. Spacer is a reservoir into which drug particles from the inhaler device is released. From the spacer, the drug is slowly inhaled over 1–2 minutes.

Beclomethasone dipropionate, budesonide, triamcinolone, fluticasone, ciclesonide and **mometasone** are available as inhalers.

Beclomethasone dipropionate is available as metered dose inhaler (MDI) and as rotacaps. It is also available in combination with salbutamol.

Preparations: Dose: 100–400 mcg 2–4 puffs a day.

BECLATE 50, 100, 200, 250 μg/puff MDI. 100, 200, 400 μg R-cap. BECORIDE, BEVENT 100 μg/puff MDI.

Budesonide has the advantage of having high topical activity and the absorbed portion is rapidly metabolised. Budesonide is used in the prophylaxis of bronchial asthma and as a nasal spray in allergic rhinitis.

Dose: 100–400 μg 2–4 times a day, BUDATE F-Resp 100 μg cap. 0.5, 1 mg/2 ml. BUDECORT 100, 200, 400 μg R-cap. 0.25, 5, 1 mg respules.

Flunisolide is available as nasal spray for allergic rhinitis.

Fluticasone has the advantages that it is poorly absorbed from the gut and also undergoes high first pass metabolism. Hence even when swallowed from an inhaled dose, systemic adverse effects are unlikely with fluticasone. It is not recommended in children below 4 years of age.

Dose: 25–100 μg twice daily. FLOHALE 25, 50, 125 μg/metered dose—2–3 puffs twice daily. Floease 50, 125 μg/puff MDI.

Ciclesonide is a recently developed inhalational steroid with a unique way of reducing toxicity. It is a prodrug and is converted by esterases to the active drug in the bronchial epithelial cells. If absorbed, the plasma protein tightly binds the active metabolite. Such bound drug is unable to bind the glucocorticoid receptors in several tissues like the skin, eye and bone, thereby avoiding toxicity to these structures. Further studies are needed to prove its benefits.

Dose: 80–160 μg OD inhalation. CALCICLEZ, OSMODE 160 μg/MDI.

Status of Glucocorticoids in Asthma

GINA guidelines now recommend inhalational steroids for all patients of asthma.

1. **Acute exacerbation:** A short course (5–7 days) of oral prednisolone 30–60 mg/day for 7 days is given in addition to β_2 agonists.
2. **Chronic asthma:** Steroid inhalation (2–4 times a day) for a long period for prophylaxis.
3. **Status asthmaticus:** Intravenous hydrocortisone hemisuccinate 100–200 mg followed by another dose every 8 hr; may be switched over to oral prednisolone as soon as possible.

Mast Cell Stabilizers

Cromolyn sodium (disodium cromoglycate) prevents bronchospasm and inflammation following exposure to allergens and decreases bronchial hyper-reactivity. It is, therefore, used for prophylaxis. It is not a bronchodilator—hence **not useful in acute episodes**.

Mechanism of Action

The exact mechanism of action is not known.

- Cromolyn inhibits the degranulation of mast cells and thereby inhibits the release of mediators of inflammation—particularly histamine.
- Cromolyn depresses the exaggerated neuronal reflexes probably by alteration in the function of chloride channels in the cell membrane leading to inhibition of cell activation. The action is responsible for inhibition of cough reflex.
- Cromolyn also inhibits the release of cytokines.

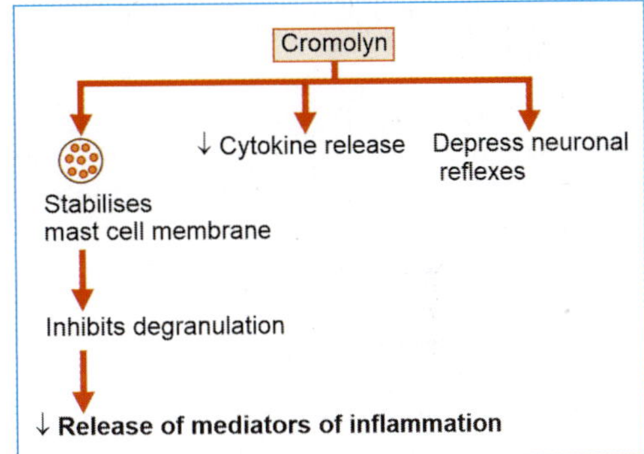

Cromolyn sodium is used as an inhaler—as microfined powder. It takes 2–4 weeks of treatment for the beneficial effects to develop. All patients do not respond—children are more likely to respond.

Pharmacokinetics

Cromolyn is poorly absorbed from the gut. Following inhalation, peak plasma concentration (~1%) is seen within 15 min.

Adverse Effects

Adverse effects are uncommon (<1 in 10,000 patients). Throat irritation, cough and sometimes bronchospasm can occur on inhalation due to deposition of the fine powder. Allergic reactions are rare.

Uses

1. **Prophylaxis of bronchial asthma:** Cromolyn sodium used over a long period—2 puffs 3–4 times daily reduces episodes of acute asthma. Cromolyn can also be used for prophylaxis before exposure to a known allergen—acute

prophylaxis. **The use of cromolyn in bronchial asthma has declined** to a large extent since we now know that inhaled steroids are safe and effective for the prophylaxis of asthma.

2. **Allergic rhinitis:** Prophylactic nasal spray can be used.
3. **Allergic conjunctivitis:** Eye drops are used prophylactically—1–2 drops, 3–4 times a day.

Preparations: Dose: 1–2 puffs 3–4 times a day. FINTAL inhaler 1 mg, eye drops 2%, nasal spray 2%, CROMAL inhaler 1, 2 and 5 mg/metered dose, eye drops 2%, nasal spray 2%.

Nedocromil is similar to cromolyn sodium in its actions and uses. It is given twice daily.

Ketotifen is an antihistaminic with actions like cromolyn sodium. It inhibits airway inflammation but it is not a bronchodilator. It is given orally. Beneficial effects are seen after 6–12 weeks of use. It is used for the prophylaxis of bronchial asthma and other allergic disorders like allergic rhinitis, atopic dermatitis, urticaria and conjunctivitis. Ketotifen is effective orally, bioavailabilty is about 50%, has a t½ of 22 hr.

Drowsiness and **dry mouth** are common side effects. It can also cause dizziness and weight gain.

Dose: 1–2 mg BD. KETAZMA, KETOVENT 1 mg tab.

Leukotriene Receptor Antagonists

Leukotrienes (LT) are important mediators of inflammation. They bring about bronchospasm, mucosal oedema, increase the influx of inflammatory cells and respiratory mucus production by their actions on leukotriene receptors particularly LTC_4 and LTD_4. **Montelukast** and **zafirlukast** are highly selective and competitive antagonists of leukotriene receptors . They block the effects of leukotrienes and thereby reduce mucosal oedema and relieve bronchospasm. They decrease the response to allergens. They inhibit exercise-induced and aspirin-induced bronchospasm.

Montelukast and **zafirlukast** can be used in the prophylaxis of mild to moderate asthma as alternatives or as add-on drugs. The oral route of administration is an advantage particularly in children. They also reduce the dose of the steroid required. Bronchodilator effect is additive with β_2 agonists. Some patients respond well to leukotriene blockers for unknown reason (responders). LT antagonists are particularly useful in aspirin-induced asthma as excess production of leukotrienes is thought to be responsible for bronchospasm. Of the two, **montelukast is more commonly used because of its once daily administration**. Leukotriene antagonists may be used as alternatives to low-dose inhaled steroids in mild but chronic asthma in 'responders'.

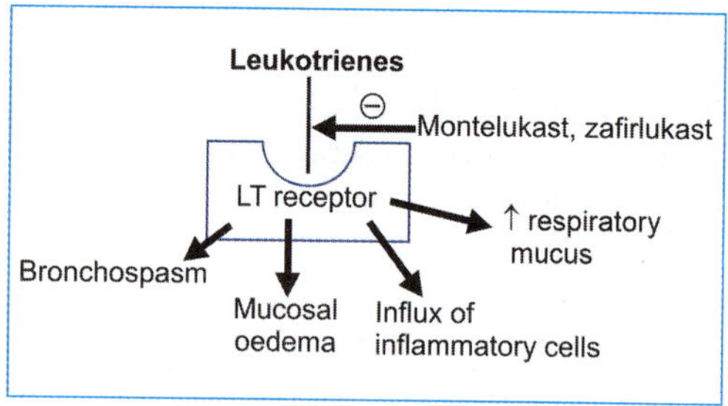

Montelukast Dose: 10 mg OD. MONTEK, MONTELAST 4, 5, 10 mg tab.

Adverse effects are rare and similar to placebo in clinical trials—headache, rashes, gastrointestinal disturbances and hepatic dysfunction can occur. Very rarely a systemic vasculitis affecting the heart, kidney and nerves with eosinophilia has been reported **(Churg-Strauss syndrome)** but is thought to be not directly related to the drug.

Zileuton inhibits leukotriene synthesis by inhibiting the enzyme lipoxygenase but causes a rise in liver enzymes not preferred.

Antihistamines: Antihistamines are indicated in patients who also have hay fever—

histamine release brings about episodes of bronchospasm in such patients. In the routine management of asthma, antihistamines have no role because the pathophysiology involves many other inflammatory mediators apart from histamine.

PDE4 Inhibitors

Roflumilast is a long-acting PDE4 inhibitor effective orally. It has anti-inflammatory properties and may be used in COPD.

ANTI-IgE ANTIBODY

Omalizumab is a monoclonal antibody against IgE. Omalizumab binds to IgE to form a complex and such bound IgE antibodies cannot bind to IgE receptors on mast cells and basophils. Thus the development of allergic response and the allergic process itself is inhibited. Omalizumab is given subcutaneously once in 2–4 weeks, has a long elimination t½ of 26 days. It is well tolerated but can occasionally cause pain at the site of injection and allergic reactions. Omalizumab can be given in asthmatics (above 12 years of age) with moderate to severe asthma for the **prophylaxis** as it reduces the frequency and severity of acute exacerbations. Omalizumab is also useful in patients with:

- **Allergic rhinitis** to reduce the frequency and severity of acute episodes.
- **Chronic urticaria**
- **Peanut allergy**.

TREATMENT OF ASTHMA

Mild Asthma

Acute episodes: Occasional acute episodes of bronchospasm need rapidly acting, inhaled β_2 stimulants like salbutamol as and when required but should preferably be taken at the onset of bronchospasm. Regular prophylaxis is not required, but a course of ICS is given to reduce the risk of exacerbations. Mild chronic asthma is characterised by episodes of mild bronchospasm once a day. It requires long-term inhaled steroids. **GINA (Global Initiative for Bronchial Asthma) guidelines** updated in 2022 have revised the treatment strategy for asthma to include an inhalational steroid (ICS) in all asthma patients. Acute bronchospasm is managed with β_2 agonist inhalation – a SABA + ICS.

Moderate Asthma

Regular prophylaxis with inhaled steroids are given. Acute episodes are managed with inhaled long-acting β_2 agonists. If inhaled steroids are contraindicated, leukotriene antagonists may be tried.

Severe Asthma

Repeated episodes of bronchospasm with frequent exacerbations and the symptoms almost continuously present so as to interfere with day-to-day activities.

a. Regular inhaled steroids
b. Inhaled β_2 agonists 3–4 times a day—β_2 agonists may be used.
c. Oral steroids may be considered
d. Additional inhaled ipratropium bromide or oral theophylline may be given.
e. *Biologicals:* Long term use of omalizumab may be considered.

Acute Severe Asthma or Status Asthmaticus

It is an acute exacerbation. It is a medical emergency; may be triggered by an acute respiratory infection, abrupt withdrawal of steroids after prolonged use, by drugs, allergens or emotional stress.

Treatment

1. Nebulization of a β_2 agonist and ipratropium alternately—every 30 minutes.

Key Box 31.3: Drugs that can cause bronchospasm

- NSAIDs (like aspirin)
- Morphine
- β-blockers (like propranolol)
- Cholinergic drugs (e.g., bethanechol, acetylcholine, organophosphorus compounds)
- Tubocurarine
- Zanamivir inhalation.

Additional salbutamol 0.4 mg IM/SC may be given. Severe tachycardia should be watched for.
2. Hydrocortisone hemisuccinate IV 100 mg stat followed by 100 mg every 8 hours infusion (till the crisis is overcome) followed by a course of oral prednisolone.
3. Oxygen inhalation is needed in most patients. An oxymeter is clipped over the finger to determine oxygen saturation.
4. Antibiotics—if infection is present.
5. IV fluids to correct dehydration and acidosis.
6. Artificial ventilation may be required in extreme cases particularly in presence of respiratory failure.
7. Magnesium sulphate may be given IV or as inhalation as adjuvant to bronchodilators but not routinely recommended.
8. K^+ supplementation may be needed as repeated use of salbutamol may result in hypokalaemia.

Drugs used in Chronic Obstructive Pulmonary Disease (COPD)

COPD is an abnormal inflammatory response of the respiratory tract to noxious gases with airflow limitation which is not fully reversible. It is mostly seen in chronic smokers. Chronic exposure to dust and respiratory infection are other factors. GOLD grading (Global initiative for chronic obstructive Lung Disease) classifies COPD depending on severity into 4 groups viz. mild, moderate, severe and very severe based on FEV1 values with mild being FEV 1 >80% and very severe <30%.

Drugs used in asthma also help COPD but the response is not as good. Smoking should be stopped. For bronchospasm, inhalation of a β_2 agonist or **ipratropium** is needed. **Tiotropium** or long-acting β_2 agonists may be used for day-long bronchodilation. Patients with repeated exacerbation may require inhaled steroids for controlling the frequency and severity of episodes. **Theophylline** may also relieve bronchospasm. PDE4 inhibitor **roflumilast** is particularly effective in COPD. Acute exacerbations need a course of antibiotics as respiratory infections are common in these patients.

DRUGS USED IN TREATMENT OF COUGH

Competency achievement: The student should be able to:
PH 1.33 Describe the mechanism of action, types, doses, side effects, indications and contraindications of the drugs used in cough (antitussives, expectorants/ mucolytics).[1]

Cough is a protective reflex that clears the irritant matter and secretions from the respiratory tract. It could be due to infection, allergy, pleural diseases and malignancy. The cause for cough should be detected and treated whenever possible. Since it is a protective mechanism, undue suppression of cough can cause more harm than benefit. In some conditions, as in dry annoying cough, it may serve no useful purpose and repeated coughing also causes exhaustion. In such situations, antitussives or cough suppressants may be used. Antitussive is a cough suppressant and only provides symptomatic relief and do not alter the cause.

Drugs for Cough

1. *Central cough suppressants (antitussives)*
   Codeine, pholcodeine, noscapine, dextromethorphan, antihistamines, benzonatate.
2. *Pharyngeal demulcents*
   Lozenges, cough drops, linctuses
3. *Expectorants*
   Drugs that increase secretions: Potassium iodide, guaiphenesin, ammonium chloride, ipecacuanha.
   Liquify secretions: Mucolytics
4. *Bronchodilators:* Salbutamol, terbutaline

Central Cough Suppressants

Central cough suppressants act by inhibiting cough centre in the medulla.

Codeine is a good antitussive with less addiction liability. It suppresses the cough centre. Codeine acts on μ opioid receptors and it suppresses cough in subanalgesic doses. However, nausea, constipation and drowsiness are common (*see* page 261). Abuse liability is low, it should be avoided in pateints with bronchial asthma since it is a respiratory depressant.

Dose: 10–15 mg every 6 hours, CODINE 15 mg tab, 15 mg/5 ml linctus.

Noscapine is a natural opium alkaloid which is a potent antitussive. No other CNS effects are prominent in therapeutic doses (*see* page 261). Nausea is the only occasional side effect.

Dose: 15–30 mg every 6 hours.

Dextromethorphan and **pholcodeine** are synthetic opioid derivatives with antitussive actions like codeine but with lesser side effects. They do not cause constipation and have no addiction liability but can cause nausea and drowsiness. **Pholcodeine** is longer-acting.

Dextromethorphan. Dose: 10–20 mg 3–4 times a day.

Pholcodeine. Dose: 10–15 mg given twice daily.

Benzonatate is chemically related to the local anaesthetic procaine. It acts on the cough receptors in the lungs and also has a central effect. It is given orally—100 mg thrice daily.

Local anaesthetics, like lignocaine, may be administered through nebulization to temporarily suppress coughing by anaesthetising the respiratory tract. They are used to facilitate bronchoscopy.

Antihistamines are useful in cough due to allergy except that due to bronchial asthma. They thicken the secretions which may be difficult to cough out. An antihistamine is generally one of the components of cough syrups. Their sedative property may be of additional value in suppressing cough. Chlorpheniramine, promethazine and diphenhydramine are the commonly used antihistamines.

Other centrally acting antitussives include **carbetapentane, chlophedianol, oxeladine** and **caramiphen**. More extensive studies are required to prove their efficacy.

Pharyngeal Demulcents

Pharyngeal demulcents (*demulcere* = to caress soothingly, in Latin) increase the flow of saliva which produces a soothing effect on the pharyngeal mucosa and reduces afferent impulses arising from the irritated mucosa. Dry cough due to irritation of the pharyngeal mucosa is relieved. Candy sugar or a few drops of lemon also serve this purpose.

Expectorants

Expectorants (Latin, *expectorare* = to drive from the chest) increase the production of respiratory tract secretions which coats and cover the irritated mucosa. As the secretions become thin and less viscid, they can be easily coughed out. Expectorants are also called mucokinetic agents and are used to treat cough that results from irritation of the respiratory mucosa. Expectorants may increase the secretions directly or reflexly.

- *Direct stimulants:* Volatile oils like eucalyptus oil; creosotes, alcohol, cidar wood oil—when administered by inhalation with steam can increase respiratory secretions. Some of them are also effective when taken orally.
- *Reflex expectorants* are given orally, they are gastric irritants and reflexly increase respiratory secretions. However, they cause gastric irritation resulting in nausea. Ipecacuanha, an emetic, is also a reflex expectorant.

Potassium iodide acts both directly and reflexly to increase airway secretions. Ammonium salts, like ammonium chloride and ammonium carbonate, can cause nausea and anorexia and, therefore, are not preferred.

Ipecacuanha is an emetic. In sub-emetic doses, it is used as an expectorant. **Guaiphenesin,** a plant product, also enhances respiratory secretions.

Mucolytics

Normally, the respiratory mucus is watery. The glycoproteins in the mucus are linked by disulphide bonds to form polymers making it slimy. In respiratory diseases, the glycoproteins form larger polymers with plasma proteins present in the exudate and the secretions become thick and viscid. Mucolytics liquefy the sputum making it less viscid so that it can be easily expectorated.

The following are mucolytics

Bromhexine a semisynthetic compound related to vasicine (an alkaloid from the plant *Adhatoda vasica),* is a good mucolytic. It depolymerises the mucopolysaccharides in the mucus. It also liberates lysosomal enzymes which breaks the thick tenacious sputum. It is given orally— 8–16 mg thrice daily. It is useful when respiratory secretions are thick or when mucus plugs make coughing strainous. Side effects are minor—may cause rhinorrhoea and lacrimation. Bromhexine is highly bitter and therefore, tablet may be preferred to syrup. It is the most commonly used mucolytic.

Dose: 8–16 mg TDS. BROMHEXINE 8 mg tab. 4 mg/5 ml syr.

Ambroxol is a metabolite of bromhexine with actions similar to it. Ambroxol may be given orally or by inhalation. It can be used as an alternative to bromhexine.

Dose: 15–30 mg TDS. AMBROLITE, MUCOLITE 30 mg tab, 30 mg/5 ml liquid.

Acetylcysteine opens disulfide bonds in mucoproteins of the sputum reducing its viscosity. It is given by aerosol. It may cause gastric irritation as the gastric mucosal barrier may be penetrated.

Carbocysteine is similar to acetylcysteine and is used orally. It can cause gastrointestinal irritation and rashes.

Dose: 250–750 mg TDS. MUCODYNE 350 mg cap, 250 mg/ml syrup.

Pancreatic dornase: Pancreatic dornase is a deoxyribonuclease obtained from the beef pancreas. It breaks the deoxyribonucleic acid (DNA) into smaller parts thus making the secretions thin and less viscid. It is administered by inhalation. Pancreatic dornase can cause allergic reactions–not preferred.

Bronchodilators

Bronchodilators, like salbutamol and terbutaline, relieve cough that results from bronchospasm.

The antitussive preparations generally have a combination of a central cough suppressant, an expectorant, an antihistaminic and sometimes a bronchodilator and a mucolytic agent.

Steam Inhalation

Steam inhalation offers an effective and inexpensive alternative to drugs. It humidifies the sputum as well as respiratory mucosa. This helps in reducing the irritation and for easier expectoration of the sputum. In presence of dehydration, just rehydrating the patient is found to be beneficial.

Drug-induced cough: Drugs like ACE inhibitors, amiodarone and beta blockers can induce cough. Certain drugs delivered to the respiratory tract like ether vapours, cromolyn, desflurane and acetylcysteine induce cough. In case of ACE inhibitors, many patients may need discontinuation of the drug. Beta-blockers are contraindicated in asthmatics.

Analeptics

Analeptics are respiratory stimulants (*see* page 275). They are CNS stimulants—also stimulate the respiratory centre. They may be used in respiratory failure. However, availability of artificial ventilators and the inconvenience of side effects of CNS stimulation like convulsions has made them less often used. **Doxapram** is the only analeptic in use currently.

Clinical Pharmacology

Bronchial asthma

- Salbutamol is the most commonly used bronchodilator.
- Beta-2 agonists may cause muscle cramps in some patients—requires reduction of dose. Unnecessary analgesics should be avoided.
- Theophylline should be avoided in patients with cardiac diseases and in those prone to seizures.
- Montelukast is particularly effective in patients with sinobronchial allergy.
- Cromolyn sodium is suitable for acute prophylaxis in exercise-induced asthma.
- Glucocorticoids should be tapered after long-term use.

Cough

- Only dry cough should be suppressed.
- Allergic cough responds to antihistamines.
- Sugar-free preparations should be prescribed for patients with diabetes mellitus.
- Most cough syrups are combinations and can cause many side effects; overdose is common as some patients tend to take 2–3 tsps at a time.

[1–2] From Medical Council of India, *Competency based Undergraduate Curriculum for the Indian Medical Graduate*, 2018;1:136–144.

Unit X

Gastrointestinal Tract

CHAPTER 32

Drugs used in Peptic Ulcer and GERD

Competency achievement: The student should be able to:

PH 1.34 Describe the mechanism/s of action, types, doses, side effects, indications and contraindications of the drugs used as below:

1. Acid-peptic disease and GERD.[1]

Acid-peptic disease is common in the present days that are full of tension and anxiety. Peptic ulcer is thought to result from an imbalance between acid-pepsin secretion and mucosal defense factors. The stomach secretes about 2.5 litres of gastric juice daily. The chief cells secrete pepsinogen while the parietal cells secrete HCl and intrinsic factor. The factors that protect the mucosa are its ability to secrete mucus, bicarbonate and prostaglandins. The mucus and bicarbonate form a layer which protects the gastric mucosa from gastric acid. Prostaglandins (PGE_2 and PGI_2) stimulate the secretion of mucus and bicarbonate, bring about vasodilation and also inhibit acid secretion. They act on the PG receptors present on the parietal cell.

Gastric acid secretion is regulated by three pathways—vagus (ACh), gastrin and local release of histamine—each acting through its own receptors (Fig. 32.1). These activate H^+, K^+-ATPase (proton pump) on the parietal cells resulting in the secretion of H^+ into the gastric lumen where it combines with Cl^- (drawn from plasma) and HCl is formed. Acetylcholine and gastrin act both directly on the parietal cells and indirectly by releasing histamine from the enterochromaffin cells. Histamine acts through H_2 receptors on parietal cells while acetylcholine through M_1 muscarinic and gastrin through G receptors. The exact etiopathogenesis of peptic ulcer is not known. Infection of the stomach mucosa with *Helicobacter pylori* is now known to be associated with chronic gastritis, peptic ulcers and their recurrence.

Drugs used in peptic ulcer may be classified as follows:

Classification

1. Drugs that neutralise gastric acid	– ***Antacids***—magnesium hydroxide, aluminium hydroxide, calcium carbonate, sodium bicarbonate
2. Drugs that reduce gastric acid secretion	
a. H_2 receptor blockers	– Cimetidine, ranitidine, famotidine, roxatidine, nizatidine
b. Proton pump inhibitors	– Omeprazole, esomeprazole, lansoprazole, dexlansoprazole, pantoprazole, rabeprazole,
c. Muscarinic antagonists	– Pirenzepine, telenzepine, propantheline
3. Ulcer protectives	– Sucralfate, bismuth compounds
4. Other drugs	– Carbenoxolone, cisapride, misoprostol, vonoprazan
5. Anti-*H. pylori* drugs	– Amoxicillin, clarithromycin, metronidazole, tinidazole

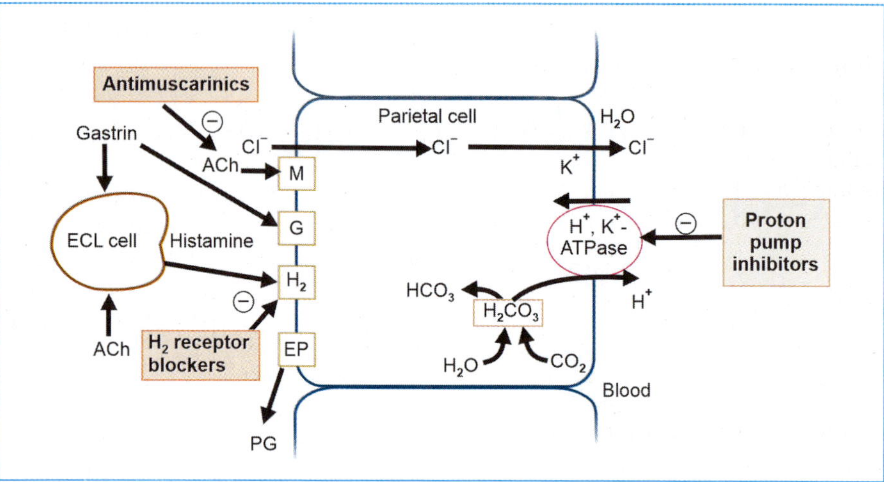

Fig. 32.1: Regulation of gastric secretion and sites of action of drugs. ECL: Enterochromaffin cell; M: Muscarinic receptor (chiefly M_1); G: Gastrin receptors; H_2: Histamine H_2 receptor, EP: Prostanoid receptor

ANTACIDS

Antacids are basic substances. Given orally they neutralize the gastric acid and raise the pH of gastric contents. Peptic activity is also reduced, as pepsin is active only below pH 4. Thus antacids provide rapid relief of symptoms in hyperacidity as they chemically neutralise the acid that is already present in the stomach but, do not reduce the acid secretion. Since the pH rises >5 there could be rebound hyperacidity due to raised gastrin levels. The duration of action of antacids is generally 30–60 min when taken on an empty stomach.

Types of Antacids

Antacids are of two types: (i) Systemic—which are absorbed and (ii) nonsystemic—which act only in the stomach and are not absorbed into the circulation.

They are as follows:

1. **Systemic antacids**
   - Sodium bicarbonate
2. **Nonsystemic antacids**
   - Aluminium hydroxide
   - Magnesium trisilicate
   - Magnesium hydroxide
   - Calcium carbonate.
3. **Others**
   - Simethicone

Systemic Antacids

Sodium bicarbonate is rapid but short-acting. CO_2 that is released in the stomach escapes as eructation.

$$NaHCO_3 + HCl \longrightarrow NaCl + H_2O + CO_2$$

Sodium bicarbonate gets absorbed from the intestines leading to systemic alkalosis. There is 'rebound' hyperacidity as gastrin levels increase due to raised gastric pH. Sodium load may increase which may be particularly troublesome in patients with cardiovascular diseases.

When higher doses of sodium bicarbonate or calcium carbonate are given with calcium rich dairy products, a syndrome known as **milk–alkali syndrome** can result—characterized by hypercalcaemia, metabolic alkalosis and renal dysfunction. Sodium bicarbonate is not preferred for long-term use because of the above disadvantages.

Uses

1. Sodium bicarbonate is used with other antacids in peptic ulcer and hyperacidity for short periods.
2. To alkalinise the urine in the treatment of poisoning due to acidic drugs.
3. To treat metabolic acidosis.

Sodium citrate is another antacid absorbed systemically and can be used in place of sodium bicarbonate.

Nonsystemic Antacids

Nonsystemic antacids are insoluble compounds that react in the stomach with HCl to form a chloride salt and water. They are not absorbed.

For example:

(i) $Mg(OH)_2 + 2HCl \longrightarrow MgCl_2 + 2H_2O$

(ii) $CaCO_3 + 2HCl \longrightarrow CaCl_2 + H_2O$

Aluminium hydroxide is slow acting. Food further slows its neutralizing capacity. It is also an astringent and demulcent—forms a protective coating over the ulcers. The aluminium ions relax the smooth muscles resulting in delayed gastric emptying and constipation. Aluminium hydroxide binds phosphate and prevents its absorption resulting in hypophosphataemia on prolonged use.

Magnesium salts include magnesium hydroxide, magnesium trisilicate, magnesium oxide and magnesium carbonate. Magnesium salts are osmotic purgatives because magnesium chloride is formed in the stomach which is an osmotic purgative and the dose used as antacid may cause mild diarrhoea. Their action is quick and prolonged. Rebound acidity is mild. A small percentage of magnesium trisilicate gets absorbed systemically. Prolonged use may cause hypermagnesaemia in presence of renal dysfunction. **Magaldrate** is a hydrated complex of hydroxymagnesium aluminate. The complex reacts with acid to release aluminium hydroxide which has a prolonged effect. Aqueous suspension of magnesium hydroxide is called **milk of magnesia.**

Calcium carbonate acts quickly and has prolonged action but liberates CO_2 which may cause discomfort. Calcium salts also have a chalky taste. They may cause constipation and hypercalcaemia. Increased plasma calcium levels may result in rebound hyperacidity. Calcium ions released in the stomach may directly reach gastric mucosa resulting in increased acid secretion. Long-term use may also result in renal calcium stones and milk–alkali syndrome.

Antacid combinations are given to obtain maximum effects with least adverse effects as follows (Table 32.1):

1. *Quick and prolonged effect:* Fast-acting [$Mg(OH)_2$] and slow as well as long acting [$Al(OH)_3$] compounds are combined.
2. *Neutralising side effects:* Magnesium salts have a laxative effect while aluminium salts are constipating—combination neutralizes each other's side effects.
3. *Gastric emptying:* Magnesium salts hasten while aluminium salts delay gastric emptying.
4. *Additive effect:* Given together, aluminium and magnesium salts have additive effect and the dose of each compound required is lower.

Uses: Antacids are used as adjuvants in hyperacidity, peptic ulcer and reflux oesophagitis. For more severe acid peptic disease however, PPIs are preferred over H_2 blockers.

- All antacid tablets should be chewed and swallowed as they do not disintegrate well in the stomach.
- Gels are more effective than tablets.
- One dose given 1 hr after food neutralizes the acid for 2 hours.
- Given on an empty stomach the effects of antacids remain for a shorter period than when given after food.
- Most antacids are available as over the counter preparations.

Table 32.1: Antacids—some examples

Brand name	*Combination*
1. GELUSIL LIQUID	Aluminium hydroxide gel 312 mg + Magnesium trisilicate 625 mg in every 5 ml
2. GELUSIL TABLET	Aluminium hydroxide gel 250 mg + Magnesium trisilicate 500 mg
3. DIGENE GEL	Magnesium hydroxide 185 mg + Aluminium hydroxide gel 830 mg + Carboxymethyl cellulose sodium 100 mg + Methylpolysiloxane 25 mg—in every 10 ml
4. DIGENE TABLET	Dried aluminium hydroxide gel 30 mg + Magnesium silicate 50 mg + Magnesium hydroxide 25 mg + Methylpolysiloxane 10 mg

- Acid neutralising capacity (ANC) of an antacid is the number of milliequivalents of 1 N HCl that can be brought to pH 3.5 in 60 minutes by a unit dose of the antacid. ANC is used to describe the potency of an antacid preparation. Thus ANC of 1 g sodium bicarbonate is 12 mEq while that of 1 g $Mg(OH)_2$ is 30 mEq and 1 g $CaCO_3$ is 20 mEq.

Drug Interactions

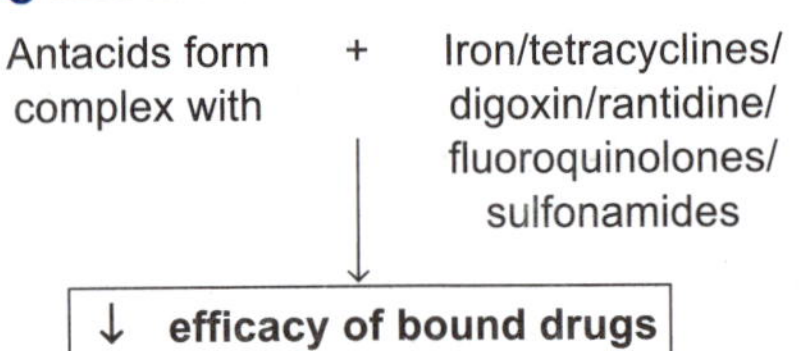

Antacids form complexes with iron, tetracyclines, digoxin, ranitidine, fluoroquinolones, sulfonamides and antimuscarinic drugs. To avoid these, antacids should be taken 2 hours before or 2 hours after other drugs.

Simethicone or dimethylpolysiloxane is a silicone polymer. It is pharmacologically inert, repels water and helps in proper dispersion of antacids in the gastric contents. It is also an antifoaming agent as it reduces surface tension and thereby decreases gastric flatulence. Simethicone may be used in combination with antacids.

Oxethazaine is a local anaesthetic that can act even at acidic pH. It anaesthetises the sensory nerve endings in the stomach and oesophagus which inhibits gastrin release and also relieves pain. Oxethazaine is available in combination with antacids. It can cause drowsiness and dizziness.

Solacid-O liquid contains oxethazaine 10 mg/ 5 ml with Aluminium hydroxide 300 mg, Magnesium hydroxide 100 mg; Magnesium trisilicate 150 mg and Simethicone 25 mg.

H_2 RECEPTOR BLOCKERS

Cimetidine, ranitidine, famotidine, roxatidine and nizatidine are the H_2 receptor blockers available.

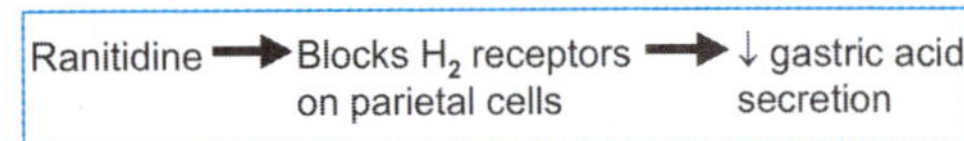

These drugs bind to the histamine H_2 receptors on the parietal cells and competitively inhibit the action of histamine on these receptors and thereby reduce gastric secretion. Both **volume and acidity** of basal, nocturnal and food induced secretion are reduced. The inhibition is **dose dependent and a single dose can cause 60–70% reduction in gastric secretion for 12 hr**. Secretion of intrinsic factor, gastrin-induced HCl secretion and pepsin are also reduced. These actions, particularly their ability to suppress nocturnal acid secretion, hasten the healing of peptic ulcers (Table 32.2).

Pharmacokinetics

H_2 blockers are rapidly and well-absorbed (~50% bioavailability) but undergo first pass metabolism. Food does not interfere with their absorption. Cimetidine acts for 5–8 hours,

Table 32.2: Dosage and frequency of administration of drugs used in peptic ulcer

Drug	*Dose and frequency*
Ranitidine	150 mg BD/300 mg HS
Famotidine	20 mg BD/40 mg HS
Roxatidine	75 mg BD/150 mg HS
Cimetidine	200 mg QID/800 mg HS
Omeprazole	20–40 mg OD
Lansoprazole	15–30 mg OD
Rabeprazole	20–40 mg OD
Sucralfate	1 g 1 hr before each meal
Colloidal bismuth subcitrate	120 mg 1 hr before meals and at bedtime
Carbenoxolone	50–100 mg TDS
Misoprostol	200 μg BD-QID

ranitidine and famotidine for 12 hours. They are partly metabolised in the liver and excreted by the kidneys. In renal impairment, dose of H_2 blockers should be reduced.

Adverse Effects

The H_2 blockers (except cemetidine) are well-tolerated with minor side effects (in <3% of patients) like diarrhoea, dizziness, muscle pain and headache. Because the H_2 receptors do not have any significant functions in other tissues (except stomach), H_2 receptor blockers are fairly selective and thereby safe drugs. They cross the placenta and are also secreted in the milk. Hence they should be avoided in pregnancy and lactation. H_2 blockers may also cause blood dyscrasias though rarely.

Cimetidine

- Cimetidine can cause **antiandrogenic effects** because it inhibits binding of testosterone to androgen receptors, displaces testosterone from its binding sites on the androgen receptors; it increases plasma prolactin levels and inhibits oestrogen metabolism in the liver. On prolonged use, it may result in **gynaecomastia,** decreased sperm count, **impotence** and loss of libido in men and **galactorrhoea in women**.
- CNS effects include confusion, restlessness, delirium and hallucinations in the elderly.
- Headache, dizziness, rashes and diarrhoea can result. Elevation of liver enzymes is transient. Cardiovascular effects, like bradycardia, AV block, cardiac arrest, atrial fibrillation, ventricular extrasystoles and ventricular tachycardia, have been reported with cimetidine and ranitidine.
- Cimetidine inhibits microsomal enzymes (cytochrome P450) and interferes with the metabolism of many drugs. This can result in several drug interactions.
- Cimetidine or other H_2 blockers should be given IV as a slow infusion because rapid injection can cause bradycardia, hypotension and cardiac arrest.

Cimetidine is **not preferred** due to the adverse effects, risk of drug interactions and also the availability of safer derivatives.

Preparations CIMET—200 mg, 400 mg tab.

Ranitidine is the preferred H_2 blocker as it has several advantages over cimetidine.

- Ranitidine is more potent and longer acting than cimetidine.
- Has no antiandrogenic effects, does not increase prolactin levels and does not influence oestrogen metabolism—hence no antiandrogenic side effects.
- No CNS effects as it does not cross BBB. Intravenous ranitidine (and other newer agents) can occasionally cause CNS effects including confusion, and hallucinations in the elderly patients and in patients with renal or hepatic dysfunction.
- Does not inhibit microsomal enzymes significantly and thereby no related drug interactions.
- Only adverse effects are headache and dizziness.

  RANTAC, ACILOC 150, 300 mg tab; 50 mg/2 ml inj.

Famotidine is similar to but more potent and longer acting than ranitidine as it firmly binds to the H_2 receptors. Apart from this, famotidine shares all the advantages of ranitidine over cimetidine. Adverse effects are mild, and include occasional headache, dizziness, bowel disturbances and skin rashes. QT prolongation has been reported.

FAMOCID, FAMONITE, 20, 40 mg tab; 20 mg/inj.

Roxatidine is similar to ranitidine in actions and advantages but is twice as potent as ranitidine and is also longer acting.

ROTANE 75, 150 mg tab.

Nizatidine is similar to ranitidine. About 90% of the dose is excreted through the kidneys.

Ebrotidine is a recent addition to the group of H_2 blockers.

Uses of H_2 Blockers

1. **Peptic ulcer:** H_2 blockers bring about rapid relief from pain and the ulcers heal in 80–90% of patients with 6–8 weeks of treatment. Since there is a risk of recurrence, a bedtime dose of an H_2 blocker may be continued for long periods.
2. **Gastritis:** H_2 blockers are the first-line drugs for nonulcer dyspepsia. They are often used as over-the-counter preparations.
3. **Prevention of stress-induced ulcers:** Stress-induced ulcers and erosive gastritis can occur in critically ill patients. They can be prevented by administration of H_2 blockers for short periods. They may be used intravenously as an infusion for better results.
4. **Zollinger-Ellison syndrome:** This condition with high circulating gastrin levels due to gastrin secreting tumour is known to cause peptic ulcers. High doses of H_2 blockers may be used as alternatives to PP inhibitors to reduce hyperacidity in these patients till surgical resection of the tumour is done.
5. **Preanaesthetic medication:** Ranitidine or other H_2 blockers may be used to reduce gastric acid secretion in order to prevent damage to the respiratory mucosa, if aspiration occurs during surgery.
6. **GERD:** H_2 blockers may be used as alternatives to PPIs in mild GERD. Though antacids may also be used, the effects are short lasting (1–2 hr).

PROTON PUMP INHIBITORS

Dr. George Sachs putforth the idea that proton pump is the final common pathway in acid secretion and drugs that inhibit the proton pump could control acid secretion. Omeprazole was discovered in 1978 and was approved for use in 1989 after clinical trials. Proton pump inhibitors (PPIs) are the most efficacious inhibitors of the gastric acid secretion (Key Box 32.1). **Omeprazole** was the first to be developed and we now have **pantoprazole, lansoprazole, dexlansoprazole, rabeprazole** and **esomeprazole** with minor pharmacokinetic variations. All are benzimidazoles.

Omeprazole is the most commonly used PP inhibitor and is considered the prototype.

Mechanism of Action

The parietal cells of the stomach secrete H^+ with the help of an enzyme H^+, K^+-ATPase (proton pump) present in its plasma membrane. This is the final step in gastric acid secretion due to any stimuli. Proton pump inhibitors are inactive **prodrugs,** they accumulate in the parietal cells where they quickly get activated in the acidic environment to sulfenamide. The active form firmly binds H^+, K^+-ATPase (SH groups) by covalent bonds and specifically and irreversibly inhibits H^+, K^+-ATPase. It thereby inhibits gastric secretion. The binding is irreversible and a single dose can almost totally (90–95%) inhibit gastric secretion. However, it requires 3–4 days of PPI

Key Box 32.1: Proton pump inhibitors

- PPIs require acid for their activation in the parietal cells and, therefore, should be given with or before food as food stimulates the secretion of acid.
- Antacids, H_2 receptor blockers and other durgs which reduce gastric acidity reduce the efficacy of proton pump inhibitors.
- Omeprazole inhibits the microsomal enzyme activity which can result in many drug interactions.

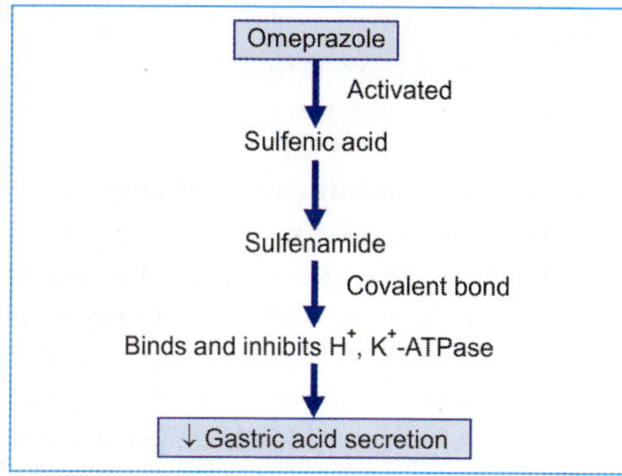

therapy for maximum efficacy to develop. In the same way, the acid secretion resumes completely only after 3–4 days after stopping the PPI, that is only after new H^+, K^+-ATPase enzyme is synthesized. IV formulation should be given continuously for the first 2–3 days as infusion or as repeated injection to obtain maximum effect. Ulcer heals rapidly even in resistant cases.

Pharmacokinetics

All PPIs are given orally—as granules in enteric-coated or delayed release capsules or tablets to avoid degradation by the acid in the stomach. PPIs are lipid-soluble, weak bases and get rapidly absorbed from the intestines. After the enteric coating is dissolved, the prodrug reaches the parietal cell canaliculi because of its acidic nature. Though it also reaches other acidic tissues, the concentration in parietal cell canaliculi is 1000 times more as it gets trapped.

Pantoprazole and esomeprazole are available for IV use.

Omeprazole is highly protein bound and is metabolised in the liver by the microsomal enzymes (cytochrome P450). PPIs also undergo first pass metabolism. Though the t½ of omeprazole is 1–2 hours, the effect of a single dose remains for 2–3 days because of its accumulation in the parietal cell canaliculi (hit and run drug). Food interferes with the absorption—reduced by 50%. **Because the maximum number of proton pumps are active by about one hour after food, and can be inhibited PPIs should be taken 1 hr before food** so that their peak levels are reached with the highest number of active proton pumps.

PP inhibitors are microsomal enzyme inhibitors and can result in many drug interactions—they may enhance the plasma levels of drugs like benzodiazepines, warfarin and phenytoin—precipitating toxicity.

Dose: 20–40 mg OD, OMEZ, LOMAC 20, 40 mg cap

Adverse Effects

Omeprazole and other PPIs are well-tolerated and are largely safe drugs.

1. Prolonged acid suppression may allow bacterial over growth in the stomach resulting in increased risk of gastrointestinal infections.
2. Dizziness, headache, diarrhoea, abdominal pain, nausea, arthralgia and rashes are rare.
3. Long-term administration may result in:
   - Vitamin B_{12} deficiency due to its reduced absorption—because acid is necessary for vitamin B_{12} to be released from the food.
   - Acid is also needed for the absorption of magnesium, calcium and iron. Elderly patients receiving PPIs for a long time need to check the calcium levels and bone density as they may have an increased rick of osteoporosis.
   - ↑ Gastrin levels due to reduced gastric acidity. On discontinuing the PPI, this raised gastrin could result in hyperacidity for some days.
   - Atrophic changes in the stomach have been noticed after 3–4 years of use.

Drug Interactions

1. PPIs decrease the absorption of certain drugs which need gastric acidity for absorption, e.g. itraconazole.
2. Enzyme inhibition—omeprazole and esomeprazole inhibit the microsomal

enzymes CYP3A4 and CYP2C19 and thereby inhibit the metabolism of drugs like diazepam, phenytoin and warfarin.

3. Clopidogrel, being a prodrug, needs CYP2 C19 for its activation. PPIs should be avoided but if needed, pantoprazole or rabeprazole may be given.

Lansoprazole and dexlansoprazole are similar to omeprazole but have higher oral bioavailability, faster onset of action and are longer-acting.

LANZOL, LANZAP 15, 30 mg cap.

Dexlansoprazole—30 mg OD

Pantoprazole is more acid stable, has higher oral bioavailability and an intravenous formulation is also available for use. When given as a continuous IV infusion for 24 hours, inhibition of acid secretion is maximum. Microsomal enzyme inhibition is milder compared to omeprazole and lansoprazole and, therefore, the drug interactions are fewer. All other features are similar to omeprazole.

Dose: 40 mg OD, PANTODAC, PANTOCID, 40 mg enteric-coated cap; 40 mg vial.

Rabeprazole has the fastest onset of action but efficacy is similar to omeprazole with milder inhibition of microsomal enzymes like pantaprazole.

RABELOC, RABICAP 10, 20 mg cap.

Esomeprazole is the S-enantiomer of omeprazole. It has a bioavailability of >80% and is given in the dose of 20–40 mg once daily.

RACIPER, ESOZ 20, 40 mg tab 40 mg vial.

Uses of PP inhibitors: Introduction of PP inhibitors revolutionised the treatment of peptic ulcer. The more severe cases were largely managed by surgical line of treatment about 2–3 decades ago but are now effectively managed by medical line of treatment.

1. ***Peptic ulcer:*** In peptic ulcer patients not responding to H_2-blockers, PPIs are used for faster and more efficient ulcer healing and pain relief. Most duodenal ulcers heal in 4–6 wk while gastric ulcers require somewhat longer time of 6–8 wk. Bleeding peptic ulcer patients run the risk of rebleeding. Higher dose of omeprazole (40 mg BD) or other PPI for 5–7 days reduce the risk of bleeding. PPIs may also be given as a continuous IV infusion.
2. ***GERD:*** Severe gastroesophageal reflux disease needs PPIs for 6–8 wk. Ulcers heal fast and pain is relieved. However, symptoms recur and many require long-term acid suppression with PPIs. Patients with symptomatic disease even without ulcers are treated with PPIs.
3. ***Dyspepsia:*** Generally, H_2-blockers are preferred for non-ulcer dyspepsia, but PPIs may also be used.
4. ***Drug-induced ulcers:*** Patients who need to continue NSAIDs would require a PPI once daily. If the NSAID is stopped, PPI may be given for 4–6 weeks and withdrawn after the ulcer heals.
5. ***H. pylori regimen:*** PPIs also form a component in *H. pylori* treatment regimen.
6. ***Zollinger-Ellison syndrome:*** PPIs are useful in Zollinger-Ellison syndrome associated with gastrin secreting tumours.
7. ***Gastrinoma:*** Gastrinomas which cannot be surgically removed could cause peptic ulceration due to excessive gastric acid secretions. PPIs are useful in such patients.
8. ***Preanesthetic medication:*** To reduce gastric acid secretion and reduce damage to gastric mucosa if aspiration occurs.

MUSCARINIC ANTAGONIST

Though atropine reduces gastric secretion, the dose needed results in several adverse effects. A derivative of atropine—**pirenzepine** selectively blocks gastric M_1 receptors and inhibits gastric secretion by 40–50% without significant side effects. It also inhibits the secretion of gastrin, mucus and bicarbonate. As it does not cross the BBB, it does not cause CNS side effects unlike atropine. Dryness of mouth and blurring of vision can occur. Pirenzepine is used as an adjuvant. **Telenzepine** is more potent than pirenzepine.

ULCER PROTECTIVES

Sucralfate

Sucralfate is a salt of sucrose and sulfated aluminium hydroxide. In acidic medium (pH <4) or water, sucralfate polymerizes to form a sticky, viscid gel which firmly adheres to the base of the ulcers (Flowchart 32.1). The negatively charged sucralfate gets attracted to the positively charged proteins in the ulcer base. It remains there for over 6 hours acting as a physical barrier and prevents contact with acid and pepsin. It also stimulates the PG synthesis in gastric mucosa. It thus promotes healing by protecting the ulcer. Sucralfate is not absorbed, is excreted in the faeces and is well-tolerated.

Uses

1. *Peptic ulcer:* One tablet (1 g) is given 1 hr before each meal and one at bedtime for 4–8 weeks and then 1 g BD is continued for 6 months to prevent recurrence.
2. Prevention of stress-induced ulcers and bleeding in critically ill patients.

Side effects are rare and include constipation (due to aluminium), abdominal discomfort and dryness of mouth. It interferes with absorption of several drugs. Long-term use may cause toxicity due to aluminium absorption.

Dose: 1 g 1 hr before each meal and at bedtime for 4–8 weeks, SUCRASE, ULCERFATE 1 g tab.

Topical, with lignocaine for anal fissures and haemorrhoids.

Drug Interactions

- Sucralfate needs acidic pH for activation. Hence antacids should not be given with it.
- Sucralfate adsorbs and interferes with the absorption of tetracyclines, digoxin, phenytoin and cimetidine.

Rabamipide enhances mucosal defense by temporarily activating genes coding for cyclo-oxygenase 2 and also acting as a free radical scavenger—it protects the gastroduodenal mucosa and promotes the healing of gastroduodenal ulcers.

Bismuth Salts

Colloidal bismuth subcitrate and bismuth subsalicylate—on oral administration chelate proteins in the ulcer base and form a protective coating over the gastric mucosa. They also inhibit the growth of *H. pylori* on gastric mucosa and stimulate the production of mucus and PGs. By these actions, they promote ulcer healing in 4–8 weeks. Bismuth subsalicylate dissociates in the stomach—bismuth is excreted through the gut while salicylate is absorbed. Bismuth salts may cause constipation, black stools, darkening of the tongue and dizziness.

Bismuth compounds are used occasionally in combination regimens for *H. pylori*

Flowchart 32.1: Mechanism of action of sucralfate

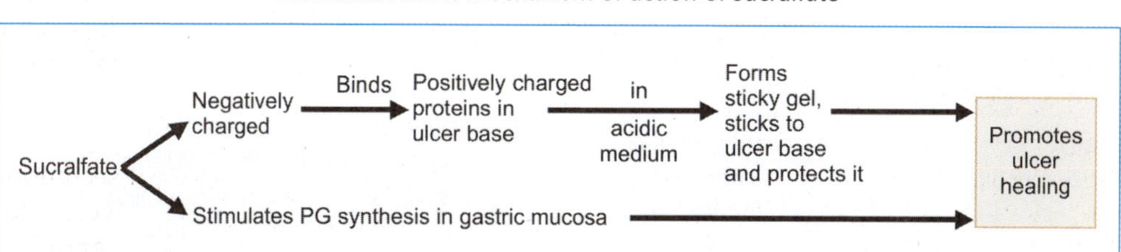

infections. They are also used for prevention of traveller's diarrhoea. Bismuth compounds should be used only for short periods.

Dose: 120 mg 1 hr before meals and at bedtime. PYLOCID, DENOL 120 mg tab.

OTHER DRUGS

Carbenoxolone is a steroid like compound obtained from glycyrrhizic acid found in the root of liquorice. On ingestion, it alters the composition of mucus so that it is more viscid and adheres to gastric mucosa to protect the ulcer base. It also inhibits pepsin activity and prolongs the life of PGs. Because of its steroid like effects, it causes salt and water retention leading to oedema and weight gain. It is, therefore, not preferred.

Prostaglandins: PGE_2 and PGI_2 synthesized by the gastric mucosa inhibit gastric secretion, enhance mucus production, mucosal blood flow and exert a **cytoprotective effect.** They act by binding to the PG receptor (EP_3) present on the parietal cells and inhibit cAMP production. Synthetic PGE_1 analog **misoprostol** and PGE_2 analogs, like **enprostil, arbeprostil,** and **rioprostil,** are used in acid peptic disease. They are all given orally and are of special value in preventing **NSAID-induced gastric ulceration** because NSAIDs are PG synthesis inhibitors—but the PG analogs are expensive. Diarrhoea, muscle cramps and oxytocic effects are common—they should be avoided in pregnancy (Key Box 32.2).

Dose: Misoprostol 200 µg qid.

Enprostil, rioprostil are PGE_2 analogs that are more stable and longer acting compared to natural PGs. They are to be avoided in pregnancy because they are ecbolics.

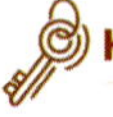

Key Box 32.2: Some ulcerogenic drugs

NSAIDs	Theophylline
Glucocorticoids	Caffeine
Iron	Tetracyclines
Alendronate	

Vonoprazan is a novel potassium competitive acid blocker which reduces gastric acid secretion. Clinical trials have shown it to be effective in acid peptic disease and as a component of anti-*H. pylori* triple drug regimen.

Gastrin Inhibitors

Proglumide is a competitive antagonist at the gastrin receptors. It is also a cholecystokinin antagonist. Clinical trials have shown it to be as effective as H_2-blockers with no reported side effects.

TREATMENT OF *H. PYLORI* INFECTION

The gram-negative bacterium *H. pylori* is adapted to living in the stomach. Infection with *H. pylori* is associated with gastroduodenal disease including gastritis and peptic ulcer. It is also thought to be responsible for recurrence of peptic ulcer disease and is considered as a major risk factor for stomach cancer. Eradication of *H. pylori* with drugs that reduce acid secretion has shown to reduce the relapse rate.

Various combination regimens of 2–4 drugs are tried with efficacy up to 95%. Combination of clarithromycin, amoxicillin or tetracyclines; metronidazole and omeprazole or an H_2 receptor blocker are given for 1–2 weeks. Use of a PP inhibitor in the regimen improves the efficacy of the antibiotics in eradicating *H. pylori* by raising gastric pH and enhancing antibiotic stability—activity of amoxicillin and clarithromycin are pH dependent. Some regimens are:

One week regimen

1. Clarithromycin 250 mg BD + Metronidazole 400 mg BD + Omeprazole 20 mg BD.
2. Amoxicillin 1000 mg BD + Tinidazole 500 mg BD + Lansoprazole 30 mg BD.

Two weeks regimen

1. Clarithromycin 500 mg TDS/Amoxicillin 750 mg TDS + OMEPRAZOLE 20 mg BD.
2. Amoxicillin 750 mg/Tetracycline 500 mg qid + Tinidazole 500 mg + Omeprazole 20 mg—all twice daily.

COMPARE AND CONTRAST

Promethazine and Ranitidine

Features	***Promethazine (H_1-blocker)***	***Ranitidine (H_2-blocker)***
Antagonist of	Histamine	Histamine
Subtype of receptor blocked	H_1	H_2
Other receptors blocked	M_1 muscarinic	Nil
Effect on sleep	*Sedative*	No sedation
Anticholinergic effects	Present	Absent
Gastric HCl secretion	Not affected	Decreased
Antiemetic property	Present	Absent
Primary use	Allergic disorders	Acid peptic disease
CNS effects of alcohol	Potentiated	No effect

3. Clarithromycin 500 mg + Amoxicillin 750 mg + Omeprazole 20 mg—all twice daily.
4. Amoxicillin 750 mg + Clarithromycin 250 mg + Lansoprazole 30 mg—all twice daily.
5. Amoxicillin 1000 mg + Lansoprazole 30 mg + Clarithromycin 500 mg—all twice daily.

Treatment of gastroesophageal reflux disease (GERD): Reflux of acidic gastric contents into the oesophagus results in 'heart burn' due to oesophagitis. The reflux could be due to anatomical (hiatus hernia) or functional causes. Most cases are functional and result from loss of tone of the lower oesophageal sphincter. The reflux of acidic contents will result in inflammation, erosion and ulcers in the esophagus. Chronic oesophagitis can result in changes in the oesophageal mucosa which could be a premalignant condition (Barrett's oesophagus).

Severity may vary from mild nonerosive GERD with occasional heart burn to severe ones with regular disturbing oesophagitis and erosive GERD. Uncomplicated, mild GERD with occasional dyspepsia may be treated with antacids. They may be combined with **sodium alginate** which reacts with acid to form a layer and floats on the top of contents in the stomach, acts as a mechanical barrier and prevents contact of the oesophageal mucosa with acids—thus protects the mucosa. H_2-blockers may be used but are less efficacious in more severe GERD.

In all patients with moderate to severe GERD, PPIs are the drugs of choice. They afford rapid relief of symptoms and promote healing of oesophageal lesions in 4–8 weeks. Treatment may have to be continued for a long period—may be years.

Prokinetic agents may be used as adjuvants, if needed. Symptoms may recur on stopping the medication in many patients.

Nonpharmacological measures like **avoiding**—heavy meals, late night dinner, smoking and alcohol—all help.

Clinical Pharmacology

- Magnesium-containing antacids should be avoided in renal failure.
- Antacids should be avoided in CCF (except occasionally because they contain sodium salts).
- PPIs should be given 30 min before food.
- Sucralfate may be used only in proven peptic ulcer—also more expensive—generally not preferred.
- Most antiulcer drugs particularly ranitidine are available as over-the-counter medication and often irrationally used. History of such drug use should be elicited.

[1] From Medical Council of India, *Competency based Undergraduate Curriculum for the Indian Medical Graduate*, 2018;1:136–144.

CHAPTER 33

Emetics, Antiemetics and Prokinetic Agents

Competency achievement: The student should be able to:

PH 1.34 Describe the mechanism/s of action, types, doses, side effects, indications and contraindications of the drugs used as antiemetics and prokinetics.[1]

PHYSIOLOGY OF VOMITING

Stimulation of the vomiting centre in the medulla oblongata results in vomiting. The vomiting centre receives afferents from the chemoreceptor trigger zone (CTZ), vestibular apparatus, GI tract and centres in the brain (Fig. 33.1). CTZ is not protected by the blood–brain barrier and is stimulated by various drugs (Key Box 33.1), chemicals and radiation (Fig. 33.2). We now know of many neurotransmitters involved in the act of vomiting.

Cytotoxic drugs/radiation

↓

Damage cells, irritate the gut mucosa

↓

Release mediators from gut mucosa

↓

Activation of vagal afferents in the gut

↓

Emetogenic impulses to NTS, CTZ

↓

Stimulate emetic centre

↓

Vomiting

Fig. 33.1: Pathophysiology of cytotoxic drug-induced vomiting

Drugs that influence these have been developed as antiemetics.

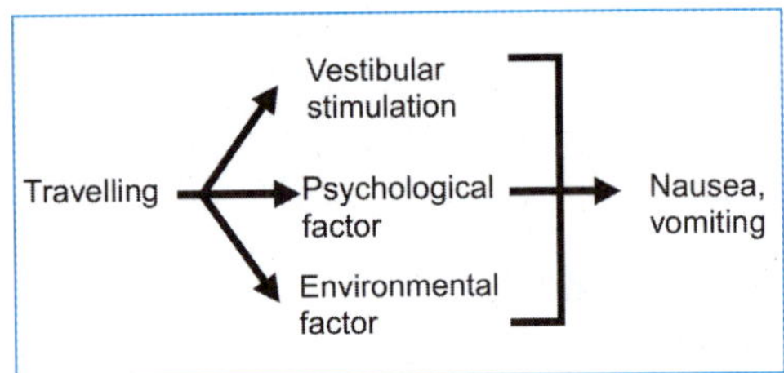

EMETICS

Emetics are drugs that produce vomiting. When a noxious substance is ingested, vomiting has to be induced. Emetics may act directly by stimulating the CTZ or reflexly by irritating the stomach mucosa. Mustard powder (1 teaspoon) with water or hypertonic salt solution can evoke vomiting reflexly.

Apomorphine is a derivative of morphine. Given SC/IM, it produces vomiting in 5–10 minutes. It acts by stimulating the dopaminergic receptors in the CTZ. Apomorphine can depress respiration and should, therefore,

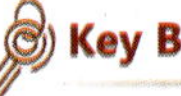

Key Box 33.1: Some emetogenic drugs

- Most anticancer drugs—cisplatin, methotrexate
- Levodopa, bromocriptine and other dopamine agonists
- Morphine and other opioids
- Cholinomimetic drugs
- Metronidazole
- Ergot alkaloids
- Chloroquine, emetine

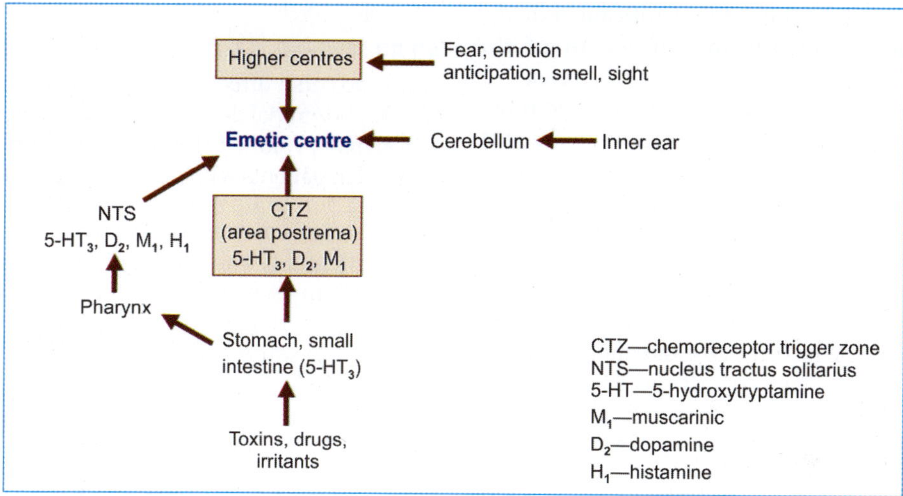

Fig. 33.2: The stimuli, pathways and centres mediating emetic reflex and the receptors involved

be avoided in presence of respiratory depression.

Ipecacuanha obtained from the dried root of *Cephalis ipecacuanha* contains an alkaloid emetine. Given as a syrup **(Ipecac syrup, dose: 15–20 ml)**, it produces vomiting in 15 minutes. It acts both directly on the CTZ and reflexly by irritating the gastric mucosa. It is safe even in children.

ANTIEMETICS

Antiemetics are drugs used in the prevention and treatment of vomiting. Vomiting is a protective mechanism aimed at eliminating the unwanted harmful material from the stomach. But in some situations, vomiting may not serve any useful purpose and may only be troublesome. It can cause dehydration, weakness and electrolyte imbalance. In such circumstances, vomiting needs to be suppressed with antiemetics—classified as:

Classification

1. **Dopamine D_2 antagonists (prokinetics)**
   Metoclopramide, domperidone, trimethobenzamide
2. **5-HT_3 antagonists**
   Ondansetron, granisetron, dolasetron
   Tropisetron, palanosetron
3. **Antimuscarinics**
   Hyoscine, promethazine
   Cyclizine, diphenhydramine
4. **Neuroleptics**
   Chlorpromazine, prochlorperazine
   Haloperidol
5. **Neurokinin receptor antagonists**
   Aprepitant
   Fosaprepitant
6. **Other agents**
   Glucocorticoids
   Cannabinoids—dronabinol, nabilone

Dopamine D_2 Antagonists

Metoclopramide and domperidone act centrally by blocking dopamine D_2 receptors in the CTZ and thereby prevent vomiting. They enhance the tone of the lower oesophageal sphincter and increase gastric peristalsis—they are prokinetics (*see* page 430). **Trimethobenzamide** has antihistaminic activity in addition to dopamine blockade.

5-HT_3 Antagonists

Ondansetron: 5-Hydroxytryptamine released in the gut is an important inducer of emesis and the nerve endings including vagal affarents in the gut are rich in 5-HT_3

receptors. It is believed that anticancer drugs, radiation therapy and infection of the gastrointestinal mucosa induce the release of 5-HT in the gut which initiates emetic reflex through 5-HT_3 receptors present in the gut, nucleus tractus solitarius (NTS) and area postrema in the brain. Ondansetron blocks 5-HT_3 receptors in the GI tract, CTZ and nucleus tractus solitarius and prevents vomiting. It is a powerful antiemetic and can be given orally or intravenously (4–8 mg). Ondansetron has an oral bioavailability is 60–70%, t½ of 3–5 hr and a duration of action of 4–12 hr (Key Box 33.2).

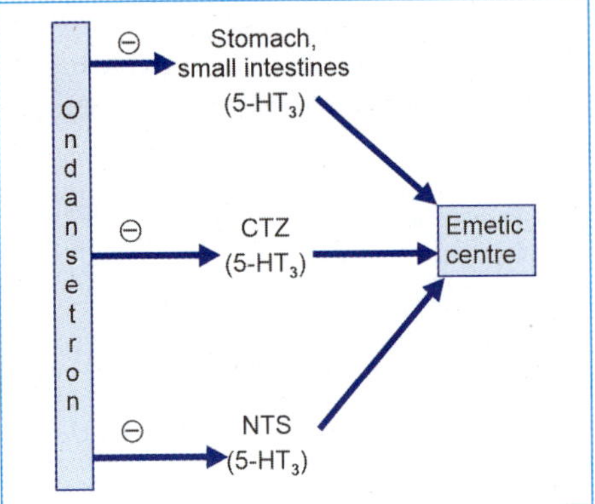

Pharmacokinetics

5-HT_3 antagonists are well absorbed from the gut. They are metabolised by the liver by microsomal enzymes and are excreted by the kidneys and partly through the gut. They can be given orally, IM and IV. Dose reduction may be required in liver dysfunction.

Dose: 4–24 mg in one or 2 divided doses, EMESET, OSTERON 4, 8 mg tab, 2 mg/ml inj.

 **Key Box 33.2: 5-HT_3 antagonists**

- Block 5-HT_3 receptors in the gut, CTZ and NTS.
- Efficient antiemetics.
- Effective both orally and parenterally.
- Largely safe—no sedation or other CNS/autonomic side effects.
- Adverse effects minor—headache, GI disturbances.
- Drugs of choice in postoperative and anticancer drug-induced vomiting.

Adverse Effects

All 5-HT_3 antagonists are well tolerated with minor adverse effects like headache, constipation, abdominal discomfort and rashes. Dolasetron may prolong QT interval and should be avoided in patients with prolonged QT interval.

Granisetron is more potent than ondansetron as an antiemetic. Though granisetron, **dolasetron** (100 mg once daily) and **tropisetron** have longer t½, their biological effect t½ remains the same and they can all be given once daily.

Dose: 1–2 mg once daily: 10 μg/ kg IV, GRANISET 1, 2 mg tab, 1 mg/ml/ inj.

Palanosetron has a higher affinity for the 5-HT_3 receptors and a longer half-life.

Uses

5-HT_3 antagonists are used to control vomiting induced by anticancer drugs or radiotherapy. They should be given intravenously 30 min before (ondensetron 8 mg infusion over 15 min) or orally 1 hr before starting chemotherapy. From second day, ondansetron may be given orally 8 mg twice daily for 3–7 days.

They are also useful in postoperative vomiting and other drug-induced vomiting (but not in motion sickness).

To prevent postoperative vomiting, a 5-HT_3 blocker is given IV (4–8 mg ondansetron) before induction and the dose may be repeated after 8 hr or as required.

Antimuscarinics

Hyosine is a labyrinthine sedative very effective in motion sickness. Motion sickness or travelling sickness is due to over stimulation of the vestibular apparatus along with psychological and environmental factors. Hyoscine also relaxes the gastrointestinal smooth muscle. Taken 30 minutes before journey, hyoscine (0.4–0.6 mg oral) acts for 6 hours and the dose should be repeated, if the journey is longer than that. A transdermal

Table 33.1: Preferred drugs for vomiting due to various causes

Conditions	*Drugs*
Motion sickness	Hyoscine, cyclizine, promethazine, cinnarizine
Vomiting due to cytotoxic drugs	1. Ondansetron + dexamethasone + aprepitant 2. Metoclopramide + dexamethasone + diphenhydramine + lorazepam.
Vomiting due to other drugs	Chlorpromazine, metoclopramide
Postoperative vomiting	Ondansetron, metoclopramide
Vomiting in pregnancy	Doxylamine, dicyclomine, pyridoxine, cyclizine, meclizine, metoclopramide

patch delivers hyoscine constantly over 3 days and is to be applied behind the ear. Sedation and dry mouth are common side effects.

Dicyclomine is used to control vomiting in morning sickness and motion sickness—orally in the dose of 10–20 mg (Table 33.1).

H_1 antihistamines like promethazine, diphenhydramine, doxylamine, cyclizine and cinnarizine have anticholinergic properties. Antihistamines block H_1 receptors in the area postrema as well as muscarinic receptors in the CNS. They probably also act on the GI tract. Some of them are useful in motion sickness and postoperative vomiting.

Doxylamine is available in combination with pyridoxine for 'morning sickness' in some countries. Though some studies have shown it to be free of teratogenic potential, its safety is not proved and, therefore, not used for the purpose in countries like USA and England.

Dose: Doxylamine 10 mg + Pyridoxine 10 mg tab, GRAVIDOX, DOXINATE 10 mg tab.

Neuroleptics

Neuroleptics (*see* page 236) also block D_2-receptors in the CTZ and are useful in vomiting due to most causes except motion sickness. Sedation and extrapyramidal symptoms are the common side effects. Prochlorperazine is mainly used as an antiemetic in vomiting and is also effective in vertigo associated with vomiting.

Prochlorperazine Dose: 5–25 mg. STEMETIL 5, 25 mg tab, 12.5 mg/ml inj.

Neurokinin Receptor Antagonists

These drugs bind to neurokinin (NK_1) receptor in the area postrema and act as antiemetics. **Aprepitant** has recently completed clinical trials and is available for oral use while **fosaprepitant** is given IV and gets converted to aprepitant in the body. Aprepitant has a t½ of 12 hr. It is metabolised in the liver by microsomal enzymes CYP3A4 and may compete with other drugs metabolised by the same pathway. NK_1 antagonists may cause dizziness, weakness and diarrhoea. NK_1 antagonists may be used for the prevention of chemotherapy induced vomiting in combination with a 5-HT_3 antagonist and a glucocorticoid. The efficacy of the combined regimen is more than the individual drugs.

Dose: APREPITANT 125 mg 1 hr before chemotherapy followed by 80 mg daily for next two days.

Other Antiemetics

1. **Glucocorticoids** are used in combination with other antiemetics like ondansetron or metoclopramide. Glucocorticoids control delayed vomiting following anticancer drug therapy. Their mode of action is not clear but may act by activating the glucocorticoid receptors in the NTS.

2. **Pyridoxine (vitamin B_6)** is used in the prevention of vomiting in pregnancy without any known pharmacological basis. The proposed rationale is that pyridoxine serves as a cofactor in GABA synthesis and GABA acting as the inhibitory neurotransmitter at CTZ may suppress vomiting. Dose: 20–60 mg.

3. **Cannabinoids:** Dronabinol, a cannabinoid is Δ9 tetrahydrocannabinol. It has antiemetic properties. It may act by the stimulation of the cannabinoid receptors (CB_1) in the vomiting centre. It also increases appetite. Dronabinol is orally effective and almost completely absorbed on oral administration. Dose 5 mg/m^2, 2 hr before chemotherapy and the dose may be repeated every 4 hr to complete 4–6 hr. Dronabinol can cause hallucinations, euphoria, dysphoria, behavioural abnormalities, dependence, increased appetite, dryness of mouth and hypotension. It can be used as an alternative in the prevention of anticancer drugs induced vomiting in combination with other antiemetics—when other drugs are ineffective. Dronabinol has also been prescribed to enhance appetite—as an appetite stimulant.

Nabilone is another Δ9THC analog used as an antiemetic.

4. **Sedative hypnotics:** Barbiturates and benzodiazepines may raise the threshold for vomiting by depressing the CNS. Their anxiolytic and sedative properties also help. Sedative hypnotics are used as adjuvants to other antiemetics in treating anticancer drug-induced vomiting.

5. **Propofol:** The general anaesthetic propofol has useful antiemetic properties.

Antiemetic Combinations

Severe retching and vomiting like that induced by anticancer drugs are treated with a combination of antiemetics including ondansetron, metoclopramide, glucocorticoids and sedative-hypnotics. Later cycles of anticancer drug regimens can cause 'anticipatory' vomiting, i.e. vomiting at the sight or even the thought of receiving anticancer drugs. This can be avoided by using appropriate antiemetics even in the earlier cycles of anticancer therapy.

PROKINETIC AGENTS

Drugs that enhance gastroduodenal motility and hasten gastric emptying are called **prokinetic agents.** The following are prokinetic agents.

Prokinetics

1. D_2 antagonists
   - Metoclopramide, domperidone
2. Others
   - Cisapride, mosapride, itopride
   - Cholinomimetics—bethanechol
   - Anticholinesterases—neostigmine
3. Motilin receptor agonist—erythromycin

Metoclopramide

Metoclopramide was introduced in 1970s. It is structurally related to procainamide but is not a local anaesthetic.

Actions

GIT: Metoclopramide promotes forward movement of contents of the upper GI tract—increases oesophageal and gastric peristalsis. It raises lower oesophageal sphincter pressure, speeds up gastric emptying and prevents the reflux of stomach contents into the oesophagus. It thus prevents reflux oesophagitis. Prokinetics have no significant effects on the motility of the small intestine and the colon.

CNS: Metoclopramide acts as an antiemetic by blocking the D_2 dopamine receptors on the CTZ. The effect on the gut, i.e. speeding up gastric emptying also contributes.

Mechanism of Action

Metoclopramide acts through both dopaminergic and serotonergic receptors (Fig. 33.3).

1. *D_2 blockade:* Stimulation of dopamine receptors in the gut particularly upper GIT, inhibits cholinergic stimulation of the gastrointestinal smooth muscle—relaxes the stomach, lower oesophageal sphincter (LES) and delays gastric emptying. Metoclopramide blocks the D_2 receptors causing a reversal of these effects, i.e. it enhances gastric peristalsis, LES tone and hastens gastric emptying.

   Blocking the D_2 receptors in the CTZ is responsible for antiemetic actions.

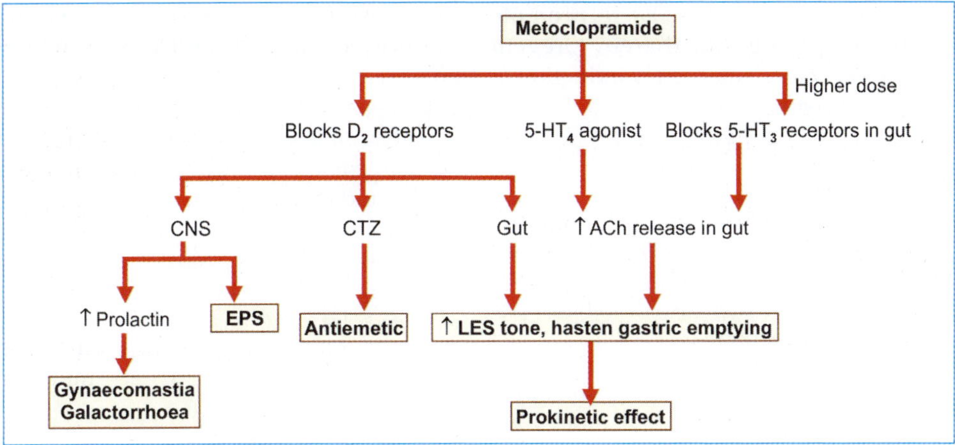

Fig. 33.3: Mechanism of action and actions of metoclopramide

2. *Serotonergic receptors*
   a. 5-HT_4 agonist—metoclopramide stimulates the 5-HT_4 receptors on the excitatory interneurons of the gut which enhances the release of acetylcholine from myentric motor neurons. This action is more important in the prokinetic activity of metoclopramide. It is augmented by bethanechol and antagonised by atropine.
   b. 5-HT_3 antagonist—in high doses-metoclopramide blocks 5-HT_3 receptors on inhibitory myentric interneurons which can enhance ACh release in the gut. Blockade of $5HT_3$ receptors in the NTS and CTZ adds to the antiemetic effects.

Pharmacokinetics

Metoclopramide is rapidly absorbed on oral administration. It crosses the blood–brain barrier, placenta and is also secreted in the milk. It has a half-life of 3–6 hr. Onset of action is almost immediate (1–2 min) after IV injection while it takes 30–60 mins following oral intake (*see* Fig. 33.2).

Dose: 10 mg TDS for chemotherapy induced vomiting 0.3–1 mg/kg. IM or slow IV, PERINORM, REGLAN 10 mg tab, 5 mg/ 5 ml syrup, 10 mg/ 2 ml. inj.

Adverse Effects

Adverse effects are sedation, restlessness, anxiety and diarrhoea. Dopamine receptor blockade results in gynaecomastia, galactorrhoea and **extrapyramidal symptoms** with dystonia, tardive dyskinesia and on long-term use, symptoms of parkinsonism can occur.

Drug Interactions

1. Metoclopramide blocks the D_2 receptors and hence blocks effects of levodopa.
2. Hastens gastric emptying and thereby hastens absorption of drugs like diazepam.

Uses

1. *Gastro-oesophageal reflux disease (GERD)* 'heart burn' due to reflux of acid into the oesophagus is benefited by prokinetic agents. They may be used as adjuvants to drugs that reduce acid secretion because the latter are safer drugs. Prokinetics also help some patients with non-ulcer dyspepsia.
2. *As antiemetics* in postoperative period and in vomiting due to anticancer drugs (along with ondensetron) and radiotherapy, in nausea and vomiting due to gastrointestinal disorders and migraine—metoclopramide is an effective antiemetic.

3. *As preanaesthetic medication* to promote gastric emptying and thereby prevent aspiration before emergency induction of general anaesthesia.
4. *In endoscopy* to assist passage of tubes into the duodenum.
5. *Delayed gastric emptying:* In patients undergoing surgeries like vagotomy and antrectomy and in diabetic gastroparesis, gastric emptying may be delayed. Prokinetics are useful in such patients.

Domperidone is a D_2 dopamine receptor blocker like metoclopramide. It blocks the dopamine receptors in the CTZ and thereby acts as an antiemetic. Advantages over metoclopramide are—domperidone does not cross the blood–brain barrier and hence extrapyramidal and neuropsychiatric side effects are rare. Because CTZ is outside the BBB, domperidone can produce its antiemetic effects.

Dose: 10–40 mg TDS, DOMSTAL, DOMPERON 10 mg tab, 1 mg/ml suspension.

Side effects are rare and include headache, dryness of mouth, diarrhoea and rashes—domperidone is well tolerated.

Uses: Domperidone can be used in place of metoclopramide and is **preferred** over it by many clinicians.

Cisapride enhances gastric motility by promoting the release of acetylcholine in the gut wall. However, it is now **banned** because it can cause cardiac arrhythmias.

Mosapride and **renzapride** are similar to cisapride but do not produce cardiac arrhythmias and do not prolong QT interval—hence preferred.

Itopride blocks dopamine D_2 receptors like metoclopramide and also enhances ACh levels in the gut (cholinesterase inhibitor). It promotes gastric motility and also has antiemetic effects. It is given in the dose of 50 mg TDS. Adverse effects include headache, dizziness and gastrointestinal disturbances. Itopride can be used in the treatment of gastroperesis, GERD and dyspepsia.

Tegaserod, a 5-HT_4 partial agonist which promotes gastric emptying, also causes cardiotoxicity and has been **withdrawn** from the market in many countries (*see* page 439).

Cholinomimetic Drugs

Cholinergic agonists, like bethanechol, enhance gastrointestinal motility by activating M_3 muscarinic receptors in the gut. They were earlier used in gastroparesis but are not preferred due to cholinergic side effects. Anticholinesterase drug neostigmine also enhances gastrointestinal motility and promotes colonic evacuation. It is used in the dose of 2 mg IV in acute colonic pseudo-obstruction (Ogilvie's syndrome) to empty the colon.

Motilin Receptor Agonists

Motilin is a peptide hormone which promotes motility in the upper gastrointestinal tract. **Erythromycin** is a motilin receptor agonist and promotes gastric and intestinal motility. It has been tried in diabetic gastroparesis and in decreased small bowel motility.

Clinical Pharmacology

- Ondansetron is the most powerful antiemetic.
- Combination of antiemetics may be used in cancer chemotherapy induced vomiting.
- Doctors should be able to identify extrapyramidal symptoms due to metoclopramide and also be familiar with its management—injection promethazine (25 mg IM).

[1] From Medical Council of India, *Competency based Undergraduate Curriculum for the Indian Medical Graduate*, 2018;1:136–144.

Drugs for Constipation, Diarrhoea, Irritable Bowel Disease, Inflammatory Bowel Disorders, Biliary and Pancreatic Diseases

CHAPTER 34

Competency achievement: The student should be able to:

PH 1.34 Describe the mechanism/s of action, types, doses, side effects, indications and contraindications of the drugs used as: Antidiarrhoeals, laxatives, inflammatory bowel disease, irritable bowel disorders, biliary and pancreatic diseases.[1]

LAXATIVES

Purgatives are drugs that promote defaecation. They are also called laxatives or cathartics. **Laxatives** or aperients have milder action while cathartics or purgatives are more powerful evacuants. **Carminatives** are drugs that promote expulsion of gases from the gut.

Purgatives may be classified as:

Classification

1. **Bulk laxatives**
   Bran, plantago seeds, agar, methylcellulose, ispaghula husk.
2. **Faecal softeners**
   Docusate sodium (DOSS),
   liquid paraffin (emollients)
3. **Osmotic purgatives**
   Magnesium sulphate, magnesium hydroxide, sodium phosphate, sodium sulphate, magnesium citrate, sodium potassium tartrate, lactulose, sorbitol, polyethylene glycol.
4. **Stimulant purgatives**
   Phenolphthalein, bisacodyl, castor oil,
   Anthraquinones—cascara sagrada, senna.
5. **Others**
   5-HT$_4$ agonists—prucalopride, cisapride
   Opioid antagonists—methylnaltrexone, alvimopan.
   Chloride channel activator—lubiprostone.

Bulk Laxatives

Bulk laxatives include indigestible vegetable fibre and hydrophilic colloids that increase the volume and lower the viscosity of intestinal contents forming a large, soft, solid stool. Dietary fibre consists of cell walls and other parts of fruits and vegetables that are unabsorbable. They add to the bulk of the intestinal contents, resulting in the formation of semisolid to solid stools. Adding fibre to the diet is a safe and natural way of treating constipation in persons on low-fibre diet. Long-term administration of bulk laxatives or fibre rich diet can itself overcome the prominent symptoms of IBS, viz. constipation and diarrhoea because the bulk of the intestinal contents reduces pressure development within the intestines (Table 34.1, Flowchart 34.1). Adequate water intake should be stressed with all bulk laxatives. All of them need 1–3 days to act and all can cause allergy. **Bran** is the residue left when flour is made from cereals and contains 40% fibre—but is unpalatable. Large quantities need to be consumed and can cause flatulence. Bulk laxatives may interfere with the absorption of other drugs.

Ispaghula and **plantago** seeds (psyllium) contain natural mucilage which absorbs water to form a gelatinous mass and are more palatable than bran. Ispaghula husk is available as powder but should not be swallowed as dry powder to avoid oesophageal impaction–may be mixed with water or milk.

Dose: 3–12 g/day. NATURE CURE, ISPAGHULA 49/100 g, ISOVAC-Psyllium 65/100 g granules—to be

Table 34.1: Choice of purgatives

Drug	Site
1. Functional constipation	Increasing dietary fibre and adequate fluid intake
2. Elderly patients	Increasing dietary fibre and adequate fluid intake
3. Pregnancy	Dietary fibre
4. To avoid straining at stools—as in hernia, piles, fissure, cardiovascular diseases like myocardial infarction	Bulk laxatives or faecal softeners
5. Irritable bowel syndrome—chronic constipation	Bulk laxatives
6. Food or drug poisoning	Osmotic purgatives
7. Bowel preparation before surgery, endoscopy and radiological examination	Bisacodyl, osmotic purgatives

Flowchart 34.1: Mechanism of action of bulk laxatives

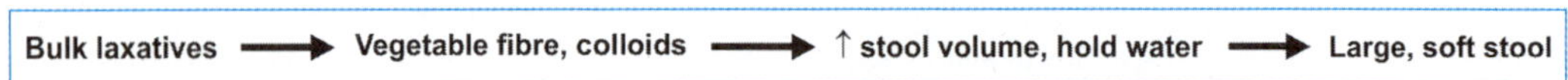

swallowed with adequate water (never dry) at the beginning of meals.

Methylcellulose is a semisynthetic hydrophilic derivative of cellulose given in the dose of 4–6 g/day.

Agar obtained from marine algae is a mucilagenous substance and contains indigestible hemicellulose. Dose: 4–5 g mixed with water.

Uses

Bulk laxatives are used in:

i. Functional constipation—adequate intake of dietary fibre is the best measure to prevent functional constipation. Additional benefit with certain dietary fibres like pectin is that they bind bile acids and prevent their absorption. Thus plasma cholesterol levels get lowered. Bulk laxatives should be avoided in patients with stenosis or adhesions in the gut.
ii. Conditions where straining at stools is to be avoided as in haemorrhoids and fissures and myocardial infarction.
iii. Irritable bowel syndrome—bulk laxatives are also useful in diarrhoea since they help forming almost solid to 'formed' stools.

Faecal Softeners

Docusate sodium (dioctyl sodium sulphosuccinate, DOSS) is an anion detergent, softens faeces by lowering the surface tension of the intestinal contents which allows more water to be retained in the faeces.

It requires 1–3 days for action; enhances the absorption of many drugs due to its detergent action. It is unpalatable (bitter) and can cause nausea and abdominal pain.

Dose: 100-400 mg/day. DOSLAX 150 mg cap; LAXICON 100 mg tab.

Liquid paraffin is a chemically inert mineral oil that is not digested. It lubricates and softens faeces. It is unpalatable; aspiration may cause lipoid pneumonia; small amounts absorbed in intestines may cause paraffinomas; it may leak out of the anus causing discomfort. Long-term use can result in deficiency of fat-soluble vitamins due to impaired absorption—hence not preferred.

Osmotic Purgatives

Osmotic purgatives are solutes that are not absorbed in the intestine, osmotically retain water and increase the bulk of intestinal contents. They increase peristalsis to evacuate a fluid stool (Flowchart 34.2). They produce soft liquid stools in 1–3 hours. Osmotic purgatives include:

- Nonabsorbable salts (saline purgatives)
- Nonabsorbable sugars—lactulose
- Polyethylene glycol.

Flowchart 34.2: Mechanism of action of osmotic purgatives

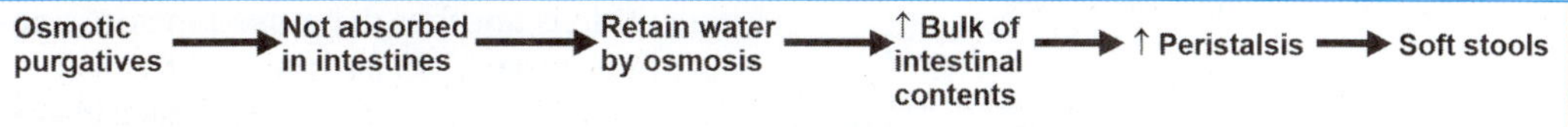

Nonabsorbable Salts

Magnesium hydroxide, magnesium sulphate, sodium potassium tartrate (Rochelle's salt), sodium sulphate and phosphate are some inorganic salts used as osmotic or **saline purgatives.** They are used to prepare the bowel before surgery and in food poisoning.

Nonabsorbable Sugars

Lactulose is a synthetic disaccharide that is not absorbed, holds water and acts as an osmotic purgative. Flatulence and cramps may be accompanied. In the colon, lactulose is fermented to lactic and acetic acids which inhibit the growth of colonic ammonia-producing bacteria. It also inhibits the absorption of ammonia by lowering pH and lowers blood ammonia levels. It is used in hepatic coma for this effect (hepatic coma is worsened by ammonia).

DUPHALAC liquid 100 ml, 450 ml.

Sorbitol is similar to lactulose. **Lactilol** is another synthetic disaccharide more palatable than lactulose.

Glycerine is used as rectal suppository or as enema (with an oil). By an osmotic effect, it softens and lubricates the stools.

Polyethylene glycol is a nonabsorbable sugar. Balanced isotonic solution containing PEG with sodium sulphate, sodium chloride, sodium bicarbonate and potassium chloride is given orally. The solution is balanced in such a way that it avoids electrolyte imbalance or fluid shift into the gut. Large volumes are rapidly ingested 3–4 litres over 2 hours—for cleaning the bowel before endoscopic examination of the bowel. PEG powder may be taken with water for chronic constipation. It has the advantage that there is no associated flatulence or abdominal cramps.

PEG electrolyte—137.15 g powder.

Stimulant Purgatives

Stimulant purgatives increase intestinal motility and increase the secretion of water and electrolytes by the mucosa. They may cause abdominal cramps.

When anthraquinones, like **cascara sagrada** and **senna** (source: plants), are given orally, active anthraquinones are liberated in the intestines and stimulate the myenteric plexes in the colon. Evacuation takes 6–8 hr. Long-term use causes melanotic pigmentation of the colon.

Phenolphthalein, an indicator, acts on the colon after 6 to 8 hours to produce soft, semi-liquid stools with some griping. It undergoes enterohepatic circulation which prolongs its actions. Allergic reactions including pink-coloured skin eruptions, other severe forms of allergy and risk of cardiac toxicity and colic limit its use.

Bisacodyl related to phenolphthalein is converted to an active metabolite in the intestines which stimulates the colon. It can be given orally (5–10 mg enteric coated tab—takes 8–12 hr for stools to be passed) but usually is used as rectal suppositories (10 mg) which results in defaecation in 15–40 minutes. There is wide variation in the dose needed. It is a popular laxative and is safe except that prolonged use may cause mild local inflammation (proctitis) and burning sensation in the rectum since it is an irritant. Hence bisacodyl should not be used for more than 10 days at a time. Leakage of the suppository can sometimes result in anal soreness.

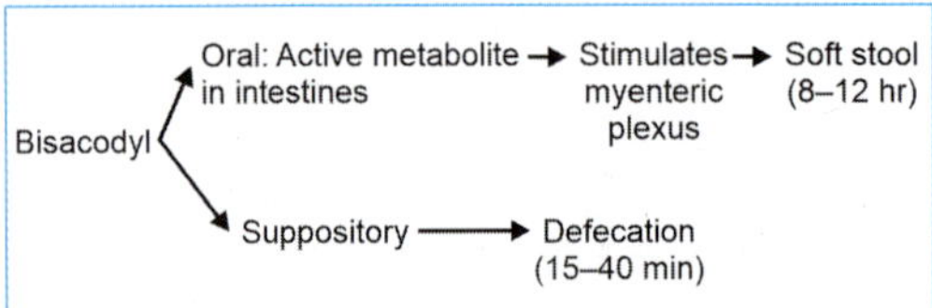

DULCOLAX 5 mg tab, 10 mg suppository. CONLAX 5–10 mg suppository.

Sodium picosulfate, related to bisacodyl is similar to it, gets hydrolysed by the colonic bacteria to the active metabolite which irritates and stimulates the colon for evacuation in 6–12 hr after oral administration. Adverse effects are similar to bisacodyl.

CREMALAX, LAXICARE 10 mg tab.

Castor oil is hydrolysed in the upper small intestine to ricinoleic acid, a local irritant that increases intestinal motility. It is a powerful and one of the oldest purgatives. Stool is semiliquid and is accompanied by griping. It is not preferred.

OTHER LAXATIVES

1. 5-HT$_4$ Receptor Agonists

Prucalopride is a 5-HT$_4$ agonist which does not have affinity for 5-HT$_{1B}$ receptor. It is approved for use in chronic constipation as a second-line drug.

2. Chloride Channel Activators

Lubiprostone is a derivative of prostanoic acid. It stimulates opening of the chloride channels in the small intestine leading to secretion of a fluid rich in chloride. This in turn stimulates intestinal motility and promotes evacuation within 24 hours. Lubiprostone may cause nausea and headache and is contraindicated in pregnant women. Lubiprostone is indicated in chronic constipation and irritable bowel syndrome.

3. Linaclotide

Linaclotide is another drug used in constipation-predominant IBS (*see* page 439).

4. Opioid Antagonists

Opioid-induced constipation can be troublesome in cancer patients and terminally ill patients receiving opioids for pain relief over long periods. **Methylnaltrexone** and **alvimopan** are opioid antagonists which block the opioid receptors in the gut. They do not cross the blood–brain barrier and, therefore, do not antagonise the analgesic effects of opioids. Methylnaltrexone (0.15 mg/kg) may be given subcutaneously once in 2 days in patients with opioid-induced constipation. Alvimopan is effective orally and is used to overcome postoperative ileus. Alvimopan is only approved for short-term use (<1 week) for the risk of cardiovascular toxicity.

ENEMA

Enema produces defaecation by softening stools and distending the bowel. Evacuant enema is used to prepare the gut for surgery, endoscopy and radiological examination (*see* page 12).

Use of Laxatives in Constipation

Fibre-rich diet, adequate fluid intake and physical activity are the best measures to prevent and treat constipation in the otherwise normal subjects. If these measures are inadequate, a laxative may be given (Table 34.2).

Drug-Induced Constipation

Drugs, like **anticholinergics, NSAIDs, opioids, clonidine, iron, calcium channel blockers; antihistamines** and **tricyclic antidepressants** (due to anticholinergic effect), can cause constipation. When withdrawal of the causative agent is not possible, a laxative may be used.

Laxative Abuse

Habitual use of laxatives, especially stimulant laxatives, may lead to various gastrointestinal disturbances like irritable bowel syndrome, loss of electrolytes, loss of calcium in the stool and malabsorption. Misconceptions regarding bowel habits should be cleared. The patient should be convinced that normal bowel habits may vary between 3 stools daily and 2 stools per week.

Contraindications

Laxatives are contraindicated in:

i. Intestinal obstruction
ii. Patients with undiagnosed acute abdomen.

DRUGS USED IN THE TREATMENT OF DIARRHOEA

Diarrhoea is the frequent passage of liquid stools. It can be due to a variety of causes like infection, toxins, anxiety and drugs (Key Boxes 34.1 and 34.2). Acute diarrhoea is one of the major causes of death in infants specially in the developing countries.

In diarrhoea, there is an increase in motility and secretions in the gut with reduced absorption of water and electrolytes. Hence the approaches in the treatment of diarrhoea include:

1. Replacement of fluid and electrolytes;
2. Treatment of the cause;
3. Antidiarrhoeal agents.

1. Replacement of Fluid and Electrolytes

Correction of fluid and electrolyte disturbances can be life saving in most cases especially infants. Oral rehydration with sodium chloride, glucose and water is useful. In the ileum, glucose and sodium citrate enhance sodium absorption and water follows. **Oral rehydration powders** are available (Table 34.2) to be mixed with water to make oral rehydration solution (ORS). ORS with sodium bicarbonate or sodium citrate are available. Trisodium citrate is used in place of bicarbonate because use of citrate makes ORS more stable, absorption of glucose is better and stool output is lower. If the ORS ready-made powder is not available, a mixture of 5 g table salt (a pinch) with 20 g sugar dissolved in one litre of boiled and cooled water may be used till regular ORS is available. Adequate oral rehydration is needed in mild to moderate cases. In severe degrees of dehydration, prompt intravenous rehydration is vital.

Table 34.2: Composition of oral rehydration salt/solution (ORS)

Sodium chloride	—	3.5 g
Potassium chloride	—	1.5 g
Sodium citrate	—	2.9 g
Glucose	—	20 g

To be dissolved in 1 litre of boiled and cooled water

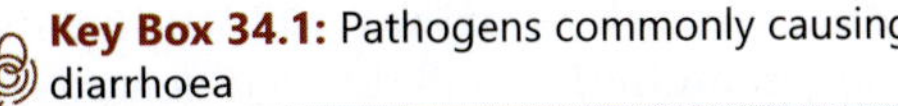

Key Box 34.1: Pathogens commonly causing diarrhoea

Virus	Bacteria	Others
Rotavirus	*E. coli*	*E. histolytica*
Astrovirus	*Salmonella*	*Glardia lambia*
Adenovirus	*Shigella*	
Coronavirus	*V. cholerae*	
Enterovirus	*C. jejuni*	

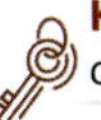

Key Box 34.2: Some drugs that produce diarrhoea

- Ampicillin
- Colchicine
- Emetine
- Cisapride
- Digitalis
- Erythromycin
- Prostaglandins and their analogs
- Anticholinesterase
- Some anticancer drugs
- Lithium
- Magnesium sulphate (oral)

Dose and Frequency of Administration

The aim of treatment is to achieve almost complete rehydration in about 5–6 hr. In children, the dose is 5 ml/kg/hr.

Mild dehydration: 50 ml/kg over 4–6 hr in multiple small divided doses.

Moderate dehydration: 100 ml/kg over 4–6 hr in multiple small divided doses.

Adequate maintenance dose should be given based on the severity.

WHO-ORS new formula: Standard ORS has Na^+ 90 mM, Cl^- 80 mM, citrate 10 mM and glucose 110 mM making up a total of 310 mOsm/l. Extensive research sponsored by WHO has shown that ORS with lower osmolality has improved efficacy with a 30% reduction in the incidence of vomiting and stool volume. WHO and UNICEF have, therefore, recommended new modified ORS solution with 245 mOsm/l osmolarity in place of the standard preparation with a decreased concentration of sodium and glucose.

The only disadvantage is that it can cause hyponatraemia in adults suffering from cholera.

The contents are as follows.

New formula (WHO)

NaCl	2.6 g
KCl	1.5 g
Trisodium citrate	2.9 g
Glucose	13.5 g
Water	1 L
Total osmolarity	245 mOsm

Super ORS: The content of ORS is modified to reduce the frequency and severity of diarrhoea. Amino acids are added which could promote sodium absorption. However, they are expensive and the benefit provided is marginal. Studies have shown that parboiled rice powder 40–50 g/litre is a good and simple glucose supplement. Since the rice also has some proteins (7%), it is a source of amino acids which stimulates the absorption of salt and water. The starch content adds to the calories. Rice is easily available, is relatively inexpensive and has good efficacy-rice based ORS may be preferred particularly in developing countries. Wheat, maize or potato may be used instead of rice.

Uses

Apart from diarrhoea, rehydration may also be needed in heat stroke, burns, following surgery or trauma. ORS is useful in all these conditions.

2. Treatment of the Cause

Acute diarrhoea could often be due to viral, bacterial or protozoal infection. The pathogen should be identified whenever possible and treated accordingly. Gastroenteritis is often due to virus and does not require antibiotics. Mild bacterial gastroenteritis is also self-limiting but some infections like typhoid, cholera and amoebic dysentery need chemotherapy.

3. Antidiarrhoeal Drugs

Antidiarrhoeal drugs afford only symptomatic relief.

Classification

Adsorbants: Kaolin, pectin, chalk, activated charcoal.

Antimotility drugs:
- Opioids—codeine, diphenoxylate, loperamide
- Other drugs—racecodotril, lactobacillus preparations

Antispasmodics: Atropine derivatives, drotaverine, mebeverine, octreotide.

Adsorbents

Adsorbents include **kaolin, pectin, chalk and activated charcoal.** Kaolin is a natural compound containing hydrated magnesium and aluminium silicate while pectin is the sugar obtained from apples. These adsorb intestinal toxins and microorganisms by coating them. They are not absorbed and have no prominent side effects. They bind to and interfere with the absorption of other drugs because of which a two-hour interval is required after administration of other drugs.

Antimotility Drugs

Opioid agonists: Codeine an opium alkaloid, stimulates the opioid receptors on the gastrointestinal smooth muscles to reduce peristalsis. This delays passage of intestinal contents and facilitates the absorption of food.

Diphenoxylate is an opioid related to pethidine. It is given with a small dose of atropine in order to discourage abuse. If taken repeatedly at short intervals, side effects of atropine would appear. In therapeutic doses, CNS effects are not prominent and is used only in diarrhoeas. Nausea, drowsiness and abdominal pain may occur. In children disturbing side effects like respiratory depression, paralytic ileus and even toxic megacolon have been reported—hence contraindicated in children below 6 years (Table 34.3).

Loperamide is an opiate. It has selective action on the GI tract with additional antisecretory activity. CNS effects are negligible. It is less sedating, less addicting and is the most commonly used antimotility drug. Loperamide is a μ receptor agonist and is longer acting than diphenoxylate; it also has weak anticholinergic properties. Its low solubility in water discourages abuse by injection.

Loperamide is poorly absorbed and is excreted through the gut. Onset of action is in 1–2 hr and duration of action is almost 12–18 hr. Loperamide may cause nausea, vomiting and abdominal cramps.

Loperamide use has resulted in paralytic ileus, abdominal distension, toxic megacolon and several fatalities are reported in children. Hence loperamide is contraindicated in children below 4 yr of age.

Dose: 4 mg followed by 2 mg after each stool up to a maximum of 10 mg/day.

Uses

Antimotility drugs are used for symptomatic treatment of non-infective diarrhoeas (as adjuvants). Antimotility drugs should be avoided in infective diarrhoeas due to invasive pathogens for the following reasons:

- They increase the risk of systemic invasion by the pathogen.
- Risk of intestinal perforation.
- Delayed clearance of the infecting organisms.
- Risk of megacolon.

Other Drugs

Racecadotril: Racecadotril, a newly introduced antidiarrhoeal agent is a prodrug. It is converted in the body to the active compound thiorphan which is a selective inhibitor of enkephalinase. The enzyme enkephalinase degrades enkephalins—the endogenous opioids. Thiorphan inhibits enkephalinase in the gut and peripheral tissues and thereby acts as an antidiarrhoeal. Enkephalins are neurotransmitters in the gut—they have antisecretory activity on the intestines (act on opioid receptors)—thus correct the hypersecretion of water and electrolytes seen in diarrhoea **without reducing intestinal motility.** The onset of action is quick, pain and distension subsides. It has the advantage over loperamide that it is not contraindicated in children.

Racecadotril is well tolerated with minor adverse effects like drowsiness, skin rashes, nausea and flatulence. Racecadotril is useful in the symptomatic treatment of acute secretory diarrhoea—should be used for short term—not >7 days.

Dose: 100 mg TDS. RACE, CADOTRIL, 100 mg Cap, 10 mg Sachet.

Table 34.3: Antimotility drugs—some preparations and dosage

Drugs	Trade names	Dose
Diphenoxylate 2.5 mg + Atropine 0.025 mg	LOMOTIL	2–4 tablets stat; 1 every 6 hr
Loperamide	LOPESTAL	4 mg stat; 2 mg every 6 hr

Lactobacillus Preparations

Lactobacillus acidophilus and *Lactobacillus sporogenes* are available as powders and tablets and are useful in some diarrhoeas. They colonise the intestines and promote the growth of saccharolytic flora and alter the gut pH so that the growth of pathogenic organisms is inhibited. They are called **probiotics** and are found to be useful in reducing the incidence of antibiotic-induced diarrhoea (*see* page 540). Curd and butter-milk are cheaper alternatives to lactobacillus commercial preparations.

Antispasmodics

Diarrhoea is often associated with abdominal colic and pain. Antispasmodics may be required to relieve the pain. **Atropine derivatives,** like propantheline and dicyclomine, relax gastrointestinal smooth muscles and relieve abdominal colics.

Drotaverine is a directly acting smooth muscle relaxant related to papaverine and also has analgesic properties. It acts by inhibiting the enzyme PDE and thereby increasing cAMP/cGMP levels which cause smooth muscle relaxation. It is used as an antispasmodic in **renal, biliary and intestinal colic and also in IBS, dysmenorrhoea and in labour for cervical dilatation.** Adverse effects are headache, dizziness, flushing and constipation.

Dose: 40–80 mg TDS DOTARIN, DOVERIN 40, 80 mg tab, 20 mg/ml inj.

Mebeverine, a reserpine derivative, is an antispasmodic. It acts both directly on the gut smooth muscle and indirectly to reduce colonic hypermotility. It reduces the permeability of smooth muscles for sodium ions and also decreases the efflux of potassium ions. Mebeverine is orally effective and is rapidly and completely absorbed. Adverse effects include dizziness, headache, constipation and some gastritis but is devoid of anticholinergic side effects. Mebeverine may be used in IBS and in dysentry as an antispasmodic. Mebeverine is also a useful antispasmodic in IBS.

Dose: 135 mg TDS; COLOSPA MEBRIN 135 mg tab, 200 mg SR tab – taken 20 min before food

Octreotide is a long-acting, synthetic analog of somatostatin. It has the following actions on the gut.

- Reduces GI motility and fluid secretion.
- Inhibits the secretion of various hormones like gastrin, secretin, cholecystokinin, growth hormone, insulin, glucagon, 5-HT, pancreatic polypeptide and vasoactive intestinal peptide.

Octreotide is used subcutaneously in gastrointestinal secretory tumours causing diarrhoea and in diarrhoea due to vagotomy, dumping syndrome and AIDS.

Traveller's Diarrhoea

Infection is the most common cause of traveller's diarrhoea and should be treated with suitable antimicrobials like doxycycline or ciprofloxacin. Oral rehydration salts may also be used.

IRRITABLE BOWEL SYNDROME

Irritable bowel syndrome (IBS) is a common condition characterised by abnormal bowel functions with no specific organic cause. Diarrhoea or constipation with abdominal pain may be present. Causes could be stress, lack of dietary fibre, food allergy or emotional disturbances.

When constipation is prominent, soluble dietary fibre like ispaghula is recommended while loperamide is preferred for diarrhoea. Benzodiazepines are given for the treatment of anxiety and other appropriate measures are taken depending on the symptoms and probable cause. Newer antidepressants have shown good response in several studies.

Aloesetron is a selective 5-HT_3 receptor antagonist. Blocking the 5-HT_3 receptors in the gut can influence intestinal motility and afferent pain impulses from the gastrointestinal tract. Aloesetron inhibits reflex activation of the GI smooth muscle and thus reduces colonic motility. It is longer acting than other 5-HT_3 antagonists like ondansetron used in vomiting.

Aloesetron is approved for use in women having IBS with prominent diarrhoea—not responding to other drugs. Adverse effects include constipation and colitis.

Tegaserod, a partial agonist at 5-HT_4 receptors, promotes gastric emptying resulting in soft stools. However, due to 10-fold increase in the risk of heart attack and stroke when tegaserod was used in IBS patients, it has now been **withdrawn** in most countries.

Linaclotide is a guanylate cyclase C agonist which reduces activation of colonic sensory neurons thereby reducing pain. It also activates motor neurons in the intestines resulting in chloride-rich intestinal secretions. It is tried as a second-line drug in constipation associated with IBS but is expensive.

Antispasmodics: For relief of pain associated with food intake, antispasmodics may be needed. Anticholinergics, like **dicyclomine,** act by inhibiting gastrocolic reflex and may be used occasionally but not regularly. **Mebeverine** is also a useful antispasmodic in IBS.

INFLAMMATORY BOWEL DISEASES

Inflammatory bowel diseases (IBD) like **ulcerative colitis** and **Crohn's disease,** are treated with glucocorticoids, sulphasalazine and immunosuppressants.

Glucocorticoids: In active IBD, treatment is initiated with **prednisolone** 40–60 mg per day and the dose is tapered after 2 weeks. If the part involved is rectum or sigmoid colon, prednisolone retention enema or other rectal preparations may be used. **Budesonide** controlled-release oral formulations which release the drug in the distal bowel (distal ileum and colon) are now being tried. They have a bioavailability of 10%. For IBD involving the rectum and the sigmoid colon, rectal route is preferred for glucocorticoid administration to minimize the side effects.

Sulphasalazine is split by flora in the colon to 5-aminosalicylate (5-ASA) and sulfapyridine. Adverse effects are common and are mostly due to sulfapyridine. Nausea, vomiting, fever, headache, diarrhoea, megaloblastic anaemia and various allergic manifestations ranging from skin rashes to Stevens-Johnson syndrome can occur.

Mesalamine is 5-ASA which is better tolerated with minor side effects. Mesalamine retention enema and suppositories are used. Other compounds in this group are ***olsalazine*** and ***balsalazide***. Balsalazide contains mesalamine linked to an inert carrier which is split by colonic bacteria and 5-ASA is released in the colon. It provides remission in mild to moderate IBD (1.5–4 g daily).

Immunosuppressants, like azathioprine, 6-mercaptopurine and methotrexate, are used for induction and maintenance of remission in patients with active IBD.

Antitumour necrosis factor (anti-TNF) therapy: In IBD, TNF is an important proinflammatory cytokine. **Infliximab, adalimumab and certolizumab** are monoclonal antibodies to TNF. They are indicated in moderate to severe Crohn's disease and ulcerative colitis not responding adequately to other drugs.

Anti-integrin therapy: Integrins are adhesion molecules on the surface of leukocytes which bind to another set of adhesion molecules on the vascular endothelium. **Natalizumab** is a monoclonal antibody that binds many integrins on the circulating inflammatory cells and block the migration and subsequent inflammatory process. Natalizumab is tried in Crohn's disease not responding to other drugs.

BILIARY DISEASES

Cholelithiasis or gall stones: **Ursodeoxycholic acid** is used orally for dissolution of stones but it can dissolve only small radiolucent stones in 50% of patients which may take 6–24 months. Hence in most cases surgery, i.e. cholecystectomy is the option.

Acute cholecystitis: Gall stones obstructing the cystic duct is the common cause of acute inflammation of the gall bladder. Signs and symptoms include nausea, vomiting, anorexia, fever and biliary colic. Murphys's sign is positive.

Treatment: Analgesics like pethidine or NSAIDs and antibiotics to treat the associated infection helps suppress the acute episode in most patients. Surgical removal of the stone or cholecystectomy may be required sooner or later.

Chronic cholecystitis: Continued presence of the gall stones with repeated acute cholecystitis results in chronic inflammation - needs surgical removal.

Cholangitis is inflammation of the bile duct and is generally due to presence of gall stones in the common bile duct (choledocholithiasis) leading to infection. Surgical removal of the stone is done.

PANCREATIC DISEASES

Pancreatitis is the most common pancreatic disease. ***Acute pancreatitis*** mostly results from gall stones though alcohol, trauma, surgery (postoperative complication), drugs (like sulphonamides, oestrogens, mercaptopurine, valproate, tetracyclines) hypercalcemia and infections are some other causes. Treatment-

1. Opioid analgesics like pethidine
2. IV fluids
3. Antibiotics—appropriate parenteral antibiotics are started.

Chronic pancreatitis follows repeated acute inflammation leading to malabsorption and pain. Opioid analgesics, low fat diet and drugs like pantoprazole to reduce gastric acidity (pancreatic enzymes are destroyed by acid) may be given.

Clinical Pharmacology

- Increasing dietary fibre itself is a good remedy for constipation. Adequate water intake is equally important.
- Habitual use of laxatives should be discouraged.
- Patients in convalescence, post-MI patients should avoid straining and laxatives may be freely given. Occasional use of laxatives is generally safe.
- In infants receiving artificial feeds, constipation is common.
- Patients should be educated regarding proper bowel habits.
- Patients receiving a powerful purge or enema require a few days for recovery of regular bowel habits.

[1] From Medical Council of India, *Competency based Undergraduate Curriculum for the Indian Medical Graduate*, 2018;1:136–144.

Unit XI

Drugs used in Haematological Disorders

35. Haematinics

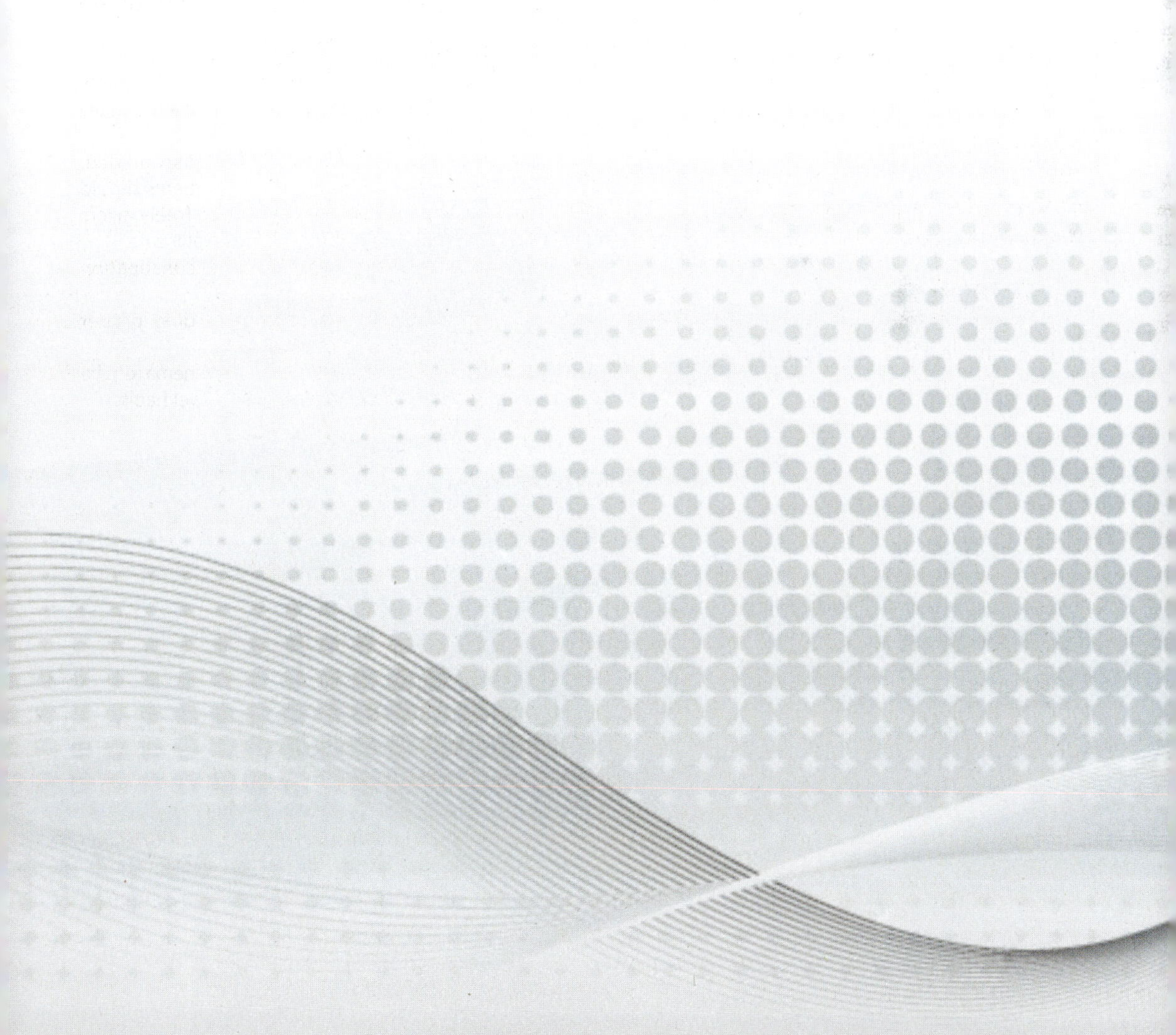

CHAPTER 35

Haematinics

> *Competency achievement:* The student should be able to:
>
> **PH 1.35** Describe the mechanism/s of action, types, doses, side effects, indications and contraindications of drugs used in hematological disorders like: Drugs used in anemias and colony stimulating factors.[1]

DRUGS USED IN ANEMIAS

Haematinics are compounds required in the formation of blood and are used in the treatment of anaemias. Haematinics include iron, vitamin B_{12} and folic acid. Haematopoietic growth factors are also discussed here.

IRON

Iron, vitamin B_{12} and folic acid are essential for normal erythropoiesis.

Iron is essential for haemoglobin production. Total body iron is about 2.5 to 5 grams, two-thirds of which is present in haemoglobin. Each molecule of haemoglobin has 4 iron-containing residues. It is also present in myoglobin, the cytochromes and other enzymes.

Distribution of iron in the body:

- Haemoglobin 66%
- Ferritin, haemosiderin 25%
- Myoglobin (in muscles) 03%
- Enzymes (cytochromes, etc.) 06%

Daily requirement of iron:

- Adult male 0.5–1 mg
- Adult female 1–2 mg
- Pregnancy and lactation 3–5 mg

Dietary Sources of Iron

Food items that are rich in iron are liver, egg yolk, meat, fish, chicken, spinach, dry fruits, wheat and apple.

Absorption

The average Indian diet provides about 10–20 mg of iron. Ten per cent of this iron is absorbed. Dietary iron may be present as heme or as inorganic iron. Heme iron (iron in meat) is absorbed better and faster since it can be absorbed as such and does not need to be dissociated into elemental iron. Iron in vegetables and grains is inorganic iron and is relatively poorly absorbed because it is tightly bound to organic compounds from which it needs to be dissociated. Such non-haeme iron should be reduced to ferrous form by a ferro reductase enzyme before absorption. It is mostly absorbed from the upper gut in the ferrous form. Absorption of iron across the intestinal mucosa takes place by an active transport process and also in a form that is bound to heme. Absorbed iron is transported into the blood by a protein called ferroportin and is soon oxidized by the help of an enzyme ferroxidase into ferric iron. Iron is better absorbed in iron deficiency states and is quickly transported to the bone marrow for the synthesis of haemoglobin.

Factors that Influence Iron Absorption

Factors	Effect
Ascorbic acid, amino acids, meat, ↑gastric acidity	Increase absorption

Antacids, phosphates, phytates, tetracyclines, presence of food in the stomach	Decrease absorption

Transport and Storage

Iron is transported with the help of a glycoprotein transferrin which has two binding sites for ferric iron. Transferrin forms a complex with two molecules of ferric iron and the complex is taken into the proliferating RBCs by endocytosis. In iron deficiency, the concentration of serum transferrin increases. In the absence of deficiency, excess iron is stored as **ferritin** in the intestinal epithelial cells and as **haemosiderin** in liver, spleen and bone marrow. The synthesis of apoferritin is regulated by free iron levels—when it is low, apoferritin synthesis is inhibited while more of it is produced when free iron levels are high.

Excretion: Daily 0.5–1 mg of iron is excreted. A large part is lost in shedding of intestinal mucosal cells and small amounts in the bile, desquamated skin and urine. In females, iron is also lost in menstruation.

Preparations of Iron

Iron is generally given orally—but can also be given parenterally.

Oral Iron Preparations

- Iron preparations are available as ferrous sulphate, ferrous fumarate, ferrous gluconate, ferrous succinate, ferric ammonium citrate and iron calcium complex. The last three preparations are claimed to be better tolerated.
- Ferrous salts are better absorbed than ferric salts and are also cheaper.
- Expensive preparations of iron with vitamins, liver extract, amino acids, etc. are available but offer no obvious benefits.
- Preparations of iron hydroxyl polymaltose have been extensively marketed and are claimed to be better tolerated with no metallic taste, direct gastrointestinal absorption and higher iron content. These are expensive preparations and their superiority over other preparations has not been proved.
- Though absorption is better when taken on an empty stomach, gastric irritation is more. Hence oral iron can be given along with or immediately after meals.
- Spansules containing tiny pellets are designed to be absorbed from the intestines to avoid gastric irritation. They are claimed to have better bioavailability. However, sustained release preparations of iron are not preferred because:
  - Iron is absorbed from the duodenum and SR preparations may release iron in large intestines.
  - Iron absorption is better in acidic environment
  - SR preparations are expensive.
- *Dose:* Ferrous sulphate 200 mg—3–4 tablets daily. The elemental iron content of different salts varies and is important. For adults, a maximum of 200 mg and for children 3–5 mg/kg of elemental iron in 2–3 divided doses can be given daily in deficiency.
- Iron therapy should be continued for 3–6 months after the correction of deficiency in order to replenish the iron stores.

Preparations

Ferrous Fumarate + Folic acid, FEBROGEN, HBACT, LIVOGEN FC cap

Iron polymaltose: FERRO HEPTANE, 3-UP, FERRON 50 mg/5 ml syr.

Ferrous ascorbate 30 mg + Folic acid 550 μg/5 ml OROFER XT susp.

Adverse Effects of Oral Iron

Epigastric pain, nausea, vomiting, gastritis, metallic taste, constipation (due to astringent effect) or diarrhoea (irritant effect) are the usual adverse effects. Liquid preparations of iron cause staining of the teeth. Patient should be informed that there would be blackening of stools.

Parenteral Iron

Iron can be administered parenterally as deep IM injection or intravenously. Iron is given parenterally only in the following indications.

Indications

1. When oral iron is not tolerated.
2. Failure of absorption—as in malabsorption, chronic bowel disease.
3. Noncompliance.
4. Severe deficiency with bleeding.
5. Pateints who have undergone gastrectomy.
6. Patients receiving erythropoietin—oral iron absorption may be insufficient as the demand increases.

Preparations

Intramuscular injection of iron is given deep IM into the gluteal region using 'Z' technique to avoid staining of the skin. Intravenous iron is given slowly over 5–10 minutes or as infusion **after a test dose**.

1. **Iron dextran** has 50 mg elemental iron/ml—it is the only preparation that can be given intravenously. It can also be given deep IM. Iron dextran is a stable complex of ferric iron and dextran polymers. Hypersensitivity reactions to iron dextran can be serious though uncommon. Incidence of allergy to iron dextran is more in patients who were previously exposed to iron dextran and those with a history of other allergies. Hypersensitivity is also more common with high molecular weight iron dextran than the low molecular weight preparations.

   A test dose of 0.5 ml of iron dextran is injected IV slowly over 5–10 min. If no obvious allergic reponse is observed, the IV preparation may be infused diluting in 500 ml of glucose. Patients should be constantly monitored for signs of allergy.

   INFED 50 mg/ml inj.
2. **Iron-sorbitol-citric acid complex** contains 50 mg elemental iron/ml; it is given only IM. This preparation should not be given IV because it quickly saturates the transferrin stores. As a result, free iron levels in the plasma rise and can cause toxicity.
3. **Iron sucrose and sodium ferric gluconate** can be given only by intravenous route. Allergy to this form of iron is seen to be lower than with iron dextran.
4. **Ferric carboxymaltose and ferumoxytol:** Two parenteral preparations enclosed in a carbohydrate shell have been introduced. Ferric carboxymaltose contains iron embedded in a carbohydrate polymer. Ferumoxytol is an aqueous preparation containing super paramagnetic iron oxide nanoparticle, which is coated with a carbohydrate. However, it interferes with MRI for 3 months after the last dose and the patient should be educated to inform the radiologist, if any MRI is required.

Serum concentration of ferritin and transferin should be monitored to avoid iron overload. Dose is calculated using a formula.

Formula:

Iron requirement (mg) = 4.4 × body weight (kg) × Hb deficit (g/dl)

This also includes iron needed for replenishment of stores.

Adverse Effects

Local: Pain at the site of injection, pigmentation of the skin and sterile abscess.

Systemic: Fever, headache, joints pain, palpitation, difficulty in breathing, urticaria, flushing, light headedness, nausea, vomiting, lymph node enlargement and rarely, anaphylaxis. Deaths have been reported due to bronchospasm.

Acute Iron Poisoning

Acute iron poisoning (*see* Chapter 60) is common in infants and children in whom about 10 tablets (1–2 g) can be lethal. Manifestations include vomiting, abdominal pain, haematemesis, bloody diarrhoea, shock, drowsiness, cyanosis, acidosis, dehydration, cardiovascular collapse and coma. Immediate diagnosis and treatment are important as death may occur in 6–12 hr.

Treatment

- Gastric lavage with sodium bicarbonate solution.
- **Desferrioxamine** is the **antidote.** It is instilled into the stomach after lavage, to prevent iron absorption; injected IV/IM.
- Correction of acidosis and shock.

Uses of Iron

Iron deficiency anaemia—both for the prophylaxis and treatment. The cause for iron deficiency should be identified. Treatment should be continued depending on the response for 3–6 months to replenish iron stores. Prophylactically, iron is given in conditions with increased iron requirement as in pregnancy, infancy and professional blood donors.

VITAMIN B_{12} AND FOLIC ACID

Vitamin B_{12} and folic acid are water-soluble vitamins, belonging to the B-complex group. They are essential for normal DNA synthesis. Their deficiency leads to impaired DNA synthesis and abnormal maturation of RBCs and other rapidly dividing cells. This results in megaloblastic anaemia, characterised by the presence of red cell precursors in the blood and bone marrow. Vitamin B_{12} and folic acid are, therefore, called maturation factors (Table 35.1). Other manifestations of deficiency include glossitis, stomatitis and malabsorption. Neurological manifestations can also result.

Vitamin B_{12}

Vitamin B_{12} (cyanocobalamin) is synthesized by microorganisms. Liver, fish, egg yolk, meat, cheese and pulses are the dietary sources of B_{12}.

Vitamin B_{12} or extrinsic factor is absorbed with the help of intrinsic factor, a protein secreted by the stomach. It is carried in the plasma by B_{12}-binding proteins called **transcobalamin** and is stored in the liver.

Functions

Vitamin B_{12} is converted in the tissues to the active coenzyme form. It is involved in several vital metabolic reactions and is essential for the synthesis of purine which is needed for the DNA synthesis.

Vitamin B_{12} acts as cofactor in the following important enzymatic reactions:

1. *Homocysteine + methyl FH_4*

   $$\xrightarrow[\text{Vitamin } B_{12}]{\text{Methionine synthase}}$$

   Methionine + FH_4

2. *Methylmalonyl CoA*

   $$\downarrow DAB_{12}$$

   Succinyl CoA

FH_4 – tetrahydrofolate DAB_{12}—deoxyadenosyl B_{12}

The above reactions show that vitamin B_{12} and folic acid metabolism are linked. Tetrahydrofolate is essential for the biosynthesis of purines.

Table 35.1: Daily requirement of vitamin B_{12} and folic acid

	Adults	*Pregnancy and lactation*	*Preparations*
Vitamin B_{12}	1–3 µg	3–5 µg	Nervijen L Vit12
Folic acid	50–100 µg	200–400 µg	FOLVITE, 0.4, 0.8 and 1.5 mg tab FORICH

As 50% of ingested drug is lost, double the amount is recommended for daily dietary intake.

Deficiency

Vitamin B_{12} deficiency may be due to:

1. *Addisonian pernicious anaemia:* Thomas Addison first described cases of anaemia not responding to iron. There is deficiency of intrinsic factor due to destruction of parietal cells resulting in failure of B_{12} absorption.
2. *Other causes:* Gastrectomy, chronic gastritis, malabsorption and fish tapeworm infestation (fish tapeworm consumes B_{12}).

Manifestations of Deficiency

- Manifestations result from abnormal maturation of RBCs and defective DNA synthesis. Megaloblastic anaemia with hypercellular marrow, weakness, lethargy, palpitations, angina, vertigo and neurological manifestations with paraesthesias of hands and feet, and in more severe cases spasticity, ataxia, loss of memory, confusion, delusions, hallucinations and psychosis can occur.

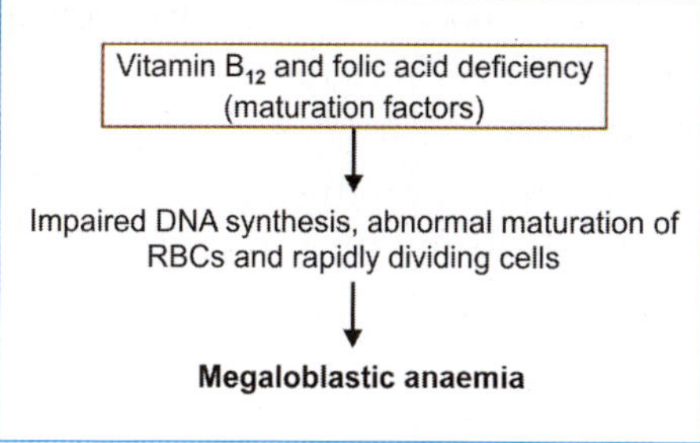

- Diagnosis of megaloblastic anaemia may be made by peripheral smear and confirmed by measuring vitamin B_{12} levels in the plasma.

Preparations

- **Cyanocobalamin:** 100 µg/ml injection may be given IM or deep SC—hypersensitivity reactions can occur. LVit$_{12}$ 500 µg inj.
- **Hydroxocobalamin:** 100, 500, 1000 µg/ml injection is preferred as it has longer lasting effect because of its high protein binding but hydroxocobalamin administration can result in the formation of antibodies.
- Sublingual vitamin B_{12} preparation is now available and is claimed to have good bioavailability.
- Multivitamin preparations contain variable amounts of vitamin B_{12} with or without intrinsic factor for oral use.

Uses

1. **Vitamin B_{12} deficiency**
   - *Treatment of megaloblastic anaemia due to B_{12} deficiency:* If B_{12} deficiency is due to lack of intrinsic factor, vitamin B_{12} is given IM or SC. **Pernicious anaemia** needs lifelong treatment with parenteral B_{12} because, in pernicious anaemia, orally given vitamin B_{12} cannot be absorbed due to intrinsic factor deficiency. Patients with severe deficiency and with neurological manifestations require immediate treatment with cyanocobalamin 100 µg IM and 5 mg folic acid. Cyanocobalamin 100 µg should be given daily with 5 mg oral folic acid for the next two weeks and then continued over three to four weeks but neurological improvement depends on the severity. Though there is a feeling of overall subjective improvement with better appetite, complete neurological recovery particularly of the mental functions may not be seen at all. Oral folic acid should be added because B_{12} induced brisk haemopoiesis also increases the demand for folic acid. It is also essential to supplement iron because such active haemopoiesis generally precipitates iron deficiency as available iron is used up.
   - *Prophylaxis of B_{12} deficiency:* Prophylactic dose of vitamin B_{12} is 3–10 µg daily.
2. **Neuropathies:** Neuropathies thought to be due to B_{12} deficiency like tropical neuropathy respond to vitamin B_{12} but the mechanism is not clear. Vitamin B_{12} is also

given in many other conditions like trigeminal neuralgia, multiple sclerosis, some psychiatric disorders and even for general weakness. There is no evidence to recommend such use for vitamin B_{12}.

Folic Acid

Folic acid is pteroylglutamic acid. It was first isolated from spinach and, therefore, named as folic acid (from leaf).

Dietary source: Green vegetables, liver, yeast, egg, milk and some fruits. Prolonged cooking with spices destroys folic acid.

Absorption takes place in the duodenum and jejunum and is transported in the blood by active and passive transport, widely distributed in the body and is stored in the liver.

Functions: Folic acid is converted to dihydrofolic acid and then to tetrahydrofolic acid which serves as a coenzyme for many vital (one-carbon transfer) reactions necessary for DNA synthesis.

Deficiency: Folate deficiency may be due to dietary folate deficiency, malabsorption and other diseases of the small intestine or drug induced. Phenytoin, phenobarbitone, oral contraceptives, methotrexate and trimethoprim can induce folate deficiency. Increased requirement, as in growing children, pregnancy and lactation, can also cause deficiency. Manifestations include megaloblastic anaemia, glossitis, diarrhoea and weakness.

Uses

1. Megaloblastic anaemia due to folate as well as B_{12} deficiency—folic acid 2–5 mg/day is given orally along with vitamin B_{12}. In folic acid deficiency due to malabsorption syndromes, folic acid is given IM.
2. Prophylactically in pregnancy, lactation, infancy and other situations with increased requirement of folic acid—500 μg daily orally.

Folinic acid (citrovorum factor, leucovorin) is N-formyl tetrahydrofolic acid and is the active coenzyme form which overcomes methotrexate toxicity (*see* page 577).

CALCIUM LEUCOVORIN 3 mg/ml inj, RECOVORIN 15 mg tab, 15, 50 mg inj.

HAEMATOPOIETIC GROWTH FACTORS

Haematopoietic growth factors are hormones that regulate erythropoiesis. Many of these glycoproteins have now been produced for clinical use by recombinant DNA technology. Frequent blood counts are needed to monitor therapy with these growth factors.

- Erythropoietin
- Myeloid growth factors
  - GM-CSF
  - G-CSF
  - M-CSF
- Megakaryocyte growth factors
  - Thrombopoietin
  - Interleukin II

Erythropoietin

Erythropoietin is produced by the kidney in response to hypoxia and anaemia. It binds to erythropoietin receptors on red cell progenitors and stimulates red cell production.

Epoetin alpha (rHuEPO) is human recombinant erythropoietin. It is given thrice weekly to treat anaemia in chronic renal failure and is not cleared by dialysis. **Darbepoetin alpha** is a modified EPO with longer half-life—given once a week. Both epoetin and darbepoetin can be given SC as well as IV. **Epoetin beta** attached to polyethylene glycol polymer is much more longer acting to be given once in 2–4 weeks.

Preparations: EPREX 2000, 4000, 10,000 IU in 1 ml prefilled syringes.

Adverse effects: If the rise in hematocrit is too rapid, thrombotic complications with increased mortality and cardiovascular events like myocardial infarction, stroke and venous thrombosis can complicate erythropoietin therapy. The drugs can rarely cause allergic reactions. To avoid adverse reactions, it is recommended that the haemoglobin level should be monitored not to exceed 12 g/dl and the lowest effective dose should be used. They can also cause hypertension and hypertensive encephalopathy, headache, tachycardia, arthralgias and myalgia.

Uses

1. Erythropoietin and its modified forms are used in the treatment of anaemia due to the following conditions:
   - Chronic renal failure
   - Zidovudine treatment in AIDS patients
   - Cancer chemotherapy
   - Aplastic anaemia
   - Multiple myeloma and cancers of bone marrow
2. To reduce the need for blood transfusion in high-risk patients undergoing certain surgeries.
3. Treatment of iron overload.
4. Anaemia of prematurity.

Myeloid Growth Factors

Myeloid growth factors include **granulocyte-macrophage colony-stimulating factor** (GM-CSF), granulocyte colony-stimulating factor (G-CSF) and monocyte colony-stimulating factor (M-CSF).

Sargramostim is recombinant human GM-CSF and this glycoprotein binds to specific receptors on the myeloid progenitor cells and stimulates the proliferation and differentiation of neutrophils and monocytes.

Sargramostim is given as SC or IV infusion. There is an increase in leucocyte count over 7 to 10 days. On stopping the drug, the count returns to baseline in 2–7 days. **Molgramostim** is another recombinant GM-CSF preparation.

Dose: 300–500 μg daily infusion for 7–14 days depending on the response, LEUKOMAX 150, 300, 400 μg inj.

Adverse effects include bone pain, fever, arthralgia, myalgia and dyspnoea. Higher doses sometimes can cause a capillary leak syndrome with oedema, pericardial and pleural effusion and heart failure.

Filgrastim is human recombinant G-CSF. It stimulates the production of neutrophils. Filgrastim is given as SC injection or IV infusion.

Dose 1–20 μg/kg/day for 7–14 days, GRAFEEL, NEUPOGEN 300 μg inj.

Adverse effects: Filgrastim is better tolerated than sargramostim. It can cause bone pain and rarely allergic reactions.

Uses: Sargramostim and filgrastim are used to shorten neutropenia in bone marrow transplantation, following cancer chemotherapy, aplastic anaemia, congenital neutropenia, myelodysplasia and in AIDS patients with neutropenia.

Pegfilgrastim is a form of filgrastim made by attaching polyethylene glycol (PEG) to filgrastim. It is long acting and can be administered once every cycle of chemotherapy. Dose 6 mg SC.

Lenograstim is an analog of filgrastim and is similar to it.

M-CSF: Stimulates the production of monocytes and macrophages. It can cause splenomegaly and thrombocytopenia.

Haematopoietic stem cell mobilizer—**plerixafor** is a novel molecule which increases CD_{34} counts in the peripheral blood.

Megakaryocyte Growth Factors

Thrombopoietin: Thrombopoietin increases the production of platelets by binding to the receptors on the platelet progenitor cells. Recombinant thrombopoietin is available for therapeutic use. It is being tried in severe thrombocytopenia that occurs following cancer chemotherapy.

Interleukins: Oprelvekin is the recombinant form of interleukin-II. It stimulates the production of megakaryocytes and platelets by activating the interleukin-II receptors on the platelet progenitor cells. Oprelvekin is used for the secondary prevention of thrombocytopenia in patients receiving cancer chemotherapy. Oprelvekin can cause sodium retention resulting in oedema.

Romiplostim belongs to a new class of therapeutic agents called 'peptibodies' where peptides are linked to antibody fragments. It increased platelet count in clinical trials in patients with chronic idiopathic thrombocytopenic purpura (ITP) who have not responded to the conventional drugs and splenectomy. It is given SC once a week and maintained at the lowest possible dose. It has been well tolerated with mild headache.

Eltrombopag is a thrombopoietin agonist which is orally effective. It is used to treat chronic ITP and in thrombocytopenia in hepatitis C.

Clinical Pharmacology

- Gastric irritation is the most common adverse effect with oral iron.
- With optimum oral iron therapy, haemoglobin levels begin to increase—a rise of about 1–2 g in 2–3 weeks is the optimum response.
- Use of parenteral iron should be strictly restricted to recommended indications only. For IV administration, the patient should be hospitalized.
- Initially, the rate of infusion should not exceed 10 drops per minute—may be increased if uneventful for about 30 minutes. Excess free iron is excreted in the urine.
- Urine of the patient receiving iron sorbitol turns dark on standing which could be due to the formation of iron sulfide.

[1] From Medical Council of India, *Competency based Undergraduate Curriculum for the Indian Medical Graduate*, 2018;1:136–144.

Unit XII

Drugs used in Endocrine Disorders

36. Hypothalamus and Anterior Pituitary Hormones
37. Thyroid Hormones and Antithyroid Drugs
38. Corticosteroids
39. Estrogens, Progestins, Hormonal Contraceptives and Drugs used in Infertility
40. Oxytocin and Drugs Acting on the Uterus
41. Androgens and Anabolic Steroids
42. Insulin and Oral Antidiabetic Drugs
43. Agents Affecting Bone Mineral Turnover and Osteoporosis

CHAPTER 36

Hypothalamus and Anterior Pituitary Hormones

Competency achievement: The student should be able to:

PH 1.37 Describe the mechanisms of action, types, doses, side effects, indications and contraindications of the drugs used as sex hormones, their analogues and **anterior pituitary hormones.**[1]

The pituitary gland, under the influence of the hypothalamus, secretes many hormones which either control the secretion of other glands or directly act on the target tissues. These are peptides and act by binding to specific receptors present on the target cells (Table 36.1). The hypothalamic and anterior pituitary hormones are used in the respective deficiency states for replacement and as diagnostic tools to detect their deficiency states. Their analogs are now available and are preferred for use as they are more convenient to use. Posterior pituitary hormones (*see* page 296).

Table 36.1: Hormones secreted by the hypothalamus and anterior pituitary and their chief functions

Hypothalamic hormone	*Anterior pituitary hormone*	*Chief actions*
1. a. Growth hormone releasing hormone (GHRH)	Growth hormone (GH)	Regulates growth
b. Growth hormone release-inhibiting hormone (somatostatin, GHRIH)		Inhibits GH release
2. Corticotropin-releasing hormone (CRH)	Corticotrophin (ACTH)	Stimulates adrenal cortex to secrete glucocorticoids, mineralocorticoids and androgens
3. Thyrotrophin-releasing hormone (TRH)	Thyroid-stimulating hormone (TSH) (Thyrotrophin)	Stimulates release of T_3 and T_4
4. Gonadotrophin-releasing hormone (GnRH)	• Follicle-stimulating hormone (FSH)	Stimulates growth of ovum and graafian follicle in the female and gametogenesis in the male
	• Luteinising hormone (LH) or (ICSH)	Stimulates ovulation in females and regulates testosterone secretion in males
5. Prolactin-releasing peptide	Prolactin (PRL)	Development of breast and lactation
6. Dopamine (prolactin-release-inhibiting hormone)	—	Inhibits prolactin-release
7. Melanocyte stimulating hormone—releasing factor	Melanocyte-stimulating hormone (MSH)	Promotes melanin synthesis causing darkening of skin; regulates feeding

HYPOTHALAMIC HORMONES

Growth hormone-releasing hormone (GHRH) stimulates the anterior pituitary to secrete growth hormone. Sermorelin is an analog of GHRH used in diagnostic tests of growth hormone deficiency (Table 36.2).

Somatostatin is growth hormone release-inhibiting hormone present in the hypothalamus, parts of the CNS, pancreas and in gastrointestinal tract. It inhibits the secretion of GH, TSH, PRL, insulin, glucagon and gastrointestinal secretions, but it is very short-acting. Steatorrhoea, diarrhoea, nausea and dyspepsia are due to its effects on the gut.

Octreotide is the synthetic analog of somatostatin which is longer-acting, more potent and useful in acromegaly, some hormone-secreting tumours, the carcinoid syndrome, diarrhoea associated with diabetes and in bleeding oesophageal varices. It is given subcutaneously in the dose of 50–500 μg every 8 hr. Depot preparations to be injected to the gluteal region every 4 wk are also available. Octreotide has a weak effect on pancreatic beta cells—hence hyperglycaemia is not common. It can cause nausea, vomiting, abdominal cramps, flatulence and vitamin B_{12} deficiency.

Lanreotide is another somatostatin analog which is longer acting than octreotide and is also used in acromegaly, TSH secreting tumours and neuroendocrine tumors.

Pegvisomant is a recently developed growth hormone receptor antagonist. Clinical trials in patients with acromegaly have shown it to be useful in it.

Thyrotrophin-releasing hormone (TRH) secreted by the hypothalamus stimulates the release of TSH from the anterior pituitary.

Protirelin is a synthetic analog of TRH used in the diagnosis of thyroid disorders.

Corticotrophin-releasing factor (CRF) releases ACTH and β-endorphins from the anterior pituitary. It is used in diagnostic tests in Cushing's disease.

Gonadotrophin-releasing hormone and its analogs: Gonadotrophin-releasing hormone (GnRH) secreted in a pulsatile manner, regulates the secretion of gonadotrophins, i.e. enhances FSH and LH production. Gonadorelin is synthetic GnRH. leuprolide, goserelin, buserelin, nafarelin, histrelin and triptorelin are synthetic analogs of GnRH which are more potent and longer acting. On the other hand continuous secretion or exogenous adminis-

Table 36.2: Analogs of hypothalamic and pituitary hormones

Hormones	*Analogs*	*Uses*
Growth hormone releasing hormone	Sermorelin	Diagnosis of GH deficiency
Somatostatin	Octreotide	Acromegaly, hormone-secreting tumours, bleeding oesophageal varices, carcinoid syndrome
TRH	Protirelin	Diagnosis of thyroid disorders
CRF		Diagnostic tests in Cushing's disease, tests of hypothalamic and pituitary function, infertility
GnRH	Gonadorelin Buserelin Leuprorelide Goserelin Nafarelin	• Controlled ovarian hyperstimulation • Endometriosis • Uterine fibroids • Prostatic cancer • Precocious puberty • Diagnostic tests of hypogonadism
ADH	Desmopressin Terlipressin Felypressin	

tration of GnRH or its analogs inhibit the secretion of gonadotrophins by the pituitary gland (Flowchart 36.1) and is used in prostatic cancers, precocious puberty and endometriosis.

Preparations

Leuprolide: LUPRIDE 1,4 mg/ml inj. LEUPROFACT 0.5 mg/ml inj.

Nafarelin: NASAREL spray 200 µg per acivation.

Goserelin: ZOLADEX 3.6 mg inj.

Triptorelin: TRYPLOG 2.5 mg/5 ml vial.

Uses

A. *Pulsatile Administration*

1. *Infertility*
   a. *Infertility in women:* Pulsatile administration of a GnRH agonist may be used in women to induce ovulation. The risk of ovarian hyperstimulation and multiple pregnancy is lesser than with gonadotrophins. A pump is available to deliver gonadorelin in pulses every 90 mins. However, because of the inconvenience in using it with an IV pump and due to the higher cost, these are not preferred.
   b. *Infertility in men:* Hypothalamic hypogonadotrophic hypogonadism resulting in infertility responds to pulsatile administration of gonadorelin.
2. *Diagnosis of hypogonadism:* Rise in LH levels following gonadorelin indicates that hypogonadism is of hypogonadotrophic aetiology (GnRH stimulation testing).

B. *Continuous Administration*

3. *To control ovarian hypostimulation:* In vitro fertilization requires induction and timing of ovulation so that multiple mature oocytes are available but the endogenous LH surge can result in premature ovulation. This can be suppressed by daily GnRH administration. Subcutaneous leuprolide or nasal application of nafarelin may be used.
4. *Endometriosis:* Continuous administration of GnRH agonist reduces oestrogen and progesterone levels, alters the cyclical changes in their levels and reduces the pain of endometriosis. **Leuprolide, goserelin** or **nafarelin** may be used for a maximum of 6 months.
5. *Uterine fibroids:* A GnRH agonist (leuprolide, goserelin or nafarelin) administered for 3–6 months reduces the size of the fibroid.

Flowchart 36.1: Actions and uses of GnRH analogs

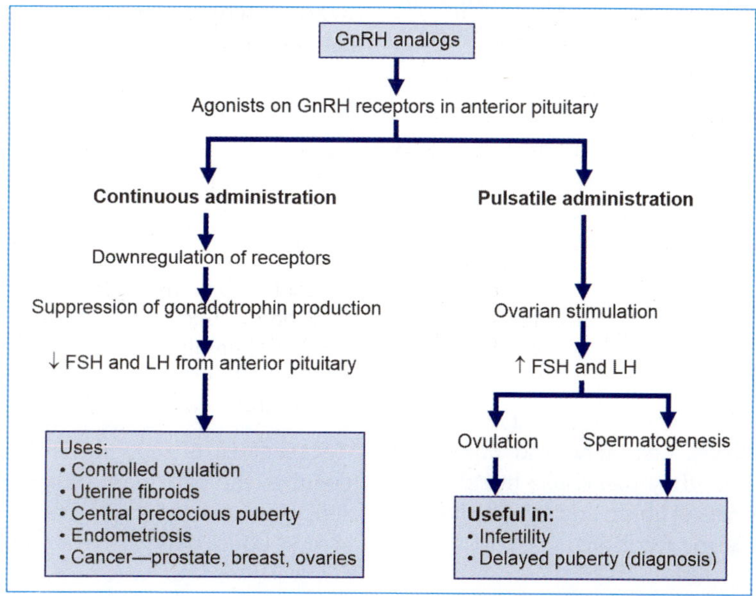

Used for 3 months prior to hysterectomy, they facilitate easy removal of the uterus and also reduce blood loss.

6. *Central precocious puberty:* Leuprolide SC 0.05 mg/kg or nafarelin, nasal spray-800 µg BD daily continued till 11 yr of age stops development of gonads. The development process resumes after stopping the drug.
7. *Prostatic cancer:* Continuous administration of GnRH agonist with an androgen receptor antagonist like flutamide induces pharmacological castration. GnRH agonists cause flare up of the disease in the first two weeks (due to increase in testosterone levels). Hence, an androgen antagonist is added.
8. *Other cancers:* Continuous administration of GnRH agonists is also useful in breast and ovarian cancers.

Adverse effects include flushing, sweating, headache—symptoms resemble menopause; allergic reactions, depression, loss of libido may also occur in women. In men, continuous GnRH administration can cause flushing, loss of libido and gynaecomastia.

Danazol is a synthetic steroid. It inhibits the release of GnRH and thereby inhibits the midcycle surge of FSH and LH (*see* page 485).

GnRH Antagonists

Cetrorelix, ganirelix, abarelix and degarelix are synthetic GnRH antagonists. They bind to and block pituitary GnRH receptors—therefore, suppress the secretion of LH, FSH and delay ovulation.

Cetrorelix and ganirelix are given subcutaneously, 0.25 mg daily; abarelix is given IM and has a long t½ of 13 days.

Adverse effects: GnRH antagonists can cause allergic reactions, headache and nausea in women. In men, they can cause hot flushes, sweating, decreased libido and gynaecomastia apart from allergic reactions.

Uses

1. *In vitro fertilization:* GnRH antagonists prevent LH surge and are used in in vitro fertilization. They are preferred over GnRH analogs because of the following advantages:
   - Less ovarian hyperstimulation.
   - Duration of treatment required is lesser.
   - Less dose of gonadotrophins required.
2. *Cetrorelix* is also useful in reducing uterine fibroids and endometriosis.
3. *Prostatic cancer:* Abarelix and degarelix control the symptoms in advanced prostatic cancer.

ANTERIOR PITUITARY HORMONES

Growth hormone (GH) is a peptide which stimulates the growth of all organs except brain and eye. It increases the uptake of amino acids by the tissues, promotes protein synthesis and positive nitrogen balance. It causes lipolysis and reduces glucose uptake by skeletal muscles. It brings about linear growth. These anabolic actions are mediated by somatomedins or insulin-like growth factors (IGF) produced in the liver.

The secretion of growth hormone is regulated by GHRH and somatostatin (GHIH).

GH deficiency in children results in dwarfism while excessive production results in gigantism in children and acromegaly in adults.

Uses (Table 36.3)

- *GH deficiency:* Replacement therapy with GH in deficient children brings about normal growth. It can also be used in GH deficient adults.
- *Other conditions:* GH has been tried in chronic renal failure and in catabolic states—like severe burns and AIDS. It is liable for abuse by athletes to promote growth.

Mecasermin is recombinant human IGF-1 useful in the treatment of severe IGF-1 deficiency not responding to GH. The common adverse effect is hypoglycaemia which should

Table 36.3: Uses of anterior pituitary hormones

Anterior pituitary hormones	*Uses*
1. Growth hormone	GH deficiency, chronic renal failure, burns
2. Corticotrophin	Diagnosis of adrenocortical insufficiency
3. Thyrotrophin	To test thyroid function, increase radioiodine uptake in thyroid
4. Gonadotrophins	Infertility—ovulation induction, *in vitro* fertilization. FSH-LH deficiency, undescended testes, amenorrhoea.

be avoided by carbohydrate meals along with mecasermin.

Corticotrophin (adrenocorticotrophic hormone, ACTH): Controls the synthesis and release of glucocorticoids, mineralocorticoids and androgens from the adrenal cortex. It is used in the diagnosis of adrenocortical insufficiency.

Thyroid-stimulating hormone (TSH, thyrotrophin): Stimulates the production and secretion of thyroid hormones and thus regulates thyroid function. Recombinant TSH is used to test thyroid function and to increase the uptake of radioactive iodine in thyroid carcinoma.

Gonadotrophins

Follicle-stimulating hormone (FSH) and luteinizing hormone (LH): Produced by the anterior pituitary, regulate gonadal function. They stimulate follicular development in women and also stimulate ovarian steroidogenesis (oestrogen and progesterone synthesis). In men, they promote spermatogenesis.

Recombinant forms of FSH available are follitropin alpha and follitropin beta; recombinant LH is leutropin alpha.

Uses

Menotropins or human menopausal gonadotrophins (HMG) are the combination of FSH-LH obtained from the urine of postmenopausal women. Menotropins are used in:

1. *Infertility in women*
   a. *For ovulation and then conception:* A definite pattern of FSH and LH release is required in women. In women with anovulation, gonadotrophins are used to induce ovulation as alternatives to clomiphene citrate—gonadotrophins are more expensive.
      Leutropin alpha can be used with FSH in infertility associated with severe LH deficiency in women.
   b. *Controlled ovarian hyperstimulation:* For assisted reproduction, FSH is given from 3rd day for 7–12 days. LH may also be needed in LH deficient women. Once the follicle has developed, HCG is given to support follicular maturation and then ovulation. This may be followed by insemination and then retrieval of the oocyte for assisted reproduction. Several regimens are now available. However, the disadvantages include multiple pregnancies and **ovarian hyperstimulation syndrome** (OHSS).
   c. *For in vitro fertilization:* To time the ovulation.
2. *Infertility in men:* Infertility associated with low sperm count in hypogonadal men due to hypothalamopituitary cause is treated with FSH and LH.
3. *Gonadotrophin deficiency in men* for replacement.
4. *Undescended testes:* Surgery is the preferred option now. Earlier, in order to stimulate the descent of testes, LH was administered which inturn would stimulate the production of androgens.
5. *Delayed puberty:* HCG may be tried as an alternative to testosterone to stimulate testosterone synthesis in boys with delayed puberty.

Preparations

1. **Menotropins:** FSH + LH-Pregnorm 75 IU FSH + 75 IU LH, Ovulate-M 150 IU FSH +150 IULH/amp for IM inj.

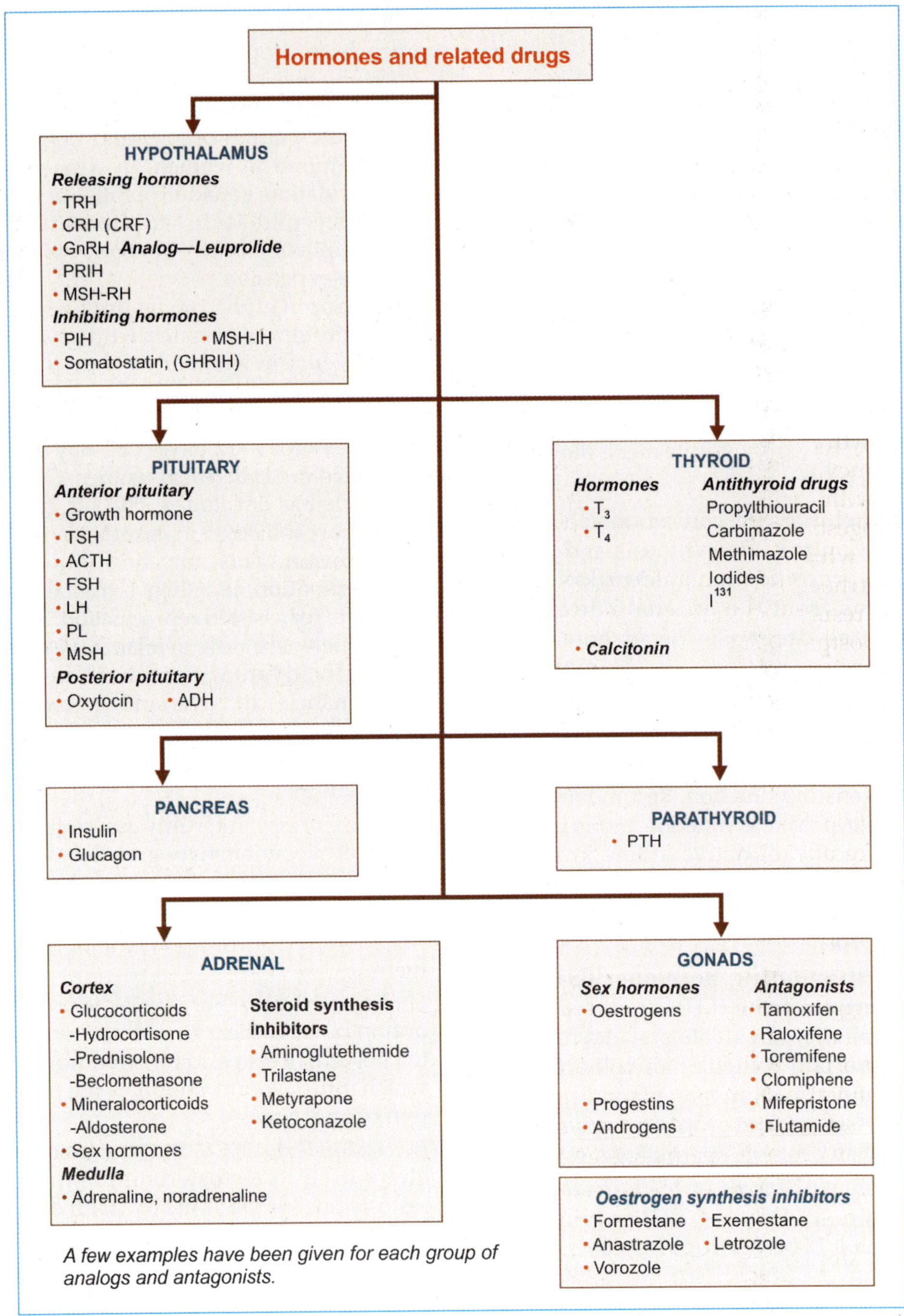

2. **Follitropin:** Materna-FSH 75 IU Foliculin 75, 150 IU/amp for IM inj.

3. **HCG:** CHORIOMON, OVIDAC, 2000, 5000 IU as dry powder with solvent for inj.

Adverse effects include hyperstimulation of the ovaries with polycystic ovary, abdominal pain, bleeding in the ovaries and shock described as OHSS. They can also cause allergic reactions.

Human chorionic gonadotrophin is a glycoprotein similar to LH. Recombinant HCG or choriogonadotrophin alpha, is now available.

Clomiphene, an estrogen antagonist, inhibits the negative feedback of endogenous oestrogens and thereby stimulates gonadotrophin release. It is, therefore, useful in the treatment of infertility (*see* page 483).

Prolactin: This peptide hormone promotes the growth and development of breast during pregnancy. It stimulates milk production along with other hormones like oestrogens and progestins. Deficiency results in lactation failure while excess prolactin results in galactorrhoea. Prolactin also inhibits GnRH release resulting in lactational amenorrhoea in the postpartum period.

Regulation of secretion: Suckling is the principal stimulus for prolactin secretion. Suckling stimulates the release of prolactin-releasing factor from hypothalamus. Oestrogens and dopamine antagonists also stimulate prolactin-release. Prolactin is not used clinically (Fig. 36.1).

Dopamine agonists like **bromocriptine, cabergoline, pergolide** and **quinagolide** inhibit prolactin release from the pituitary by acting directly on dopamine receptors.

Bromocriptine is an ergot derivative with dopamine agonistic properties. It reduces the secretion of prolactin by activating DA receptors in the pituitary. In patients with acromegaly, it reduces GH release. Stimulation of dopamine receptors in CTZ leads to nausea and vomiting.

Bromocriptine is used:

1. *To suppress lactation:* Bromocriptine and other dopamine agonists stimulate the dopamine receptors in the pituitary to inhibit the release of prolactin. Bromocriptine is used to suppress lactation and breast engorgement after delivery (like in stillbirth) and following abortion.
2. *In galactorrhoea* due to excess prolactin, bromocriptine or cabergoilne may be used.
3. *Prolactin-secreting tumours* or prolactinomas.
4. *Acromegaly:* In normal subjects, dopamine agonists stimulate the release of growth hormone by the pituitary but in patients with acromegaly, they suppress growth hormone release by a paradoxical effect. Bromocriptine is, therefore, used in acromegaly also but the response is seen only in a few patients. Bromocriptine also helps to reduce prolactin release. Octreotide, pituitary surgery and radiation therapy may be needed in acromegaly.
5. *Parkinsonism:* Bromocriptine is used as an adjunct and also to treat on off phenomenon (*see* page 230).

Cabergoline has actions similar to bromocriptine but is longer acting (twice weekly dose) and more selective for D_2 receptors—hence preferred over bromocriptine for acromegaly and to suppress lactation.

Quinagolide is a nonergot DA agonist with high affinity for D_2 receptors.

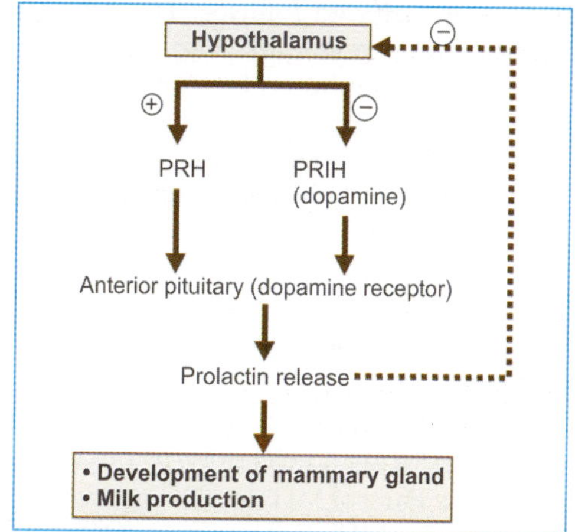

Fig. 36.1: Actions and regulation of prolactin release

[1] From Medical Council of India, *Competency based Undergraduate Curriculum for the Indian Medical Graduate*, 2018;1:136–144.

CHAPTER 37

Thyroid Hormones and Antithyroid Drugs

Competency achievement: The student should be able to:

PH 1.36 Describe the mechanism of action, types, doses, side effects, indications and contraindications of drugs used in endocrine disorders (diabetes mellitus, **thyroid disorders** and osteoporosis).[1]

THYROID HORMONES

Thyroxine (tetraiodothyronine, T_4) and triiodothyronine (T_3) are the hormones secreted by the thyroid gland. T_4 is the less active precursor of T_3. The other hormone, calcitonin is secreted by the parafollicular cells (*see* page 682).

Synthesis, Storage and Secretion

The thyroid hormones are synthesized and stored in the thyroid follicles. The principal source of iodine is diet. The main steps involved in the synthesis of thyroid hormones are as follows (Fig. 37.1).

1. *Uptake* of plasma iodide by thyroid cells by an active transport process with the help of sodium iodide symporter.
2. *Oxidation* of iodide to I^+ (iodinium ions) by a thyroperoxidase enzyme with the help of hydrogen peroxide.
3. *Iodination:* These bind to tyrosine residues of thyroglobulin (Tg) to form monoiodotyrosine (MIT) and diiodotyrosine (DIT).
4. *Coupling:* Pairs of MIT and DIT are coupled to form T_3 (MIT+DIT) and T_4 (DIT+DIT) catalyzed by the same peroxidase enzyme.

Storage: Tg containing iodinated tyrosine residues are stored in the follicles.

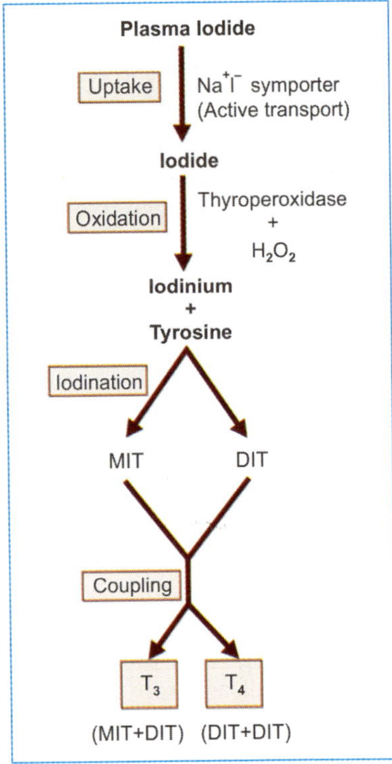

Fig. 37.1: Steps in thyroid hormone synthesis

Release: The hormones T_4 and T_3 are released into the circulation.

Regulation

The thyroid secretion is regulated by TSH secreted by the anterior pituitary and TRH from the hypothalamus (Fig. 37.2). Normally about 70–90 μg of T_4 and 15–30 μg of T_3 are secreted daily. In the peripheral tissues, most

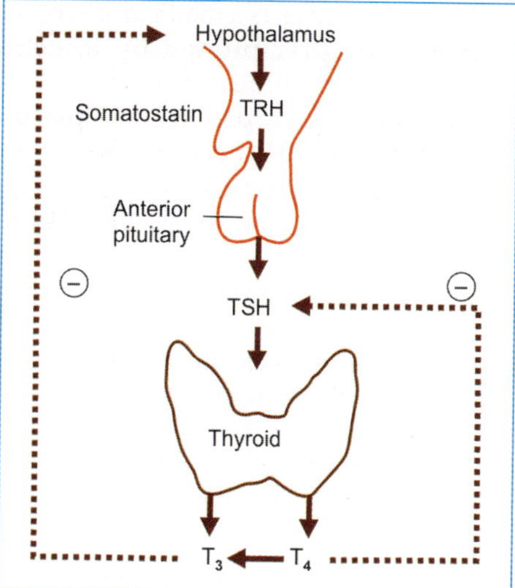

Fig. 37.2: Regulation of thyroid hormone secretion

of the secreted T_4 is converted to T_3 which is the active hormone.

Actions

Thyroid hormones influence several body functions.

- Thyroid hormones are essential for normal growth, development, function and maintenance of all body tissues. Congenital deficiency results in cretinism.
- Thyroid hormones have important metabolic functions—they increase metabolic rate—BMR is increased, body temperature rises (calorigenesis), enhance carbohydrate metabolism with increased utilization of sugars by the tissues, glycogenolysis and gluconeogenesis. Therefore, in hyperthyroidism, hyperglycaemia is seen.
- *Protein metabolism:* Excess thyroid hormones are catabolic and proteins are used to generate energy. In hyperthyroidism, there is negative nitrogen balance, tissue wasting and weight loss.
- Stimulate lipolysis by potentiating the effect of lipolytic hormones.
- They facilitate erythropoiesis.
- Thyroid hormones are essential for normal functioning of the CNS (mental retardation is seen in cretinism), skeletal muscles (muscle weakness in myxoedema), cardiovascular system, reproductive system and gastrointestinal system (hypothyroid patients are constipated while hyperthyroid have diarrhoea).

Mechanism of Action

Thyroid hormones act on specific receptors. Thyroid receptors are nuclear receptors like the steroid receptors. T_3 enters into the cells, bind to the receptor and the T_3 receptor then changes conformation, activates gene transcription and regulates synthesis of proteins involved in thyroid hormones functions (*see* Fig. 38.4, page 471).

Pharmacokinetics

T_4 and T_3 are well absorbed with oral bioavailability of 80% for T_4 and 95% for T_3. Both T_4 and T_3 are extensively bound to plasma proteins. The free hormone is metabolized in the liver and excreted in the bile. Hepatic microsomal enzyme inducers hasten the metabolism of thyroid hormones. The t½ of T_4 is 6–7 days and that of T_3 is 1–2 days. In hyperthyroidism, both T_3 and T4 are metabolised faster and their half lives get shorter. T_3 is 3–5 times more potent than T_4 and acts faster.

Preparations

Both T_3 and T_4 are given orally. Leothyronine is also available for IV administration for use in myxoedema coma. T_3 is reserved for emergencies because of its fast onset of action, and shorter half-life. T_4 is preferred to T_3 for therapeutic use except in emergencies because:

i. T_3 has a rapid onset of action with the risk of precipitating angina, arrhythmias or cardiac failure.

ii. T_4 is longer acting (used once daily) and also gets slowly converted to T_3—thus provides both T_3 and T_4.

iii. Stability of the T_4 preparation.
iv. Lower cost.

L-thyroxine: ELTROXIN, THYRONORM 25, 50, 100 mcg tab. L-THYROXINE SODIUM 200, 500 µg inj.

Stored in dark bottles to avoid spontaneous deiodination.

Uses

Both thyroxine and triiodothyronine are available but T_4 is more commonly used. Levothyroxine is synthetic T_4 and leothyronine is synthetic T_3 and both are given orally.

1. *Replacement therapy*
   - *Cretinism* may be sporadic or endemic. Congenital absence of thyroid or defective thyroid hormone synthesis cause sporadic cretinism. Extreme deficiency of iodine can result in endemic cretinism. Treatment should be started immediately to avoid mental retardation. Early detection and treatment produce dramatic results with normal physical and mental development. Levothyroxine 25 µg/day is started and treatment monitored by clinical response and TSH levels. The requirement increases with age—50 µg/day from 6 to 12 months, to 75 µg/day up to 5 yr, 100 µg/day up to 18 yr and 100–200 µg/day in adults. Replacement should be continued lifelong.
   - *Hypothyroidism* in adults results from decreased thyroid activity and can be reversed by appropriate activity and treatment. Treatment is started with levothyroxine 50 µg daily and increased gradually every 2–3 weeks, depending on the plasma TSH levels. A daily maintenance dose of 100–200 µg may be required in most patients. In patients with ischaemic heart disease, treatment is started with much smaller doses to avoid angina and myocardial infarction. Larger doses are required in pregnancy.
   - *Myxoedema coma* is a medical emergency. It may be precipitated by infection, trauma, inadequate treatment or exposure to cold. Clinical features include hypothermia, bradycardia, hypotension, hypoglycaemia, hypoventilation, lactic acidosis and coma.

     Treatment: Blood may be drawn for hormone estimation but treatment should be started immediately. IV thyroxine 300–500 µg or liothyronine 100 µg thrice daily should be given with prophylactic corticosteroids to avoid adrenal insufficiency. Gradual warming, prophylactic antibiotics, ventilatory support, correction of fluid and electrolyte balance are all important.
   - *Myxoedema with coronary artery disease:* If myxoedema is rapidly corrected in patients with coronary artery disease, the sudden increase in myocardiac workload could result is angina, arrhythmias or even myocardial infarction. Hence hypothyroidism should be gradually corrected in these patients. Whenever, possible, coronary artery disease should be treated before hypothyroidism.
   - *Subclinical hypothyroidism* with elevated TSH and normal thyroid hormone levels is often seen. They need constant TSH monitoring and in patients with very high levels of TSH (>10) or in certain conditions like pregnancy dyslipidemia, psychiatric disorders and infertility, thyroxin replacement is recommended.
2. *Non-toxic goitre:* Could be endemic or sporadic goitre. Decrease in production of thyroid hormones results in elevated TSH levels stimulating the thyroid gland enlargement. Administration of T_4 suppresses TSH production and the goitre regresses (though the extent varies). Iodine deficiency should be corrected.
3. *Thyroid carcinoma:* Postoperatively higher dose of T_4 induces TSH suppresion which in turn reduces the risk of tumour cell proliferation.

4. *Miscellaneous:* Thyroxine is tried in refractory anaemias, infertility and non-healing ulcers.

HYPERTHYROIDISM AND ANTITHYROID DRUGS

Hyperthyroidism is due to an excess of circulating thyroid hormones and could be due to various causes. Graves' disease, an autoimmune disorder, is the most common cause. It is characterized by hyperthyroidism, diffuse goitre and IgG antibodies that activate TSH receptors. Antithyroid drugs may act by interfering with the synthesis, release or actions of thyroid hormones.

Antithyroid drugs:

1. *Inhibit hormone synthesis*
   Thioureylenes
   Propylthiouracil, methimazole, carbimazole
2. *Inhibit hormone release*
   Iodine, iodides
   Iodinated radiocontrast media.
3. *Ionic inhibitors*
   Thiocyanate, perchlorate.
4. *Destroy thyroid tissue*
   Radioactive iodine
5. *Others:* Lithium, cholestyramine

Thioureylenes

Thioureylenes are thionamides and include propylthiouracil, methimazole and carbimazole.

Actions

Thioureylenes reduce the synthesis of thyroid hormones by inhibiting iodination of tyrosine residues and coupling of iodotyrosine residues. They bring about these effects by inhibiting the peroxidase enzyme. Propylthiouracil also inhibits peripheral conversion of T_4 to T_3. T_3 and T_4 levels gradually fall. Large doses may stimulate the release of TSH resulting in thyroid enlargement. Over 3–4 weeks of treatment, the signs and symptoms of hyperthyroidism subside. Propylthiouracil is faster acting while carbimazole is longer acting. Carbimazole is a prodrug of methimazole (*see* Compare and Contrast: Propylthiouracil and Methimazole).

Key Box 37.1: Drugs that influence thyroid function

Amiodarone	Phenytoin
Sulfonamides	Carbamazepine
Lithium	Sodium nitroprusside

Pharmacokinetics

Thioureylenes are effective orally and well absorbed; about 75% propylthiouracil is firmly bound to plasma proteins—hence very little crosses the placenta and a negligible fraction reaches the milk; but carbimazole and methimazole cross the placenta and are secreted in the milk. Thioureylenes are concentrated in the thyroid and, therefore, their effects persist even when plasma levels fall (their plasma t½ is short). They are metabolised in the liver.

Preparations

Carbimazole: Start with 5-15 mg TDS; maintenance 5-10 mg/day. NEOMERCAZOLE, ANTITHYROX 5, 10, 20 mg tab.

Methimazole: Start with 5-10 mg TDS. maintenance dose 2.5-5 mg/day OD.

Propylthiouracil: Start with 50-150 mg TDS; maintenance 25-50 mg TDS. Generic PTU : 50 mg tab.

Adverse Effects

Adverse effects include allergic reactions like skin rashes, urticaria, dermatitis and arthralgia. Hepatitis, cholestatic jaundice, headache, can occur. Agranulocytosis is a rare but serious adverse effect which occurs in about 0.1% of patients. It is reversible on stopping the antithyroid drug but patient should be monitored with frequent WBC counts. Thioureylenes can also cause arthralgia, myalgia, lymphadenopathy and rarely, psychosis.

Uses

Antithyroid drugs are used in hyperthyroid states like:

Compare and Contrast
Propylthiouracil and Methimazole

Features	***Propylthiouracil***	***Methimazole***
Onset of action	Faster acting	Slower acting
t½	1–2 hours	6 hours
Additional action	Prevents peripheral convertion of $T_4 \rightarrow T_3$	No such effect
Protein binding	75%, Firmly protein bound	Nil
Placental transfer	Negligible amount crosses placenta	Easily crosses
Secretion in milk	Negligible	Significant
Pregnancy	Preferred	Not preferred
Lactating mothers	Drug of choice	Not used
Dose frequency	tid-qid	OD–BD
Potency	Less potent	10 times more potent

(Carbimazole is a prodrug, converted to methimazole in the body)

1. *Graves' disease* or diffuse toxic goitre needs long-term (1–15 years) treatment with antithyroid drugs. One of the thiourelyenes is continued till remission sets in—which may take a long time. Thyroid hormone levels return to normal in about 12 weeks but treatment should be continued. Smaller maintenance doses are then sufficient. Younger patients with mild disease are likely to respond. Remission may not be seen in all patients. Radioactive iodine therapy is now considered definitive therapy in most patients with Graves' disease.
2. *Toxic nodular goitre:* As an alternative—when surgery cannot be done as in the elderly—antithyroid drugs are used.
3. *Preoperatively:* Hyperthyroid patients are made euthyroid with antithyroid drugs and then operated.
4. *Hyperthyroidism in pregnancy:* It is rare but when severe, requires treatment. Propylthiouracil is the preferred drug in 1st trimester as it poorly crosses the placental barrier. During 2nd and 3rd trimesters, patient is switched to carbimazole. In lactating mothers, though only negligible amount of propylthiouracil is secreted in the milk due to toxicity and lack of specific advantage, methimazole (10–30 mg/day) is used.
5. *With radioiodine:* Radioiodine treatment requires about 3 months for the response. Antithyroid drugs may be employed till then to control hyperthyroidism. They may then be gradually withdrawn.
6. *Thyroid storm* or thyrotoxic crisis is sudden, severe exacerbation of thyrotoxicosis and can be life-threatening. It is precipitated by factors like stress, infections, trauma, surgery, etc. Inadequately treated thyrotoxic patients may go into thyroid storm. Symptoms include fever, tachycardia, nausea, vomiting, diarrhoea, profuse sweating, confusion, restlessness, pulmonary oedema, CCF and may lead on to coma and death.

Treatment of thyroid storm

- Propylthiouracil 400–600 mg stat orally or as an enema rectally to block the hormone synthesis (alternative carbimazole 20 mg).
- 6–10 drops of oral/rectal potassium iodide or Lugol's iodine inhibit the release of hormones from the thyroid gland.
- IV hydrocortisone 50 mg inj repeated every 6 hr helps to combat shock and also blocks the conversion of T_4 to T_3.
- Propranolol 1–2 mg slow IV or 40–60 mg oral QID may be used to rapidly control the symptoms particularly cardiovascular symptoms. It also impairs conversion of T_4 to T_3 which may be of value.

- If propranolol is contraindicated, diltiazem 60–120 mg TDS may be given orally to control hypertension and tachycardia.
- Radiocontrast media: Iodine containing radiocontrast media like iopanoic acid or ipodate inhibit thyroid hormone release and peripheral conversion of T_4 to T_3.
- Tepid sponging, sedation, IV fluids and supportive therapy are needed immediately.
- Peritoneal dialysis may rarely be required to clear the plasma thyroxine.

Iodides

Administration of iodides inhibit the release of thyroid hormones described as **Wolff-Chaikoff effect**. It is an autoregulatory effect and iodides inhibit synthesis (organification) and release of thyroid hormones. The T_3 and T_4 levels fall and in thyrotoxic patients the symptoms subside in 1–2 days. The gland becomes firm, less vascular and shrinks in size over a period of 10–14 days. These effects are transient and may be used to quickly reduce thyroid hormone levels as in thyroid storm but the effect decreases after 14–15 days (known as **thyroid escape**). If radioactive iodine or other antithyroid drug administration is intended, iodides may be avoided because treatment with iodides increases the intra-glandular stores of iodine due to which thioureylenes and radioiodine may not be effective for several weeks.

Jod-Basedow effect is iodine-induced hyperthyroidism seen in patients with thyroid abnormalities. It may also be seen following the administration of iodine-containing drugs like amiodarone.

Iodides are administered orally as Lugol's iodine or as potassium iodide solution—3 drops 3 times a day. Iodine is converted into iodides in the intestine which is then absorbed.

Uses

1. *Preoperative preparation for thyroidectomy:* Iodine is started just 10 days prior to surgery to make the thyroid gland firm and less vascular.
2. *Thyroid storm:* Iodides act rapidly to reduce the release of thyroid hormones.
3. *Prophylaxis:* Iodide or iodate is added to common salt to prevent endemic goitre.
4. *Protection against radioactivity:* Potassium iodide administered prophylactically following a nuclear accident protects the thyroid from radioactive iodine (by Wolff-Chaikoff effect)
5. *Antiseptic* (*see* page 688).
6. *Expectorant:* Potassium iodide is used in cough.

Preparations

Lugol's iodine (5% iodine in 10% potassium iodide solution), collosol liquid—8 mg iodine/ 5 ml.

For topical use: Povidone iodine (5–10% solution), tincture of iodine (2% iodine with 2.4% sodium iodide).

Adverse effects

Adverse effects include allergic reactions like skin rashes, conjunctivitis, rhinitis, vasculitis, swelling of the lips and salivary glands, fever and lymphadenopathy. Chronic overdose can cause iodism with metallic taste, excessive salivation, lacrimation, burning sensation in oral cavity and throat, running nose, sore throat, cough, headache and rashes.

Iodine Overdosage

Acute toxicity with iodine can be fatal (3–4 grams is the fatal dose) (*see* page 710).

Signs and Symptoms

Iodine is a powerful irritant and vesicant.

- Nausea, vomiting, diarrhoea, and an unpleasant metallic taste.
- Vesication, desquamation and corrosion of skin and mucous membrane with brownish yellow stains.
- Corrosion and perforation of mouth, throat and GI tract can occur.

- Nephritis and renal failure.
- Delirium, stupor.
- Inhalation produces oedema of glottis and pulmonary oedema.
- Anaphylactic reactions can occur.

Treatment

- Administer starch or flour solution orally (30 g per litre of water). Milk is also helpful.
- Sodium thiosulphate is the antidote. A solution of 1 to 5% sodium thiosulphate is given orally. This will convert iodine to iodide which is relatively harmless.
- Skin lesions can be treated with 20% alcohol.
- Supportive therapy.
- Induction of vomiting or stomach wash are contraindicated.

Iodism is a term used to denote chronic poisoning with iodide salts and is characterized by erythema, urticaria, acne, stomatitis, conjunctivitis, rhinorrhoea, parotid swelling, lymphadenopathy, anorexia and insomnia. Treatment involves liberal intake of sodium chloride which promotes excretion of iodides. This is because chloride competes with iodide for excretion at the level of the renal tubules.

Radioactive Iodine

^{131}I given orally as a solution is rapidly absorbed and is concentrated by the thyroid in the follicles. It emits both γ and β rays. The γ rays pass through the thyroid tissue while β particles penetrate only 0.5 to 2 mm of the tissue due to which it destroys only the thyroid tissue without damaging the surrounding structures. ^{131}I has a half-life of 8 days but the radioactivity is present up to 2 months. It is given as a single dose; clinically the effect is seen after 1–2 months but the peak effect is from about 3–6 months.

Radioactive iodine is used in the treatment of hyperthyroidism as due to Graves' disease and toxic nodular goiter and in thyroid carcinoma. It is available as a solution of Na ^{131}I and is given in the dose of 3–10 millicuries on an empty stomach for thyrotoxicosis. The dose depends on the size of the thyroid with higher doses needed for toxic nodular goiter. In thyroid carcinoma, 80–100 millicurie ^{131}I is given after thyroidectomy to ablate the remaining thyroid tissue. Patient should be instructed to dispose the urine carefully in the toilet and flush it with enough water. Patient should be kept away from children and pregnant women for 2–3 days. Thyroid function should be assessed after 3 months and if required the dose may be repeated. Small dose—in microcurie doses (25–100 microcuries) is used for diagnostic purpose in thyroid function tests.

Advantages of ^{131}I

i. Administration is simple
ii. Convenient—can be given as out patient.
iii. Surgery and its associated risks and morbidity can be avoided.
iv. Less expensive when compared to surgery.

Disadvantages of ^{131}I

i. The long time (3 months) taken for maximum response.
ii. The risk of hypothyroidism—40–60% of people may develop hypothyroidism after months or even years. The patient needs to be followed up for the symptoms of hypothyroidism and replacement therapy with thyroid hormones should be promptly given.
iii. Risk of thyroid carcinoma—since radiation can be carcinogenic, the risk of secondary carcinoma exists (though uncommon). Hence, its use is restricted to adults and is **avoided in children**.

Iodine Containing Radiocontrast Media

Radiocontrast media are used in diagnostic radiology for better visualization of body structures. Most of them are iodinated because iodine has several suitable properties like it can be easily incorporated into an organic compound and is nonionisable making it least toxic. Some examples are iopodate, iopamidol, iotrolon and iodixanol. They are also useful in thyroid storm as they inhibit the release of thyroid hormones as well as inhibit the conversion of T_4 to T_3.

β-adrenergic Blockers

Many of the symptoms of hyperthyroidism are of sympathetic overactivity as there is increased tissue sensitivity to catecholamines in hyperthyroidism. β-adrenergic blockers like propranolol relieve symptoms like palpitation, tremors, nervousness, sweating and myopathy. They also inhibit the peripheral conversion of T_4 to T_3 in higher doses. They only afford symptomatic relief and are used as adjuvants. They are particularly useful in controlling the symptoms of thyroid storm.

Ionic Inhibitors

Ionic inhibitors interfere with the concentration of iodine by the thyroid gland. Thiocyanate and perchlorate inhibit the organification of iodine but are not used now due to the adverse effects. Potassium perchlorate has been tried in hyperthyroidism in patients allergic to thionamides. Food items like cabbage; drugs like sodium nitroprusside and cigarette smoking increase the concentration of thiocyanate in the blood and may result in hypothyroidism.

Drugs that Influence Thyroid Function

Apart from antithyroid drugs, several drugs can influence thyroid function.

- Amiodarone, an antiarrhythmic drug contains iodine. It can cause hypothyroidism or hyperthyroidism, chemical thyroiditis and thyrotoxicosis. Amiodarone may have to be withdrawn in some patients.
- Phenytoin, carbamazepine, phenobarbitone, rifampicin and protease inhibitors cause microsomal enzyme induction—increase metabolism of T_3 and T_4.
- Cholestyramine and cholestipol bind and decrease the absorption of thyroid hormones in the gut.
- Proton pump inhibitors, ciprofloxacin and sucralfate—interfere with T_4 absorption.
- Lithium and amiodarone inhibit the synthesis and release of thyroid hormones.
- Sulfonamides inhibit the coupling reaction.
- Drug-induced hypothyroidism or hyperthyroidism is best treated by stoping the drug.

Clinical Pharmacology

- Thyroxine tablets need to be taken on empty stomach in the morning.
- Patients on long-term thyroid supplements may need calcium and iron. However, calcium needs to be given at a separate time since it may interfere with absorption of thyroxine.
- Increments in thyroxine dosage need to be made until TSH is suppressed to <2.5 IU/ml.

[1] From Medical Council of India, *Competency based Undergraduate Curriculum for the Indian Medical Graduate*, 2018;1:136–144.

CHAPTER 38

Corticosteroids

> *Competency achievement:* The student should be able to:
>
> **PH 1.38** Describe the mechanism of action, types, doses, side effects, indications and contraindications of corticosteroids.[1]

Corticosteroids are hormones produced in the cortex of the adrenal gland. They are glucocorticoids, mineralocorticoids and a small amount of androgens. Cortisol is the major glucocorticoid while aldosterone is the major mineralocorticoid. The secretion of adrenal cortex is under the control of ACTH, secreted by the anterior pituitary and this is in turn regulated by CRF and plasma corticosterone levels (Fig. 38.1). This is termed hypothalamic-pituitary-adrenal axis.

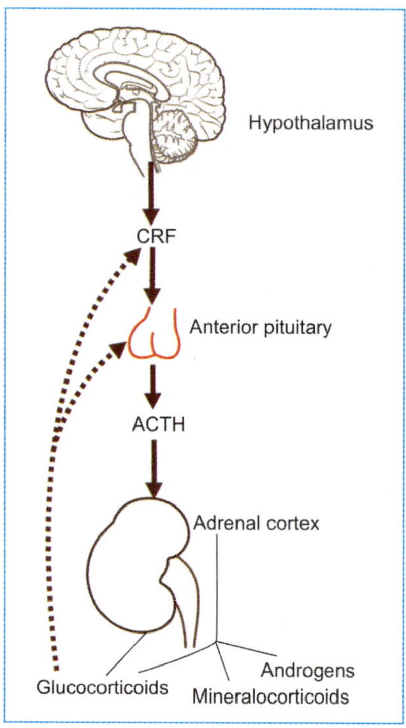

Fig. 38.1: Hypothalamic-pituitary-adrenal axis. Regulation of synthesis and secretion of adrenal corticosteroids

Structure and Biosynthesis

The corticosteroids have a cyclopentanoperhydrophenanthrene (steroid) ring (Fig. 38.2). They are synthesized in the adrenal cortex from cholesterol (Fig. 38.3) under the influence of ACTH.

In a normal person, every day about 10–20 mg of hydrocortisone (maximum in the early morning) and 0.125 mg of aldosterone are secreted. They are also released in response to stress.

GLUCOCORTICOIDS

Hydrocortisone (cortisol) is the natural glucocorticoid while prednisolone, triamcinolone, dexamethasone, paramethasone and betamethasone are synthetic derivatives. Hydrocortisone has both glucocorticoid and mineralocorticoid activity.

Actions

A. *Glucocorticoid Actions*

Glucocorticoids have a wide range of effects influencing several systems in the body. They enable the body to handle stress. Apart from direct effects, glucocorticoids also have other actions in coordination with other hormones or regulators and are called permissive effects.

Fig. 38.2: Structure of hydrocortisone and the steroid nucleus

1. *Metabolic effects:* Carbohydrate, protein and fat metabolism: Glucocorticoids promote gluconeogenesis and glycogen deposition in the liver and also inhibit peripheral utilization of glucose resulting in increased blood glucose levels.

They enhance protein breakdown and nitrogen is excreted leading to negative nitrogen balance. Glucocorticoids are catabolic hormones. They reduce muscle mass.

Glucocorticoids promote lipolysis and redistribution of fat takes place—fat is mobilised from the extremities and is deposited over the face, neck and shoulder and these features of excess glucocorticoid activity is described as 'moon face', 'fish mouth' and 'buffalo hump', respectively.

2. *Anti-inflammatory and immunosuppressive effects:* Glucocorticoids have profound anti-inflammatory properties which is the basis for their beneficial effects in several conditions. They are also immunosuppressants by following actions:

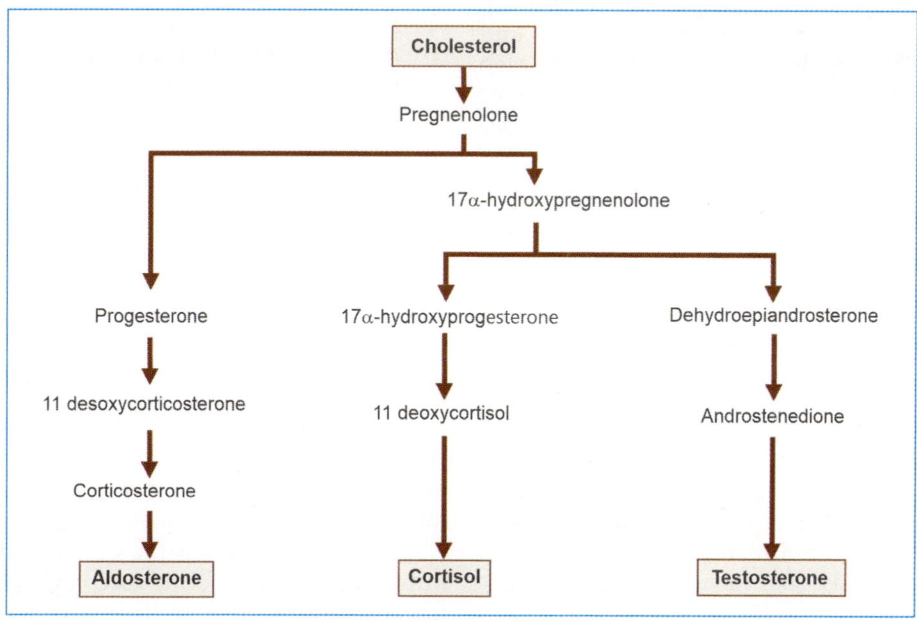

Fig. 38.3: Synthesis of adrenal steroids

i. Glucocorticoids suppress the development of inflammatory response to all types of stimuli like the chemical, mechanical and immunological stimuli.
ii. They inhibit both early and late manifestations of inflammation. Inhibition of late response like capillary proliferation, collagen deposition, fibroblastic activity and scar formation may delay wound healing.
iii. They inhibit migration and depress the function of the leukocytes and macrophages and inhibit the release of chemical mediators of inflammation. The ability of these cells to respond to antigens is decreased.
iv. Glucocorticoids—even a single dose brings about a decrease in the number of WBCs—lymphocytes, monocytes, eosinophils and basophils decline.
v. Metabolites of arachidonic acid, like prostaglandins and leukotrienes, are important mediators of inflammation. Glucocorticoids induce the synthesis of a protein—lipocortin, which inhibits phospholipase A2, thereby decreasing the production of prostaglandins and leukotrienes. Glucocorticoids also suppress the production of cyclo-oxygenase-2 (COX-2) in the inflammatory cells.
vi. They also suppress the production of cytokines (IL-6 and IL-b) which play a key role in inflammation.

Glucocorticoids thus suppress cell-mediated immunity, prevent manifestations of allergy and inflammation and prevent homograft rejection. Large doses also inhibit antibody production.

3. *Other actions*

i. *CVS:* Glucocorticoids reduce capillary permeability, thereby reducing fluid exudation and maintain the tone of arterioles. They have a positive inotropic effect on the heart. Prolonged use can cause hypertension.
ii. *Skeletal muscle:* They are essential for normal muscular activity.
iii. *CNS:* They are required for normal functioning of the central nervous system. Deficiency results in apathy and depression while large doses result in restlessness, anxiety and sometimes, psychosis. Large doses may increase intracranial pressure.
iv. *GIT:* Glucocorticoids enhance the secretion of gastric acid and pepsin in the stomach and may aggravate acid peptic disease.
v. *Calcium metabolism:* Glucocorticoids inhibit absorption and enhance the renal excretion of calcium—they antagonise the effect of vitamin D on calcium absorption. Bone resorption takes place.
vi *Formed elements of blood:* Glucocorticoids have a lympholytic effect which is very prominent in lymphomas; but they increase the number of platelets and RBCs.
vii *Kidney:* They are essential for maintaining normal GFR.
viii. *Fetal lungs:* They have a vital role in the development of fetal lungs and stimulate the production of surfactants.

B. *Mineralocorticoid Actions*

Glucocorticoids have a weak mineralocorticoid action—cause some salt and water retention and potassium excretion. Some synthetic glucocorticoids are devoid of this activity.

Mechanism of Action

Glucocorticoids bring about their effects by activating the glucocorticoid receptors which are widely distributed in the body. They are nuclear receptors but in an inactivated state, they are found in the cytoplasm.

Corticosteroids enter the cells by simple diffusion, bind to specific receptors present in the cytoplasm (Fig. 38.4) and activate them. The drug–receptor complex is then

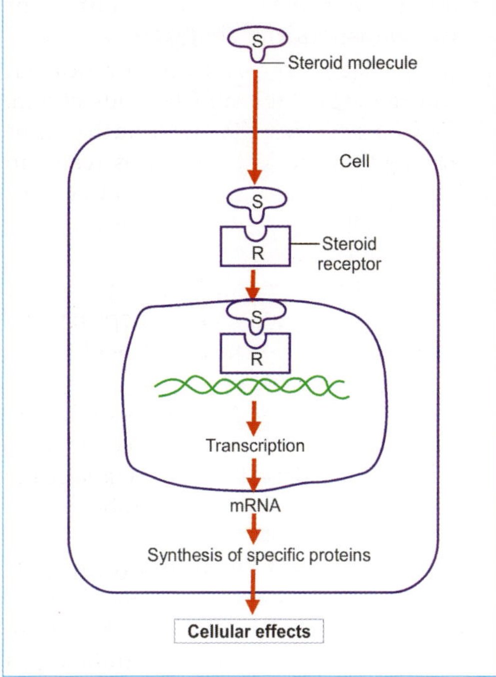

Fig. 38.4: Mechanism of action of corticosteroids

transported into the nucleus where it binds to specific sites on DNA (called glucocorticoid response elements or GRE) and induces the synthesis of specific mRNA. Such mRNA are transferred to the cytoplasm where they regulate the synthesis of new proteins that bring about the hormone effects. The glucocorticoid receptor is made up of 800 amino acids and has 3 domains—the glucocorticoid-binding domain, the DNA-binding domain and the transcription-activating domain.

PHARMACOKINETICS

Most glucocorticoids including natural and synthetic ones are well-absorbed orally. Hydrocortisone undergoes high first pass metabolism but synthetic corticoids have good bioavailability. Hydrocortisone is 90–95% bound to plasma proteins—corticosteroid binding globulin (CBG) or **transcortin** synthesized by the liver. Once the CBG is saturated, free plasma cortisol levels start increasing. The CBG levels increase in pregnancy and hyperthyroidism. The synthetic steroids have a greater affinity for albumin than CBG. Biological half-life is longer because of their mechanism of action. Glucocorticoids are metabolised by microsomal enzymes in the liver. They first undergo oxidation and reduction followed by conjugation. Sulphate and glucuronide **conjugation** produce inactive water-soluble compounds which are excreted by the kidneys. The t½ varies with each agent and we have short- intermediate- and long-acting agents (Table 38.1). Prednisone is a prodrug converted to prednisolone in the liver.

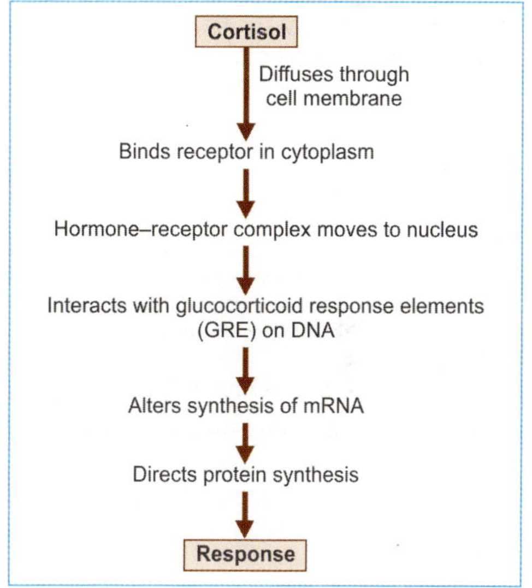

Preparations

Glucocorticoids are given by many routes—orally, parenterally, topically, by inhalation and nasal spray. They may also be injected intra-articularly. The synthetic analogs are more potent than hydrocortisone and have less or no mineralocorticoid activity.

- *Hydrocortisone*, the chief natural glucocorticoid is used orally and parenterally; in emergencies hydrocortisone hemisuccinate is used intravenously.

Table 38.1: Relative potency of some corticosteroids

Drug	*Glucocorticoid activity*	*Mineralocorticoid activity*	*Equivalent dose*
Short-acting (8–12 hr)			
Hydrocortisone	1	1	20 mg
Cortisone	0.8	0.8	25 mg
Intermediate-acting (18–36 hr)			
Prednisolone	4	0.8	5 mg
Methylprednisolone	5	0.5	4 mg
Triamcinolone	5	0	4 mg
Fludrocortisone	10	125	2 mg
Long-acting (36–54 hr)			
Paramethasone	10	0	2 mg
Dexamethasone	25	0	0.75 mg
Betamethasone	30	0	0.6 mg

Dose: For replacement, 20 mg in the morning, 10 mg in the afternoon orally. Pharmacotherapy—100 mg IV solution followed by 100 mg infusion every 8 hr. Efcorlin, Primacort 100, 200, 400 mg. Lycor Cream 1%.

- *Prednisolone* has potent glucocorticoid with mild mineralocorticoid activity. It is the most commonly used preparation.

  Dose: 5-60 mg WYSOLONE, EMSOLONE 5, 10, 20 mg tab. MEPSONATE, 0.5, 1 g inj. Pree-M 5, 10 mg/ml inj. 1% eye drops. MPA 40 mg/1 ml inj. RENISONE, SANPRED 1% eyedrops.

- *Prednisolone acetate*, RENISOL 1% eye drops.
- *Methylprednisolone* is similar to prednisolone and is used as retention enema in ulcerative colitis and for high dose pulse therapy. Depot preparation is available for the purpose.

  Dose: 4-32 mg 0.1%, MSLONE 4, 16 mg tab. SOLUMEDROL 4 mg tab, 80,160 mg inj OMNACORTIL Cream.

- Triamcinolone, dexamethasone and betamethasone have no mineralocorticoid activity but have selective and potent glucocorticoid effects.

  Triamcinolone: Dose: 4-20 mg KENACORT 4 mg tab 10 mg/ml inj.

  Dexamethasone: Dose: 0.5-5 mg oral, 4-20 mg IV/IM inj. DEXONA 0.5 mg tab, 4 mg/ml inj. LOSONE eye drops 0.01% w/v 5 ml.

- *Betamethasone:* Dose: 0.5-5 mg oral, 4-20 mg IV/IM. BETNESOL 0.5, 4 mg/ml inj, BETAMINE, SYNCORT 0.5 mg tab.

Deflazacort is a newer glucocorticoid with **no** mineralocorticoid activity. It is particularly useful in children as some studies have shown it to be better suited for them with fewer adverse effects (less growth retardation) on long-term use. DEFZA, DEFLAR 1, 6, 30 mg tab.

Special Preparations

Glucocorticoids are administered by local routes to deliver the drug directly to the site of action so that the dose requirement is reduced.

- *Topical preparations:* Several glucocorticoid preparations are available for topical use as creams, ointments, nasal and eye drops. Some of them also contain antibiotics (Table 38.2).
- *Inhalation:* Glucocorticoids are also available for inhalation (Table 38.3). Beclomethasone dipropionate, budesonide, fluticasone, mometasone furoate are available as aerosols for inhalation in bronchial asthma (*see* page 401).
- *Nasal spray:* Beclomethasone, triamcinolone acetonide, budesonide, flunisolide and mometasone are available as nasal spray for use in allergic rhinitis.

  BUDANASE 100 μg/actuation

- *Ophthalmic preparations:* Should be used carefully as immunosuppression may herald the growth of microorganisms.

  RENISOL 1% eye drops

- *Enema:* Hydrocortisone is available as enema for use in ulcerative colitis.

ADVERSE EFFECTS OF GLUCOCORTICOIDS

Adverse effects of glucocorticoids (Fig. 38.5) are dependent on the dose, duration of therapy and the relative potency of additional mineralocorticoid effects. Whenever possible, they should be used topically to avoid systemic effects. Single doses are harmless while short courses are well-tolerated. Prolonged use is associated with toxicity. Adverse effects include:

1. *Cushing's syndrome:* With characteristic appearance of moon face, supraclavicular hump, truncal obesity, muscle wasting, myopathy, thinning of the limbs and skin, easy bruising and purple striae. Cutaneous atrophy at the site can occur on prolonged topical use.

   Fine hair grows over the face, trunk and thighs; weight gain, acne may appear.
2. *Hyperglycaemia:* Increased protein breakdown and neoglucogenesis result in hyperglycaemia and sometimes diabetes mellitus may be precipitated.
3. *Susceptibility to infections:* Glucocorticoids increase the susceptibility and the severity of any infection may be more because of immunosuppression. Opportunistic infections—bacterial and fungal may occur. Previously dormant tuberculosis may become active.
4. *Osteoporosis:* Especially of the vertebrae is more common in the elderly.
5. *Avascular necrosis* of the bone due to restriction of blood flow through bone capillaries may cause joint pain, stiffness and restriction of movement. Head of the femur, humerus and distal part of femur may be affected. Growth in children may be suppressed.
6. *Peptic ulceration:* It may sometimes occur on prolonged therapy especially when other ulcerogenic drugs (e.g. NSAIDs) are used concurrently.
7. *Mental disturbances:* Alterations in behaviour can occur with high doses of steroids. Symptoms may range from insomnia, anxiety, nervousness, mood changes, euphoria, psychosis or depression.
8. *Cataract* and glaucoma may follow long-term use of glucocorticoids even as eye drops. Patients receiving long-term steroids should undergo eye examinations for these.
9. *Delayed wound healing:* Steroids may delay wound healing. If prolonged topical use is required this should be considered.
10. *Other effects:* Include raised intracranial pressure, convulsions, hypercoagulability of the blood and menstrual disorders.

Table 38.2: Some topical glucocorticoid preparations

Preparation	Strength
Hydrocortisone acetate (LYCORTIN oint)	1%
Hydrocortisone oral paste (ORABASE)	0.5%
Triamcinolone (LEDERCORT oint)	0.1%
Dexamethasone (DECADRON cream)	0.1%
Flucinolone acetonide (FLUCORT oint)	0.025%
Betamethasone dipropionate/valerate (BETNOVATE oint, cream)	0.025%
Beclomethasone dipropionate (BECLATE cream)	0.025%
Clobetasol propionate (TOPIFORT cream)	0.05%

Table 38.3: Steroids for inhalation

Drug	Dose
Beclomethasone (BECLATE INHALER)	50, 100 μg
Budesonide (BUDECORT)	200 μg/metered dose
Fluticasone (FLOHALE)	25, 50, 150 μg/metered dose

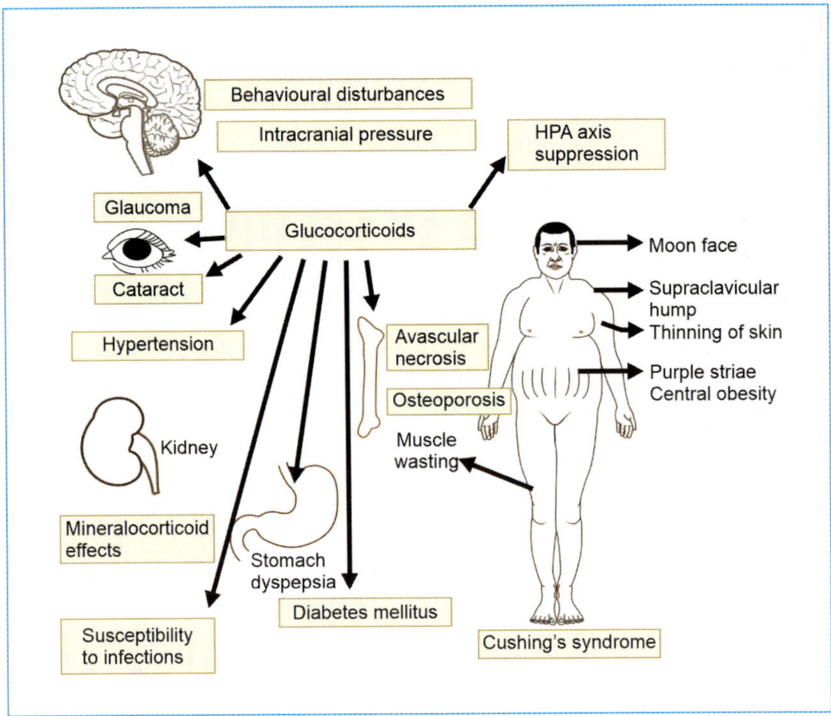

Fig. 38.5: Adverse effects of glucocorticoids

11. *HPA axis suppression:* Depends on the dose, duration and time of administration. After administration of steroids for >2 weeks, HPA axis suppression is likely to develop and on continued use adrenal cortex gradually atrophies due to feedback inhibition. If steroid administration is suddenly stopped, acute adrenal insufficiency results. Hence after prolonged administration, steroids should be tapered before withdrawal to allow HPA axis to recover. Prior to surgery or general anaesthesia, it is advisable to elicit proper drug history. If the patient has received long-term glucocorticoids within the previous six months, it is prudent to administer prophylactic hydrocortisone to avoid shock. If the patient is exposed

Compare and Contrast

Hydrocortisone and Dexamethasone

Features	***Hydrocortisone***	***Dexamethasone***
Source	Natural	Synthetic
Mineralocorticoid activity	Present	Absent
Potency	Less potent	More potent
Equivalent dose	20 mg	0.75 mg
Plasma t½	8–12 hr	36–54 hr
Duration of action	Short	Long
Production in the body	Endogenous	Not produced (exogenous administration)

to minor stress, steroid supplements should be given. Two weeks of use of >20 mg hydrocortisone/day needs tapering of the dose.

In order to minimize HPA axis suppression, lowest effective dose of a glucocorticoid for the shortest possible period should be used. The drug should be given in a single morning dose. Administration on alternate days is found to be associated with least/no HPA axis suppression and whenever possible this measure should be followed, especially when long-term steroids are needed.

12. *Mineralocorticoid effects:* Salt and water retention and oedema add to weight gain; hypokalaemia and hypertension are rare with drugs having selective glucocorticoid activity.

Uses

A. **Replacement therapy**

i. Acute adrenal insufficiency is an emergency condition that could be precipitated by an infection, trauma, stress or sudden withdrawal of steroids. Symptoms include nausea, vomiting, weakness, hypotension, dehydration, hyponatraemia and hyperkalaemia. Intravenous hydrocortisone hemisuccinate 100 mg bolus is given immediately followed by infusion 100 mg every 4–6 hours. The dose may be repeated depending on the patient's condition. Once the patient recovers, to be switched over to oral preparations. Immediate correction of fluid and electrolyte balance is important. When acute adrenal insufficiency is not confirmed, dexamethasone (4 mg IV) should be used in place of hydrocortisone because dexamethasone does not interfere with the estimation of cortisol levels for diagnosis.

ii. Primary adrenal insufficiency (Addison's disease). Oral hydrocortisone 20–40 mg daily is given with additional fludrocortisone (a mineralocorticoid).

iii. Congenital adrenal hyperplasia is characterised by impaired synthesis of corticosteroids due to deficiency of some enzymes involved in synthesis. As a result, ACTH levels rise resulting in adrenal hyperplasia. It is a familial disease. Excess amounts of the precursor of adrenal hormone are released. Depending on the deficient enzyme, there could be production of more androgens leading to virilization or mineralocorticoid excess leading to hypertension. Hydrocortisone is given daily 0.6 mg/kg/day in divided doses and if mineralocorticoids are also deficient, fludrocortisone (0.2 mg/day) may be added. If a member of such family gets pregnant, it may be associated with a risk for congenital adrenal hyperplasia.

B. **For diagnostic purpose:** Glucocorticoids can be used for many diagnostic tests. **Dexamethasone suppression test** is used in the diagnosis of Cushing's syndrome. Dexamethasone inhibits the release of corticotrophin-releasing hormone (by negative feedback) but does not interfere with the measurement of endogenous glucocorticoid levels in the plasma. Suppression of cortisol production indicates that HPA axis is intact.

C. **Pharmacotherapy:** Glucocorticoids have been used in a variety of nonendocrine conditions where they are of palliative value, but may even be life saving. Their **anti-inflammatory activity** is the basis for their use in many of these conditions while immunosuppressive effects help in some.

1. *Rheumatoid arthritis:* In progressive disease, steroids are given with NSAIDs. If 1–2 joints are involved, intra-articular injections are preferred. If multiple joints are involved, systemic steroids are given.
2. *Osteoarthritis:* Steroids are given as intra-articular injections in acute exacerbations

with strict aseptic precautions. A minimum of 3 months interval should be given between two injections of steroids into the joint. Repeated injections can result in joint destruction.

3. *Rheumatic carditis:* Severely ill-patients with fever and carditis not responding adequately to NSAIDs require glucocorticoids in addition.
4. *Acute gout:* When treatment with NSAIDs has not been successful and colchicine is not tolerated, a short course of prednisolone is used as an adjuvant orally or as intra-articular injection.
5. *Allergic diseases:* Allergic diseases like angioneurotic oedema, hay fever, serum sickness, contact dermatitis, urticaria, drug reactions and anaphylaxis—steroids are indicated. Steroids are slow acting and in less severe cases, antihistamines should be preferred. For allergic reactions on the skin, topical steroids may be used.
6. *Shock:* Severe inflammatory reaction may be the cause for septic shock. An infusion of hydrocortisone 100 mg over 8 hr for 5–7 days may be life saving in such patients. Glucocorticoids act directly on the vascular smooth muscle and indirectly by sensitizing the adrenergic receptors to the effects of sympathomimetics.
7. *Bronchial asthma*
   - Acute exacerbations—a short course of oral prednisolone
   - Status asthmaticus—intravenous hydro-cortisone hemisuccinate 100–200 mg repeated after 8 hr or methyl-prednisolone 60 mg every 6 hours followed by oral prednisolone 40–60 mg per day for 5 days till the patient recovers. Prednisolone should then be tapered.
   - *Chronic asthma:* Steroids are used as supplements to bronchodilators. Inhalational steroids are used and in more severe cases low dose oral prednisolone is indicated. COPD exacerbation may be treated with short courses of prednisolone.
8. *Collagen diseases:* Like polyarthritis nodosa, lupus erythematosus, polymyositis, Wegener's granulomatosis and other rheumatoid disorders respond to glucocorticoids—the first-line drugs and may be life saving. Higher doses of prednisolone is given for 6 weeks and tapered over another 6 weeks.
9. *Eye diseases:* Allergic conjunctivitis, uveitis, optic neuritis and other inflammatory conditions are treated with glucocorticoid eye drops or ointment. Long-term glucocorticoid administration can increase IOP which should be monitored. In ocular infections, steroids are contraindicated.
10. *Renal diseases:* Renal diseases, like nephrotic syndrome, are treated with steroids. Glucocorticoids are the first-line drugs. Prednisolone is given for 6 weeks and tapered over another 6 weeks.
11. *Skin diseases:* Atopic dermatitis, seborrhoeic dermatitis, inflammatory dermatoses and other local skin conditions are treated with topical steroids. Systemic steroids are **life-saving** in serious infections like pemphigus, exfoliative dermatitis and Stevens-Johnson syndrome.
12. *Gastrointestinal diseases:* Mild inflammatory bowel diseases, like ulcerative colitis, and Crohn's disease, are treated with steroid retention enema while severe cases need oral prednisolone. **Budesonide** may be given as retention enema or as oral enteric coated capsule so that it is released in the ileum and colon. It causes fewer side effects when compared to other glucocorticoids.
13. *Liver diseases:* Steroids are useful in conditions like autoimmune chronic active hepatitis and may be tried in alcoholic hepatitis.
14. *Haematologic disorders:* Like purpura and haemolytic anaemia having immunological aetiology respond to steroids.

15. *Cerebral oedema:* Large doses of dexamethasone or betamethasone reduce cerebral oedema occurring in some malignancies.
16. *Malignancies:* Because of their lympholytic effects and inhibition of cell proliferation, steroids are used in the treatment of acute lymphocytic leukaemia and lymphomas-as a component of combination chemotherapy. Steroids are used for rapid symptomatic relief in other malignancies like breast cancer.
17. *Lung diseases:* Apart from bronchial asthma, steroids are used in other diseases like aspiration pneumonia and prevention of infant respiratory distress syndrome. Glucocorticoids hasten the lung maturation and production of surfactant and, therefore, may be given in late pregnancy. Betamethasone 12 mg IM to the mother and repeated the next day (if premature delivery is expected) reduces the incidence of respiratory distress at birth. It is also used for the treatment of acute respiratory distress syndrome (ARDS).
18. *Organ transplantation:* For prevention and treatment of graft rejection, high doses of prednisolone are started at the time of surgery with immunosuppressive agents.
19. *Thyroid storm:* Glucocorticoids inhibit the peripheral conversion of T_4 to T_3 and may be of additional value.
20. *Others:* Glucocorticoids are useful in:
    - Sarcoidosis to induce remission.
    - *Pneumocystis jiroveci* pneumonia in patients with AIDS—glucocorticoids reduce the risk of respiratory failure and decrease mortality.
    - Haemolytic anaemia—glucocorticoids reduce the autoimmune destruction of erythrocytes in haemolytic anaemia.

Precautions and Contraindications

Glucocorticoids should be used with caution in several conditions and are contraindicated in some of them. They should be monitored particularly on long-term use for the development of diabetes mellitus, peptic ulcer, hypertension, osteoporosis and exacerbation of dorment tuberculosis. Contraindications are given in Table 38.4.

Drug Interactions

- Drugs like erythromycin, ketoconazole, cyclosporine and isoniazid inhibit the metabolism of glucocorticoids resulting in an increase in the plasma levels of glucocorticoids.
- Microsomal enzyme inducers, like phenobarbitone and rifampicin, enhance the rate of metabolism of glucocorticoids.

MINERALOCORTICOIDS

The most important natural mineralocorticoid is aldosterone, synthesized in the zona glomerulosa of the adrenal cortex. Small amounts of desoxycorticosterone is also released which also has some glucocorticoid activity.

Actions: Mineralocorticoids promote sodium and water retention by distal renal tubules with loss of potassium. They act by binding to the mineralocorticoid receptor.

Adverse effects include weight gain, oedema, hypertension and hypokalaemia.

Table 38.4: Precautions and contraindications to glucocorticoid therapy

Steroids should be used with caution in
1. Peptic ulcer
2. Hypertension
3. Infections like tuberculosis and varicella
4. Diabetes mellitus
5. Ocular infections particularly viral infections
6. Osteoporosis
7. Psychoses
8. Epilepsy
9. CCF
10. Glaucoma
11. Renal failure
12. Myopathy
13. Pancreatitis
14. Hepatic diseases

Fludrocortisone has predominantly mineralocorticoid properties and is used for replacement therapy in aldosterone deficiency as in Addison's disease. Although aldosterone is the principal natural mineralocorticoid, it is not used therapeutically since it is not effective orally. FLORICORT 100 mg tab.

Mineralocorticoid antagonists include spironolactone and eplerenone (*see* page 291).

INHIBITORS OF ADRENAL STEROIDS SYNTHESIS

Certain drugs inhibit the synthesis of adrenal steroids by inhibiting certain enzymes involved in steroid synthesis. They are used in Cushing's syndrome and some prostatic and breast cancers.

- **Aminoglutethimide:** Blocks the first step in the synthesis of steroids, i.e. it inhibits the conversion of cholesterol to pregnenolone (*see* Fig. 41.3) and thus inhibits the synthesis of all corticosteroids.
- **Ketoconazole,** an antifungal drug, inhibits adrenal and gonadal steroid synthesis by inhibiting several enzymes involved in it. The dose needed is higher than the antifungal dose.
- **Metyrapone** inhibits the enzyme 11 beta hydroxylase and thereby inhibits the synthesis of cortisol and corticosterone. The fall in cortisol levels stimulates compensatory increase in ACTH secretion by negative feedback.
- **Mitotane:** Produces atrophy of the zona fasciculata and zona reticularis leading to reduced plasma levels of corticoids.
- **Trilostane:** Inhibits the enzyme beta-17-hydroxysteroid dehydrogenase and thereby inhibits the synthesis of adrenal and gonadal steroid hormones.
- **Abiraterone:** It is an irreversible inhibitor of 17-alpha-hydroxylase and CYP 17 activity—reduces the synthesis of cortisol and gonadal steroids.
- **Mifepristone**—a progesterone receptor antagonist also blocks glucocorticoid receptors (*see* page 486).

Adverse effects of glucocorticoid synthesis inhibitors include hirsutism and water retention leading to oedema and weight gain.

Uses

1. *Diagnostic tests:*
   a. To test for adrenal function (HPA-axis)—a normal response to metyrapone indicates normal HPA-axis.
   b. To test for pituitary function—ACTH levels are measured after (8 hr after) metyrapone to estimate the ability of the pituitary to produce ACTH.
2. *Cushing's syndrome:* While the cause for Cushing's syndrome is being detected, metyrapone can be used to relieve the symptoms. It is the only drug in this group to be found safe in pregnant women with Cushing's syndrome.
3. *Cancer:* Abiraterone is used in refractory prostatic cancers to produce medical castration. Trilastane may be used in breast cancer in post-menopausal women.

Clinical Pharmacology

- Short courses of glucocorticoids are safe.
- 3–4 weeks of prednisolone 20–30 mg or equivalent daily can cause HPA axis suppression—glucocorticoids should be tapered.
- Prednisolone is the most commonly used glucocorticoid.
- Glucocorticoids should be used with great caution on the eye.
- Other gastric irritant drugs, like NSAIDs, should be avoided with glucocorticoids.

[1] From Medical Council of India, *Competency based Undergraduate Curriculum for the Indian Medical Graduate*, 2018;1:136–144.

CHAPTER 39

Estrogens, Progestins, Hormonal Contraceptives and Drugs used in Infertility

Competency achievement: The student should be able to:

PH 1.37 Describe the mechanisms of action, types, doses, side effects, indications and contraindications of the drugs used as **sex hormones, their analogues** and anterior pituitary hormones.[1]

PHYSIOLOGICAL CONSIDERATION

At puberty, the ovary begins its cyclic function which stretches over 30–40 years characterised by regular episodes of uterine bleeding.

The hypothalamus releases the GnRH in pulses which stimulates the release of FSH and LH from the anterior pituitary (Fig. 39.1). At the beginning of each cycle, a number of follicles begin to enlarge in response to FSH. After 5–6 days, one of the follicles begin to develop more rapidly. The granulosa cells of this follicle multiply and under the influence of LH and FSH, synthesize estrogens. Estrogen inhibits FSH release, resulting in regression of the smaller follicles. The ovarian follicle consists of an ovum surrounded by a fluid-filled antrum, lined by granulosa and theca cells. Just before the midcycle, the oestrogen secretion reaches a peak, stimulating a brief surge in FSH and LH levels which results in ovulation by around the 14th day of the cycle.

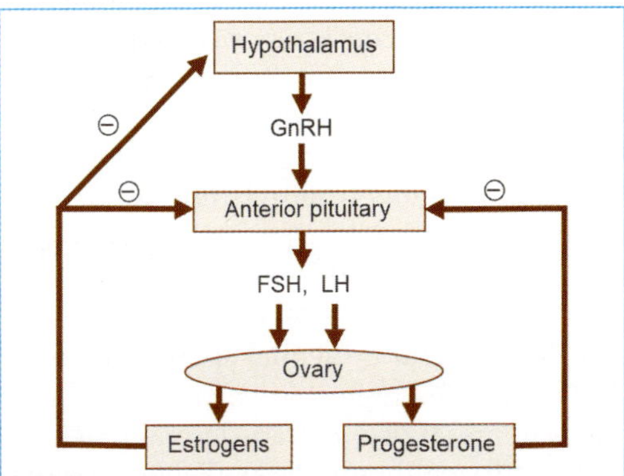

Fig. 39.1: Regulation of secretion of gonadal hormones

ESTROGENS

The estrogens are produced by the ovaries, placenta and in small amounts by the adrenals, testes and by peripheral aromatisation of the androgens. During the first part of the menstrual cycle, estrogens are produced by the granulosa cells by aromatisation of the androgens derived from theca cells in the ovarian follicle. The major estrogens are estradiol, estrone and estriol (Fig. 39.2). Estradiol is converted to estrone and estriol by the liver and other tissues. Some chemical alterations have been made in the structure of natural estrogens to produce synthetic estrogens. Some nonsteroidal compounds with estrogenic activity have also been synthesized—like diethylstilbestrol, dienestrol and hexestrol.

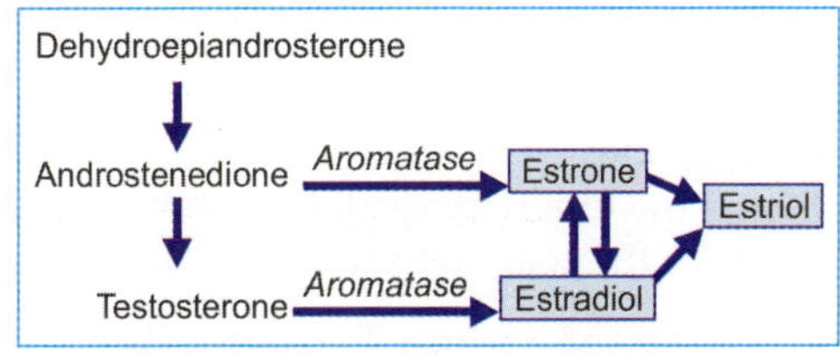

Fig. 39.2: Biosynthesis of estrogens

Estrogens include:
1. *Natural estrogens*
   - Estradiol, estrone, estriol.
2. *Synthetic estrogens*
   - Systemic—ethinyl estradiol, stilbestrol, mestranol.
   - Topical—dienestrol.
3. *SERMs*
   - Tamoxifen, Raloxifene, Toremifene, Ormeloxifene
4. *SERDs*
   - Clomiphene, Fulvestrant.

Estrogen receptors are nuclear receptors and are of two types. ERα and ERβ.

Distribution: ERα—female reproductive tract, breast, blood vessels and hypothalamus. ERβ—ovaries and prostate.

Selective agonists of these receptor subtypes are being developed. Selective estrogen receptor modulators (SERMs) are now available for clinical use. Selective estrogen receptor down regulators (SERDs) have also been developed.

Actions: Estrogens are required for:
1. The normal maturation of the female reproductive tract.
2. Development of secondary sexual characters in the female.
3. Stimulation of preovulatory endometrium.
4. *Metabolic effects:* Estrogen promotes retention of sodium, nitrogen and fluid in the tissue.
5. *Integrity of skeleton:* Estrogens inhibit the resorption of bone and maintain the bone mass. They promote the fusion of epiphyses.
6. Estrogens are important for the maintenance of normal structure of the skin and blood vessels in women.
7. Estrogens decrease plasma LDL cholesterol and raise HDL cholesterol and triglycerides.
8. Effect on blood coagulation—estrogens enhance the coagulability of the blood.

Mechanism of action: Estrogens bind to estrogen receptors. Estrogens bring about their effects by stimulating the specific estrogen receptors on the target cells. The estrogen—receptor complex moves to the nucleus and binds to the estrogen response elements (ERE) which are present on the target gene and bring about the synthesis of specific proteins involved in the effects of estrogen. Some of the quick actions may be mediated by other mechanisms not related to the genomic mechanisms.

Pharmacokinetics: Natural estrogens are metabolised rapidly in the gut—hence are not effective orally; they have a short t½. Synthetic oestrogens are orally effective and are longer-acting. All estrogens get absorbed through the skin and mucous membrane. They are largely bound to plasma proteins (globin). Estrogens are metabolised by glucuronide and sulfate conjugation in the liver. They also undergo enterohepatic circulation.

Adverse Effects

- Nausea, breast tenderness, migraine headaches, hyperpigmentation, hypertension and cholestasis (gallstones are common) may be seen. In men, gynaecomastia and feminization can occur.
- Estrogen therapy can cause postmenopausal uterine bleeding and endometrial hyperplasia. Estrogen should be given cyclically and a progesterone added—to allow withdrawal bleeding and also to avoid endometrial hyperplasia.
- *Cancers:* Increased incidence of endometrial and breast cancers is reported on long-term use of only estrogens. Therefore, it should be combined with progesterone.
- *Teratogenicity:* When given to a pregnant lady, estrogens (diethylstilbesterol) may cause:
  - In female child—increased risk of vaginal and cervical cancers.
  - In male child—genital abnormalities.

Preparations: Estrogens are available for oral and parenteral use. A transdermal patch for cyclic estrogen therapy is available. Estrogen vaginal cream and vaginal pessaries are also available. Conjugated estrogens are available as tablets, injections and vaginal cream.

Cenestin is a synthetic conjugated estrogen available as tablets (0.625 mg) for control of menopausal symptoms.

CONJUGASE, ESPAUZ, PREMARIN 0.625 mg, 1.25 mg, 0.3 mg, 25 mg inj, 0.625 mg/g VG cream.

Uses

Estrogens are used for replacement in deficiency states, to suppress endogenous production of related hormones as in contraception and in estrogen responsive states (Table 39.1).

1. *Replacement therapy*
   - *In primary hypogonadism:* Estrogen started at 11–13 years of age on diagnosis of hypogonadism stimulates the development of secondary sexual characters and menstruation. It also requires supplementation with progestins at appropriate times to induce menstruation.
   - *Postmenopausal syndrome:* Due to decreased estrogen production at menopause, hot flushes, anxiety, fatigue, sweating, muscle and joints pain are common. Other longer-lasting changes including osteoporosis, genital atrophy, skin changes, increased risk of cardiovascular disease, sleep disturbances and psychological disturbances may be seen. Estrogens given in low doses are highly effective in reversing most of the changes.

Table 39.1: Uses of estrogens and progestins

Estrogens	*Progestins*
1. HRT • *Primary hypogonadism* • *Postmenopausal syndrome*	1. HRT
2. Contraception	2. Contraception
3. Senile vaginitis	3. Dysmenorrhoea
4. Osteoporosis	4. DUB
5. Carcinoma prostate	5. Endometriosis
6. DUB	6. Premenstrual syndrome
7. Dysmenorrhoea	7. Endometrial cancer
	8. Endometrial hyperplasia

2. *Senile vaginitis:* It is common in elderly women due to reduced estrogen synthesis by the ovary. Estrogen cream is used topically. It reverts the changes in vaginal cytology to premenopausal pattern.
3. *Osteoporosis:* In postmenopausal osteoporosis, estrogens restore calcium balance and need to be given for a long time. SERMs are preferred over estrogens for this purpose.
4. *Hormonal contraceptives:* Estrogens are used with progestins; Estrogen was used as monotherapy for postcoital contraception but not used now.
5. *Dysmenorrhoea:* Estrogens combined with progestins suppress ovulation and such anovulatory cycles are painless.
6. *Dysfunctional uterine bleeding:* Estrogens are used as adjuvants to progesterone.
7. *Carcinoma prostate:* It is an androgen dependent tumour. Estrogens antagonise the action of androgens, suppress androgen production and are useful for palliative therapy.
8. *Acne:* Secretion of androgens at puberty results in acne. Though estrogen helps to reduce acne, it should be avoided since safer topical drugs are available.

Contraindications: Estrogen-dependent tumours, liver disease and thromboembolic disorders.

SELECTIVE ESTROGEN RECEPTOR MODULATORS (SERMs) AND ANTI-ESTROGENS

Tamoxifen was earlier considered to be an estrogen antagonist (Table 39.2). However now it is understood that it acts as an agonist, antagonist or partial agonist depending on the site. Raloxifene, toremifene and ormeloxifene have actions similar to tamoxifen and are all termed selective estrogen receptor modulators (SERMs). SERMs include **tamoxifen, raloxifene, toremifene, ormeloxifene, clomiphene** and

Table 39.2: Antagonists of sex hormones and their uses

Hormone	*Receptor antagonist*	*Uses of antagonist*
Estrogen	Tamoxifen	Breast cancer
	Raloxifene	Osteoporosis
	Clomiphene citrate	• Infertility • *In vitro* fertilization
	Fulvestrant	Breast cancer
	Ormeloxifene	DUB, contraception
Progesterone	Mifepristone	Termination of pregnancy
Androgen	Flutamide Cyproterone	• Carcinoma prostate • Hypersexuality in men • Female hirsutism

fulvestrant. SERMs have tissue-selective estrogenic activities, i.e.

- They have agonistic effects on bone, lipid metabolism, brain and liver.
- Antagonists at breast, pituitary and endometrium.
- Partial agonists at genitourinary epithelium, bone remodelling and cholesterol metabolism.

Tamoxifen is a nonsteroidal agent. By its tissue selective activity on the estrogen receptor, tamoxifen has the following actions:

- Inhibits the proliferation of tumour cells in the breast.
- Stimulates the proliferation of the endometrium.
- Reduces bone resorption.
- Decreases total cholesterol and LDL cholesterol but has no effect on HDL or triglycerides.
- Increases the risk of deep vein thrombosis and pulmonary embolism.

Tamoxifen is effective orally. It has two elimination phases with half lives of 7–14 hr and 4–11 days and, therefore, a long duration of action. It is metabolized by microsomal enzymes in the liver and undergoes enterohepatic circulation.

Preparations: TOMIFEN, MAMOFEN 10, 20 mg tab.

Side effects include hot flashes, nausea, vomiting, anorexia,vaginal dryness, bleeding, cataract and skin rashes. Tamoxifen increases the risk of endometrial cancer because of its agonistic activity on the uterus. Also it almost doubles the risk of thromboembolism.

Uses

Breast cancer: Tamoxifen is used in the palliation of advanced breast cancer in postmenopausal women with estrogen receptor positive tumours.

Tamoxifen has also been tried for the prophylaxis of breast cancer in women with a high risk for it.

Raloxifene a nonsteriodal SERM, acts as an estrogen receptor agonist in the bone. It also improves the bone density in postmenopausal women. In women with postmenopausal osteoporosis, raloxifene has antiresorptive effects on the bone. It reduces bone loss and may even help to gain bone mass. Raloxifene also lowers LDL and total cholesterol.

It acts as an estrogen antagonist in the breast due to which it reduces the incidence of breast cancer. Raloxifene does not stimulate the uterine endometrial proliferation hence no risk of carcinoma.

Raloxifene has poor oral bioavailability, has a t½ of 28 hr, metabolised by glucuronidation and excreted through the gut.

Dose: 60 mg/day. RALOX, RALOFEN, 60 mg tab.

Adverse effects include hot flushes, leg cramps and an increased risk of deep vein thrombosis and pulmonary embolism.

Uses: Raloxifene is indicated for the prevention and treatment of postmenopausal osteoporosis.

Toremifene has actions similar to tamoxifen and is indicated in the treatment of metastatic breast cancer in postmenopausal women.

Ormeloxifene or centchroman (*see* page 493) has antagonistic effects on the estrogen receptors in the uterus and breast tissue. It prevents the endometrial proliferation. It prevents excessive bleeding in anovulatory cycles at the time of menopause. Ormeloxifene can cause headache, nausea, weight gain, rise in BP, and prolonged menstrual cycles. It has been tried in dysfunctional uterine bleeding and is a popular contraceptive.

Dose: 120 mg twice a week for 2-3 months followed by 60 mg weekly for the next 3 months.

CENTRON 30 mg, SEVISTA 60 mg tab.

Clomiphene citrate binds to the estrogen receptors ERα and ERβ and acts as a competitive inhibitor of endogenous oestrogens. Like tamoxifen, it is also a partial agonist. Clomiphene opposes the negative feedback of endogenous oestrogens on the hypothalamo-pituitary axis resulting in increased gonadotrophin secretion (FSH and LH levels increase) and thereby induces ovulation. Thus in women with polycystic ovarian syndrome and anovulatory cycles, clomiphene effectively induces ovulation.

Side effects include ovarian hyperstimulation resulting in multiple pregnancy, ovarian cysts, hot flushes, headache and skin rashes. It could also increase the risk of ovarian tumours.

Uses

1. *Infertility:* Clomiphene citrate is used in infertility due to ovarian disorders. It is given orally, 50 mg daily for 5 days starting from 2 to day 6 of the cycle; course may be repeated for a few cycles till ovulation occurs.
2. *In vitro fertilization:* Clomiphene-induced ovulation is also useful in *in vitro* fertilization.
3. *PCOS:* Polycystic ovarian syndrome is often associated with infertility. Clomiphene may be used to induce ovulation.

Cyclofenil is structurally similar to clomiphene and can be used to induce ovulation. Given orally 200 mg BD for 10 days starting on the third day of menstruation and the cycles may be repeated, if required.

Fulvestrant is an estrogen receptor antagonist. It has affinity for both ERα and ERβ and blocks these receptors. It acts as an antagonist at all tissues with estrogen receptors. The estrogen receptors are also degraded and down regulated because of which it is also called a **selective estrogen receptor down** (SERD) **regulator**. It is given as IM depot preparation of 250 mg once a month.

It can cause headache, hot flushes and nausea.

Fulvestrant is indicated in breast cancer resistant to tamoxifen.

Preparation: FULVENAT 250 mg inj—once a month.

ESTROGEN SYNTHESIS INHIBITORS

1. *GnRH agonists* administered continuously suppress the biosynthesis of estrogens.
2. *Aminoglutethimide* inhibits the synthesis of all steroids by inhibiting the activity of aromatase—an enzyme involved in steroidogenesis.
3. *Aromatase inhibitors*

Aromatase is the enzyme which catalyses the final step in the synthesis of estrogen from testosterone. **Formastane** and **exemastane** are steroid compounds which irreversibly inhibit aromatase while **anostrozole, letrozole, vorozole** and **fadrozole** are not steroids and the aromatase inhibition is reversible. Both circulatory and local estrogen levels drastically decline—they are very effective in suppressing the growth of breast cancer cells even in patients with tamoxifen resistant tumours. Moreover, they have the advantage over tamoxifen that they do not increase the risk of thromboembolism or endometrial cancer. Hence aromatase inhibitors are the preferred drugs in the treatment of breast cancer.

Anastrozole, letrozole and fadrozole are orally effective. Anastrazole is longer acting and may be given once daily. Exemastane in addition has weak androgenic activity.

Uses

1. Aromatase inhibitors are used as first-line drugs or as adjuvants following mastectomy as well as for palliation in advanced breast cancers in postmenopausal women.
2. They are also used as ovulation-inducing agents in infertility.

Letrozole: Dose: 2.5 mg BD. FEOFER, LETZOL, ONCOLET 2.5 mg tab

Anastrozole: Dose: 1 mg OD. ALTRAZ, ARMOTRAZ, ALTROL 1 mg tab.

PROGESTINS

Natural progestins: Progesterone is the natural progestin synthesized in the ovary and placenta. It is also synthesized by the testis and adrenals where it acts as a precursor of various steroid hormones (*see* under corticosteroids).

Synthetic progestins: Several progesterone compounds have been synthesized which differ from natural progesterone in some properties. Third generation synthetic progestins include desogestrel, norgestimate and gestodene. They have very weak or no androgenic activity.

Progestins

- *Natural*
  - Progesterone
- *Synthetic*
  - Medroxyprogesterone acetate
  - Allylestrenol, megestrol
  - Norethisterone acetate
  - Lynestrenol, norethindrone
  - Levonorgestrel
- *Newer synthetic progestins* (third generation progestins with no androgenic activity)
  - Norgestimate, desogestrol, gestodene

Actions

1. *Uterus:* The secretory changes in the endometrium like increased tortuosity of the glands are due to progesterone. In pregnancy, decidual changes in the endometrium take place under the influence of progesterone. Progesterone is very important for the maintenance of pregnancy (Progestin = favours pregnancy).
2. *Cervix:* The watery cervical secretions are changed to a viscid scanty secretion by progesterone.
3. *Vagina:* Vaginal epithelium changes to that seen in pregnancy.
4. *Mammary gland:* Along with estrogen, progesterone is responsible for the development of the secretory apparatus in the breast and prepares the gland for lactation.
5. *Body temperature:* Increase in the body temperature by 1°C during luteal phase beginning at ovulation is due to progesterone.

Pharmacokinetics

Natural progesterones are rapidly absorbed but undergo high first pass metabolism. Synthetic progestins are orally effective, are bound to globulins and have a longer t½. They are metabolised in the liver and the active metabolites pregnenalone and pregnanediol undergo glucuronide conjugation and are excreted in the urine.

Preparations

1. Progesterone Dose: 100–400 mg OD oral, 10–100 mg IM. LUPIGESTRONE 50 mg/4 ml inj. GESTONE 100 mg, 200 mg Cap. 50 mg/ml inj. NATUROGEST 100, 200, 400 mg cap.
2. Medroxyprogesterone acetate 5–20 mg OD-BD oral, 50–150 mg IM every 1–3 months. PROVERA, MODUS 2.5, 10 mg tab. Depot-Provera 150 mg/ml inj
3. Allyl Estrenol 10–40 mg/day. GESTANIN, MAINTANE 5 mg tab.
4. Norethindrone 5–10 mg OD-BD oral. NORGEST, PRIMOLUT-N 5 mg tab.

Adverse Effects

Headache, breast engorgement, rise in body temperature, oedema, acne and mood swings may be seen. Progesterone is teratogenic. Some progestins (nortestosterone derivatives) can cause virilisation of the female foetus.

Progestins with androgenic activity are more likely to cause weight gain, acne and hirsutism. If these are significant, the preparation can be changed to one with no androgenic activity.

Uses

1. *Contraception* (*see* page 488).
2. *Hormone replacement therapy (HRT):* Progestins are combined with estrogens in HRT of postmenopausal women (given cyclically). Estrogen administration increases the risk of endometrial cancer—supplementing it with progestin counters this risk.
3. *Ovarian suppression:* Progestins are used to suppress ovulation in dysmenorrhoea, endometriosis, dysfunctional uterine bleeding (DUB) and premenstrual syndrome. After stoping the treatment, ovulatory function resumes but often may take a long time.
4. *Threatened or habitual abortion:* Efficacy in this condition is not proved. Most such patients have no deficiency of progesterone—yet have been used quite often for this indication.
5. *Endometrial carcinoma:* High doses of progestins are used as a palliative measure in cases with metastasis.
6. *To delay premature labour:* Progestins have been tried and the results are encouraging.
7. *Endometrial hyperplasia:* Progesterone administration for long time—up to 1 year is used to suppress endometrial hyperplasia.
8. *Diagnostic:* To test for estrogen secretion in women with amenorrhoea, progesterone for 5 days should be followed by withdrawal bleeding, if estrogen levels are normal.
9. *Postponement of menstruation:* Administration of progesterone in the 2nd half of menstrual cycle prolongs the luteal phase and thereby postpones the begining of menstruation. Norethisterone 5 mg is given orally—started early in the second half of the menstrual cycle. Higher doses are needed, if started in the latter part of the second half of the cycle.

Other Progesterone Derivatives

Danazol is a derivative of ethisterone (17α ethinyl testosterone). It has weak progestational, androgenic and glucocorticoid activities. It inhibits the midcycle surge (but not the basal secretion) of FSH and LH in women. This reduction of ovarian function results in atrophic changes in the endometrium.

Danazol is primarily used in the treatment of endometriosis. It is also used in menorrhagia, fibrocystic disease of the breast, gynaecomastia and is tried in some disorders of allergic aetiology like idiopathic thrombocytopenic purpura, angioedema, haemophilia and Christmas disease.

Danazol can cause side effects like hot flushes, oedema, weight gain, acne, headache, adrenal suppression and hepatotoxicity.

ANTIPROGESTINS AND PROGESTERONE RECEPTOR MODULATORS

Mifepristone

Mifepristone (RU 486) has antiprogestational as well as antiglucocorticoid activity. It binds to the progesterone receptors and blocks the actions of progesterone. It is a progesterone receptor modulator—acts as both a competitive antagonist and a partial agonist of progesterone receptors. When given in early pregnancy—abortion occurs (Fig. 39.3).

Mechanisms of Action

- Mifepristone blocks the progesterone receptors in the uterus which causes decidual breakdown; blastocyst gets detached, HCG and progesterone secretions fall. This in turn increases prostaglandin levels and stimulate uterine contractions. It also softens the cervix and facilitates expulsion of the blastocyst.
- If given during the follicular phase—mifepristone prevents the midcycle surge of gonadotrophins and delays ovulation.
- Mifepristone has leuteolytic properties and may act as an emergency contraceptive.
- Mifepristone also binds to glucocorticoid receptors and acts as an antagonist at these receptors because of which it may be useful in Cushing's syndrome, endometriosis and breast cancer.

Pure antagonists at the progesterone receptors are being studied.

Pharmacokinetics

Though mifepristone is absorbed on oral use, bioavailabilty is about 25%. It is metabolised in the liver by CYP3A4, undergoes entero-hepatic circulation and is excreted through the gut. As the metabolites are also active, the t½ is long—20–40 hr.

Preparations: MT PILL, UNDO, 200 mg tab.

Adverse Effects

Nausea, vomiting, headache and uterine cramps are common. Severe bleeding and infection can occur and require caution and immediate treatment. When used for

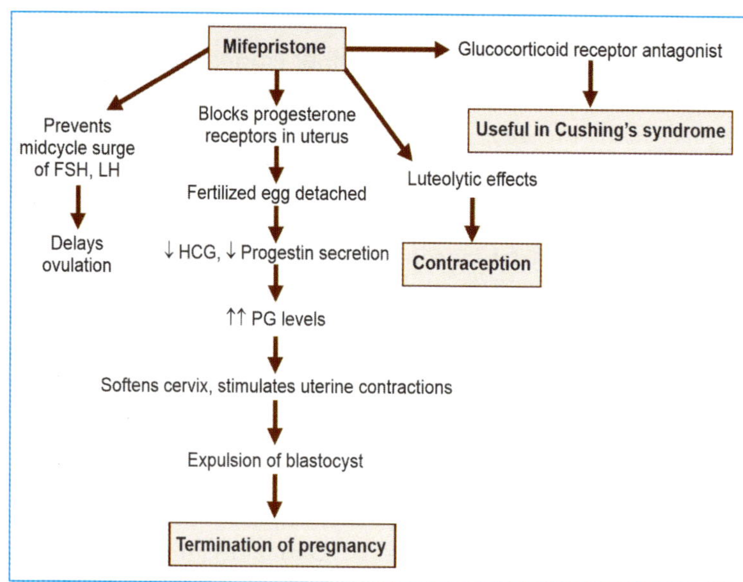

Fig. 39.3: Actions and uses of mifepristone

termination of pregnancy, there is about 1% chance of failure—curettage should be done in such cases.

Uses

1. ***Termination of pregnancy:*** Early pregnancy up to 9 weeks can be terminated with a single oral dose—600 mg of mifepristone followed 48 hr later by a prostaglandin to increase uterine contractions and facilitate expulsion of the blastocyst. The prostaglandin used may be oral misoprostol 400 mg or gemeprost 1mg vaginal pessary or sulprostone IM inj. The combination has a success rate of >90%.

   Adverse effects include vaginal bleeding for 1–2 weeks, nausea, diarrhoea and abdominal pain. A small percentage of patients may have heavy vaginal bleeding requiring medical attention.
2. ***Postcoital contraception:*** Mifepristone prevents implantation when given within 72 hours after coitus and thus is a good postcoital contraceptive.
3. ***Monthly contraception***
   - When mifepristone is used regularly in late luteal phase—200 mg for 2 days after mid-cycle—it acts as a contraceptive.
   - A single dose of 600 mg mifepristone taken on 27th day of the cycle every month acts as a contraceptive. This should, however, not be used for long periods as a regular method of contraception.
4. ***Uterine fibroids:*** Low dose mifepristone 25–30 mg daily for 3 months reduces the size of the fibroid. This can be used to minimize blood loss when surgery has to be postponed for some reason.
5. ***Ectopic pregnancy:*** Mifepristone is injected into the unruptured sac of ectopic pregnancy to discourage the growth.
6. ***Cervical ripening:*** Given orally 1 day prior, mifepristone facilitates cervical ripening and softening of the cervix used for terminating intrauterine death.
7. ***Cushing's syndrome:*** Due to its antiglucocorticoid effects, mifepristone is useful in Cushing's syndrome.

Contraindications

Mifepristone is contraindicated in women on long-term glucocorticoid therapy because it has antiglucocorticoid activity.

Caution is required in women having anaemia or those receiving anticoagulants because it can cause heavy bleeding which could be dangerous.

Onapristone is almost a pure progesterone antagonist with very little antiglucocorticoid activity. Lilopristone is similar to mifepristone.

Ulipristal, a selective progesterone receptor modulator (SPRM), inhibits ovulation and has been approved for use as an emergency contraceptive.

DRUGS USED IN THE TREATMENT OF MENOPAUSAL SYMPTOMS

Signs and Symptoms

Decreased production of estrogen at menopause results in symptoms like hot flushes, vaginitis, vaginal dryness, anxiety, fatigue, sweating, muscles and joints pain; longer lasting changes include osteoporosis, urogenital atrophy, dysparunia, skin changes, increased risk of cardiovascular disease and psychological disturbances.

Drugs used include:

- *Hormonal agents*
  - Estrogen
  - Progesterone
  - Tibolone
- *Nonhormonal agents*
  - Clonidine
  - Veralipride
  - Propranolol
  - SSRIs

Hormonal Agents

Hormone replacement therapy (HRT) or menopausal hormone replacement with estrogen reverses the menopausal symptoms and reduces the risk of osteoporosis and cardiovascular disease, but using estrogen alone can increase the risk of endometrial carcinoma and may stimulate the growth of uterine fibroids. Addition of a progestin counters these unwanted effects. Hence a combination of estrogen and progestin has been recommended for HRT at menopause. Various regimens with cyclic and continuous estrogens and progestins have been tried. If withdrawal bleeding is undesirable, the hormones are given continuously. They may be given orally or as transdermal patches or subcutaneous implants.

Management of postmenopausal women depends on the symptoms and presence of other risk factors.

- Treatment should be started as far as possible at the onset of menopause itself.
- Smallest dose of estrogen that can relieve symptoms should be used for the shortest duration of time for vasomotor symptoms. For vaginal dryness, topical preparations of estrogens are preferred. Conjugated estrogens 0.3–1.25 mg/day or ethinyl estradiol 0.01–0.02 mg/day may be used.
- All postmenopausal women should receive calcium supplements.
- Since estrogen administration increases the risk of endometrial cancer, a progestin should be added.
- Addition of a progestin is not required in women who have undergone hysterectomy.
- Estrogen is given for first 21–28 days and a progestin is added for the last 10–12 days of the cycle (medroxy progesterone 2.5–10 mg/day). If breakthrough bleeding is undesirable, the hormones may be given daily 0.625 mg of conjugated estrogens + 2.5–5 mg medroxy progesterone.
- HRT effectively controls the symptoms of menopause. The endometrium undergoes atrophy and by about 4 months most women are amenorrhoeic.
- A large study has shown that HRT in postmenopausal women does not afford any benefit but may increase the risk of cardiovascular diseases and breast cancer. Other studies have disproved the increased risk of breast cancer. Estrogen may be given transdermally or topically to reduce the risk of cardiovascular diseases to avoid biotransformation in the liver.
- HRT is now recommended only for women who undergo premature menopause and for the treatment of vasomotor symptoms of menopause.

Tibolone is a synthetic steroid, which has effects like both estrogen and progesterone with weak androgenic properties. It is found to reduce the symptoms of estrogen deficiency in menopause with endometrial stimulation. Osteoporosis and vasomotor symptoms subside but it can cause weight gain. It is given in the dose of 2.5 mg daily throughout the cycle.

Nonhormonal Agents

Clonidine, an α-adrenergic agonist and veralipride, a dopamine antagonist, can reduce hot flushes. Propranolol can be used to overcome palpitations. SSRIs like fluoxetine or sertraline may be tried for vasomotor symptoms.

HORMONAL CONTRACEPTIVES

Competency achievement: The student should be able to:

PH 1.39 Describe mechanism of action, types, doses, side effects, indications and contraindications the drugs used for contraception.[1]

Millions of women around the world use hormonal contraceptives making them one of the most widely used drugs. When properly used, they are the most effective spacing methods of contraception. Hormonal contraceptives have greatly contributed to the control of population throughout the world.

Two types of preparations are available—Estrogen + progesterone combination and progesterone only preparations.

They are available for oral and parenteral use. Hormonal contraceptives include:

1. *Combined hormonal contraceptives* (estrogen with a progestin)
   - Oral pills
     - Monophasic
     - Biphasic
     - Triphasic
   - Parenteral combined contraceptives
     - Injectable
     - Transdermal patches
     - Vaginal rings
2. *Progestin only contraceptives*
   - Oral—mini pill
   - Parenteral
     - IM inj
     - SC implants
3. *Postcoital contraceptives*
   - Estrogen + progestin
   - Levonorgestrel
   - Mifepristone
   - Ulipristal
   - Non-hormonal—methotrexate

1. Combined Hormonal Contraceptives

Combined pills contain low doses of an estrogen and a progestin. They are highly efficacious (success rate 98%).

Ethinylestradiol and mestranol (in the dose of 20–50 μg) are the estrogens used. Newer progestins, like desogestrel and norgestimate, cause least side effects, ensure prompt withdrawal bleeding and also counter the increased risk of endometrial cancer due to estrogen.

Oral Pills

Monophasic: The pill is started on the 5th day of the menstrual cycle, taken daily for 21 days followed by a gap of 7 days, during which, bleeding occurs. This is monophasic regimen.

Biphasic: Oral contraceptives are also available as biphasic or triphasic preparations (Table 39.3). This reduces the amount of hormones needed and more closely mimics menstrual cycles. Biphasic pills consist of estrogens given for 10 days followed by a progestin for the next 11 days. Because of the risk of endometrial cancer following such biphasic use of the hormones, biphasic pills are not preferred.

Triphasic: Triphasic pills with low doses of an estrogen with a progestin are very effective with least side effects.

If a woman misses a pill, she should take 2 pills the next day and continue the course. If more than 2 pills are missed, then that course should be withdrawn, should follow an alternative method of contraception for that particular cycle and restart the course on the 5th day of the next menstrual cycle.

If the woman has conceived, the pregnancy should be terminated as these hormones are teratogenic. However, recent studies have shown that in such low doses, the hormones are **not** teratogenic.

Parenteral Combined Contraceptives

Combined injectable contraceptives containing an estrogen with a progestogen are injected at monthly intervals. They are highly effective with side effects similar to progesterone-only implants. They are better tolerated but further reports of long-term effects on reversal of ovulation are yet to be available.

Transdermal contraceptives: A transdermal patch containing a progestin and ethinyl estradiol is available. It is to be applied once a week for 3 weeks and the next week withdrawal bleeding follows. It has the advantage of better compliance.

Vaginal rings containing levonorgestrel are now available. They are placed in the vagina for 3 weeks of the cycle and then removed for one week. The hormone is absorbed gradually through the vaginal mucosa. The advantage is the need for a low dose of the hormone because the first pass metabolism is avoided.

2. Progestin Only Contraceptives

Mini pill: A low dose progestin is taken daily without a gap (75 μg norgestrel). Estrogen and

Table 39.3: Hormonal contraceptive preparations—oral

Regimen	*Estrogen + Progestin dose*	*Duration in days and Trade name*
1. Combined pills		
a. *Monophasic*	1. EE 50 μg + Norgestrel 500 μg	21 days from day 5 of the menst. cycle (OVRAL-G)
	2. EE 30 μg + Levonorgestrel 150 μg	21 days from day 5 of the menst. cycle (OVRAL-L)
	3. EE 30 μg + Levonorgestrel 300 μg	21 days + 7 days of ferrous sulphate tab (MALA-D)
	4. EE 20 μg + Desogestrel 150 μg	21 days + 7 days of ferrous sulphate tab (FEMILON)
b. *Biphasic*	1. EE 35 μg + Norethindrone 500 μg	10 days
	EE 20 μg + Desogestrel 150 μg	Next 11 days
c. *Triphasic*	1. EE 30 μg + Levonorgestrel 50 μg	Day 1–6
	EE 40 μg + Levonorgestrel 75 μg	Day 7–11
	EE 30 μg + Levonorgestrel 125 μg	Day 12–21 (TRIQUILAR)
	2. EE 35 μg + Norethindrone 50, 75 and 100 μg	7+7+7 days (ORTHONOVUM)
2. Progestin only pill (Mini pill)		1. Norgestrel 75 μg (OVRAL) daily 2. Norethindrone 350 μg
3. Postcoital pills	1. Combined pill - EE 50 μg + levonorgestrel 250 μg	2 stat. and 2 after 12 hr
	2. Levonorgestrel 1.5 mg	Single dose within 72 hr of coitus (iPILL)
	3. Mifepristone 600 mg	Within 72 hrs of coitus followed 48 hr later by 400 mg misoprostol
	4. Ulipristal 30 mg	Single dose within 120 hr of coitus
	5. Methotrexate 50 mg/m^2	Oral/IM
	6. Diethylstilbesterol 25 mg/day	5 days (STILPHOSTROL): Not prefered

All tablets (except post-coital) started on day 5 of menstrual cycle. EE: Ethinyl estradiol

its accompanied long-term adverse effects are thus avoided, but efficacy is lower, menstrual cycles may be irregular and is, therefore, not popular.

Progestin injections: Depot preparations contain a progestin and are given as:

1. *Intramuscular injections* at 3–6 months intervals, e.g. depot medroxyprogesterone acetate (DMPA) 150 mg every 3 months injected IM or Norethisterone enantate 200 mg (NETEN).

   Ovulation is inhibited for about 14 weeks. Long-term use of DMPA reduces menstrual blood loss. The risk of endometrial carcinoma is also reduced.

2. *Subcutaneous implants:* They are implanted under the skin. Capsules containing norgestrel are (NORPLANT capsules) implanted subcutaneously in the forearm or upper arm. Low dose of the progestin is released and the effect can last up to 5 yr. Since the progestin levels are low, adverse effects like altered lipoprotein and carbohydrate metabolism are insignificant.
3. *Intrauterine device:* A progestasert impregnated with progesterone is introduced into the uterus. It releases a low dose of progesterone locally for up to 5 years.

Disadvantages of Parenteral Progestins

i. Amenorrhoea is common.
ii. Unpredictable bleeding or spotting.
iii. Disruption of menstrual cycle.
iv. Suppression of ovulation may sometimes continue up to 18 months after the last injection. Thus long time is required for return of fertility.

v. Suppression of estrogen secretion may result in a reduced bone density—but is reversible.

3. Postcoital Contraceptives

The following may be used for postcoital contraception:

1. Combination of low doses of estrogen and progestins is used as lesser side effects are reported. Two tablets containing ethinyl estradiol (50 µg) and a progestin levonorgestrel 0.5 mg are given as soon as possible (within 72 hours of coitus 2 tablets of OVRAL-G). They can cause nausea and vomiting and have an efficacy of 90–98%. The dose is repeated after 12 hours. It is called YUZPe method.
2. Levonorgestrel 0.75 mg 2 doses 12 hours apart has also been found to be effective and commonly used (iPILL—1.5 mg single dose within 72 hrs after coitus).
3. Mifepristone (RU486) 600 mg prevents implantation when given within 72 hours after coitus followed 48 hrs later by 400 mg misoprostol improves success rate.
4. Methotrexate in the dose of 50 mg/m^2 given orally or IM effectively induces abortion in the first trimester. Being a folic acid antagonist and also because its active metabolite gets concentrated in the placenta, methotrexate acts as an abortifacient. Misoprostol is added to promote uterine motility.
5. Ulipristal 30 mg orally within 5 days of coitus is effective.
6. Insertion of an intrauterine device (IUD) like copper-T within 5 days of coitus can also prevent implantation and thereby prevent pregnancy.
7. High dose of an estrogen (stilbestrol—25 mg daily for 5 days) was used earlier but this may cause severe nausea and vomiting and hence generally not preferred. If the pills are expelled in vomiting, they need to be repeated.

- Postcoital pills act by preventing implantation. The earlier they are started the better is their efficacy.
- If postcoital pills fail, pregnancy should be terminated by other methods because oral contraceptives are likely to be teratogenic.
- Postcoital contraception is advocated as an emergency method in situations following rape or contraceptive failure.

Mechanism of Action of Hormonal Contraceptives

Combined pills act by multiple mechanisms (Fig. 39.4).

1. They prevent ovulation—by a negative feedback on the hypothalamus. Progesterone decreases GnRH pulses and thereby LH release which is essential for ovulation.
2. Estrogens suppress FSH release by negative feedback on the pituitary. As a result, the ovarian follicle fails to develop.
3. Progesterone also inhibits estrogen-induced mid-cycle LH surge.
4. Progesterone renders the cervical mucus thick and unfavourable for sperm penetration.
5. OCs alter the uterine endometrium making it unfavourable for implantation.
6. OCs also adversely influence the coordinated contractions of the cervix, uterus and fallopian tubes which are required for transport of the ovum, sperm as well as for fertilisation and implantation.

Pharmocological Effects

- Hormonal contraceptives inhibit gonadotrophin secretion, suppress ovarian function and on prolonged use the size of the ovaries may be reduced. However, on stopping the hormonal contraceptives, 95% patients have regular cycles in about 2–3 months. Cervical hypertrophy may be present and the cervical mucus gets thick

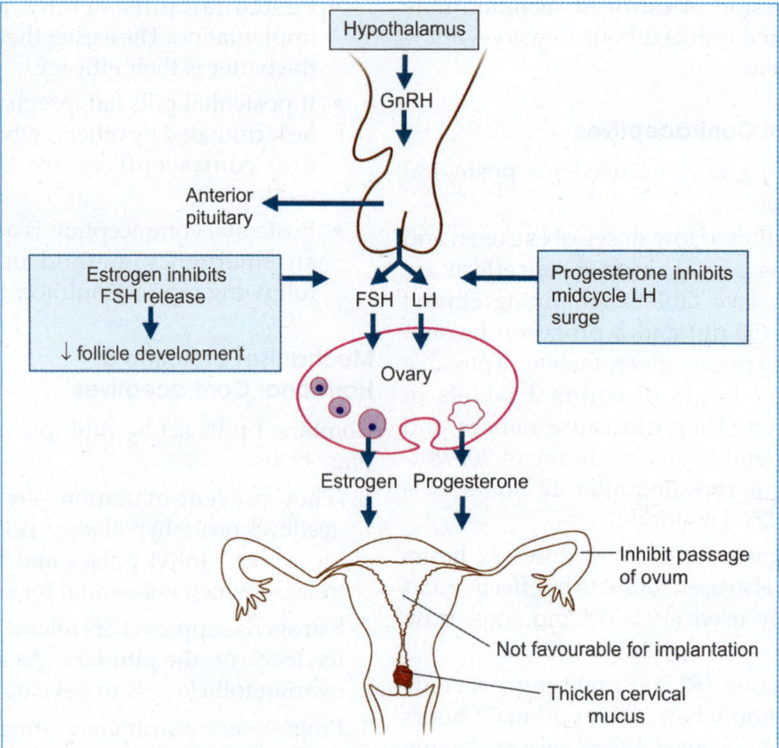

Fig. 39.4: Mechanism of action of hormonal contraceptives

and scanty. The endometrium shows glandular atrophy and, therefore, less menstrual bleeding. Slight enlargement of the breasts may be seen.

- An increase in the clotting factors VII, VIII, IX and X and a derease in antithrombin III are noted.
- Carbohydrate absorption from the gut is slower while insulin levels are slightly increased.
- There is a slight increase in cardiac output, heart rate and BP. Increased plasma renin activity with salt and water retention contribute to hypertension.
- All changes are reversible or cessation of hormonal contraceptives.
- Skin pigmentation particularly on exposure to sun may be seen in some women.

Adverse Effects

Milder effects

- Headache, may be mild and may subside on continued treatment. Migraine headache in some women, can be troublesome and may require discontinuation of hormonal contraceptives. Nausea, vomiting, edema, breast tenderness, amenorrhoea and irregular menstrual cycles may occur.
- Weight gain, acne, mood swings and hirsuitism may occur.

More severe side effects

1. *Cardiovascular effects*
   a. In women above 35 years, HCs may increase the risk of venous thrombosis and pulmonary embolism. HCs may also increase the coagulability of blood. The risk of thromboembolism is more in

women with predisposing factors like genetic susceptibility and altered antithrombin III and platelet function. Antithrombin III levels are decreased by hormonal contraceptives but are reversible on cessation of therapy. But the newer low-dose preparations are found to be safer when used in healthy women with no other risk factors for MI, stroke or thromboembolism.

b. *Myocardial infarction:* Women with other risk factors for myocardial infarction like cigarette smoking, obesity, diabetes mellitus increased lipoproteins and hypertension have a slightly higher chance of developing myocardial infarction.

c. *Cerebrovascular disease:* Risk of stroke is marginally higher among older women.

d. *Hypertension:* The high dose preparations may precipitate hypertension in some women and hormonal contraceptives should be withdrawn. But the newer low dose preparations are safer.

2. *Cancers:* OCs may increase the incidence of cervical, breast cancers—but the risk is not significant. Long-term use of combination hormonal contraceptives may increase the risk of cervical cancers in women.
3. *Cholestatic jaundice and gallstones:* Incidence may be higher in high dose preparations. Genetically, predisposed women particularly those who had cholestatic jaundice during pregnancy may develop cholestatic jaundice on using hormonal contraceptives. Hormonal contraceptives have to be discontinued and jaundice disappears gradually. The incidence of cholecystitis, gallstones, cholangitis and hepatic adenomas is reported to be higher.
4. *Impaired glucose tolerance:* OCs may impair glucose tolerance—but the newer low dose preparations do not carry such risk.
5. *Depression:* Mood swings may be noted; depression can occur in a small percentage of women and when significant, hormonal contraceptives may have to be withdrawn.

Contraindications to Combined Pill

- Thromboembolic and cerebrovascular disease
- Breast cancers
- Liver disease
- OCs should be used with caution in diabetes, hypertension, convulsive disorders, oedema and CCF.

Other uses of Combined Preparations

1. *Hormone replacement therapy:* Discussed earlier.
2. *DUB:* Though progestin is the mainstay of treatment for DUB, low dose combined preparations may also be used as cyclic therapy or as continuous administration.
3. *Endometriosis:* Combined pills may be used continuously to induce atrophy of the endometriotic tissues. Amenorrhoea is produced.
4. *Postponement of menstruation:* Combined pills are started 2 tablets daily 3–6 days prior to the expected date of menstruation and continued till desired. Menstruation occurs 2–3 days after stopping the drug. Such use in higher dose may cause nausea and vomiting. Another way of using the hormones is to start low dose combined pill on day 7–10 (1 tab daily) and continue throughout the cycle and stop it when menstruation is desired.
5. *Premenstrual syndrome:* Oral contraceptive pills are used to suppress ovulation and continued for 3–6 cycles.
6. *Dysmenorrhoea:* If analgesics cannot be used, oral contraceptive pills may be given for 3–4 cycles.
7. *Idiopathic hirsutism:* Cyclic therapy with combined pills is useful in hirsutism (Key Box 39.1).

Centchroman: Centchroman or **ormeloxifene** (a SERM) a chroman derivative, is a non-steroidal, nonhormonal, oral contraceptive developed in India. It has antioestrogenic and antiprogestogenic activity and acts by

Key Box 39.1: Benefits of combined pills

1. Effective and convenient method of contraception.
2. Reduced risk of ovarian cancers (reduced ovarian stimulation by gonadotrophins as ovulation is also suppressed)
3. Reduced risk of endometrial cancers (progesterone antagonises the endometrial proliferation induced by estrogens)
4. Reduced incidence of pelvic inflammatory disease and ectopic pregnancy.
5. Menstrual benefits—less menstrual blood loss, less iron-deficiency; premenstrual tension and dysmenorrhoea are less intense.

preventing implantation. Onset of action is quick (<60 minutes) and duration of action is 7 days.

Preparations and dose: 30 mg twice a week for 3 months followed by once a week till contraception is desired (the tablet should be continued without withdrawing for menstruation).

SAHELI, CENTRON 30 mg tab

Centchroman has the following:

Advantages

1. Success rate claimed is 97–99%.
2. It is devoid of the side effects of hormonal contraceptives including nausea and effects on blood coagulation.
3. Long t½ allows once a week administration.
4. No teratogenicity, carcinogenicity or mutagenicity reported.
5. Return of fertility is faster.
6. It is well tolerated.

Disadvantages

1. Centchroman may cause prolongation of menstrual cycles in 10% of women.
2. It may cause ovarian enlargement and should be avoided in polycystic ovaries.
3. It should also be avoided in renal and hepatic dysfunction, tuberculosis and in lactating mothers.

Clinical Pharmacology

- For most indications, a combination of estrogen and progesterone is used.
- Several contraceptive methdos are available, but the right one to suit each couple should be chosen.
- Fertility returns within 1–2 months of discontinuing oral contraceptives. However, with injectable contraceptives, the return of fertility takes several months.
- Routine use of mifepristone—misoprostol as a regular method of contraception is not advisable.
- Birth control vaceines (hCG vaccines) are under trial.

DRUGS FOR INFERTILITY

Competency achievement: The student should be able to:

PH 1.40 Describe mechanism of action, types, doses, side effects, indications and contraindications of: (1) Drugs used in the treatment of infertility, and (2) Drugs used in erectile dysfunction.[2]

Infertility is generally of multifactorial origin. Ovulatory dysfunction can often be corrected with drugs like ovulation inducing agents.

Drugs used for ovulation induction:

- Clomiphene citrate
- Aromatase inhibitors—Letrozole
- Gonadotrophins—recombinant FSH
- Drugs that facilitate ovulation induction—insulin senitizers like metformin.

Clomiphene citrate*—see page 483*

Aromatase inhibitors (page 483) Letrozole is considered the first line drug in women with higher body weight—2.5 to 5 mg for 5 days from day 3 to 7 of the cycle. Anastrozole is not preferred.

Gonadotrophins may be used as 2nd line or along with clomiphene citrate. HCG has LH activity. Start with 50–75 IU IM from day 5. Ultrasound monitoring of ovulation is done and when follicular size is optimum, 5000 units is given IM to trigger ovulation.

Insulin sensitizers: Insulin resistance is seen in PCOS. Correction of insulin resistance with metformin (500 mg TDS daily) helps and is used along with clomiphene.

DRUGS USED IN ERECTILE DYSFUNCTION

Sexual impotence is the inability of a man to have satisfactory sexual intercourse due to inability to have and maintain an erection. Very often it is psychological while in some cases there could be an organic cause.

During erection, there is relaxation of the nonvascular smooth muscle of the corpora covernosa. As a result blood flows into the sinuses of the cavernosa at a high pressure which is responsible for erection. Several drugs have been tried including testosterone, yohimbine, papaverine and antidepressants in the treatment of erectile dysfunction. The recent introduction—sildenafil has been a success in a large percentage of them.

Nitric oxide is released which activates guanylyl cyclase leading to increased synthesis of cGMP resulting in smooth muscle relaxation.

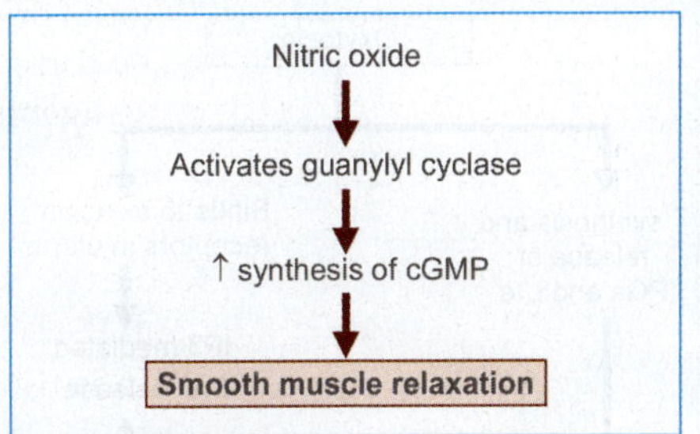

Hence drugs that enhance cGMP are useful in patients with erectile dysfunction.

Sildenafil (Viagra)

Sildenafil is the first agent to be effective orally for the treatment of erectile dysfunction. Sildenafil inhibits the enzyme phosphodiesterase in the penis and thus prolongs the life of cyclic-GMP. This causes relaxation of smooth muscle in the corpus cavernosum and vasodilation—both resulting in cavernosal engorgement and penile erection. Sildenafil is given orally.

Preparations

Dose: 50–100 mg 1 hour before sexual activity. SUHAGRA, ANDROZ 25, 50, 100 mg tab. ADAMS DELITE 50, 100 mg tab. TADALAFIL 10, 20 mg tab.

Adverse Effects and Precautions

Due to vasodilation—headache, dizziness and nasal stuffiness can occur. It potentiates the hypotensive action of nitrates and is contraindicated in patients on nitrates and in patients with coronary artery disease. Elderly men above 60 years need less dose (25 mg). Patients with liver and kidney disease, bleeding disorders and elderly people are at a higher risk of toxicity. Several deaths have been reported in such patients. Two other derivatives **tadalafil** and **vardanafil** have properties similar to sildenafil.

Other uses of Sildenafil

Sildenafil has found several indications in cardiology. It has been shown to be beneficial in patients with **pulmonary arterial hypertension** and **systemic hypertension**. It could prevent cardiac remodelling in patients with **IHD**. Sildenafil has also been tried in patients with **cystic fibrosis** and **benign prostatic hyperplasia**.

Alprostadil: Alprostadil is PGE_1 analog that can be injected directly, into the cavernosa. It can also be used as a minisuppository placed in the urethra and it diffuses into the cavernosal tissue. Alprostadil is used in patients who do not respond to sildenafil or in whom sildenafil cannot be used.

Phentolamine, an alpha blocker, can also be injected into the cavernosa with or without papaverine—called phentolamine/papaverine induced penile erection (PIPE therapy). However, it is not preferred because of the inconvenience of the route of administration and complications.

[1–2] From Medical Council of India, *Competency based Undergraduate Curriculum for the Indian Medical Graduate*, 2018;1:136–144.

CHAPTER 40

Oxytocin and Drugs Acting on the Uterus

Competency achievement: The student should be able to:

PH 1.41 Describe the mechanisms of action, types, doses, side effects, indications and contraindications of uterine relaxants and stimulants.[1]

UTERINE STIMULANTS

Drugs which stimulate the uterine contractions are **oxytocin, ergometrine** and **prostaglandins.** They are also called **oxytocics** or **ecbolics.** These drugs are useful in obstetrics.

Oxytocin

Oxytocin is a peptide hormone secreted by the posterior pituitary along with ADH. It is synthesized in the supraoptic and paraventricular nuclei of the hypothalamus, transported along the axon and stored in the neurohypophysis. It is released by stimuli such as suckling, coitus and parturition.

Actions

Uterus: Oxytocin contracts the uterus. The fundus and the body contract, while the lower segment is relaxed. Both force and frequency of contractions are enhanced and there is full relaxation in between the contractions. This relaxation allows adequate blood supply to the foetus.

Mechanism of Action

Oxytoxin brings about its effects by acting on oxytocin receptors which are G-protein-coupled receptors. At full term, the uterus is highly sensitive to the effects of oxytocin as there is an increase in the number of oxytocin receptors. Estrogen enhances the synthesis of oxytocin receptors and sensitizes the uterus to the effects of oxytocin. The effects are dose dependent. High doses produce sustained contractions with no relaxation in between, resulting in reduced blood flow to the foetus, foetal distress and death. Synthetic oxytocin is used for therapeutic purpose.

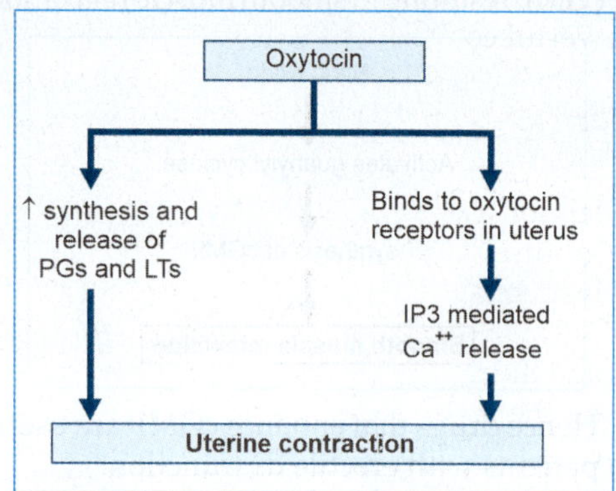

Mammary gland: Oxytocin facilitates milk ejection by contraction of the myoepithelium in the mammary alveoli. Suckling stimulates the release of oxytocin.

Kidney: Oxytocin has mild antidiuretic effects.

Pharmacokinetics

Oxytocin is given as IV infusion. It is metabolised by the liver and kidneys by the enzyme oxytocinase.

Preparations

5 IU diluted in 500 ml glucose/saline infusion. PITOCIN, SYNTOCINON 5 units/ml inj.

Table 40.1: Comparison between oxytocin and ergometrine

	Oxytocin	*Ergometrine*
Source	Synthetic (for commercial use)	Natural *(Claviceps purpurea)*
Chemistry	Peptide	Alkaloid
Acts on:	Oxytocin receptors	5-HT receptors
Occurrence	Produced in the body (endogenous)	Exogenous
Administration	• Not effective orally • Given as IV drip	• Effective orally • Both IM and IV
Duration of action	Short	Longer
t½	15 minutes	1–2 hours
Action on uterus	• Contracts body and fundus • Relaxes lower segment	• Contracts whole uterus • No relaxation • Tone increased.
Uses	• Induction of labour • Milk ejection	• PPH • To ensure uterine involution after delivery

Adverse Effects

Large doses cause water intoxication and very powerful contractions.

Uses

1. *Induction of labour:* Oxytocin is used to induce labour as in postmaturity or to augment labour when uterine contractions are inadequate. Given as an infusion 5 units in 500 ml glucose solution, slowly to begin with and the rate gradually increased depending on the response. Oxytocin is the ecbolic of choice because of the following advantages:
   i. Upper segment contracts while the lower segment relaxes which facilitates foetal expulsion.
   ii. Relaxation in between contractions allows adequate blood supply to the foetus.
   iii. Oxytocin has a short t½ which means action can be easily controlled by monitoring the drip rate.
2. *PPH:* Oxytocin is now the prefered drug for the prevention and treatment of PPH.
3. *Milk ejection:* When milk ejection is impaired in nursing mothers, intranasal oxytocin spray can be used.
4. *Abortion:* As an alternative to induce midtrimester abortion.

Ergometrine

Ergometrine and its derivative methylergometrine are used as uterine stimulants. Ergot has been used by midwives to quicken labour since centuries. Ergot alkaloids (*see* page 147).

Actions on the Uterus

Ergometrine is a powerful uterine stimulant. The force and frequency of uterine contractions are enhanced. All parts of the uterus including the fundus, body and the lower segment contract. There is no relaxation in between contractions. Full-term uterus is more sensitive to the actions of ergometrine. Ergometrine also causes some vasoconstriction which helps to reduce bleeding from the uterus in post partal state. It brings about its effects by binding to serotonin receptors.

Pharmacokinetics: Ergometrine is rapid and short acting. It can be given orally, IM or IV.

Methylergometrine in addition can be given SC.

Preparations

Ergometrine 0.25, 0.5 mg tab; 0.5 mg/ml inj. ZOTARGINE 0.125 mg tab. ERINMET 0.5 mg inj.

Methylergometrine, ERGOGIN, METHERGIN, UTERGIN 0.125 mg tab, 0.2 mg/ml inj.

Adverse effects include nausea, vomiting vasospasm visual disturbances and rarely hypertension.

Uses

1. Postpartum haemorrhage: Ergometrine was used to control and prevent PPH. However, because of adverse effects of ergometrine, oxytocin is now the preferred drug.
2. To hasten uterine involution: Ergometrine was used earlier.
3. To prevent uterine atony—after caesarean section.

Prostaglandins

Prostaglandins are synthesized by the uterus and play a significant role in menstruation as well as parturition. PGE_2 and PGF_{2a} stimulate the contraction of both pregnant and nonpregnant uterus though sensitivity is higher during pregnancy. They also soften the cervix and hasten dilatation (cervical ripening). PGs produced by foetal tissues mediate initiation and progression of labour.

PGs used in obstetrics are:

- Dinoprostone (PGE_2) intravaginal or extra-amniotic
- Carboprost (15 methyl PGF_{2a}) deep IM
- Misoprostol (Gemeprost, PGE1) intravaginal

Prostaglandins are also involved in the pathogenesis of dysmenorrhoea and menorrhagia. Hence NSAIDs are useful in relieving dysmenorrhoea and probably menorrhagia.

Adverse effects include nausea, vomiting, headache, fever and diarrhoea.

Preparations

Dinoprostone (PGE_2): CERVIPRIME, DINORIPE gel 0.5 mg/syringe, PG TAB, PRIMIPROST 0.5 mg tab.

Carboprost: DEVIPROST, PROSTODIN 250 µg/ml.

Misoprostil: MESOPIL, PRESTAKIN D, MISOPROST 250 µg/ml.

Uses

1. *Abortion:* PGs are used as vaginal suppositories to induce mid-trimester abortion. Dinoprostone is given intravaginally or by the extra-amniotic route. PGs are also used with mifepristone in the termination of pregnancy up to 9 weeks. Gemeprost is given as vaginal pessary following mifepristone.
2. *PPH:* As an alternative to ergometrine carboprost can be used.
3. *Cervical priming:* Gels are used intravaginally to soften the cervix and for cervical ripening prior to induction of labour.
4. *Induction of labour:* PGs are used as alternatives to oxytocin.

UTERINE RELAXANTS (TOCOLYTICS)

Tocolytics are drugs that reduce uterine motility and relax the uterus. They are:

- β_2-adrenergic agonists: Salbutamol, terbutaline, ritodrine and isoxsuprine.
- Oxytocin receptor antagonist: Atosiban.
- Cycloxygenase inhibitors: Aspirin, indomethacin and sulindac.
- Miscellaneous: Magnesium sulfate, ethylalcohol, calcium channel blockers, nitroglycerine.

Salbutamol: Selective β_2 adrenergic agonists ritodrine and salbutamol relax the uterus and thereby suppress premature labour in a large number of cases. IV infusion is started 10 mg per minute and the dose may be gradually increased up to 40 mg per minute. Alternatively ritodrine IV infusion may be started—50 mg per minute and gradually increased to 100 mg per minute till the contractions stop.

Adverse effects include anxiety, palpitation, restlessness, headache, hypotension, arrhythmias and hyperglycaemia. β_2-agonists should be avoided in pregnant women with diabetes and heart diseases.

RITROD, RITODINE 10 mg tab, 10 mg/ml inj.

Atosiban is an oxytocin receptor antagonist. It has been found to be effective as a tocolytic to delay preterm labour. It may be used as an alternative to β_2-adrenergic agonists as an IV infusion. It is available in some countries.

Miscellaneous

Intravenous magnesium sulphate is used as an alternative when β_2 agonists are contra-indicated. However, high doses can cause significant CNS and respiratory depression. Magnesium sulphate is also used to suppress convulsions and control the BP in pre-eclampsia and eclampsia. A bolus dose of 2 g is infused over 10–20 min followed by 1 g/litre infusion.

Calcium channel blockers (CCBs) like nifedipine sublingual 10 mg repeated every 20 mins for 3 doses relax the uterus but can reduce placental perfusion and hence CCBs are not preferred.

Ethyl alcohol given IV is a tocolytic but produces marked CNS depression. Though cyclo-oxygenase inhibitors, aspirin and indomethacin relax the uterus, they are not preferred as tocolytics because of the risk of closure of ductus arteriosus and other adverse effects.

Uses of Tocolytics

1. *To delay premature labour:* Tocolytics may not always be successful. Uterine contractions may be controlled for 24–48 hr which should be utilised to prepare the foetus for preterm birth, i.e. by giving glucocorticoids to bring about early maturation of foetal lungs.
2. *In threatened abortion* was used to inhibit uterine contractions.

[1] From Medical Council of India, *Competency based Undergraduate Curriculum for the Indian Medical Graduate*, 2018;1:136–144.

CHAPTER **41**

Androgens and Anabolic Steroids

> *Competency achievement:* The student should be able to:
>
> **PH 1.37** Describe the mechanisms of action, types, doses, side effects, indications and contraindications of the drugs used as **sex hormones**, their analogues and anterior pituitary hormones.[1]

PHYSIOLOGICAL CONSIDERATIONS

Androgens are produced chiefly in the testis and small amounts in the adrenal cortex. In the females, small amounts of androgens are produced in the ovary and adrenal cortex. Androgens are synthesized from cholesterol (*see* Fig 38.3). Androgens include:

Natural: Testosterone, dihydrotestosterone.

Synthetic: Methyl testosterone, fluoxymesterone, testosterone enanthate, testosterone cypionate.

Anabolic steroids: Oxandralone, nandrolone decanoate, stanozolol, methandienone.

Testosterone is the most important natural androgen. In the adult male, 8–10 mg of testosterone is produced daily. Secretion is regulated by gonadotrophins and GnRH.

Physiological Actions

In the male, testosterone is essential for the development of **secondary sexual characters** and **sex organs**. It is necessary for normal spermatogenesis and is important for maintaining sexual function in men. Testosterone promotes bone growth, enhances the muscle mass, protein synthesis and positive nitrogen balance—has **anabolic actions**. It also promotes erythropoiesis by increased production of erythropoietin.

Mechanism of Action

Mechanism of action of androgens is similar to other steroids (*see* Fig. 38.4). Androgens bind to androgen receptors on the target cells, the complex moves to the nucleus where it stimulates the protein synthesis.

Pharmacokinetics

Testosterone is given parenterally as it has poor oral bioavailability. Given intramuscularly it has a t½ of 10–20 min; 98% is bound to sex hormone binding globulin. It is metabolized in the liver and excreted by the kidneys. Esters of testosterone have longer action. Testosterone pellets implanted subcutaneously can act for 6–8 months.

Preparations and Dose

1. Testosterone: AQUAVIRON 25 mg/ml inj IM
2. Testosterone Propionate 25–50 mg IM thrice a week. TESTOVIRON, TESTANON 25, 50 mg/ml inj.
3. Testosterone Enanthate 250 mg every 2–3 wk. TESTOVIRON Depot inj. 250 mg/ml inj
4. Testosterone undecanoate 40–120 mg/day. NUVIR 40 mg cap
5. Mesterolone 25–75 mg/day. MESTILON 25 mg tab.

Newer preparations: Topical preparations are available which have longer action and also bypass the liver; to be applied over the scrotum daily.

1. Gel: Dihydrotestosterone gel
2. Testosterone transdermal patch

Designer steroids

Designer steroids are developed or designed in an attempt to obtain compounds with more selective anabolic activity on the androgen receptors, e.g. norbolethone, desoxymethyl testosterone (DMT) and tetrahydrogestrinone. Some of them are nonsteroidal anabolic molecules. Designer steroids are, however, abused as they may not be detected by routine doping tests.

Adverse Effects

Masculinization and acne in females; hepatotoxicity, increased libido and precocious puberty can occur in young boys. With large doses, salt and water retention, suppression of spermatogenesis resulting in infertility can be seen. Feminizing effects like gynaecomastia in men can occur as some androgens are converted to estrogens.

Uses

1. *Testicular failure:* For androgen replacement therapy in primary and secondary testicular failure.
2. *Other uses:* Androgens may be used in senile osteoporosis and carcinoma of the breast in premenopausal women (Fig. 41.1).

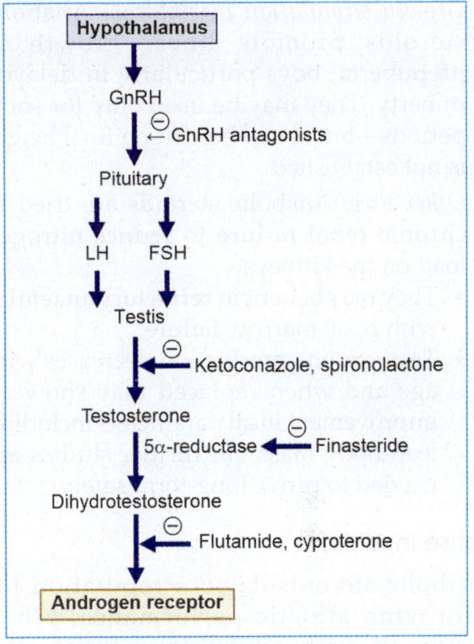

Fig. 41.1: Androgens and antiandrogens

ANABOLIC STEROIDS

Anabolic steroids are synthetic androgens with higher anabolic and low androgenic activity. These are believed to enhance protein synthesis and increase muscle mass. But with higher doses, the relative anabolic activity is lost (Table 41.1).

Adverse effects of anabolic steroids are similar to those caused by androgens.

Uses

1. *Catabolic states:* Anabolic steroids may benefit patients following surgery, trauma, prolonged illness and debilitating conditions. Given during convalescence, the negative nitrogen balance is corrected, appetite improves and there is a feeling of well-being.
2. *Senile osteoporosis* seen in elderly males respond by formation of new bone tissue.

Table 41.1: Preparations of anabolic steroids

Anabolic steroid	*Dose and route*	*Trade name*
Methandienone	2–5 mg/day, oral, IM	Pronabol, Anobolex 2,5 mg tab
Nandrolone phenylpropionate	10–50 mg/week, IM	Durabolin 10,25 mg/ml inj
Nandrolone decanoate	25–100 mg/3 weeks, IM	Decadurabolin 25, 100 mg/ml inj
Ethylestrenol	2–4 mg/day, oral	Orabolin
Oxandrolone	5–10 mg/day, oral	Anavar
Stanozolol	2–10 mg/day, oral	Stromba, Neurabol

3. *Growth stimulation in children:* Anabolic steroids promote linear growth in prepubertal boys particularly in delayed puberty. They may be used only for short periods—but actual benefit on final height is not established.
4. *Other uses:* Anabolic steroids are tried in **chronic renal failure** to reduce nitrogen load on the kidneys.
   - They may benefit in **refractory anaemias** with bone marrow failure.
   - Testosterone production decreases with age and when replaced may show an improvement in all parameters including lean body mass but further studies are needed to prove long-term safety.

Abuse in Athletes

Anabolic steroids enjoy a reputation for improving athletic performance. When combined with adequate exercise, the muscle mass increases. But the dose used by athletes is very high and is associated with serious adverse effects like testicular atrophy, sterility and gynaecomastia in men and virilizing effects in women; increased aggressiveness, psychotic symptoms and increased risk of coronary heart disease in both sexes. Moreover, there is no evidence that athletic performance improves. Hence the use of anabolic steroids by athletes has been banned and is medically not recommended. Contraindications for the use of androgens:

1. Pregnancy
2. Carcinoma of prostate/breast in males
3. Infants and chlidren
4. Renal/cardiac/liver disease.

ANTIANDROGENS

Cyproterone acetate a derivative of progesterone competitively binds to androgen receptors and thus blocks the actions of androgens. It also has progestational activity. Cyproterone is used:

i. To treat severe hypersexuality in males,
ii. In carcinoma prostate and
iii. In female hirsutism—used along with an estrogen.

Flutamide, bicalutamide, nilutamide and **enzalutamide** are potent competitive antagonists at androgen receptors.

Flutamide can cause gynecomastia, mastalgia and hepatotoxicity. It is given thrice daily in the dose of 250 mg. FLUTIDE 250 mg tab.

Bicalutamide is longer acting given once daily and is more hepatotoxic than flutamide. Bicalutamide is better tolerated than flutamide and affords good sympatomatic relief.

Dose: 50–150 mg/day. BIPROSTA 25 mg tab.

Nilutamide is similar to bicalutamide but appears to produce more adverse effects than it. It is used following surgical castration.

Enzalutamide is a pure androgen receptor antagonist with higher affinity for it.

These antiandrogens are used with a GnRH analog/leuprolide in the treatment of carcinoma prostate.

Finasteride inhibits the enzyme 5-alpha reductase (type II isozyme) and thus inhibits the convertion of testosterone to its active metabolite dihydrotestosterone which acts mainly in the male urogenital tract. Finasteride is used in benign prostatic hypertrophy (BPH) to reduce the prostate size. The symptoms of obstruction also decrease and there is an

Rationale for combining tamsulosin and finasteride in BPH

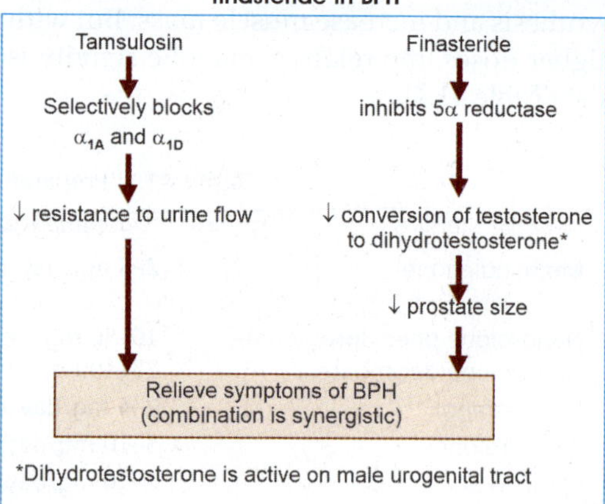

improvement in the urine flow. It may be combined with tamsulosin or other alpha blockers for **synergistic effect**.

Finasteride is also tried in the treatment of male pattern baldness with fairly good results but it requires continued use as the effect may be reversed in 6–12 months after stopping the drug. Side effects include decreased libido and impotence. Finasteride may be used along with estrogen and cyproterone in the treatment of hirsutism.

Dose: BPH 5 mg OD. Baldness: 1 mg OD. FINARA 5 mg tab. FINPECIA 1 mg tab

Dutasteride inhibits both type I and type II isoforms of 5 alpha reductase. Dutasteride has a slow onset but longer duration of action. It is useful in BPH, male pattern baldness and for the prevention of prostatic cancer.

Dose: 0.5 mg OD. AVODART, DUPROST 0.5 mg cap.

Inhibitors of Androgen Synthesis

- Gonadotrophin releasing hormone or its agonist like leuprolide when given continuously inhibits LH and testosterone secretion resulting in pharmacological castration—used in men with prostatic cancer.
- Danazol—*see* page 485
- Antifungal agent ketoconazole also inhibits steroid hormone synthesis and thereby inhibits androgen synthesis. Cimetidine and spironolactone compete with dihydrotestosterone for the androgen receptors in the target tissues–have antiandrogenic properties which are responsible for their antiandrogenic side effects (Fig. 41.1).

MALE CONTRACEPTIVES

The requirement of a safe and effective chemical contraceptive in men has not been fulfilled largely because it is difficult to totally suppress spermatogenesis. Various compounds including testosterone with progestin, oestrogens with progestins, antiandrogens like cyproterone acetate have been tried, but are neither reliable nor safe.

GnRH agonists and antagonists along with testosterone inhibit gonadotrophin secretion and are being studied.

Gossypol, a cotton seed derivative, has shown to produce oligozoospermia and impair sperm motility in Chinese studies. This effect is reversible in a few months. Hypokalaemia is the major adverse effect.

Lifestyle Drugs

Drugs used for non-health-related indications or for indications other than illnesses, to meet the 'lifestyle' requirements are termed 'lifestyle' drugs. Examples include cosmetics, anti-obesity drugs, food supplements, anabolic steroids, drugs for erectile dysfunction and oral contraceptives.

[1] From Medical Council of India, *Competency based Undergraduate Curriculum for the Indian Medical Graduate*, 2018;1:136–144.

CHAPTER 42

Insulin and Oral Antidiabetic Drugs

Competency achievement: The student should be able to:

PH 1.36 Describe the mechanism of action, types, doses, side effects, indications and contraindications of drugs used in endocrine disorders (**diabetes mellitus**, thyroid disorders and osteoporosis).[1]

DIABETES MELLITUS

Diabetes mellitus is a chronic metabolic disorder characterised by hyperglycaemia and altered metabolism of carbohydrates, lipids and proteins. It is a common condition affecting 1–2% of population with a strong hereditary tendency.

Diabetes mellitus (DM) was earlier grouped into two types but most researchers now classify them into four types.

Type I previously called insulin-dependent diabetes mellitus (IDDM) is an autoimmune disorder where antibodies destroy the β cells of the islets of Langerhans leading to absolute insulin deficiency. It usually occurs in the young children and adolescents (hence called juvenile onset diabetes mellitus). The incidence of this type of DM is fortunately low.

Type II was earlier called non-insulin-dependent diabetes mellitus (NIDDM). Most patients are obese. There is both reduced sensitivity of tissues to insulin and impaired regulation of insulin secretion.

Type III or secondary diabetes is due to causes like pancreatectomy, drugs and nonpancreatic diseases.

Type IV is gestational diabetes which manifests around 20–24 weeks of pregnancy during which rising placental hormones are responsible for insulin resistance.

Prolonged exposure of tissues to hyperglycaemia results in various complications including premature atherosclerosis, retinopathy, nephropathy and gangrene of the limbs. It is thought to be due to reduced blood supply to these structures—because of thickening of the capillary walls. Accumulation of glycosylated products in the vessel walls may be responsible for the thickening. Moreover, intracellular glucose is converted to sorbitol by the enzyme aldose reductase. This sorbitol exerts osmotic effect resulting in tissue damage particularly in the retina and peripheral nerves. Hence, it is necessary to maintain normal blood glucose levels though diabetes mellitus as such does not cause significant troublesome symptoms. It helps to prevent or delay the onset of complications of diabetes. The haemoglobin becomes glycosylated and forms HBA_{1C} and its concentration indicates the severity and duration of the hyperglycaemic state.

Administration of glucose by oral route stimulates insulin secretion better than by IV route because orally given glucose evokes the release of gastrointestinal hormones and also stimulates vagal activity.

INSULIN

In 1921, Banting and Best first obtained insulin in the form of pancreatic extract. In 1922, an extract containing insulin was first used on a 14-year-old boy suffering from severe diabetes mellitus with excellent response. Insulin was then purified in a few years.

Chemistry, Synthesis and Secretion

The islets of Langerhans are composed of 4 types of cells—β (B) cells secrete insulin, α (A) cells glucagon, δ (D) cells somatostatin and P cells secrete pancreatic polypeptide. Glucose enters the pancreatic β cells with the help of glucose transporters. Insulin is released from the granules by a process of exocytosis. Natural insulin is a polypeptide synthesized from the precursor preproinsulin which is cleaved to get proinsulin. Proinsulin is processed in the secretory granules to get insulin. It has two peptide chains—A chain (21 amino acids) and B chain (30 amino acids) linked by disulphide bridges. Human insulin differs from bovine insulin by 3 amino acids and from porcine insulin by 1 amino acid. Hence porcine insulin is closer to human insulin.

Insulin is stored in granules in the β islet cells of the pancreas. Normal pancreas releases about **40 to 50** units of insulin everyday. Basal insulin secretion is 0.5–1 U/hr and increases after meals up to 6 U/hr. The secretion is regulated by factors like food, hormones and autonomic nervous system. Hypokalaemia inhibits insulin release. Blood glucose concentration is the main factor which determines insulin secretion.

Insulin is metabolised in the liver, kidney and muscle.

Glucose transporters are proteins present in different tissues. They are of 5 subtypes—GLUT1 to GLUT5. They mediate various functions, e.g. GLUT4 present in muscle and adipose tissues promotes the uptake of glucose.

Actions of Insulin

1. *Carbohydrate metabolism:* Insulin stimulates the uptake and metabolism of glucose in the peripheral tissues especially skeletal muscles and adipose tissue. It inhibits glucose production in the liver by inhibiting gluconeogenesis and glycogenolysis.

   By the above actions, insulin lowers the blood glucose concentration.
2. *Lipid metabolism:* Insulin inhibits lipolysis in adipose tissue and promotes the synthesis of triglycerides. In diabetes, large amounts of fat are broken down. The free fatty acids so formed are converted by the liver to acetyl-CoA and then ketone bodies. This results in ketonaemia and ketonuria.

   Insulin indirectly enhances lipoprotein lipase activity resulting in increased clearance of VLDL and chylomicrons. In insulin deficiency, there is hypertriglyceridaemia.
3. *Protein metabolism:* Insulin facilitates amino acid uptake and protein synthesis and inhibits protein breakdown—**anabolic effect**.

   In diabetes, there is increased catabolic effect and negative nitrogen balance.

Mechanism of Action

Insulin acts by binding to specific receptors (Fig. 42.1). Insulin receptor is a glycoprotein made up of two α and two β subunits. Insulin receptors are present on almost all cells in the body. Insulin binds to the α subunit of the receptors present on the surface of target cells. This binding stimulates tyrosine kinase activity in the β subunit. This in turn activates a cascade of phosphorylation and dephosphorylation reactions which stimulate or inhibit the enzymes involved in the metabolic actions of insulin.

Side Effects

1. *Hypoglycaemia* is the most common complication of insulin therapy. It may be due to too large a dose, inappropriate time of administration, unusually small meal or vigorous exercise or simply by intensive efforts to reduce hyperglycaemia. Symptoms—sweating, palpitation, tremors, hunger, anxiety, difficulty in concentration and drowsiness are the first symptoms of hypoglycaemia and appear at blood glucose

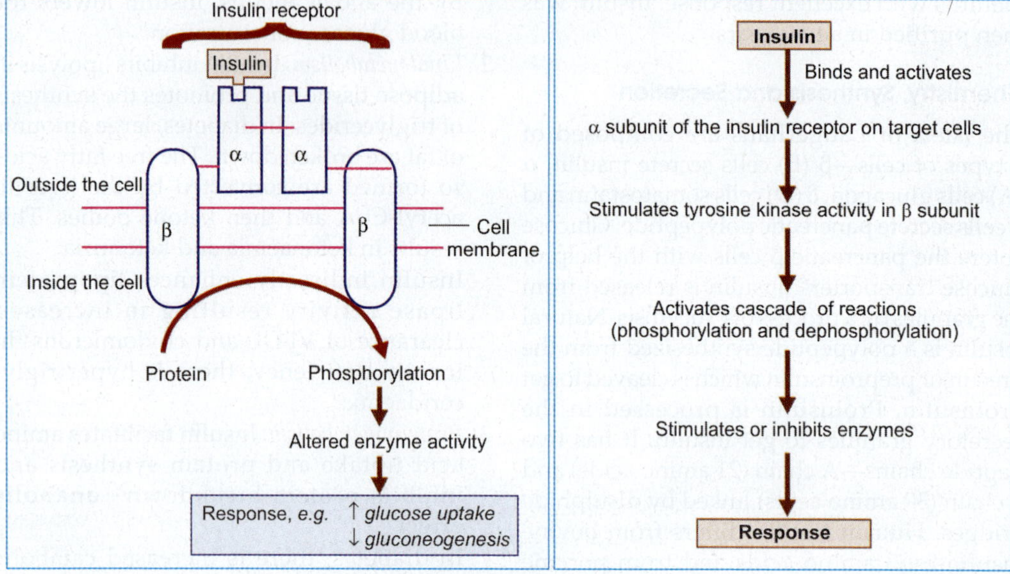

Fig. 42.1: Mechanism of action of insulin

levels of 60–80 mg/dl. These are followed by blurred vision, confusion and weakness. Severe hypoglycaemia may result in convulsions and coma due to cerebral glucopenia.

Treatment: Oral glucose or fruit juice like orange juice or in severe cases IV glucose promptly reverse the symptoms.

2. *Allergy:* This is due to the contaminating proteins. Urticaria, angio-oedema and rarely anaphylaxis can occur. It is rare with purified preparations and human insulin.

3. *Lipodystrophy:* Atrophy of the subcutaneous fat at the site of injection may be due to immune response to contaminating proteins.

Lipohypertrophy, i.e. enlargement of subcutaneous tissue, can also occur due to the local action of insulin. Insulin absorption may be irregular from such areas. This can be prevented by frequently changing the sites of injection. Lipodystrophy is rare with purified preparations.

4. *Oedema:* Some severe diabetics develop oedema which is self-limiting.

Preparations of Insulin

- Insulin preparations are classified as in Table 42.1.
- Insulins are destroyed by the acidic pH of gastric juice when given orally, hence all preparations are given subcutaneously.
- In emergencies, only regular (plain) insulin can be given IV.
- Doses are expressed as units.
- **Regular insulin** is plain/soluble insulin which is mixed with a small amount of zinc. Given SC it gets absorbed over 30–60 minutes. It is the only type of insulin **suitable for IV use.**
- Long-acting preparations are obtained by mixing regular insulin with protamine or zinc. Neutral protamine Hagedorn (NPH or isophane insulin) is neutral in pH with added protamine. It acts for 18–24 hr. Protamine zinc insulin (PZI) has both protamine and zinc complexed to insulin for a long duration of action.

Insulin zinc suspension in different ratios and particle sizes result in lente preparations.

Table 42.1: Preparations of insulin

1. ***Rapid-acting insulin analogs***
   Insulin lispro
   Insulin aspart
   Insulin glulisine
2. ***Short-acting insulins***
   Regular/plain
3. ***Intermediate-acting insulins***
   Isophane insulin (NPH)
   Insulin zinc suspension/Lente
4. ***Long-acting insulin analogs***
   Insulin glargine
   Insulin detemir
   Insulin degludec
5. ***Insulin mixtures***
   Combinations of 20–50% regular/rapid acting analogs with 80–50% NPH or longer acting analogs

Semilente is short-acting, lente is intermediate acting and ultra-lente is long-acting. However, these lente preparations are not available in most countries now.

Insulin dose: Requirement of insulin should be calculated in each patient by monitoring blood glucose and glycosylated haemoglobin levels. Several regimens including mixtures of insulins are being used. Multiple doses of insulin offer better glycaemic control as compared to single bedtime dose. In an IDDM patient, the daily requirement of insulin varies from 0.2 to 1 IU/kg. In obese patients, the requirement is higher. In type II diabetes, patients insulin requirement varies from 0.2 to 1.6 IU/kg/day.

Based on the duration of action, insulin preparations (Table 42.2) may be grouped as:

1. Rapid-acting Insulins

Some insulin analogs act much faster than regular insulin. When injected, natural insulin forms hexamers which are absorbed slowly while rapid-acting insulin analogs form monomers which are absorbed faster and rapidly attain peak levels. Such rapid peaks resemble physiological release of insulin. They are absorbed 3 times faster than human insulin—therefore, can be given subcutaneously 10 minutes before food; have lesser chances of hypoglycaemia.

Insulin lispro, insulin aspart and insulin glulisine are rapid- and short-acting with a maximum duration of action of 4–5 hours. Their absorption is more reliable compared to other insulins stored in the form of hexamers.

i. *Insulin lispro* differs from human insulin by the transposition of two amino acids—proline and lysine in the β chain (at

Table 42.2: Onset and duration of action of insulin preparations

Insulin	*Onset*	*Duration (hr)*
Rapid acting insulin analogs		
Lispro	5–15	2–5
Aspart	5–15	3–5
Glulisine	5–15	1–2
Short-acting insulin		
Regular (plain, soluble)	30–60 min	5–8
Intermediate-acting		
Insulin zinc suspension	2 h	18–24
NPH (neutral protamine hagedorn) or Isophane insulin	2 h	18–24
Long-acting		
Glargine	2–5 h	18–24
Detemir	1–2 h	6–24
Insulin mixtures		
Insulin zinc suspension crystalline	6 h	20–36
PZI (protamine zinc insulin)	6 h	24–36

position B28 and 29)—hence the name lispro. On SC administration, onset of action is in 5–15 min and peak effect in 1 hr. It offers better glycaemic control and 20–30% lesser incidence of hypoglycaemia compared to regular insulins.

HUMALOG 100 U/ml inj.

ii. *Insulin aspart* is obtained by substituting aspartic acid in place of proline in the β chain. It has similar effects as insulin lispro.

NOVORAPID FLEXPEN 100 IU/ml inj.

iii. *Insulin glulisine* is similar to insulin lispro. It is formed by substituting glutamic acid for lysine (at position B29) and lysine for asparagine (at position B23). It is the analog used in insulin pump.

2. Short-acting Insulins

Regular insulin is soluble or plain insulin which is mixed with a small amount of zinc. It can be given by SC, IV and IM injection. Though rapid acting insulins can be given IV, regular insulin is the only insulin preparation that is preferred for IV use. The insulin molecules bind to form hexamers in the vial which on injection gradually dissociate into monomers to get absorbed. Hence regular insulin should be administered 30 minutes before food. On IV use, the hexamers immediately dissociate into monomers and are, therefore, useful in emergencies.

3. Intermediate-acting Insulins

NPH or isophane insulin is neutral in pH and combined with protamine to delay the absorption. Onset of action is about 2 hours but acts for 18–24 hours. It is generally mixed with regular or rapid-acting analogs for fast and long-action. Since the long-acting insulin analogs have more predictable actions, NPH is the less preferred form of insulin.

4. Long-acting Insulin Analogs

Insulin glargine is a long-acting analog which acts for 24 hr. The effect is peakless but attains a broad plasma concentration plateau. Obtained by adding 2 arginine molecules to carboxyl terminal of beta chain and placing glycine for asparagine (at A 21 position). On SC injection, glargine molecules dissolve gradually and provide a low but steady concentration of insulin in the plasma over 24 hr—the best among long-acting insulins. Insulin glargine should not be mixed with any other insulin in the syringe because it is acidic and there is a risk of loss of efficacy of the other drugs.

LANTUS 100 U/ml in 3 ml pen injector.

Insulin detemir is another long-acting insulin analog. Myristic acid, a fatty acid, is attached to the terminal lysine and from B30 position, the terminal threonine is removed to get the analog insulin detemir. It has an onset of action of 1–2 hr—however, it is given twice daily for smoother control of blood sugar and lower incidence of hypoglycaemic episodes. It should not be mixed with any other insulins.

Insulin degludec is similar to human insulin with a minor modification like deletion of last amino acid from the B-chain and addition of a glutamyl link from Lys B29. It is long acting (>40 hr) and also is compatible with rapid-acting insulins—it can be mixed with them.

5. Insulin Mixtures

Mixtures of short-, intermediate- and long-acting preparations are given for a rapid onset and long duration of action. Such ready-made mixtures may be available in vials or may be mixed by the patient in the syringe just before injecting. NPH insulin may be mixed with regular insulin before use. Example of one such regimen that offers good glycemic control is one dose of glargine once a day and 2–3 injections of a rapid-acting insulin like insulin lispro—one dose before each meal.

Types of Insulin

Insulin preparations differ in their source and duration of action. Based on the source they may be grouped as:

1. ***Animal insulins or conventional insulins*** are obtained from bovine and porcine pancreas and are no more used because human insulins are now available. Though they are cheaper, they have the disadvantages of being allergenic and poorly stable (Table 42.2).
2. ***Highly purified insulins*** are mostly porcine insulins purified by more developed purification techniques. Though they are less antigenic, they are not used now because human insulins are better.
3. ***Human insulins*** are the insulins used now. They are produced by recombinant DNA technology. Human proinsulin gene is introduced into *E. coli*, which is cultured and proinsulin is extracted. This is modified to get human insulin. It can also be obtained by enzymatic treatment of porcine insulin. Human insulin is available as regular and long-acting (NPH) preparations. Human insulin is less immunogenic and is absorbed more rapidly; dose needed is lesser (~10%).
4. ***Insulin analogs:*** Minor modifications of the position of amino acids in the insulin molecule can yield insulin analogs. Such genetically engineered recombinant analogs have certain advantages over original insulins as:
   - Favourable pharmacokinetic profile
   - Better blood glucose control than with natural insulins
   - Rapid-acting analogs produce rapid insulin peaks which closely mimic physiological insulin release.

Rapid- and short-acting analogs include insulin lispro, aspart and glulisine while insulin glargine, determir and degludec are long-acting insulin analogs given as follows.

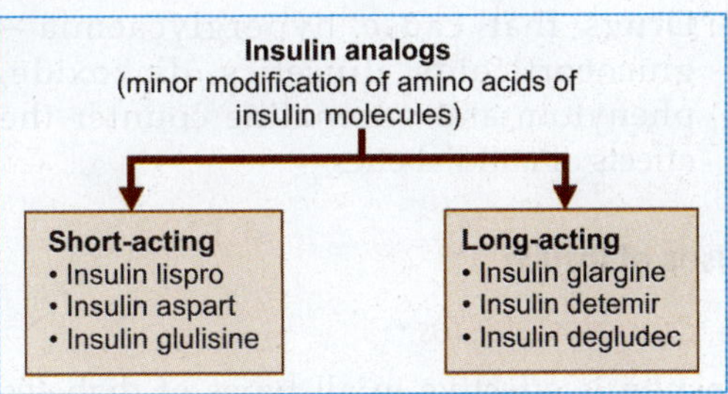

Insulin Delivery Devices

Devices have been designed which make insulin administration more convenient. Portable **pen injectors** are small pen-size devices containing multiple doses of insulin and retractable needles. They can be carried while travelling and to the place of work. Insulin pumps (also called continuous subcutaneous insulin infusion or CSII) deliver appropriate doses of insulin on the basis of self-monitored blood glucose results. The set is inserted subcutaneously.

Alternative routes of insulin delivery have been tried—by inhalation, nasal spray, orally, rectally and as subcutaneous pellet implants.

Insulin is inhaled through the mouth with a special inhaler device which delivers human insulin powder. Inhaled insulin is absorbed through lungs and attains therapeutic levels. However, very soon after its launch, it was withdrawn from the market because of safety concerns.

Orally insulin is tried with liposomes as carriers. Orally delivered insulin is yet to make a breakthrough. Subcutaneous pellets deliver insulin over weeks.

Drug Interactions

1. β adrenergic blockers mask tachycardia, the important warning symptom of hypoglycaemia. They also prolong hypoglycaemia by inhibiting compensatory mechanisms acting through β_2 receptors.
2. Salicylates, lithium and theophylline precipitate hypoglycaemia by enhancing insulin secretion and β cell sensitivity to glucose.

3. Drugs that cause hyperglycaemia—glucocorticoids, diuretics, diazoxide, phenytoin and adrenaline counter the effects of antidiabetics.

Uses of Insulin

1. *Diabetes Mellitus*

Insulin is effective in all types of diabetes mellitus. The dose should be adjusted as per the needs of each patient—guided by blood sugar and glycosylated Hb levels.

2. *Diabetic Ketoacidosis*

Diabetic ketoacidosis is a medical emergency and can be life-threatening. It is more common in patients with IDDM. Ketoacidosis may be precipitated by infection, trauma, stress or high doses of glucocorticoids. Insulin deficiency results in severe hyperglycaemia (600–800 mg/dl) and excessive production of ketone bodies.

Clinical features include metabolic acidosis, dehydration with loss of sodium and potassium in the urine causing electrolyte imbalance, nausea, vomiting, abdominal pain, confusion, impaired consciousness and hyperventilation—may proceed to coma. Ketone bodies in blood and urine are increased.

Treatment

- *Correction of hyperglycaemia:* Intravenous regular (plane) insulin 0.1U/kg bolus followed by 0.1 U/kg/hour by continuous IV infusion till the patient recovers. Once the patient has fully recovered, SC insulin should be administered 30 minutes before stopping the infusion.
- *Correction of dehydration:* Fluid and electrolyte replacement is important. Normal saline infusion—1 litre in the first hour and then 1 litre over the next 4 hours. The dose can then be titrated based on the severity of dehydration.
- *Correction of acidosis:* Sodium bicarbonate may be needed in some patients with severe acidosis.
- *Potassium:* Rapid correction of hyperglycaemia may result in the movement of potassium into the cells resulting in hypokalaemia. 10–20 mEq/hour potassium chloride is added to the drip. When serum phosphate is also low, potassium biphosphate may be given to supplement both potassium and phosphorus.
- *Blood glucose* may come down to normal but ketosis requires a longer time to be corrected and requires adequate insulin. Hence when the blood glucose comes down to about 300 mg/dl it may be needed to administer glucose with insulin while we wait for the clearance of ketone bodies.

3. *Hyperglycaemic, Hyperosmolar, Nonketotic Coma*

Severe hyperglycaemia and glycosuria result in severe dehydration and increased plasma osmolarity leading to mental confusion, sometimes convulsions and coma and has a high mortality rate.

The treatment is similar to ketoacidosis with immediate correction of fluid and electrolyte balance and plain insulin.

4. *Other Uses of Insulin*

Insulin has been tried in the past for other indications like in *hyperkalaemia* as insulin promotes movement of potassium into the cells. Insulin 5–10 units with 50 ml of 50% glucose slow infusion may be tried.

Insulin resistance is said to be present when the insulin requirement is increased to >200 U/day. Many consider insulin requirement of >100 U/day as resistance. Acute resistance develops quickly but it is also of short duration and reversible. It may be precipitated by factors like infection, stress including emotional and physical stress (trauma, surgery) or drugs that cause hyperglycaemia (like thiazides, Key Box 42.2). Once the precipitating factor is treated, requirement of insulin decreases.

Chronic resistance develops over years of insulin use. It is due to the antibodies to insulin which partly neutralise it. This is rare with purified preparations and human insulin. Antibodies may also develop to contaminants and other added constituents like protamine. Hence in presence of resistance, it is necessary to change over to highly purified/human insulin, if the patient is receiving conventional insulin. Most patients need regular insulin for some time till the resistance is overcome. Other precipitating factors should be corrected. In some patients, immunosuppression with glucocorticoids, like prednisolone, may help. Pregnancy and hormonal contraceptives can induce insulin resistance.

ORAL ANTIDIABETIC DRUGS

The main disadvantage of insulin is the need for injection. The advent of oral antidiabetics came as a boon to millions of NIDDM patients with early and mild diabetes. Sulfonylureas were the first oral antidiabetics (OAD) to be made available in 1950s. We now have several groups of oral antidiabetics. Many newer drugs are also being introduced. Though all orally active antidiabetic drugs are often called oral hypoglycaemics, all of them do not cause hypoglycaemia. Therefore, 'oral antidiabetic drugs' is a more appropriate terminology for them.

Classification

1. **Insulin secretogogues**
   A. *Sulfonylureas (K_{ATP} channel blockers)*
      I generation
      Tolbutamide
      II generation
      Glibenclamide, glipizide
      gliclazide, glimepiride
   B. *Meglitinides*
      Repaglinide, nateglinide
   C. *GLP-1 analogs* (subcutaneous)
      Exenatide, Liraglutide, albiglutide
      dulaglutide
   D. *DPP-4 inhibitors*
      Sitagliptin, Vildagliptin, Saxagliptin,
      Linagliptin, alogliptin
2. **Biguanide**
   Metformin
3. **Thiazolidinediones**
   Troglitazone, pioglitazone
4. **α-glucosidase inhibitors**
   Acarbose, miglitol, voglibose
5. **Amylin analog**
   Pramlintide (subcutaneous)
6. **SGLT-2 inhibitors**
   Dapagliflozin, remogliflozin

1. INSULIN SECRETAGOGUES

A. Sulfonylureas

A sulfonamide derivative used for its antibacterial effects in typhoid patients produced hypoglycaemia. This observation led to the development of sulfonylureas. These drugs **enhance insulin release**—insulin secretogogues.

Mechanism of Action

Sulfonylureas reduce the blood glucose level by:

1. Stimulating the release of insulin from the pancreatic β cells.
2. Increasing the sensitivity of peripheral tissues to insulin.
3. Increasing the number of insulin receptors.
4. Suppressing hepatic gluconeogenesis.
5. Prolonged administration of sulfonylureas in Type II DM patients reduces the glucagon levels probably due to negative feedback from raised insulin levels.

Sulfonylureas bind to the sulfonylurea receptors (SUR) which are nothing but the ATP sensitive K^+ channels (K_{ATP}) present on the cell membrane of the pancreatic beta cells. Sulfonylureas bind to the SUR1 subunit on the K_{ATP} and bring about closure of these K^+ channels (prevent K^+ efflux) causing

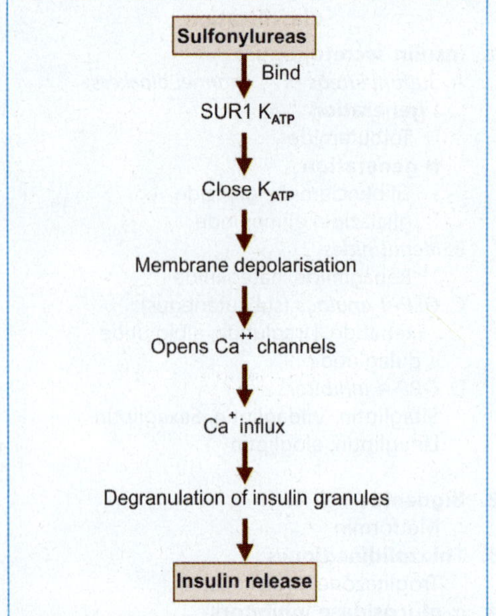

depolarisation of the membrane. This inturn opens the voltage-dependent calcium channels, thereby leading to calcium influx. This calcium brings about release of insulin that is stored in the granules of the beta cells.

Pharmacokinetics

Sulfonylureas are well-absorbed orally, extensively bound to plasma proteins (>90%), metabolised in the liver and some are excreted in the urine. Hence they should be avoided in patients with renal or liver dysfunction.

Adverse Effects

- Second generation agents have fewer adverse effects. Hypoglycaemia is the most common adverse effect, least with tolbutamide due to short t½ and low potency.
- Nausea, vomiting, jaundice, and allergic reactions can occur (Table 42.3).
- Sulfonylureas can precipitate a **disulfiram-like reaction** on consumption of alcohol. Patients should be warned to abstain from alcohol while on sulfonylureas.

Drug Interactions

I. Drugs that augment hypoglycaemic effect.
  - NSAIDs, warfarin, sulfonamides—displace sulfonylureas from protein binding sites.
  - Alcohol, chloramphenicol, cimetidine—inhibit metabolism

II. Drugs that reduce the effects of sulfonylureas
  - Diuretics and glucocorticoids—increase blood glucose levels.

First Generation Agents

First generation agents include tolbutamide and chlorpropamide but after the synthesis of second generation agents which have certain advantages, first generation agents are not preferred.

Tolbutamide is short acting as it is rapidly metabolised in the liver, t½ 4–5 hr and is therefore, associated with lesser risk of hypoglycaemia but is rarely used now.

Dose: 500 mg BD-TDS. RASTINON 500 mg tab

Second Generation Agents

Second generation agents are more potent, have fewer side effects and drug interactions as compared to first generation agents. They can cause hypoglycaemia because of which they should be used cautiously particularly in the elderly. Utmost caution is also required in patients with cardiovascular diseases. They are all contraindicated in renal and hepatic impairment.

Glibenclamide (gliburide) is a commonly used sulfonylurea. It is longer acting—can be given once a day (Table 42.4). It can cause hypoglycaemia and rarely, flushing after alcohol consumption. It may be started with a low dose of 2.5 mg in the morning and increased to 5–10 mg once daily. Different formulations are available for controlled release and extended release.

Dose: 2.5–5 mg OD. DAONIL, EUGLUCON 2.5, 5 mg tab

Table 42.3: Mechanism of action and adverse effects of oral antidiabetics

Oral antidiabetics (example)	*Major mechanism*	*Adverse effects*
1. Sulphonylureas (glipizide)	↑insulin release from pancreas ↑tissue sensitivity to insulin	Hypoglycaemia, cholestatic jaundice Disulfiram-like reaction
2. Meglitinides (repaglinide)	↑insulin release from pancreas	Hypoglycaemia
3. GLP-1 analogs/incretin analogs (liraglutide)	↓glucagon release, delay gastric emptying ↓appetite	Nausea, vomiting, diarrhoea, weight loss, haemorrhagic pancreatitis
4. DPP-4 inhibitors (linagliptin)	↑insulin secretion ↓glucagon levels ↓appetite	Headache, allergy ↑ incidence of URI
5. Biguanides (metformin)	↓hepatic gluconeogenesis ↑tissue sensitivity to insulin	Diarrhoea, metallic taste, rarely lactic acidosis.
6. Thiazolidinediones (pioglitazine)	PPAR γ agonist ↑glucose transport into tissues ↓hepatic gluconeogenesis	Weight gain, oedema, may precipitate CCF, Risk of hepatotoxicity
7. α glucosidase inhibitors (acarbose)	↓glucose absorption ↓hydrolysis of disaccharides	Flatulence, diarrhoea, abdominal distension
8. Amylin analogs (pramlintide)	↓glucagon release, delay gastric emptying ↓appetite	Nausea, vomiting, anorexia
9. SGLT-2 inhibitors (dapagliflozin)	Inhibit sodium glucose cotrans-porter-2 in kidneys→ ↑glucose excretion	↑urinary frequency ↑UTI (↑glucose in urine) electrolyte imbalance

Table 42.4: Duration of action of oral antidiabetics

Drug	*Duration of action*
Tolbutamide	6–8 hr
Chlorpropamide	36–48 hr
Glibenclamide	18–24 hr
Glipizide	12–18 hr
Gliclazide	12–24 hr
Glimepiride	12–24 hr
Metformin	6–8 hr
Repaglinide	4–5 hr
Nateglinide	3–4 hr
Pioglitazone	12–24 hr

Glipizide has a short t½; food delays its absorption, hence should be taken 30 min before breakfast. It is less likely to cause hypoglycaemia because of its short t½. Started with 5 mg/day the dose may be increased to 15 mg/day. It is metabolized in the liver; contraindicated in renal and hepatic dysfunction.

Dose: 5–15 mg OD-BD. GLYNASE, GLIBETIC, D-GLIP 5 mg tab

Gliclazide can be used in diabetes with renal dysfunction. It is found to delay the onset of retinopathy in diabetics.

Dose: 40–240 mg OD. D-GLIC, GLIX

Glimepiride is longer acting and can be given as a single morning dose—started with 1 mg, the dose may be increased to 4 mg daily but a maximum of 8 mg has also been given.

Dose:1–4 mg OD. GLYPRIDE, GLIMZ, AMARYL-1, 2 mg tab.

B. Meglitinides

Repaglinide and nateglinide are insulin secretogogues and like sulphonylureas, meglitinides enhance the release of insulin by **blocking the ATP-dependent K⁺ channels** (sulfonylurea receptors) in the pancreatic β cells.

Repaglinide is rapidly absorbed, has a rapid onset of action, peak effect in 1 hr and a t½ of 1 hour. It is metabolised in the liver by microsomal enzymes. Gastrointestinal disturbances are common with repaglinide. Both drugs can cause hypersensitivity reactions and hypoglycaemia—but the incidence is relatively lower with nateglinide.

Dose: 0.5–4 mg. TDS-QID 30 min before food.
RAPLEN 0.5, 1, 2 mg tab. EUREPA 0.5, 2, 4 mg.

Nateglinide is a D-phenylalanine derivative. It is rapidly absorbed with peak effect in 60 min and a duration of action of 3–4 hr. It is metabolised by microsomal enzymes in the liver. It can be given even in patients with renal dysfunction and hypoglycaemia is least with it. Nausea, dizziness, joints pain can occur. Nateglinide is administered just before meals in the dose 60–120 mg two-three times a day.

GLINATE 60, 120 mg tab.

Uses: Meglitinides can be used in type II diabetes mellitus either alone or with biguanides. They can also be used as alternatives to sulfonylureas—a dose before each major meal.

- May be useful in patients allergic to sulfonylureas, they do not have sulfur in their structure.
- Meglitinides enhance insulin release in presence of glucose—therefore, the incidence of hypoglycaemia is least with their use.
- In patients who have significant post-prandial hyperglycaemia (fast action and less hypoglycaemia) but the basal insulin secretion is not altered by meglitinides.

C. Glucagon Like Peptide-1 (GLP-1) Analogs/Incretin Analogs

Glucagon like peptides (also called incretins) are released from the gut following oral glucose administration and GLP-1 inturn enhances insulin secretion. However, GLP-1 cannot be used therapeutically due to its rapid degradation by the enzyme dipeptidyl peptidase-4 (DPP-4). Exenatide is a synthetic GLP-1 analog which acts on the GLP-1 receptors. It enhances the glucose-1-mediated insulin secretion, suppresses glucagon release, delays gastric emptying and reduces appetite. Studies have shown it to increase the beta cell mass and reduce HdA1c levels.

Exenatide is given SC 30–60 min before food in the dose of 5–10 µg twice daily in type II DM. Long-acting preparations are available for once weekly injection.

Liraglutide, a longer-acting analog, is given once daily. Started with a low dose of 0.6 mg and doubled after a week, liraglutide may be used as an add-on drug.

Albiglutide is GLP-1 fused to human albumin and **dulaglutide** is another GLP-1 analog and both have a longer t½ for once weekly injection. Semaglutide and lixisenatide are other GLP-1 analogs.

GLP-1 analogs can cause nausea, vomiting (self-limiting), diarrhoea and weight loss. One adverse effect of concern though rare is the **haemorrhagic pancreatitis** which can be fatal. Should be avoided in patients with renal impairment as it can be worsened.

D. Dipeptidyl Peptidase 4 (DPP-4) Inhibitors

Dipeptidyl peptidase is an enzyme which degrades incretins. **Sitagliptin** is a DPP-4 inhibitor and thereby enhances incretin levels. It enhances insulin secretion and decreases glucagon levels. Sitagliptin is orally effective (dose: 100 mg OD) and may be used alone or along with other antidiabetic drugs. Adverse effects include headache, increased susceptibility to upper respiratory infections and allergic reactions. Saxagliptin (2.5–5 mg OD) and linagliptin (5 mg OD) are longer acting DPP-4 inhibitors.

2. BIGUANIDES

Biguanides lower blood glucose level by insulin-like effects on the tissues (Key Box 42.1).

Key Box 42.1: Biguanides

- Have insulin-like effects
- Do not cause hypoglycaemia
- Weight reduction—due to anorexia
- Nausea, diarrhoea, metallic taste are transient
- Preferred in obese diabetics
- Suitable for combination therapy
- **Off label uses**—obesity, hirsutism, infertility in PCOD patients.
- **Contraindications:** Renal, hepatic and unstable cardiac diseases

Mechanism of action is not clear but could act as follows:

- Suppress hepatic gluconeogenesis by activation of an enzyme (AMP-activated protein kinase or AMPK)—this is the principal effect.
- Inhibit glucose absorption from the intestines.
- Stimulate peripheral uptake of glucose in tissues in the presence of insulin.
- Stimulate glycolysis in the tissues.
- Reduce plasma glucagon levels.
- Decrease appetite

Pharmacokinetics: Metformin is well-absorbed from the gut, has a duration of action of 6–8 hr, is not metabolised but excreted unchanged in the urine.

Dose: 500 mg OD-BD. GLYCIPHAGE, DIAFORMIN 500 mg tab.

Adverse effects: Though phenformin is also a biguanide, it is not used therapeutically as it causes lactic acidosis. Metformin is safer with lower incidence of **lactic acidosis**. It does not cause hypoglycaemia since it is an **euglycaemic** (or antihyperglycemic) **agent**.

Nausea, diarrhoea, and metallic taste are self-limiting. Rarely lactic acidosis can occur particularly in patients with renal and hepatic dysfunction. **Anorexia** is advantageous as it helps in reducing body weight. Long-term use may interfere with vitamin B_{12} absorption—leading to vitamin B_{12} deficiency—B_{12} levels should be checked once a year.

Uses: Other than in diabetes, metformin is tried in a variety of conditions (off-label uses) like obesity, hirsutism and infertility in PCOD patients. Metformin reduces androgen levels and increases chances of ovulation.

3. THIAZOLIDINEDIONES (TZDs)

Thiazolidinediones (TZDs) or glitazones are agonists at the PPAR-γ receptors (gamma subtype of peroxisome proliferator-activated receptors). These are nuclear receptors present mostly in adipose tissue and also in muscle, liver and other tissues. TZDs activate the PPAR-γ receptors and modulate the expression of insulin-sensitive genes, i.e. they induce the synthesis of genes which enhance insulin action.

TZDs increase insulin-mediated glucose transport into muscle and adipose tissue. They also promote glucose utilization.

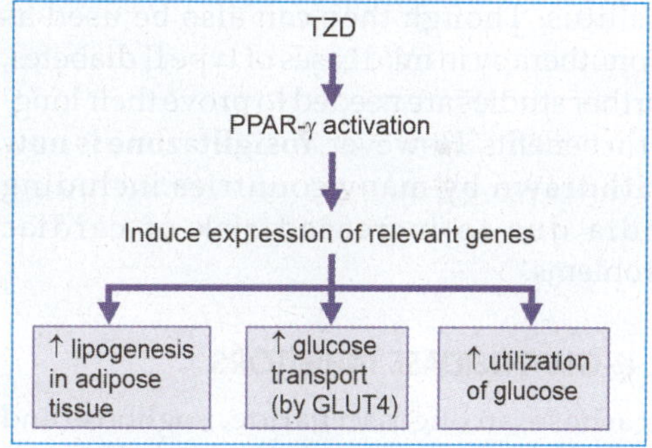

Advantages

- Reduce hepatic gluconeogenesis
- Once a day administration
- Low potential for hypoglycaemia
- Increase HDL cholesterol
- No clinically significant drug interactions known so far.
- Reduce mortality.

Disadvantages

- 6–12 weeks of treatment is required to establish maximum therapeutic effect.

- May cause weight gain and anaemia.
- May cause oedema and precipitate or worsen CCF.
- Liver function should be monitored regularly.
- Increased risk of bone fracture in post-menopausal women.
- Troglitazone causes severe hepatotoxicity and, therefore, is not used.

Pioglitazone is an agonist at PPAR-α and PPAR-γ receptors. It lowers plasma triglyceride levels and raises HDL cholesterol—could be due to its action on PPAR-α receptors. It is absorbed over 2 hr after oral administration and absorption is further delayed by food. It is metabolised by hepatic microsomal enzymes and the metabolites are also active.

Dose: 15–45 mg once daily. PIONORM, PIOREST 15, 30 mg tab.

Uses: TZDs are used as adjuvants to sulfonylureas/biguanides/insulin in Type II diabetes mellitus. Though they can also be used as monotherapy in mild cases of type II diabetes, further studies are needed to prove their long-term benefits. However, **rosiglitazone is now withdrawn** by many countries including India due to increased risk of cardiac problems.

4. α-GLUCOSIDASE INHIBITORS

Acarbose, an oligosaccharide, voglibose and miglitol competitively inhibit the enzymes α-glucosidases present in the intestinal brush border and thereby prevent the absorption and delay the digestion of carbohydrates. Monosaccharides like glucose and fructose are absorbed from the intestines while disaccharides and oligosaccharides are broken down into monosaccharides before being absorbed. This 'breaking down' is done by the enzymes α-glucosidases (e.g. sucrase, maltase, glycoamylase) and α-amylase present in the intestinal wall. Alpha glucosidase inhibitors inhibit the hydrolysis of disaccharides and decrease carbohydrate absorption.

- Alpha-glucosidase inhibitors reduce the glucose absorption from upper intestines, thereby reducing postprandial blood glucose levels.
- Miglitol also inhibits isomaltase and beta glucosidases.

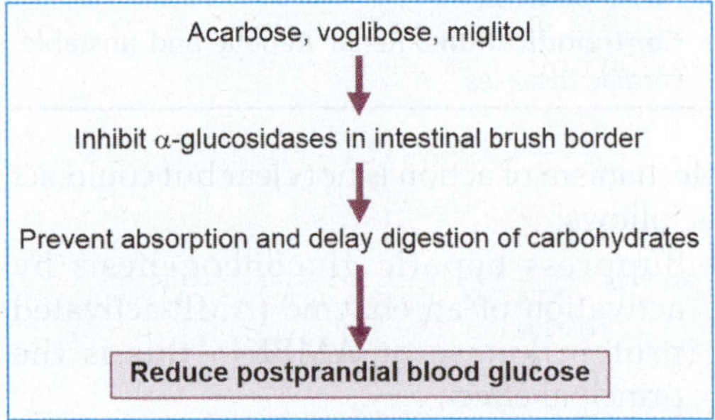

- Alpha-glucosidase inhibitors do not cause hypoglycaemia. When used with other antidiabetics—if hypoglycaemia occurs, glucose should be given and not sucrose because sucrase is also inhibited.
- They may cause gastrointestinal disturbances including abdominal distention and pain, flatulence and diarrhoea because of undigested carbohydrates reaching the colon and then getting fermented to fatty acids and in the process gas is released.
- They can be used alone in patients with predominantly postprandial hyperglycaemia or in combination with other oral anti-diabetics or insulin.
- They are contraindicated in patients with inflammatory bowel disease and in renal failure.

5. AMYLIN ANALOGS

Amylin is a polypeptide produced by the pancreatic beta cells. It inhibits glucagon secretion, delays gastric emptying and suppresses appetite. **Pramlintide,** a synthetic amylin analog, modulates postprandial glucose levels like amylin.

Pramlintide has beneficial effects on HbA_{1C} levels. Given subcutaneously it is rapidly absorbed and has a duration of action around 2–3 hr. Started with a low dose of 15 μg just before meals; dose may be increased to 60–120 μg but the concurrent dose of insulin or other antidiabetics may be reduced to avoid hypoglycaemia. It should not be mixed with other drugs in the syringe. It can cause nausea, vomiting and anorexia. Pramlintide can be used in both type I and type II DM.

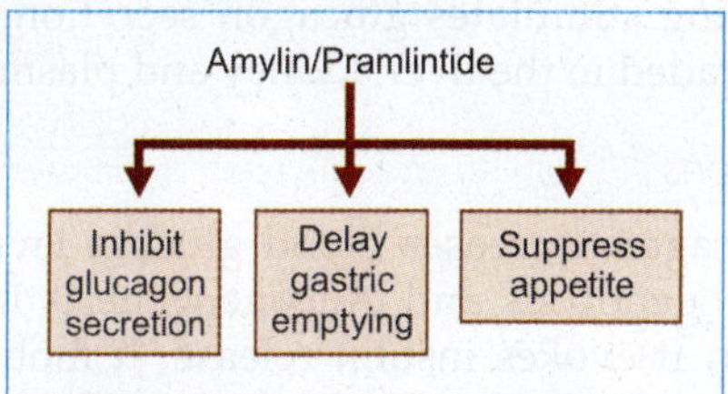

6. SGLT-2 INHIBITORS

A large amount of glucose is reabsorbed from the proximal tubule by **sodium-glucose cotransporter-2** (SGLT-2). Inhibition of SGLT-2 reduces the absorption of glucose and sodium and causes glycosuria. Dapagliflozin, remogliflozin, canagliflozin, empagliflozin and sergliflozin are SGLT-2 inhibitors found to be useful in patients with diabetes. They are particularly useful when the patients also have hypertension. They do not cause hypoglycaemia but could cause hypotension and increase the risk of urinary infection due to the presence of glucose in the urine. They should be avoided in presence of low GFR.

Metabolic syndrome

Metabolic syndrome is a prediabetic state and is associated with an increased risk of developing coronary heart disease.

Criteria for metabolic syndrome:

- Triglycerides, >150 mg/dl
- HDL cholesterol, <40 mg/dl in men
- BP >130/85 mm Hg
- Fasting glucose >110 mg/dl
- Waist circumference: >90 men; >85 cm women.

TREATMENT OF DIABETES MELLITUS

The aim of treatment is to keep the blood sugar within normal limits and prevent complications of diabetes. For patients with type I, insulin is the only treatment as there is insulin deficiency due to destruction of pancreatic β cells. Sulfonylureas need functional β cells for their action and, therefore, are not useful in them.

Mild type II may be controlled by diet, exercise and weight reduction. When not controlled, an oral hypoglycaemic should be given. Most patients may require insulin sometime later in life.

Status of Oral Antidiabetics

Uncomplicated type 2 diabetes mellitus patients not controlled by diet and exercise are given oral anti-diabetics, patients with recent onset diabetes, age above 40 years at the onset of diabetes, obese with fasting blood sugar <200 mg/dl are candidates for OAD. They are convenient to use. Sulfonylureas and metformin are first-line drugs. Metformin is generally are preferred. **Metformin** has the advantages of

- Reducing appetite
- Being euglycaemic
- Suitable for combination with other drugs.

Therefore, can be considered first-line drug in mild diabetics.

If uncontrolled or if metformin not tolerated, sulfonylurea or any other OAD may be added depending on the patient's need may be added. In conditions like stress, surgery or complications of diabetes, insulin should be used. TZDs, meglitinides, α-glucosidase inhibitors or SGLT-2 inhibitors may be used as monotherapy in mild diabetes patients or as adjuvants along with sulfonylureas or biguanides.

Therapeutic Failure

If patients are not responding to OAD from the very beginning, it is called primary failure and is rare. Secondary failure of sulfonylureas may result from poor diet control, progression of the disease, or from desensitization of the receptors or dug-induced (Key Box 42.2). In

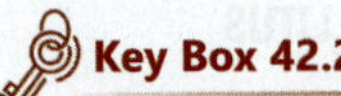

Key Box 42.2

Drugs that can cause hyperglycaemia

- Diazoxide, phenytoin, thiazides, β-adrenergic agonists
- Hormones–adrenaline, glucagon, thyroid hormones, glucocorticoids

Drugs that can cause hypoglycaemia

- Quinine
- Lithium
- Alcohol
- Pentamidine

such cases, it is necessary to change over to another sulfonylurea or add metformin and if still not controlled, switch over to insulin. In some patients, insulin may be supplemented with sulfonylureas as the latter increase the tissue sensitivity to insulin.

Sugar Substitutes

Sugar substitutes are non-sugars which are sweet but have minimum or no caloric value.

Saccharin sodium is an artificial sweetener, 500 times sweeter than sugar and can be used as a dilute (1%) solution. It is excreted unchanged within 24 hours and has no caloric value. Therefore, it can also be used in preparations for diabetes and in slimming diets. It is stable and non-toxic. It can also be used in tooth pastes because it is less likely to encourage the development of caries when compared to other carbohydrates. Saccharin has an unpleasant after-taste while sodium saccharine does not have this disadvantage.

Aspartame is a sugar substitute which is 200 times sweeter than sugar. It is metabolized in the body like proteins and does not have the metallic after-taste of saccharin.

Sugar-free tablets and powder.

Neotame, an analog of aspartame, is sweeter than it and has better heat stability and can be used while cooking.

Sucralose is a trichlorinated sucrose 600 times sweeter than sucrose. It is not absorbed and is excreted through the gut.

Sugarfree gold-powder.

GLUCAGON

Glucagon is synthesized in the alpha (A) cells of the pancreatic islets of Langerhans; like insulin, the secretion of glucagon is regulated by nutrients—chiefly glucose, paracrine hormones and autonomic nervous system. Fasting stimulates glucagon secretion. It is degraded in the liver, kidney and plasma.

Actions

Glucagon increases blood glucose level by glycogenolysis and gluconeogenesis in the liver. It evokes insulin release. It mobilises stored fat and carbohydrates. Glucagon increases heart rate and force of contraction. It also relaxes the intestinal smooth muscles.

Uses

1. Severe hypoglycaemia—glucagon can be used in the emergency treatment of severe hypoglycaemia due to insulin.
2. Diagnostic uses—for diagnosis of IDDM.
3. Radiology of the bowel—as glucagon relaxes the intestinal smooth muscles.

Clinical Pharmacology

- Metformin is the most commonly used drug particularly in obese diabetics.
- Metformin advantages-reduces weight, regulates lipids, lowers blood pressure-beneficial in cardiovascular risk reduction.
- Sulfonylureas are well tolerated and are widely used.
- Pioglitazone or DPP-IV inhibitors and incretins are used as adjuvants.
- Acarbose, voglibose may be added for postprandial hyperglycemia particularly in patients on carbohydrate rich diet.
- Insulin may be used after sulfonylurea failure.

[1] From Medical Council of India, *Competency based Undergraduate Curriculum for the Indian Medical Graduate*, 2018;1:136–144.

Agents Affecting Bone Mineral Turnover and Osteoporosis

CHAPTER 43

Competency achievement: The student should be able to:

PH 1.36 Describe the mechanism of action, types, doses, side effects, indications and contraindications of drugs used in endocrine disorders (diabetes mellitus, thyroid disorders and **osteoporosis**).[1]

Calcium and phosphorus are the most important minerals of the bone with 1–2 kg of calcium and 1 kg of phosphorus stored in it. Calcium and phosphorus metabolism is chiefly regulated by vitamin D, parathormone and we now know of fibroblast growth factor 23 (FGF 23). Other hormones that also influence calcium and phosphorus metabolism are calcitonin, growth hormone, insulin, thyroid hormone, prolactin, glucocorticoids and sex hormones (Key Box 43.1).

CALCIUM

Calcium is essential for tissue excitability, muscular excitation–contraction coupling, secretion from glands, myocardial contractility and formation of bone and teeth. It also maintains the integrity of mucous membranes and cell membrane. Calcium is essential for normal blood coagulation.

Calcium is absorbed from the small intestine by a carrier-mediated active transport. Normally, about 30% of the dietary calcium is absorbed, while in Ca^{++} deficiency, the absorption increases under the control of vitamin D (Fig. 43.1). About 40% of calcium is bound to plasma proteins, about 50% of absorbed Ca^{++} circulates in ionized form. FGF23 influences the Ca^{++} and phosphate metabolism by stimulating the excretion of phosphate by the kidney and inhibiting the production of 1,25 $(OH)_2D_3$ by the kidneys. The normal plasma calcium level is 9–11 mg/dl. It is excreted in the faeces, urine and sweat.

Key Box 43.1: Hormones that influence bone metabolism

- Vitamin D
- Parathormone
- Calcitonin
- Glucocorticoids
- Estrogens

Preparations

Shelcal: Calcium carbonate 625 mg, vit D_3 125 IU tab and syrup.

Osteocalcium: Calcium phosphate 380 mg + Vit D_3 400 IU tab, Calcium phosphate 240 mg/5 ml containing Vit D_3 200 IU and B_{12}.

Calcium sandoz: Calcium glucobionate 137.5 mg/ml inj. Calcium carbonate 650 mg.

Adverse Effects

Oral calcium can produce constipation.

Uses

1. To prevent and treat calcium deficiency. Calcium supplements are given orally in children, pregnant and lactating women and in postmenopausal osteoporosis to prevent calcium deficiency.

   Tetany: 5–10 ml IV calcium gluconate followed by 50–100 ml slow IV infusion promptly reverses the muscular spasm. The injection produces a sense of warmth. This is followed by oral calcium 1.5 g daily for several weeks.

2. *Osteoporosis:* Calcium + vitamin D is given along with other drugs in the prevention and treatment of osteoporosis.
3. Vitamin D deficiency rickets—calcium is given along with vitamin D.
4. As an antacid—calcium carbonate is used.
5. For placebo effect—IV calcium is used in weakness, pruritus and some dermatoses. The feeling of warmth produced by the injection could afford psychological benefit.

PHOSPHORUS

Phosphorus is present in many food items including milk, cereals, fish, meat, pulses and nuts.

Daily requirement of phosphorus is about 900 to 1000 mg in adults. Human body contains about 500–600 grams of phosphorus of which 75% is present in bones. In bones and teeth, phosphorus is in the form of orthophosphates while in soft tissues it is in the form of organic esters. When plasma phosphate is measured it is nothing but the plasma inorganic phosphate measured. Phosphorus is absorbed by the small intestine. Excretion of phosphorus is under the control of parathormone. The renal excretion of phosphorus is increased by parathormone.

Physiological Function

1. Phosphorus is necessary for the formation of bones and teeth.
2. Phosphorus is essential for phosphorylation reactions.
3. Phosphorus is present in the nuclei and cytoplasm.
4. Phosphorus is important in maintaining the acid–base balance in the plasma and the cells—phosphates are buffers.
5. Phosphates play a vital role in various enzymatic reactions and are important for the structure and function of the cells.

Hypophosphataemia

Causes

1. Dietary phosphorus deficiency
2. Long-term intake of aluminium containing antacids
3. Vitamin D deficiency
4. Hyperparathyroidism
5. Chronic alcoholism
6. Diabetic ketoacidosis.

Signs and symptoms: Anorexia, muscular weakness and pain, abnormal bone mineralization, haemolysis, decreased myocardial contractility and respiratory failure.

Hyperphosphataemia

Causes: Hypoparathyroidism, acromegaly and renal failure.

Clinical features: Hypocalcaemia, bone resorption and calcification of soft tissues.

Uses of Phosphorus

1. Phosphorus deficiency
2. Chronic hypercalcaemia (without hyperphosphataemia)

PARATHYROID HORMONE (PARATHORMONE6PTH)

Parathormone is a peptide secreted by the parathyroid gland. Secretion of PTH is regulated by plasma Ca^{++} concentration—low plasma Ca^{++} stimulates PTH release, while high levels inhibit secretion (Fig. 43.1). Parathormone maintains plasma calcium concentration by mobilising calcium from the bone, promoting reabsorption of Ca^{++} from the kidneys and by stimulating the synthesis of calcitriol which in turn enhances calcium absorption from the intestines. PTH stimulates the osteoblasts to induce a protein (RANK ligand) which enhances the number as well as activity of osteoclasts and stimulates bone modelling. PTH also promotes phosphate excretion.

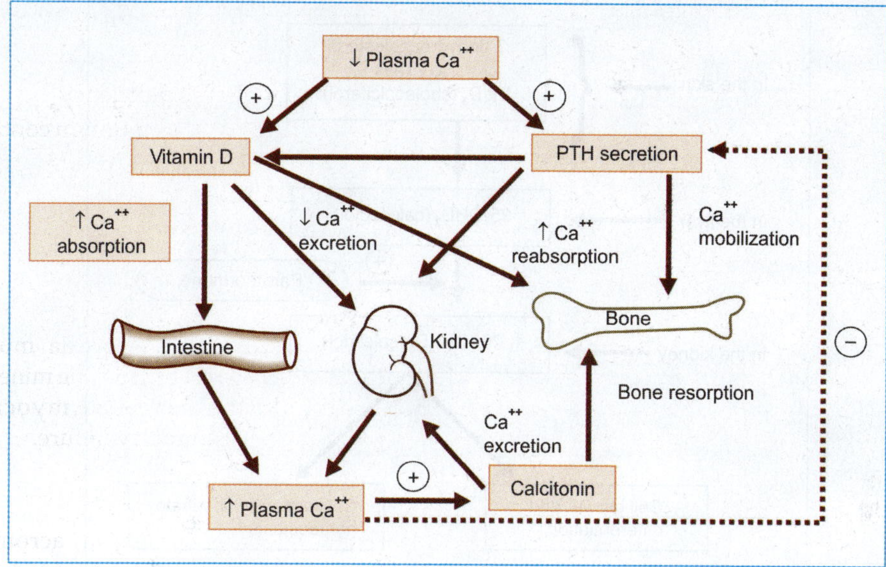

Fig. 43.1: Regulation of plasma calcium level

Hypoparathyroidism is characterised by low plasma calcium levels with its associated manifestations. Hyperparathyroidism which is most commonly due to parathyroid tumour produces hypercalcaemia and deformities of the bone.

PTH is not therapeutically used. It is used for the diagnosis of pseudohypoparathyroidism.

Teriparatide is recombinent PTH found to be useful in the treatment of osteoporosis.

VITAMIN D

Vitamin D, a fat-soluble vitamin, is a prehormone produced in the skin from 7-dehydrocholesterol under the influence of ultraviolet rays. It is converted to active metabolites in the body which regulate plasma calcium levels and various functions of the cells.

Source

- Diet—as ergocalciferol (vitamin D_2) from plants.
- Fish, liver, fish liver oils (cod, shark liver oil); milk.
- Cholecalciferol (vitamin D_3) is synthesized in the skin from 7-dehydrocholesterol.

Cholecalciferol (vitamin D_3) is converted to 25-OHD_3 (calcifediol) in the liver (Fig. 43.2) which is in turn converted to 1, 25-dihydroxycholecalciferol (calcitriol) in the kidneys. Calcitriol is the active form of vitamin D while calcifediol is the main metabolite in circulation. Conversion of calcifediol to calcitriol is influenced by PTH and plasma phosphate concentration.

Mechanism of action of vitamin D is similar to glucocorticoids—it binds to the vitamin D receptors, the complex moves to the nucleus where it enhances the synthesis of specific mRNA and regulates protein synthesis.

Actions

The chief actions of calcitriol are:

- It stimulates calcium and phosphate absorption in the intestine. Calcitriol enhances the synthesis of calcium channels

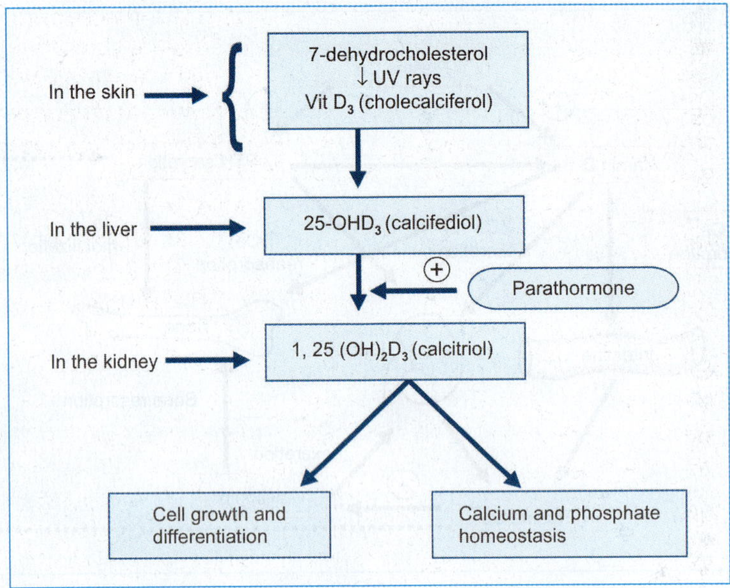

Fig. 43.2: Synthesis and functions of vitamin D

and the calcium binding protein called 'Calbindin' in the gut which is a carrier protein for calcium.

- Mobilises calcium from the bone by promoting osteoclastic activity.
- Increases reabsorption of Ca^{++} and phosphate from the kidney tubules.

Calcitriol is essential for normal bone mineralization. It is essential for skeletal muscles as well as for cellular growth and differentiation. Calcitriol may also act directly on the gastrointestinal mucosa to enhance Ca^{++} uptake from the gut.

Vitamin D deficiency results in low plasma calcium and phosphate levels with abnormal mineralization of the bone; causes rickets in children and osteomalacia in adults.

Daily requirement—400 IU (10 mg).

Pharmacokinetics

Given orally, vitamin D is well-absorbed from the small intestines in the presence of bile salts. It is converted to $25\text{-}OHD_3$ in the liver and circulates in the plasma, bound to a protein and is stored in the adipose tissue. Vitamin D is also degraded in the liver and the metabolites are excreted in the bile.

Preparations

- **Calciferol capsules** 25000; 50,000 IU.
- **Cholecalciferol granules** oral 60,000 IU in IG; 3,00,000 IU/ml; 6,00,000 IU/ml inj.
- **Shark liver oil with vit D** 1000 IU/ml, vit A: 6000 IU/ml.
- **Calcifediol ($25(OH)D_3$),** alpha-calcidiol ($1\text{-}\alpha(OH)D3$) and calcitriol ($1,25(OH)_2D_3$) are synthetic vitamin D analogs available for use.

Adverse Reactions

High doses of vitamin D used for long periods result in hypervitaminosis D manifesting as generalised decalcification of the bones, hypercalcaemia, hyperphosphataemia resulting in weakness, drowsiness, nausea, abdominal pain, thirst, renal stones and hypertension. Hypervitaminosis D in children is most often due to unnecessary vitamin D supplementation by parents.

Uses

1. **Prophylaxis:** 400 IU daily or 3,00,000 IU every 3–6 months IM prevents vit D deficiency. Adequate dietary calcium and phosphate intake is necessary. In the breastfed infants, from the first month onwards oral vit D supplements are needed. In obstructive jaundice, prophylactic 6,00,000 units vit D given IM prevents deficiency.
2. **Nutritional rickets and osteomalacia** 6,00,000 units IM repeated after 4–6 weeks is needed in rickets and osteomalacia along with calcium supplements.
3. **Vitamin D resistant rickets** is a hereditary disorder with abnormality in renal phosphate reabsorption. Phosphate with vitamin D is found to be useful.
4. **Vitamin D dependent rickets** is due to calcitriol deficiency (inability to convert calcifediol to calcitriol) and is treated with calcitriol.
5. **Senile osteoporosis:** Oral vitamin D supplements with calcium may be tried.
6. **Hypoparathyroidism:** Calcitriol with Ca^{++} supplements are beneficial.

Other Drugs

- **Thiazides** enhance calcium reabsorption and reduce renal calcium excretion. Thiazides are used in the treatment of renal stones with hypercalciuria.
- **Plicamycin** or mithramycin is an anticancer antibiotic which reduces plasma calcium levels by its action on the osteoclasts. It is used in the treatment of Paget's disease and hypercalcaemia.
- **Fluoride** is taken up by the bones and teeth. It prevents dental caries and is being tried for the treatment of osteoporosis.
- **Calcimimetics** (calcium sensor mimetics) are drugs that activate calcium sensing receptor (Ca R) and mimic the action of calcium. Cinacalcet is a calcimimetic which blocks the PTH secretion by activating the CaR in the parathyroid gland.

Cinacalcet is effective orally, has t½ of 30–40 hr, is metabolised by microsomal enzymes in the liver and is eliminated by the kidneys. Started with the dose of 30 mg once daily, dose may be increased to 180 mg/day. The most common side effect is hypocalcaemia. Cinacalcet is given orally in the treatment of secondary hyperparathyroidism due to chronic renal disease and in parathyroid carcinoma.

CALCITONIN

Calcitonin is a peptide hormone secreted by the parafollicular 'c' cells of the thyroid gland. Secretion is regulated by plasma calcium concentration and high plasma calcium stimulates calcitonin release.

Actions

The chief effects of calcitonin are to lower serum calcium and phosphate by its actions on the bone and kidney. It inhibits osteoclastic bone resorption and in the kidney, it reduces both calcium and phosphate reabsorption.

In general, the effects are opposite to that of PTH. Calcitonin is used to control hypercalcaemia, Paget's disease, metastatic bone cancer and osteoporosis and to increase bone mineral density.

Other hormones that regulate bone turnover are glucocorticoids and oestrogens. Glucocorticoids antagonise vitamin D stimulated intestinal calcium absorption and enhance renal Ca^{++} excretion. Oestrogens reduce bone resorption by PTH and also enhance calcitriol levels. Estrogen receptors are found in bone which suggests that they may also have a direct effect on bone remodelling.

DRUGS USED IN THE DISORDERS OF BONE

Drugs used in the disorders of bone are:

- Bisphosphonates: Alendronate, etidronate, pamidronate, residronate

- Raloxifene (selective estrogen receptor modulator)
- Other drugs:
  - Vitamin D
  - Calcium
  - Denosumab

Bisphosphonates

Bisphosphonates are analogs of pyrophosphate; they inhibit bone resorption.

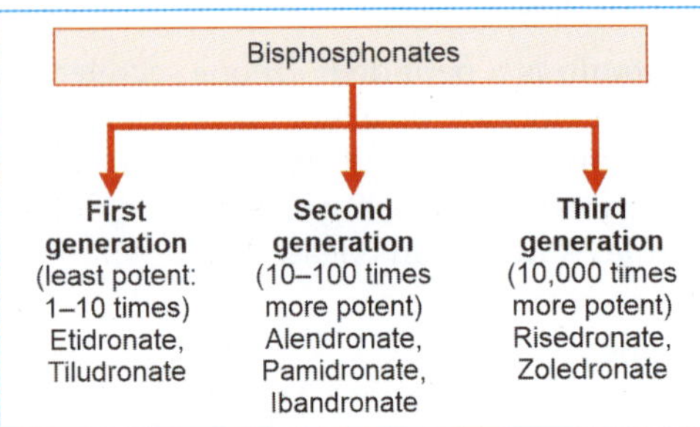

Mechanism of Action

- Bisphosphonates concentrate at sites of acute bone remodelling. They have a high affinity for calcium, get incorporated into bone matrix, are imbibed by osteoclasts and then incapacitate the osteoclasts resulting in reduced bone resorption. They also slow the formation and dissolution of hydroxyapatite crystals.
- Some bisphosphonates interfere with the mevolonate pathway which plays an important role in the functions of osteoclasts.

Adverse Effects

The most common adverse effect is gastroesophagitis due to irritation—should be taken with a full glass of water. Fever, flu-like symptoms and hypocalcaemia can occur. Headache, bodyache, thrombophlebitis on IV infusion are common. Long-term use can lead to osteomalacia due to inhibition of bone mineralization. Higher doses can rarely cause osteonecrosis of the jaw.

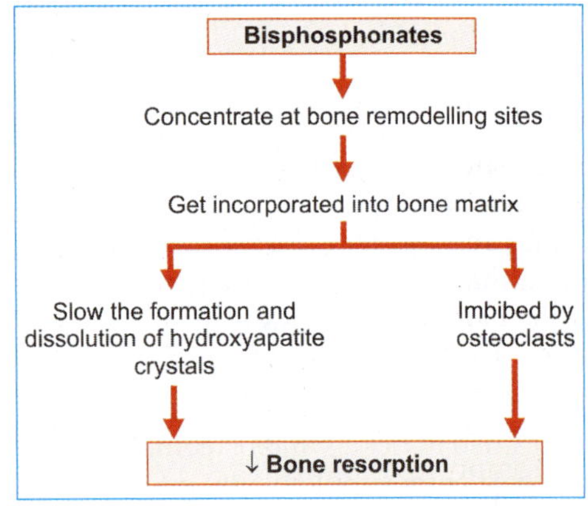

Pharmacokinetics

Bisphosphonates are poorly absorbed—bioavailability ~10%. Food interferes with their absorption—hence given on empty stomach.

Uses

Bisphosphonates are used in osteoporosis, Paget's disease of the bone and hypercalcaemia.

1. *Osteoporosis:* Alendronate, residronate and ibandronate are the most effective agents for the prevention of postmenopausal osteoporosis in women. They are also used in osteoporosis in elderly men. They improve bone mineral density and reduce the risk of bone fractures. Bisphosponates are given along with calcium and vitamin D. Though bisphosponates are generally well tolerated, gastrointestinal symptoms may be a limiting factor. For such patients, a parenteral bisphosphonate like ibandronate 3 mg intravenously once every 3 months or zolendronate 4 mg every month may be given.
2. *Paget's disease:* Bisphosphonates relieve pain and induce remission.
3. *Hypercalcaemia of malignancies:* Some malignancies are associated with hypercalcaemia. Severe hypercalcaemia can be life-threatening and requires immediate treatment. Intravenous pamidronate 4 mg IV infusion over 15 min is useful in reducing

plasma Ca^{++} levels. IV fluids and frusemide may be added.

Individual Agents

Etidronate was the first bisphosphonate to be available but due to certain disadvantages it is not preferred now. **Tiludronate** is more potent than etidronate but is not available in India. **Pamidronate** is used only as an IV infusion as it is a gastric irritant but can cause thrombophlebitis in the vein that is used for infusion. **Alendronate** is orally effective-given on an empty stomach with a full glass of water 30 min before breakfast. The patient should be instructed to avoid oesophagitis. **Risedronate** has good potency but poor oral bioavailability. It is given in the dose of 35 mg/ week. **Zoledronate** is the most potent of bisphosphonates and is the preferred agent for hypercalcaemia as it rapidly corrects it. **Zoledronate** is given parenterally and causes less irritation of the veins compared to other bisphosphonates.

Preparations

Pamidronate: Dose: 60-90 mg IV infusion over 2-4 hr. PAMIDRIA, PAMIFOS 30, 60, 90 mg inj.

Alendronate: 5-10 mg OD or 35-70 mg once weekly. ALENE, DRONAL 10 mg tab. BIFOSA, Osteophos 5, 10, 35, 70 mg tab.

Risedronate: 35 mg oral weekly 30 min before breakfast with a full glass of water. RESTOFOS, ACTONEL 35 mg tab.

Zoledronate: 4 mg in 100 ml saline infusion over 15 min. ZOLENDRON, ZOLTER 4 mg inj.

Raloxifene is a SERM useful in women for the prevention of postmenopausal osteoporosis.

Vitamin D: Enhances absorption of calcium and is useful in the prevention and treatment of osteoporosis.

Calcium: Supplementation of calcium in combination with vitamin D in the post-menopausal women and in the elderly suppresses bone turnover, improves bone mineral density and decreases the incidence of fractures.

Denosumab: Denosumab an inhibitor of RANK ligand (RANKL) reduces bone resorption in patients with osteoporosis. RANK ligand with a protein produced by osteoblasts which enhances the activity of osteoclasts.

AGENTS USED IN THE PREVENTION AND TREATMENT OF OSTEOPOROSIS

Drugs may be used either to prevent bone resorption or promote bone formation or a combination of both in the prevention and treatment of osteoporosis. These agents reduce the risk of fractures in patients with osteoporosis.

Drugs that Prevent Bone Resorption

- Calcium (↑ BMD)*
- Vitamin D (↑ absorption of calcium)
- Estrogen (prevents osteoporosis)
- Raloxifene—SERM (↑ BMD)
- Calcitonin prevents bone resorption (↑ BMD)
- Bisphosphonates—bone resorption (↑ BMD)
- Denosumab

*BMD—Bone mineral density

Drugs that Promote Bone Formation

- Fluoride in small doses—osteoblastic activity—increases bone mass—but generally not preferred.
- Testosterone—in hypogonadal men
- Anabolic steroids—in postmenopausal women.
- PTH analogs are being tried.

SPORTS MEDICINE

Drugs are used in sports to treat sports ailments. Unfortunately many drugs are also abused in sports.

Drugs of Abuse in Sports

Several drugs like anabolic steroids and growth hormone, are used by sports persons for improving performance in competitions. However, such use of performance-enhancing drugs is officially prohibited. **World Anti-Doping Agency (WADA)** has defined doping as the occurrence of one or more of the anti-**doping** rule violations mentioned in the WADA code. Drugs and methods prohibited include (as per WADA code).

Prohibited Substances

Anabolic agents are used extensively by athletes and body builders.

Though use of anabolic steroids could bring about some increase in muscle mass, there is no evidence that they improve athletic performance. They could cause serious adverse effects and are not medically recommended.

Other Banned Substances

1. **Erythropoietin** stimulates the synthesis of erythrocytes leading to increased oxygen carrying capacity but can increase blood viscosity, hypertension and increase the risk of stroke and coronary thrombosis.
2. **Insulin-like growth factors** influence skeletal muscle growth when infused into target muscles
3. **Chorionic gonadotrophin and luteinizing hormone in males and corticotrophins:** HCG enhances the production of testosterone by stimulating the Leydig cells of the testis.
4. **Growth hormone:** Promotes muscle development, increases lean body mass and reduces body fat. However, it can cause gigantism, acromegaly, cardiac hypertrophy and cardiomyopathy.
5. **Beta-2 adrenergic agonists** like salbutamol used by athletes to produce bronchodilation and cardiac stimulation with the intention of improving performance is prohibited except in patients with exercise-induced asthma.
6. **Hormones**, aromatase inhibitors (e.g. anastrozole), SERMs, other anti-estrogenic and metabolic modulators like peroxisome proliferator activated receptor γ (PPARγ) agonists are banned by WADA.
7. **Various CNS stimulants** like ephedrine, amphetamines and other sympathomimetics, nikethamide, caffeine and cocaine, have shown to improve performance in some of the sports like weight lifting. Use of all stimulants is banned except some of them for topical use.

   Narcotics (opioids) used as protection against pain from injuries in sports and cannabinoids are prohibited substances.

   Glucocorticoids: Used for their anti-inflammatory and euphoric effects are banned except when medically indicated.
8. **Diuretics, and other masking agents:** Diuretics are used for rapid weight reduction so that they could fit into lower weight categories. Diuretics also counter the fluid retention brought about by anabolic and other steroids. Moreover, as diuretics modify the urinary excretion of drugs including banned drugs, they could **mask** their presence in the urine. Therefore, diuretics are abused in sports for multiple reasons but such use is prohibited.

Other drugs used as masking agents include epitestosterone (mask testosterone in urine samples), alpha reductase inhibitors like finasteride (mask steroid excretion), probenecid (alters excretion of acidic drugs), plasma expanders (mask erythropoietin use) and desmopressin.

Blood doping: Athletes get IV infusion of RBCs, RBC products in order to increase the oxygen delivery to the tissues particularly muscles. This is associated with the risk of thrombosis due to increased viscosity of the blood.

Substances Prohibited in Particular Sports

Alcohol: Consumption of alcohol is prohibited in aeronautic events, archery, automobile competitions, karate, motorcycling, power boating.

Beta blockers: Beta adrenergic blockers, like propranolol, are used to overcome anxiety in some sports like shooting. They also reduce benign essential tremors. Use of β blockers is restricted in sports like archery, billiards, golf, shooting and aeronautic events.

[1] From Medical Council of India, *Competency based Undergraduate Curriculum for the Indian Medical Graduate*, 2018;1:136–144.

Unit XIII

Chemotherapy

CHAPTER 44

General Considerations

Competency achievement: The student should be able to:

PH 1.42 Describe general principles of chemotherapy.[1]

PH 1.43 Describe and discuss the rational use of antimicrobials including antibiotic stewardship program.[2]

Chemotherapy can be defined as the use of a chemical substance in infectious diseases to destroy microorganisms without damaging the host tissues.

Antibiotics are substances produced by microorganisms which suppress the growth of or destroy other microorganisms at low concentrations.

Pasteur and Joubert were the first to identify that microorganisms could destroy other microorganisms. **Paul Ehrlich** 'The **Father of Modern Chemotherapy'** coined the term 'chemotherapy'. He showed that certain dyes can destroy microbes and demonstrated that methylene blue can be used in malaria. He synthesized many arsenical compounds for the treatment of syphilis and sleeping sickness. Paul Ehrlich was awarded Nobel Prize for his work on chemotherapy. The evolution of chemotherapy can be studied in three periods.

i. Pre-Ehrlich era—before 1891
ii. The period of Paul Ehrlich
iii. Post-Ehrlich era—after 1935

Domagk in 1935 demonstrated that prontosil, a sulfonamide dye, is effective in some infections. Domagk was awarded Nobel Prize for his work. **Sir Alexander Fleming** discovered penicillin in 1928. He was studying different variants of staphylococci and found that a fungus was contaminating one of the culture plates. This fungus, *Penicillium notatum,* produced a substance which inhibited the growth of a variety of microorganisms. The substance was named Penicillin. It needed extensive research and purification for clinical use. In 1941, penicillin was first used therapeutically on a policeman. The discovery of penicillin is described as the beginning of the 'golden era' of antibiotics. In the last 60 years, several powerful antibiotics and their semisynthetic derivatives have been produced.

Many infectious diseases, which were earlier incurable, can now be treated with just a few doses of antimicrobial drugs. Thus the development of antimicrobial drugs is one of the important advances of modern medicine. In fact, antimicrobials are one of the most commonly prescribed drugs but are often the most over used or misused drugs.

Mechanisms of Action of Antimicrobials

The structure and composition of the bacterial cell differs from the mammalian cells in many aspects. This has made it possible to some extent to design antibacterials to act on such structures, enzymes, etc. to make them more selective to bacteria and less toxic to the human beings. Thus, antibiotics target different sites on the bacterial cell like:

1. *Cell wall:* Beta lactams and glycopeptides (vancomycin) inhibit the synthesis of bacterial cell wall. As a result, bacteria with

Classification

Based on the site of action

Antimicrobials may be classified (Fig. 44.1) as drugs that:

1. ***Inhibit cell wall synthesis***
   Penicillins, cephalosporins, carbapenems, monobactam, vancomycin, teicoplanin, bacitracin, cycloserine.
2. ***Damage cell membranes***
   (causing leakage of cell contents)
   Polymyxins, amphotericin B, nystatin.
3. ***Bind to ribosomes and inhibit protein synthesis***
   50S—erythromycin, chloramphenicol
   clindamycin, streptogramins, linezolid
   30S—tetracyclines, aminoglycosides
4. ***Inhibit DNA gyrase***
   Fluoroquinolones
5. ***Inhibit DNA function***
   (↓DNA dependent RNA polymerase)
   Rifampicin
6. ***Interfere with metabolic steps***
   (Antimetabolite action)
   Sulfonamides, sulfones, trimethoprim, pyrimethamine

weak cell walls are formed which swell and burst due to difference in tonicity.

2. *Cell membrane:* Polymyxins alter the permeability of the cell membrane leading to leakage of cell contents followed by cell death. Amphotericin B causes leakage of fungal cell contents to damage the cell membrane leading to cell death.
3. *Protein synthesis:* Several antimicrobials act by interfering with the protein synthesis. The bacterial ribosome has a 50S and a 30S subunit and mammalian ribosome has 60S and 40S subunits which are involved in protein synthesis. Antimicrobials like amino glycosides, tetracyclines, chloramphenicol and macrolides bind to and interfere with the activity of 30S or 50S ribosomal subunits in the bacteria and thereby inhibit protein synthesis.

   Antibacterials may interfere with nucleic acid synthesis either by inhibitng DNA or RNA polymerase (e.g. rifampicin) or by inhibiting the enzyme DNA gyrase (quinolones).
4. *Metabolic pathway:* Drugs like sulfonamides interfere with the metabolic pathway of the bacteria, block the enzymes involved in

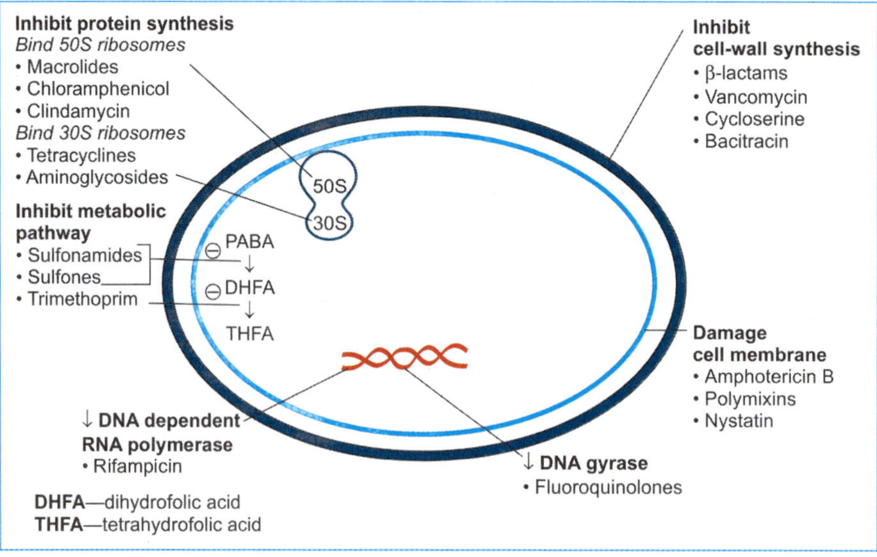

Fig. 44.1: Classification of antimicrobials based on their mechanisms of action

Antimicrobials may also be classified as:

Bacteriostatic agents that suppress the growth of bacteria, e.g. sulfonamides, tetracyclines, linezolid, chloramphenicol and clindamycin

Bactericidal agents that kill the bacteria, e.g. penicillins, cephalosporins, aminoglycosides, fluoroquinolones, rifampicin, metronidazole and vancomycin.

folic acid synthesis and thereby interfere with bacterial growth and multiplication.

However, some drugs may be bacteriostatic at low doses and bactericidal at higher doses, e.g. erythromycin; also, some drugs may be bacteriostatic to some microorganisms and 'cidal' to others, e.g. chloramphenicol is bactericidal to *H. influenzae, S. pneumoniae* and *N. meningitidis,* while it is bacteriostatic to other microorganisms. Similarly, otherwise bactericidal drugs, like vancomycin and penicillin, suppress the growth of enterococci and are not bactericidal to them. For most patients, use of bacteriostatic or bactericidal agents may not make much difference except in patients with impaired host defence. For the treatment of **infections in neutropenic patients, meningitis and endocarditis, bactericidal drugs must be used.**

Antibacterial Spectrum

An antimicrobial may have a narrow or broad-spectrum of activity. Antimicrobials may be classified based on their antibacterial spectrum as:

- *Narrow spectrum antibiotics,* e.g.
  - Penicillin G - gram-positive organisms
  - Aminoglycosides - gram-negative organisms
- *Broad-spectrum antibiotics*
  - Tetracyclines, Chloramphenicol - gram-positive and gram-negative organisms, rickettsiae, chlamydiae, mycoplasma.

Broad-spectrum antibiotics are so-called because in addition to suppression of gram-positive and gram-negative bacteria, they also inhibit the growth of other microorganisms like rickettsiae, chlamydiae, mycoplasma and some protozoa. However, in practice, the term 'broad-spectrum' is often used to include all antimicrobials with a wide-spectrum of activity, i.e. those effective against both gram-positive and gram-negative organisms, e.g. ampicillin.

Factors that influence the successful chemotherapy of an infection are:

- *Site:* The drug should reach the site of infection.
- *Concentration:* It should attain adequate concentration at the site.
- *Host defence:* Active host defences reduce the antibiotic requirement.
- *Sensitivity:* The microorganism should be sensitive to the antimicrobial agent.

RESISTANCE TO ANTIMICROBIAL AGENTS

Resistance is the unresponsiveness of a microorganism to the antimicrobial agent. Resistance may be natural or acquired.

Natural resistance: In natural resistance, the organisms have never responded to the antimicrobial—may be due to the absence of the particular enzyme or target site affected by the drug, e.g. gram-negative bacilli are not sensitive to pencillin G. However, this type of resistance is clinically not a problem as alternative drugs are available.

Acquired resistance: Here, the microbes which were previously sensitive to the antimicrobial agents become resistant to it. Clinically, this poses a problem.

Bacteria acquire resistance by a change in their DNA. Such DNA changes may occur by:

i. *Mutation*

ii. *Transfer of genes.*

- *Mutation:* Mutation is a genetic change that occurs spontaneously. In any population of bacteria, a few resistant mutants may be present. When the sensitive organisms are destroyed by the antibiotic, the resistant mutants freely multiply. Mutation may take place in a single step (e.g. *Staph. aureus* to rifampicin) or multiple steps where several gene modifications are made, e.g. gonococci to penicillin G.

- *Transfer of genetic material:* Many bacteria contain extrachromosomal genetic material called **plasmids** in the cytoplasm. These carry genes coding for resistance (called R-factors). These R-factors are transferred to other bacteria and spread resistance (Fig. 44.2).

Transfer of genetic material may take place by:

1. *Transduction:* Plasmid DNA is transferred through bacteriophage, i.e. virus which infects bacteria.
2. *Transformation:* Resistant bacteria may release genetic material into the medium which is taken up by other bacteria.
3. *Conjugation* is the most important mode of spread of resistance. The R-factor is transferred from cell-to-cell by direct contact through a sex pilus or bridge and the process is known as conjugation.

The resistance acquired by the bacteria may be exhibited in the following ways:

- Production of enzymes that inactivate the drug, e.g. β-lactamase by staphylococci; aminoglycoside inactivating enzymes by *E. coli.*
- Decreased accumulation of the drug in the bacterium, e.g. resistance to tetracyclines by gram-positive and gram-negative bacteria.
- Altered target for the drug—the binding site may be altered, e.g. binding sites for aminoglycosides on the ribosomes may be altered.
- Altered metabolic pathway—bacteria may produce folic acid by an alternative pathway.

Cross-resistance is the resistance seen among chemically related drugs. When a microorganism develops resistance to one drug, it is also resistant to other drugs of the same group, even when not exposed to them, e.g. resistance to one tetracycline means resistance to all other tetracyclines.

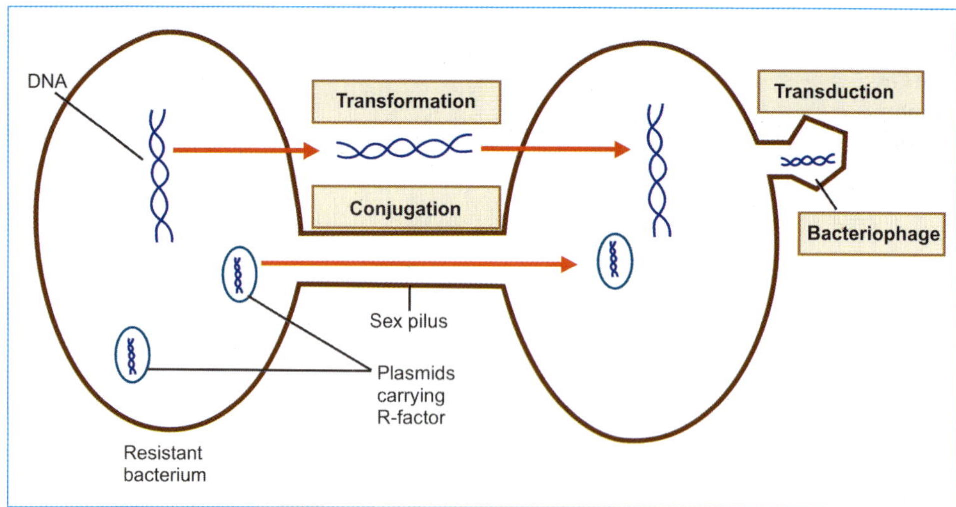

Fig. 44.2: Mechanisms of transfer of resistance

Prevention of Resistance to Antimicrobials

Development of resistance to drugs can be avoided to some extent by the following measures:

- Antibiotics should be used only when necessary.
- Selection of the appropriate antibiotic is absolutely important.
- Correct dose and duration of treatment should be followed.
- Combination of drugs should be used as in tuberculosis to delay the development of resistance.

ANTIBIOTIC STEWARDSHIP PROGRAM

Antimicrobial stewardship is a program to promote appropriate use of antimicrobials by the prescriber, to reduce their overuse and prevent resistance. The program is meant to control and supervise the use of antibiotics in order to decrease the emergence and spread of infections due to multidrug resistant organisms.

Selection of an Antimicrobial Agent

Various factors should be considered in the selection of an antibiotic like: (i) Patient factors, (ii) microbe factors, and (iii) drug factors.

Patient Factors (Flowchart 44.1)

a. *Age of the patient:* Chloramphenicol can cause Grey baby syndrome in the newborn; sulfonamides can cause kernicterus in the newborn because they displace bilirubin from the binding sites which reaches the CNS due to the weak BBB in the neonate. Ototoxicity due to aminoglycosides could be troublesome in the elderly because of their pre-existing hearing impairment due to old age which may be further worsened. Their weaker kidney function may further raise the aminoglycoside levels.

b. *Host defence status:* If host defence is impaired, more powerful antibiotics or higher doses of them are needed. Bactericidal drugs are preferable to bacteriostatic drugs in such patients.

c. *Site of infection:* It is the prime factor that guides the choice of the drug and its route of administration. Presence of pus, necrotic material, clots and anaerobic environment interfere with the activity of most antibiotics. It should be ensured that the antibiotic reaches the site of infection in adequate concentrations. Drugs that cross the BBB should be used for infections of the meninges.

d. *Renal and hepatic function:* Impairment of kidney and liver functions mean higher plasma levels and more toxicity. Drugs like nalidixic acid, cephalothin, tetracycline (except doxycycline) are to be avoided in renal impairment (Table 44.1).

e. *Allergy*: Since many antibiotics are obtained from microorganisms, allergic reactions are expected. Previous exposure to antibiotics can result in allergy and history of allergy

Flowchart 44.1: Factors affecting selection of antimicrobials

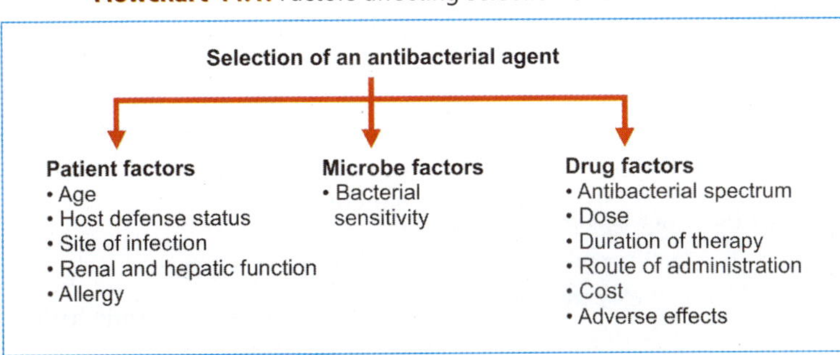

Table 44.1: Antibacterials for which dose has to be reduced in renal failure

Ampicillin	Vancomycin
Aminoglycosides	Cloxacillin
Cephalosporins	Ethambutol
Carbenicillin	Imipenem
Meropenem	Aztreonam
Fluoroquinolones	

should be taken. If allergy is known, such an antibiotic should be avoided and an alternative one used.

Microbe Factors

The infecting microorganism should be sensitive to the antibacterial to be used.

Whenever possible, bacteriological culture report should guide the drug selection. When not available, empirical therapy should be started to cover all the likely organisms.

Antibiotics are used in two ways

1. *Empiric therapy:* The antibiotic must cover all the likely pathogens. A combination or a broad-spectrum agent may be used. This therapy should be employed only in some situations. When the culture report is available, antimicrobial agents should be changed accordingly.
2. *Definitive therapy:* When the microorganism is identified, specific antibacterial agents are given.

Drug Factors

The drug should be effective against the particular microorganisms. Narrow spectrum antibiotics are preferred. Bactericidal drugs may be needed for patients with poor host defence. Adequate dose and duration of therapy should be emphasized. The antimicrobial should be safe. Least toxic drugs like penicillins should be preferred to avoid adverse effects and poor patient compliance.

Antimicrobials not eliminated by the kidney

Doxycycline	Rifampicin
Erythromycin	Cefoperazone
Chloramphenicol	Ceftriaxone

Whenever possible, orally effective antibiotics with long enough action to permit once daily administration should be preferred.

Cost of treatment should be borne in mind and less expensive ones should be chosen. Newer ones are more expensive and should, therefore, be used only when absolutely necessary.

Dose of the Antimicrobials

The dose of the antimicrobial should be adequate enough for the drug to attain plasma concentrations above the **minimum inhibitory concentration** (MIC). MIC is the lowest concentration of the antimicrobial agent that prevents visible growth of the microorganism after 18 to 24 hours of incubation.

The bactericidal activity of most antimicrobials is based on two factors:

i. Concentration in the plasma
ii. Time for which drug is in the plasma.

Concentration-dependent killing: Higher the antibacterial concentration attained, better is the killing, that is, as the concentration of the antimicrobial agent increases in the plasma above the MIC, the rate and extent of bactericidal activity also increases, e.g. aminoglycosides, quinolones. Thus, aminoglycosides may be given as single daily doses instead of thrice daily dosing.

Time-dependent killing: For some drugs, the longer the presence of the drug in the plasma, greater is the bactericidal effect. For such drugs, the presence of the drug in the concentration above MIC for a longer period is needed and thus the drug levels need to be maintained as long as the bactericidal activity is required, e.g. beta-lactam antibiotics, vancomycin.

Postantibiotic Effect

Some antibiotics continue to suppress the bacterial multiplication even after their plasma concentration falls below the MIC known as postantibiotic effect (PAE). Most antibiotics exhibit some postantibiotic effect against many microorganisms. The PAE indicates the time taken for bacteria to return to normal growth, e.g. aminoglycosides, carbapenems, chloramphenicol have such effect against gram-negative bacteria.

Mechanism of Development of Postantibiotic Effect

The exact mechanism is not known but may be due to:

a. Persistence of the drug in the periplasmic space or at the binding site.
b. Time needed for suppressed enzymes in the microbes to be resynthesized, e.g. DNA gyrase.

Though most antibiotics have a short PAE *in vitro*, the *in vivo* PAE is longer. Many antibiotics have good PAE against gram-positive cocci while PAE against gram-negative bacilli is possessed by only a handful of them. The concentration- and time-dependent killing effects exhibited by antimicrobial agents also influence the PAE.

Aminoglycosides and quinolones exhibit concentration-dependent killing and also have a PAE. Hence, the dosage interval may be kept longer. Thus, gentamicin may be given as a single daily dose—this allows good bactericidal activity because the entire dose is given in one injection and also has the convenience of single daily injections.

Some antibiotics also have a postantibiotic leukocyte enhancement (PALE) effect which could account for the longer *in vivo* post-antibiotic effect.

COMBINATION OF ANTIMICROBIALS

Use of a combination of antimicrobials may have synergistic, antagonistic or indifferent (no change) effects. Hence, appropriate drugs should be used for combination.

Two bactericidal drugs given together (e.g. penicillin + aminoglycosides) are generally synergistic.

Combination of a bacteriostatic with a bactericidal drug is not useful because bacteriostatic drugs inhibit the multiplication of bacteria and thereby antagonize the effects of bactericidal drugs (as bactericidal drugs act on actively multiplying bacteria). Hence, such combinations should be avoided.

A combination of antimicrobial agents is indicated in certain specific situations. The combination serves one of the following purposes:

1. *To obtain synergism:* Combination of antibiotics to attain synergism is recommended in:
   - *Bacterial endocarditis*
     Penicillin + streptomycin/gentamicin is synergistic.
   - *Pseudomonas infections*
     Carbenicillin + gentamicin
   - *Pneumocystis jiroveci pneumonia*
     Trimethoprim + sulfamethoxazole
   - *β-lactamase producing organisms* like *H. influenzae*
     Amoxicillin + clavulanic acid
   - *Tuberculosis*
     INH + rifampicin.
2. *Treatment of mixed infections:* Intra-abdominal infections, brain abscesses, genitourinary infections are often mixed infections. Aerobic and anaerobic organisms may be involved. Two or more antimicrobials can be used depending on the culture and sensitivity report.
3. *Initial treatment of severe infections:* Drugs covering both gram-positive and gram-negative pathogens may be used initially till the culture report is available, e.g. penicillin + aminoglycoside; cephalosporin + aminoglycoside. If anaerobes are likely to be present, metronidazole may be added. Samples for culture should, however, be taken before starting the antibiotics.

4. *To prevent the emergence of resistance:* In the treatment of tuberculosis and leprosy, combination of drugs is used to prevent the development of resistance.
5. *To reduce the adverse effects:* The doses needed may be lower when a combination is used. This may reduce the incidence and severity of adverse effects, e.g. amphotericin B + flucytosine in cryptococcal meningitis.

Disadvantages of Antimicrobial Combinations

1. Risk of toxicity from each agent—especially if toxicity is overlapping—may get added up, e.g. many antitubercular drugs are hepatotoxic.
   Toxicity of one drug may be enhanced by another, e.g.
   Vancomycin + aminoglycosides → more severe renal toxicity
2. *Selection of resistant strains:* The few resistant mutants that remain may multiply unchecked.
3. Emergence of organisms resistant to multiple drugs.
4. Increased cost of therapy.

CHEMOPROPHYLAXIS

Chemoprophylaxis is the use of antimicrobial agents to prevent infection. This is recommended in the following situations:

1. *To protect healthy persons*
   - Penicillin G is given for prevention of gonorrhoea or syphilis in patients after contact with infected persons—post-exposure prophylaxis.
   - For preventing meningococcal infection in healthy children during an epidemic, rifampicin or sulfonamides may be used.
   - Malaria in healthy individuals visiting an endemic area—chemoprophylaxis with chloroquine or pyrimethamine + sulfadoxine is given.
   - HIV prophylaxis in needle stick injury (tenofovir + emtricitabine)
2. *To prevent infection in high-risk patients*
   - In neutropenic patients, like patients receiving anticancer drugs, immunosuppressive agents and patients with AIDS, penicillin or fluoroquinolones or cotrimoxazole may reduce the incidence of bacterial infection.
   - In patients with valvular heart diseases, even minor procedures like dental extraction, tonsillectomy or endoscopies may result in bacterial endocarditis (damage to mucosa results in bacteraemia). Penicillin is used for prophylaxis.
   - In patients with contaminated or exposed wounds as in road traffic accidents.
   - Catheterisation of urinary tract—norfloxacin is used.
   - In burns, to prevent colonisation by bacteria.
3. *In close contacts:* Chemoprophylaxis is recommended particularly in children when infectious (open) cases of leprosy or tuberculosis are in close contact.
4. *Surgical prophylaxis:* Prevention of surgical wound infection is vital to limit the morbidity as well as for the success of the surgery. Surgical wound infection accounts for a large percentage of nosocomial infections. The surgeon needs to take strict aseptic precautions perioperatively to prevent surgical wound infection.

The classification of wounds indicates their chances of being infected and can be considered as a guideline for designing chemoprophylaxis (Table 44.2).

Guidelines for Surgical Prophylaxis

1. Surgical prophylaxis is important for dirty, contaminated, clean-contaminated wounds, procedures in immunocompromised host, and in patients requiring prosthetic implants.
2. Clean surgical procedures which do not require any implants like the low-risk caesarean section are unlikely to have infection as a problem. Hence, surgical prophylaxis may not be of much help in such patients.

Table 44.2: Wound classification (US National Research Council Guidelines)

Wound type	*Features*	*Infection rate*
Clean	No acute inflammation, no break in technique, elective, primarily closed procedure, no entry into gastrointestinal, respiratory, genitourinary or biliary tract, no infection at site	<5%
Clean contaminated	Emergency surgery, elective cases, controlled opening of GI, respiratory or biliary tract with minimum spillage or break in sterile technique	<10%
Contaminated	Penetrating trauma less than 4 hr old, major technique break or major spillage from GI tract, acute purulent inflammation, chronic open wounds to be covered	15–20%
Dirty	Penetrating trauma more than 4 hr old, purulence or abscess, preoperative perforation of viscera, respiratory, gastrointestinal or biliary tract	~40%

3. Selection of the antibiotic for surgical prophylaxis.
   - The antibiotic should be effective against most of the microorganisms that are likely to infect the surgical wound.
   - Toxicity should be low and the antibiotic should be inexpensive.
   - The antibiotic must achieve adequate concentration well above the MIC at the site of infection and must be present before incisions and throughout the procedure. If the antibiotic is short-acting, a dose may be repeated for long surgical procedures.
   - Cefazolin 1 g injected IV at the induction of anaesthesia (or 60 min prior to incision) is the agent of choice for most clean procedures. In caesarean section, the antibiotic is injected after umbilical cord clamping.
   - *Duration:* The antibiotic should be used for the shortest period and in most cases as a single dose.
   - Hospitals with high prevalence of MRSA or in patients with serious allergy for beta-lactams—vancomycin is the preferred agent.
4. When appropriate surgical prophylaxis is given, it can significantly decrease the incidence of infection. However, the benefit should be balanced against the risk of adverse effects and chances of emergence of resistant strains.
5. For most procedures, a single dose of an antibiotic given preoperatively may be sufficient. For some cases, another dose may be repeated. The antibiotic should not be continued beyond 24 hours because it can result in unwanted effects like superinfection, selection of resistant strains and is also of no benefit to the patient.
6. For contaminated and dirty wounds, the antibiotic is continued for 5 days. The recommended drugs for such cases would be one of the following given for 5 days:
   - Cefazolin 1 g IV 8 hrly + Vancomycin 1 g IV 12 hrly.
   - Cefotetan 1 g IV 12 hly.
   - Ceftizoxime 1g IV 12 hrly.
   - Cefoxitin 1 g IV 6 hrly.
   - Clindamycin 600 mg IV 8 hourly + Gentamicin 1.5 mg/kg IV 8 hourly.
7. Cat and human bites may be contaminated by aerobic and anaerobic microorganisms from the oral cavity and need prophylaxis with one of the following for 5 days—amoxicillin 750 mg with clavulanic acid 125 mg twice a day (oral) or doxycycline 100 mg (oral) twice a day.

SUPERINFECTION

Superinfection/suprainfection is the appearance of a new infection resulting from the use of antimicrobials. Use of antibacterials alter the normal microbial flora of the intestinal,

Table 44.3: Common causative organisms, manifestations and treatment of superinfection

Microorganisms	*Manifestations*	*Treatment*
Candida albicans	Oral thrush, diarrhoea, vaginitis	Clotrimazole/nystatin
Staphylococci	Enteritis	Cloxacillin
Clostridium difficile	Pseudomembranous colitis	Metronidazole/vancomycin
E. coli	UTI	Norfloxacin
Pseudomonas	UTI	Carbenicillin/piperacillin
Proteus	UTI, enteritis	Cephalosporin/gentamicin

respiratory and genitourinary tracts. The normal flora contribute to host defence mechanisms as follows:

- They inhibit the colonisation of pathogenic organisms by producing antibacterial substances called bacteriocins.
- By competing for nutrients.

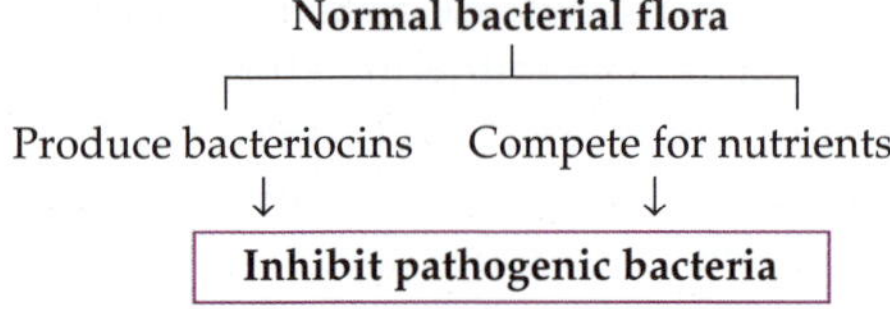

When the normal flora are destroyed by antibacterials, there can be dangerous infections due to various organisms especially the normal commensals which become pathogenic. The broader the antibacterial spectrum of a drug, the more are the chances of superinfection, as the alteration of the normal flora is greater (Table 44.3).

Sites involved: Gastrointestinal, respiratory and genitourinary tracts.

Superinfection is likely to occur in the following situations:

- Use of broad-spectrum antibiotics
- Immunocompromised patients
- Diabetes mellitus
- AIDS patients.

Measures for Prevention of Superinfection

a. Narrow spectrum and specific antibiotics should be used.
b. Antibiotics to be used only when absolutely necessary.
c. Appropriate drug to be used for the right duration because superinfection is more common with prolonged antibiotic use.

Misuse of Antibiotics

Antibiotics are one of the most overused or misused drugs. Faulty practices like the use of antibacterials in viral infections which are self-limiting, using too low doses or unnecessarily prolonged treatment, using antibiotics in all fever cases—are all irrational and can do more harm than any benefit. Since most of the vulnerable sites in the microorganisms have already been targeted by various antibiotics, we are left with very few or no targets for the development of antibiotics in future. Hence, it is absolutely necessary that we do not encourage the development of resistance by microbes due to inappropriate use of the available antimicrobials (Table 44.4). Successful treatment of infections will then be beyond imagination, considering the methods and speed with which bacteria are developing resistance to antimicrobials at present.

Antibiotics in Pregnancy

As far as possible, antibiotics are to be avoided in pregnancy. Very few of them have been known to be safe in pregnancy like **penicillins** and **some cephalosporins**. Many of them including tetracyclines, chloramphenicol, sulfonamides and aminoglycosides should be avoided in pregnancy.

Probiotics

Probiotics are products containing viable, nonpathogenic micro-organisms administered orally to alter the intestinal microflora (Greek: For life). *Lactobacillus, Bifido bacterium, Streptococcus salivarius,* some *enterococci* and *Saccharomyces boulardii* are some of the

Table 44.4: Choice of antibiotics recommended in the treatment of some common infections

Microorganisms	*Clinical diagnosis*	*Drug of first choice*	*Alternative drugs*
Gram-positive organisms			
Group A Streptococcus	Pharyngitis, Otitis media, sinusitis, cellulitis, erysipelas, impetigo, bacteraemia	Penicillin or amoxicillin	Erythromycin, A first generation cephalosporin
Group B Streptococcus	Bacteraemia, endocarditis, meningitis	Ampicillin or penicillin + an aminoglycoside	A first generation cephalosporin
Staphylococcus aureus	Furuncle, cellulitis, bacteraemia, osteomyelitis, pneumonia		
• *Methicillin-sensitive*		Cloxacillin or dicloxacillin	A first generation cephalosporin or vancomycin
• *Methicillin-resistant*		Vancomycin	Linezolid Quinupristine-dalfopristine, minocycline, daptomycin, tigecycline
Pneumococcus	Pneumonia, sinusitis, otitis, endocarditis, meningitis	Penicillin G	A first generation cephalosporin Amoxicillin
• *Penicillin-resistant*		Ceftriaxone Cefotaxime Vancomycin	Clindamycin Cotrimoxazole Chloramphenicol
Enterococcus	Endocarditis	Penicillin G + gentamicin	Vancomycin + gentamicin
Corynebacterium diphtheriae	Diphtheria	Erythromycin	A first generation cephalosporin Clindamycin
Clostridium tetani	Tetanus	Penicillin G	Clindamycin Doxycycline
Clostridium difficile	Pseudomembranous colitis	Metronidazole	Vancomycin Bacitracin
Clostridium perfringens	Gas gangrene	Penicillin G	Ceftizoxime Cefoxitine Chloramphenicol Doxycycline
Bacillus anthracis	Malignant pustule, pneumonia	Penicillin G	Erythromycin Doxycycline A first generation cephalosporin
Gram-negative organisms			
Gonococcus	Gonorrhoea, pelvic inflammatory disease	Ceftriaxone Cefixime	Ampicillin, amoxicillin Doxycycline Erythromycin Azithromycin
Meningococcus	Meningitis	Ceftriaxone Cefotaxime	Penicillin G Chloramphenicol
	Carrier state	Rifampicin	Minocycline

Contd...

Table 44.4: Choice of antibiotics recommended in the treatment of some common infections *(Contd.)*

Microorganisms	*Clinical diagnosis*	*Drug of first choice*	*Alternative drugs*
Escherichia coli	Urinary tract infection	Norfloxacin Ciprofloxacin Cotrimoxazole	Ampicillin + gentamicin; Amoxicillin + clavulinic acid; aztreonam
Proteus mirabilis	Urinary tract infection	Ampicillin	Cephalosporin I or II generation
	Bacteraemia and other infections	Ciprofloxacin Amoxicillin	A cephalosporin Gentamicin/cotrimoxazole
Pseudomonas aeruginosa	Urinary tract infection	Piperacillin/carbenicillin aminoglycoside Ciprofloxacin/imipenem	Aztreonam, Cefepine Ceftazidime
Klebsiella pneumoniae	Urinary tract infection Pneumonia	A cephalosporin + gentamicin	Mezlocillin/piperacillin Imipenem, an aminoglycoside A fluoroquinolone Piperacillin Aztreonam Amoxicillin + clavulinic acid
Salmonella	Typhoid fever, bacteraemia	Ciprofloxacin Ceftriaxone	Chloramphenicol Ampicillin Cotrimoxazole
Shigella	Gastroenteritis	Ciprofloxacin or norfloxacin	Cotrimoxazole Ampicillin Azithromycin, ceftriaxone
Haemophilus influenzae	Sinusitis, pneumonia, otitis media	Amoxicillin + clavulinic acid Cotrimoxazole	Amoxicillin Ciprofloxacin Azithromycin A cephalosporin
	Meningitis	Ceftriaxone	Chloramphenicol Ampicillin + sulbactam
Haemophilus ducreyi	Chancroid	Ceftriaxone Cotrimoxazole	Ciprofloxacin Erythromycin Doxycycline
Brucella	Brucellosis	Doxycycline + rifampicin	Cotrimoxazole Gentamicin Chloramphenicol
Yersenia pestis	Plague	A tetracycline + streptomycin	Doxycycline Chloramphenicol Ciprofloxacin
Vibrio cholerae	Cholera	Doxycycline	Cotrimoxazole
Compylobacter jejuni	Enteritis	Ciprofloxacin erythromycin azithromycin	Tetracycline
Treponema pallidum Ceftriaxone		Syphilis	Penicillin G Doxycycline
Leptospira	Weil's disease Meningitis	Penicillin G	Doxycycline
Helicobacter pylori	Peptic ulcer	Clarithromycin + amoxicillin + omeprazole	Omeprazole + amoxicillin + tetracycline + metronidazole + bismuth

Contd...

Table 44.4: Choice of antibiotics recommended in the treatment of some common infections *(Contd.)*

Microorganisms	*Clinical diagnosis*	*Drug of first choice*	*Alternative drugs*
Legionella	Pneumonia	Azithromycin + rifampicin Quinolone	Erythromycin Clarithromycin Doxycycline
Other agents			
Mycoplasma pneumoniae	Atypical pneumonia	Erythromycin Doxycycline	Azithromycin Clarithromycin, quinolone
Rickettsiae	Typhus fever Q fever Rocky mountain spotted fever	Doxycycline	Chloramphenicol
Chlamydia trachomatis	Lymphogranuloma venereum, Trachoma, Inclusion conjunctivitis, Urethritis	Doxycycline Azithromycin	Erythromycin Clindamycin ofloxacin
Chlamydia psittaci	Psittacosis	Doxycycline	Chloramphenicol
Chlamydia pneumoniae	Pneumonia	Doxycycline Erythromycin	Clarithromycin Azithromycin
Pneumocystis jiroveci	Pneumonia	Cotrimoxazole	Atovaquone Trimethoprim + dapsone

presently tried probiotics. A mixture of strains have greater efficacy.

Mechanism of Action

Probiotics act by:

- Production of bacteriocins and organic acids
- Blocking the binding sites of pathogens and competing with them for nutrients
- Modulation of immune response

Uses

Studies have shown them to be useful in:

1. Acute infectious diarrhoea and rotavirus diarrhoea
2. Antibiotics associated diarrhoea
3. Irritable bowel syndrome
4. Inflammatory bowel disease, ulcerative colitis

Side Effects

Well tolerated → can cause GI distress like bloating.

VIBACT 500 mg cap 1 BD.

Prebiotics are non-digestible substances which stimulate the growth of intestinal flora and thereby prevent the colonisation by pathogenic bacteria. There are non-digestible carbohydrates which provide nutrition to probiotics and include soybeans, raw oats, unrefined sugars, wheat, barley, lactulose and inulin. The prebiotics help the growth and survival of probiotic flora. **Synbiotics** are probiotics combined with prebiotics.

[1] From Medical Council of India, *Competency based Undergraduate Curriculum for the Indian Medical Graduate*, 2018;1:136–144.

CHAPTER 45

Sulfonamides, Cotrimoxazole, Quinolones and Chemotherapy of Urinary Tract Infection

Competency achievement: The student should be able to:

PH 1.43 Describe and discuss the rational use of antimicrobials including antibiotic stewardship program.[1]

PH 1.48 Describe the mechanisms of action, types, doses, side effects, indications and contraindications of the drugs used in UTI/STD and viral diseases including HIV.[2]

SULFONAMIDES

Sulfonamides were the first effective antibacterial agents to be used systemically in man. They were introduced by Domagk in 1935 and in the next few years several of them were synthesized and widely used. Currently, their role in therapeutics is limited because of their toxicity, development of resistance and availability of safer drugs.

Chemistry

Sulfonamides are structural analogs of p-aminobenzoic acid (PABA). They are synthetic agents that contain a sulfonamide group.

Antibacterial Spectrum

Sulfonamides inhibit many gram-positive and some gram-negative bacteria including *streptococci, H. influenzae, H. ducreyi, Nocardia, E. coli, Salmonella, Shigella, Proteus, V. cholerae,* a few strains of *staphylococci, gonococci, meningococci* and *pneumococci*. They are also effective against *chlamydiae, P. falciparum and Toxoplasma gondii.*

Mechanism of Action

Folic acid is essential for the synthesis of nucleic acids. Bacteria synthesize their own folic acid from PABA with the help of the enzyme folic acid synthetase. Sulfonamides are structurally similar to PABA and competitively inhibit the enzyme folic acid synthetase. This results in folic acid deficiency and thereby inhibition of bacterial growth as well as injury to the bacterial cell. Sulfonamides are **bacteriostatic.** Other folate antagonists, *see* Table 3.2 on page 56.

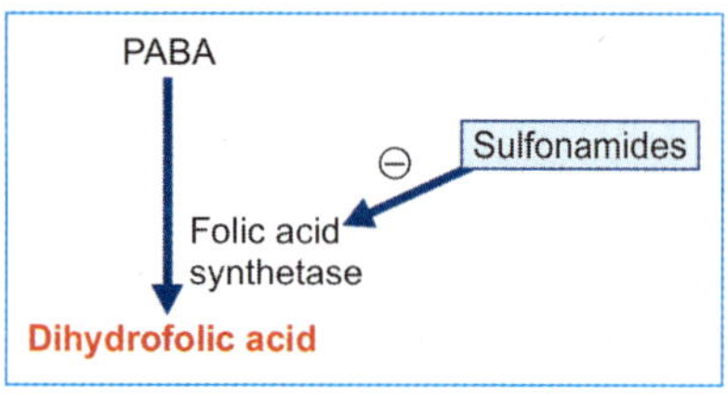

Human cells are not affected because they require preformed folic acid supplied from the diet and cannot synthesize folic acid by themselves.

Presence of **pus**, **blood** and **tissue breakdown products** make sulfonamides ineffective because these are rich in PABA.

Classification

1. ***Short-acting***
   • Sulfisoxazole, sulfadiazine
2. ***Intermediate-acting***
   • Sulfamethoxazole
3. ***Long-acting***
   • Sulfamethoxypyridazine, sulfadoxine
4. ***Poorly absorbed***
   • Sulfasalazine
5. ***Topical***
   • Sulfacetamide, mafenide, silver sulphadiazine

Resistance: Bacteria acquire resistance to sulfonamides by:

1. Mutations—resulting in over production of PABA.
2. Using alternative metabolic pathway for folic acid synthesis producing folate synthetase which has a low affinity for sulfonamides.
3. Low permeability to sulfonamides.

Pharmacokinetics

Sulfonamides (except sulfasalazine) are well-absorbed from the stomach and small intestine, extensively bound to plasma proteins and are well distributed to all tissues and body fluids including CSF. They are metabolized in the liver by acetylation and glucuronidation. The metabolites are excreted through the kidney. The dose of sulfonamides should be reduced in renal failure.

Preparations

1. Sulfadiazine; 0.5–2 g BD
   Sulphadiazine-500 mg tab
   Silver sulfadiazine, BURN AID CREAM 1%, SILVERINE CREAM 1%, SILVINDON CREAM 1%
2. Sulfasalazine: 0.5–1 g BD, SAAZ 500 mg tab, SALAZAR EC tab 500 mg
3. Sulfamethoxazole 0.5–1 g BD, GANTANOL 500 mg tab
4. Sulfacetamide, ALEKTRA 20% eye drops, ALBUCID 10, 20, 30% eyedrops, 6% eye ointment.

Adverse Effects

1. Renal irritation, haematuria, albuminuria and crystalluria—due to precipitation of the drug in acidic urine. This can be avoided by intake of large volumes of fluids and by alkalinising the urine with sodium bicarbonate. Nephrosis and allergic nephritis can also occur.
2. *Allergic reactions:* Sulfonamides can produce a range of **hypersensitivity reactions** like rashes, fever, anaphylactoid reactions, urticaria, photosensitivity and rarely, **Stevens-Johnson syndrome** (SJS) and exfoliative dermatitis. Stevens-Johnson syndrome can be fatal and should be watched for. Nephritis may also be of allergic aetiology.
3. Anorexia, nausea, stomatitis, abdominal pain, conjunctivitis and arthritis can occur.
4. Sulfonamides can cause **haemolytic anaemia** and decreased granulocyte and thrombocyte count. Haemolytic anaemia may be precipitated in patients with G6PD deficiency.
5. *Kernicterus:* Sulfonamides displace bilirubin from the plasma protein binding sites which crosses the BBB and may cause **kernicterus** in the newborn. Hence, sulfonamides are contraindicated in pregnancy and in infants.

Uses

Because of the development of resistance and availability of better antimicrobials which are more effective and less toxic, sulfonamides are not commonly used now except in a few cases. They are given in combination with other drugs like trimethoprim and pyrimethamine.

1. ***Urinary tract infections:*** Uncomplicated acute UTI can be treated with sulfonamides in areas where resistance is not high. Sulfisoxazole (1 g QID) or sulfamethoxazole (1 g TDS).
2. ***Nocardiosis:*** High doses of sulfonamides can be used as alternatives.
3. ***Toxoplasmosis:*** Sulfadoxine with pyrimethamine is the treatment of choice in *T. gondii* infection. They block sequential steps in folate synthesis and are synergistic. Sulfadoxine is given in the dose of 4 g/day while pyrimethamine is given as a bolus dose of 75 mg followed by 25 mg daily. The treatment is continued for 4–6 weeks. Such doses require leucovorin rescue (10 mg folinic acid daily) to prevent severe folic acid deficiency (*see* page 672).
4. ***Trachoma, inclusion conjunctivitis, lymphogranuloma venereum and chancroid:*** Sulfonamides are used as alternatives to tetracyclines.

5. ***Malaria:*** Sulfadoxine is used with pyrimethamine in chloroquine-resistant malaria.
6. ***Prophylactic use:*** In patients allergic to penicillins, sulfonamides may be used for prophylaxis of streptococcal pharyngitis in rheumatic fever.
7. ***Topical:*** Sulfacetamide eye drops are used in bacterial conjunctivitis—sulfacetamide also readily penetrates into the aqueous humour; mafenide and silver sulfadiazine (preferred) ointments are used in burns to prevent infection.
8. ***Ulcerative colitis:*** Sulfasalazine is useful in ulcerative colitis (*see* page 439) and rheumatoid arthritis.

COTRIMOXAZOLE

The combination of trimethoprim and sulfamethoxazole is cotrimoxazole. Trimethoprim is effective against several gram-positive and gram-negative organisms. However, when used as a sole agent, resistance develops rapidly.

Antibacterial spectrum: Cotrimoxazole is effective against several gram-positive and gram-negative organisms like *Staph. aureus, streptococci, meningococci, C. diphtheriae, E. coli, Proteus, H. influenzae, Salmonella, Shigella,* and *Pneumocystis jiroveci.*

Mechanism of action: Sulfonamides inhibit the conversion of PABA to dihydrofolic (DHF) acid and trimethoprim (Fig. 45.1) inhibits dihydrofolate reductase (DHFR) and thus prevents the reduction of DHF to tetrahydrofolic (THF) acid. The two drugs thus **block sequential steps** in folic acid synthesis and the combination is ***synergistic***. Given alone, both trimethoprim and sulfonamides are bacteriostatic but the combination is bactericidal.

Trimethoprim has a high degree of selective affinity for bacterial DHFR compared to the human enzyme.

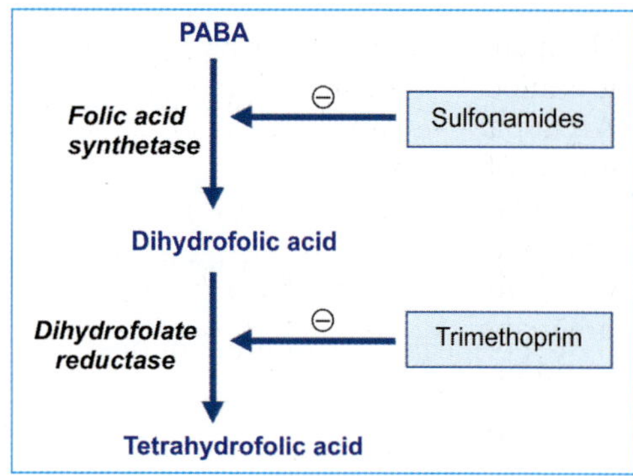

Fig. 45.1: Sequential blockade by sulfonamides and trimethoprim in folic acid synthesis

The ratio of 'trimethoprim: sulfamethoxazole' used is 1:5 to attain the right plasma concentration. The optimal peak plasma concentration of the combination is in the ratio 1:20 (trimethoprim: sulfamethoxazole). Among sulfonamides, sulfamethoxazole is chosen since its pharmacokinetic properties closely match with that of trimethoprim.

Resistance: Development of resistance to the combination is slower when compared to either drugs given alone. Bacteria may acquire resistance by mutation or by acquisition of a plasmid coding for an altered DHFR.

Pharmacokinetics: Both trimethoprim and sulfamethoxazole have similar t½. They are given orally but may also be given IV. Both are well absorbed from the gut and widely distributed in the body. Trimethoprim has good distribution into the tissues including prostatic and vaginal fluids. Because of its basic nature, trimethoprim concentrates in the acidic fluids. Both the drugs are excreted by the kidneys to an extent that in renal failure the dose has to be reduced.

Adverse Effects

- Nausea, vomiting, headache, glossitis, stomatitis and allergic skin rashes are relatively common.
- In patients with folate deficiency, cotrimoxazole may precipitate megaloblastic anaemia.

- Haematological reactions like anaemia and granulocytopenia are rare.
- AIDS patients are more prone to adverse effects of cotrimoxazole.
- Patients with renal disease may develop uraemia.
- Cotrimoxazole should not be given in pregnancy as it is an antifolate drug and could be teratogenic.

Preparations

Trimethoprim	Sulfamethoxazole
80 mg	400 mg
160 mg	800 mg—double strength (DS)

CIPLIN, SEPTRAN, SEPMAX, BACTRIM

Dose: Single to double strength 1 tab BD.

Uses

1. *Urinary tract infection*
    - *Uncomplicated acute UTI:* It is treated for 7–10 days with cotrimoxazole (DS, twice a day). Both drugs attain good concentration in the urine.
    - *Chronic and recurrent UTI:* Small doses are given for prophylaxis (1 tab single strength thrice a week).
    - *Bacterial prostatitis:* Trimethoprim attains high concentration in prostatic fluid. Cotrimoxazole DS twice daily.
2. *Respiratory tract infections:* Upper and lower respiratory infections including bronchitis, sinusitis and otitis media respond.
3. *Bacterial gastroenteritis:* Due to *Shigella* and *E. coli* respond to cotrimoxazole.
4. *Typhoid:* Cotrimoxazole is used as an alternative to fluoroquinolones.
5. *Pneumocystis jiroveci infection:* Cotrimoxazole is used for the prophylaxis and high doses (trimethoprim 20 mg/kg + sulfamethoxazole 100 mg/kg daily) for the treatment of *Pneumocystis jiroveci* pneumonia (*see* page 649) in neutropenic and AIDS patients. It also protects against infections with other gram-negative bacteria.
6. *Chancroid:* Cotrimoxazole (DS, BD for 7 days) is the drug of choice.
7. *Melioidosis:* It is caused by *Burkholderia pseudomallei*. An outbreak has been reported recently in South India. Cotrimoxazole may be tried in mild infection but severe infection and septicaemia requires combination of antibiotics. Initial intensive phase needs 2 weeks of ceftazidime or meropenem and eradication requires 3 months of cotrimoxazole ± doxycycline.
8. *Toxoplasmosis*: As an alternative to pyrimethamine + sulfadiazine.
9. *Intravenous cotrimoxazole:* Generally cotrimoxazole is used orally. In serious illness and when it cannot be taken orally as in pneumocystis pneumonia, typhoid, and UTI caused by susceptible microbes, cotrimoxozole may be given intravenously.

Clinical Pharmacology

- Cotrimoxazole is inexpensive and hence has been widely used.
- Currently cotrimoxazole use is restricted to the treatment of pneumocystosis and toxoplasmosis. It is the first-line treatment in UTI before culture–report is available.
- Gram +ve organisms have demonstrated resistance to cotrimoxazole because of extensive use and its use has declined in the last few years. It is likely to make a 'come back' as many cultures are now sensitive to cotrimoxazole.
- Use of sulfonamide monotherapy is uncommon.
- Allergic reactions must be borne in mind while using sulfonamides.

The quinolones are a group of synthetic antimicrobial agents. Nalidixic acid is the older agent in the group. Oxalinic acid and cinoxacin are other quinolones.

NALIDIXIC ACID

Nalidixic acid is bactericidal against various gram-negative organisms like *E. coli, Shigella, Enterobacter, Proteus* and *Klebsiella*. Its mechanism of action is the same as that of fluoroquinolones—by inhibition of DNA gyrase in the bacteria (*see* on the next page).

Though nalidixic acid is well absorbed orally, the plasma concentration of the free drug is inadequate to produce systemic effects because it is **too rapidly excreted**. However, it **attains high concentrations in the urine** (*see* Compare and Contrast).

Adverse Effects

Adverse effects are uncommon; haemolytic anaemia, particularly in G6PD deficient individuals, allergic reactions and CNS effects like headache, myalgia, drowsiness and visual disturbances may be encountered.

Uses

UTI: Nalidixic acid is an urinary antiseptic used in uncomplicated UTI due to *E.coli, Shigella* and *Proteus.*

Diarrhoea: Nalidixic acid is useful in the treatment of diarrhoea due to proteus, *E. coli* and *Shigella.*

Dose: 0.5–1 g 3–4 times a day. GRAMONEG, URODIC 500 mg tab 0.3 g/5 ml liquid.

Oxalinic acid and **cinoxacin** have properties and uses similar to nalidixic acid.

FLUOROQUINOLONES

The fluorinated quinolones were synthesized and the fluoroquinolones have many advantages over quinolones:

- Wider spectrum of activity
- Fewer side effects
- Lesser chances of resistance
- Attain therapeutic blood levels
- Have better tissue penetration.

The fluoroquinolones (FQs) include:

1. *First generation agents:* Norfloxacin, ciprofloxacin, pefloxacin, ofloxacin.
2. *Second generation agents:* Levofloxacin[1], lomefloxacin, sparfloxacin, prulifloxacin[2], moxifloxacin[2], gemifloxacin[2].

Note

[1]*Levofloxacin is grouped by some workers as third generation FQ*

[2]*Respiratory FQs*

Mechanism of Action

Fluoroquinolones are **bactericidal**. They inhibit the bacterial enzymes DNA gyrase and topoisomerase IV which are required for DNA replication and transcription (Fig. 45.1).

During DNA replication, there is excessive positive supercoiling of the DNA (Fig. 45.2). This is corrected by the enzyme DNA gyrase by continuously introducing negative supercoils and, therefore, this enzyme is necessary for DNA replication. By inhibiting the enzyme **DNA gyrase**, fluoroquinolones inhibit DNA replication. Instead of DNA gyrase, human cells have topoisomerase II which functions as DNA gyrase. Topoisomerase II is also inhibited by FQs but only at 500–1000 times higher concentrations. Hence, FQs are reasonably safe drugs.

Topoisomerase IV is essential for separation of the daughter cells following replication. FQs also inhibit topoisomerase IV and block the separation of daughter cells. This activity of FQs is primarily responsible for inhibiting the gram-positive bacteria while DNA gyrase inhibition suppresses gram-negative bacteria.

Bacteria with damaged DNA are formed which are degraded by nuclease enzymes. Thus FQs are ***bactericidal***.

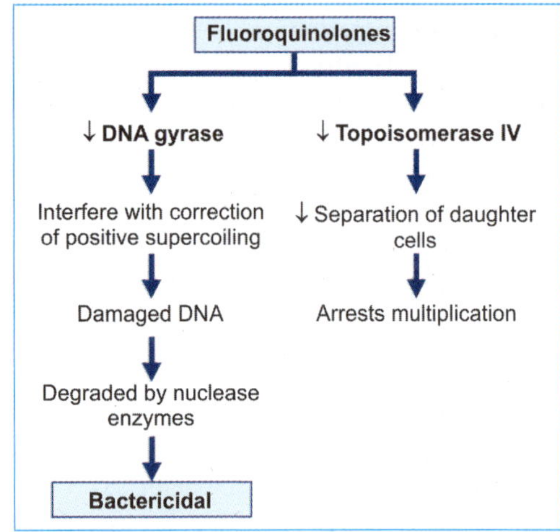

Fig. 45.2: Mechanism of action of fluoroquinolones

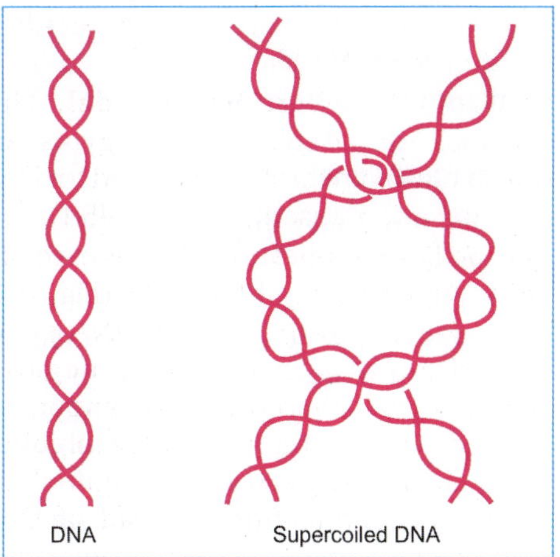

Fig. 45.3: Schematic diagram showing DNA and supercoiled DNA

Resistance to FQs could be due to

- Mutations in the target enzyme—the drug loses affinity for it.
- A change in the permeability of the organism to the drug. Several strains of *E. coli, staphylococci, gonococci, Salmonella, Pseudomonas* and *Serratia* have now developed resistance. Cross-resistance among FQs may be present.
- Protection of DNA gyrase by some proteins—plasmid mediated.

Antibacterial Spectrum

Gram-negative organisms like *gonococci, meningococci, H. influenzae, E. coli, Salmonella, Shigella, enterobacteria, Proteus, H. pylori and Vibrio cholerae* and gram-positive organisms like *staphylococci* are susceptible; *legionella, chlamydiae, mycoplasma and mycobacteria* including *M. tuberculosis* and *M. avium* complex also respond to FQs. Some of the newer fluoroquinolones are effective against some anaerobic organisms and *Streptococcus pneumoniae.*

Pharmacokinetics

On oral administration, fluoroquinolones are well-absorbed and widely distributed. Food, antacids and other cations interfere with their absorption—therefore, FQs should be **taken 2 hr before** or 4 hr after the administration of these. Pefloxacin and ofloxacin cross the BBB. All FQs are metabolised by hepatic microsomal enzymes and FQs are ***microsomal enzyme inhibitors***—can result in related drug interactions. These drugs are excreted by the kidneys. Hence dose should be reduced in renal failure except for moxifloxicin. Plasma t½ varies from 3 hr (norfloxacin), 10 hr (pefloxacin) to 18–20 hr (sparfloxacin given once daily).

Adverse Reactions

Fluoroquinolones are well-tolerated.

- ***GI adverse effects:*** Nausea, vomiting, abdominal discomfort, and diarrhoea
- ***Allergic reactions:*** Skin rashes may be seen.
- **Musculoskeletal effects: Tendonitis** with associated risk of tendon rupture has been reported. Fluoroquinolones **damage the growing cartilage** resulting in arthropathy and arthralgia and are, therefore, to be avoided up to 18 years of age.
- ***CNS effects*** include headache, dizziness and insomnia. In patients receiving NSAIDs and other epileptogenic drugs, like theophylline, fluoroquinolones, can precipitate seizures.
- **CVS:** Levofloxacin, gatifloxacin, moxifloxacin and gemifloxacin can cause QTc prolongation.
- Grepafloxacin causes cardiac arrhythmias, trovafloxacin causes hepatotoxicity and clinafloxacin—phototoxicity due to which all three have been **withdrawn**.

Uses

1. *Urinary tract infections:* FQs are very effective in UTI even those caused by multidrug resistant bacteria—norfloxacin is generally used (400 mg BD for 5–10 days).
2. *Typhoid:* Ciprofloxacin is the drug of choice (500 mg BD–10 days)—it also eradicates the carrier state.

3. *Diarrhoea:* Due to *Shigella, Salmonella, E. coli* and *Campylobacter* respond.
4. *Gonorrhoea:* Single dose 250 mg ciprofloxacin is curative but resistance in many countries has now emerged and ciprofloxacin is now not the first-line treatment of gonorrhoea.
5. *Chancroid:* As an alternative to cotrimoxazole, ciprofloxacin is used for 3 days.
6. *Respiratory tract infections* due to *H. influenzae, Legionella and Mycoplasma* can be treated with fluoroquinolones. Gemifloxacin, moxifloxacin, gatifloxacin and levofloxacin are called **respiratory fluoroquinolones** as they are effective against most respiratory pathogens including gram-positive bacteria as well as **Legionella, Chlamydia** and **Mycoplasma**.
7. *Bone, joint, soft tissue and intra-abdominal infections:* Osteomyelitis and joint infections require prolonged treatment. Soft tissue infections due to sensitive bacteria can be treated with fluoroquinolones.
8. *Tuberculosis:* Ciprofloxacin is one of the drugs in multi-drug regimens used for **resistant tuberculosis**. It is also useful in **atypical mycobacterial infections**.
9. *Bacterial prostatitis and cervicitis:* FQs are useful. Chlamydial urethritis and cervicitis also respond—ciprofloxacin or sparfloxacin can be used as alternatives to tetracyclines.
10. *Eye infections:* Ciprofloxacin and ofloxacin may be used topically in the treatment of eye infections.
11. *Anthrax:* Ciprofloxacin is the DOC for anthrax. It is also useful for prophylaxis.
12. *Neutropenic patients:* FQs may be used for prophylaxis of infection in neutropenic patients.
13. *Gram-negative septicaemias:* FQs may be combined with a III generation cephalosporin/aminoglycosides in the treatment of gram-negative septicaemia.
14. *Meningococcal carrier state:* FQs eradicate carrier state; they are also used in meningitis.

Contraindications

1. Fluoroquinolones are contraindicated in **pregnancy.**
2. To be avoided in boys and girls less than 18 years of age because FQs damage the growing cartilages and cause **arthropathy**. However, since the effect is reversible, FQs are being used in some selected infections even in children.
3. To be avoided in patients with **prolonged QTc interval**, in those receiving other drugs that prolong QTc interval (e.g. mefloquine, erythromycin) and class I and II antiarrhythmics.
4. Toxicity due to theophylline (and other epileptogenic drugs) may be precipitated by FQs due to **microsomal enzyme inhibition**.
5. Calcium, iron and other preparations containing **divalent cations** should be avoided as they reduce FQ absorption.
6. Dose adjustment should be done in **renal failure** (except for moxifloxacin).

Individual Agents (Table 45.1)

Ciprofloxacin is the most commonly used FQ; has a bioavailability of 60–70% and t ½ 3–4 hr. It is the drug of choice in typhoid fever but many strains of Salmonella have now developed resistance and should be treated with a third generation cephalosporin like ceftriaxone.

Dose: Oral 250–750 mg BD. IV 200–400 mg over 30–60 min twice daily, CIFRAN, CIPLOX 250, 500 mg tab, 200 mg/100 ml inj.

Norfloxacin has a relatively narrow spectrum of activity compared to ciprofloxacin; has a bioavailability of 35–40%, t½ 5 hr. Since higher amounts are present in the gut, norfloxacin is useful in diarrhoea including traveller's diarrhoea and cholera. It is partly excreted unchanged by the kidneys and is useful in UTI—given

Table 45.1: Salient features of some FQs

Drug	*Salient features*
Norfloxacin	Does not achieve adequate plasma concentration; used in urinary and genital infections
Ciprofloxacin	Most widely used FQ
Pefloxacin	Penetration into CSF is good—used in meningeal infections
Ofloxacin	Long-acting; used in urinary, respiratory tract infections, gonorrhoea; chlamydial infections, but with drawn in some countries
Lomefloxacin	Has a long t½
Sparfloxacin	Gram +ve organisms, atypical pneumonia, chlamydial infections, TB and MAC infections, but withdrawn in some countries.
Gatifloxacin	Active against gram-positive and atypical pneumonia pathogens.
Levofloxacin	Better activity against gram-positive organisms and atypical pneumonia pathogens; excreted mainly through kidneys; long-acting—used OD.

for 2–3 weeks. Norfloxacin is also used in prostatitis.

Dose: 400 mg BD, NORFLOX, NORBACTIN 200, 400, 800 mg tab.

Pefloxacin is a highly lipid-soluble derivative of norfloxacin—almost completely absorbed—bioavailabilty >90%, higher blood levels and better tissue penetrability, higher concentration in the CSF—therefore, preferred in meningeal infection. Pefloxacin is metabolized in the liver, has a longer t½ of 8–14 hr. Dose should be readjusted in hepatic impairment.

Dose: 400 mg BD, IV —400 mg over 1 hr twice daily, PELOX 400 mg tab, 400 mg/5 ml inj.

Ofloxacin has good activity against some gram-positive organisms, some anaerobes, *M. tuberculosis, M. leprae,* atypical mycobacteria, other chlamydiae and mycoplasma. Its efficacy against *M. leprae* and *M. tuberculosis* makes it suitable for use in multidrug regimens in leprosy and tuberculosis (300–800 mg/day). Ofloxacin has also been used in the treatment of chlamydial infections, gonorrhoea (single 200 mg dose), pelvic inflammatory disease (along with metronidazole) and in infections of the respiratory tract.

Ofloxacin is well absorbed with bioavailability >95%; food does not interfere with its absorption. It crosses the BBB. Dose reduction is needed in renal failure as it is largely excreted unchanged by the kidneys.

Dose: 200–400 mg OD, OFLOX, TARIVID 100, 200, 400 mg tab. 200 mg/100 ml for infusion. ZANOCIN, Oflox 0.3% eye drops.

Levofloxacin is the levoisomer of ofloxacin with oral bioavailability ~100%. It is widely distributed, has a t½ 6–8 hours, excreted unchanged slowly over 24 hours in the urine. It is used in respiratory infection including community acquired pneumonia and in urinary, skin and soft tissue infections.

Dose: 500 mg OD, LEVOCIDE—250, 500, 750 mg tab 500 mg in 100 ml inj.

Lomefloxacin is a difluorinated quinolone with good oral bioavailabililty (>90%). It is longer acting, t½ 6–8 hr and also remains in the tissues for a longer period—given once a day. It is largely excreted unchanged by the kidneys and the dose should be reduced in renal failure. It is used in the treatment of urinary tract and respiratory tract infections.

Dose: 400 mg BD for 7–14 days, LOMADAY, LOMEDON 400 mg tab LOX 0.3% eye drops.

Sparfloxacin: Another difluorinated quinolone with good activity against several gram-positive organisms and some gram-negative organisms including streptococci, staphylococci, *H. influenzae, B. fragilis,* Moraxella, Mycoplasma, Chlamydia and Legionella. Sparfloxacin is particularly useful in *M. tuberculosis, M. avium complex* and *M. leprae.* Sparfloxacin has a good oral bioavailability of about 90%, long t½ of 15–21 hr—given once daily; it is metabolized in the liver. It can cause photosensitivity and the patients should be advised to avoid exposure to sun. Though QTc prolongation is not very significant, concurrent administration of other drugs that prolong QTc including antiarrhythmics should be avoided. Sparfloxacin is indicated in the treatment of respiratory infections including pneumonia (S. *pneumoniae* pneumonia and atypical pneumonia), sinusitis, bronchitis and in otitis. It is also used in chlamydial infections, tuberculosis, MAC infections in AIDS patients and in leprosy.

Dose 100–200 mg OD SPARDAC, SPARTA 100, 200 mg tab

Prulifloxacin, a prodrug of ulifloxacin is effective against several gram positive and gram negative microbes. It has good efficacy in UTI and chronic bronchitis.

Dose: 600mg OD upto 10 days. PRULIFACT 600 mg tab

Moxifloxacin is another second generation FQ effective against gram-positive bacilli and some anaerobes. It is used in respiratory and soft tissue infections. It also causes QTc prolongation and necessary precautions are to be taken.

Dose: 400 mg OD, MOXICIP 400 mg tab, 200 mg in 250 ml inj , MOXIF 400 mg tab.

CHEMOTHERAPY OF URINARY TRACT INFECTION

Infection of the urinary tract is quite common and may be acute or chronic. **Urinary antiseptics** are drugs which exert antibacterial activity only in the urinary tract (and no systemic activity). They include nitrofurantoin and methenamine mandelate.

Nitrofurantoin

Nitrofurantoin, a synthetic nitrofuran, is bacteriostatic, but at higher concentrations, it may be bactericidal. It is effective against many gram-positive and gram-negative bacteria.

Mechanism of action is not exactly known. Nitrofurantoin is rapidly reduced by the bacteria to highly reactive derivatives which damage DNA and affect DNA and RNA synthesis. Since human cells require a long time to reduce nitrofurantoin, toxicity is not significant. Moreover, the development of resistance is slow.

It is rapidly and completely absorbed from the gut. Plasma t½ is 0.3–1 hr; attains high concentration in the urine.

Nitrofurantoin may cause nausea,vomiting, diarrhoea, allergic reactions and rarely chronic-active hepatitis. Haemolytic anaemia can occur in G6PD deficient individuals. Nitrofurantoin turns the urine dark brown by its metabolites. Pneumonitis and interstitial pulmonary fibrosis may occur after long term which may be due to generation of oxygen radicals in the lung. Long-term treatment can also result in neurological disorders due to the formation of toxic metabolites in the body.

Dose: 50–100 mg 6 hrly, FURADANTIN 50, 100 mg tab 25 mg/5 ml susp.

Uses

1. Nitrofurantoin is an useful alternative in acute UTI, if the microorganisms are found to be sensitive to it. Since alkalinity of the urine can reduce the antimicrobial activity, **acidification of urine** with ascorbic acid or other organic acids is useful.
2. Long-term suppression of chronic UTI (single dose 100 mg at bedtime) and for prophylaxis of UTI.

Methenamine Mandelate

Methenamine (hexamine) mandelate, a salt of mandelic acid and methenamine, releases formaldehyde in acidic urine below pH 5.5. Formaldehyde is bactericidal and resistance does not develop to it. **Acidic pH** of the urine should be maintained by using ascorbic acid, mandelic acid or hippuric acid. Acidic pH itself is bacteriostatic—an added advantage of maintaining low pH. Urea splitting microorganisms like proteus may counter the effects of methenamine by raising the urinary pH. Hence, it is important to keep a watch on urinary pH for such organisms. *E. coli* and gram-negative bacteria are suppressed.

COMPARE AND CONTRAST

Nalidixic acid (quinolone) and Ciprofloxacin (fluoroquinolone)

Features	***Nalidixic acid***	***Ciprofloxacin***
Chemistry	Quinolone	Fluorinated quinolone
Potency	Low	High
Antibacterial spectrum	Narrow Gram-negative organisms	Wide—both gram-positive and gram-negative organisms
Plasma concentration attained	Poor (just near MIC value)	Very high
Tissue penetrability	Poor	Very high—attains high concentration in most tissues
Resistance	Frequent	Slow to develop
Therapeutic use	Limited to UTI, bacterial diarrhoea	Useful in several systemic infections
Frequency of administration	3–4 times a day (more)	Twice a day (less)

Dose: 1 g 3–4 times a day. MANDELAMINE 0.5 g, 1 g tab.

High doses can cause nausea and epigastric distress due to release of formaldehyde in the stomach—given as enteric-coated tablets to prevent this. Long-term use can cause haematuria, chemical cystitis and painful micturition. Methenamine mandelate should be avoided in renal failure as mandelic acid adds to acidosis.

Drug interactions: Methenamine binds sulfonamides and neutralises their action. Also, sulfonamides are precipitated in the acidic urine. Hence, the combination should be avoided.

Uses

Methenamine mandelate is used orally in chronic UTI that is resistant to other drugs.

Other Drugs

Other drugs used in UTI are sulfonamides, cotrimoxazole, nalidixic acid, fluoroquinolones, ampicillin, cloxacillin, carbenicillin, aminoglycosides, tetracyclines and cephalosporins.

Urinary Analgesic

Phenazopyridine, an azo dye, has analgesic actions on the urinary tract (not an antibacterial) and relieves burning symptoms of dysuria and urgency in cystitis and UTI. It can cause nausea and gastric irritation. It colours the urine **orange red**.

Dose: 200–400 mg TDS, PYRIDIUM 200 mg tab.

Clinical Pharmacology

- Fluoroquinolones are the most commonly used and overused group of antimicrobials.
- Many organisms including *S. typhi* have developed resistance to fluoroquinolones.
- Very rarely used in children below 12 yr—ofloxacin is used only in resistant typhoid and neonatal meningitis.

[1] From Medical Council of India, *Competency based Undergraduate Curriculum for the Indian Medical Graduate*, 2018;1:136–144.

CHAPTER **46**

Beta-Lactam Antibiotics

The β-lactam antibiotics have a β-lactam ring in their structure.

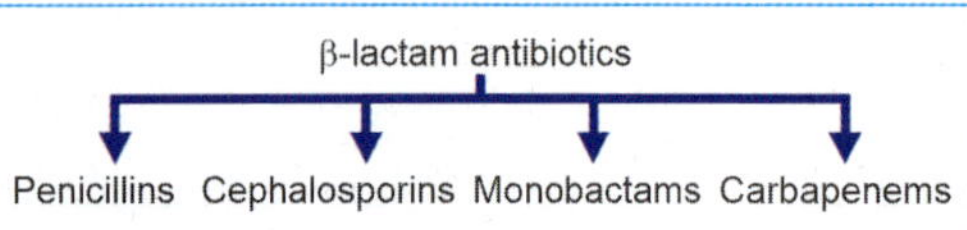

PENICILLINS

Sir Alexander Fleming discovered penicillin in 1928 from *Penicillium notatum*. In 1941, penicillin became available for therapeutic use. Though several antibiotics have been introduced since then, penicillins are one of the most important groups of antibiotics. Penicillin is now obtained from the fungus *Penicillium chrysogenum* for therapeutic use.

Chemistry

The structure of penicillin consists of a thiazolidine ring (A) attached to a beta-lactam ring (B) to which a side chain (R) is attached. A and B together is called 6-aminopenicillanic acid nucleus or **penicillin nucleus** which is essential for the antibacterial activity (Fig. 46.1). The side chains determine some of the pharmacokinetic and antibacterial properties. Modification of the side chains resulted in semisynthetic penicillins with some variations in pharmacological properties.

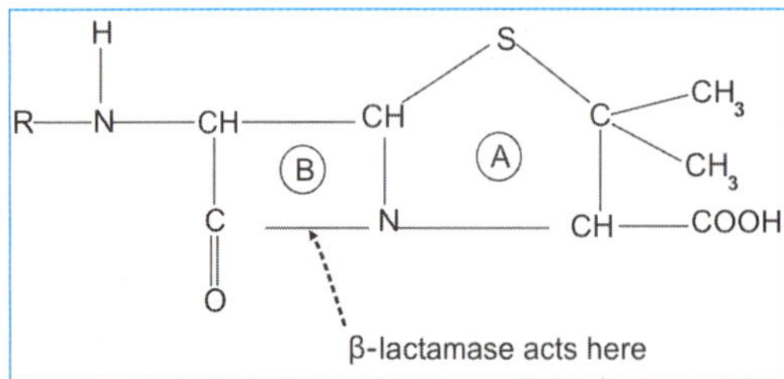

Fig. 46.1: Structure of penicillin

Unitage of penicillin: International unit (IU) of penicilllin is the specific penicillin activity present in 0.6 g of the crystalline sodium penicillin G. 1 million units of penicillin = 0.6 μg.

Mechanism of Action

The rigid cell wall of the bacterium maintains the integrity, shape and protects it from lysis due to osmotic pressure. Peptidoglycan—a complex polymer, is an important component of the cell wall. It consists of glycan chains which are cross-linked by peptide chains. The glycan chain is made up of alternating sugars N-acetylglucosamine and N-acetylmuramic acid. The glycan chain is cross-linked to peptide chain (Fig. 46.2) and the cross-linking provides strength to the cell wall. The synthesis of the peptidoglycan requires enzymes called **transpeptidases**. The last step in the

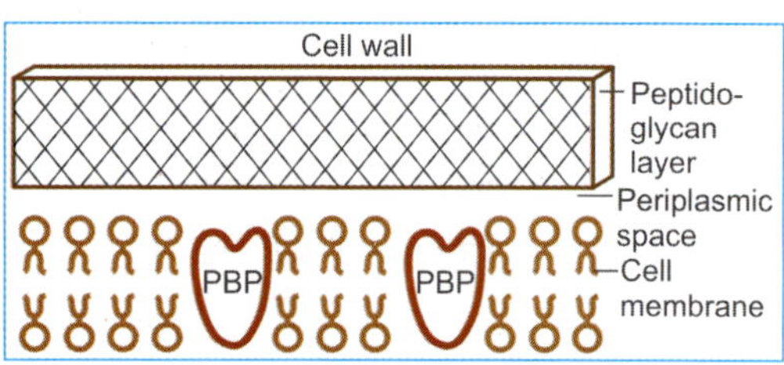

Fig. 46.2: In gram-positive bacteria; the thick peptidoglycan layer provides mechanical strength to the cell wall. Penicillins inhibit the synthesis of the peptidoglycan layer. PBP—penicillin-binding protein

synthesis of peptidoglycan chain is the process of cross-linking with the help of the enzymes transpeptidases—the penicillin binding proteins (PBPs). PBPs are enzymes present in the cell membrane which take part in cross-linking of the peptidoglycan. β-lactam antibiotics covalently bind to PBPs and inhibit the synthesis of peptidoglycans, resulting in the formation of cell wall deficient bacteria. These undergo lysis. Thus penicillins are **bactericidal** and act on actively multiplying bacteria.

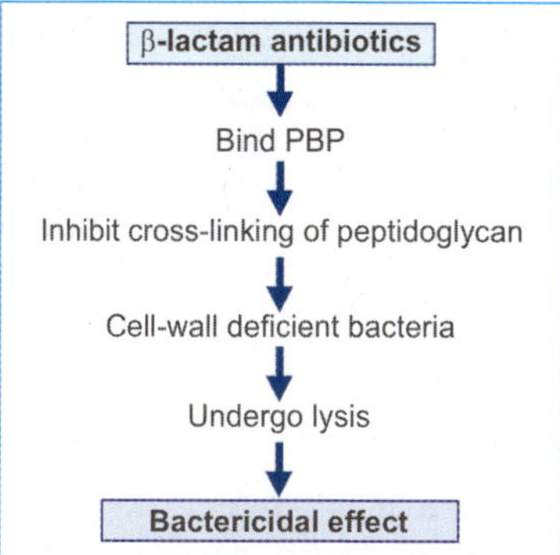

Gram-positive bacteria are more susceptible to penicillins because they have a thick cell wall which is vital for their living and is easily accessible to penicillins while gram-negative bacteria have a thin cell wall. Pencillins are highly safe because the peptidoglycan layer is unique to bacteria and is absent in higher animals.

Resistance to Beta-Lactams

Bacteria develop resistance to penicillins by one of the following mechanisms:

- Many organisms like staphylococci produce a penicillinase which is a beta-lactamase—it opens the β-lactam ring and inactivates penicillins—most common mechanism of resistance to penicillins.

  There are several types of beta-lactamases. Some of them selectively hydrolyse penicillins while others can inactivate both pencillins and cephalosporins. Carbapenems are resistant to most beta lactamases but are inactivated by carbapenemases.
- Altered target proteins (PBPs) on the bacterial cell which reduce affinity for penicillins.
- Poor penetration of the drug into the bacteria as in gram-negative bacteria.
- Efflux of penicillin from the gram-negative bacteria by an efflux pump.

Penicillin may be classified as:

Classification

A. Natural	
Regular	*Penicillin G*
Repository penicillins	*Procaine penicillin, Benzathine penicillin*
B. Semisynthetic	
• ***Acid resistant***	*Penicillin V*
• ***Penicillinase resistant***	*Methicillin, oxacillin Cloxacillin, nafcillin*
• ***Aminopenicillins***	*Ampicillin, Bacampicillin Talampicilln, pivampicillin, Amoxicillin*
• ***Antipseudomonal penicillins***	
– *Carboxypenicillins*	*Carbenicillin Carbenicillin-indanyl Ticarcillin*
– *Ureidopenicillins*	*Azlocillin Mezlocillin Piperacillin*

NATURAL PENICILLINS

Penicillin G (Benzyl Penicillin)

Antibacterial Spectrum

Penicillin G (PnG) has a narrow antibacterial spectrum and is effective against gram-positive cocci and bacilli and a few gram-negative cocci. Thus streptococci, pneumococci, gonococci, meningococci, *B. anthracis*, *C. diphtheriae*, clostridia, Listeria and spirochetes are highly sensitive. Penicillins are also effective against some anaerobes.

Pharmacokinetics

Benzylpenicillin is destroyed by gastric juice (acid lable), has a very low bioavailability—

hence given parenterally. Food interferes with its absorption—hence should be given 2 hr before or after food. Penicillins are widely distributed into most tissues and body fluids but remain mostly extracellularly as they are polar compounds. Though generally penicillins do not readily cross the BBB, **in presence of inflammation, therapeutic concentrations are attained in the CSF** because inflammation weakens the BBB and allows penicillins to reach the brain. Benzylpenicillin attains peak levels in 15–30 min, has t½ of 30–60 min and about 60% is bound to plasma albumin. Penicillin G is rapidly excreted by the kidneys ~10% by glomerular filtration and about 90% by **renal tubular secretion** as penicillins are organic acids. **Probenecid competes** for renal tubular secretion and thereby prolongs the duration of action of penicillins. In renal failure and in neonates in whom renal function is not fully developed, the duration of action of penicillins gets prolonged and the t½ may be increased to 10 hr.

Repository Penicillins

Oral penicillin can be used only in minor infections and benzylpenicillin is short-acting. Hence, repository forms like procaine penicillin and benzathine penicillin are formulated so that they are slowly absorbed with prolonged blood levels and are longer-acting. Given deep IM they release penicillin slowly from the site. Procaine penicillin is given 12–24 hourly while a single injection of benzathine penicillin is effective for 3–4 weeks.

Preparations and Dose

PnG is mainly given parenterally though orally effective form of PnG is also available. IM inj of benzyl penicillin is painful as it is an irritant and is, therefore, given intravenously. Benzyl penicillin is given IV, procaine penicillin IM and benzathine penicillin deep IM. The repository penicillins release penicillin G slowly.

1. **Sodium penicillin G:** 0.5–5 MU/IV 4–6 hrly. CRYSTAPEN, BENZYLPEN, 0.5, 1MU inj.
2. **Procaine penicillin G:** 0.5–1 MU IM 12–24 hrly. PROCAINE PENICILLIN G 0.5,1 MU dry powder vial. FORTIFIED PROCAINE PENICILLIN-PROCAINE PENICILLIN 3 lakh units + SODIUM PENICILLIN G 1 lakh units/vial.
3. **Benzathine penicillin G:** 1.2–2 MU deep IM every 3–4 weeks. PENIDURE LA, LONGACILLIN 0.6, 1.2, 2.4 MU dry powder vials.
4. **Penicillin G** POTASSIUM 200–800 mg qid PENTIDS—200, 400, 800 mg tabs.

Adverse Effects

Penicillins are highly safe drugs with a high therapeutic index; most adverse effects are not serious in therapeutic doses except hypersensitivity reactions.

Hypersensitivity: PnG is the most common cause of drug allergy. Degradation products of penicillin like penicilloic acid is antigenic. Allergic reactions range from skin rashes, urticaria, pruritus, fever, bronchospasm, serum sickness and rarely, exfoliative dermatitis and anaphylaxis. Though all forms of penicillins can cause allergy, anaphylaxis is more common following parenteral than oral preparations. Topical penicillins are highly sensitizing and their use is banned. The highest incidence of hypersensitivity is with procaine penicillin where allergy is most often due to the procaine component. There is cross-sensitivity among different penicillins.

History of allergy to penicillins should be taken before prescribing; incidence is higher among atopic individuals. A scratch test or intradermal sensitivity test with 2–10 units should be done. Even if this is negative, it does not completely rule out allergy. Penicillin should be given cautiously in all patients and **a syringe loaded with adrenaline to treat anaphylaxis should be kept ready**.

It is best to avoid penicillins in patients allergic to it as alternative drugs are now available. However, if the use of penicillin is inevitable in an individual allergic to it, desensitization/hyposensitization can be done by starting with a low dose and gradually increasing the dose—given intradermally at hourly intervals.

Other Adverse Effects

Local: Pain at the site of IM injection (due to irritation), thrombophlebitis on IV injection particularly large doses due to irritation.

CNS: Large doses of PnG >20 mega units injected IV may produce confusion, muscle twitchings, convulsions and coma particularly in the presence of renal dysfunction.

Suprainfections are rare because of narrow spectrum of activity of penicillins.

Jarisch-Herxheimer reaction: When penicillin is injected to a patient with syphilis, there is sudden destruction of spirochetes and release of their lytic products. This triggers a reaction with fever, myalgia, shivering, exacerbation of syphilitic lesions and vascular collapse.

Uses

Penicillin G is the antibiotic of choice for several infections unless the patient is allergic to it.

1. **Pneumococcal infections:** For infections like pneumonia, meningitis and osteomyelitis due to penicillin-sensitive pneumococci, PnG is the **drug of choice**.
2. **Streptococcal infections:** Pharyngitis, sinusitis, pneumonia, meningitis and endocarditis are all treated with penicillin. Infective endocarditis due to *Strep. viridans* is treated with high dose PnG in combination with an aminoglycoside.
3. **Meningococcal infections:** PnG is the drug of choice for all meningococcal infections.
4. **Staphylococcal infections:** Since most staphylococci produce penicillinase, a penicillinase-resistant penicillin should be used.
5. **Syphilis** is treated with procaine penicillin for 10 days or with benzathine penicillin.
6. **Diphtheria:** Antitoxin is the only effective treatment. PnG eliminates carrier state—PP_6 given for 10–12 days.
7. **Anaerobic infections:** Pulmonary, periodontal and brain abscesses due to anaerobes respond to PnG.
8. **Actinomycosis:** PnG is the drug of choice for all forms of actinomycosis. 12 to 20 MU should be given for 6 weeks.
9. **Tetanus and gas gangrene:** Antitoxin is the treatment for tetanus—but PnG has adjuvant value.

   Gas gangrene—PnG is the **drug of choice**.
10. **Other infections:** PnG is the **agent of choice** for infections like anthrax, trench mouth, rat bite fever and listeria infections.
11. **Leptospirosis** can be fatal when not treated on time. It responds to a course of penicillins.
12. **Prophylactic uses:**
    - ***Rheumatic fever:*** Benzathine penicillin 1.2 MU every month prevents colonisation by streptococci and thereby decreases the recurrences of rheumatic fever. It is to be continued for 5 years but most physicians prefer to use it for several more years.
    - ***Gonorrhoea and syphilis:*** Sexual contacts are effectively protected against these diseases when treated with penicillin within 12 hours of exposure.
    - ***Valvular heart diseases:*** 25% cases of bacterial endocarditis are seen following dental extractions. Patients with valvular heart diseases undergoing dental extractions, endoscopies and other minor surgical procedures that may cause bacteraemia should be given penicillin prophylaxis.

Disadvantages of Natural Penicillins

Natural penicillins have the following disadvantages:

- Narrow spectrum of activity
- Not effective orally—acid labile

Mnemonic: PADMA STOPS Syphilis & leptospirosis
- **P**neumococcal infection
- **A**naerobic infection
- **D**iphtheria
- **M**eningococcal infection
- **A**ctinomycosis
- **S**treptococcal
- **T**etanus
- **O**ther infections
- **P**rophylactic
- **S**taphylococci
- **S**yphilis
- **L**eptospirosis

- Susceptible to penicillinase
- Risk of hypersensitivity

Hence, semisynthetic penicillins were obtained in an effort to overcome these disadvantages.

SEMISYNTHETIC PENICILLINS

1. Acid-Resistant Penicillins

Penicillin V (phenoxymethyl penicillin) is acid stable and can be given orally. It is used only in mild infections as it has a low bioavailability, short action (6 hrly dosing) and a narrow spectrum of activity. It may be given in streptococcal pharyngitis, sinusitis and trench mouth.

Dose: 250–500 mg 6 hourly. PENICILLIN V POTASSIUM CRYSTAPEN-V, KAYPEN, 125, 250 mg tab.

2. Penicillinase-Resistant Penicillins

Penicillinase-resistant penicillins are resistant to hydrolysis by penicillinase produced by bacteria. However, against nonpenicillinase producing microorganisms, these are less effective than PnG. **Methicillin** is destroyed by gastric juice—hence given parenterally. Methicillin-resistant *Staph. aureus* (MRSA) are fairly common and such staphylococci are also resistant to other penicillins. Oxacillin, cloxacillin and dicloxacillin are relatively acid stable but food interferes with their absorption—to be given 1 hr before or after food. **Nafcillin** is highly resistant to penicillinase and also has useful activity against nonpenicillinase producing organisms. It requires parenteral administration because of its unreliable absorption from the gut. Nafcillin is extensively bound to plasma proteins and is primarily excreted in the bile.

Uses

Penicillinase-resistant penicillins are the drugs of choice for infections with susceptible penicillinase producing staphylococci. For more severe staphylococcal infection, nafcillin/oxacillin may be given by intermittent IV infusion. Methicillin-resistant strains have now emerged and are treated with vancomycin.

Cloxacillin, Dose: 250–500 mg qid. KLOX 250, 500 mg cap.

Dicloxacillin Dose: 250–500 mg qid BIOCLOX 250, 500 mg cap, NAFCILLIN Dose: 1–2 g 4–6 hrly (not available in India).

3. Aminopenicillins

Aminopenicillins are **extended spectrum penicillins**—cover a wider antibacterial spectrum including many gram-negative bacilli. They are orally effective but are sensitive to beta-lactamases.

Ampicillin

Antibacterial spectrum: Both gram-positive and gram-negative organisms including streptococci, meningococci, pneumococci and *H. influenzae* are sensitive. Aminopenicillins were very effective against *E. coli, Proteus*, most enterobacter, *Salmonella, Shigella* and *Klebsiella* but most strains are now resistant. The spectrum of activity can be widened by addition of beta-lactamase inhibitor.

Ampicillin is acid stable and well-absorbed orally; food interferes with its absorption. On IM inj, peak levels are attained in about 60 min. It is excreted mainly through kidneys and t½ gets prolonged in renal failure.

Dose: 0.5–2 g 6 hrly—oral or IM/IV inj AMPICIN, BIOCILIN, ROSCILLIN—250, 500 mg cap, 125, 250,

500 mg, 1 g inj. 250 mg/5 ml Dry syrup. The solution for the injection may be freshly prepared because storage results in loss of stability.

Adverse effects: Diarrhoea due to irritation of the gut by the unabsorbed drug is the most common adverse effect with ampicillin. Skin **rashes** are also fairly frequent particularly in patients with infectious mononucleosus and AIDS and in those receiving allopurinol. The rashes usually subside by themselves.

Uses

1. **Respiratory tract infections:** Bronchitis, sinusitis and otitis media respond to ampicillin.
2. **Urinary tract infections:** Though ampicillin was the drug of choice earlier, many organisms have now become resistant.
3. **Meningitis:** Ampicillin is given with a cephalosporin/chloramphenicol—but many meningeal pathogens are now resistant to ampicillin.
4. **Typhoid:** Ampicillin is an alternative to ciprofloxacin and chloramphenicol.
5. **Septicaemia due to gram-negative organisms:** Intravenous ampicillin may be used with an aminoglycoside or a third generation cephalosporin.
6. **Bacillary dysentery:** Caused by shigella used to be successfully treated with ampicillin but several strains are now resistant and is, therefore, not the preferred drug.
7. **Bacterial endocarditis:** Parenteral ampicillin can be used in place of benzyl penicillin along with gentamicin.

Bacampicillin is an ester of ampicillin. It is a prodrug that is better absorbed (hence diarrhoea is less common) and longer-acting than ampicillin.

Dose: 400 mg BD PENGLOBE 200/400 mg cap.

Talampicillin is an ester of ampicillin, hydrolysed by tissue esterases to release ampicillin in the intestines which gets absorbed into circulation.

Dose: 250–500 mg 6–8 hrly.

Pivampicillin is a prodrug of ampicillin—but pivampicillin and talampicillin are not available in India.

Amoxicillin is similar to ampicillin but differs from ampicillin in the following:

1. Amoxicillin is better absorbed orally.
2. Food does not interfere with its absorption.
3. Attains high blood levels after oral administration; it is also less protein bound.
4. Diarrhoea is rare (because it is well absorbed).
5. Given thrice daily—as it is longer-acting than ampicillin.

Amoxicillin is used in similar infections as ampicillin like respiratory infections, salmonella gastroenteritis and urinary tract infections. Amoxicillin is a component of the various regimens to eradicate *H. pylori*. Amoxicillin is preferred over ampicillin by many except for shigellosis for which amoxicillin is not very effctive.

Dose: 250–500 mg TDS. NOVAMOX, MOX—250, 500 mg cap, 125 mg/5 ml dry syr. MOXYLONG Amoxicillin 250 mg + Probenecid 500 mg tab.

4. Antipseudomonal Penicillins

A. Carboxypenicillins

Carbenicillin: In addition to activity against gram-positive and gram-negative organisms, carbenicillin is also effective against ***Pseudomonas aeruginosa*** and ***Proteus*** infections and may be combined with an aminoglycoside. Carbenicillin is given parenterally.

Dose: 2–5 g 6 hrly IM or IV CARBELIN 1, 5 g per vial inj.

Carbenicillin indanyl is effective orally as it is acid stable but is not available in India. **Ticarcillin**, an analog of carbenicillin, has better activity than carbenicillin against *P. aeruginosa*. It is often combined with an aminoglycoside for synergistic activity against Pseudomonas. It reaches the CSF, pleural fluid and sputum. Ticarcillin may be given both IM and IV. It is used in severe urinary tract infections especially due to *P. aeruginosa*. All three carboxypenicillins are susceptible to penicillinase. **Temocillin** is a penicillinase-resistant carboxypenicillin effective against *H. influenzae* and Enterobacteriaceae.

Adverse effects: Carbenicillin is used as a sodium salt and in higher doses this excess sodium may cause oedema and CCF; may also cause bleeding due to abnormal platelet aggregation.

Uses: Ureidopenicillins are preferred to carboxypenicillins in all relevant indications. Carbenicillin indanyl and ticarcillin are not marketed in India. Carbenicillin may be used in serious infections by *Pseudomonas* and *Proteus* like in burns.

B. *Ureidopenicillins*

Piperacillin, azlocillin and **mezlocillin** are ureidopenicillins. They have a wider antibacterial spectrum and are effective against a variety of gram-negative organisms including *Pseudomonas, Klebsiella, Proteus* and *H. influenzae*. Ureidopenicillins have greater activity against **Pseudomonas** than ticarcillin. Moreover, their sodium content is low. Hence, ureidopenicillins have almost replaced carboxypenicillins.

Piperacillin is administered intravenously though it can also be given IM. When combined with a beta-lactamase inhibitor, piperacillin can be considered to have the broadest antibacterial spectrum among the penicillins. It crosses the BBB and is, therefore, useful in meningitis.

Dose: 100–150 mg/kg in 3 divided doses IV. PIPRAPEN, PIPRIL 1, 2 g vials.

Uses: Piperacillin is indicated in severe infections particularly due to *Pseudomonas* and *Klebsiella*. It can be used with a beta-lactamase inhibitor tazobactam in severe infections. In serious gram-negative infections in immunosuppressed patients, an aminoglycoside may be added.

Azlocillin and mezlocillin have similar actions and uses.

5. Amidinopenicillins

Mecillinam is an amidinopenicillin with high efficacy against some gram-negative organisms (but not gram-positive bacteria) including *Salmonella, Shigella, E. coli, Proteus, Klebsiella* and *Aerobacter* (but not *Pseudomonas*). It acts by inhibiting cell wall synthesis by a mechanism that is different from that of penicillins. It is given IM as oral absorption is poor. **Pivmecillinam** is a prodrug of mecillinam that is effective orally. The two drugs are tried in urinary tract infection, typhoid and dysentery. Amidinopenicillins are not available in India.

COMPARE AND CONTRAST

Penicillin G and Amoxicillin

Features	*Penicillin G*	*Amoxicillin*
Source	Natural (*Penicillium chrysogenum)*	Semisynthetic
Acid stability	Acid labile	Acid stable
Antibacterial spectrum	Narrow (mostly Gm +ve)	Wide (Gm +ve and Gm –ve)
Route of administration	Parenteral only	Oral and parenteral
Duration of action	Short	Longer
Plasma t½	30 minutes	2 hr
Frequency of administration	QID	TID
Prominent adverse effect	Allergy	Diarrhoea
Structure	Has β-lactam ring	Has β-lactam ring

Gm +ve—Gram-positive Gm –ve—Gram-negative

BETA-LACTAMASE INHIBITORS

β-lactamases are enzymes produced by bacteria that open up the β-lactam ring and inactivate the β-lactam antibiotics. β-lactamase inhibitors bind to and inactivate β-lactamases thereby preventing the destruction of the β-lactam antibiotics. They broaden the antibacterial spectrum of penicillins to include penicillinase producing *staphylococci, gonococci, E. coli, H. influenzae* and others. The antibacterial spectrum depends on the penicillin used. There are several types of β-lactamases. Some of them are inhibited by these β-lactamase inhibitors. Three β-lactamase inhibitors are available—**clavulanic acid, sulbactam** and **tazobactam**. These are themselves β-lactam compounds but have no significant antibacterial activity. However, β-lactamase inhibitors are not effective against β-lactamases produced by *Pseudomonas*, enterobacter and MRSA. Each beta-lactamase inhibitor is combined with a penicillin having a suitable pharmacokinetic profile for combined use.

Clavulanic Acid

Clavulanic acid (CA) is obtained from *Streptomyces clavuligerus*. It binds to the β-lactamases, inactivates them and itself gets inactivated in this process. Such a compound is called a **'suicide inhibitor'.** It binds to β-lactamases produced by both gram-positive and gram-negative bacteria and the binding is irreversible—by covalent bond.

Clavulanic acid is combined with amoxicillin for both oral and parenteral administration. It extends the antibacterial spectrum of amoxicillin and the combination inhibits organisms like β-lactamase producing *staphylococci, gonococci, E. coli* and *H. influenzae.*

Pharmacokinetics: Clavulanic acid is rapidly absorbed on oral use and can also be given parenterally. It has a t½ of 60 min. Clavulanic acid is metabolised and excreted by glomerular filtration.

Adverse effects: The combination is fairly well tolerated with minor gastrointestinal disturbances and occasional superinfection with Candida.

Uses: Clavulanic acid is combined with amoxicillin for the treatment of cellulitis, diabetic foot and other skin and soft tissue infections, respiratory and genitourinary infections, mixed aerobic–anaerobic and nosocomial infections. The combination is also used in the treatment of gonorrhoea in a single dose of amoxicillin 3 g + clavulanic acid—0.5 g and probenecid 1 g. Clavulanic acid is also combined with ticarcillin for parenteral use.

Preparations

AUGMENTIN: AMOX 500/875 mg + CA 125 mg tab

AMOX 200 + CA 28.75/5 ml Syr.

AMOX 250/500/1000 mg + CA 50/100/200 mg—inj ACLAV: AMOX 500 mg + CA 125 mg tab.

Sulbactam is similar to clavulanic acid and is combined with ampicillin. Dose should be reduced in patients with renal dysfunction. It is preferably given parenterally as oral absorption is unreliable. Pain at the site of injection, thrombophlebitis and diarrhoea occur. It is suitable for use in mixed intra-abdominal and pelvic infections. Other indications are similar to clavulanic acid.

Dose: Ampicillin 1 g + Sulbactam 0.5 g IV/ deep IM 6–8 hrly. SULBACIN.

Tazobactam is suitable for combination with piperacillin for parenteral administration and has good activity against several β-lactamases.

TAZOBACT, TAZACT, Piperacillin 4 g + 0.5 g Tazobactam for inj.

They are available in fixed combinations.

Drugs	*Route*
Clavulanic acid + amoxicillin	Oral IV
Clavulanic acid + ticarcillin	IV
Sulbactam + ampicillin	IV
Tazobactam + piperacillin	IV

Though the above are the common, approved combinations, β-lactamase inhibitors with several other β-lactam antibiotics including cephalosporins are available for use.

CEPHALOSPORINS

Cephalosporins are semisynthetic antibiotics with a β-lactam ring related to penicillins. They are derived from cephalosporin-C and have a wider spectrum of activity than penicillins (Table 46.1).

Chemistry: The beta-lactam ring is fused to a dihydrothiazine ring. Modification of the side chain at position 7 of beta-lactam ring alters antibacterial activity while modification at position 3 of dihydrothiazine ring alters the pharmacokinetic properties.

Mechanism of action: Cephalosporins inhibit the bacterial cell wall synthesis similar to penicillins (*see* page 554). They are bactericidal.

Resistance: As in the case of penicillins, beta-lactamases or cephalosporinases and altered target proteins, i.e. altered PBPs determine resistance to cephalosporins. The antibiotic may be unable to penetrate the bacteria.

Cephalosporins are classified into 4 generations based on their antibacterial spectrum and stability to beta-lactamases as follows.

Classification

Parenteral	*Oral*
First generation	
Cephalothin	Cephalexin
Cefazolin	Cefadroxil
	Cephradine
Second generation	
Cefamandole	Cefaclor
Cefuroxime	Cefuroxime axetil
Cefotetan	Cefprozil
Cefoxitin	Loracarbef
Cefronide	
Third generation	
Cefotaxime	Cefixime
Ceftrioxone	Cefpodoxime proxetil
Cefoperazone	Ceftibuten
Ceftizoxime	Cefdinir
Ceftazidime	Cefditoren pivoxil
Fourth generation	
Cefepime	
Cefpirome	
Fifth generation	
Ceftaroline	
Ceftobiprole	

First Generation Cephalosporins

First generation cephalosporins are very effective against gram-positive organisms. They are used in minor infections of the respiratory and urinary tract, skin and skin structures and cefazolin for surgical prophylaxis (Table 46.1).

Cefazolin: In addition to the antibacterial spectrum of first generation agents like streptococci, staphylococci, cefazolin is also effective against some *Enterobacter* and has good activity against *Klebsiella* and *E. coli*. It is well tolerated, about 85% bound to plasma proteins, has a longer t½ to suit thrice daily use and is excreted by glomerular filtration. It is the agent of choice for **surgical prophylaxis** because (i) it is effective against most microorganisms that are likely to cause wound infection, (ii) has a longer t½ and (iii) its tissue penetrability is good.

Dose: 0.5 g–1 g, q 6–8 hrly. IM/IV. AZOLIN, ORIZOLIN 0.25, 0.5, 1 g inj.

Cephalexin is effective orally. Its antibacterial spectrum is same as that of other first generation agents (except that it is less effective against penicillinase producing staphylococci). It is metabolised and is excreted through the kidneys. Cephalexin is used for minor infections like abscesses or cellulitis.

Dose: 0.25–1 g, 6–8 hr. SPORIDEX, CEPHAXIN 250, 500 mg cap; 125 mg/ml dry syr, 100 mg/ml paediatric drops.

Cephradine is similar to cephalexin; absorbed rapidly and almost completely on oral administration, excreted unchanged in the urine.

Dose: 0.5–1 g q 6–8 hrly oral/IM.

Table 46.1: Salient features of some cephalosporins

Cephalosporin	*Salient features*
	First generation
Cephalothin	Used in staphylococcal infection; penicillinase resistant
Cefazolin	Long t½, better tissue penetration—surgical prophylaxis, also effective in *Enterobacter, Klebsiella, E. coli*
Cephalexin	Oral; minor infections—abscess, cellulitis
Cefadroxil	Oral; cephalexin analog, good concentration in urine, longer t½—BD dose, Use: UTI, respiratory, minor infections
Cephradine	Oral; completely absorbed; like cephalexin
	Second generation
Cefamandole	*E. coli, Proteus, Klebsiella, H. influenzae*, Enterobacter
Cefuroxime	Resistant to β-lactamases; good CSF concentration used in meningitis
Cefotetan	Gram-negative aerobes and anaerobes; decreased vitamin K activity—hypoprothrombinaemia, bleeding
Cefoxitin	Active against anaerobes, mixed aerobic–anaerobic infections
Cefaclor	Oral, *H. influenzae, Proteus, E. coli, Moraxella*
Cefuroxime axetil	Oral, prodrug of cefuroxime
Cefprozil	Oral, *streptococci, E. coli, Proteus, Klebsiella*
	Third generation
Cefotaxime	Good gram-negative coverage, highly resistant to β-lactamases; crosses BBB; used in meningitis, mixed infections, *B. fragilis*
Ceftriaxone	Long acting—once daily, good CSF levels—meningitis; typhoid; single dose in gonorrhoea
Cefoperazone	Very effective in Pseudomonas hypoprothrombinaemia, bleeding → vitamin K prophylaxis; disulfiram-like reaction
Ceftazidime	Very effective in Pseudomonas, Enterobacteriaceae
Ceftizoxime	Active against *B. fragilis*
Cefixime	Oral, gram +ve cocci, *H. influenzae, N. gonorrhoeae* and Enterobacteriaceae; in urinary, respiratory and biliary tract infection.
Cefpodoxime proxetil	Prodrug of cefpodoxime; used in respiratory, skin and other infections
	Fourth generation
Cefepime	Good CSF level; excreted through kidney; nosocomial, serious infections in immunocompromised host.
Cefpirome	Good penetration into gram –ve bacteria and tissues.
	Fifth generation
Ceftaroline	Effective against MRSA; used in skin and soft tissue infections and community-acquired pneumonia
Ceftobiprole	Active against MRSA and Pseudomonas; uses same as ceftaroline

Cefadroxil an analog of cephalexin is similar to it; attains good concentration in the plasma and urine. It is excreted unchanged in the urine and is used in UTI. It is also used in respiratory and other minor infections. It has a long duration of action—can be given twice daily.

Dose: 0.5–1 g BD. DROXYL, CEFADROXY 0.5, 1 g tab 250/5 ml dry syr.

Cephalothin is resistant to penicillinase, hence can be used in staphylococcal infections.

Second Generation Cephalosporins

Second generation cephalosporins are more active against some gram-negative organisms compared to first generation ones, and are also active against some anaerobes. They are more resistant to beta-lactamases and *H. influenzae, E. coli, Proteus, Klebsiella* and *Enterobacter* are inhibited (but not *P. aeruginosa)*.

Cefamandole has good activity against *H. influenzae, Enterobacter, E. coli, Proteus* and *Klebsiella*. It has a t½ of 50–60 min and is excreted unchanged in the urine.

Dose: 0.5–2 g IM/IV q 4–8 hr. KEFADOL 0.5, 1, 2 g inj.

Cefuroxime is resistant to beta-lactamases; attains good CSF concentration but is not used in meningitis because it is less effective than a III generation agent. It is effective against some gram-negative bacteria, Citrobacter, Enterobacter, community acquired pneumonia and in gonorrhoea. Cefuroxime is orally effective, t½ 1.5–2 hr.

Dose: 0.75–1.5 g IM/IV q 8hr. SUPACEF, CEFOGEN 250, 750 mg inj.

Cefuroxime axetil a prodrug is an ester of cefuroxime converted to cefuroxime in the body. It is orally effective.

Dose: 250–500 mg BD, CEFTUM, WIDECEF 125, 250, 500 mg caps. 125 mg/5 ml syr. 0.75 g, 1.5 g inj.

Cefaclor is very effective against *H. influenzae, Proteus, E. coli, Moraxella*. It is orally effective.

Dose: 0.25–1g TDS. KEFLOR, DISTACLOR 250 mg cap, 125, 250 mg dispersible tab. 125 mg/5 ml dry syr.

Cefoxitin is more active against anaerobes and is used in the treatment of anaerobic and mixed aerobic–anaerobic infections including lung abscess and pelvic inflammatory diseases.

Dose: 1–2 g q 6–8 h. MEFOXIN 1 g, 2 g inj.

Third Generation Cephalosporins

Third generation cephalosporins are highly resistant to β-lactamases; have good activity against several gram-negative organisms and anaerobes. Antibacterial spectrum includes *Citrobacter, Serratia, Enterobacteriaceae, Pseudomonas aeruginosa, N. gonorrhoeae* and β-lactamase producing *H. influenzae*; but these have weak activity against some gram-positive cocci though they are highly effective against streptococci. Many cross BBB and are useful in meningitis.

Third generation cephalosporins can be lifesaving in serious gram-negative infections including aminoglycoside resistant ones and have replaced second generation agents for these indications.

Cefotaxime is highly resistant to several beta- lactamases and it has a wide gram-negative coverage. It is metabolised in the body to a metabolite which is also active. It crosses the BBB and has been used successfully in the treatment of meningitis due to *H. influenzae, S. pneumoniae and N. meningitidis*.

Dose: 1–2 g IM/IV q 8–12 h. OMNATAX, TAXIM 0.25, 0.5, 1g inj.

Ceftizoxime is similar to cefotaxime, is more active against *B. fragilis*. It is excreted unchanged in the urine; t½ 1–2 hr.

Dose: 0.5–2 g CEFIZOX 0.25, 0.5 g; ELDOCEF 0.25, 1 g inj.

Ceftriaxone is a long-acting cephalosporin t½ ~8 hr—given once daily for most infections and twice daily for meningitis. It attains good concentration in the CSF. About 50% is excreted through the bile and no dosage adjustment is needed in renal failure. A single dose of 125–250 mg is curative in gonorrhoea. It is one of the most commonly used agents in meningitis.

Dose: 1–2 g IM/IV for 2 days; Meningitis 4 g/day; Typhoid 2 g/day for 7–10 days. MONOCEF, CEFAXONE, 0.125, 0.5, 1 g inj.

Cefpodoxime proxetil is an orally effective prodrug—ester of cefpodoxime used in respiratory and skin infections.

Cefditoren pivoxil, another prodrug, is hydrolysed to cefditoren which is excreted unchanged in the urine. It is used in uncomplicated respiratory and skin infections.

Dose: 200–400 mg BD CEFDITRAN 200 mg tab.

Cefoperazone is particularly more effective against—*Pseudomonas* while actvity against other gram-negative organisms is weaker. Majority of the drug is excreted in the bile and dose reduction is not required in renal failure. It causes hypothrombinaemia resulting in bleeding and requires vitamin K prophylaxis; also causes disulfiram like reactions.

Dose: 1–3g IM/IV q 8–12 hr. CEFOMYCIN 1 g inj, MAGNAMYCIN, MYTICEF 0.25, 1 g, 2 g inj.

Cefixime is orally effective with good activity against gram-positive cocci, *H. influenzae*, gonococci and is highly effective against Enterobacteriaceae. It is used in infections of the urinary, respiratory and biliary tract.

Dose: 200–400 mg BD. NOVACEF 50, 100, 200 mg DT-tab, 50 mg/5 ml syr.

Cefdinir is active against gram-positive cocci including beta-lactamase producing ones. It is used in the treatment of respiratory and ENT infections and in typhoid.

Dose: 300 mg BD. ADCEF 300 mg cap.

Ceftazidime has excellent activity against *Pseudomonas* and Enterobacteriaceae but weaker activity against other organisms.

Dose: 0.5–2 g IM/IV q 8 hr FORTUM, CEFZID 0.25, 0.5 and 1 g inj.

Fourth Generation Cephalosporins

Fourth generation cephalosporins—**cefepime** and **cefpirome,** are active against a variety of gram-positive and gram-negative organisms including streptococci, staphylococci, meningococci, gonococci, some enterococci, enterobacteriaecae, *H. influenzae* and *Pseudomonas aeruginosa*. They are more resistant to many of the β-lactamases. Both cefepime and cefpirome are administered parenterally, have a t½ of ~2 hr; are excreted almost completely through the kidneys. Cefepime attains good CSF levels while cefpirome has good tissue penetrability. Cefpirome is particularly effective against gram-negative organisms because it penetrates well through the porin channels.

The fourth generation agents are used in **septicaemia**, **nosocomial** and other serious infections of the **skin, respiratory** and **urinary tracts** and infections in **immunocompromised patients**.

Cefepime Dose: 1–2 g IV q 8–12 h. CEPIME, CEFPIME—0.5, 1g inj.

Cefpirome Dose: 1–2 g IM/IV q 12 h. CEPIROM, CEF-4 1g inj.

Fifth Generation Cephalosporins

Fifth generation cephalosporins include ceftaroline and ceftobiprole. They are anti-MRSA cephalosporins. Both are also effective against penicillin-resistant ***Streptococcus pneumoniae*** in addition to gram-negative microbes. They inhibit PBP_{2a} which is specific to MRSA. They are approved for use in skin and skin structure infections and community-acquired pneumonia. Ceftobiprole is also effective against *Pseudomonas*.

Ceftaroline Dose: 600 mg slow IV over 1 hour 12th hourly.

Adverse Reactions

Cephalosporins are generally well-tolerated.

1. **Hypersensitivity reactions** like skin rashes, fever, serum sickness and rarely anaphylaxis are seen. 20% of patients allergic to penicillins show cross-reactivity to cephalosporins. There are no reliable skin tests for testing allergy.
2. **Nephrotoxicity:** Mild nephrotoxicity is noted with some cephalosporins. Combination with other nephrotoxic drugs should be avoided.

3. **Diarrhoea** can result from some of the cephalosporins—more common with cefoperazone—could be because a large fraction of it is excreted through the bile.
4. **Bleeding** is due to hypoprothrombinaemia which is more common in malnourished patients. Cephalosporins with a methylthiotetrazole group like cefoperazone, cefotetan and cefamandole can cause bleeding due to hypoprothrombinaemia. This can be prevented by concurrent administration of vitamin K, 10 mg twice daily.
5. **Low WBC count** may be seen though rarely.
6. **Pain** at the injection site may occur.
7. **Disulfiram-like reaction** with alcohol is reported with the cephalosporins that contain methylthiotetrazole group, e.g. cefoperazone.

Uses of Cephalosporins

1. **Gram-negative infections:** Urinary, respiratory and soft tissue infections due to gram-negative organisms respond—a third generation agent is used.
2. **Surgical prophylaxis:** Cefazolin is preferred due to its longer t½ and better tissue penetrability.
3. **Gonorrhoea:** Ceftriaxone (single dose 250 mg) is the drug of choice.
4. **Meningitis:** Due to *H. influenzae, N. meningitidis and S. pneumoniae*—third generation agents are useful—cefotaxime or ceftriaxone may be used. *Pseudomonas meningitis*—ceftazidime + an aminoglycoside very effective.
5. **Mixed aerobic–anaerobic infections:** Common following pelvic surgeries—a third generation agent is used.
6. **Typhoid:** As alternatives to ciprofloxacin.
7. **Nosocomial infections** can be treated with 3rd generation cephalosporins.

CARBAPENEMS

Carbapenems contain a β-lactam ring fused with a five-membered penem ring. Carbapenems include **imipenem, meropenem, ertapenem, doripenem** and **faropenem.**

Antibacterial Spectrum

Carbapenems have a wide antibacterial spectrum and inhibit various gram-positive, gram-negative organisms and anaerobes including *streptococci, staphylococci, enterococci, Listeria, Enterobacteriaceae* (including cepha losporin-resistant ones), *Pseudomonas* and *B. fragilis.*

Mechanism of Action

Carbapenems inhibit bacterial cell wall synthesis similar to penicillins (*see* page 554). Carbapenems are highly resistant to most beta-lactamases.

Imipenem

Imipenem is not absorbed orally and is administered intravenously (250–500 mg every 6–8 hours); it has good tissue penetrability and attains good CSF levels. Imipenem is inactivated quickly by a dehydropeptidase in the renal tubules. Hence, it is always combined with **cilastatin**, an **inhibitor of dehydropeptidase** in order to prolong its plasma half-life. Plasma t½ of both imipenem and cilastatin is ~1 hr. Carbapenems are excreted through the kidneys—dose should be reduced in renal faliure.

Adverse effects to imipenem include nausea, vomiting, diarrhoea and allergic reactions especially in patients allergic to other β-lactam antibiotics. High doses can occasionally cause seizures in 1.5% of patients.

Uses

Imipenem-cilastatin is used in UTI, respiratory, skin, bone, soft tissue, intra-abdominal and gynaecological infections due to susceptible microorganisms that are resistant to other antibiotics. It is particularly useful in infections with penicillin-resistant pneumococci and other nosocomial infections resistant to other antibiotics. It is used with an aminoglycoside in *Pseudomonas* infections to reduce the risk of developing resistance. Since imipenem and other carbapenems are resistant to β-lactamases produced by enterococci, it is the drug of choice in enterobacter infections.

Dose: 500 mg q 6 h IV. PRIMIXAN 500 mg inj.

Meropenem has the following advantages over imipenem:

- Meropenem is not destroyed by renal dipeptidase and, therefore, does not require to be combined with cilastatin.
- Risk of seizures is less than with imipenem. Indications of meropenem are similar to imipenem.

Dose: 0.5–2 g q 8 h slow IV MERONAM, MENEM 0.5, 1 g inj.

Ertapenem is similar to meropenem except that it is not useful against *P. aeruginosa*. It is longer acting—given once daily—1 g daily IM/IV. Since ertapenem is an irritant, IM injections are painful—hence marketed in combination with 1% lignocaine.

Doripenem is similar to meropenem with better activity against gram-negative aerobes than gram-positive ones.

Dose: 500 mg q 8 h slow infusion over 4 hr.

Faropenem is another carbapenem that is orally effective with good efficacy against both gram-positive and gram-negative organisms and some anaerobes. Adverse effects are nausea, diarrhoea and abdominal pain.

Uses: Bacterial sinusitis, community-acquired pneumonia and genitourinary infections. It is not available in many countries but is marketed in India.

Dose: 100–300 mg TDS FARONEM 100, 200 mg tab.

CARBACEPHEMS

Loracarbef is a carbacephem. It is a synthetic beta-lactam antibiotic with properties similar to second generation cephalosporins (cefaclor) and is, therefore, included by some under second generation cephalosporins. It is orally effective and is largely excreted by the kidneys.

MONOBACTAMS

Monobactams are monocyclic beta-lactams, i.e. they contain a single ring—the beta-lactam ring.

Aztreonam is a monobactam active against gram-negative bacilli including *Pseudomonas aeruginosa.* Aztreonam is resistant to beta-lactamases produced by gram-negative bacteria. It is highly effective against *H. influenzae*, gonococci and Enterobacteriaceae, but it is **not** effective against gram-positive organisms and anaerobes.

Mechanism of action: Aztreonam acts by inhibiting the cell wall synthesis like penicillins. It is given parenterally.

Aztreonam is well tolerated. The adverse effects include occasional skin rashes, urticaria, bronchospasm and rarely anaphylaxis. Thrombophlebitis on IV use and pain after IM use are reported. Nausea, vomiting, diarrhoea, altered taste and raised liver enzymes have been noted.

Uses

- Aztreonam is used in *Pseudomonas* infections especially nosocomial and in other gram-negative infections.
- Aztreonam can be used in patients allergic to penicillins as there is no cross allergenicity with other β-lactams.

Dose: 0.5–2 g q 6–8 h IM/IV. AZENEM, TRAZAN 0.5, 1, 2 g inj.

Clinical Pharmacology

- Penicillins are yet the first-line drugs in many infections.
- Measures to treat anaphylaxis should be kept ready while using penicillins parenterally.
- Amoxicillin + clavulanic acid is commonly used often irrationally and should be restricted.
- Amoxicillin is the commonest penicillin in use.
- Benzathine penicillin is the commonest penicillin used for prophylaxis.
- Use of ampicillin has drastically reduced. It is used in combination with cefotaxime in meningitis.
- Piperacillin + tazobactam—effective in bacterial meningitis and other serious infections.
- None of the first 4 generations of cephalosporins are effective against MRSA.
- Cephalosporins are commonly used for gram-negative septicaemia.
- Combination of several cephalosporins with β lactamase inhibitors are available for use.
- After the introduction of meropenem, imipenem + cilastatin use has reduced.

CHAPTER 47

Broad-Spectrum Antibiotics

TETRACYCLINES

Tetracyclines are antibiotics with four cyclic rings (hence the name) in their structure (Fig. 47.1) obtained from the soil actinomycetes. Chlortetracycline was the first tetracycline to be obtained from *'Streptomyces aureofaciens'* in 1948 and was named so because the colonies appear golden yellow. (Discovered by Benjamin Duggar working under Yellapragada Subba Rao). Several semisynthetic derivatives were then produced. In addition to gram-positive and gram-negative bacteria, tetracyclines also inhibit the growth of other microorganisms like *rickettsiae, chlamydiae, mycoplasma* and some protozoa. Therefore, they are called *broad-spectrum antibiotics.*

Intermediate and long-acting agents are semisynthetic tetracyclines.

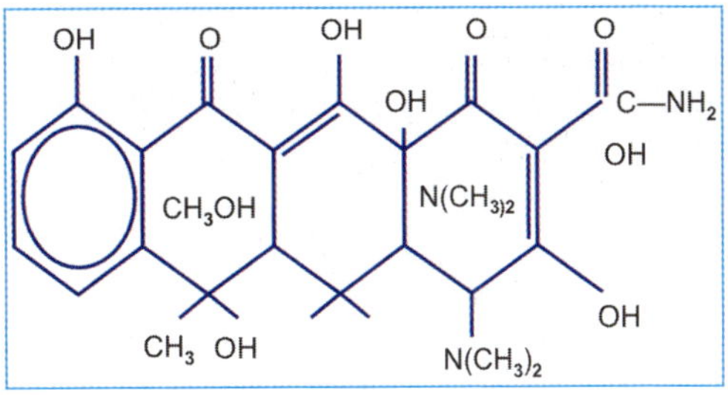

Mechanism of Action

Tetracyclines are taken up by susceptible microorganisms by active transport. Since mammalian cells lack this active transport process, tetracyclines are selectively toxic to microorganisms. Because of the differences in the ribosomes of prokaryotes and eukaryotes, it has been possible to achieve some selective targeting of the protein synthesis process in the microorganisms. The bacterial ribosome (Fig. 47.2) consists of 50S and 30S subunits and tetracyclines bind to 30S subunit. The tRNA carries amino acids to the ribosome for protein synthesis. The ribosome has three binding sites, viz. A, P and E sites. Tetracyclines bind to 'A' site and prevent the binding of tRNA to this site. As a result, amino acids cannot be added to the growing peptide chain. Thus they prevent protein synthesis and are **bacteriostatic**.

Classification

Short-acting (t½ 6 hr)
- Chlortetracycline
- Tetracycline
- Oxytetracycline

Intermediate-acting (t½ ~12 hr)
- Demeclocycline
- Methacycline

Long-acting (t½~18 hr)
- Doxycycline
- Minocycline

Newer tetracycline
- Tigecycline (t½ 36 hr)

OH O OH O O OH C—NH$_2$ OH CH_3OH $N(CH_{3})_2$ CH_3 OH OH $N(CH_3)_2$

Fig. 47.1: Structure of tetracycline

Antibacterial Spectrum

Tetracyclines have a broad antibacterial spectrum. When they were introduced, they were effective against a wide range of gram-positive and gram-negative microorgansims but many bacteria have now developed resistance to tetracyclines. The spectrum

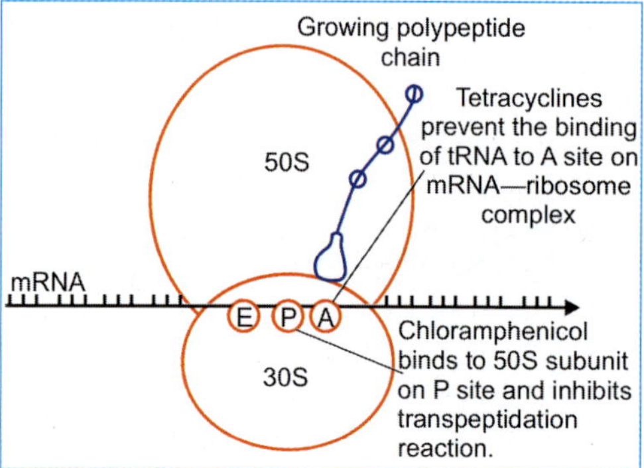

Fig. 47.2: Mechanism of action of tetracyclines and chloramphenicol

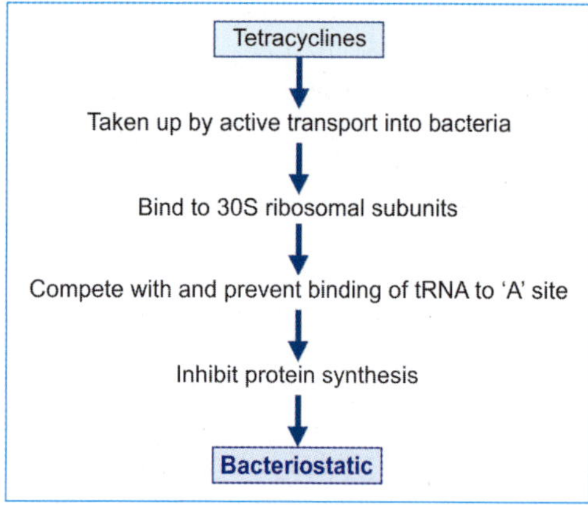

includes gram-positive and gram-negative bacteria including streptococci, staphylococci, gonococci, meningococci (particularly minocycline), clostridia, *Bacillus anthracis, Listeria, corynebacteria, Propioni bacterium acnes, H. influenzae, Vibrio cholerae, Yersinia pestis, H. ducreyi, Campylobacter, Brucella, Bordatella, Pasturella and Spirochaetes*. Many of the organisms and some strains of certain organisms have now become resistant. Rickettsiae (highly sensitive), chlamydiae, Mycoplasma, actinomycetes and the protozoa—*Entamoeba histolytica* and plasmodia are all inhibited by tetracyclines.

Resistance

Many organisms have now become resistant. The resistance has been so widespread that the usefulness of this group of drugs is largely brought down. Resistance to tetracyclines is transmitted by plasmids that contain the genes coding for resistance. Moreover, the organism may easily develop resistance to many other antibiotics because the genes that control resistance to tetracyclines also influence the resistance to many other antibiotics. Resistance is exhibited as:

1. Decreased uptake or efflux of the antibiotic from the bacterium.
2. Displacing tetracyclines from the binding site, i.e. the target ribosome.
3. Elaborating enzymes that inactivate tetracyclines.

Cross-resistance among different tetracyclines is also noted.

Pharmacokinetics

Older tetracyclines are incompletely absorbed from the gut; food interferes with their absorption, bioavailability of chlortetracycline is 30% and that of tetracycline, oxytetracycline, demeclocycline and methacycline range between 60 and 70%. Doxycycline ~95% and **minocycline is 100% absorbed** and food does not affect the absorption of these two agents. Tetracyclines **chelate calcium** and other metals which reduce their absorption. Hence, tetracyclines should **not be given with milk and milk products, iron preparations, zinc supplements and antacids.** Tetracyclines undergo enterohepatic circulation because of which they remain in the body for a long time. Tetracyclines like oxytetracycline and doxycycline can be given intravenously but they cause irritation and thrombophlebitis. **Intramuscular injections** are painful due to local irritation and should, therefore, be **avoided.**

Tetracyclines are widely distributed in the body. They accumulate in the liver, spleen, bone marrow, bone and teeth and attain a good concentration in most secretions including CSF, sinuses, synovial fluid, urine, prostate and in milk. They also cross the placenta.

All tetracyclines except doxycycline and minocycline are excreted through the kidneys. Doxycycline and minocycline are **excreted through the gut** even when given parenterally and are, therefore, safe in renal insufficiency.

Administration

- Tetracyclines are available for oral, parenteral and topical use.
- Tetracyclines may be given with food to reduce the severity of gastrointestinal irritant effects.
- Milk, dairy products, antacids, iron and sucralfate (contain aluminium) can interfere with the absorption of tetracyclines and should, therefore, not be given concurrently.
- Cholestyramine and cholestipol bind tetracyclines given orally and thereby interfere with their absorpton. A gap of 2 hours should be given between their administration.
- Intramuscular injection of tetracyclines should be avoided because:
  i. They can cause irritation.
  ii. Absorption is poor and unreliable.
- Doxycycline and minocycline are the only tetracyclines that are suitable for IV use because other tetracyclines cause thrombophlebitis.

Preparations

Dose: Tetracycline 250–500 mg QID, HOSTACYCLINE, RESTECLIN 250, 500 mg cap.

Demeclocycline 150–300 mg BD; LEDERMYCIN, DECLOMYCIN 150, 300 mg tab.

Chlortetracycline 250–500 mg QID. AUREOMYCIN 250, 500 mg cap.

Adverse Effects

1. **GIT:** Gastrointestinal irritation, leading to epigastric burning, oesophageal ulcers, nausea, vomiting and diarrhoea can occur—tetracyclines are to be given with food to minimize these effects.
2. **Hepatotoxicity** can develop on using large doses of tetracyclines *and* may result in jaundice. Acute hepatic necrosis may occur in pregnant women but is rare.
3. **Renal toxicity:** Renal failure may be aggravated because of increased levels of nitrogen due to the antianabolic effects of tetracyclines. Outdated tetracyclines cause a syndrome like **Fanconi's syndrome** with vomiting, polyuria, proteinuria, glycosuria and acidosis due to the metabolites of outdated tetracyclines.
4. **Phototoxicity:** Skin reactions and dermatitis on exposure to sun are more likely with doxycycline and demeclocycline.
5. **Effect on teeth and bones:** Tetracyclines chelate calcium. The calcium tetracycline orthophosphate complexes get deposited in the developing teeth and bones. The deformities depend on the time of tetracycline administration.

Period affected	*Structure*	*Deformity*
Mid-pregnancy to 5 months of postnatal life	Deciduous teeth	Brownish discolouration, ill formed and are more susceptible to caries
2 months to 5 yr of age	Permanent teeth	Pigmentation, discolouration
Pregnancy and childhood up to 8 yr of age	Skeleton	Depressed bone growth

Onycholysis and pigmentation of the nails may also develop. Tetracyclines are thus **teratogenic.**

6. **Suprainfections:** Since the intestinal flora are extensively suppressed by tetracyclines, these are the most common antibiotics to cause suprainfections.
7. **Hypersensitivity reactions** are not very common.
8. **Local** IV injections can cause thrombophlebitis, due to their irritant effects.
9. **Pseudotumor cerebri:** Tetracyclines may increase intracranial pressure specially in infants. This results in bulging of anterior

fontanelle in infants giving a false impression of tumour. This is described as pseudotumor cerebri. In adults, it can result in headache.

10. **Antianabolic effect:** When large doses are given for long periods, tetracyclines can increase the urinary excretion of nitrogen by an antianabolic effect.
11. **Long-term use:** May cause leukocytosis, formation of atypical lymphocytes and thrombocytopenic purpura.
12. **Nephrogenic diabetes insipidus:** Democlocycline inhibits the action of ADH in the kidney and thereby causes nephrogenic DI. The use of it is also associated with a higher incidence of **phototoxicity** because of which **demeclocycline** is not preferred as an antibiotic. However, it is used in inappropriate ADH secretion.

Mnemonic for uses of tetracyclines

After **P**ainless **CATARACT S**urgery, **P**atient **GOT B**lindness **C**ured

After—Atypical
Painless—Plague
C—Clamydia
A—Acne
T—Tubrculosis
A—Amoebiasis
R—Ricketssiae
A—ADH secretion (inappropriate)
C—Cholera
T—topical use
Surgery—STD
Patient—Protozoal infection
G—granuloma inguinale
O—Others (Lyme's, leptospira)
T—Travellers diarrhea
Blindness—Brucellosis
Cured—Chlamydia pnemoniae

Uses

Tetracyclines were earlier used as empirical therapy for all infections. However, since several organisms have lost sensitivity to them, and also because better and safer antibiotic combinations can be used (a penicillin + an aminoglycoside) tetracyclines are not preferred for empirical therapy.

A. Tetracyclines are the drugs of choice in:

1. *Rickettsial infections:* All rickettsial infections, including tick typhus, Q fever, Rocky Mountain spotted fever respond to tetracyclines—fever subsides and clinical improvement is seen in 48 hours. Hence, tetracyclines are the drugs of choice in rickettsial infections.

   Dose: 2 g 6 hourly initially and then reduced to 1 g 6 hourly.

2. *Chlamydial infections*
   a. *Lymphogranuloma venereum:* Tetracyclines are given for 2 weeks.
   b. *Trachoma:* Both topical and oral tetracyclines are needed. Tetracycline ointment is applied 3–4 times a day for 4–6 weeks and treatment should be continued up to 40 days.
   c. *Inclusion conjunctivitis:* Topical application of tetracycline ointment for 2–3 weeks 4 times a day.
   d. *Urethritis/cervicitis* due to chlamydiae is treated with tetracyclines.
   e. *Chlamydia pneumoniae:* Pneumonia due to *Chlamydia pneumoniae* responds to tetracyclines.
   f. *Psittacosis* needs 2 wks of tetracycline in a dose of 2 g/day.
3. *Atypical pneumonia* due to *Mycoplasma pneumoniae.*
4. *Granuloma inguinale* caused by *Calymmate bacterium granulomatis* responds to tetracyclines given for 3 weeks.
5. *Cholera:* Tetracyclines reduce the duration of illness and are of adjuvant value. The treatment of dehydration is lifesaving in cholera as there is loss of electrolytes particularly sodium. The *Vibrio cholerae* are killed by single dose of 200 mg doxycycline or 2 g tetracycline.
6. *Brucellosis:* Doxycycline 200 mg + rifampicin 600 mg daily for 6 weeks is the treatment of choice.

COMPARE AND CONTRAST

Tetracycline and Doxycycline

Features	***Tetracycline***	***Doxycycline***
Source	Semisynthetic	Semisynthetic
Intestinal absorption	Incomplete	Complete
Bioavailability	75%	95%
Lipid solubility	Low	High
Plasma t½	Short (8–10 hr)	Long (18–24 hr)
Dose and frequency of administration	500 mg QID	200 mg stat, 100 mg OD from day 2
Route of excretion	Kidney	Gut
Safety in renal impairment	Not safe	Safe
Inhibition of intestinal flora	Significant	Low
Phototoxicity	Low	High

7. *Plague:* Tetracyclines may be combined with an aminoglycoside. Highly effective in both types of plague.

B. *Tetracyclines* are useful in other infections, like:

1. *Traveller's diarrhoea:* Doxycycline reduces the incidence of traveller's diarrhoea.
2. *Sexually transmitted diseases* like syphilis, gonorrhoea and chancroid also respond to tetracyclines—but are not preferred.
3. *Acne:* The propioni bacteria in the sebaceous follicles metabolize lipids in the sebum into irritating free fatty acids. These cause irritation of the sebacious gland causing inflammation and forming a comedone (black head). This triggers the development of acne. Tetracyclines inhibit the propioni bacteria. Low doses are given for a long time (250 mg BD for 4 weeks).
4. *Tularaemia:* A combination of tetracycline with an aminoglycoside can be used in tularaemia.
5. *Other infections:* Tetracyclines are also useful in the treatment of Lyme disease, relapsing fever, leptospirosis and post-exposure prophylaxis of anthrax. Doxycycline is used in COVID-19 along with other drugs.
6. *Protozoal infections*
   - *Amoebiasis:* Tetracyclines are useful in chronic intestinal amoebiasis.
   - *Malaria:* Doxycycline is given with quinine in multi-drug resistant malaria.

C. *Inappropriate secretion of ADH:* Demeclocycline is used because it inhibits the action of ADH in the kidney.

D. *Topical use:* Tetracycline ophthalmic solution is used for eye infections.

Contraindications

1. Tetracyclines are contraindicated in pregnancy, lactation and in children up to 8 years of age for the following reasons:
   - Their effects on teeth and bones.
   - Risk of acute hepatic necrosis in pregnant women.
   - Risk of pseudotumor cerebri in infants.
2. Should be used cautiously in renal and hepatic impairment.

Doxycycline and minocycline are semisynthetic tetracyclines.

- Given orally they are 95% and 100% absorbed, respectively.
- Food does not interfere with their absorption.
- Both are highly lipid-soluble.
- Have long t½—can be given once daily.
- Excreted through the gut—hence can be given in usual dose even in the presence of renal impairment.

- Both can be given orally and parenterally (IV) though doxycycline is preferred for parenteral use.
- Microsomal enzyme inducers like barbiturates, phenytoin and ethyl alcohol can hasten the metabolism of doxycycline resulting in shorter t½ of doxycycline.
- Minocycline causes vestibular toxicity characterised by vertigo, dizziness, ataxia, nausea and vomiting.
- Minocycline can be used as an alternative to rifampicin to eradicate meningococcal carrier state, i.e. to eradicate the meningococci from the nasopharynx of the carriers.
- Doxycycline is preferred for post-exposure prophylaxis of anthrax.
- **Doxycycline** Dose: 100 mg BD on 1st day. 100 mg OD for next 6–14 days. DOXY 150, 100, 200 mg cap. NOVADOX 100 mg cap. **Minocycline** Dose: Same as DOXY. CYNOMYCIN, MINOLOX 50, 100 mg caps.

CHLORAMPHENICOL

Chloramphenicol is a broad-spectrum antibiotic first obtained from *Streptomyces venezuelae* in 1947.

Mechanism of Action

Chloramphenicol is bacteriostatic but to some organisms it is bactericidal. It binds to 50S ribosomal subunit and inhibits protein synthesis—by inhibiting transpeptidation reaction (Fig. 47.2).

Chloramphenicol
↓
Binds to 50S ribosomal subunit
↓
Inhibits protein synthesis
↓
Bacteriostatic

Antibacterial Spectrum

Antibacterial spectrum is broad and includes gram-negative organisms, some gram-positive organisms, anaerobic bacteria, *rickettsiae,* and *Mycoplasma.* Thus *H. influenzae, Salmonella, Shigella, Bordatella, Brucella, gonococci, meningococci, streptococci, staphylococci, Clostridium, E. coli and Klebsiella*—are inhibited apart from *Rickettsiae* and *Mycoplasma.* Chloramphenicol is bactericidal to *Neisseria meningitidis, H. influenzae* and some strains of bacteroides.

Resistance is plasmid-mediated and may be due to:

1. Inactivatng enzymes (chloramphenicol acetyltransferase which inactivates chloramphenicol)
2. Reduced permeability of the microorganisms to the antibiotic.
3. Ribosomal insensitivity.

Pharmacokinetics

Chloramphenicol is rapidly absorbed from the gut; **penetration into tissues is excellent;** attains high concentration in CSF—almost as much as in plasma. It is metabolised in the liver by reduction and glucuronide conjugation. The metabolites are excreted in the urine.

Dose: 250–500 mg QID: RECLOR 250, 500 mg cap Chloramphenicol 1 g vial.

Adverse Reactions

1. *Gastrointestinal disturbances:* Nausea, vomiting and diarrhoea.
2. *Bone marrow depression:* Chloramphenicol may cause bone marrow depression in two ways:
   - Dose-dependent anaemia, leukopenia and thrombocytopenia due to inhibition of protein synthesis. In higher doses, mammalian cells are susceptible to inhibition of protein synthesis by chloramphenicol. It is reversible.
   - *Idiosyncratic response* resulting in aplastic anaemia which may be fatal. It may be due to a toxic metabolite. Incidence is 1 in 30,000 patients and occurs in genetically predisposed individuals. This

Drugs used in the treatment of typhoid

The incidence of typhoid or enteric fever caused by *Salmonella typhimurium* has been increasing and requires prompt treatment to avoid complications. The choice of antibiotic depends on the susceptibility of the microorganism.

Drugs for empirical treatment

- Ceftriaxone—1–2 g/day i.v. for 7–14 days.
- Azithromycin 1 g/day oral for 5 days.

Other drugs (based on sensitivity report)

- Ciprofloxacin 750 mg BD for 10 days
- Amoxicillin 1 g tid oral for 14 days
- Chloramphenicol 25 mg/kg tid oral/i.v. for 14 days
- Cotrimoxazole double strength BD oral for 7–14 days

Multidrug resistant

- Ciprofloxacin 500 mg BD for 5–7 days
- Ceftriaxone 2–3 g/day IV
- Azithromycin 1 g/day oral.

toxicity has limited the use of chloramphenicol.

3. *Gray baby syndrome:* Newborn babies given high doses of chloramphenicol may show *'gray baby syndrome'* manifested as vomiting, refusal of feeds, hypotonia, hypothermia, abdominal distension, metabolic acidosis and ashen gray cyanosis. It may be fatal. As the newborn cannot metabolize (due to inadequate hepatic glucuronidation) and excrete chloramphenicol adequately, toxicity results. However, it is seen with higher doses only and can largely be avoided.
4. *Hypersensitivity reactions* like rashes and fever are uncommon.
5. *Superinfection* can occur.

Drug Interactions

Chloramphenicol inhibits hepatic microsomal enzymes and thereby prolongs the half-life of drugs metabolised by this system. This may result in enhanced toxicity of some drugs like phenytoin, warfarin, tolbutamide and dicumarol.

Uses

Because of the risk of bone marrow toxicity and availability of safer drugs, chloramphenicol is not generally preferred. Some specific indications are:

1. *Typhoid fever:* Chloramphenicol was earlier considered the drug of choice in typhoid fever. However, *S. typhi* developed resistance to it and such strains spread across the world. For the sensitive strains of *Salmonella typhi*, chloramphenicol can still be used as an alternative to fluoroquinolones and cephalosporins. It is given for 14 days (500 mg QID till fever subsides and then 250 mg QID up to 14th day).
2. *Bacterial meningitis:* In meningococcal and *H. influenzae* meningitis, chloramphenicol is an alternative to penicillin and cephalosporins.
3. *Anaerobic infections:* Chloramphenicol + penicillin + an aminoglycoside can be used in severe anaerobic infections as an alternative to metronidazole and clindamycin.
4. *Rickettsial infections:* As an alternative when tetracyclines are contraindicated.
5. *Eye and ear infections:* Chloramphenicol eyedrops are used topically because of the good penetration into aqueous humour. Eardrops are effective in infections of the external ear.
6. *Brain abscess* due to anaerobes responds to surgical drainage and a course of chloramphenicol.

TIGECYCLINE

Tigecycline, a glycylcycline, is a derivative of minocycline. It has a broad antibacterial spectrum including many methicillin and vancomycin resistant strains of staphylococci, streptococci, multidrug resistant enterococci, *S. pneumoniae,* anaerobes, Enterobacteriaceae, mycobacteria, rickettsiae, chlamydiae and legionella. Tigecycline is thus effective against many gram-positive and gram-negative aerobes and anaerobes that are resistant to tetracyclines.

Tigecycline is given only by parenteral route (IV) initial dose of 100 mg followed by 50 mg twice daily. It has a long t½ of 36 hr. Penetration and distribution into cells and tissues are very good. It is **excreted through the gut** and, therefore, does not require dose reduction in renal dysfunction. Tigecycline can cause nausea and vomiting apart from other adverse effects of tetracyclines. It is well tolerated.

Uses

Tigecycline is used as an alternative in **life-threatening infections** due to drug-resistant microorganisms and **nosocomial** pathogens including skin and skin structure infections, intra-abdominal infections and pneumonia.

Clinical Pharmacology

- Tetracyclines should **not** be given along with milk, milk products, antacids and iron.
- Doxycycline is the commonly used tetracycline.
- Tetracyclines should preferably not be given IM because of pain at infection site and unreliable absorption.
- Doxycycline, minocycline and tigecycline do not require dosage adjustment in renal failure.
- Tigecycline is not useful in urinary infection as it does not attain adequate concentration in the urine.

CHAPTER 48

Aminoglycosides

Aminoglycosides (AGs) are antibiotics with amino sugars joined by glycosidic linkages. They are derived from the soil actinomycetes of the genus Streptomyces (streptomycin, kanamycin, tobramycin, neomycin) and the genus Micromonospora (gentamicin and sisomicin)—hence the difference in spelling. Amikacin and netilmicin are semisynthetic products.

Common Properties of Aminoglycosides

1. Aminoglycosides are polycationic carbohydrates containing amino sugars in glycosidic linkages.
2. They are highly water-soluble, polar compounds.
3. Aminoglycosides are not absorbed orally (as they ionize in solution)—therefore, they are all given parenterally.
4. They remain extracellularly and penetration into CSF is very poor.
5. They are excreted unchanged by the kidneys.
6. They are more active at alkaline pH.
7. They are all bactericidal.
8. They act by inhibiting bacterial protein synthesis.
9. They are mainly effective against gram-negative organisms.
10. They produce variable degrees of ototoxicity and nephrotoxicity as adverse effects.

Aminoglycosides include:

- Streptomycin, gentamicin, tobramycin, kanamycin, paromomycin.
- Newer ones—amikacin, sisomicin, netilmicin.
- Topical—neomycin, framycetin.

Antibacterial Spectrum

Aminoglycosides have a narrow spectrum and are effective mainly against aerobic gram-negative bacilli like *E. coli, Proteus, Y. pestis, Nocardia, V. cholerae, Pseudomonas, Brucella, Salmonella, Shigella* and *Klebsiella*.

Mechanism of Action

Aminoglycosides, being water-soluble, penetrate the bacterial cell membrane through aqueous pores and reach the periplasmic spaces. They are taken up and transported across the cell membrane into the cytoplasm by an oxygen-dependent active transport process. It is observed that aminoglycosides disrupt the bacterial cell membrane and this also allows penetration of the drug into the bacterium from the periplasmic space.

Inside the cell (Fig. 48.1), aminoglycosides **bind to 30S ribosomes and inhibit bacterial protein synthesis**—block initiation of protein synthesis, cause termination of protein synthesis and cause addition of incorrect amino acids resulting in the synthesis of abnormal proteins (Key Box 48.1). Aminoglycosides are **bactericidal.** Higher the concentration, greater is the bactericidal effect (dose-dependent killing). A residual bactericidal effect—**post-antibiotic effect**—remains even after the plasma levels of aminoglycosides fall. Hence, even though they have a short t½, they can be given once a day.

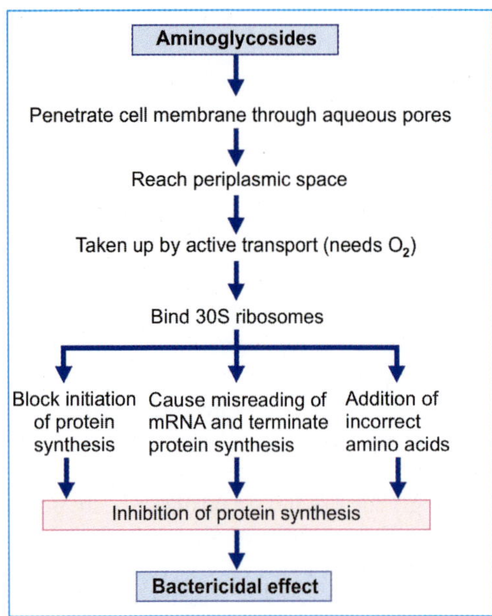

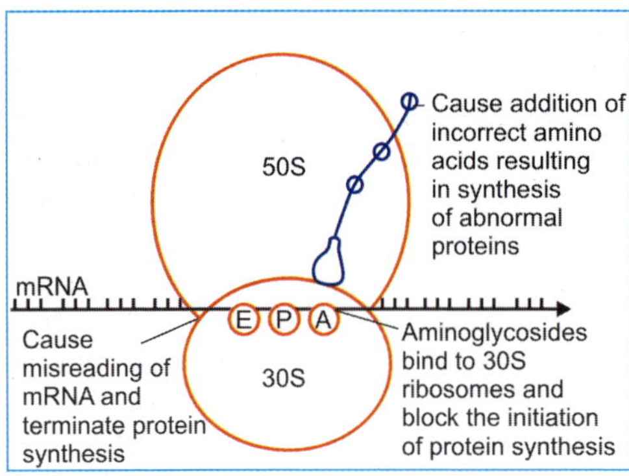

Fig. 48.1: Mechanism of action of aminoglycosides

Low extracellular pH and anaerobic environment inhibit the uptake of aminoglycosides by active transport because this is an oxygen-dependent process. Hence aminoglycosides are not effective in anaerobic infections. Drugs acting on the cell wall, like penicillins, counter this negative effect of low pH and anaerobiasis and improve penetration. Penicillins inhibit bacterial cell wall synthesis and facilitate diffusion of aminoglycosides into the bacteria. These are some of the reasons for synergism of the combination.

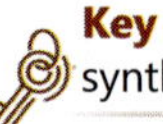

Key Box 48.1: Antibiotics that inhibit protein synthesis by binding to ribosomes

50S		***30S***
Erythromycin	Clindamycin	Tetracyclines
Chloramphenicol	Streptogramins	Aminoglycosides
	Linezolid	

Resistance to aminoglycosides is acquired by:

1. Aminoglycoside inactivating enzymes: On binding to aminoglycosides, the enzyme inactivates aminoglycosides which fail to bind to the target ribosomes.
2. Low affinity of ribosomes—acquired by mutation.
3. Decrease in permeability to the antibiotic.

There is partial **cross-resistance** among various aminoglycosides.

Pharmacokinetics

Aminoglycosides are not absorbed from the gut but when instilled into body cavities or applied over large wounds, they may get rapidly absorbed. Following IM injection, peak levels are seen in 60 minutes. They are not bound to plasma proteins and do not enter the cells or cross barriers—mostly remain in the vasculature. In patients with severe infection, plasma concentration of aminoglycosides should be determined to guide the treatment (Table 48.1). Aminoglycosides are excreted almost completely through the kidneys. Half-life is 2–3 hr but gets prolonged to 24–48 hr in renal impairment—dose should be reduced.

Adverse Effects

1. *Ototoxicity* is the most important toxicity. Both vestibular and auditory dysfunction can occur depending on the dose and duration. The aminoglycosides get concentrated in the labyrinthine fluid of the inner ear and damage both cochlear hair cells and vestibular sensory cells. The auditory nerve degenerates. As the cochlear cells cannot

Table 48.1: Dose and routes of administration of aminoglycosides

Aminoglycosides	*Doses*	*Routes*
Streptomycin	1–2 g/day	IM
Gentamicin	3–5 mg/kg/day in 3 divided doses	IM/IV
Tobramycin	3–5 mg/kg/day in 3 divided doses	IM/IV
Amikacin	15 mg/kg/day in 2–3 divided doses	IM/IV
Netilmicin	4–6 mg/kg/day in 2–3 divided doses	IM/IV

regenerate, there is progressive, **permanent deafness.** Tinnitus appears first, followed by deafness; elderly people are more susceptible. Stoping the drug can prevent further damage. Vestibular dysfunction is manifested by headache, nausea, vomiting, dizziness, vertigo, nystagmus and ataxia. Most symptoms subside in two weeks except ataxia which may persist for 1–2 years. Neomycin, amikacin and kanamycin are the aminoglycosides which are most likely to cause deafness, while streptomycin and gentamicin are most likely to cause vestibular toxicity.

2. *Nephrotoxicity:* Aminoglycosides attain high concentration in the renal cortex and cause damage to the renal tubules. This results in loss of urine concentrating capacity, low GFR and albuminuria. These effects are reversible. Gentamicin, neomycin and tobramycin are the most nephrotoxic.
3. *Neuromuscular blockade:* Aminoglycosides have curare-like effects and block neuromuscular transmission.

Precautions in using Aminoglycosides

1. Avoid concurrent use of other ototoxic drugs like loop diuretics.
2. Avoid concurrent use of other nephrotoxic drugs like amphotericin B, cephalothin and cisplatin.
3. Avoid concurrent use of curarimimetic drugs.
4. To be used cautiously in elderly, in renal dysfunction and in combination with skeletal muscle relaxants.
5. Contraindicated in pregnancy because of the risk of deafness in the child.
6. Do not mix aminoglycosides with any other drug in the same syringe.
7. Determination of plasma levels of aminoglycosides may be needed in severe infections and in patients with renal dysfunction.

Uses

1. Aminoglycosides are used in the treatment of infections due to gram-negative bacteria.
2. Aminoglycosides are also used in streptococcal and enterococcal endocarditis in combination with a penicillin. The combination is synergistic due to the following reasons:
   - Both are bactericidal.
   - Low pH and anaerobiasis reduce the uptake of aminoglycosides by active transport. This negative effect is reversed by penicillins.
   - Penicillins improve penetration of aminoglycosides by inhibiting cell wall synthesis in the bacteria.
3. Some aminoglycosides (streptomycin, kanamycin, amikacin) are also used in tuberculosis. Indications are discussed under individual aminoglycoside agents.

Streptomycin obtained from *Streptomyces griseus* is mainly effective against aerobic gram-negative bacilli. When used alone, bacteria, especially the tubercle bacillus rapidly develops resistance to it. Streptomycin is the least nephrotoxic among aminoglycosides.

Uses

1. *Tuberculosis:* Streptomycin is a second-line drug in tuberculosis (*see* page 598).

2. *Subacute bacterial endocarditis (SBE):* Combination of streptomycin and penicillin is synergistic in enterococcal and *Streptococcus viridans* endocarditis.
3. *Plague, tularaemia and brucellosis:* Streptomycin is given with a tetracycline.

Gentamicin obtained from *Micromonospora purpurea* is more potent and has a broader spectrum of action compared to streptomycin. Development of resistance has limited its use. It causes more nephrotoxicity and vestibulotoxicity.

Uses

1. *UTI:* Gentamicin is effective in uncomplicated UTI as it is released for a long time from the renal cortex.
2. *Pneumonia* due to gram-negative organisms may be treated with gentamicin + penicillin.
3. *Osteomyelitis, peritonitis, septicaemia, abscess, burns* caused by gram-negative organisms (*Pseudomonas*, *Proteus* and *Klebsiella*) can be treated with gentamicin.
4. *Meningitis due to gram-negative bacilli:* Gentamicin is used with a third generation cephalosporin.
5. *SBE:* Gentamicin may be used in place of streptomycin in SBE.
6. *Topical:* Gentamicin cream is used topically in burns and other infected wounds. Gentamicin eye drops are used in the prevention and treatment of bacterial conjunctivitis.

Tobramycin has better activity against *Pseudomonas* and is used with an antipseudomonal penicillin in such infections. It can be used in place of gentamicin.

Kanamycin: Due to its toxicity, its use is limited to multi-drug resistant tuberculosis.

Amikacin, a semisynthetic derivative of kanamycin, has **widest antibacterial spectrum among the aminoglycosides** because it is resistant to aminoglycoside inactivating enzymes.

Uses

1. *Nosocomial* infections due to gram-negative organisms.
2. *Tuberculosis:* Amikacin is useful in multidrug resistant tuberculosis in combination with other drugs. It is also used in infections due to atypical mycobacteria in patients with AIDS.

Netilmicin: Like amikacin, netilmicin is resistant to aminoglycoside inactivating enzymes. It is used in serious infections due to gram-negative bacilli. It can be used in place of gentamicin or tobramycin.

COMPARE AND CONTRAST

Amoxicillin and Gentamicin

Features	***Amoxicillin***	***Gentamicin***
Chemistry	β-lactam antibiotic	Aminoglycoside
Source	Semisynthetic	Natural—from micromonospora purpurea
Antibacterial spectrum	Wide—Gm +ve and Gm –ve microorganisms	Narrow—mostly Gm –ve
Mechanism of action	Inhibits cell wall synthesis	Inhibits protein synthesis
Intestinal absorption	Well absorbed	Not absorbed
Route of administration	Oral	Parenteral
Volume of distribution	Large	Small
Prominent adverse effects	Diarrhoea, allergic reactions	Ototoxicity, nephrotoxicity
Major action	Bactericidal	Bactericidal

Gm +ve—gram-positive, Gm –ve—gram-negative

Sisomicin has actions, toxicity and uses similar to gentamicin.

Neomycin has a wide antibacterial spectrum—effective against gram-positive and gram-negative bacteria. As it is highly ototoxic, it is not given systemically. It is used topically as ointments, creams and powder. It is also used orally for action on the gut.

Adverse effects: Neomycin can cause skin rashes on topical use. Oral use can cause diarrhoea, steatorrhoea and malabsorption due to damage to the intestinal villi. Superinfection with Candida can also occur.

Uses

1. *Topical:* Neomycin is used topically in skin infections, burns, ulcers and wounds; eye and ear infections.
2. *Orally*
   a. *Neomycin* is not absorbed when given orally. It inhibits the growth of intestinal flora and is excreted in the feces. It is used to prepare the bowel for surgery, i.e. for preoperative gut sterilization 1 g 3–4 times a day for 1–2 days with or without 1 g erythromycin.
   b. *Hepatic coma:* Ammonia produced by colonic bacteria is absorbed and converted to urea by the liver. In severe hepatic failure, as liver is unable to handle this NH_3, blood NH_3 levels rise resulting in encephalopathy. As neomycin inhibits intestinal flora, NH_3 production falls. Neomycin is given orally for this purpose. However, lactulose is now preferred for this indication.

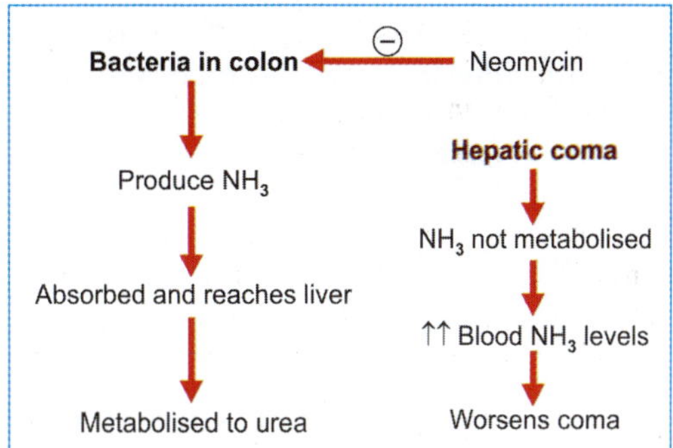

Clinical Pharmacology

- Once daily dosing has advantages of better efficacy and post-antibiotic effect.
- Therapeutic drug monitoring may be required for aminoglycosides.
- For once daily injections, plasma trough concentrations are measured which should be <1 µg/ml. Sample is collected after 2 hr and 12 hr following a dose.
- Dose of aminoglycosides should be reduced in renal impairment. *Calculation:*

$$\text{Dose in renal insufficiency} = \frac{\text{Regular therapeutic dose}}{\text{Serum creatinine value}}$$

- Neomycin, kanamycin and amikacin are the most ototoxic; neomycin, tobramycin and gentamicin are the most nephrotoxic while streptomycin and gentamicin are the most vestibulotoxic.
- Aminoglycosides should always be combined with another antibiotic for pneumonia as efficacy may not be good because of their poor penetration into infected tissue (lung), due to low oxygen tension and acidic pH.
- Purulent exudation can inactivate gentamicin to some extent.

CHAPTER **49**

Macrolides and other Antibacterial Agents

Macrolides are antibiotics with a large (macrocyclic) lactone ring to which sugars are attached. **Erythromycin** and its semisynthetic derivatives **roxithromycin**, **clarithromycin** and **azithromycin** are the macrolides currently used (Table 49.1). **Dirithromycin**, **oleandomycin**, **troleandomycin** and **spiramycin** are other macrolide antibiotics.

ERYTHROMYCIN

Erythromycin is obtained from *Streptomyces erythreus.*

Antibacterial spectrum: Erythromycin has a narrow spectrum and is effective against aerobic gram-positive bacteria and a few gram-negative organisms.

Streptococci, pneumococci, staphylococci, gonococci, legionella, *C. diphtheriae, B. pertussis, T. pallidum, C. jejuni, Mycoplasma, Chlamydiae* and some atypical mycobacteria are sensitive.

Mechanism of Action

Erythromycin is bacteriostatic at low and cidal at high concentrations. It is more effective in the alkaline pH. It binds to 50S ribosomes (Fig. 49.1) and inhibits bacterial protein synthesis. Macrolides inhibit the translocation of the growing peptide chain from A site to P site. Hence, A site is not available for binding of the next amino acid (brought by tRNA) and protein synthesis stops. Chloramphenicol and clindamycin also bind to 50S ribosomes and the three may antagonise each others activity because they compete for the same binding site. Hence, the combination should be avoided (Fig. 49.1).

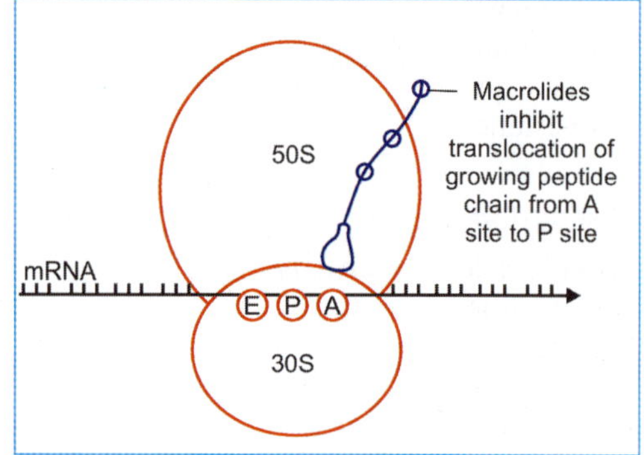

Fig. 49.1: Mechanism of action of macrolide antibiotics

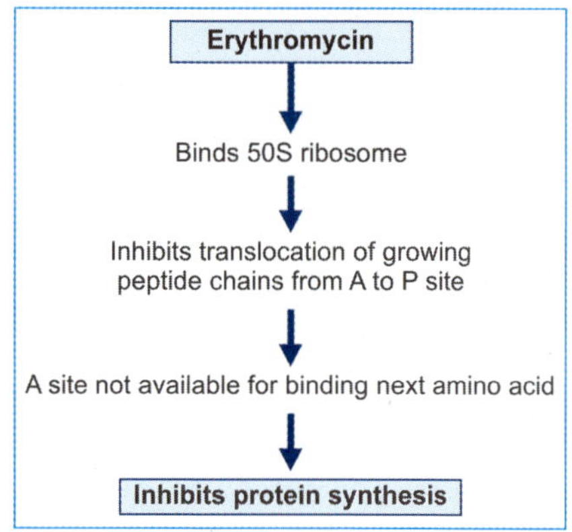

Resistance to macrolides is acquired through plasmids. The mechanism of expression of resistance may be:

- Low permeability of the bacteria to the antibiotic.
- Production of inactivating enzymes that hydrolyze macrolides.
- Low affinity of ribosomes to macrolides—such organisms are also resistant to other

Table 49.1: Adult dose and duration of treatment with macrolides

Drug	*Dose and duration*	*Preparations*
Erythromycin stearate	250–500 mg QID, 7–14 days	ERYTHROCIN 250, 500 mg cap
Erythromycin estolate	250–500 mg QID, 7–14 days	ALTHROCIN 250, 500 mg cap
Erythromycin base	0.25–1g QID, for 7–14 days	ERYSAFE 250, 500 mg cap
Erythromycin-ointment	To be applied twice daily	GERY OINT 30%
Roxithromycin	150 mg BD, for 5–10 days	ROXID 150 mg cap
Azithromycin	500 mg day 1 f/b 250–500 mg OD 3 days	AZITHRAL 250–500 mg tab
Clarithromycin	250–500 mg BD, for 7–14 days	CLARICAP 250 mg cap

drugs which bind 50s ribosomes—lincosamides and streptogramins called macrolide-lincosamide-streptogramin or MLS-type resistance.

Pharmacokinetics

Food interferes with absorption. Among the different salts, erythromycin estolate is the best absorbed, but not preferred due to risk of adverse effects. Erythromycin is destroyed by gastric acid and is, therefore, given as enteric coated tablets. Plasma t½ ~1.5 hr. Good concentration is attained in most fluids except brain and CSF. It also crosses the placenta. Erythromycin is a **microsomal enzyme inhibitor**. It is mainly excreted through the bile; dose adjustment is not needed in renal failure (Table 49.1).

Adverse Effects

1. Hepatitis with cholestatic jaundice starts after 2–3 weeks of treatment and incidence is more common with the estolate salt. The symptoms—nausea, vomiting and abdominal cramps, mimic acute cholecystitis and may be wrongly treated. These are followed by jaundice and fever. It may be an allergic response to the estolate salt. Hepatitis is self-limiting but erythromycin should be avoided in such patients as they are likely to develop hepatitis again.
2. Epigastric distress, nausea, vomiting and diarrhoea are often reported. Erythromycin is a **motilin receptor agonist** due to which it causes increased intestinal motility.
3. Allergic reactions including fever and skin rashes can occur.
4. Cardiac arrhythmias are reported in patients with cardiac diseases or on other arrhythmogenic drugs.
5. Erythromycin can also cause reversible hearing impairment in some patients.

Drug Interactions

Erythromycin and clarithromycin are **microsomal enzyme** (cytochrome P450) **inhibitors**. They inhibit the hepatic metabolism and thereby enhance the plasma levels of other drugs like carbamazepine, terfenadine, theophylline, valproate, digoxin and warfarin resulting in toxicity due to these drugs.

Uses

Erythromycin can be used as an alternative to penicillin in patients allergic to penicillin.

1. *Atypical pneumonia:* May be caused by agents like *Mycoplasma, Chlamydia* and *Legionella*. Atypical pneumonia due to *Mycoplasma pneumoniae*—erythromycin is the drug of choice—500 mg 6 hrly oral or IV.
2. *Legionnaires' pneumonia:* It is treated for 10–14 days with erythromycin. IV erythromycin is preferred. Azithromycin is now considered the drug of choice.
3. *Whooping cough:* Erythromycin is the drug of choice for the treatment and post-exposure prophylaxis of close contacts. Clarithromycin and azithromycin may also be used.

Erythromycin (!)

Mr Raju, a 42-year-old man, reported to a hospital with nausea, vomiting and abdominal cramps. After examination and investigations, a diagnosis of acute cholecystitis was made and the patient was taken for cholecystectomy. On opening the abdomen, it was found that the gallbladder was normal. The patient developed jaundice (cholestatic) after 2 days. When history was re-elicited, the patient revealed that 2 weeks back he was treated with a long course of erythromycin estolate for respiratory infection. His present symptoms were a result of an adverse effect of erythromycin. The right treatment was just to do nothing—it is self-limiting. Here the patient was subjected to unnecessary trauma of surgery because a proper history was not elicited.

4. *Streptococcal infections:* Pharyngitis, tonsillitis and scarlet fever respond to erythromycin.
5. *Staphylococcal infections:* Minor infections may be treated but now resistant strains are common.
6. *Diphtheria:* Erythromycin is very effective in acute stage though antitoxin is life saving. Erythromycin also eradicates the carrier state.
7. *Syphilis and gonorrhoea:* Erythromycin is used as an alternative to penicillins.
8. *Campylobacter gastroenteritis:* As an alternative to fluoroquinolones.
9. *Tetanus:* Erythromycin eradicates carrier state.
10. *Anthrax:* Erythromycin is an alternative to penicillin.
11. *Prophylaxis:* Erythromycin may be used as an alternative to penicillin in valvular heart disease patients undergoing dental and other minor procedures.
12. *Topical:* Erythromycin ointment (2–4%) is used for skin infections and boils, lotion for acne vulgaris.
13. *Other uses:*
    a. Erythromycin is a motilin receptor agonist and stimulates GI motility. This property can be made use of in gastroparesis in postoperative patients and in diabetic gastroparesis.
    b. Erythromycin has been found to have anti-inflammatory actions and may be of value in rheumatoid arthritis and chronic sinusitis.

Roxithromycin

Roxithromycin is longer-acting, acid-stable, more potent, better absorbed and has better tissue penetrability compared to erythromycin. It does not inhibit the metabolism of other drugs—hence no risk of related drug interactions. It is more potent against Legionella. Roxithromycin should be taken **30 minutes before food** because food can interfere with absorption and reduce bioavailability. It can be used as an alternative to erythromycin but is more expensive.

Clarithromycin

Compared to erythromycin, clarithromycin is longer-acting, acid-stable and better absorbed; it is more effective against *H. influenzae, Legionella, atypical mycobacteria, H. pylori* and some protozoa. It has also shown some activity against *M. leprae* and *T. gondii.* Clarithromycin is structurally similar to erythromycin and, therefore, its drug interactions are also similar to erythromycin. Clarithromycin is rapidly absorbed, metabolised in the liver and excreted in the urine. Dose reduction may be required in renal dysfunction.

Clarithromycin is used:

1. As a component of triple regimen for *H. pylori* infections in peptic ulcer patients.
2. For the prevention and treatment of atypical mycobacterial infections in AIDS patients.

Though clarithromycin is effective in other indications of erythromycin, its higher cost makes it less preferable.

Azithromycin

Azithromycin, an azalide, is a derivative of erythromycin with activity similar to clarithromycin. Antibacterial spectrum is similar to erythromycin except that it is also effective against *Mycobacterium avium* complex (MAC) and *T. gondii*. Advantages of azithromycin over erythromycin are:

- Azithromycin has excellent activity against *H. influenzae*.
- It is acid-stable
- Rapidly absorbed
- Has better tissue penetrability
- Longer acting–once daily. Azithromycin remains in the tissues for a long period and is gradually released from them and therefore, the elimination t½ is almost 3 days. Hence in many infections, it is effective even in a single dose.
- Better tolerated than erythromycin.
- Azithromycin is also effective against MAC, *T. gondii* and *H. influenzae*.
- Azithromycin is free of drug interactions as it does not suppress microsomal enzymes in the liver and thereby hepatic metabolism of other drugs.

Azithromycin is used in the prophylaxis and treatment of atypical mycobacterial infections in AIDS patients. Like erythromycin, it can also be used in respiratory, genital and skin infections and in pneumonias. Azithromycin is preferred in *Legionella pneumoniae* and chlamydial infections.

Other Macrolides

Dirithromycin is similar to erythromycin with some minor differences. It has better activity against *C. jejuni*, is acid-stable, longer-acting—may be given once daily. Dose: 500 mg OD.

Oleandomycin and troleandomycin are less potent but otherwise similar to erythromycin. Both are used in the dose of 200–500 mg QID.

Spiramycin is used in *T. gondii* infection to prevent transmission from the mother to the foetus.

KETOLIDES

Ketolides are modified macrolides that resemble newer macrolides and are effective against macrolide-resistant pneumococci.

Telithromycin, a ketolide, is a semisynthetic derivative of erythromycin. It is effective against *Staphylococcus aureus, S. pyogenes, S. pneumoniae, H. influenzae, H. pylori, M. catarrhalis, Mycoplasma, Chlamydia, T. gondii, Legionella, B. fragilis* and some mycobacteria.

Mechanism of action of ketolides is similar to macrolides but may be effective even against organisms that are resistant to macrolides. This is because the structure of ketolides is such that they are not destroyed by the inactivating enzymes and also bind to the 50S ribosomes with greater affinity than macrolides. The mechanisms that confers resistance to macrolides do not influence ketolides.

Telithromycin is well absorbed on oral administration with bioavailability 60% and has a t½ of 9–10 hrs—given once daily. Its penetration into tissues is good; metabolized by the liver partly by CYP3A4. Telithromycin is well tolerated—can cause nausea, vomiting, diarrhoea and pseudomembranous colitis. Raised liver enzymes and hepatic failure have been reported. Due to QTc prolongation and increased risk of ventricular arrhythmias, it should be avoided in patients with prolonged QTc or receiving other drugs that prolong QTc. Telithromycin inhibits the microsomal enzyme CYP3A4 and can result in drug interactions. It can increase the plasma levels of other drugs metabolized by CYP3A4.

Uses

Telithromycin can be used in mild to moderate community-acquired bacterial pneumonia, streptococcal pharyngitis and sinusitis.

MISCELLANEOUS ANTIBIOTICS

Spectinomycin is related to aminoglycosides and is effective against gram-negative bacteria. It is used only in gonorrhoea (2 g IM single dose) in patients allergic to penicillin and quinolones.

LINCOSAMIDES

Lincomycin and clindamycin are lincosamides. Lincomycin is no longer used clinically.

Clindamycin

Clindamycin is a congener of lincomycin. It binds to 50S ribosomal subunit and suppresses protein synthesis like erythromycin. Streptococci, staphylococci, pneumococci, many anaerobes, *T. gondii and P. jiroveci* are inhibited by clindamycin. Clindamycin is well-absorbed on oral administration and 90% bound to plasma proteins. It attains good concentration in the bone and many other tissues. It is metabolised in the liver and excreted in the urine and bile—t½ 2.5 hr.

Adverse effects include diarrhoea due to pseudomembranous colitis, skin rashes and neuromuscular blockade. Intravenous use can cause thrombophlebitis.

Dose: 150–300 mg QID. CLINCIN, DALCIN 150, 300 mg cap. ACNERIS 1% w/w gel.

Uses

1. *Anaerobic infections:* Abdominal, pelvic, bone and joints infections due to anaerobes are treated with clindamycin. It may be combined with an aminoglycoside or a cephalosporin. Pelvic infections, aspiration pneumonia may also respond to clindamycin + an aminoglycoside.
2. *Streptococcal and staphylococcal infections:* Clindamycin is effective in skin and soft tissue infections due to *Streptococcus* and *Staphylococcus* including MRSA infections
3. *P. jiroveci infection:* Along with primaquine (30 mg/day), clindamycin 300 mg QID for 21 days can be used as an alternative in *P. jiroveci* pneumonia in AIDS patients.
4. *T. gondii:* Clindamycin and pyrimethamine combination is used in toxoplasmosis in AIDS patients.
5. *Prophylaxis:* In valvular heart disease patients undergoing minor procedures like dental procedures, clindamycin may be used as an alternative to penicillin and erythromycin for prophylaxis.

GLYCOPEPTIDE ANTIBIOTICS

Vancomycin and teicoplanin are glycopeptides. and their derivatives **telavancin, dalbavancin and oritavancin** are lipoglycopeptides.

Vancomycin, produced by *Streptococcus orientalis,* is active against gram-positive bacteria particularly staphylococci including those resistant to methicillin. It acts by inhibiting the cell wall synthesis like penicillin. Vancomycin binds to the peptidoglycan chain and prevents elongation of the chain and cross-linking. Thus cell wall deficient/weak bacteria are formed which undergo lysis. It is thus bactericidal. In addition, vancomycin also weakens the cell membrane.

Resistance is due to genetic mutation changing the target protein—vancomycin fails to bind to the target, vancomycin-resistant enterococci are responsible for several nosocomial infections. Vancomycin-resistant *S. aureus* has also emerged.

Pharmacokinetics: Vancomycin is not absorbed orally—given IV. It can be given orally for pseudomembranous colitis. It is widely

COMPARE AND CONTRAST

Vancomycin and Teicoplanin

Features	***Vancomycin***	***Teicoplanin***
Source	*Streptococcus orientalis*	*Actinoplanes teicomyetius*
MOA	Inhibit cell wall synthesis	Inhibit cell wall synthesis
Route of administration	Only IV (IM painful)	Both IM and IV
Duration of action	Short	Long
Elimination	6–24 hr	70–100 hr
Frequency of administration	4 times a day	Once a day

distributed and mostly excreted through the kidneys. In renal impairment, the half-life of vancomycin gets prolonged and it accumulates in the body.

Adverse effects are skin rashes, pain at the site of injection, thrombophlebitis, ototoxicity and nephrotoxicity. Concurrent use of other ototoxic and nephrotoxic drugs should be avoided; dose should be adjusted in renal dysfunction. Intravenous infusion of vancomycin can sometimes provoke histamine release resulting in a maculopapular rash over the head, neck and back with fever and chills—described as ***'redman or red-neck syndrome'.*** This can be avoided by diluting vancomycin and injecting it as an infusion over 1–2 hr.

Dose: 30 mg/kg/day in 2–3 divided doses. CYTOVAN, VANCORIN. VANCOCARE, 0.5, 1 g inj.

Uses

1. *MRSA infections:* Methicillin-resistant staphylococci—vancomycin is given IV for serious infections like osteomyelitis, endocarditis and soft tissue abscesses.
2. *Enterococcal endocarditis:* Vancomycin with gentamicin is effective—used as an alternative to penicillin.
3. *Penicillin-resistant pneumonococcal infections:* In meningitis and other infections, vancomycin is effective and may be given with a cephalosporin.
4. *Pseudomembranous colitis due to C. difficile:* Oral vancomycin is used 125–250 mg QID as an alternative to metronidazole.

Telavancin a derivative of vancomycin is a lipoglycopeptide with better efficacy against gram +ve bacteria. In addition to inhibiting the cell wall synthesis like vancomycin, telavancin also damages cell membrane and increases its permeability. It can be given once daily.

Dose: VIBATIN 250/750 mg IV.

Teicoplanin obtained from *Actinoplanus teichomyetius* has mechanism of action and antibacterial spectrum similar to vancomycin, but teicoplanin can be safely given intramuscularly. It is also less toxic. Half life is 70 hr—given once daily (*see* Compare and Contrast).

Drugs used in MRSA*

- Vancomycin
- Tigecycline
- Teicoplanin
- Daptomycin
- Quinupristin-dalfopristin
- Linezolid
- Rifampicin

**Methicillin-resistant Staphylococcus aureus*

Pseudomonas aeruginosa

- Antipseudomonal penicillin ± aminoglycoside
- Ceftazidime or cefepime
- Antipseudomonal pencillin + ciprofloxacin
- Imipenem/meropenem + aminoglycoside
- Aztreonam + aminoglycoside

Anaerobic infections

- Metronidazole
- Clindamycin
- Chloramphenicol
- Cefotaxime, ceftizoxime
- Carbapenems
- Ampicillin + sulbactam
- Piperacillin + tazobactam

Atypical mycobacteria

- Clarithromycin + ethambutol
- Rifabutin + ethambutol + ciprofloxacin
- Amikacin
- Cotrimoxazole
- Azithromycin
- Ofloxacin

Toxoplasma gondii

- Pyrimethamine + sulfadiazine + folinic acid
- Spiramycin
- Pyrimethamine + clindamycin +folinic acid

Occasionally causes allergic reactions; can also cause fever and ototoxicity. It is used in osteomyelitis and endocarditis due to methicillin-resistant staphylococci and enterococci.

Dose: 200–400 mg/day. TARGOCID 200, 400 mg inj.

Dalbavancin, a derivative of teicoplanin, is a lipoglycopeptide which acts like teicoplanin with better efficacy against streptococci and staphylococci. It has the advantage of a very long half-life of 6–11 days—hence given IV once a week.

Ramoplanin, an analog of teicoplanin, is highly active against enterococci (*E. faecium* and *E. faecalis)* and *C. difficile*. It is given orally (but is not absorbed) to decolonize the gut of enterococci and to treat pseudomembranous colitis due to *C. difficile*. It is well tolerated.

POLYPEPTIDE ANTIBIOTICS

Polymyxin B and colistin (polymyxin E), polymyxin obtained from *Bacillus polymyxa* and colistin from *Bacillus colistinus,* are effective against gram-negative bacteria. Polypeptide antibiotics are not absorbed orally and are too toxic for systemic use. Hence, they were earlier not used systemically but were used topically. However, due to emergence of multi-drug resistant microbes, **colistin** has been used systemically (parenterally) in life-threatening infections as a last resort.

Mechanism of action: Polymyxin and colistin alter the permeability of the cell membrane resulting in leakage of the cell contents. They are **bactericidal**.

Systemic colistin causes **nephrotoxicity**, interferes with neuromuscular transmission leading to weakness and apnoea; also can cause paraesthesias, vertigo and dysarthria. Applied topically, polypeptides may rarely cause skin rashes.

Neosporin Powder—POLYMYXIN 5000 u + NEOMYCIN 3400 u + BACITRACIN 400 u, NEOSPORIN eye drops, ear drops.

COLISTIN: GDSAFE 12.5, 25 mg /5 ml syr.

Uses

1. Life-threatning infection: Colistin used as a last resort.
2. Oral colistin is used in children for diarrhoea (not absorbed) due to gram-negative bacilli.
3. Used topically for skin infections, ear and eye infections.

OTHER ANTIMICROBIAL AGENTS

Bacitracin, produced by *Bacillus subtilis,* is effective against gram-positive bacteria. It inhibits the cell wall synthesis and is bactericidal. It is too toxic to be given systemically, not absorbed orally and is, therefore, used only for topical application—in skin infections, surgical wounds, ulcers and ocular infections (Table 49.2).

NEOSPORIN powder-bacitracin + NEOMYCIN.

Sodium fusidate (fusidic acid), obtained from *Fusidium coccineum,* is effective against gram-positive organisms particularly staphylococci. It is bactericidal. It is mainly used topically as a 2% ointment. It may be given orally for resistant staphylococcal infections.

FUCIDIN 2% ointment.

Mupirocin or pseudomonic acid is obtained from *Pseudomonas fluorescens*. It is bactericidal against gram-positive and some gram-negative organisms including MRSA. Mupirocin acts by inhibiting the enzyme tRNA synthetase. It is used as a 2% ointment for minor skin infections particularly due to staphylococci and streptococci. It is also used intranasally as spray to eradicate staphylococcal carrier state.

BACTROBAN-2% w/w cream. MPOWER 2% ointment.

Fosfomycin is an analog of phosphoenol pyruvate. Fosfomycin is effective against both gram-positive and gram-negative organisms. It acts by inhibiting the enzyme endopyruvate transferase. This enzyme is required for the first step in bacterial cell wall synthesis. Thus it inhibits bacterial cell wall synthesis. The salt used is fosfomycin tetrametol which is

Table 49.2: Groups of antimicrobial agents

β-lactam antibiotics	**Quinolones**	**Sulphonamides**	**Macrolides**
• ***Penicillins*** Benzyl penicillin Ampicillin Amoxicillin Methicillin Cloxacillin Nafcillin Carbenicillin Ticarcillin Azlocillin Piperacillin • ***Cephalosporins*** Cephalexin Cephazolin Cefuroxime Cefachlor Ceftriaxone Ceftazidime Cefpirome Cefepime • ***Carbapenems*** Imipenem Meropenem Ertapenem • ***Carbacephem*** Loracarbef • ***Monobactams*** Aztreonam	Nalidixic acid Cinoxacin Oxalinic acid ***Fluoroquinolones*** Ciprofloxacin Sparfloxacin Trovafloxacin Norfloxacin Ofloxacin **Newer agents** • ***Streptogramins*** Quinupristin + Dalfopristin • ***Oxazolidinones*** - Linezolid • ***Lipopeptide*** - Daptomycin	Sulfisoxazole Sulfadiazine Sulfadoxine Sulfacetamide Sulfasalazine **Cotrimoxazole** Trimethoprim + Sulfamethoxazole **Miscellaneous** • ***Glycopeptides*** - Vancomycin - Teicoplanin • ***Lincosamides*** - Clindamycin • ***Polypeptides*** - Polymyxin - Colistin • ***Others*** - Bacitracin - Sodium fusidate - Mupirocin	Erythromycin Roxithromycin Azithromycin Clarithromycin Dirithromycin **Aminoglycosides** Gentamicin Streptomycin Neomycin Amikacin Netilmicin Sisomycin **Broad-spectrum antibiotics** Chloramphenicol Oxytetracycline Tetracycline Demeclocycline Doxycycline Minocycline

available for both oral and parenteral use. It is excreted by the kidneys and attains high concentration in the urine. Fosfomycin is approved for use in uncomplicated lower UTI in women—single 3 g dose is effective.

Dose: 3 g in 100 ml water FOSMICIN 100–200 mg tab. 2–4 g inj.

Cycloserine, obtained from *Streptomyces orchidaceus,* inhibits many gram-positive and gram-negative organisms including *M. tuberculosis*. It acts by inhibiting cell wall synthesis and is used as a second-line drug in tuberculosis.

CYCLOKOX, CYCLORIN, MYSER 250 mg cap.

Nitroimidazoles

Nitroimidazoles include metronidazole, secnidazole, ornidazole and satranidazole. They are very effective in the treatment of anaerobic microorganisms apart from amoebiasis. They are discussed under antiamoebic drugs (*see* page 645).

Newer Agents

Most of the possible sites in the bacteria have been targetted and, therefore, we now have very few newly introduced antibacterial agents. **Streptogramins, linezolid, daptomycin and fidoxomicin** are the recently introduced antimicrobials.

Streptogramins

Quinupristin and dalfopristin are (also called pristinamycin) obtained from *Streptomyces pristinaspiralis*. A combination of **quinupristin** (streptogramin B) and **dalfopristin** (streptogramin A) in the ratio 30:70 is bactericidal against gram-positive cocci including methicillin-resistant staphylococci.

Mechanism of action: Streptogramins bind to 50S ribosomal subunit and inhibit protein synthesis.

Pharmacokinetics: Streptogramins are not effective orally as they are rapidly metabolised in the liver—undergo extensive first pass metabolism. Given intravenously, streptogramins are rapidly metabolised and t½ 0.85 and 0.7 hr and are excreted largely through faeces. Hence adjustment of dose is not required in renal insufficiency but in hepatic failure dose should be reduced. Streptogramins inhibit the microsomal enzyme CYP3A4 which also metabolizes several other drugs. The dose of cyclosporine should be reduced.

Dose: 7.5 mg/kg every 8–12 hr.

Adverse effects: Adverse effects include arthralgia, myalgia, nausea, vomiting, diarrhoea and pain at the site of injection.

Uses: The combination is used intravenously in the treatment of infections due to streptococci, methicillin-resistant staphylococci, enterococci and vancomycin-resistant *E. faecium.*

Oxazolidinones

Linezolid is an oxazolidinone effective against gram-positive bacteria including methicillin-resistant staphylococci, gram-positive anaerobic organisms and tubercle bacillus. It acts by **inhibiting protein synthesis on binding to 50S ribosomes**. Linezolid binds to the 23S ribosomal RNA of the 50S subunit and prevents initiation of protein synthesis—the first step in protein synthesis. Though a bacteriostatic agent, linezolid is bactericidal against streptococci.

An advantage with linezolid is its good oral bioavailability—**completely (100%) absorbed**; food does not interfere with its absorption. It is widely distributed and has a t½ of 4–6 hr. In patients undergoing haemodialysis, linezolid should be given after dialysis because it can be excreted through dialysis. It can be given oral or IV.

Mnemonic for Salient features of Linezolid

LINES(Z)OLID Dose 600 mg CAPS

L—Linezolid
I—Inhibits protein synthesis (23S)
N—Nocardiosis, nosocomial pneumonia
E—*E. faecium* inf
S—Serotonin syndrome
O—Oral absorption 100%
L—Lactic acidosis
I—Inhibits MAO → cheese reaction
D—Diarrhoea
D—Dizziness

600—Dose
Mg—MDR TB, Myelosuppression
CAP—Community acquired pneumonia
S—SSSI, Septicemia

Dose: 600 mg BD. LIZOLID 600 mg cap. LINOX 600 mg tab, 200 mg inj.

Adverse effects include nausea, diarrhoea, dizziness and on prolonged use of >2 weeks can cause myelosuppression with **thrombocytopenia** (which is reversible), anaemia and neutropenia; peripheral neuropathy and lactic acidosis. **Cheese reaction**—linezolid is an MAO inhibitor and can cause **serotonin syndrome** with other drugs that increase serotonin levels or with tyramine-rich food.

Uses

1. Nosocomial pneumonia by *S. aureus* including MRSA—linezolid is effective; dose 600 mg BD–IV or oral.
2. Community acquired pneumonia—due to *S. pneumoniae* responds.
3. Skin and skin structure infections and septicaemia due to *Streptococcus* and *Staphylococcus*–400 mg BD.
4. *Vancomycin*-resistant *E. faecium* infections. The use of linezolid should be restricted to infections due to multi-drug-resistant gram-positive bacteria.

5. MDR tuberculosis with other drugs (*see* page 599)
6. Nocardiosis: As an alternative.

Tedizolid: Another oxazolidinone under development is similar to linezolid but longer acting (once daily dose) and has better efficacy against staphylococci.

Daptomycin

Daptomycin is a lipopeptide obtained from *Streptomyces roseosporus*. It is bactericidal for most susceptible microorganisms and multi-drug-resistant streptococci. Daptomycin appears to have a unique mechanism of action. It binds to the cell membrane, forms channels and depolarises the membrane. This results in K^+ efflux (and loss of membrane potential) which leads to outward movement of potassium ions resulting in rapid cell death. Daptomycin is thus bactericidal. It is synergistic with gentamicin.

Antibacterial spectrum is effective against aerobic gram-positive microorganisms including methicillin and vancomycin-resistant staphylococci and also against anaerobes.

Because absorption on oral administration is poor, daptomycin is given IV. It is **not** given intramuscularly as it causes direct toxicity to the muscle. Daptomycin can cause myopathy, peripheral neuropathy, headache, insomnia, dizziness, jaundice and GI disturbances. **It should not be used to treat pneumonia** because surfactant in the lungs antagonises the effects of daptomycin.

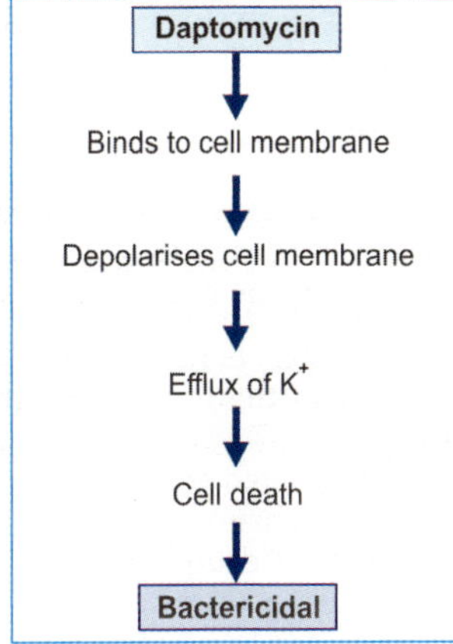

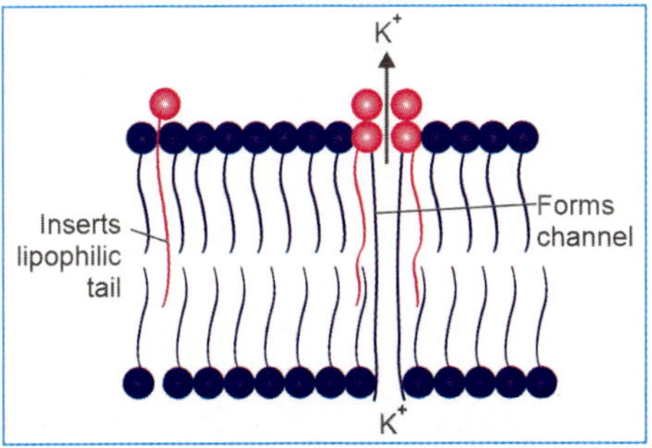

Fig. 49.2: Mechanism of action of daptomycin. It forms channels in the cell membrane, depolarises it and the K^+ efflux occurs through the channel

Uses

Daptomycin is used in complicated skin and soft tissue infections. It may be used as an alternative to vancomycin.

Dose: 4–6 mg/kg/day.

Fidaxomicin is a narrow spectrum antibiotic effective against gram-positive bacteria. It binds to RNA polymerase and inhibits protein synthesis. Given orally, it is poorly absorbed and is effective in the treatment of colitis due to *C. difficile*. Dose: 200 mg BD.

DRUGS USED IN THE TREATMENT OF SEXUALLY TRANSMITTED DISEASES

Competency achievement: The student should be able to:

PH 1.48 Describe the mechanisms of action, types, doses, side effects, indications and contraindications of the drugs used in UTI/STD and viral diseases including HIV.[1]

There has been an increase in the prevalence of sexually transmitted diseases (STD) in the recent times with changes in social outlook and practices throughout the world. Drugs used in the treatment of STDs have all been described in the respective chapters. Some of them have been summarised in Table 49.3.

Table 49.3: Drugs used in some common sexually transmitted diseases

STD	*Treatment*	*Alternative*
1. Syphilis	PP 6L units IM daily × 10 days B. Penicillin 2.4 MU IM single dose	Doxycycline 100 mg BD × 15 days Erythromycin 500 mg QID × 15 days
2. Gonorrhoea		
a. Uncomplicated	Ciprofloxacin 500 mg oral single dose Ceftriaxone 250 mg IM single dose Cefixime 400 mg oral single dose	Levofloxacin 250 mg oral single dose Spectinomycin 2 g IM single dose Cotrimoxazole 2 tab BD × 5 days
b. Complicated	Ofloxacin 400 mg BD × 14 days + Clindamycin 450 mg QID × 14 days	PP 2MU IM × 10 days + Doxy 100 mg BD × 14 days
3. Lymphogranuloma venereum	Doxycycline 100 mg BD, oral × 21 days Azithromycin 1 g oral single dose	Tetracycline 500 mg QID × 21 days
4. Chancroid	Azithromycin 1g oral single dose Erythromycin 500 mg QID × 7–10 days Ceftriaxone 250 mg IM single dose	Ciprofloxacin 500 mg BD × 3 days Cotrimoxazole 2 BD for 7 days
5. Granuloma inguinale	Doxycycline 100 mg BD × 3–4 wks Azithromycin 1 g once a wk × 4 wks	Cotrimoxazole 2 BD × 3–4 wks
6. Trichomoniasis	Metronidazole 2 g oral single dose	Secnidazole 2 g single dose

PP: Procaine penicillin B. Penicillin: Benzathine penicillin L: Lakhs Doxy: Doxycycline

Treatment of AIDS, and Herpes the viral STDs is described in Chapter 52.

Chemoprophylaxis

For the post-exposure prophylaxis of syphilis and gonorrhoea, penicillin 4–8 MU IM into the gluteal region is effective. Alternatively, doxycycline 100 mg BD for 15 days can be used for the prophylaxis of gonorrhoea, syphilis, granuloma inguinale, LGV and chancroid.

Clinical Pharmacology

- Azithromycin is often the preferred macrolide because of advantages of long action and good penetrability into tissue but it is expensive.

Linezolid

- Linezolid dose reduction is not required in renal dysfunction.
- Should be administered after dialysis as it can be excreted in the dialysate.
- Reserved for multidrug-resistant gram +ve bacteria.
- 100% bioavailability—hence same oral and IV dose.

Vancomycin

- Vancomycin—dose should be reduced in renal failure.

CHAPTER 50

Chemotherapy of Tuberculosis and Leprosy

Competency achievement: The student should be able to:

PH 1.44 Describe the first line antitubercular drugs, their mechanisms of action, side effects and doses.[1]

PH 1.45 Describe the drugs used in MDR and XDR tuberculosis.[2]

Tuberculosis (TB) is a chronic granulomatous disease caused by *Mycobacterium tuberculosis.* In developing countries, it is a major public health problem. India has the highest number of TB cases in the world. Tuberculosis is also an enormous socioeconomic burden to India with one-fifth of global TB burden borne by India alone, accounting for ~1000 deaths every day. Though the disease burden in terms of incidence, prevalence and mortality is reduced, it is yet a major public health problem in India. After the spread of AIDS, the problem has become more complex, as tuberculosis and *Mycobacterium avium complex* (MAC) infections are not only more common but also rapidly progress in these patients.

DRUGS USED IN TUBERCULOSIS

	Antitubercular drugs	
	Bactericidal	**Bacteriostatic**
First-line drugs	Isoniazid Rifampicin Pyrazinamide Streptomycin	Ethambutol
Second-line drugs	Levofloxacin Moxifloxacin Bedaquiline Delamanid Kanamycin Capreomycin Amikacin Imipenem-cilastatin Meropenem	Linezolid Ethionamide Prothionamide Cycloserine Terizidone Clofazimine Para-aminosalicylic acid

FIRST-LINE DRUGS

First-line drugs are superior in efficacy to second-line drugs. Most patients can be treated successfully with these drugs.

Isoniazid (INH)

It is the most effective and cheapest primary antitubercular drug. It is effective both in acidic and alkaline medium. INH is tuberculocidal for rapidly multiplying bacilli but static for resting bacilli. INH destroys:

i. Intracellular bacilli as it freely penetrates into the cells, i.e. tubercle bacilli in macrophages, and
ii. Bacilli multiplying in the walls of the cavities. Thus it is effective against **both intra- and extracellular organisms** (Fig. 50.1 and Table 50.1).

If used alone, mycobacteria develop resistance to it. Hence, it should be used in combination with other drugs.

Mechanism of Action

INH inhibits the synthesis of mycolic acids which are important components of the mycobacterial cell wall. The cell wall of mycobacteria differs from other bacteria in having large amounts of mycolic acids which form essential components of mycobacterial cell wall. INH, a prodrug, freely enters the mycobacteria and is converted to an active form by an enzyme catalase-peroxidase (Kat G) present in the mycobacteria. This active form covalently binds certain enzymes and thereby **inhibits mycolic acid synthesis**.

Resistance to INH is seen when there is over production of the enzymes that are inhibited by INH. Mutations of *inhA* and *Kat G* enzymes also result in resistance.

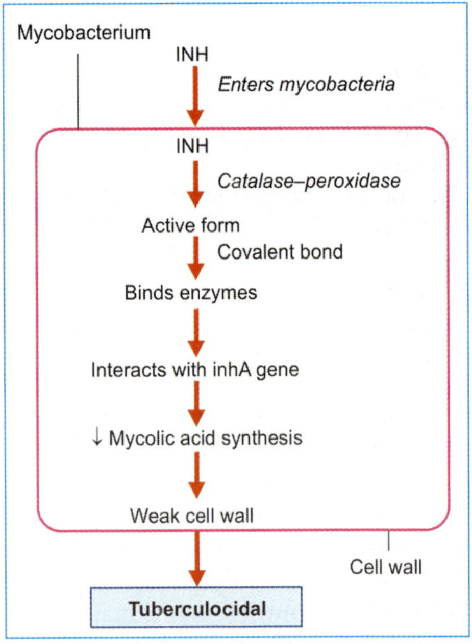

Fig. 50.1: Sites of action of antitubercular drugs

Pharmacokinetics

INH is **completely absorbed** orally, penetrates all tissues, tubercular cavities, ascitic fluid, necrotic tissues, caseous material and CSF. It is metabolised by acetylation and this is genetically determined. Patients can be **fast or slow acetylators** depending on the genetic inheritance—slow acetylators responding better. The t½ in slow acetylators is 3–5 hours while in fast acetylators it is 1 hour. Peripheral neuropathy is more common in slow acetylators while hepatotoxicity is more likely in fast acetylators. If INH is given once weekly in fast acetylators, adequate therapeutic concentrations may not be attained. Metabolites of INH are excreted in the urine (Table 50.2).

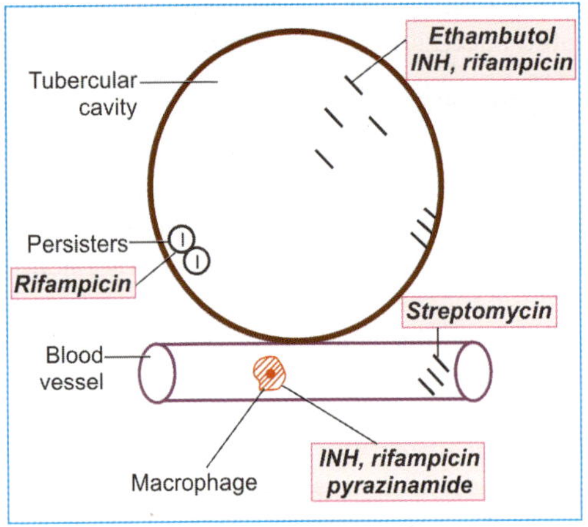

Table 50.1: Antitubercular actions and characteristic adverse effects of some antitubercular drugs

Drug	*Antitubercular action*	*Serious toxicity*
Isoniazid	Tuberculocidal; acts on intra- and extracellular organisms	Peripheral neuritis, hepatitis, seizures, psychosis
Rifampicin	Tuberculocidal; acts on intra- and extracellular organisms, persisters and drug resistant organisms	Hepatotoxicity, flu-like syndrome, nephritis; urine and secretions are coloured orange-red
Pyrazinamide	Tuberculocidal; kills intracellular organisms; more active in acidic pH	Hepatotoxicity, arthralgia, hyperuricaemia
Streptomycin	Tuberculocidal; acts on extracellular organisms	Ototoxicity, nephrotoxicity
Ethambutol	Tuberculostatic; inhibits tubercle bacilli in the walls of cavities	Optic neuritis with ↓ visual acuity and red-green colour blindness
Bedaquiline	Tuberculocidal; inhibits mycobacterial ATP synthase and interferes with generation of energy	QTc prolongation, hepatotoxicity, arthralgia

Adverse Effects

Peripheral neuritis due to interference with utilization and increased excretion of pyridoxine can be avoided by giving prophylactic **pyridoxine** (10–50 mg) with INH. However, it is uncommon with therapeutic doses and is seen in higher doses with an incidence of 10–20% and in patients with comorbid conditions like AIDS, diabetes and malnutrition.

Hepatitis is another major adverse effect, more common in alcoholics and in the elderly. If hepatitis is mild, INH may be continued, but in a small percentage of patients, INH can cause hepatic necrosis with anorexia, nausea, vomiting and jaundice—can sometimes be fatal. In such patients with the first signs of hepatic necrosis, INH should be withdrawn.

INH can cause **CNS toxicity** including psychosis and seizures but is less common—epileptics are more prone to this effect and pyridoxine helps these patients. Other minor effects like anorexia, gastrointestinal discomfort, fever and allergic reactions can occur. Haemolysis can occur in patients with G6PD deficiency.

Mnemonic on INH Salient Features

Pulmonologist Cleverly Prevented INH MISHAP

Pulmonologist—peripheral neuritis
Cleverly—CNS toxicity; Completely absorbed
Prevented—pyridoxine
INH
Mycolic acid synth inhibition
Intra- and extracellular organisms (acts on)
Seizures
Hepatitis
Acetylation—fast and slow
Psychosis

Rifampicin

Rifampicin (rifampin) is a semisynthetic derivative of rifamycin, an antibiotic obtained from *Streptomyces mediterranei*. The other rifamycins are rifabutin and rifapentine. Rifampicin is bactericidal to *M. tuberculosis*, *M. leprae* and atypical mycobacteria. It also inhibits most gram-positive and gram-negative bacteria like *Staph. aureus*, *N. meningitidis*, *E. coli*, *Proteus*, *Pseudomonas* and *Legionella*.

Table 50.2: Anti-TB drugs and their dosages as per weight band

S.No.	Drugs	16–29 kg	30–45 kg	46–70 kg	>70 kg
1.	Rifampicin (R)	300 mg	450 mg	600 mg	600 mg
2.	INH (H)	300 mg	600 mg	900 mg	900 mg
3.	Ethambutol	400 mg	800 mg	1200 mg	1600 mg
4.	Pyrazinamide (Z)	750 mg	1250 mg	1750 mg	2000 mg
5.	Kanamycin (Km)	500 mg	750 mg	750 mg	1000 mg
6.	Capreomycin (Cm)	500 mg	750 mg	750 mg	1000 mg
7.	Amikacin (Am)	500 mg	750 mg	750 mg	1000 mg
8.	Levofloxacin (Lfx)	250 mg	750 mg	1000 mg	1000 mg
9.	Moxifloxacin (Mfx)	200 mg	400 mg	400 mg	400 mg
10.	Ethionamide (Eto)	375 mg	500 mg	750 mg	1000 mg
11.	Cycloserine (Cs)	250 mg	500 mg	750 mg	1000 mg
12.	PAS	10 g	14 g	16 g	22 g
13.	Pyridoxine (Pdx)	50mg	100 mg	100 mg	100 mg
14.	Clofazimine (Cfz)	50 mg	100 mg	100 mg	200 mg
15.	Linezolid (Lzd)	300 mg	600 mg	600 mg	600 mg
16.	Amoxyclav (Amx/Clv)	875/125 mg BD	875/125 mg	875/125 mg	875/125 mg
17.	Bedaquiline	Week 0–2: 400 mg daily Week 3–24: 200 mg 3 times per week			

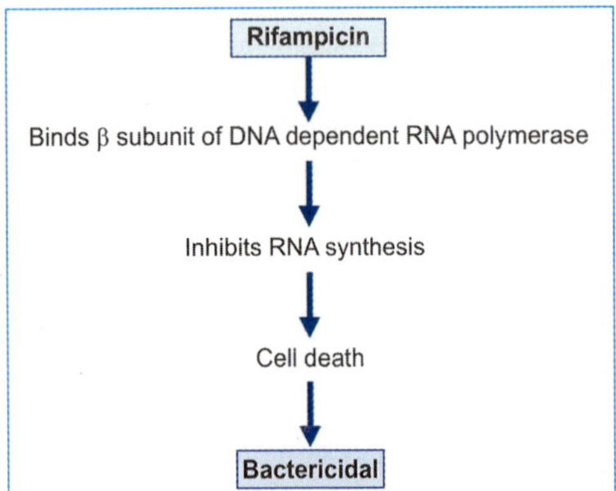

Antitubercular Action

Rifampicin is highly effective, tuberculocidal and is the only drug that acts on persisters; acts on both intra- and extracellular organisms and is effective against tubercle bacilli resistant to other drugs—it is called a **'sterilizing agent'**. If used alone resistance develops.

Mechanism of Action

Rifampicin binds to the β subunit of the DNA-dependent RNA polymerase and inhibits RNA synthesis in the bacteria. It is bactericidal. In therapeutic concentrations, rifampicin cannot bind human RNA polymerase and it, therefore, selectively destroys the bacteria. Moreover, it reaches the cavities, caseous material and penetrates macrophages.

Resistance due to genetic mutation in DNA and RNA polymerase results in reduced binding of rifampicin to RNA polymerase.

Pharmacokinetics

Rifampicin is well-absorbed and has **good tissue penetrability**—reaches caseous material, cavities and macrophages. Good CSF concentrations are reached in presence of meningitis. It also appears in saliva, tears and sweat. It is metabolised in the liver. It is a **microsomal enzyme inducer**—hence can result in many drug interactions. Rifampicin is excreted through the bile and undergoes enterohepatic circulation.

Adverse Effects

1. *Hepatotoxicity:* Rifampicin can cause hepatitis. Patients receiving other hepatotoxic drugs or those with any liver dysfunction and chronic alcoholics should be carefully monitored—deaths have been reported in such patients. However, in patients with normal liver function, hepatitis is rare.
2. *Gastrointestinal disturbances:* Epigastric distress, nausea, vomiting, abdominal cramps and diarrhoea can occur.
3. *Flu-like syndrome:* Characterised by fever, bodyache, chills and haemolytic anaemia is more common in **intermittent dosing** regimen.
4. *CNS symptoms:* Including headache, drowsiness, dizziness, ataxia, confusion and peripheral neuropathy with pain and numbness in the extremities and muscle weakness have been reported.
5. *Hypersensitivity reactions:* With fever, skin rashes and urticaria, rarely renal manifestations with nephritis, haemolysis, haematuria and renal insufficiency can occur.
6. *Staining of secretions:* Rifampicin stains the secretions including tears, saliva and sweat—an orange red colour and the patient should be informed about this. Soft contact lens may also be stained.

Drug Interactions

1. Aminosalicylic acid may delay the absorption and reduce the bioavailability of rifampicin. When both are needed in a patient, there should be a gap of 8–12 hours between them.
2. Rifampicin is a **microsomal enzyme inducer.** It hastens the metabolism of many drugs including anticoagulants, hormonal contraceptives, corticosteroids, ketoconazole, cyclosporine, some anticonvulsants, antiretroviral protease inhibitors and NNRTIs. Oral contraceptive failures can be expected—a preparation with higher doses of oestrogen should be used or alternative methods of contraception followed.

Uses

1. *Tuberculosis and atypical mycobacterial infections:* Rifampicin is given in combination with other antitubercular drugs—in both TB and atypical myobacterial infections. It can also be used for the prophylaxis as an alternative to INH.
2. *Leprosy* 600 mg once monthly supervised (*see* page 602).
3. *Prophylaxis: H. influenzae* and meningococcal meningitis in close contacts particularly children—20 mg/kg/day for 4 days.
4. *Resistant staphylococcal infections:* Rifampicin may be given in combination with a beta lactam antibiotic or vancomycin.
5. *Brucellosis:* Rifampicin 600–900 mg + doxycycline 200 mg daily for 6 weeks—drug of choice.
6. *Pneumococcal meningitis:* If pneumococci are resistant to penicillin, they can be treated with rifampicin + ceftriaxone.
7. *To eradicate carrier state:* Rifampicin eradicates the nasal carrier state of *N. meningitidis, H. influenzae* and *S. aureus*—600 mg BD for 2 days.

Rifabutin: It is similar to rifampicin except that it causes milder enzyme induction and is more active against atypical mycobacteria. Rifabutin may be used in place of rifampicin in tuberculosis patients with AIDS who are receiving antiretroviral drugs, *viz.* protease inhibitors (PIs) and NNRTIs. Since these antiviral drugs are also metabolised by microsomal enzymes and rifampicin being a powerful enzyme inducer, concurrent use can result in many drug interactions. Rifabutin is a better choice in such patients. Adverse effects to rifabutin include myalgia and anterior uveitis.

Uses: Rifabutin can be used in tuberculosis and atypical mycobacterial infections for chemoprophylaxis.

Dose: 300 mg/day.

In patients receiving protease inhibitors—150 mg/day in patients receiving NNRTIs—450 mg/day.

Mnemonic for salient features of rifampicin

RIFAMPICIN TABLETS Given in PHC

R—Resistant *Staph aureas*
I—Intracellular and extracellular bacilli killed
F—Flu like symptoms (ADR)
A—Avoid in alcoholics
M—Microsomal enzyme inducer
P—Prophylaxis of *H. influenzae*
I—Inhibits RNA synthesis
N—Neuropathy

T—TB
A—Atypical TB
B—Brucellosis
L—Leprosy
E—Eradicate carrier state
T—Tissue penetrability good
S—Staining of secretions

Given in—GI disturbances

P—Pneumococcal meningitis
H—Hypersensitivity reactions
C—CNS symptoms

Rifapentine is an analog of rifampicin and is similar to it in mechanism of action, actions, drug interactions and toxicity. Rifapentine 600 mg once weekly may be used in tuberculosis in place of rifampicin. It should, however, be avoided in AIDS patients because of the risk of development of resistance.

Pyrazinamide

Pyrazinamide, an analog of nicotinamide, was introduced in 1952.

Mechanism of Action

It is tuberculocidal. It requires an acidic pH (5.5) for its tuberculocidal activity. This is in fact advantageous because tubercle bacilli reside in the phagosomes of the macrophages where the pH is acidic. Mechanism of action is not exactly known. Pyrazinamide is converted to its active metabolite pyrazinoic acid by an enzyme pyrazinamidase present in the mycobacteria. This metabolite may inhibit the synthesis of mycolic acids by the mycobacteria. If used alone, resistance develops.

Pyrazinamide is well-absorbed and widely distributed in the tissues (achieves good concentration in the CSF).

Hepatotoxicity is the most common adverse effect. It is dose dependent—can result initially in raised serum transaminases and later jaundice and rarely hepatic necrosis. Deaths due to hepatic necrosis have been reported. Liver function tests should be done before starting pyrazinamide and it should be avoided in patients with hepatic impairment. Patient should be monitored for signs and symptoms of hepatotoxicity and if present, pyrazinamide should be stopped. **Hyperuricaemia** due to decreased excretion of uric acid may result in gouty arthritis; other effects like arthralgia, anorexia, vomiting, fever and rashes may be seen.

Streptomycin

Streptomycin is tuberculocidal, acts only against extracellular organisms due to poor penetrating power. It has to be given IM. When used alone resistance develops. Because of these disadvantages and its toxicity (oto- and nephrotoxicity), streptomycin is the least preferred of the first-line drugs.

Ethambutol

Ethambutol is tuberculostatic and acts on fast multiplying bacilli in the cavities. It is also effective against atypical mycobacteria. It inhibits the incorporation of mycolic acids into the mycobacterial cell wall by inhibiting certain enzymes (arabinosyltransferases) involved in it.

Ethambutol is well absorbed on oral administration (bioavailability ~80%). It crosses the BBB in presence of meningeal inflammation. Half the dose is excreted through the kidneys and the dose should be reduced in renal failure.

Optic neuritis resulting in decreased visual acuity and inability to differentiate red from green is an important adverse effect which needs withdrawal of the drug. Colour vision should be monitored during treatment. Ethambutol is to be avoided in children because their ability to differentiate red from green cannot be reliably tested. Other adverse effects include nausea, anorexia, headache, fever and allergic reactions.

Ethambutol decreases the renal excretion of uric acid and thereby enhances plasma urate levels.

SECOND-LINE DRUGS

Second-line drugs are generally less effective and more toxic when compared to first-line drugs. They are used only if the organism is resistant to first-line drugs.

Bedaquiline a newly introduced antibacterial is a diarylquinoline.

Mechanism of action: Bedaquiline has a unique mechanism of action. It binds to and inhibits mycobacterial ATP synthase and thereby interferes with the generation of energy. It is tuberculocidal.

Fatty food increases its bioavailability, is extensively bound to plasma proteins and is metabolized by microsomal enzymes (cytochrome P450). Co-administration of other microsomal enzyme inducers like rifampicin and also enzyme inhibitors should be avoided.

Adverse effects: Since bedaquiline can cause QTc prolongation, other drugs that prolong QTc should be avoided along with it. Hepatotoxicity, nausea, arthralgia and headache are reported.

Bedaquiline may be used in the treatment of MDR tuberculosis in combination with other antitubercular drugs.

Dose: 400 mg OD for 2 weeks increased to 200 mg TDS for 22 weeks with food.

Delamanid is a nitroimidazole recently approved for the treatment of tuberculosis. It acts by inhibiting the synthesis of mycolic acid, an important component of mycobacterial cell wall. Presence of food improves absorption and is therefore taken with food. It is approved for MDR TB in adults and adolescents (6–17 yr). Dose: 100 mg orally twice a day for 24 weeks.

Thiacetazone is tuberculostatic with low efficacy; it delays the development of resistance to other drugs and its low cost makes it a suitable drug in combination regimens. Hepatotoxicity, dermatitis, allergic reactions and GI side effects may occur.

Ethionamide and Prothionamide: These tuberculostatic drugs are effective against both intra- and extracellular organisms. They are also effective in atypical mycobacteria.

Anorexia, nausea, vomiting and metallic taste in the mouth are the most common adverse effects. They can also cause hepatitis, skin rashes and peripheral neuritis (needs prophylactic pyridoxine).

Para-aminosalicylic acid (PAS) related to sulfonamides is tuberculostatic. Gastrointestinal effects like nausea, anorexia, epigastric pain and diarrhoea make it a poorly tolerated drug. Allergic reactions and hepatitis are also seen. It is rarely used.

Amikacin, kanamycin and capreomycin need parenteral administration and are oto- and nephrotoxic. Amikacin has good antitubercular activity and is also effective against atypical mycobacteria. The other two are not preferred.

Cycloserine is an antibiotic that inhibits cell wall synthesis, is tuberculostatic and is also effective against some gram +ve organisms. It causes CNS toxicity including headache, tremors, psychosis and sometimes seizures. It is used only in resistant tuberculosis.

Fluoroquinolones inhibit tubercle bacilli as well as atypical mycobacteria in addition to gram-positive and gram-negative bacteria. They enter into the cells and destroy intracellular mycobacteria. Levofloxacin and Moxifloxacin are the FQs used in tuberculosis resistant to first-line drugs.

Fluoroquinolones have been used along with second-line drugs in multidrug-resistant TB.

Linezolid. Its penetrability into cells is good and is lethal to intracellular bacilli. It can be used in a single daily dose of 600 mg along with second-line drugs.

TREATMENT OF TUBERCULOSIS

Tuberculosis is one of the most difficult infections to cure. The properties of the mycobacteria like slow division, development of resistance, ability to remain as persisters for years and intracellular location of the bacilli have enhanced the problem. Moreover, the caseous material makes it difficult for the drugs to reach. The need for long-term treatment, drug toxicity, cost and thereby poor patient compliance have all added to further complicate the problem. However, with the availability of effective drugs, most patients can now be treated as outpatients.

The aim of treatment is to kill the dividing bacilli thus making the patient sputum negative and to destroy the persisters in order to prevent relapse and ensure complete cure.

A combination of drugs is used in tuberculosis to:

1. Delay the development of resistance
2. Reduce toxicity
3. Shorten the course of treatment.

Majority of cases are sensitive to first-line drugs. Initial treatment should be intensive and include drugs that have maximum effect. Good patient compliance and cost of therapy should also be considered.

Chemotherapy is given in two phases:

1. *Intensive phase* is the first phase of 1–3 months duration aimed at killing as many bacilli as possible.
2. Continuation phase is second phase to destroy the dormant or persisters—duration 4–9 months.

Table 50.3: Treatment categories of tuberculosis as per NTEP recommendation

Type of patient	*Regimen*	
	Intensive phase (IP)	*Continuation phase (CP)***
New/Previously treated*	8 wk 2HRZE (56 doses)	16 wk 4HRE (112 doses)

**Should be evaluated for DRTB. H: INH, R: Rifampicin, Z: Pyrazinamide, E: Ethambutol. ** CP extended by 12–24 wks more for CNS, skeletal and disseminated TB if required.*

The treatment should be constantly monitored (Table 50.3).

Directly Observed Treatment, Short Course (DOTS) Chemotherapy

Though many effective antitubercular drugs are available, the success of chemotherapy depends on regular intake of appropriate drugs by the patients. Directly Observed Treatment, Short Course (DOTS) chemotherapy is a strategy that is found to be effective and is recommended throughout the world. DOTS was launched in 1997 and is the fastest expanding health programme in India. It involves providing most effective medicine and confirming that it is taken—a DOTS provider ensures that the drug is taken by the patient in his presence.

RNTCP and NTEP

The Government of India along with WHO and World Bank reviewed national TB programme and revised the strategy as Revised National Tuberculosis Control Programme (RNTCP) which was introduced in 1993. After launching the RNTCP programme, the death rate has been reduced from 29 to 4% in smear-positive cases. The revised program (2016) in now being implemented throughout the country (Table 50.4). The RNTCP has revised the treatment schedule in 2016 with 2 major changes—(i) introduction of daily dose regimen and (ii) supply of fixed dose combinations (FDC). The program also takes the help of information technology to monitor the regular intake of tablets, i.e. to ensure better patient compliance. Under the RNTCP program, antitubercular drugs are available as 4-drug FDC and 3-drug FDC. A single tablet of 4 FDC contains isoniazid 75 mg, rifampicin 150 mg, pyrazinamide 400 mg and ethambutol 275 mg. The number of tablets to be taken daily depends on the patient's body weight. From 2020, RNTCP is changed to **National TB elimination program** (NTEP) with an aim of tuberculosis elimination in the country and the program is being implemented throughout the country.

Table 50.3a: Daily dose schedule for adults (as per NTEP weight bands)

Weight band	*Number of tablets*	
	Intensive phase HRZE (4FDC)	*Continuation phase HRE (3FDC)*
	75/150/400/275 mg	*75/150/275 mg*
25–34 kg	2	2
35–49 kg	3	3
50–64 kg	4	4
65–74 kg	5	5
≥75*kg	6	6

Resistant Tuberculosis

If sputum remains positive even after 6 months of treatment, organisms are likely to be resistant. Such patients should be treated with 4–5 drugs, of which 3 are first-line drugs and treatment is continued for at least 1 year after the sputum becomes negative.

Resistance may be to one or multiple drugs. As per WHO, a **multidrug-resistant (MDR)** strain is one that is at least resistant to isoniazid and rifampicin. **Extensively drug-resistant tuberculosis (XDR-TB)** is resistant to almost all second-line drugs like FQs, amikacin, capreomycin and kanamycin. Resistance could develop due to inadequate treatment, irregular supply of drugs or poor compliance. Impaired host defence as in AIDS patients also contributes to resistance. Resistant cases are more difficult to treat and require more vigorous and longer periods of treatment. If the sensitivity of the bacilli is known, effective drugs may be used. The patient should be hospitalized or isolated to prevent spread of resistant strains to others including health care workers.

End TB Strategy

In 2015, End TB strategy has been launched to end the global TB epidemic. The aim is to reduce TB incidence by 95% and TB deaths by 90% by 2035 as compared to 2015.

Role of Glucocorticoids

As glucocorticoids depress host defense mechanisms, they should be used only in conditions like tubercular meningitis, miliary tuberculosis, pleural effusion, renal tuberculosis and rapidly progressing pulmonary tuberculosis. In these conditions, steroids suppress inflammatory reaction which can lead to extensive fibrosis and damage.

Chemoprophylaxis is given only in:

i. Contacts of open cases especially children. INH is used daily (5 mg/kg) for 6–12 months. Rifampicin can be used as an alternative to INH.
ii. HIV-infected patients exposed to multi-drug-resistant tuberculosis—rifampicin and pyrazinamide are given daily for 2 months.

Tuberculosis in AIDS Patients

Due to depressed immunity, AIDS patients are at a higher risk (25–30 times) of contracting tuberculosis. AIDS patients are likely to have more severe and rapidly progressing tuberculosis. Moreover, adverse effects to antitubercular drugs are more common in them. They should be given more vigorous and supervised chemotherapy as per the guidelines. Antiretroviral therapy has to be started within 2–8 weeks of starting anti-TB treatment. If a TB patient who has been on treatment is diagnosed to be having HIV infection **2 HRZES + 1 HRZE + 5 HRE regimen** is recommended.

Drugs for *Mycobacterium avium* Complex (MAC)

Infection with MAC is more common in HIV patients and is more severe in them. With the use of prophylactic regimens, the incidence of MAC infections has greatly decreased. In non-HIV patients, MAC infection causes milder disease with chronic productive cough.

The drugs effective are:

- Rifabutin, clarithromycin
- Azithromycin, fluoroquinolones
- Ethambutol, clofazimine
- Amikacin, ethionamide.

The **macrolides,** clarithromycin and azithromycin, are highly effective, and are the first choice drugs in MAC therapy. Clarithromycin (500 mg twice a day) or azithromycin (500 mg once daily) with ethambutol is the preferred regimen (rifabutin may be added) for MAC infection and needs lifelong treatment. **Fluoroquinolones,** like ciprofloxacin, ofloxacin and sparfloxacin, have useful activity against *M. tuberculosis* and MAC bacteria. Ciprofloxacin 1500 mg in two or three divided doses is used in combination therapy in HIV patients with MAC infections (4 drug regimen with ciprofloxacin + clarithromycin + rifabutin + amikacin). Rifabutin, clarithromycin or azithromycin may be used for prophylaxis.

DRUGS USED IN THE TREATMENT OF LEPROSY

Competency achievement: The student should be able to:
PH 1.46 Describe the mechanisms of action, types, doses, side effects, indications and contraindications of antileprotic drugs.[3]

Leprosy caused by *Mycobacterium leprae* is a chronic infectious disease affecting skin, mucous membranes and nerves. Hansen discovered lepra bacillus in 1873. As lepra bacillus does not grow on artificial media and cannot be transmitted to all animals, it is difficult to culture this organism and study the effect of drugs.

In India, leprosy is a major public health problem affecting millions of people.

Drugs used in Leprosy

- Sulfones: Dapsone
- Rifampicin
- Clofazimine
- Ethionamide and protionamide.

Dapsone

Dapsone is diaminodiphenylsulfone (DDS) and is related to sulfonamides.

Mechanism of Action

Like sulfonamides, dapsone inhibits the incorporation of para-amino benzoic acid (PABA) into folic acid. The lepra bacillus develops resistance to dapsone on prolonged use. Hence, it should be used with other drugs in leprosy. It is also well distributed to other tissue fluids.

PABA
↓ ⇠⊖ Dapsone
Folic acid

Actions

Dapsone is leprostatic. Though it inhibits the growth of many other bacteria, the dose needed is high and is, therefore, not used.

Dapsone is completely absorbed on oral administration and reaches high concentrations in the skin. It attains higher levels in the skin infected with lepra bacillus than the normal skin. It is metabolised in the liver and excreted in the bile.

Adverse Effects

Dapsone is well-tolerated—anorexia, nausea and vomiting are common. Fever, pruritus, rashes and dermatitis can occur. Haemolytic anaemia is the most important dose-related toxicity (more common in patients with G6PD deficiency). Iron preparations should be given to prevent anaemia. Hepatitis and agranulocytosis are seen. Patients with lepromatous leprosy may develop lepra reactions.

Uses

1. *Leprosy:* Dapsone is the primary drug in leprosy (*see* below) used for both treatment and chemoprophylaxis.
2. *P. jiroveci:* Dapsone is used along with trimethoprim as an alternative in *P. jiroveci* infections in patients with AIDS—both for the prevention and treatment.

   Dose: Dapsone 100 mg + Trimethoprim 15–20 mg/kg/day for 3 weeks. Prophylaxis: Dapsone 100 mg/daily.

Clinical Pharmacology

- Resistance develops to all antitubercular drugs, if used as monotherapy—hence all antitubercular drugs should be used only in combination regimens.
- Most first-line drugs cause hepatotoxicity and liver function should be watched for.
- Patient should be convinced about the importance of compliance.
- In India, antitubercular drugs are supplied by the government.

3. *Dermatitis herpetiformis,* a chronic blistering skin disease seen in patients with coeliac disease, can be treated with gradually increasing dose of dapsone 50–300 mg/day.

Rifampicin is rapidly bactericidal to *M. leprae* and is highly effective—a single dose of 1500 mg can kill 99% of the lepra bacilli. It can be conveniently given once monthly. Used in combination with dapsone, it shortens the duration of treatment. Given alone—resistance develops. Rifampicin is now an important drug in multidrug regimens for leprosy.

Clofazimine a dye, has weak bactericidal actions against *M. leprae.* It also has anti-inflammatory property which is useful in suppressing lepra reactions. It is used orally in multi-drug regimens.

Clofazimine imparts a reddish-black discolouration to the skin specially on the exposed parts which remains for several months. It can also cause dryness of skin, itching and phototoxicity. It can rarely cause gastrointestinal disturbances.

Ethionamide is bactericidal to lepra bacilli but is more expensive and more toxic than dapsone. It can cause gastric irritation, peripheral neuritis and hepatotoxicity. Ethionamide can be used in multidrug regimen in patients who cannot tolerate clofazimine. **Prothionamide** is similar to ethionamide.

Other Drugs

Fluoroquinolones: Ofloxacin is lepricidal and is suitable for use in multi-drug regimens in leprosy along with rifampicin. Ofloxacin 400 mg + rifampicin 600 mg daily for 28 days has been used in short-term clinical trials.

Minocycline a tetracycline, has been found to have useful activity against *M. leprae* and is being tried in combination regimens to shorten the duration of treatment. It is given in the dose of 100 mg daily but should not be used in children and pregnant women.

Clarithromycin a macrolide antibiotic, has bactericidal activity against *M. leprae.* Given 500 mg daily for 28 days can kill 99% of viable bacilli.

Treatment of Leprosy

For the sake of treatment, leprosy is divided into paucibacillary (non-infectious) and multibacillary (infectious) leprosy (Table 50.4). Several alternative and short-term regimens including drugs like ofloxacin, minocycline and clarithromycin are under evaluation.

WHO has recommended a combination of drugs in leprosy to:

1. Eliminate persisters
2. Prevent drug resistance
3. Reduce the duration of therapy.

Lepra Reactions

Lepra reactions are immunologically mediated acute inflammatory reactions that occur in leprosy. They are acute exacerbations triggered by acute infections, stress, anxiety and treatment with dapsone. Lepra reactions need to be suppressed promptly because they can result in permanent neurological changes. Early detection and prompt treatment are essential.

Type I reactions (reversal reactions) seen in tuberculoid leprosy are cell-mediated, delayed hypersensitivity reactions to the antigens of *M. leprae.* Cutaneous ulcerations occur and existing lesions show more erythema; nerves may be painful and tender. If untreated, there could be permanent damage to the nerves. It should be differentiated from relapse. They are treated with glucocorticoids or clofazimine while in mild cases aspirin suffices.

Dose: Prednisolone 40–60 mg daily for 2 weeks and gradually tapered over next 8–10 weeks by reducing 10 mg every 2 weeks.

Type II reactions are seen in lepromatous leprosy (are known as **erythema nodosum leprosum** or ENL). New lesions appear and the existing lesions become worse. Fever, lymphadenitis, myositis and neuralgia may occur. The severity varies; it is a hypersensitivity reaction to the antigens of *M. leprae* an arthus type reaction. Mild ENL is treated with aspirin or clofazimine which is effective due to its anti-inflammatory properties but has weak and slow effects—may require several weeks. Chloroquine, corticosteroids and thalidomide are also effective. All severe ENL cases are treated with prednisolone. Dapsone should be continued throughout.

Chemoprophylaxis

Only about 1% of contacts develop clinical disease. Dapsone 100 mg daily and rifampicin 600 mg once a month for 6 months or till the contact case becomes noninfectious are reco-

Table 50.4: Multidrug regimen for leprosy

Drugs	*Multibacillary leprosy (for 12 months)*	*Paucibacillary leprosy (for 6 months)*
Rifampicin	600 mg once monthly supervised	600 mg once monthly supervised
Dapsone	100 mg daily self-administered	100 mg daily self-administered
Clofazimine	300 mg once monthly supervised	—
	50 mg daily self-administered	—

All drugs are given orally

Table 50.5: Source of some antibiotics

Antibiotic	*Source*
Penicillin G	*Penicillium notatum, Penicillium chrysogenum*
Cephalosporin	*Cephalosporium acrimonium*
Imipenem	*Streptomyces cattleya*
Aztreonam	*Chromobacterium violaecium*
Streptomycin	*Streptomyces griseus*
Gentamicin	*Micromonospora purpurea*
Erythromycin	*Streptomyces erythreus*
Quinupristin + dalfopristin	*Streptomyces Pristinaespiralis*
Spectinomycin	*Streptomyces spectabilis*
Polymyxin	*Bacillus polymyxa*
Colistin	*Bacillus colistinus*
Vancomycin	*Streptomyces orientalis*
Teicoplanin	*Actinoplanus teichomyceticus*
Daptomycin	*Streptomyces roseosporus*
Rifampicin	*Streptomyces mediterranei*
Chloramphenicol	*Streptomyces venezuelae*
Tetracycline	*Streptomyces aureofaciens*
Mupirocin	*Pseudomonas fluorescens*
Fusidic acid	*Fusideum coccineum*

mmended for child contacts. Acedapsone is found to be advantageous for chemoprophylaxis as a single IM injection every 10 weeks. All contacts should be examined every 6 months.

Vaccine: BCG vaccine has been shown to afford some protection against leprosy but the extent is variable. Hence it has been modified and is undergoing evaluation for use.

[1–3] From Medical Council of India, *Competency based Undergraduate Curriculum for the Indian Medical Graduate*, 2018;1:136–144.

CHAPTER **51**

Antifungal Drugs

There has been an increase in the incidence and severity of fungal infections in the recent years. Several unusual and drug-resistant organisms have emerged. This may be consequent to the use of broad-spectrum antibiotics, anticancer drugs and HIV infections all of which impair host defense mechanisms. Fungal infections may be systemic or superficial. Superficial fungal infections include infections of the skin, mucous membrane, hair and nails. They require prolonged treatment. Some of the systemic fungal infections may be life-threatening, particularly in immunocompromised patients.

Sites of Action

Antifungal drugs may act (Fig. 51.1) on the fungal cell wall (pneumocandins), cell membrane (polyenes, azoles) or on the nucleus (griseofulvin, flucytosine). Antifungal drugs may be classified into:

Classification

1. ***Drugs acting on cell membrane***
   i. **Polyene antibiotics**
   Amphotericin B, Nystatin, Hamycin, Natamycin
   ii. **Azoles**
   - **Imidazoles**
     Clotrimazole, Econazole, Miconazole, Ketoconazole, Butaconazole, Oxiconazole, Sulconazole, Sertaconazole, Isoconazole
   - **Triazoles**
     Fluconazole, Itraconazole, Terconazole Voriconazole, Posaconazole, Ravuconazole Isavuconazole.

   iii. **Allylamines**
   Terbinafine, naftifine
2. ***Drugs acting on cell wall*** *(inhibit* cell wall synthesis)
   - Pneumocandins/echinocandins—caspofungin, micafungin, anidulafungin.
3. ***Drugs acting on nucleus*** *(inhibit protein synthesis)*
   - Griseofulvin
   - Flucytosine
4. ***Other topical agents***
   - Tolnaftate, undecylenic acid, benzoic acid, salicylic acid, naftifine, selenium sulfide, ciclopirox olamine.

DRUGS ACTING ON CELL MEMBRANE

Polyene Antibiotics

Amphotericin B: Amphotericin B obtained from *Streptomyces nodosus* is a polyene antibiotic containing many double bonds.

Antifungal spectrum: Amphotericin B has a wide antifungal spectrum. It inhibits the growth of *Candida albicans, Histoplasma capsulatum, Cryptococcus neoformans, Coccidioides, Aspergillus* and *Blastomyces dermatitidis*. It is fungistatic at low and fungicidal at high concentrations. Amphotercin B also has activity against leishmania.

Mechanism of action: Amphotericin B binds to ergosterol present in fungal cell membrane and forms pores in the cell membrane. Through these pores, cell contents leak out resulting in cell death. Since amphotericin has greater affinity for the fungal membrane sterol, i.e. ergosterol and also because cholesterol is the main sterol in human cells, the action of amphotericin is selective for the fungi.

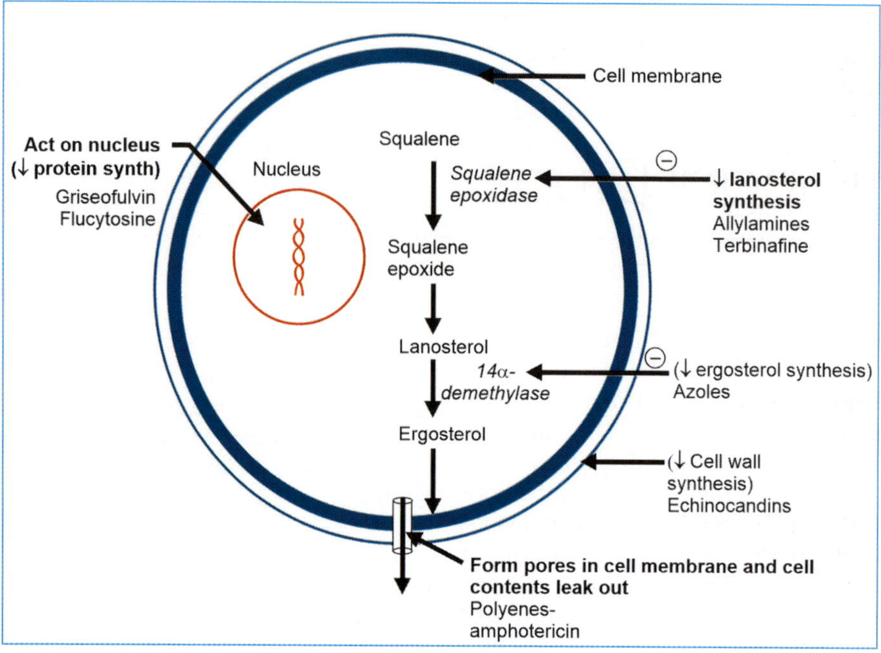

Fig. 51.1: Sites of action of antifungal drugs

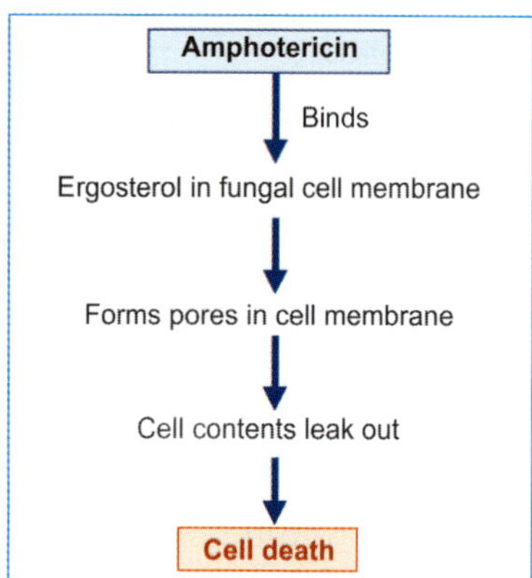

Pharmacokinetics: Amphotericin is not absorbed orally. Given IV, it is >90% bound to plasma proteins, widely distributed in the body and has a long t½ of 15 days. It is not soluble in water and hence it is dispensed as a colloidal suspension for IV use.

Lipid formulations of amphotericin B have been developed to reduce toxicity. Lipid formulation of amphotericin B is less likely to bind the human cell membrane and is thereby **less toxic.** In these preparations, amphotericin binds to lipids which act as reservoir and this avoids binding to human cells, thus reducing toxicity and it is possible to use larger doses of the drug. However, the preparations are very **expensive** and the benefit afforded is only moderate. Hence, they are used only in patients who do not respond to conventional preparations.

Adverse Effects

Fever, chills, muscle spasms, vomiting, dyspnoea, headache and hypotension can be encountered on IV infusion. Fever and chills subside in about 30 minutes. Administration of paracetamol (oral) or hydrocortisone (IV) prior to the infusion of amphotericin B can reduce the severity of these reactions. Amphotericin should be injected slow IV, cautiously—to avoid arrhythmias; anaphylaxis is rare. Allergic reactions are less common with lipid formulation.

Nephrotoxicity: Renal impairment is a common adverse effect of amphotericin use. It is associated with renal tubular acidosis along with the loss of potassium and magnesium. Infusion of normal saline before each dose of amphotericin can reduce these toxic effects to some extent. Prerenal renal failure is reversible but prolonged use can cause irreversible nephrotoxicity. Concurrent administration of other nephrotoxic drugs should be avoided.

Mnemonic (Salient features of amphotericin)

I **L**ove **AMPHOTERICIN**
L—Lipid formulation
A—Anemia
M—Muscle spasms
P—Paracetamol before ampho
H—Hepatotoxicity, headache, hypotension
O—Orally given in gut infection
T—Topical use: rashes
E—↓ erythropoietin
R—Renal impairment
I—Irreversible nephropathy (long-term use)
C—Chills
I—IV (used)
N—Neurotoxicity

Anaemia due to decreased production of erythropoietin by injured renal tubular cells and bone marrow depression can also occur.

Neurotoxicity and abnormal liver function tests have also been reported. Neurotoxicity depends on the dose and duration of treatment.

Topical use can cause skin rashes.

Dose: 0.5 mg/kg infusion AMFOTEX, FUNGIZONE IV 50 mg vial.

Uses

- Amphotericin B is the drug of choice for all life-threatening mycotic infections because it is fungicidal and has a broad antifungal spectrum. 0.5 mg/kg in 5% dextrose infused over 4 hr is the usual therapeutic dose. Amphotericin B is given intravenously in the treatment of mucormycosis, invasive aspergillosis, cryptococcosis, sporotrichosis, trichosporanosis, blastomycosis, histoplasmosis, coccidioidomycosis and paracoccidioidomycosis.
- In cystitis due to Candida, amphotericin B is used to irrigate the bladder.
- Amphotericin B is also used to prevent relapse of cryptococcosis and histoplasmosis in patients with AIDS.
- Amphotericin B can be given orally in fungal infections of the gut.
- It is used topically in candidiasis (3% lotion, cream, ointment).
- *Leishmaniasis:* In kala-azar and mucocutaneous leishmaniasis, amphotericin is used as an alternative.

Nystatin obtained from *Streptomyces noursei* has actions similar to amphotericin B. Because it is too toxic for systemic use, it is used topically. It is used for local candidial infections like oral thrush and vaginal candidiasis. 5 ml oral nystatin suspension should be swished in the mouth and then swallowed 4 times a day to treat the candida in the oesophagus.

MYCOSTATIN 5 lakh unit tab

Hamycin is similar to nystatin. It is used topically for cutaneous candidiasis and otomycosis.

AZOLES

***Imidazoles*:** Ketoconazole, clotrimazole, econazole, miconazole, butaconazole, oxiconazole, sulconazole, sertaconazole, isoconazole.

***Triazoles*:** Fluconazole, itraconazole, terconazole, voriconazole, posaconazole, ravuconazole.

The older antifungals need to be given intravenously and are quite toxic. Azoles are newer synthetic antifungals that are effective orally and are **less toxic**. Azoles include imidazoles and triazoles. The **triazoles have more selective effect** on fungal sterol synthesis than imidazoles. Triazoles are also **longer-acting**. Ketoconazole, miconazole and clotrimazole are the commonly used imidazoles—of them clotrimazole and miconazole are used only topically.

Antifungal spectrum have a broad-spectrum antifungal activity. They inhibit *dermatophytes, Blastomyces dermatitidis, Candida, Cryptococcus neoformans, H. capsulatum, coccidioides, some paracoccidioides* and other deep mycoses.

Mechanism of Action

Azoles inhibit the synthesis of ergosterol, an important component of the fungal cell membrane.

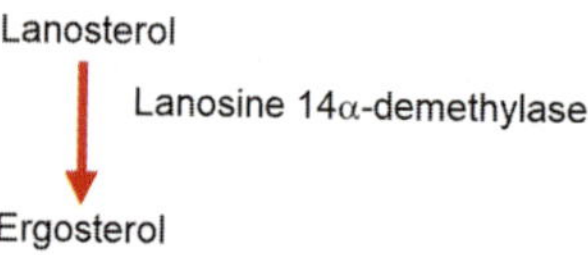

Azoles inhibit the fungal cytochrome P450 enzyme lanosine 14α-demethylase which catalyses the convertion of lanosterol to ergosterol. Thus it results in ergosterol deficiency which results in weak fungal cell membrane and fungal replication. They also interfere with the function of some fungal enzymes and inhibit the growth of the fungi.

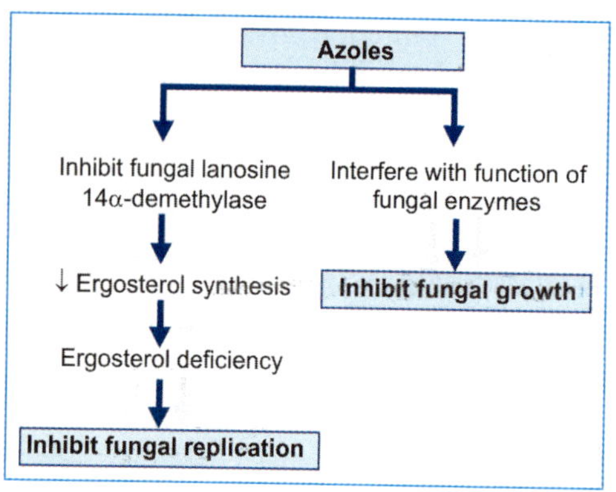

Since azoles have higher affinity to fungal than human CYP 450 enzymes, some selective activity is attained. Resistant strains are now common in AIDS patients and is due to genetic mutations resulting in altered enzyme 14α-demethylase.

Ketoconazole (KTZ) is the first oral azole to be made available. It is well-absorbed from the gut. Food and low gastric pH enhance absorption.

Adverse reactions include gastric irritation, nausea, vomiting, headache, allergic reactions, and rarely fatal hepatotoxicity. In large doses, KTZ inhibits the biosynthesis of adrenal and gonadal steroids in humans—resulting in gynaecomastia, infertility, decreased libido, azoospermia, menstrual irregularities and hypertension. This steroid suppression effect of KTZ limits its use.

Preparations

FUNGICIDE, NIZRAL-ointment, shampoo, 20 mg tab. DERM-KETA 20 MG/1 G CREAM.

Drug Interactions

- Antacids, H_2-receptor blockers, and proton pump inhibitors reduce the bioavailability of KTZ because acidic medium is necessary for KTZ dissolution.
- Rifampicin and phenytoin induce KTZ metabolism and decrease its efficacy.
- KTZ inhibits CYP450 (CYP3A4) and increases the plasma levels of several drugs, like sulfonylureas leading to hypoglycaemia, phenytoin toxicity, cycloserine induced nephrotoxicity and warfarin toxicity, viz. bleeding.

Uses (Table 51.1)

- Mucocutaneous candidiasis and dermatophytosis can be treated with ketoconazole.
- It is useful in Cushing's syndrome.
- KTZ is also useful in deep mycoses but is not preferred in them because of slow response, toxicity and long duration of treatment (6 to 12 months) required.
- Effective in cutaneous leishmaniasis.

Fluconazole a flourinated triazole is water-soluble, well absorbed from the gut, reaches all body fluids and attains good CSF concentration. Hence it is useful even in fungal

Table 51.1: Drugs used in systemic fungal infections

Fungal infection	*Drug of choice*	*Alternative drugs*
Invasive aspergillosis	Voriconazole	Amphotericin Itraconazole
Blastomycosis	Amphotericin Itraconazole	Ketoconazole/Fluconazole
Candidiasis	Fluconazole Voriconazole Caspofungin	Amphotericin Flucytosine/Itraconazole
Coccidioidomycosis	Amphotericin Itraconazole Fluconazole	Ketoconazole
Cryptococcosis	Amphotericin + Flucytosine Fluconazole	Itraconazole
Histoplasmosis	Itraconazole Amphotericin	Fluconazole
Mucormycosis	Amphotericin	Posaconazole/isavuconazole
Paracoccidioidomycosis	Itraconazole	Amphotericin
Sporotrichosis	Itraconazole	Amphotericin

meningitis. Fluconazole is eliminated by the kidneys, has a t½ of 25 hr. Fluconazole is available for oral and IV use.

Adverse effects are mild gastrointestinal disturbances, headache and rashes. Since it has very little effect on hepatic microsomal enzymes, drug interactions are less common.

ADCON 150 mg tab; FUSYS 50 mg DT-tab, 150, 200 mg tab

Uses

1. *Cryptococcal meningitis:* Fluconazole is used in cryptococcal meningitis after initial treatment with amphotericin B. Dose: 400 mg/day for 8 weeks followed by 200 mg/day—continued depending on the patient's condition. Fluconazole can also be used for prophylaxis.
2. *Coccidioidal meningitis:* Fluconazole is the drug of choice. Higher doses (400–800 mg/day) are required.
3. *Candidiasis:* Fluconazole is effective in oropharyngeal and oesophageal candidiasis. Dose: 200 mg on 1st day followed by 100 mg/day for 2 weeks. Given IV to treat candidaemia in ICU patients. Fluconazole is also effective in other mucocutaneous candidal infections.
4. *Other fungal infections:* Fluconazole is also useful in tinea infections but in other systemic fungal infections like histoplasmosis, itraconazole is preferred because of better efficacy.
5. *Leishmaniasis (off label use).* Oral fluconazole is effective in leishmaniasis 200 mg daily for 6 weeks.

Itraconazole is the most potent azole. Given orally, its absorption is increased by food and gastric acid. It does not have much effect on hepatic microsomal enzymes when compared to KTZ and does not affect steroid synthesis. Thus it is preferred over ketoconazole. Itraconazole is >99% bound to plasma proteins and does not reach the CSF. It has a t½ of 30–36 hours. It is available both for oral and IV use.

Interactions with several drugs which are metabolised by CYP450 enzymes are expected with itraconazole and other triazoles.

COMPARE AND CONTRAST

Ketoconazole (Imidazole) and Fluconazole (Triazole)

Features	***Ketoconazole***	***Fluconazole***
Chemistry	Imidazole	Triazole
Water solubility	Low	High
Bioavailability	Low	High
CSF levels	Low	High
t½	Short (~ 7 hr)	Long (~ 25 hr)
Antifungal spectrum	Narrow	Wide
Elimination	Hepatic	Renal
Route of administration	Only oral	Oral and parenteral (IV)
In fungal meningitis	Not effective	Effective
Corticosteroid suppression	Yes	No
Uses	Limited to fungal skin infections	Systemic and dermatological fungal infections

Preparations

Dose: 100 mg BD. ITASPOR, 100 mg cap.

Adverse effects include headache, dizziness, GI disturbances and allergic reactions. It can rarely cause hepatitis and hypokalaemia. It should not be used in pregnant women.

Uses

Itraconazole is the drug of choice in most systemic mycoses (without meningitis) 100 mg BD with food. It can be given IV in severe infections. Itraconazole oral solution is used in oropharyngeal and oesophageal candidiasis—10 ml (100 mg) to be swished vigorously in the mouth before swallowing on an empty stomach—twice a day for 2–4 weeks.

Itraconazole can also be used in onychomycosis, candidiasis and dermatophytoses but is expensive.

A carrier molecule **cyclodextran** has been used in new formulations of itraconazole.

Preparations: CANDITRAL, FULCOVER 100 mg cap.

Voriconazole has a wider spectrum and better efficacy than fluconazole. It is almost completely absorbed (>90% bioavailability) widely distributed in the tissues and metabolised by microsomal enzymes in the liver. Voriconazole is a microsomal enzyme inhibitor (inhibits CYP3A4) resulting in drug interactions with concurrently administered medication.

Adverse effects: Skin rashes, visual disturbances, hepatic toxicity and QTc prolongation have been reported. IV formulation can rarely cause anaphylaxis. It is contraindicated in pregnancy.

Uses: Voriconazole is the drug of choice in invasive aspergillosis where it has been found to have better efficacy and less toxicity than amphotericin B. Voriconazole can also be used in oesophageal candidiasis.

Posaconazole is a recent addition to the group of triazoles. It is a lipophilic triazole similar to itraconazole but with the broadest spectrum of antifungal activity among azoles including zygomycosis and mucormycosis. It is available as a liquid only for oral use. Fatty food enhances the absorption. It attains high levels in the tissues.

Posaconazole is indicated in the treatment of refractory invasive aspergillosis, chromoblastomycosis, fusariosis and coccidioidomycosis. It is also indicated for the prophylaxis of fungal infection in patients receiving chemotherapy in leukaemia and in bone marrow transplantation. Drug interactions due to inhibiton of CYP3A4 can occur.

Ravuconazole is a new triazole with longer action and broader spectrum of activity. It has

Table 51.2: Drugs used in superficial mycosis

	Topical	*Oral*
Ringworm	An azole Terbinafine	Terbinafine Itraconazole Griseofulvin
Candidiasis		
• ***Cutaneous***	Amphotericin An azole Ciclopirox Nystatin	Fluconazole
• ***Oropharyngeal***	An azole Nystatin Amphotericin Fluconazole	Itraconazole
• ***Vaginal***	An azole Nystatin	Fluconazole

been found to be effective in candidiasis, in antifungal prophylaxis, in immunocompromised patients and in onychomycosis.

Isavuconazole is another recently approved triazole useful in systemic fungal infections including invasive aspergillosis.

Topical Azoles

Clotrimazole, miconazole and econazole (Table 51.2) are poorly absorbed from the skin (<1%). Absorption from the vaginal mucous membrane is not significant—used topically in dermatophytic infections (ringworm) and mucocutaneous candidiasis. Miconazole penetrates the cutaneous layer—stratum corneum and remains at this site for 3–4 days. It has better efficacy. Clotrimazole troche is available for oral thrush. They can cause mild irritation at the site of application—particularly on mucous membrane. Skin preparations can rarely cause rashes, oedema and pruritus. Econazole cream may also cause burning or stinging sensation.

Preparations

- *Clotrimazole:* CANDID, CLODERM Lotion, cream, vaginal pessary 100 mg inserted into the vagina at bed time for 7 days or 200 mg daily for 3 days or 500 mg single dose.
- *Miconazole:* DAKTARIN, ZOLE 2–4% ointment, gel, cream, lotion and vaginal suppository (100, 200 mg)
- *Econazole:* ECANOL, VAGINAL (R) 150 mg tab.

Fenticonazole, terconazole, tioconazole, butaconazole, oxiconazole, sulconazole and **sertaconazole** are all azoles available for topical use as creams and lotions for use in dermatophytoses and mucocutaneous candidiasis.

ALLYLAMINES

Terbinafine is a synthetic antifungal that is effective against dermatophytes and Candida. It is orally effective and is fungicidal. It gets concentrated in the keratin like griseofulvin. Terbinafine inhibits an enzyme (squalene epoxidase) needed for the biosynthesis of ergosterol by fungi.

Terbinafine is well absorbed, undergoes extensive first pass metabolism and >99% bound to plasma proteins. On attaining steady state, the t½ increases to 200–400 hr.

Adverse effects are rare—gastrointestinal disturbances, rashes and headache can occur.

Terbinafine is used in dermatophytosis, pityriasis, onychomycosis and candidiasis. It is particularly preferred in onychomycosis.

Dose: 250 mg OD for 3 months—where it is superior to azoles and griseofulvin. SEBIFIN-250 mg daily; 1% cream. DASKIL, TERBEST 250 mg tab.

Naftifine is used topically for superficial fungal infections.

DRUGS ACTING ON CELL WALL

Echinocandins or Pneumocandins

Echinocandins are a newly introduced group of fungicidal drugs that are effective against candidiasis and *Aspergillus* species including those resistant to azoles. *Caspofungin, micafungin* and *anidulafungin* are the echinocandins currently available. Caspofungin also has activity against *Pneumocystis jiroveci* infections.

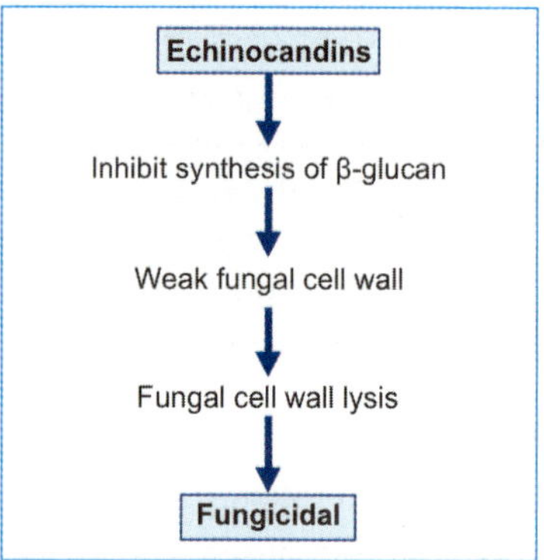

Echinocandins inhibit the formation of the fungal cell wall. They inhibit the synthesis of an important component of the fungal cell wall—a glucose polymer β-glucan as a result of which the fungal cell lysis occurs.

Echinocandins are given IV as they are not absorbed on oral use. Caspofungin has a t½ of about 13 hr while anidulafungin is longer acting with t½ 24–48 hr.

Adverse Effects

Adverse effects are minor and echinocandins are well tolerated—can cause histamine release on rapid infusion and thrombophlebitis.

Dose: CASPOFUNGIN 70 mg: IV over 1 hr—followed by 50 mg/day.

Uses

1. *Candida infections:* For treatment and for antifungal prophylaxis in febrile neutropenia, caspofungin, micafungin and anidulafungin may be used.
2. *Invasive aspergillosis:* Patients who have not responded to amphotericin—caspofungin has been approved for use.

DRUGS ACTING ON NUCLEUS

Griseofulvin

Griseofulvin is a fungistatic derived from *Penicillium griseofulvum.* It is effective in superficial dermatophytosis (caused by *Trichophyton, Microsporum and Epidermophyton).* Griseofulvin is the antifungal given orally for superficial dermatophytosis.

Mechanism of Action

Griseofulvin binds to microtubular protein in the nucleus, disrupts the mitotic spindle and inhibits mitosis in the fungus. It gets deposited in the newly forming skin, binds to keratin and protects the skin from getting newly infected.

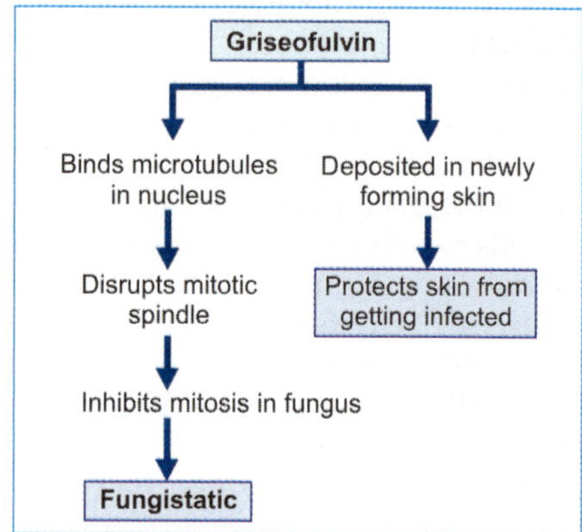

Pharmacokinetics: Griseofulvin is poorly water soluble with poor bioavailability. Absorption can be enhanced by using microfined drug particles and by giving it with fatty food. Griseofulvin is a microsomal enzyme inducer.

Adverse effects include allergic reactions, hepatitis and neurotoxicity.

Dose: 125–250 mg QID GRISONORM 250 mg tab. DERMONORM 250, 500 mg tab.

Drug Interactions

- Phenobarbitone reduces the absorption of griseofulvin—may result in therapeutic failure.
- Griseofulvin enhances warfarin metabolism by inducing microsomal enzymes.
- Alcohol should be avoided because griseofulvin can cause intolerance to alcohol (disulfiram-like reaction).

Uses

Griseofulvin is used orally in superficial dermatophytosis. It gets particularly concentrated in the tinea-infected cells and, therefore, suitable for ringworm infection of skin and nail. Dose: 1 g daily. It is particularly preferred when a larger area is involved when topical antifungals are not suitable. Duration of treatment varies from 3 weeks to 1 year depending on the site of infection. Nail infections require 6–12 months of treatment.

Flucytosine is a fluorinated pyrimidine effective against *Cryptococcus neoformans* and some strains of *Candida*. It is a prodrug taken up by the fungal cells and converted to 5-fluorouracil which inhibits DNA synthesis.

Because the drug cannot be converted by human cells to active metabolites, flucytosine is toxic only to the fungal cells. Flucytosine has synergistic activity with amphotericin B and azole antifungals. Amphotericin damages the fungal cell membrane which increases the penetration of flucytosine and this could be responsible for the synergistic effect. Flucytosine is well absorbed, reaches all body fluids including CSF and is excreted by the kidneys.

Bone marrow depression and gastrointestinal disturbances are the most common adverse effects.

Uses

Flucytosine is used with amphotericin B in cryptococcal meningitis and systemic candidiasis because:

i. Used alone, resistance develops rapidly
ii. It is synergistic with other drugs

Flucytosine is also used with itraconazole in chromoblastomycosis.

Dose: 100 mg/kg/day in 4 divided doses.

OTHER TOPICAL ANTIFUNGAL AGENTS

Apart from nystatin, clotrimazole, miconazole and terbinafine, some drugs like salicylic acid, benzoic acid, tolnaftate, naftifine, haloprogine and ciclopirox olamine are used topically for dermatophytosis and pityriasis versicolor.

Ciclopirox olamine is effective against Candida, dermatophytes and *Malassezia furfur*. When applied to the skin it does not get absorbed systemically but penetrates the skin to reach the dermis and no adverse effects are reported.

BATRAFAN 10 mg/g cream. OLAMIN 1.5% solution, 1% w/w cream.

Selenium sulfide is useful in tinea versicolor caused by *Malassezia furfur*, and also in dandruff. It is an irritant to the eyes and the odour is unpleasant.

SELSUN 2.5% suspension in a shampoo base.

Newer Drugs

Nikkomycins are a class of antifungals which inhibit chitin synthesis which is another important component of fungal cell wall and is under development.

Sordarins are a new class of antifungal agents that selectively inhibit fungal protein synthesis. They block the elongation factor 2 which is important in protein synthesis. Sordarin and its semisynthetic derivatives have been studied in clinical trials and have shown good activity against a variety of Candida species, some filamentous fungi and also against *Pneumocystis jiroveci*.

Clinical Pharmacology

- Most of the azoles are microsomal enzyme inhibitors and result in many drug interactions.
- Ketoconazole is now mostly used for topical application.
- Voriconazole is superior to amphotericin B and safer in invasive aspergillosis.
- Posaconazole attains higher levels in tissues than in blood.
- Fatty food increases the absorption of ketoconazole, itraconazole and posaconazole.
- Nikkomycins and sordarins are newer groups of antifungal agents under development.

CHAPTER **52**

Antiviral Drugs

Competency achievement: The student should be able to:
PH 1.48 Describe the mechanisms of action, types, doses, side effects, indications and contraindications of the drugs used in UTI/ STD and viral diseases including HIV.[1]

Viruses are intracellular parasites and depend on the host cells for their food, growth and multiplication. The virus attaches (Fig. 52.1) itself to the host cell membrane and penetrates it (entry), DNA/RNA is released in the host cell (uncoating) where it is duplicated. The viral components are assembled (assembly) and the mature viral particle is then released from the host cell (budding and release). Chemotherapy can interfere with any of these steps (Table 52.1). However, drugs that interfere with viral replication may also interfere with host cell function. Currently, efforts are being made to develop drugs that selectively inhibit the virus without affecting the host cell function. Antiviral drugs may be classified as follows:

There are two types of viruses—DNA and RNA viruses and there are minor differences in their replicative cycles. The DNA virus depends on host cell enzymes (mRNA polymerase) to synthesize mRNA while RNA viruses use their own enzymes for mRNA synthesis.

Classification

1. **Anti-herpes virus agents**
   Acyclovir, ganciclovir, famciclovir, penciclovir, valaciclovir, idoxuridine, trifluridine, foscarnet, fomivirsen, cidofovir
2. **Anti-CMV agents:** Ganciclovir, valganciclovir, foscarnet, cidofovir
3. **Anti-influenza virus agents**
   Amantadine, rimantadine, oseltamivir, zanamivir
4. **Anti-hepatitis agents**
   Anti-hepatitis B agents: Adefovir, entecavir, telbivudine, lamivudine, tenofovir interferons
   Anti-hepatitis C agents: Ribavirin, interferons, sofosbuvir, protease inhibitors—Boceprevir, simeprevir, telaprevir.
5. **Antirhinovirus/antienterovirus agent**
   Pleconaril
6. **Others**
   Palivizumab, imiquimod
7. **Anti-retroviral agents**
   a. ***Nucleoside and nucleotide reverse transcriptase inhibitors (NRTIs)***
   Zidovudine, didanosine, stavudine, emtricitabine, zalcitabine, lamivudine, abacavir, tenofovir
   b. ***Non-nucleoside reverse transcriptase inhibitors (NNRTIs)***
   Nevirapine, efavirenz, delavirdine, etravirine, rilpivirine.
   c. ***Protease inhibitors (PIs):*** Saquinavir, indinavir, ritonavir, nelfinavir, amprenavir, lopinavir, atazanavir, darunavir, fosamprenavir, tipranavir
   d. ***Entry inhibitors:*** Enfuvirtide, maraviroc
   e. ***Integrase inhibitors (INSTIs):*** Raltegravir, elvitegravir, dolutegravir.

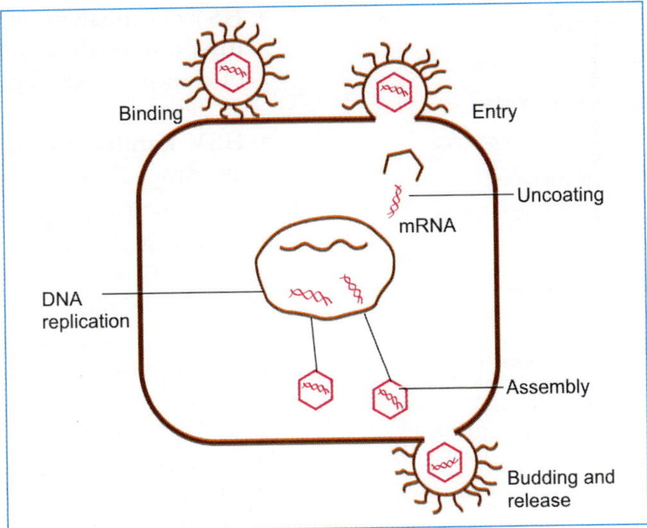

Fig. 52.1: Stages of viral replication and sites of action of antiviral drugs

Table 52.1: Drugs acting on viral replication steps

Viral replication steps	*Drugs effective*
Viral attachment and entry	Enfuvirtide, maraviroc, docosanol, palivizumab
Uncoating	Amantadine, rimantadine
Transcription	Interferons
Translation of viral proteins	Fomivirsen, interferons
Nucleic acid synthesis, DNA and RNA replication	Acyclovir, cidofovir, famciclovir, ganciclovir, foscarnet, idoxuridin, NRTIs, NNRTIs, PIs, ribavirin, sorivudine
Assembly	Interferons
Budding and release	Zanamivir, oseltamivir

Retroviruses

Retroviruses, a type of RNA viruses, are known to cause AIDS. In retroviruses, a viral enzyme reverse transcriptase is involved in replication. Two groups of antiviral drugs inhibit this enzyme. The immature virion formed undergoes maturation with the help of the enzyme protease. Inhibitors of this protease prevent maturation of the virions.

ANTI-HERPES VIRUS AGENTS

Acyclovir

Acyclovir is effective against herpes simplex virus (HSV) type 1 and type 2, varicella zoster virus (VZV) and Epstein-Barr virus (EBV).

Mechanism of Action

Acyclovir (Fig. 52.2) is taken up by the virus infected cell, converted to acyclovir triphosphate (by viral thymidine kinase) and this inhibits viral DNA synthesis by inhibiting viral DNA polymerases and causing DNA chain termination. Like acyclovir, valaciclovir, ganciclovir, valganciclovir, famciclovir, penciclovir and idoxuridine get converted to their respective monophosphate, diphosphate and then triphosphate derivatives which are the active metabolites. The active metabolite inhibits viral DNA/RNA polymerases and interferes with viral replication.

Resistance to acyclovir is due to reduced production of viral kinases, or altered viral DNA polymerases due to mutation.

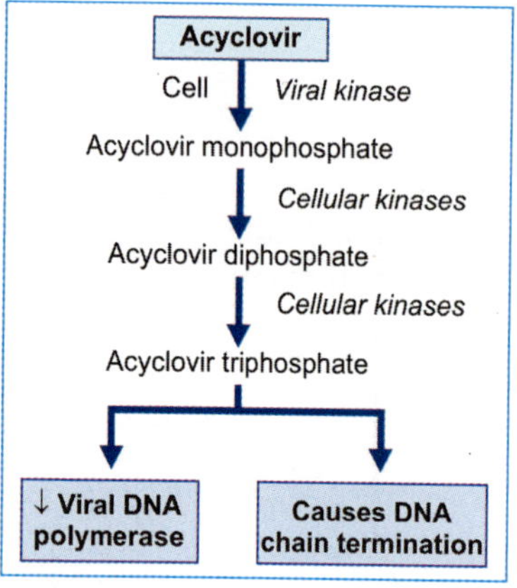

Fig. 52.2: Mechanism of action of acyclovir

Pharmacokinetics

Oral absorption of acyclovir is poor with bioavailability 15–20%; it is well distributed—attains good concentration in the CSF and aqueous humour. It is eliminated by the kidneys and the t½ is prolonged in renal faiure.

Preparations: ACIVIR 200, 400, 800 mg DT-tab, 3% oint, 25 mg inj. HERPEX 200 mg tab, 800 mg DT-tab

Adverse Effects

Acyclovir is well-tolerated; nausea, diarrhoea, headache and rashes may occur occasionally. Topical acyclovir can cause burning and irritation. Given IV, it may cause renal and neurotoxicity but are uncommon.

Uses

1. *HSV infections:* Infection with HSV-1 causes diseases of the mouth, face, skin, oesophagus or brain. HSV-2 usually causes infections of the genitals, rectum, skin, hands or meninges.
   - Oral acyclovir is effective in **primary and recurrent genital and labial herpes** (400 mg TDS for 10 days). In mild cases, topical acyclovir (5% oint) can be tried. In recurring genital herpes, parenteral acyclovir is needed—IV 5 mg/kg every 8 hr for 10 days. For long-term suppression, oral acyclovir is given for (400 mg BD) 1 year.
   - **HSV encephalitis** and other severe HSV infections—IV acyclovir is the drug of choice—10–20 mg/kg every 8 hr for 10 days.
   - **HSV keratoconjunctivitis**—acyclovir eye drops (3–5%) are effective.
2. *Herpes zoster:* Acyclovir shortens the duration of illness. In immunodeficient patients—IV acyclovir is used—10 mg/kg 8 hourly for 7 days.
3. *Chickenpox:* In adults and in immunodeficient patients (15 mg/kg/day IV for 7 days), acyclovir reduces duration and severity of illness. In children, routine use is not recommended. In close contacts, acyclovir 400 mg QID for 7 days given during the incubation period may prevent chickenpox.

Valacyclovir is a prodrug of acyclovir and is rapidly converted to it in the liver. High plasma levels of acyclovir are attained. It is well tolerated but high doses used in AIDS patients can cause confusion, seizures and hallucinations. Valacyclovir is used in herpes simplex, including genital and orolabial herpes, herpes zoster and CMV disease like acyclovir.

Dose: 0.5–1 g BD for 3–10 days. VALCIVIR 0.5, 1 g tab

Penciclovir and Famciclovir

Famciclovir is the prodrug of penciclovir and is rapidly converted to it on oral administration. Penciclovir triphosphate inhibits viral DNA polymerase. It is well tolerated with occational GI symptoms. Famciclovir is used orally in the treatment of primary and recurrent genital herpes, herpes labialis, herpes zoster, EBV and HSV. 250-500 mg BD- TDS 5-10 days. FAMIRAX 250, 500 mg tab.

Penciclovir, the active metabolite of famciclovir, is used topically for recurrent herpes labialis and in VZV infections.

Idoxuridine is effective in DNA viruses. It acts by inhibiting viral DNA synthesis. Idoxuridin is used topically in HSV keratitis (it is too toxic for systemic use). Eyelid oedema, itching, allergic reactions may occur.

Dose: TOXIL 0.1% eye drops, eye ointment.

Docosanol suppresses viral replication by inhibiting the viral entry into the cell. It is used topically in the treatment of orolabial herpes. It should be used early at the onset of lesion.

Trifluridine is used topically in HSV eye infections.

DRUGS USED IN CYTOMEGALOVIRUS (CMV) INFECTIONS

Ganciclovir and Valganciclovir

Ganciclovir is a guanosine analog effective against herpes viruses especially cytomegalovirus. Valganciclovir, is the prodrug of ganciclovir, it is orally effective. It is converted like acyclovir to ganciclovir, triphosphate in the cells. Ganciclovir triphosphate inhibits viral DNA polymerase and interferes with DNA chain elongation. This convertion to active metabolite takes place to a large extent in the CMV infected cells than in the normal cells. The active drug remains in the CMV infected cells for a longer time and is suitable for **once a day** administration. Given IV, ganciclovir attains high concentration in the vitreous humour.

Toxicity includes myelosuppression and gonadal toxicity (Table 52.2).

Uses

1. Intravenous ganciclovir and oral valganciclovir are used in the treatment and chronic suppression of CMV retinitis in immunocompromised patients.
2. They are also used to prevent CMV disease in organ transplant patients.
3. Topical ganciclovir may be used for herpetic keratitis.

Ganciclovir: GANGUARD 250, 500 mg cap.

Penciclovir Triphosplate inhibits viral DNA polymerase. It is well tolerated with occasional gastrointestinal symptoms.

Foscarnet is a pyrophosphate analog that directly inhibits viral DNA polymerase and RNA polymerase. It is given IV because of low bioavailabilty. It attains good concentrations

Table 52.2: Indications of some antiviral drugs

Drugs	*Route*	*Indications*
Acyclovir	Topical	Herpes genitalis, HSV eye infections
	Oral	Herpes genitalis, mucocutaneous HSV, chickenpox
	IV	HSV encephalitis, severe herpes genitalis, chickenpox/ herpes zoster in immunocompromised patients
Idoxuridine } Trifluridine }	Topical	HSV keratitis
Ganciclovir	IV/oral	CMV infections
Valganciclovir	Oral	CMV retinitis
Famciclovir	Oral	Genital, orolabial herpes infection
Valaciclovir	Oral	Herpes genitalis, herpes zoster
Amantadine	Oral	Influenza A
Rimantadine	Oral	Influenza A
Foscarnet	IV	CMV retinitis, acyclovir-resistant HSV infections
Cidofovir	Oral	CMV retinitis, HPV skin infections
Ribavirin	Aerosol	RSV bronchiolitis
	Oral/IV	Severe influenza and measles
Interferon α	IV	Chronic hepatitis B and C, genital warts, Kaposi's sarcoma
Zidovudine	Oral	HIV infection

Key Box 52.1: Drugs used in CMV infections

Treatment of CMV retinitis

Valacyclovir	Oral: Induction 900 mg, BD for 10–21 days followed by 900 mg/day
Ganciclovir	IV: Induction 5 mg/day Q12h maintenannce: 5 mg/kg/day. Oral induction: 1 g TDS. Intraocular implant induction: 4.5 mg once in 5–8 months
Foscarnet	IV induction: 90 mg/kg Q 12h Maintenance: 90 mg/kg/days
Cidofovir	IV induction: 5 mg/kg once in 7 days Maintenance 5 mg/kg once in 14 days

Prophylaxis of CMV retinitis (in transplant patients)

Valacyclovir Oral 900 mg/day

Ganciclovir Oral 1 g TDS.

in the CSF, has a t½ of about 6 hr and is excreted by the kidneys. Foscarnet is given intravenously to treat **CMV retinitis** as an alternative to ganciclovir. It may be effective in **CMV colitis** and **oesophagitis**. It may be used in other infections like acyclovir resistant **herpes infections** (Key Box 52.1).

Adverse effects: Foscarnet chelates divalent cations resulting in hypocalcaemia, hypokalaemia and hypomagnesaemia.

Fomivirsen is effective against cytomegalovirus. It is given by intravitreal injection in severe cases of CMV retinitis which do not respond to other drugs.

Cidofovir is a cytidine analog effective against herpes viruses, VZV, CMV, EBV, human papillomavirus (HPV) and adenoviruses—has a broad-spectrum of activity. Cidofovir acts by inhibiting viral DNA synthesis. It is given intravenously to prevent the progression of CMV retinitis in AIDS patients. It can also be used topically in HPV skin infections.

ANTI-INFLUENZA VIRUS AGENTS

Amantadine and Rimantadine

Amantadine and its derivative rimantadine inhibit the replication of influenza A viruses. Rimantadine is more active than amantadine. These drugs inhibit uncoating of viral RNA and thereby prevent viral replication. Given orally, both of them are well absorbed and attain good concentrations in the nasal secretions and CSF. They are generally well-tolerated; nausea, vomiting, diarrhoea, anorexia, dizziness, insomnia, difficulty in concentrating and ankle oedema are reported, but are seen with only higher doses. Both are teratogenic. Rimantadine is longer-acting and has fewer adverse effects.

Uses (Table 52.2)

1. *Treatment of influenza A:* When started at the onset of symptoms, amantadine and rimantadine reduce the fever, duration and severity of influenza by 1–2 days.

   Dose: 200 mg/day for 5 days OD of Amantadine/Rimantadine.
2. *Prophylaxis of influenza A:* During an epidemic especially in high-risk patients and also for seasonal prophylaxis in high-risk patients, these drugs are effective.
3. *Parkinsonism:* Amantadine enhances the release of dopamine and is beneficial in parkinsonism.

Oseltamivir and Zanamivir

Oseltamivir and zanamivir gained wide popularity in the recent H1N1 pandemic that spread across different countries including India. They inhibit viral replication by **inhibiting the neuraminidase** activity which is essential for the release of daughter virions. Oseltamivir and zanamivir are effective against both influenza A including H1N1 and influenza B. To be effective, these drugs should be administered within a few hours after the onset of symptoms (in 36–48 hr). They reduce both the duration and severity of illness.

Oseltamivir is given orally. It is a prodrug, well absorbed from the gut and activated in the liver by esterases. Oseltamivir is well tolerated—can cause nausea, vomiting, headache, diarrhoea and abdominal discomfort. It should not be given in children < 1 yr of

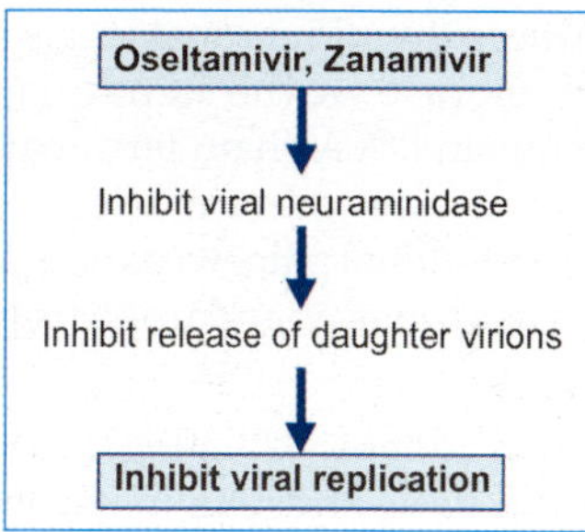

age. Zanamivir is given by inhalation which can occasionally cause respiratory distress.

Uses

Oseltamivir and zanamivir are used in the prevention and treatment of influenza including H1N1 infection.

Dose: Oseltamivir 75 mg BD for 5 days. Tamiflu 75 mg tab. Zanamivir 10 mg inhalation twice daily for 5 days. RELENZA inhaler.

Ribavirin has broad-spectrum antiviral activity. Its active metabolite ribavirin triphosphate is effective against many DNA and RNA viruses including influenza A and B, respiratory syncytial virus (RSV), HCV and HIV. It is used as an aerosol in RSV bronchiolitis in children. Ribavirin is also used in severe influenza and measles in immunocompromised patients and in HCV. Adverse effects include haemolytic anaemia, fatigue, nausea and allergic reactions.

Dose: 200 mg QID. REBETOL 200 mg cap. RIBAVIN 100, 200 mg cap, 50 mg/ 5 ml syrup.

ANTI-HEPATITIS AGENTS

Anti-Hepatitis B Agents

Adefovir is effective against hepatitis B virus. It is available as adefovir dipivoxil which is a prodrug of adefovir and is rapidly converted to adefovir by the esterases in the blood and intestines. Adefovir is phosphorylated by viral kinase to adefovir diphosphate which inhibits viral DNA polymerase. It is incorporated into viral DNA and causes DNA chain termination.

Once in the cells, adefovir remains up to 18 hours and therefore, can be given once daily. Adefovir is well tolerated. It can cause headache, diarrhoea, weakness and abdominal pain. Nephrotoxicity has been reported. Adefovir is used orally in the treatment of chronic HBV infection and is particularly useful in lamivudine-resistant HBV patients (Key Box 52.2).

Dose: 10 mg OD. ADFOVIR, ADESERA 10 mg tab.

Key Box 52.2: Drugs for viral hepatitis

Chronic hepatitis B	*Chronic hepatitis C*
Lamivudine	Ribavirin
Adefovir	
Entecavir	
Tenofovir	
Telvibudine	
Interferon alpha	

Note: Interferon alpha is also used in acute hepatitis

Entecavir is a guanosine nucleoside analog that inhibits DNA polymerase. It is completely absorbed on oral administration, but should be given on an empty stomach. It is well tolerated. Entecavir is useful in chronic HBV infection.

Interferons (IFN) are cytokines produced by host cells in response to viral infections. They also have immunomodulating and antiproliferative properties. There are three types—α, β and γ interferons in man. Interferons α and β are produced in response to viral infections. Interferon-γ is produced by T lymphocytes in response to antigens and some cytokines. They inhibit the multiplication of many DNA and RNA viruses. Interferons are given parenterally (SC/IM).

Mechanism of action: Interferons bind to specific receptors and activate JAK-STAT pathway and thereby stimulate the synthesis of certain proteins which inhibit viral protein synthesis. Interferon-α acts on multiple stages of viral replication including inhibition of viral penetration, protein synthesis, maturation and release.

Adverse effects include flu-like syndrome which starts in about 6 hours but may resolve in 12–24 hr. Pretreatment with antipyretics reduces the febrile response. Other adverse effects including myelosuppression, hypotension, arrhythmias, depression, transient elevation of enzymes, hepatotoxicity, weight loss, alopecia, pneumonitis, ototoxicity, retinopathy, thyroiditis, headache and arthralgia are reported on long-term use. It can also cause neurotoxicity resulting in confusion, sedation and, rarely seizures.

Pegylated interferons alpha –2a and 2b have better efficacy and are longer-acting than interferons and have, therefore, replaced interferons for most indications.

Uses

1. *Chronic hepatitis B:* Interferons administered for 4–6 months afford significant benefit in about half the number of patients—there is an overall improvement and plasma HBV activity declines.
2. Chronic hepatitis C infection: IFNs bring about sustained remission in chronic hepatitis C infection. When combined with ribavirin, the response is better and longer lasting, and therefore, always given in combination.
3. Kaposi's sarcoma in AIDS patients.
4. Genital warts caused by papilloma can accumulate virus—interferons are injected into the lesion.
5. Hairy cell leukaemia, some lymphomas, mutiple myeloma and CML
6. Multiple sclerosis: Interferon β can be used to reduce severity, HSV, herpes zoster and CMV infections in immunocompromised patients.
7. *Rhinovirus cold:* Interferon α is given intranasally for prophylaxis.

Lamivudine: Lamivudine used in antiretroviral therapy has the following advantages in HBV:

1. Long intracellular t½ in HBV infected cells.
2. It can be given even in patients with liver disease.
3. It has shown efficacy in prevention of vertical transmission from mother to fetus.
4. Adverse effects are mild and lamivudine is well tolerated by HBV patients.

Telbivudine, a thymidine analog, also inhibits DNA polymerase in the hepatitis B virus which results in DNA chain termination. It is well tolerated—can cause nausea, vomiting, headache, abdominal pain, weakness, myalgia, peripheral neuropathy and upper respiratory infection.

Tenofovir an adenosine analog used in AIDS is also found to be effective in chronic hepatitis. Tenofovir has activity against lamivudine-resistant strains.

TAVIN, TENTIDE 300 mg tab.

Antihepatitis C agents

Hepatitis due to infection with hepatitis C virus can vary in severity from mild infection of few weeks to serious life long disease. Hepatitis C related liver diseases include cirrhosis and liver cancer. Drugs used to treat HCV infection include:

- Interferons
- Ribavirin
- Newer drugs—sofosbuvir
- Protease inhibitors—boceprevir, simeprevir and telaprevir.

HCV is treated with a combination of interferon alpha and ribavirin or newer drugs.

Sofosbuvir is activated to its triphosphate derivative which when given orally inhibits RNA-dependent RNA polymerase. Sofosbuvir is used in combination with peg IFN-α and ribavirin to attain high cure rates. It is given orally and is well tolerated; fatigue and headache are reported.

Protease inhibitors boceprevir, simeprevir and telaprevir inhibit HCV protease and are used in combination with IFNs and ribavirin. All are orally effective, are to be taken with food and are metabolized by CYP3A4 which could result in drug interactions.

ANTIRHINOVIRAL DRUG

Pleconaril binds to viral capsid and prevents attachment and/or viral uncoating. It is found to be effective in picorna viruses like rhinovirus and entero-virus and is indicated in enteroviral meningitis and rhinoviral cold.

OTHER ANTIVIRAL DRUGS

Palivizumab is a monoclonal antibody effective against respiratory syncytial virus. It is used in high-risk children <2 years of age who also have chronic lung disease. **Imiquimod** is an immunomodulating agent effective topically in the treatment of genital warts (condylomata acuminata). It stimulates the immune system by inducing the cytokines, interferon α, TNF α and interleukins. It is used as a 5% cream applied thrice a week for 16 weeks. It can also be used for actinic keratosis.

ANTI-RETROVIRAL AGENTS

Acquired immunodeficiency syndrome (AIDS) results from infection with human immunodeficiency virus (HIV)—a retrovirus. The spread of HIV infection is alarmingly high with prolonged, significant morbidity and mortality resulting in death of millions every year. Two types of HIV have been identified HIV-1 and HIV-2.

Drugs used in the treatment of AIDS are of five groups (Flowchart 52.1).

The goal of treatment is to suppress the multiplication of HIV as long as possible.

HIV has a high mutation rate and, therefore, easily develops resistance to the drugs. Multi-drug-resistant strains have emerged which further complicate the treatment. A combination of drugs is used in AIDS to improve prognosis—known as **highly active antiretroviral therapy** (HAART). Each HAART regimen includes two NRTIs as backbone drugs with a third drug from another group. Using a HAART regimen suppresses HIV replication, plasma HIV RNA levels are greatly reduced and prolongs patient survival. Newer regimens are being regularly introduced to tackle resistance and improve efficacy as well as quality of life. With good treatment adherence and follow up, it has been possible to achieve prolonged survival, almost comparable to non infected humans and also prevent vertical transmission of infection from mother to the newborn. National AIDS Control Organisation (NACO) is working towards controlling spread of AIDS in India (Fig. 52.4).

NUCLEOSIDE AND NUCLEOTIDE REVERSE TRANSCRIPTASE INHIBITORS (NRTIS)

Zidovudine is the first drug to be used in the treatment of HIV infection. Others including didanosine, stavudine, zalcitabine, lamivudine, emtricitabine, abacavir, tenofovir and were developed later (Table 52.3).

Flowchart 52.1: Drugs used in the treatment of AIDS

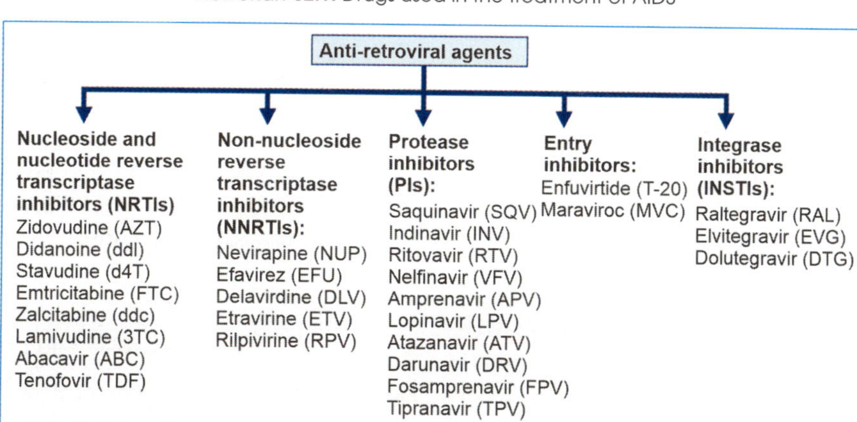

Table 52.3: Nucleoside reverse transciptase inhibitors—salient features

Drug	Analog of	Dose	Adverse effects
Zidovudine	Thymidine	200 mg BD	Myelosuppression, headache, nausea, insomnia
Didanosine	Adenosine	200 mg BD	Pancreatitis, peripheral neuropathy, diarrhoea, hyperuricaemia
Stavudine	Thymidine	30 mg BD	Peripheral neuropathy, stomatitis
Zalcitabine	Cytidine	0.75 mg TID	Peripheral neuropathy, stomatitis, pancreatitis
Lamivudine	Cytidine	150 mg BD	Headache, nausea
Abacavir	Guanosine	300 mg BD	Hypersensitivity syndrome
Emtricitabine	Cytosine	200 mg QID	Nausea, diarrhoea
Tenofovir	Adenosine	300 mg QID	Renal dysfunction

Mechanism of Action

NRT inhibitors enter the cells and are converted to their corresponding triphosphate derivatives which have a high affinity for reverse transcriptase, an enzyme specific to HIV and required for DNA synthesis. The NRT inhibitors are nucleoside analogs. They competitively inhibit reverse transcriptase, are incorporated into viral DNA chain and terminate DNA chain elongation.

Tenofovir is a nucleotide analog and competitively inhibits HIV reverse transcriptase similar to nucleoside analogs.

Pharmacokinetics: The NRT inhibitors are well absorbed when given orally. Their plasma t½ varies from 1 to 4 hours. All NRT inhibitors (except abacavir) are excreted by the kidneys.

Common adverse effects to NRTIs include- anaemia, granulocytopenia, myopathy, peripheral neuropathy and pancreatitis. Lactic acidosis and hepatic steatosis are rare but can be fatal. Toxicity is due to inhibition of DNA polymerase in human cells though to a small extent.

Zidovudine (Azidothymidine, AZT)

Zidovudine is a thymidine analog, active against HIV infections and other retroviruses.

Adverse Effects

Bone marrow suppression is the most prominent adverse effect of zidovudine. It is more common in patients with advanced AIDS. Anaemia can be treated with erythropoietin while neutropenia needs G-CSF or GM-CSF. Headache, nausea, anorexia, myalgia, fatigue and insomnia can occur. High doses cause myopathy, dyslipidaemia and neurotoxicity.

Uses

AIDS: Given along with other antiviral drugs. Treatment with AZT results in prolonged survival, decreased opportunistic infections, weight gain and in early cases, it delays disease progression.

Given during pregnancy to reduce the risk of transmission to the baby with other antiretroviral drugs.

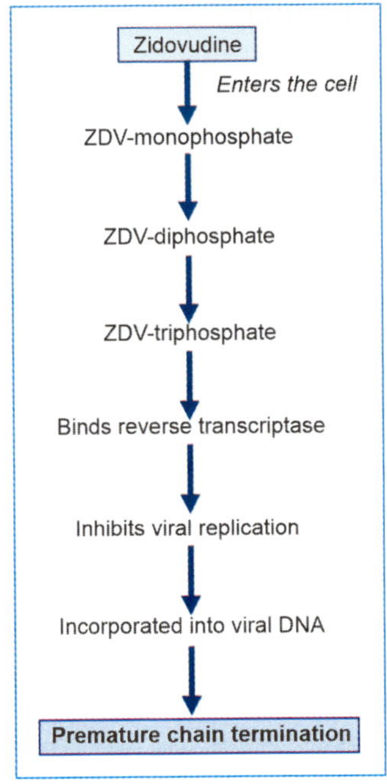

Fig. 52.3: Mechanism of action of zidovudine and other NRTIs

Didanosine (ddI), zalcitabine (ddc), stavudine (d4T), lamivudine (3TC), emtricitabine (FTC), abacavir (ABC) and tenofovir (TDF) are other reverse transcriptase inhibitors (Table 52.3) used as alternatives to AZT or with AZT in patients with advanced HIV.

Didanosine an adenosine analog is destroyed by acid and is, therefore, given with an antacid but this may interfere with the absorption of many other drugs including antiviral drugs—hence should be given separately. Food reduces its absorption. It can be given once daily because the drug remains intracellularly for a long time. Pancreatitis is dose-dependent.

Zalcitabine a cytosine analog has good bioavailability of 90% but short t½—to be given 8 hrly. It can cause peripheral neuropathy.

Stavudine is well absorbed (bioavailability 90%) and attains good CSF levels.

Lamivudine is a cytidine analog. Apart from HIV, lamivudine is also effective against hepatitis B virus as it inhibits DNA polymerase in the HBV. It requires long-term treatment and discontinuation of lamivudine, can, result in recurrence and emergence of lamivudine-resistant strains.

Lamivudine is well absorbed and well tolerated with no serious adverse effects in therapeutic doses. It can cause insomnia, fever, headache and diarrhoea.

Emtricitabine (ETC) an analog of lamivudine has the advantages of good bioavailability (93%) and long intracellular t½ of >24 hr given once daily. It can cause nausea, diarrhoea, headache, fatigue and rarely pigmentation of palms and soles.

Tenofovir (TDF) is an adenosine analog. It is converted to tenofovir diphosphate which is incorporated into reverse transcriptase and causes termination of the chain. Tenofovir is used as an alternative in the treatment of HIV infections in combination with other drugs.

Tenofovir is orally effective and well tolerated with occasional nausea, vomiting and diarrhoea. It can cause osteoporosis and is contraindicated in renal failure. Tenofovir alafenamide (TAF) is safer in patients with osteoporosis and renal dysfunction.

Abacavir (ABC), has the advantages of good oral bioavailability and slow development of resistance. A drug interaction with alcohol may need attention as abacavir is metabolised by alcohol dehydrogenase and alcohol competes for the metabolism.

Abacavir can cause a hypersensitivity syndrome with fever, rash and bronchitis, which can be fatal. Hence, abacavir should be withdrawn at the onset of such symptoms. Peripheral neuropathy, pancreatitis, rash, fever and headache can occur. It is also effective against HBV.

Drug Interactions of NRT Inhibitors

- Since AZT causes myelosuppression, it should not be combined with other myelosuppressants.
- Stavudine competes with zidovudine for activation pathway. Zidovudine decreases efficacy of stavudine. Hence, the combination should be avoided.
- Combination of zalcitabine and didanosine should be avoided due to overlapping toxicity, i.e. pancreatitis and peripheral neuropathy.
- Zalcitabine and lamivudine may antagonise each other—combination should be avoided.
- Plasma levels of abacavir is increased by alcohol.
- AZT toxicity increased by paracetamol may be due to competition for glucuronidation.
- AZT metabolism is inhibited by azoles as they are microsomal enzyme inhibitors.

NON-NUCLEOSIDE REVERSE TRANSCRIPTASE INHIBITORS

The NNRT inhibitors nevirapine, delavirdine, efavirenz and etravirine are synthetic compounds.

Mechanism of Action

The NNRT inhibitors bind to reverse transcriptase (are not converted to triphosphate derivatives) and bring about a change in the enzyme thereby inactivating the enzyme. NNRT inhibitors are effective only against HIV-1 (not against HIV-2 and other retroviruses).

When used as monotherapy resistance develops rapidly.

Adverse Effects

NNRTIs can cause GI disturbances and allergic reactions. These drugs are metabolised by cytochrome P450 enzymes (CYP3A4) and can result in related drug interactions.

Nevirapine (NPV) is well absorbed orally >90% bioavailability, attains high levels in CSF and has a long t½. **Fatty food enhances the absorption and also toxicity—hence, it should be taken on empty stomach.** It is metabolised by the microsomal enzymes CYP3A4 in the liver. Allergic reactions ranging from skin rashes, pruritus to Stevens-Johnson syndrome and toxic epidermal necrolysis can occur. It should be started with a low dose and gradually increased. If allergic reactions are severe, nevirapine should be withdrawn. Fever, nausea, headache and drowsiness are common. Occasionally, fulminant hepatitis can occur.

Nevirapine is used in the treatment of HIV-1 infections in combination with other drugs. Nevirapine is effective in a single dose (200 mg) at the onset of labour and in newborn 2 mg/kg single dose within 3 days of birth to prevent vertical transmission from the mother to the newborn.

Delavirdine is an NNRTI but not preferred.

Efavirenz (EFV) has an oral bioavailability of 50%, it is 99% bound to plasma proteins, is long acting and can be given once daily. It is metabolised by the microsomal enzymes.

Side effects include headache, dizziness, drowsiness, nightmares, confusion, vomiting diarrhoea and skin rashes. Efavirenz has teratogenic effects in monkeys and is contraindicated in pregnant women.

Efavirenz is used in the treatment of HIV-1 infection in combination with other antiretroviral drugs.

Etravirine is effective in HIV-1 that is resistant to other NNRTIs. It is well tolerated—can cause nausea, diarrhoea, skin rashes and raised liver enzymes. Etravirine is also metabolised by microsomal enzymes, inhibits some (like CYP 2C9 and CYP 2C19) and induces some others like CYP3A4 (Key Box 52.3).

Rilpivirine is effective against HIV-1 resistant to other NNRTIs. Its use with other drugs needs caution as drug interactions are likely and is therefore less preferred.

Drug Interactions of NNRT Inhibitors

- Nevirapine is a microsomal **enzyme inducer**. Concurrent administration of rifampicin and ketoconazole should be avoided. Oral contraceptives can fail, hence alternative methods of contraception should be followed.
- Delavirdine is a microsomal **enzyme inhibitor**. It also increases plasma levels of protease inhibitors like saquinavir and indinavir.

Key Box 52.3: NNRT inhibitors

- Nevirapine, delavirdine, efavirenz and etravirine.
- Directly bind reverse transcriptase of HIV-1 and inactivate it.
- They are well absorbed and extensively bound to plasma proteins.
- Metabolised by microsomal enzymes. Nevirapine and efavirenz are enzyme inducers; delavirdine and etravirine are enzyme inhibitors—drug interactions are common.
- Allergic reactions particularly skin rashes, headache and nausea are common.
- Used in HIV-1 infections in combination with other antiretroviral drugs.

- Efavirenz is a microsomal enzyme inducer and inhibitor of CYP3A4 and thereby induces its own metabolism.
- Etraverine is an inducer of CYP3A4 and inhibitor of others like CYPC9. Drug interactions are common.

PROTEASE INHIBITORS (PI)

Protease inhibitors have been used with other antiretroviral drugs. **Saquinavir** is the first agent to be used in this group but we now have 10 protease inhibitors. Since all of them are metabolized by microsomal enzymes, a small dose of ritonavir (100 mg) which is a microsomal enzyme inhibtor is used with other PIs to increase or 'boost' their levels (Table 52.4).

Mechanism of action: HIV protease activity is essential for the activation of viral enzymes and HIV replication. It is needed for the production of mature virion and for viral infectivity. The protease inhibitors bind competitively to HIV protease and block viral maturation. This makes the daughter viral particles immature and non-infectious.

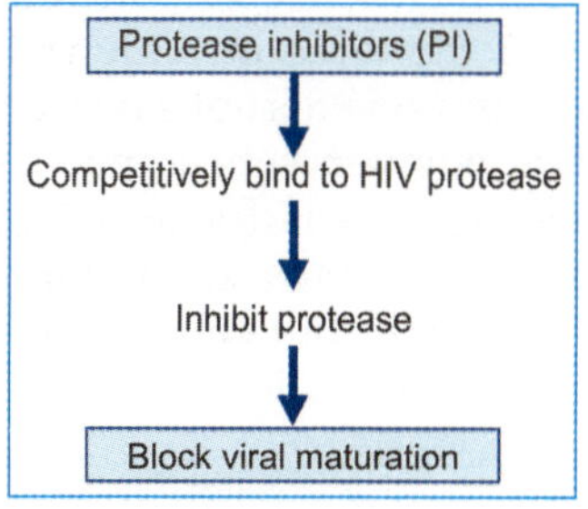

Pharmacokinetics: Except saquinavir, other protease inhibitors are well absorbed. All PIs are extensively bound to plasma proteins. They are all metabolised by hepatic microsomal enzymes (cytochrome P450) and are also microsomal enzyme inhibitors. Hence many drug interactions can occur.

Adverse effects: Protease inhibitors are well tolerated. **Gastrointestinal symptoms** like nausea, vomiting and diarrhoea can occur. Drug interactions are common due to microsomal enzyme induction and inhibition. Other adverse effects are given in Table 52.4.

Uses: Protease inhibitors are used in combination with other antiretroviral drugs in the treatment of HIV infections. Ritonavir inhibits microsomal enzymes and thereby prolongs the plasma half-life of other protease inhibitors. This beneficial drug interaction permits use of lower doses of other PIs with ritonavir and is used to **boost**—their drug levels.

Ritonavir is well absorbed and metabolised by microsomal enzymes like CYP3A4. It is a powerful enzyme inhibitor. Gastrointestinal disturbances are significant but may gradually subside. Hence, it is started with a low dose and is gradually increased. Ritonavir is used in low doses 100–200 mg BD along with other protease inhibitors to

Table 52.4: Protease inhibitors

Drug	*Recommended dose*	*Adverse effects*
Saquinavir	1200 mg TID	GI disturbances
Ritonavir	100 mg BD (booster)	GI disturbances, taste perversion, perioral and peripheral paraesthesias, ↑serum cholesterol, ↑TG
Indinavir	800 mg TID	GI disturbances, crystalluria, nephrolithiasis (advise lot of fluid intake), ↑serum bilirubin, alopecia, dry skin
Nelfinavir	750 mg TID	GI disturbances, ↑blood glucose, ↑serum lipids
Amprenavir	1200 mg BD	GI disturbances, rash, ↑blood glucose, avoid high-fat meals
Lopinavir	400 mg BD	GI disturbances, ↑serum lipids
Atazanavir	300 mg OD	GI disturbances, peripheral neuropathy, jaundice

Key Box 52.4: Protease inhibitors

- Bind HIV protease and prevent viral maturation
- All except saquinavir are well absorbed.
- All PIs are extensively bound to plasma proteins.
- All are metabolised by microsomal enzymes and inhibit these enzymes—drug interactions are common.
- Gastrointestinal disturbances are the common side effects
- Used in combination with other antiretroviral drugs in HIV infections.
- Ritonavir is used to boost the plasma levels of other PIs like lopinavir, darunavir, tipranavir and atazanavir.

'boost' the plasma levels of other protease inhibitors (microsomal enzyme inhibitor) so that lower doses of them are sufficient and are better tolerated.

Amprenavir is now replaced by its prodrug **fosamprenavir** which is converted rapidly to amprenavir in the intestines. It can cause rash—has highest propensity to cause allergic reactions among protease inhibitors and could be because of sulfonamide group in its structure.

Atazanavir is long-acting to permit once-a-day use. Common adverse effects are gastrointestinal disturbances, peripheral neuropathy and skin rashes. Raised liver enzymes, jaundice and QTc prolongation are also noted. It is a microsomal enzyme inhibitor—drug interactions are expected. Ritonavir enhances plasma levels; omeprazole should be avoided as it largely reduces bioavailability of atazanavir.

Saquinavir has low (4–10%) bioavailability but fatty food increases absorption by >5 times. Ritonavir boosts its plasma levels. GI disturbances are common.

Darunavir is another protease inhibitor to be given along with ritonavir. Allergic reactions are common apart from other adverse effects and drug interactions common to protease inhibitors.

Indinavir is absorbed in presence of acidic medium and should be given on an empty stomach. It can cause GI disturbances and renal stones—enough water intake needed. Not a preferred drug.

Lopinavir is given along with ritonavir (LPV/r)—effective against both HIV-1 and HIV-2. It should be given with food. Lopinavir should not be given concurrently with fosamprenavir, rifampicin and alcohol.

Nelfinavir is similar to other protease inhibitors.

Tipranavir is a recent addition to the group of protease inhibitors. It is effective in HIV-1 that is resistant to other PIs—given along with ritonavir. It can cause hepatitis and some fatalities have been reported.

ENTRY INHIBITORS

a. Fusion Inhibitor

Enfuvirtide binds to a glycoprotein on the virus and inhibits the binding of the virus to the host cell membrane, and thereby blocks the entry of the virus into the cell (fusion inhibitor) thus prevents transmission of HIV. Enfuvirtide is given subcutaneously twice daily; metabolism is by hydrolysis and microsomal enzymes are **not** involved. It can cause **local injection site** reactions (common), pneumonia and lymphadenopathy.

Enfuvirtide requires parenteral administration—therefore, used only as an add-on drug twice daily in patients not responding to other antiretroviral drugs in HIV-1 infected patients.

b. CCR5 Receptor Antagonist

Maraviroc CCR5 is a coreceptor involved in fusion and entry of the virus into the CD4 cells. Maraviroc selectively binds to CCR5 receptors and blocks the entry of HIV into the cells. It is effective orally, metabolized by hepatic microsomal enzymes CYP3A4 and excreted through the gut. Microsomal enzyme inducers and inhibitors can alter the plasma levels of maraviroc. It can cause diarrhoea, sleep disturbances, cough, myalgia, arthralgia, respiratory infections and raised liver enzymes. Maraviroc is indicated in HIV-1 infection not responding to other drugs.

Combinations to be avoided	*Reason*
1. Stavudine + Didanosine	Increased risk of lactic acidosis and pancreatitis
2. Stavudine + Zidovudine	Zidovudine decreases activation of stavudine
3. Lamivudine + Zalcitabine	Inhibit each other's activation (phosphorylation)
4. Lamivudine + emtricitabine	Common mechanism of action and resistance

INTEGRASE INHIBITORS OR INTEGRASE STRAND TRANSFER INHIBITORS (INSTIs)

Raltegravir

Integrase is a viral enzyme necessary for viral replication in both HIV- 1 and HIV- 2 viruses. Raltegravir, **elvitegravir** and dolutegravir bind to integrase and prevent integration of HIV—DNA into the chromosomes of host cells. Raltegravir is effective on oral administration, metabolised in the liver but **not** by CYP450 system. It can cause nausea, diarrhoea, headache and dizziness.

Dolutegravir (DTG)

Prevents integration of viral DNA into the host chromosome.

Advantages

- DTG is highly effective in HIV-1 and HIV-2
- Well tolerated
- Effective in HIV resistant to other drugs.
- Convenient to use (once daily)
- Drug interactions are low

Adverse Reactions

Hypersensitivity reactions, raised serum creatinine.

Uses

DTG is now the first line drug along with abacavir and lamivudine in the treatment of HIV infection.

Treatment of HIV Infection

Currently several drugs are available for the treatment of HIV infection and with appropriate medication it is possible to control the disease and prolong the life to a large extent. Combination of drugs is used to improve efficacy and delay the development of resistance. WHO recommends fixed dose combination (FDC) to improve compliance (Table 52.5). Two NRTIs form the backbone drugs and a third drug added may be an INSTI or efavirenz, these form the first-line drugs. If first-line therapy fails, alternative first line drugs are given.

Cobicistat is a microsomal enzyme inhibitor– it inhibits cytochrome P450 enzymes like CYP 3A4 and thereby increases the plasma levels of drugs metabolised by these enzymes. It also inhibits intestinal transport protein resulting in better absorption of drugs like atazanavir and darunavir.

Cobicistat is used in anti HIV combination regimens to enhance the plasma levels of drugs like elvitegravir, atazanavir, darunavir and tenofovir alafenamide. However, creatinine levels should be monitored as cobicistat increases renal secretion of creatinine.

Post-exposure prophylaxis (PEP): Accidental exposure to potential blood-borne infections including HIV, HBV and HCV among health care workers including doctors needs immediate attention. Post-exposure prophylaxis should be initiated at the earliest possible. The risk assessment is done based on the severity of the source of infection. Counselling, risk assessment, first aid and short-term (4 wk) antiretroviral drugs with appropriate follow-up would help prevent the disease.

First dose of PEP should be given at the earliest, preferably within 2 hours but at least

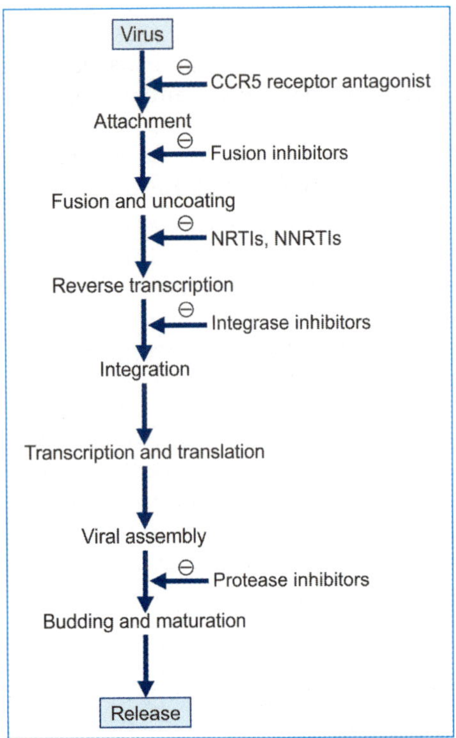

Fig. 52.4: Steps in HIV replication and the drugs acting at different stages

before 72 hours and the complete course is 28 days.

***PEP regimen:* Three-drug regimen-WHO recommendation**

Two drugs (TDF+3TC) have been used for PEP but now WHO and other updated guidelines recommend three drug regimen (Table 52.5).

For children <10 yr

Zidovudine (AZT) and lamivudine (3TC) are backbone drugs

Ritonavir boosted lopinavir (LPVr) or atazanavir (ATV/r) is the third drug (Table 52.6).

Pre-exposure prophylaxis

Persons at high risk for acquiring HIV infection can now be given pre-exposure prophylaxis (PrEP) with tenofovir + emtricitabine or topical use of tenofovir gel. WHO recommends such PrEP for high risk groups.

Table 52.5: Antiretroviral drug regimen

Adults, Adolescent, Pregnant	TDF + 3TC (or FTC) + DTG/EFV
Children	ABC + 3TC + DTG
Neonates	AZT + 3TC +RAL

As per NACO guidelines 2021

Table 52.6: Post-exposure prophylaxis

Adults and adolescents	TDF + 3TC/FTC + DTG
Children	AZT + 3TC + DTG ABC + 3TC + DTG

as per NACO guidelines 2021

PHARMACOTHERAPY OF COVID-19

COVID-19 is a viral infection caused by SARS CoV2, mostly affecting the respiratory tract. It is said to be a zoonotic disease first started in China but spread rapidly worldwide because of its high degree of contagiousness. WHO declared it to be a pandemic on 11th March 2020. The numbers kept increasing worldwide every passing day. Majority of patients could be asymptomatic, but it can be severe and fatal in symptomatic patients. Though around 2–3% mortality rate is generally seen, various factors determine the mortality and could be higher. Comorbidities like bronchial asthma, COPD, cardiovascular diseases, immunosuppression, diabetes mellitus and old age increase the risk of death. Transmission is through aerosolised respiratory droplets and also through direct person to person contact though other routes of transmission are yet to be better known.

Clinical features include fever, cough, sore throat, myalgia and fatigue. Other features include anosmia, altered taste sensation, headache and gastrointestinal disturbances. Skin rashes, petechiae, conjunctival redness and irritation, tachycardia, hypotension and renal failure may occur. Difficulty in breathing, chest pain and hemoptysis may progress to severe respiratory distress and shock resulting in death. Cytokine storm is a dreaded feature of COVID which could be fatal. Diagnosis is by RT-PCR identification of the COVID viral RNA in the respiratory secretions or serum. Detection of antibodies is also definitive.

Treatment

Since it is a viral infection and specific antiviral is not yet available, treatment is largely symptomatic. Cases progressing to severe acute respiratory illness need ICU care with ventilator support. Regular and frequent oxygen saturation monitoring is vital and life-saving in all patients tested positive for COVID-19. Several drugs are tried:

- **Chloroquine and hydroxychloroquine** have been shown to be useful in some limited studies. HCQS is better tolerated of the two and has been widely used both for treatment and prophylaxis.
- **Azithromycin** has been used with HCQS but added cardiotoxicity, particularly prolonged QTc has led to increased mortality in some patients.
- **Doxycycline** is a useful alternative to azithromycin.
- **Antiretroviral drugs lopinavir-ritonavir** used in other corona viruses like SARS and MERS have been tried in COVID also. Interferon-alfa has been added to this combination in China but there are views for and against such use.
- **Ivermectin,** an anthelmintic has good antiviral activity *in vitro* but its antiviral activity *in vivo* is yet to be proved. Many clinicians claim excellent response to ivermectin. Moreover it is fairly well tolerated.
- **Remdesivir (IV)** has been reported to be useful in patients with severe disease. It should be started early to be effective in moderate to severe disease. ICMR guidelines allow its usage even in moderate disease with normal saturation.
- **Immunotherapy** with monoclonal antibody and **tocilizumab** have been tried in some centres. **Sarilumab** 200 mg to 400 mg IV or SC is being evaluated as add-on with antiviral therapy. All patients also receive **zinc** 50 mg daily and **vitamin C** 500 mg TID, **Vitamin D** 2000–4000 units per day, to be given if there is deficiency. **Melatonin** 6–12 mg at night and **famotidine** 20–40 mg daily may help.
- **Glucocorticoids** are **not** to be used routinely but in patients with cytokine storm, immunosuppression with steroid in low dose has reportedly saved many lives. However, timing is very important.
- **Convalescent plasma** obtained from patients recovered from COVID has been used with some success by a few physicians. Combination of antibodies also has been tried with some success.
- **High flow oxygenation, mechanical ventilation** and fluid management are needed in more severe cases.
- Comorbidities need special attention as they could contribute to increased mortality.

Symptomatic treatment: Fever and body ache are treated with **paracetamol** (but other NSAIDs are contraindicated) an initial dose of **heparin** is used to prevent microthrombi formation which have been implicated in fatality.

Prophylaxis: Some of the drugs have been tried with the hope of preventing infection, reducing severity and avoiding cytokine storm particularly in health care workers. HCQS and ivermectin have been used. **Immune boosters** including vitamin C, zinc, vitamin D and multiple household remedies like some spices, *tulsi*, amla, ginger have been tried with the hope of improving immunity.

Prevention of transmission: Since there is neither cure nor vaccine for COVID-19 which shook the whole world, prevention of transmission is key to managing the disease. Patients with asymptomatic infection may spread infection and this

Treatment protocols for COVID-19

Mild	***Moderate***	***Severe***
Antiviral HCQS—400 mg BD day 1 200 mg BD next 4 days Or Favipiravir 1800 mg BD day 1 800 mg BD next 6 days Or Ivermectin 12 mg OD 3 days + Doxycycline 100 mg BD—5 days	*Antiviral* Inj Remdesivir IV 200 mg day 1 100 mg daily for next 4 days Or HCQS if Remdesivir not available. Avoid Remdesivir + HCQS combination	*Antiviral* Inj Remdesivir IV (if not received) 200 mg day 1, 100 mg next 4 days Inj Tocilizumab 8 mg/kg IV infusion over 1 hour. Repeat after 12–24 hr Or Italizumab—1.6 mg/kg IV 1st dose 0.8 mg/kg weekly infusion if required
	Immunosuppression Inj Methylprednisolone 0.5–1 mg/kg or Inj Dexamethasone 0.1–0.2 mg/kg for 3–5 days	*Immunosuppression* Inj Methylprednisolone 0.5–1 mg/kg or Inj Dexamethasone 0.10–0.2 mg/kg for 3–5 days
Anticoagulation (if X-ray/D-dimer necessitates) Inj Enoxaparin 40 mg SC × 7 days	*Anticoagulation* Inj enoxaparin 40 mg SC × 7 days	*Anticoagulation* Inj enoxaparin 1 mg/kg SC twice daily × 7 days
Others Supportive therapy Tab Zinc 50 mg × 7 days Tab Vit C 500 mg TDS Tab N acetylcysteine 600 mg TDS if patient has cough	*Others* • Suitable antibiotics • Awake proning • Convalescent plasma 200 ml slowly over 2 hr • Supportive therapy	*Others* • Oxygen • Antibiotics • Awake proning • Supportive therapy • Diuretics—in presence of heart failure

Protocols are subject to change as more experience is gained. Supportive therapy is same for all groups

makes effective prevention even more challenging. Isolation of infected patients, quarantine of exposed persons, perfect hand hygiene, social distancing, use of proper personal protective equipment, all help to a large extent to prevent transmission. Greeting others without handshake or hugging, maintaining physical distance of 6 ft and effective social distancing, all go a long way in preventing the spread. Health care workers are at greater risk, particularly when the viral load is more as in surgeries on infected patients. They require to follow strict aseptic measures to avoid infection. Knowledge about this disease is yet in its infancy. The viruses are well known to mutate which poses a great challenge in vaccine development. However, vaccine or an effective antiviral drug is needed to contain the pandemic.

Clinical Pharmacology

- NNRT inhibitors, PIs and maraviroc are subject to drug interactions by microsomal enzyme inducers and inhibitors. However, most NRTIs, enfuvirtide and raltegravir are devoid of such drug interactions as they are not metabolised by CYPs.
- Currently available antiretroviral drugs prevent infection of susceptible normal cells but do not affect the cells that are already infected with HIV.
- Lactic acidosis and hepatic steatosis are more common with stavudine.
- Nevirapine dose should be gradually built up to avoid skin rashes. If systemic symptoms of allergy appear, nevirapine should be withdrawn.

CHAPTER **53**

Antimalarial Drugs

Competency achievement: The student should be able to:

PH 1.47 Describe the mechanisms of action, types, doses, side effects, indications and contraindications of the drugs used in malaria, kala-azar, amebiasis and intestinal helminthiasis .[1]

Malaria was so named because it was thought to be due to bad air (*'mala'*—bad *'aria'*—air in Italian). Malaria caused by protozoa of the genus *Plasmodium* is most commonly transmitted through the bite of a female Anopheles mosquito, though malaria can also be transmitted by blood transfusion and vertically from mother to the foetus across the placenta. Every year about 250 million cases of malaria occur throughout the world with 2 million deaths. However, the incidence as well as the death rates have fallen since 2000 due to extensive control programms and active role of WHO with about 228 million cases and 4 lakh deaths in 2018. It is a major public health problem in most of the developing countries including India with about 4.3 lakh confirmed cases of malaria reported in 2018 with 96 deaths. There are primarily 5 species of the malarial parasite. They are:

- *P. falciparum* causes the most severe form of malaria **(malignant tertian)** which can be fatal. 90% of deaths due to malaria is due to *P. falciparum.* The parasite in the RBCs requires about 48 hours to complete its life cycle and ruptures every 3rd day (hence the name tertian) and this results in fever. In later stages of the erythrocytic cycle of the parasite, the **infected erythrocytes get sequestered in capillaries**, i.e. they pack the capillaries of various tissues resulting in tissue anoxia particularly cerebral anoxia making it lethal malaria. However, relapses do not occur because *P. falciparum* has no exoerythrocytic stage in its life cycle.
- *P. vivax* causes less severe malaria **(benign tertian)** with a lower mortality rate. Relapses can occur because of the exoerythrocytic forms or hypnozoites.
- *P. ovale* is mostly seen in Africa, causes milder form of malaria similar to *P. vivax* and relapses can occur.
- *P. malariae* also causes malaria of milder type similar to *P. vivax* **(benign quartan)** with no exoerythrocytic cycle. Febrile attack is seen every fourth day because 72 hours are needed for the maturation of the parasite in the RBCs and it is, therefore, called quartan malaria.
- A fifth species of the malaria parasite is now known. *P. knowlesi* is a zoonotic malaria acquired from macaque monkeys and has been increasingly reported from South-East Asian countries like Thailand, Malaysia and Vietnam. It has a 24-hr erythrocytic cycle with fever occurring everyday.

LIFE CYCLE OF THE MALARIA PARASITE

The bite of an infected female anopheles (meaning worthless) mosquito introduces the sporozoites into the bloodstream of man (Fig. 53.1). These sporozoites enter the liver cells where they develop and multiply and the

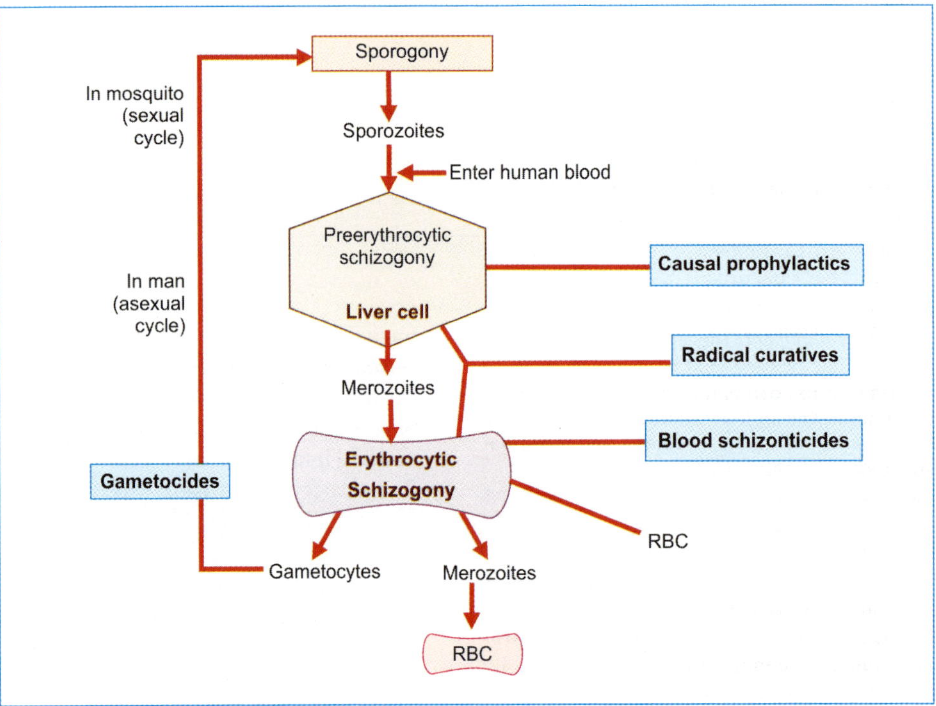

Fig. 53.1: Stages of life cycle of the malaria parasite and drugs acting on these stages

cells rupture to release merozoites (pre-erythrocytic stage). The merozoites enter red blood cells to develop and mature (erythrocytic stage/erythrocytic schizogony) for which it needs 48 hours (72 hours in *P. malariae*) and then the RBCs rupture releasing merozoites which invade fresh RBCs and continue to multiply. The material that is released when the RBCs rupture induces the release of cytokines and other mediators of inflammation which is responsible for fever and other symptoms of malaria. In *P. vivax* and *P. ovale* species, some sporozoites in the liver cells enter a dormant stage (hypnozoites or sleeping forms) which can multiply later (even after several months) resulting in relapse (exoerythrocytic stage). Some merozoites entering the RBCs, differentiate into male and female sexual forms or gametocytes. These forms enter the mosquito when they suck the blood and undergo sexual cycle in the mosquito. Antimalarial drugs can be classified therapeutically and chemically as follows.

Clinical Features

Signs and symptoms of malaria include fever with chills, myalgia, arthralgia, headache, vomiting and fatigue—these symptoms mimic viral fever and malaria may often go undiagnosed for sometime and by this time it could assume a more severe form. Diarrhoea, abdominal pain, dizziness, hypotension and in more severe forms convulsions may occur. Mild anaemia and splenomegaly and in some of them mild hepatomegaly are the expected findings.

CHLOROQUINE

Chloroquine (CQ) is a synthetic 4-aminoquinoline. It was synthesized separately in America and by Germans. It has been the

A. Therapeutic Classification

1. **Causal prophylactics** (primary tissue schizonticides) (destroy parasite in liver cells and prevent invasion of erythrocytes)	Primaquine, pyrimethamine
2. **Blood schizonticides** (suppressives, destroy parasites in the RBCs and terminate clinical attacks of malaria.)	Chloroquine, quinine, artemisinin and derivatives mefloquine, halofantrine, pyrimethamine, atovaquone, chloroguanide,
3. **Tissue schizonticides** used to prevent relapse (hypnozoitocidal drugs—act on hypnozoites of *P. vivax* and *P. ovale* that produce cause relapses)	Primaquine, tafenoquine
• Radical curatives (eradicate all forms of *P. vivax and P. ovale* that cause relapses)	Blood schizonticides+ hypnozoitocidal drugs
4. **Gametocidal drugs** (or gametocytocides destroy gametocytes and prevent transmission)	Primaquine, chloroquine, quinine.

B. Chemical Classification

1. **4-aminoquinolines**
   Chloroquine, amodiaquine
2. **8-aminoquinolines**
   Primaquine, bulaquine, tafenoquine
3. **Quinoline methanols**
   Quinine, quinidine, mefloquine
4. **Sesquiterpene lactones**
   Artemisinin, artesunate, artemether, arteether
5. **Folate antagonists**
   Proguanil, sulfadoxine, pyrimethamine
6. **Phenanthrene methanol**
   Halofantrine, lumefantrine
7. **Naphthaquinone**
   Atovaquone
8. **Antibiotics**
   Tetracycline, doxycycline, ciprofloxacin, clindamycin, azithromycin

primary drug in the treatment and prevention of malaria since 1940.

Antimalarial Actions: Chloroquine is a highly effective blood schizonticide with activity against all 5 species of the plasmodia. It completely cures sensitive falciparum malaria. It is rapidly acting—patients become afebrile in 24–48 hr. Chloroquine also destroys gametocytes of *P. vivax, P. ovale* and *P. malariae,* but has no effect on the hypnozoites in the liver. Chloroquine is safe in pregnancy.

Mechanism of action is not clear. Chloroquine is specifically taken up by the parasite in the erythrocytes by a specific uptake mechanism. Chloroquine is a base. It concentrates in the acidic food vacuoles of the parasite. Malarial parasites digest the host haemoglobin (which is their source of amino acids) and transports it into their acidic food vacuoles. In this process, a toxic product 'haeme' is formed. This haeme is converted to nontoxic 'haemazoin' a malarial pigment, by the enzyme haeme polymerase. Chloroquine, quinine and mefloquine inhibit the enzyme haeme polymerase resulting in accumulation of haeme which causes lysis of the parasite membrane and thereby death of the parasite. Chloroquine also prevents the digestion of haemoglobin by the parasite thereby disrupting the parasite's amino acid supply.

Chloroquine-resistant strains of *P. falciparum* are now common throughout the world. Chloroquine is rapidly transported out of the food vacuoles by the resistant strains. In *P. falciparum,* the resistance is due to mutations in the gene that encodes a chloroquine-resistance transporter. Chloroquine resistant *P. vivax* strains are also increasing and posing a problem in controlling malaria. In vivax, the resistance may be modulated by P-glycoprotein and other transporters which

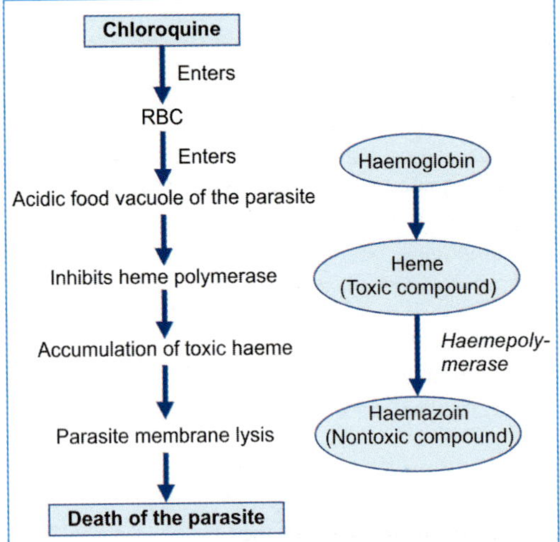

transport chloroquine out of the parasite. Several studies have shown that resistance to chloroquine can be reversed by using drugs like verapamil, chlorpheniramine and desipramine. These drugs prevent the efflux of chloroquine from the parasite. However, the benefits of their clinical application need to be established (Dose: Table 53.1).

LARIAGO, RESOCHIN 250 MG TAB, 500 mg DT-tab, 40 mg/ml inj.

Other Actions

Chloroquine has activity against *Giardia lamblia and Entamoeba histolytica.* Chloroquine attains a high concentration in the liver and is useful in hepatic amoebiasis. Chloroquine has local anaesthetic properties. It also has **anti-inflammatory** properties because of which it is used in rheumatoid arthritis as a disease-modifying antirheumatic drug.

Pharmacokinetics: Chloroquine may be given both orally and parenterally, but following parenteral administration toxic concentration may be attained in the plasma in a very short time. Hence parenteral chloroquine should be used only when definitely needed and it should be given as a **slow infusion** in divided doses. Chloroquine is rapidly and almost **completely absorbed** from the gut. It is widely distributed in the tissues and it has a **large apparent volume of distribution of >100 litres/kg.** It has a high affinity for melanin rich tissues and nuclear chromatin. It thus **accumulates in retina** and long-term use can result in retinopathy. Chloroquine has a half-life of 6 to 7 days. It is metabolized by hepatic microsomal enzymes and is largely excreted in the urine. Its terminal elimination **t½ is 1–2 months** as it is bound to the tissues.

Adverse effects: Though chloroquine in therapeutic doses is considered a reasonably safe drug, doses used for the treatment of malaria are often poorly tolerated as compared to prophylactic doses.

Nausea and **vomiting** may be quite severe in some patients. Prior treatment with an antiemetic 30 minutes before chloroquine is generally practiced.

Anorexia, pruritus, headache, dizziness, visual disturbances, insomnia and skin rashes may occur. IV chloroquine may cause hypotension, **widening of QRS complex** and **arrhythmias**, respiratory and cardiac arrest—hence parenteral chloroquine should be avoided.

High doses can also cause cardiomyopathy, peripheral neuropathy, ototoxicity, convulsions and psychiatric disturbances.

Long-term suppressive therapy can cause blurring of vision, confusion, bleaching of hair, myopathy and rarely blood dyscrasias.

Prolonged treatment with high doses can cause **irreversible retinopathy**—as chloroquine accumulates in retina and can result in blindness. Corneal deposits are also known but are reversible (Table 53.1).

Uses

1. *Malaria:* Chloroquine is highly effective in the treatment of malaria due to sensitive strains of all 4 species—chloroquine phosphate 250 mg tablet contains 150 mg base. Dose: CHLOROQUINE 1 g (600 mg base) at 0 followed by 0.5 g at 6, 24 and 48 hr. It is also

Table 53.1: Preferred antimalarials in the treatment and prophylaxis of malaria

Treatment

1. **Uncomplicated chloroquine-sensitive vivax malaria**
   Chloroquine: Oral 1 g (600 mg base) at 0 hr (stat) followed by 0.5 g at 6, 24 and 48 hr or 1 g (4 tabs) at 0 and 24 hr followed by 500 mg (2 tabs) after 48 hr (4+ 4+2 regimen) + Primaquine 15 mg/day for 14 days
2. **Uncomplicated chloroquine-sensitive falciparum malaria**
   Chloroquine (dose as above) + Primaquine 45 mg single dose
3. **Uncomplicated chloroquine-resistant falciparum malaria**
   Treatment choices are:
   a. Artesunate 100 mg BD for 3 days + Pyrimethamine 75 mg, Sulfadoxine 1500 mg—single dose.
   b. Artesunate 100 mg BD for 3 days + Mefloquine 750 mg on day 2 and 500 mg on day 3.
   c. Artemether 80 mg BD + Lumefantrine 480 mg twice a day for 3 days.
   d. Quinine 600 mg TDS for 3 days followed by one of the following:
      Doxycycline 100 mg BD for 7 days or Clindamycin 600 mg BD for 7 days.
   e. Atovaquone 1 g + Proguanil 100 mg daily for 3 days.
4. **Severe or complicated falciparum malaria**
   Treatment choices are:
   i. Artesunate: 2.4 mg/kg IV or IM, followed by 2.4 mg/kg after 12 and 24 hr, and then once daily for 7 days. Switched over to 3 day oral ACT in between whenever the patient can take and tolerate oral medication.
   ii. Artemether 3.2 mg/kg IM on 1st day followed by 1.6 mg/kg daily for next 4 days. Whenever possible switch over to oral artesunate.
   iii. Quinine 20 mg/kg loading dose diluted in dextrose and infused over 4 hr followed by 10 mg/kg maintenance IV over 4 hr thrice daily. Switch over to oral quinine as soon as possible—600 mg TDS for 7 days + Doxycycline 100 mg BD for 7 days or Clindamycin 600 mg BD for 7 days.
5. **Mixed infection (*P. vivax* + *P. falciparum*)**
   Full course of ACT and Primaquine 15 mg/day for 14 days.

Prophylaxis

- *Areas with chloroquine-sensitive strains*
  Chloroquine 2 tabs/ wk; start 1 wk before and continue for 4 wk after leaving the endemic area
- *Areas with chloroquine-resistant P. falciparum like India*
  Choices are:
  1. Mefloquine 250 mg/wk start 1–2 wks before departure and continue for 4 wk after leaving the endemic area
  2. Atovaquone 250 mg + proguanil 100 mg—1 tab daily start 2 days before journey and continue for 1 week after leaving the endemic area.
  3. Doxycycline 100 mg/day start two days before and continue for 4 wk after leaving the endemic area

Terminal prophylaxis

Prophylaxis given to travellers after leaving endemic area to eradicate hypnozoites.
Primaquine 30 mg /day for 14 days after travel.

Based on recommendation by WHO and NVBDCP

used for prophylaxis—300 mg base per week. WHO has simplified the chloroquine regimen as chloroquine 1 g (600 mg dose) at 0, 24 hr and 0.5 g at 48 hr (2-2-1 regimen).

2. Extraintestinal amoebiasis (*see* page 648)
3. Rheumatoid arthritis
4. Photogenic reactions
5. Lepra reactions.
6. Discoid lupus erythematosus
7. Infectious mononucleosis

The rationale for uses listed under 3–7 is the anti-inflammatory action of chloroquine.

Precautions and Contraindications

- Chloroquine should be avoided or used carefully in patients with myopathy and hepatic, gastrointestinal or neurological disorders, psoriasis and porphyria.
- Parenteral administration of chloroquine should be avoided but when required, it should be given as a slow infusion.
- Concurrent use of gold or d-penicillamine with chloroquine can cause more severe dermatitis.
- Chloroquine, quinine and mefloquine should not be given concurrently because they compete for accumulation in the parasite and may result in therapeutic failure. Also, chloroquine + mefloquine increase the risk of seizures.
- Chloroquine + halofantrine → increased risk of arrhythmias. Hence, a gap of at least 12 hours should be given, if patients have to be switched over from chloroquine to quinine/mefloquine/halofantrine.
- Chloroquine should be avoided in patients with retinal diseases. When chloroquine is given in high doses for a long time, regular neurological and eye examination should be done.
- Magnesium containing antacids and kaolin interfere with the absorption of chloroquine— hence concurrent use should be avoided.

Amodiaquine is similar to chloroquine in actions and adverse effects but is somewhat better tolerated. It may be used in uncomplicated falciparum malaria.

QUININE

Quinine (QN) is an alkaloid obtained from the bark of the cinchona tree. The name cinchona probably comes from the name of a Countess *'Chinchon'*— the wife of the Viceroy of Peru who was cured of her fever by quinine in 1638. She introduced quinine to European medicine in 1640. In the next two centuries, quinine enjoyed the place of a popular medicine. It was extensively used for treating the soldiers of their fevers during the world wars. At a particular time, the bark powder was worth its weight in gold. It was grown in many countries including South America, India, Sri Lanka and Java. When the Japanese occupied Java and cut off the world's quinine supply, an extensive research followed and quinine was synthesized.

Actions

Quinine destroys erythrocytic forms of the parasite similar to chloroquine and is useful as a suppressive. It is rapidly acting and is often effective even in chloroquine-resistant strains of *P. falciparum*. It is also gametocytocidal for three species of the malarial parasite except for *P. falciparum*.

Quinidine, the d-isomer of quinine, can be used in place of quinine.

Mechanism of action is not exactly known. Quinine may act like chloroquine by inhibiting the enzyme haeme polymerase. Resistance to quinine is now known in some parts of South East Asia.

Other Actions

- Quinine also has mild analgesic and antipyretic activity.
- Like quinidine, it is a myocardiac depressant. IV administration can cause significant hypotension.
- It has local anaesthetic properties (sodium channel blocker).
- Quinine is a skeletal muscle relaxant.
- Quinine stimulates the uterus and is an abortifacient.

Pharmacokinetics

On oral administration, quinine is rapidly and well absorbed, with peak plasma levels in 1 to 4 hr. It is widely distributed in the body tissues. The half-life of quinine is longer in patients with malaria because of increased protein binding (to alpha 1 acid glycoprotein) in malaria; it also attains higher plasma levels in them. It is metabolized in the liver and excreted in the urine.

Dose: 600 mg TDS 3–7 days.

Adverse Effects

Adverse effects are many and some are serious.

- Quinine is highly bitter and is a gastric irritant—causes nausea, vomiting and epigastric pain—hence poorly tolerated.
- Hypoglycaemia can be quite profound to result in coma. Hypoglycaemic coma should be distinguished from cerebral malaria. Hypoglycaemia may be because:
  i. Quinine stimulates the pancreatic beta cells to release insulin.
  ii. Parasite consumes glucose.
  iii. Decrease in food intake due to malaria.
- Cinchonism with ringing in the ears, high tone deafness, headache, nausea, visual disturbances and vertigo may be encountered.
- Quinine produces neurotoxicity particularly in higher doses and can cause convulsions.
- Quinine can cause hypotension (this can be profound, if injected rapidly), widening of QRS complex, AV block and arrhythmias. Hence constant monitoring of cardiovascular functions is a must while administering quinine intravenously.
- In more severe poisoning, hypoglycaemia, fever, delirium, confusion, hypotension, cardiac arrhythmias and coma may develop. Fatal dose of quinine is 2–8 g. Death is due to respiratory arrest.
- Allergic reactions:
  i. Black water fever—quinine can precipitate acute haemolytic anaemia with renal failure, haemoglobinuria and fever, which can be fatal. Fortunately, this complication is uncommon and is thought to be a hypersensitivity reaction.
  ii. Quinine can also cause skin rashes, urticaria and angioedema. Idiosyncratic reactions where the patient develops symptoms of cinchonism with a single dose of quinine is not very common.

Precautions and Contraindications

1. Intravenous quinine should be injected as slow infusion and cardiac function should be monitored. Quinine should preferably be given orally but in situations where it needs to be given parenterally, adequate monitoring is needed.
2. Hypoglycaemia should be watched for—adequate glucose supplementation should be given.
3. Quinine should never be combined with mefloquine for the risk of cardiotoxicity. If the patient has received mefloquine earlier (even up to 20–30 days) and if quinine is needed, it should be used with great caution.

Uses

1. *Malaria:*
   a. *Uncomplicated falciparum malaria:* Quinine is given orally in the dose of 600 mg TDS for 3–7 days. Doxycycline 100 mg BD for 7 days may be added to reduce the duration of quinine treatment to 3 days.
   b. *Complicated falciparum malaria and cerebral malaria:* As an alternative to artemisinin, quinine is given IV as a slow infusion 15 mg/kg over 4 hr followed by 7.5 mg/kg over 4 hr—three times a day. Quinine is used in the treatment of resistant falciparum malaria and cerebral malaria (Dose: Table 53.1). Quinidine can be used in place of quinine. Quinine is usually given in combination with a second drug like doxycycline in order to shorten the treatment with quinine.
2. *Babesiosis:* A combination of quinine and clindamycin is considered the first line treatment of babesiosis.
3. *Nocturnal muscle cramps:* Low dose quinine-200–300 mg at night relieves nocturnal muscle cramps. However, safer muscle relaxants are now available.
4. *Myotonia congenita:* Quinine is useful in relieving the muscle spasms.

MEFLOQUINE

Mefloquine (MQ) is a quinoline methanol. In a single dose given orally mefloquine is highly effective against erythrocytic forms of the malaria parasite including the multi-drug-resistant (MDR) strains of *P. falciparum.*

Mefloquine gets concentrated in the acidic vacuoles of the parasite. Mechanism of action is not exactly known but it is thought to act like chloroquine by inhibiting heme polymerase in the parasite. Some strains of *P. falciparum* have developed resistance to mefloquine in parts of Asia.

It is well absorbed when given orally and has a long t½ of nearly 20–30 days—as it undergoes extensive enterohepatic circulation; since it causes severe local irritation at the site, it is not given parenterally. It is excreted through the gut.

Dose: 20 mg/kg single dose or in 2 divided doses

Adverse effects: Nausea, vomiting, dizziness, confusion, headache, abdominal pain, sleep disturbances are common. CNS effects like ataxia, disorientation, visual and auditory disturbances, seizures, encephalopathy and psychotic manifestations are rare and reversible, particularly when given IV. Mefloquine can depress cardiac conduction resulting in bradycardia and arrhythmias.

Contraindications

Mefloquine should be avoided in patients with arrhythmias, conduction defects in the heart, epileptics, and in psychiatric patients. Mefloquine should not be combined with quinine and halofantrine.

Though mefloquine is considered safe in pregnancy (based on the information currently available), it may be avoided in first trimester as its safety in first trimester is yet to be proved.

Uses

- Uncomplicated MDR strains of falciparum malaria—mefloquine used with artesunate.
- Prophylaxis of MDR malaria in travellers—mefloquine 250 mg/week.

HALOFANTRINE AND LUMEFANTRINE

Halofantrine and lumefantrine are schizontocidal against erythrocytic forms of all *Plasmodium* species including MDR strains of *P. falciparum.* Actions are similar to mefloquine. They are given orally but absorption is erratic. Food enhances their absorption and are excreted in the stools. The disadvantages are:

- The response to oral dosage is unpredictable due to variable absorption. Toxicity due to good absorption or therapeutic failure due to poor absorption may result. Absorption is enhanced by fatty food.
- Halofantrine cannot be given parenterally—a disadvantage in emergencies.

Adverse effects: Halofantrine can cause gastrointestinal disturbances, headache, rashes, pruritus and cardiotoxicity including prolongation of QT interval and arrhythmias. It is also contraindicated in pregnancy. Lumefantrine is less toxic.

Uses

- Though halofantrine was used as an alternative in MDR strains of falciparum malaria it is now not preferred.
- Artemisinine—lumefantrine is used in the treatment of MDR falciparum malaria and the combination should be given with fatty food to ensure good bioavailability. Lumefantrine is 99% bound to plasma proteins and has a t½ of 3–4 days when given in combination. Though it can cause some prolonged QTc, it is not as profound as halofantrine.

The combination is well tolerated with side effects like gastrointestinal disturbances, headache, dizziness and rashes.

PRIMAQUINE

Primaquine is effective against all forms of the malarial parasite except erythrocytic forms.

- **Causal prophylactic:** It destroys the parasite in the liver cells and prevents the invasion of erythrocytes—but it is generally not used for this purpose.
- **Hypnozoitocide:** Primaquine destroys the hypnozoites (exoerythrocytic form) in the liver and thereby prevents relapse of *P. vivax* and *P. ovale* malaria.
- **Gametocide:** Destroys the gametocytes of all four species of the malarial parasite.
- **Schizontocide:** It has weak activity against the erythrocytic forms.

Mechanism of action of primaquine is not known.

Resistance: In certain parts of South-East Asia and America, relative resistance of some strains of *P. vivax* has been noted. Hence in such areas, the dose of primaquine has been revised to 30 mg (instead of 15 mg) daily for 14 days for radical cure of vivax malaria.

Pharmacokinetics: Primaquine is completely absorbed when given orally and is widely distributed. The metabolites induce haemolysis more than the parent compound.

Adverse effects: Primaquine is well tolerated in therapeutic doses. Epigastric distress can occur.

Most Caucasians tolerate primaquine well. In individuals with **G6PD deficiency**, the therapeutic doses of primaquine can induce **haemolysis**. G6PD deficiency is more common in African-Americans and would require evaluation of G6PD levels before administration of primaquine. Normal erythrocytes have several enzymatic and nonenzymatic mechanisms to protect the membrane from damage due to chemicals and drugs. These mechanisms require G6PD. Primaquine can induce the generation of free radicals and create oxidative stress in G6PD deficient erythrocytes leading to haemolysis.

Dose: 15 mg daily for 14 days. PQUINE 7.5 mg tab. MALIRID, PRIMALAP 7.5, 15 mg tab

Uses

1. *Radical cure of P. vivax and P. ovale malaria:* Primaquine is used for radical cure along with a blood schizonticide in vivax and ovale—it also destroys gametocytes. Dose: 15 mg/day for 14 days.
2. *Gametocidal effects:* Primaquine is used for its gametocidal effect in *P. falciparum* malaria—45 mg single dose.
3. *Terminal prophylaxis:* After a visit to an endemic area (along with regular chloroquine prophylaxis), a course of primaquine is recommended by some workers for prophylaxis to destroy the liver forms and gametocytes—15–30 mg for 14 days. This may be particularly relevant when the exposure is significant.
4. *Chemoprophylaxis of malaria:* As an alternative to mefloquine/doxycycline, primaquine may be used in the dose of 30 mg daily for chemoprophylaxis, found to be effective against vivax and falciparum malaria. Since it has to be given daily, its routine use is not recommended. Available data have shown it to be well tolerated up to 1 year of use (except in G6PD deficiency).
5. *Pnumocystis jiroveci:* In mild to moderate pneumocystosis, as an alternative to cotrimoxazole, a combination of clindamycin with primaquine may be used—better tolerated than cotrimoxazole.

Bulaquine is an analog of primaquine developed in India and is claimed that patients require fewer days (5 days) of antirelapse therapy and is better tolerated when compared to primaquine. However, further extensive clinical trials are required to prove its clinical benefits.

Dose: 25 mg/day for 5 days.

Etaquine and **tafenoquine** are other longer acting analogs of primaquine being tried.

FOLATE ANTAGONISTS

Pyrimethamine

Pyrimethamine related to trimethoprim is effective against the erythrocytic forms of all 4 species of plasmodia but it is slow acting when given alone. Pyrimethamine is combined with **sulfadoxine,** a sulfonamide and the combination acts faster. It is slowly absorbed from the gut, reaches peak levels in 2–6 hr and is bound to plasma proteins. It has a long t ½ of 3.5–4 days thereby permiting once a week administration for prophylaxis.

Mechanism of Action

Pyrimethamine is a dihydrofolate reductase inhibitor. Pyrimethamine preferentially binds plasmodial dihydrofolate reductase with about 2000 times higher affinity than mammalian enzymes (Fig. 53.2). When sulfadoxine is given with pyrimethamine, together they produce sequential blockade resulting in inhibition of nuclear division. This mode of action makes them slow acting. The **combination** (SP) **is synergistic** and the development of resistance is slower. (However, given alone, sulfadoxine has weak activity aganist erythrocytic forms of *P.vivax*.) Pyrimethamine can also be combined with dapsone which acts like sulfonamides.

Resistance *P. falciparum* has to a large extent and *P. vivax* to some extent developed resistance to pyrimethamine + sulfadoxine and the resistance is quite widespread. (However, in Africa, most strains are still susceptible to the combination.) Mutation in DHFR and folate synthetase leads to resistance.

Pyrimethamine is quite safe; the combination may cause nausea, rashes and in high doses megaloblastic anaemia. Sulfadoxine may cause serious allergic reactions including Stevens-Johnson syndrome.

Preparations

- Sulfadoxine 500 mg + Pyrimethamine 25 mg
- Dapsone 100 mg + Pyrimethamine 25 mg

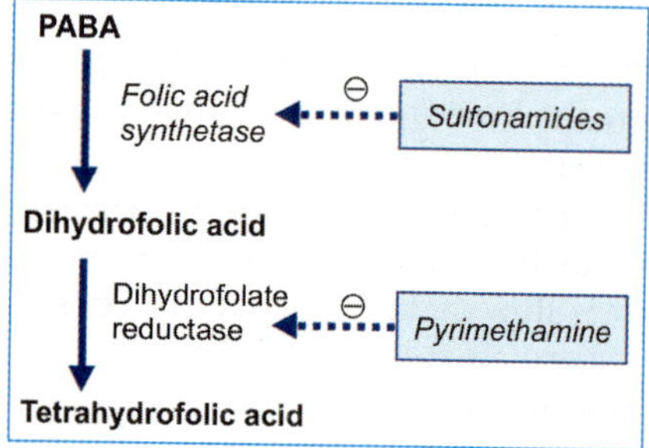

Fig. 53.2: Sequential blockade in folic acid synthesis

Uses

1. *Malaria*
   i. *Treatment:* Sulfadoxine-Pyrimethamine combination is now used with artemisinine derivative in ACT and with quinine.
   Dose: 3 tablets as a single dose.
   ii. *Chemoprophylaxis:* 1–2 tablets once weekly for prophylaxis against MDR falciparum malaria when a person is visiting an endemic area but now not preferred.
   iii. *Intermittent preventive therapy:* In high risk patients including pregnant women, intermittent preventive therapy with 2 or more doses of SP during the second or third trimister is being practiced in Africa.

   Seasonal chemoprophylaxis is considered in areas known to harbour SP-sensitive strains.
2. *Toxoplasmosis:* Sulfadoxine-Pyrimethamine combination is the treatment of choice for *Toxoplasma gondii* infection. Pyrimethamine is given as 200 mg bolus dose followed by 50 mg daily for 4 to 6 weeks along with sulfadoxine 4 g/day. Leucovorin (folinic acid) should be given 10 mg daily to prevent severe folate deficiency.
3. *Pneumocystosis:* Caused by *P. Jiroveci*, pyrimethamine-sulfadoxine combination may be used as an alternative to cotrimoxazole.

CHLOROGUANIDE (PROGUANIL)

Proguanil is a biguanide. It is an erythrocytic schizonticide which also has causal prophylactic activity against the pre-erythrocytic forms of the malaria parasite. The onset of action is slow and when used as monotherapy resistance develops rapidly. Hence, it is always used in combination with atovaquone in malaria.

Mechanism of action: Proguanil, a prodrug, is converted to cycloguanil in the body. This metabolite is an inhibitor of dihydrofolate reductase in the *Plasmodium*.

Adverse effects: Adverse effects are minor including nausea, vomiting, diarrhoea, abdominal pain and rarely haematuria.

Uses

- Along with atovaquone, proguanil is used in the treatment of MDR falciparum malaria (*see* atovaquone).
- For causal prophylaxis of falciparum malaria.
- As an alternative to sulfadoxine-pyrimethamine for the prophylaxis of MDR falciparum malaria.

ATOVAQUONE

Atovaquone is a naphthaquinone, effective against the erythrocytic forms of plasmodia. When combined **with proguanil**, the activity is synergistic and development of resistance is less common.

Mechanism of action: Atovaquone inhibits the mitochondrial electron transport leading to the collapse of the mitochondrial membrane potential in the malarial parasite. Proguanil potentiates this action. Atovaquone also interferes with pyrimidine synthesis in the parasite because pyrimidine (and ATP) synthesis in the parasite is dependent on mitochondrial electron transport.

Atovaquone is also effective against *T. gondii* and *P. jiroveci* infections.

Atovaquone is effective orally, but the bioavailability is low and fatty food increases its absorption. It is extensively bound to plasma proteins and has a long t½ of 2–3 days. It is excreted through the gut.

Adverse effects include vomiting, headache, abdominal pain, diarrhoea, skin rashes and insomnia. Atovaquone is contraindicated in pregnancy.

Uses

1. Atovaquone + Proguanil can be used in the treatment of chloroquine-resistant and MDR falciparum malaria. Atovaquone 250 mg + proguanil 100 mg 4 tabs daily for three days—it is not used in India.
2. Atovaquone 250 mg + Proguanil 100 mg may be used for chemoprophylaxis of falciparum malaria (one tablet daily).
3. Atovaquone may also be used in *P. jiroveci* infection as an alternative to cotrimoxazole—750 mg BD with food for 3 weeks.

ARTEMISININ AND DERIVATIVES

Artemisinin

Artemisinin, a highly bitter compound, is a sesquiterpene lactone obtained from the plant *Artemisia annua* which has been used in the Chinese traditional medicine 'Quinghaosu' for almost 2000 years. Several semisynthetic analogs have been obtained with better efficacy and improved pharmacokinetic profile including—**artesunate, dihydroarte-**

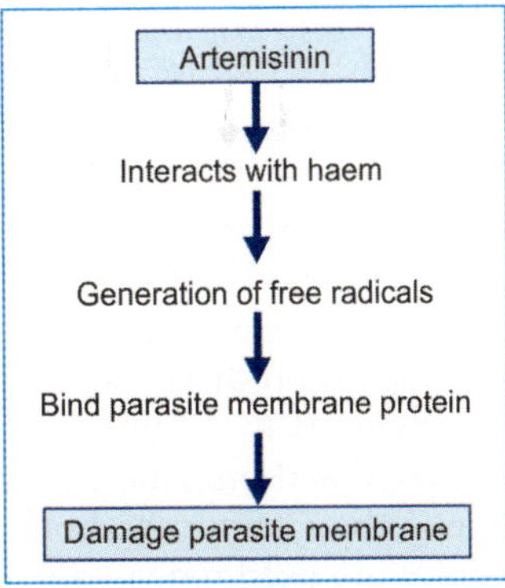

misinin, artemether and arteether. Artemisinin derivatives are now the first line drugs in the treatment of falciparum malaria.

Mechanism of action: Artemisinin interacts with haem resulting in the generation of free radicals that bind to the macromolecules as well as membrane proteins and damage the macromolecules and the parasite membrane. It could also inhibit calcium ATPase in the parasite. Though resistance does not develop readily, strains of *P. falciparum* which are less susceptible to artemether and treatment failures have been reported. Hence **monotherapy with these drugs should be avoided**.

Actions: Artemisinin is a potent, rapidly acting, erythrocytic schizonticide effective against all the 5 plasmodial species, including MDR *P. falciparum*. It is also effective against gametocytes (but not the liver stages). It is useful in cerebral malaria. No resistant strains are known so far. Recrudescence is common due to its short t½. Combining with mefloquine avoids this. Though artemisinin is thought to be safe in pregnancy, it has been shown to be teratogenic in animals.

Artemisinin has activity against other organisms like *T. gondii, Leishmania major* and *schistosomes.*

Pharmacokinetics: Artemisinin is poorly soluble in water and oil. The derivatives are suitable for administration by different routes.

- Artesunate—water soluble—oral, IM, IV, rectal.
- Artemether—lipid soluble—oral, IM and rectal.
- Dihydroartemisinin—water soluble—oral.
- Arteether—longer—IM.

Oral bioavailability of artemisinin compounds is poor (<30%) but they are rapidly absorbed. Artemisinin and artemether may be considered prodrugs because both of them are converted to dihydroartemisinin; they are microsomal enzyme inducers and both enhance their own metabolism when multiple doses are used repeatedly.

Adverse Effects

Artemisinin and its derivatives are the **best tolerated antimalarials**—mild gastrointestinal symptoms, fever, and bradycardia are reported—these could be due to malaria itself. They can also cause itching, rashes, other allergic reactions and rarely raised serum transaminases. Bone marrow toxicity with anaemia, haemolysis, neutropenia and decrease in reticulocyte count are rare and reversible. Though artemisinin compounds are embryotoxic in animals, studies have not shown any such toxicity in human subjects. Hence artemisinin can be used in pregnant women during the 2nd and 3rd trimesters.

Dose: Artesunate; Oral 100 mg BD on first day and 50 mg BD for the next 4 days. IV 120 mg on the first day and 60 mg daily for the next 4 days; Mefloquine (25 mg/kg) is given on the second day. ARNET, ARTESA, ARTESTAR 50 mg tab. 60 mg inj.

Artemisinin Orally 100 mg BD on first day, 50 mg next 4 days.

Artemisinin-based Combination Therapy

Artemisinin-based combination therapy (ACT) is the WHO recommended treatment for all confirmed cases of falciparum malaria.

In the treatment of chloroquine/MDR falciparum malaria, when compared to monotherapy with any of the antimalarials, combination of drugs has been shown to have:

- Rapid action
- Better efficacy
- High cure rates
- Reduced risk of development of resistance
- Fewer toxic effects and thereby better tolerated
- In some cases, shorter duration of treatment.

Hence, WHO now recommends the use of combination of drugs and has particularly listed some ACT regimens to be used in falciparum malaria. Such combination regimens are better tolerated. Artemisinin compounds act quickly to produce rapid clinical response and parasite clearance. However, they have a short t½ and this is compensated by the addition of a second drug like mefloquine, lumefantrine or pyrimethamine-sulfadoxine. For uncomplicated MDR falciparum malaria, drugs are given orally while for complicated and severe infections parenteral regimens are recommended. Intravenous artesunate is highly effective and reduces mortality in severe falciparum malaria and is, therefore, preferred over quinine in such patients. Some of them are:

1. Artesunate-sulfadoxine + pyrimethamine (AS + SP)
2. Artemether + lumefantrine (AL)
3. Artesunate + mefloquine (AS-MQ)
4. Artesunate + Amodiaquine (AS + AQ)
5. Dihydroartemisinin + piperaquine (DHA + PPQ)

Pyronaridine was synthesized in China. It is effective against erythrocytic forms of the malaria parasite.

ANTIBIOTICS IN MALARIA

- **Tetracycline** has weak activity against erythrocytic forms of the malaria parasites.
- **Doxycycline** is used along with quinine or artesunate in the treatment of falciparum malaria. Doxycycline can also be used in the chemoprophylaxis of falciparum malaria.
- **Sulfadoxine** is used in combination with pyrimethamine.
- **Clindamycin** has activity against erythrocytic forms of the malarial parasite—may be used as an alternative to doxycycline following administration of quinine or artemisinin.
- **Fluoroquinolones** and **azithromycin** have also been found to have antimalarial activity.

MALARIA IN PREGNANCY

1. *P. vivax* malaria—chloroquine
2. *P. falciparum* malaria
   a. *Uncomplicated:*
      - 1st trimester—quinine + clindamycin (7 days)
      - 2nd and 3rd trimesters—ACT (artemether + lumefantrine)

      Alternatives
      1. ACT with mefloquine
      2. Quinine

   b. *Complicated:* ACT

Immunity in malaria: People residing in an endemic area can develop antibodies to erythrocytic forms of the malaria parasite. Immunity infact can be both humoral and cell-mediated. Immunity is specific to the species and strain prevalent in that particular area.

Recommended drugs for treatment of malaria in India (as per NVBDCP)

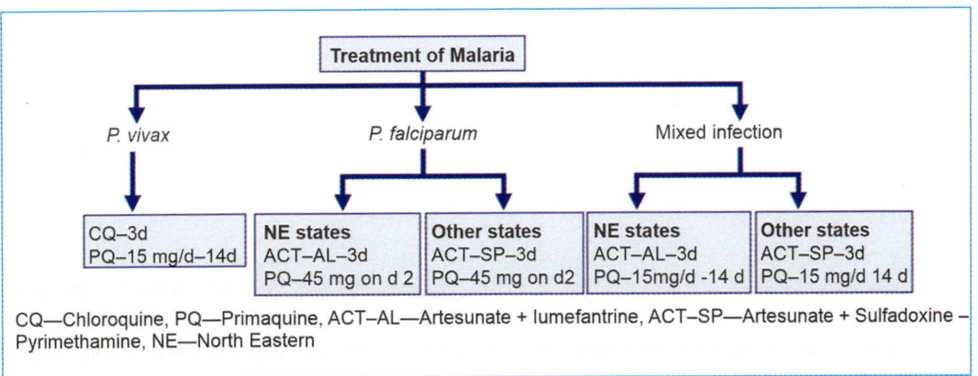

CQ—Chloroquine, PQ—Primaquine, ACT–AL—Artesunate + lumefantrine, ACT–SP—Artesunate + Sulfadoxine – Pyrimethamine, NE—North Eastern

Immunity could be the reason why many people do not suffer from malaria though they live in an endemic area. Passive immunity with IgG antibodies has shown to be effective in children. The transfer of maternal antibodies protects the infants from the disease up to a few months of life. If a person who has acquired immunity to malaria is away from the endemic area for a period of 6–12 months, his immunity is lost.

Malaria vaccine: Vaccines have been developed against the different stages of the parasite, viz sporozoite vaccine, merozoite vaccine and gametocyte vaccine. Studies are on to evaluate the efficacy of vaccines in malaria. Presence of multiple strains of the malaria parasite has been a major problem in the development of an effective vaccine for malaria.

Clinical Pharmacology

- *P. falciparum* attacks RBCs of all ages resulting in severe malaria and severe anaemia which can be fatal.
- Most antimalarials including chloroquine and quinine do not destroy gametocytes of *P. falciparum*. Hence patients with *P. falciparum* need primaqune 45 mg single dose to destroy the gametocytes and prevent the spread of malaria.
- Hepatic forms of *P. falciparum* and *P. malariae* rupture simultaneously and no hypnozoites.
- Both mefloquine and halofantrine are effective only orally—a problem in severely ill patients.
- Presumptive treatment with chloroquine is no more recommended.
- WHO now recommends ACT for most forms of malaria except uncomplicated, chloroquine-sensitive strains.
- ACT regimens have better efficacy and are better tolerated.

[1] From Medical Council of India, *Competency based Undergraduate Curriculum for the Indian Medical Graduate*, 2018;1:136–144.

Drugs used in Amoebiasis, Pneumocystosis, Leishmaniasis (Kala-Azar) and Trypanosomiasis

CHAPTER **54**

Competency achievement: The student should be able to:

PH 1.47 Describe the mechanisms of action, types, doses, side effects, indications and contraindications of the drugs used in malaria, **Kala-Azar**, **amebiasis** and intestinal helminthiasis .[1]

DRUGS USED IN AMOEBIASIS

Amoebiasis caused by the protozoan *Entamoeba histolytica* is a tropical disease common in developing countries. It spreads by faecal contamination of food and water. Though it primarily affects colon, other organs like liver, lungs and brain are the secondary sites. Acute amoebiasis is characterised by bloody mucoid stools and abdominal pain. Chronic amoebiasis manifests as anorexia, abdominal pain, intermittent diarrhoea and constipation. Cyst passers or carriers are usually symptom free—they are asymptomatic carriers.

Classification

1. **Drugs effective in both intestinal and extra-intestinal amoebiasis**
   Nitroimidazoles: Metronidazole, tinidazole, secnidazole, ornidazole, satranidazole
   Alkaloids: Emetine, dehydroemetine.
2. **Drugs effective only in intestinal amoebiasis (Luminal amoebicides)**
   Diloxanide furoate, Nitazoxanide, quiniodochlor, iodoquinol, tetracyclines, paromomycin.
3. **Drugs effective only in extraintestinal amoebiasis**
   Chloroquine.

Metronidazole

Metronidazole, a nitroimidazole, is a powerful amoebicide. It is amoebicidal, kills the trophozoites and is effective in both intestinal and extraintestinal amoebiasis. Apart from this, it also inhibits *Trichomonas vaginalis, Giardia lamblia and Balantidium coli.*

Anaerobic bacteria are also sensitive to metronidazole. Other actions include—radiosensitization, mutagenesis, and depressed CMI.

Mechanism of Action

Metronidazole is a prodrug. Susceptible microorganisms including anaerobic bacteria and certain protozoa reduce the nitro group of metronidazole by **a nitroreductase** and convert it to a cytotoxic derivative. This derivative binds to DNA and inhibits protein synthesis. **Aerobic bacteria lack this nitroreductase** and are, therefore, not susceptible to metronidazole.

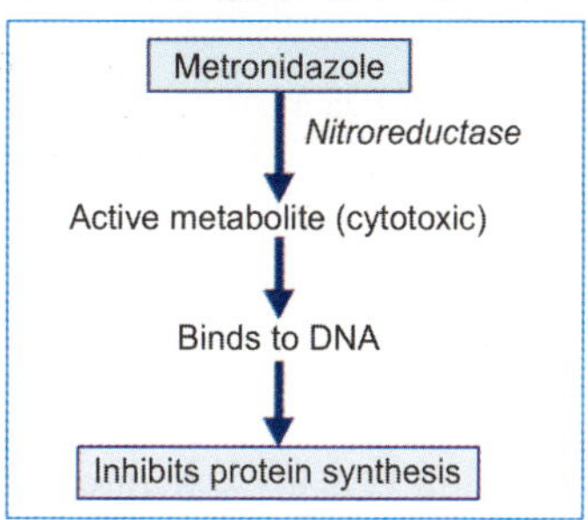

Pharmacokinetics

Metronidazole is well-absorbed, is widely distributed, penetrates all tissues and reaches adequate concentrations in the CSF. It has a plasma t½ of 8 hr. It is metabolised in the liver by oxidation and glucuronide conjugation.

Dose: 400–800 mg TDS FLAGYL 200, 400 mg tab, 200 mg/5 ml suspension.

Adverse Effects

Gastrointestinal effects like nausea, anorexia, abdominal pain and metallic taste in the mouth are the most frequent. Headache, stomatitis, glossitis, furry tongue; dizziness, insomnia, ataxia, vertigo and rarely, on IV use, peripheral neuropathy can occur. Pruritus, urticaria and skin rashes can also occur. High doses given IV can cause convulsions. Hence, metronidazole should be cautiously used in patients with neurological diseases and severe hepatic dysfunction. On long-term administration, metronidazole is carcinogenic in mice though such an effect is not yet seen in human beings. However, it is contraindicated in pregnancy. Intravenous injection can cause thrombophlebitis. This can be avoided by adequate dilution of the drug solution.

Drug Interactions

- Metronidazole can produce a **disulfiram-like reaction** in patients taking alcohol. Hence patients should be advised to avoid alcohol while on metronidazole.
- Drugs like cimetidine which are microsomal enzyme inhibitors, enhance the plasma levels of metronidazole resulting in toxicity.

Dose: 400–800 mg TDS. FLAGYL, METROGYL 200, 400 mg tablets; 200 mg/5 ml suspension; 500 mg/100 ml inj and 1% gel and ointment.

Uses

1. *Amoebiasis:* Metronidazole is the drug of choice in all forms of amoebiasis in the dose of 400–800 mg TDS for 7–10 days but it does not eradicate the cysts.
2. *Trichomonas vaginitis:* Metronidazole 200 mg TDS for 7 days or a single 2 g dose is the drug of choice (Table 54.1).
3. *Giardiasis:* Metronidazole given 200 mg TDS for 7 days is the treatment of choice.
4. *Anaerobic infections:* Metronidazole is given intravenously for serious anaerobic infections. It is also useful for surgical prophylaxis of abdominal and pelvic infections. It is particularly useful in *C. difficile* enteritis.

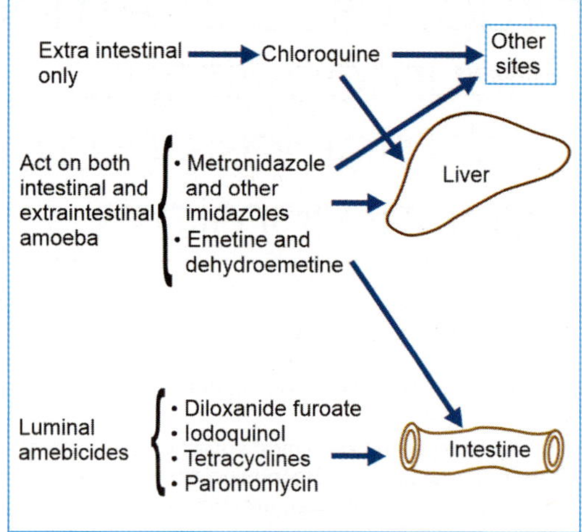

Fig. 54.1: Sites of action of antiamoebic drugs

5. *H. pylori infections:* In peptic ulcer patients, *H. pylori infection* can be treated with a combination of metronidazole, clarithromycin and omeprazole/ranitidine.
6. *Pseudomembranous colitis:* Due to *Clostridium difficile,* responds to metronidazole. 250–500 mg TDS for 7 to 14 days is the preferred line of treatment. Oral vancomycin is the alternative.
7. *Acute ulcerative gingivitis:* Metronidazole can be used as an alternative to penicillin G.
8. *Dracunculosis:* Metronidazole facilitates extraction of the guinea worm.
9. *Topical preparations:* 1% Gel is used in skin infections and acne.

Tinidazole is **longer-acting** and is **better tolerated** than metronidazole due to lesser side effects. It can be given 2 g once daily for 3 days in amoebiasis and as a single dose for most other indications of metronidazole.

Dose: 2 g OD AMEBA, MAGMA, TINIBA 300 mg tab.

Secnidazole is longer-acting and can be given as a **single 2 g dose** for most indications of metronidazole.

Dose: 2 g. AMBIFORM 500 mg, 1 g tab.

Table 54.1: Drugs used in giardiasis and trichomoniasis

Drugs of choice	*Route*	*Dose*	
Giardiasis	Metronidazole/tinidazole	Oral	250 mg TDS for 5 days
	(or other nitroimidazoles)	Oral	2 g single dose
	Alternative drugs		
	1. Secnidazole	Oral	2 g single dose
	2. Furazolidone	Oral	100 mg QID for 7 days
	3. Nitazoxanide	Oral	500 mg BD for 3 days
	4. Albendazole	Oral	400 mg OD for 5 days
Trichomoniasis	Metronidazole	Oral	2 g single dose
	Tinidazole	Oral	2 g single dose
	Secnidazole	Oral	2 g single dose
	Alternative drugs		
	1. Clotrimazole	Vaginal	100 mg vaginal pessary for 6–12 days
	2. Hamycin	Vaginal	4–8 lakh units/day vaginal pessary for 15 days
	3. Diiodohydroxyquinoline	Vaginal	200 mg vaginal pessary for 1–2 weeks
	4. Quiniodochlor	Vaginal	200 mg vaginal pessary for 1–3 weeks

Ornidazole is longer acting with a t½ of 12–14 hr. Other aspects including dose is similar to tinidazole.

Dose: 2 g ORNI, ZIL 500 mg tab

Satranidazole is more potent than tinidazole and also does not cause disulfiram-like antabuse reactions. It is better tolerated as it is unlikely to cause nausea, metallic taste and peripheral neuropathy.

SATRANIDAZOLE 300 mg FC-tab

Benznidazole is also effective in American typanosomiasis and needs to be given for a long time, 5–7 mg/kg in 2 divided doses for 60–90 days. Other effects and pharmacokinetic profile are similar to tinidazole.

Nimorazole has actions and efficacy similar to metronidazole.

Emetine and Dehydroemetine

Emetine is an alkaloid, derived from Ipecac (Brazil root) while dehydroemetine is a semi-synthetic analog. They directly affect the trophozoites but not the cysts. As oral absorption is improper, they are given parenterally (SC or IM but not IV). Emetine or dehydroemetine can be used only in severe amoebiasis for 3–5 days in patients in whom metronidazole cannot be used but are generally not preferred due to toxicity. Adverse effects include pain at the injection site, thrombophlebitis, nausea, vomiting and diarrhoea. Cardiotoxicity including arrhythmias, hypotension and cardiac failure can occur. These drugs should be avoided in patients with cardiac dysfunction. Dehydroemetine is preferred over emetine as adverse effects are milder.

Diloxanide Furoate

Diloxanide furoate is directly amoebicidal. It is split in the intestines to diloxanide and furoic acid. It acts on the parasite in the intestines but not in the tissues.

Diloxanide is metabolised by conjugation. It is given orally—500 mg TDS for 10 days. It is also available in combination with metronidazole. Flatulence, nausea and occasionally abdominal cramps and rashes can occur.

Uses

With amoebicide: Diloxanide is used along with a nitroimidazole for the cure of amoebiasis, as diloxanide eradicates cysts.

Eradication of cysts: It can be used alone in asymptomatic cyst passers, mild intestinal amoebiasis.

Dose: 500 mg TDS DYRADE-M-500 mg.

Nitazoxanide

Nitazoxanide is a congener of niclosamide effective against *E. histolytica, T. vaginalis,* Giardia and also some intestinal helminths like *Ascaris* and *H. nana*. Nitazoxanide and its active metabolite interfere with the PFOR enzyme-dependent electron transfer reaction in anaerobic metabolism.

Given orally, nitazoxanide is rapidly converted to tizoxanide which is highly protein bound (>99%) and is metabolized in the liver.

It is well tolerated as adverse effects are rare. It imparts a **greenish tint to the urine**; should be avoided in pregnancy.

Uses

Nitazoxanide is indicated in giardiasis, diarrhoea due to cryptosporidia, *C. parvum, H. nana, Ascaris, T. trichura* and *E. vermicularis.*

Dose: 500 mg BD for 3 days. NITACURE, NITARID 200, 500 mg tab, 100 mg/5 ml dry syrup.

Iodoquinol and Quiniodochlor

These 8-hydroxyquinolines are directly acting luminal amoebicides. The exact mechanism of action is not known. They are effective orally. Adverse effects include headache, nausea, vomiting, abdominal pain and diarrhoea. Iodine present in these compounds may result in thyroid enlargement, pruritus and skin rashes. Prolonged use of some of these compounds like clioquinol can produce neurotoxicity including subacute myelo-optic neuropathy in which there may be an irreversible loss of vision.

Iodoquinol appears to be safe at therapeutic doses and can be used for asymptomatic amoebiasis—requires treatment for 20 days. However, diloxanide furoate which is safer and needs shorter duration of administration (10 days) is now preferred.

Paromomycin is an aminoglycoside antibiotic given orally. It is poorly absorbed from the gut and acts as an intestinal amoebicide. Adverse effects are mild and include diarrhoea and abdominal discomfort. Paromomycin is used as a luminal amoebicide.

Tetracyclines: The older tetracyclines, like chlortetracycline, are not well-absorbed and large amounts reach the colon—hence these are useful in intestinal amoebiasis. They inhibit the intestinal flora and break the symbiosis between them and the amoebae. Tetracyclines are used as adjuvants in chronic cases.

Chloroquine attains high concentration in the liver, is directly toxic against trophozoites and is, therefore, useful in hepatic amoebiasis. As chloroquine is completely absorbed from the small intestines, it is not effective against amoebae in the colon. It is used (300 mg base/ day for 21 days) as an alternative to metronidazole in hepatic amoebiasis. A luminal amoebicide should also be given.

Treatment of Different Forms of Amoebiasis

1. *Acute intestinal amoebiasis:* One of the following can be given.
   - *Metronidazole* 400–800 mg TDS for 5–7 days or 2.4 g OD for 3 days
   - *Tinidazole* 2 g OD for 3 days or
   - *Secnidazole* 2 g single dose

   Alternatively ornidazole/satranidazole/ benznidazole may be used. All of the above should be followed by diloxanide furoate 500 mg TDS for 10 days to eradicate the cysts.
2. *Chronic amoebiasis and asymptomatic cyst passers:* Diloxanide furoate 500 mg TDS for 10 days or tetracycline 250 mg qid for 10 days. The alternatives are iodoquinol (650 mg TDS for 21 days) or paromomycin (10 mg/kg TDS for 7 days).
3. *Hepatic amoebiasis:* Requires intensive treatment for the complete eradication of the parasite from the liver in order to avoid relapses. A course of metronidazole 600–800 mg TDS for 10 days or tinidazole are

the first-line drugs. In addition, chloroquine may be given to ensure complete destruction of the liver forms. A course of diloxanide furoate 500 mg TDS for 10 days should follow in order to eradicate the cysts.

TREATMENT OF PNEUMOCYSTOSIS

Pneumocystis jiroveci is a micro-organism having features of both protozoa and fungi though now considered to be a fungus. Recent studies have shown that pneumocystosis in human beings is caused by *Pneumcystis jiroveri* while *P.carinii* causes pneumocystosis in animals. It is now known to cause opportunistic infections particularly pneumonia in patients with AIDS which can often be fatal.

Drugs used in the treatment of pneumocystosis include:

- *Cotrimoxazole:* High oral dose of trimethoprim 20 mg/kg + sulphamethoxazole 75 mg/kg daily in 3–4 divided doses to be continued for 21 days. Folinic acid should be added to prevent toxicity.
- *Pentamidine:* 4 mg/kg daily for 14 days parenterally.
- *Atovaquone:* As an alternative to cotrimoxazole.
- *Pyrimethamine-sulfadoxine:* It is an alternative. The combination may also be used for chemoprophylaxis against *P. jiroveci* in immunocompromised patients—one DS tab/day.

TREATMENT OF LEISHMANIASIS

Leishmaniasis is caused by protozoa of the genus leishmania. **Kala-azar** or visceral leishmaniasis is caused by *Leishmania donovani;* oriental sore by *L. tropica* and mucocutaneous leishmaniasis by *L. braziliensis.* The infection is transmitted by the bite of the female sandfly phlebotomus. It is endemic in Bihar.

Drugs used in leishmaniasis include

Antimony compounds	Sodium stibogluconate Meglumine antimonate
Diamidines	Pentamidine
Other drugs	Amphotericin B, ketoconazole, Miltefosine, allopurinol, paromomycin.

Antimony Compounds

Sodium stibogluconate a pentavalent antimonial is the most effective drug in kala-azar. It is also effective in mucocutaneous and cutaneous leishmaniasis. It is given as a 4% solution in the dose of 10–20 mg/kg IM (gluteal region) or IV for 20 days. Mechanism of action is unknown.

Adverse effects include a metallic taste in the mouth, nausea, vomiting, diarrhoea, headache, myalgia, arthralgia, pain at the injection site, bradycardia, skin rashes, haematuria and jaundice. Some cases of sudden death due to shock have occurred. ECG should be monitored as arrhythmias can occur during the later days of therapy.

Though sodium stibogluconate is quite effective, resistance has been encountered in endemic areas like Bihar and, therefore, miltefosine and amphotericin are more commonly used presently.

Meglumine antimonate and **ethyl stibamine** can also be used in all forms of leishmaniasis.

Pentamidine is an aromatic diamidine effective against *Leishmania donovani,* trypanosomes, *Pneumocystis jiroveci* and some fungi. Given intramuscularly the drug is rapidly absorbed but very little reaches the CNS.

Dose: 4 mg/kg deep IM/slow IV on alternate days for 5–25 weeks.

Adverse effects: Pentamidine **liberates histamine** which is responsible for vomiting, diarrhoea, flushing, pruritis, rashes, tachycardia and hypotension apart from pain at the injection site. Other effects include hepatotoxicity, renal impairment, ECG changes and in some patients diabetes mellitus may be precipitated.

Uses

1. *Leishmaniasis:* Pentamidine can be used in kala-azar as an alternative to sodium stibogluconate.

2. *Trypanosomiasis* (sleeping sickness): Pentamidine can be used as an alternative to suramin or along with suramin in trypanosomiasis. It can also be used for chemoprophylaxis against African trypanosomiasis.
3. *Pneumocystosis:* Pentamidine is an alternative in *Pneumocystis jiroveci* infections in patients unable to tolerate cotrimoxazole.

Miltefosine

Miltefosine is the first drug that can be used orally in leishmaniasis. It has a high efficacy against both visceral and cutaneous leishmaniasis. It is effective also in leishmania resistant to stibogluconate. It is approved for use in India in visceral leishmaniasis—700 mg/kg/day for 4 weeks. Miltefosine is safe—vomiting and diarrhoea are common while raised liver enzymes and creatinine are reversible. It is contraindicated in pregnancy.

Other Drugs

Amphotericin B has been tried in leishmaniasis in the endemic areas where antimonials may be ineffective.

Ketoconazole inhibits ergosterol synthesis in the leishmania and is effective in cutaneous leishmaniasis.

Allopurinol (*see* page 174): In leishmania, allopurinol is converted to a metabolite which inhibits protein synthesis. It may be used along with antimonials.

Dose: 300 mg 3–4 times a day for 2–4 weeks.

Paromomycin (aminosidine) is an amoebicidal, aminoglycoside drug which is also found to be effective in leishmaniasis. It is useful in all forms of leishmaniasis. It can be used alone or in combination with antimonials.

Drugs for Oriental Sore (Dermal leishmaniasis)

Sodium stibogluconate may be injected around the sore: 2 ml solution containing 200 mg is infiltrated. Alternatively, paromomycin ointment may be applied topically on the sore.

TREATMENT OF TRYPANOSOMIASIS

Trypanosomiasis is caused by protozoa of the genus Trypanosoma. African trypanosomiasis or sleeping sickness is caused by *T. gambiense* and *T. rhodesiense* while South American trypanosomiasis is caused by *T. cruzi.* Drugs used in trypanosomiasis are suramin, pentamidine, melarsoprol, eflornithine, nifurtimox and benznidazole.

Suramin sodium is the drug of choice for early stages of trypanosomiasis. It does not cross the BBB and, therefore, cannot be used in later stages of the disease. It is also useful for the prophylaxis but pentamidine is preferable. Suramin is given IV; it is extensively bound to plasma proteins and may be traced for nearly 3 months in the plasma. Suramin is also effective in eradicating adult forms of *Onchocerca volvulus*.

Toxicity is high; vomiting, shock and loss of consciousness may follow IV injections. Rash, neuropathies, haemolytic anaemia and agranulocytosis may also occur.

Melarsoprol is the preferred drug in later stages of trypanosomiasis which is associated with encephalitis and meningitis.

Eflornithine is used as an alternative in CNS trypanosomiasis. **Nifurtimox** and **benznidazole** are useful in Chagas' disease (American trypanosomiasis).

Clinical Pharmacology

- Metallic taste is a common complaint while on metronidazole.
- Single dose preparations of secnidazole, tinidazole and ornidazole are preferred.
- Metronidazole (or any other imidazole) is the first-line drug in anaerobic infections.
- In pneumocystosis, folinic acid should be given with high dose cotrimoxazole.

[1] From Medical Council of India, *Competency based Undergraduate Curriculum for the Indian Medical Graduate*, 2018;1:136–144.

CHAPTER 55

Anthelmintics and Drugs used in Scabies and Pediculosis

Competency achievement: The student should be able to:

PH 1.47 Describe the mechanisms of action, types, doses, side effects, indications and contraindications of the drugs used in malaria, Kala-Azar, amebiasis and **intestinal helminthiasis.**[1]

Worm infestations are more common in the developing countries. It is seen in people with poor hygiene. Anthelmintics are deworming agents. A **vermicidal** kills while a **vermifuge** promotes expulsion of worms. Several deworming agents are now available and it is possible to successfully treat many worm infestations.

BENZIMIDAZOLES

Benzimidazoles include thiabendazole, mebendazole and albendazole. Thiabendazole the first agent of this group was discovered in 1961 but now the newer ones, mebendazole and albendazole are more commonly used due to milder toxicity and better anthelmintic effect.

Mebendazole

Mebendazole a broad-spectrum anthelmintic cures roundworm, hookworm, pinworm and strongyloides infestations. The eggs and larvae are also destroyed. The dead parasites are slowly expelled from the gut over several days.

Mechanism of action: Benzimidazoles bind to β-tubulin of the parasite with high affinity (~400 times more than for humans) and inhibit the synthesis of microtubules. These microtubules are essential for several metabolic processes in the parasite. Benzimidazoles also inhibit glucose uptake in the parasite (*see* Fig. 55.1).

Pharmacokinetics: Mebendazole is poorly absorbed (10%) from the gut and also undergoes first pass metabolism. Fatty food enhances absorption. Mebendazole is extensively bound to plasma proteins and is metabolised by the liver.

Dose: 100 mg BD for 3 days or 500 mg single dose, HELMINTOL, MEBAZOLE 100 mg tab

Adverse effects: Mebendazole is well-tolerated; nausea, abdominal pain and diarrhoea may be seen in heavy infestations. Large doses may cause headache, dizziness, loss of hair and granulocytopenia. Rarely, it may provoke abnormal migration of the roundworms which may come out through the mouth or nose. It should be avoided in pregnancy and in children <2 yr.

Uses

Mebendazole is used in the treatment of roundworm, hookworm, pinworm, tapeworm, trichuriasis and hydatid disease. It is of special value in multiple worm infestations (Table 55.1).

Albendazole

Albendazole a congener of mebendazole is a broad-spectrum anthelmintic. It is a prodrug and the active metabolite (albendazole sulfoxide) has good efficacy against roundworm, hookworm, pinworm, threadworm,

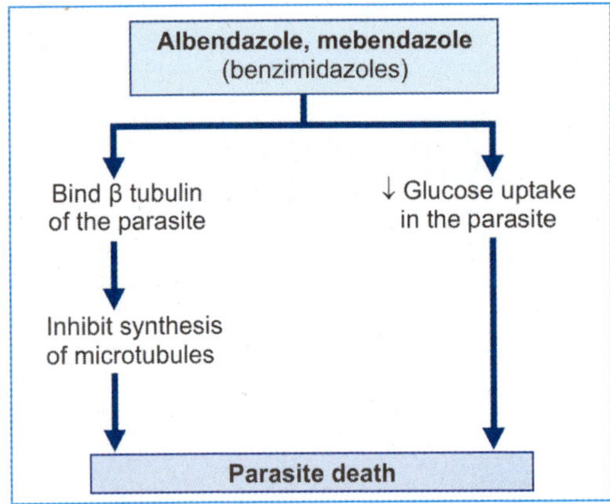

Fig. 55.1: Mechanism of action

tapeworm and trichuriasis. It is also useful in hydatic disease as the active metabolite penetrates the hydatic cyst. Albendazole has actions and mechanism of action similar to mebendazole but it has several advantages over mebendazole because of which it is the preferred benzimidazole.

Advantages Over Mebendazole

- The active metabolite of albendazole achieves a higher concentration (100 times more) than mebendazole.
- Albendazole is better tolerated.
- Effective in single dose in most infections.
- Superior to mebendazole in hookworm and threadworm infections, hydatid disease and neurocysticercosis.
- Albendazole also has some activity against *Trichomonas vaginalis, Giardia lamblia* and *W. bancrofti.*

Pharmacokinetics

Albendazole is rapidly absorbed from the gut and **fatty food enhances its absorption.** Hence it should be given on an empty stomach for treating intestinal worms while for parasites in the tissues, albendazole is given with a fatty meal. It penetrates well into tissues including CSF and hydatid cyst. It is rapidly metabolised in the liver and excreted in urine.

ZENTEL, BANDY 400 mg chewable tab, 200 mg/5 ml susp.

Table 55.1: Preferred drugs for helminthiasis infections

	Worms	*Drugs of choice*	*Alternative drugs*
1.	Roundworm *(Ascaris lumbricoides)*	Mebendazole/albendazole/pyrantel	Piperazine
2.	Hookworms *(Ancylostoma duodenale, Necator americanus)*	Mebendazole/albendazole	Pyrantel
3.	Pinworm *(Enterobius vermicularis)*	Mebendazole/albendazole/pyrantel	Piperazine
4.	Whipworm *(Trichuris trichura)*	Mebendazole	Albendazole
5.	*Threadworm (Strongyloides stercoralis)*	Albendazole	Thiabendazole
6.	Guineaworm *(Dracunculus medinensis)*	Metronidazole	Mebendazole
7.	Tapeworms *(Taenia saginata, Taenia solium, H. nana, D. latum)*	Niclosamide/praziquantel	Albendazole
	Neurocysticercosis	Albendazole	Praziquantel
8.	Hydatid disease *(E. granulosus, E. multilocularis)*	Albendazole	Mebendazole
9.	Filaria *(Wuchereria bancrofti, Brugia malayi)*	Diethylcarbamazine + albendazole	Ivermection + albendazole
10.	Schistosomes	Praziquantel	—
11.	*Onchocerca volvulus*	Ivermectin	—
12.	*Fasciola hepatica* (Sheep liver fluke)	Bithionol	—

Table 55.2: Salient features of anthelminthics

Drug	*MOA*	*Uses*	*Other salient features*
Albendazole } Mebendazole	Bind tubulin → inhibit microtubules ↓ parasite death	Roundworm, Pinworm, Hookworm, Tapeworm, Trichuriasis, Stongyloidosis Neurocysticercosis	ABZ taken on: Empty stomach → for intestinal worms With fatty food → for tissue parasites
Pyrantel pamoate	Depolarizing NMB → ↓cholinesterase enzyme →Expels paralyzed worms	Roundworm, Hookworm, Pinworm	Repeat dose after 2 weeks for pinworm
Piperazine citrate	GABA receptor agonist→ flaccid paralysis → worms expelled	Roundworm, Pinworm	To be avoided with pyrantel
Levamisole	Paralyses the worms → expelled	Roundworm, Hookworm	Immunomodulator
Niclosamide	Stimulation of ATPase activity	Tapeworms: *T solium, T sagina, H nana and D latum*	Alternative to ABZ
Praziquantel	↓cell membrane permeability to Ca^{++} → contraction followed by paralysis → worms expelled	Schistosomiasis Tapeworms Neurocysticercosis Other flukes (TONS mnemonic)	Contraindication Ocular cysticercosis
Diethylcarbamazine (DEC)	Immobilizes microfilaria, alters their surface structure → Susceptible to host defence	Filariasis Tropical eosinophilia Loa loa	Contraindications: • Onchocerciasis • Severe reaction
Ivermectin	Binds glutamate gated chloride channel → ↓ permeability of cell membrane to chloride ions → hyperpolarization of neuronal membrane → paralysis	Onchocerciasis, lymphatic filariasis, strongyloidiasis, cutaneous larva migrans, Ascariasis, Scabies, Lice infestation	Mazotti reaction Avoid with other drugs acting on GABA

ABZ: Albendazole; NMB: Neuromuscular Blocker

Adverse Effects

Adverse effects are minor and similar to mebendazole. Nausea, diarrhoea, abdominal pain, headache, dizziness and allergic reactions can occur. High doses used over a long time can cause jaundice, fever, weakness, alopecia and granulocytopenia. Albendazole is teratogenic in animals and, therefore, should not be given in pregnancy.

Uses

1. *Roundworm, pinworm:* Albendazole is the drug of choice in roundworm, and pinworm infestations in a single dose of 400 mg. Dose should be repeated after 2 weeks in pinworm infestation to prevent reinfection from ova that mature later.
2. *Trichinosis, hookworm, tapeworms and strongyloidosis* require 400 mg daily for 3 days.
3. *Neurocysticercosis:* Albendazole is the drug of choice in a dose of 400 mg twice daily but the duration depends on the number of cysts and may vary from 8 to 30 days. **Glucocorticoids** should be given before starting albendazole to prevent immunological reactions to the dead parasite.

4. *Hydatid disease:* Albendazole is the drug of choice; 400 mg twice daily is given for 4 weeks. If needed, the course may be repeated after 2 weeks. When the cysts are removed by surgery, albendazole is more effective in providing cure.
5. *Filariasis:* Combination of albendazole (400 mg) with DEC (6 mg/kg) or ivermectin (0.3 mg/kg) given as a single dose is found to be effective in *W. bancrofti* in suppressing microfilariae for one year. This also prevents the spread of filariasis and may be continued once a year for 5–6 years.

Thiabendazole is a benzimidazole and acts like mebendazole but due to. But due to frequent side effects, it is not preferred. Dizziness, anorexia, vomiting, diarrhoea, drowsiness, paraesthesia, bradycardia, hypotension, convulsions and liver dysfunction can occur. It is used as an alternative to albendazole in strongyloidosis and cutaneous larva migrans.

PYRANTEL PAMOATE

Pyrantel pamoate is effective against roundworm, hookworm and pinworms. Since it is poorly absorbed from the gut, it acts on the worms in the gut. It stimulates the release of acetylcholine which activates the nicotinic cholinergic receptor in the worm leading to persistent depolarisation and spastic paralysis **(depolarising neuromuscular blocker)**. It also inhibits cholinesterase enzyme. The paralysed worms are expelled.

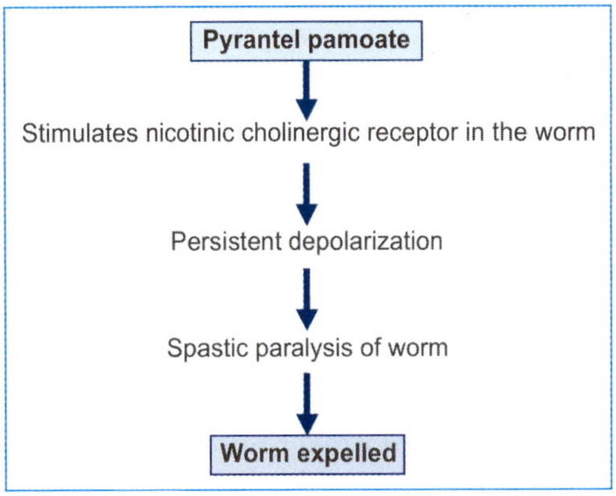

Pyrantel pamoate
↓
Stimulates nicotinic cholinergic receptor in the worm
↓
Persistent depolarization
↓
Spastic paralysis of worm
↓
Worm expelled

It is well-tolerated; occasional abdominal pain, headache, rashes, weakness and dizziness may occur. Single dose yields high cure.

Uses

Pyrantel is used as a single oral dose (11 mg/kg) in the treatment of roundworm, hookworm and pinworm infestations. For pinworm, the dose is repeated after 2 weeks.

Oxantel pamoate an analog of pyrantel pamoate is effective in the treatment of trichuriasis infection.

PIPERAZINE CITRATE

Piperazine citrate is effective in roundworm and pinworm infestations. It competitively blocks the action of acetylcholine and thereby contractions in the worms. Flaccid paralysis results and the worms are expelled through the gut by peristalsis. It is also a GABA receptor agonist.

Adverse effects are mild—gastrointestinal symptoms, headache and dizziness are seen occasionally. Piperazine citrate is indicated for roundworm infestation. It is also safe in pregnancy.

Dose: 4 g OD for 2 days.

LEVAMISOLE

Levamisole is effective against roundworms and hookworms and can be used as an alternative drug in these infestations. It causes paralysis of the worms which are expelled live. It is well-tolerated and is effective in a single dose of 150 mg in roundworm and 2 doses of 150 mg at an interval of 12 hr in hookworm infection. It is also an immunomodulator.

NICLOSAMIDE

Niclosamide is effective against most tapeworms. The segments of the dead tapeworms are partly digested and in case of *T. solium*, the ova released from these segments may develop into larvae and reach various organs resulting in visceral cysticercosis. **Purge** may be given 2 hours after niclosamide to wash off the worms and avoid cysticercosis. The scolex detected in the stool ensures eradication.

Niclosamide is well-tolerated. Abdominal discomfort and rarely pruritus and rashes may occur.

Uses

Niclosamide is an alternative drug in infestations by tapeworms like *T. solium, T. saginata, H. nana* and *D. latum* and in intestinal fluke infestations.

Dose: 2 g in the morning on empty stomach, to be chewed and swallowed.

PRAZIQUANTEL

Praziquantel is effective against all schistosomes and most other trematodes and cestodes including cysticercosis. It is effective as a single oral dose in most infestations. It increases cell membrane permeability to calcium resulting in contraction followed by paralysis and the worms are expelled.

Adverse effects are mild and include GI disturbances, headache, dizziness, **drowsiness**, rashes, myalgia and arthralgia.

Praziquantel is contraindicated in ocular cysticercosis since the host response can cause irrepairable damage.

Dose: 10 mg/kg CYSTICIDE 500 mg tab. PRAZI PLUS 500 mg with 400 mg Albendazole.

Uses

1. *Schistosomiasis:* Praziquantel is the drug of choice in all forms of schistosomiasis. 20 mg/kg 3 doses at 6 hr intervals.
2. *Tapeworms:* Single dose (10 mg/kg) of praziquantel is effective in all tapeworm infestations. In *T. solium,* it has the advantage that it kills the larvae and, therefore, visceral cysticercosis is avoided.
3. *Neurocysticercosis:* Praziquantel is an alternative to albendazole. Inflammatory reactions to the dying parasite may result in worsening of neurological symptoms. Hence glucocorticoids may be used along with praziquantel to suppress the inflammatory response. Unfortunately, the bioavailability of praziquantel is reduced when taken with glucocorticoids.
4. *Other flukes:* Praziquantel is also effective in cestodes like *H. nana, D. latum, Clonorchis sinensis, Paragonimus westermani.*

DIETHYLCARBAMAZINE (DEC)

Diethylcarbamazine is the drug of choice in filariasis, *W. bancrofti, B. malayi and B. timori.* It immobilizes the microfilariae resulting in their displacement in the tissues and also alters their surface structure making them more susceptible to the host defense mechanisms. Microfilariae rapidly disappear from the blood except those present in hydrocele and nodules. It also kills the adult worms of *Loa loa* and prolonged treatment can kill the adult *B. malayi* and probably *W. bancrofti.*

DEC is rapidly absorbed on oral administration and is also rapidly metabolised. Alkalinizing the urine enhances the plasma levels and prolongs the action of DEC. Dose should be reduced in renal dysfunction.

Dose: 100 mg TDS DDICAB 100 mg tab, EOFIL 150 mg tab

Adverse effects are mild; anorexia, nausea, vomiting, dizziness and headache; allergic reactions with itching, rashes and fever due to release of proteins and antigens from the dying worms may occur. Antihistamines are given with DEC to minimize these reactions. DEC is contraindicated in onchocerciasis as it can cause severe reaction to products of destroyed microfilaria.

Pregnancy: To be avoided in pregnancy as animal studies have shown DEC to be an abortifacient by increased production of PGs.

Uses

- *Filariasis:* DEC is the drug of choice (2 mg/kg TDS for 21 days). In 7 days, patients are rendered non-infective to mosquitoes as microfilariae rapidly disappear. However, adult worms may need repeated courses. Antihistamines should also be started to reduce allergic reactions and continued for a few days. If reactions are noted, glucocorticoids may be given. In patients with renal dysfunction, DEC should be used cautiously. Mass treatment with DEC in endemic areas has been effective in reducing filaria transmission. DEC (0.2–0.4%) incorporated into table salt or given as a single annual dose (6 mg/kg) with albendazole (400 mg) reduces microfilaria in the blood.
- *Tropical eosinophilia* (2 mg/kg TDS for 7 days). Symptoms rapidly disappear.
- *Loa loa:* DEC is effective in loiasis. A test dose should be given 50 mg/day for 3 days followed by 150 mg TDS for 2–3 weeks.

IVERMECTIN

Ivermectin is a semisynthetic analog of avermectin B obtained from *Streptomyces avermitilis*. Ivermectin is effective against many nematodes, arthropods and filariae that infect animals and human beings. Ivermectin is very effective against the microfilaria of *Onchocerca volvulus*. It is microfilaricidal and also blocks the release of microfilariae from the uterus of adult worms. There is a rapid decrease in the microfilarial count in the skin and eyes.

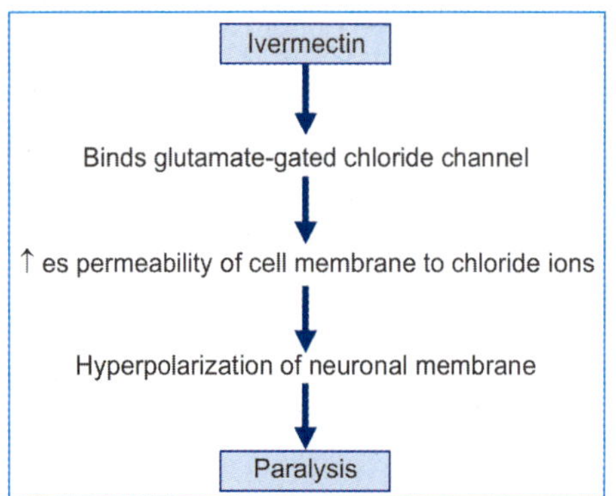

Ivermectin acts by paralysing the worms by binding to glutamate-gated chloride channels and also enhancing GABA activity. It binds to the channels and enhances the permeability of the cell membranes to chloride ions leading to hyperpolarization and paralysis. It also enhances the GABAergic transmission in the nerves of the nematodes.

Ivermectin is as effective as DEC against *W. bancrofti* and *B. malayi*. It is also effective against *Strongyloides stercoralis, Ascaris lumbricoides, cutaneous larva migrans, Sarcoptis scabii* and lice.

Dose: 10–15 mg single dose ASCAPIL 6 mg DT-tab. MECTIN 3 mg, 6 mg tab

Adverse Effects

Ivermectin is well tolerated. Apart from nausea and vomiting, allergic reactions can result due to hypersensitivity to the dying microfilarial proteins (**Mazzotti reaction**).

Ivermectin should not be used with other drugs that influence GABA activity (e.g. benzodiazepines, valproic acid) and in patients with meningitis and sleeping sickness as these conditions impair the BBB.

Uses

1. *Onchocerciasis:* Ivermectin is the preferred drug in the treatment of onchocerciasis. Single dose 150 μg/kg given orally once or twice a year is safe and effective. Single dose is repeated once every year till the adult worms die. Microfilariae in the anterior chamber may need prior glucocorticoids to avoid inflammatory reactions in the eye.
2. *Lymphatic filariasis:* Ivermectin is also useful in the treatment of lymphatic filariasis. A single dose of 400 μg/kg ivermectin with 400 mg albendazole is given once a year for mass chemotherapy of lymphatic filariasis.
3. *Strongyloidiasis:* A single dose of 200 μg/kg is curative in strongyloidiasis. However, the dose is to be repeated after 2 weeks.

4. Ivermectin is also useful in **cutaneous larva migrans, ascariasis**, in **scabies** and **lice infestations** in a single dose of 200 µg/kg.
5. *COVID-19:* Ivermectin is found to have anticovid activity *in vitro* and is being used in COVID-19 along with other drugs both for the treatment and prophylaxis.

Doxycycline has been found to be lethal to the adult worms of *W. bancrofti* and *Onchocerca volvulus*. It has a unique mechanism of action—it kills the bacterium Wolbachia which exists in symbiosis with filaria. It may have a role in the treatment of filariasis.

Metrifonate is a prodrug that is converted to dichlorovas—an organophosphorus insecticide. Metrifonate is used as an alternative to praziquantel in the treatment of *Schistosoma haematobium* infections. By anticholinesterase activity, it paralyses the adult worm which move to the lungs and are killed by the immune system. However, the eggs are not destroyed. It may even be used for prophylaxis in children in endemic areas since it is a fairly safe drug.

Oxamniquine is effective against *S. mansoni* and is used as an alternative to praziquantel in the treatment of *S. mansoni* infections. It is well absorbed when given orally (15 mg/kg single dose) and it is safe and effective.

Bithionol is the drug of choice in the treatment of *Fasciola hepatica* infections.

Resistance to Anthelmintic Drugs

Resistance is now widespread. The extensive use of anthelmintic drugs in farming could be considered one of the contributory factors for the development of resistance. Resistance can result from:

- Efflux of the drug by P-glycoprotein transporter.
- Reduced affinity for binding of drug as in benzimidazoles to the beta tubulin.
- Modification of the structure of the binding site.

Hence, anthelmintic drugs should not be indiscriminately used.

DRUGS USED IN SCABIES AND PEDICULOSIS

Scabies is caused by *Sarcoptes scabiei* or *Acarus scabiei* (itch mite). Scabies is more common in people with poor hygiene. It is transmitted by close body contact with an infected person and spreads easily in overcrowded housing conditions. Drugs used in scabies are as follows.

Permethrin a synthetic pyrethroid, is an insecticide effective against scabies and lice. The insects are paralysed and a single application is sufficient in most patients. 5% cream is applied all over the body below the chin and washed after 12 hours. It is safe, effective, convenient to use and well tolerated with nearly 100% cure rates—hence preferred for the treatment of scabies and pediculosis.

Ivermectin, an anthelmintic, is also found to be effective in scabies and pediculosis. It differs from all other scabicides in that it is given orally. A single dose of 200 µg/kg is highly effective and cure rates have been 91–95%. It is well tolerated but should be avoided in pregnant and lactating women and in children.

Benzyl benzoate is a liquid applied in the form of 25% emulsion. After a hot scrub bath, the emulsion should be applied over the entire body below the chin including the soles of the feet. The application should be repeated after 12 hours and after the next 12 hours the hot scrub bath should be repeated. Benzyl benzoate can cause irritation, specially when repeated frequently.

Lindane or Gamma Benzene Hexachloride (Gammexane, BHC): 1% Lindane in a vegetable oil/cream is applied over the body and the treatment repeated after 2–3 days. It is found to be an effective scabicide as well as pediculocide and causes milder irritation when compared to other drugs. But resistance to lindane is common and this can be prevented by combining it with benzyl benzoate which improves efficacy. Another disadvantage is that lindane is highly lipid-soluble because of which it can be absorbed through intact skin resulting in systemic toxicity. Lindane can cause arrhythmias and seizures—it is a CNS stimulant. It can rarely cause aplastic anaemia.

Other Drugs

Crotamiton is effective against both lice and scabies. It needs to be applied as a 10% cream 2–3 times at an interval of 24 hours followed by a wash. It is unlikely to cause irritation because of which it may be preferred in children.

Sulfur: 10% sulfur ointment was used earlier but it is now not preferred because it is inconvenient to use, has an unpleasant smell and needs to be applied repeatedly.

DDT is applied as a 2% lotion for pediculosis and scabies. It paralyses the insects. It is now not preferred because of the availability of better scabicides and pediculocides.

Tetmosol (monosulphiram) is related to disulfiram. 5% solution is applied three times in 24 hours for scabies. It is an effective sarcopticide. It can cause mild irritation. Alcohol consumption should be avoided and tetmosol should not be used in children below 5 years of age.

PEDICULOSIS

Pediculosis is caused by the louse *Pediculus humanus.* Lice can infest scalp, body or pubic region. Drugs used in lice infestations include:

1. Permethrin 1% lotion or cream is rubbed over the scalp, allowed to remain for 10 minutes and then washed off. Permethrin is preferred for topical use
2. Ivermectin (200 µg/kg) may be used orally as a single dose.
3. DDT 2% lotion, gammaxane 2% shampoo, malathion 0.5% lotion or any of the other drugs for scabies including benzyl benzoate (not preferred because of weak ovicidal action).

Clinical Pharmacology

- Single dose (400 mg) albendazole is the most commonly used deworming agent.
- Albendazole should not be given in children below 2 years and in pregnancy.
- Periodic deworming every 3–6 months may be needed.
- Hookworm infection should be considered in patients with iron deficiency anaemia.
- Praziquantel absorption is increased by high carbohydrate meal and by cimetidine.

[1] From Medical Council of India, *Competency based Undergraduate Curriculum for the Indian Medical Graduate,* 2018;1:136–144.

CHAPTER 56

National Health Programmes

Competency achievement: The student should be able to:

PH 1.55 Describe and discuss the following National Health Programmes including immunisation, tuberculosis, leprosy, malaria, HIV, filaria, kala Azar, diarrhoeal diseases, anaemia and nutritional disorders, blindness, non-communicable diseases, cancer and Iodine deficiency.[1]

National health programmes are part of the healthcare system of the country which are designed to improve the health status of the population. They take into account the various socio-cultural, political, economic and local factors, for providing essential preventive, promotive, curative and rehabilitative services. Currently there are 3 major health policies in India, i.e. National Health Policy 2017, National Population Policy 2000 and National Nutrition Policy 1998. As covering all the national health programmes in detail is beyond the scope of this book, only applied aspects of the programmes have been dealt with in brief.

The major emphasis of the health programmes is to provide healthcare to vulnerable sections of the society. Hence National Rural Health Mission (NRHM) was launched in 2005 for rural population and National Urban Health Mission (NUHM) in 2013 for urban poor and together they constitute National Health Mission (NHM). All the existing national health programmes come under the National Health Mission.

Community based outreach services are provided to door step of the people, by ASHA/ANM/AWW and include preventive and promotive services.

Fixed facility services are those which are curative and provided by doctors.

Referral services are needed when patients cannot be managed at a primary facility. Such patients are stabilized and referred to a unit which can provide specialist care.

1. Reproductive, Maternal, Newborn, Child Plus Adolescent Health (RMNCH+A)

This program is based on "Life cycle approach", i.e. from birth of a woman till she gives birth to a child. Package of services includes:

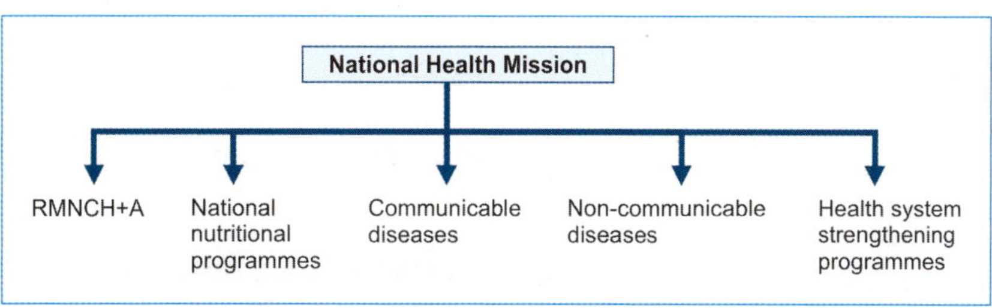

Fig. 56.1: Broad classification of health programmes under NHM. RMNCH+Aóreproductive, maternal, newborn, child plus adolescent health

Table 56.1: Major health programmes under each of the categories

RMNCH+A	*National Nutrition Programmes*	*Communicable diseases*	*Non-communicable diseases*	*Health system strengthening*
Janani Shishu Suraksha Karyakram (JSSK)	Umbrella ICDS including poshan abhiyan	National TB Elimination Program (NTEP): (earlier RNTCP)	National Tobacco Control Program (NTCP)	Ayushman Bharat-PM JAY
Rashtriya Kishor Swasthya Karyakram (RKSK)	Anemia Mukht Bharat (AMB)	National Leprosy Elimination Program	National Mental Health Program	LaQshya
Rashtriya Bal Swasthya Karyakram (RBSK)	Mothers Absolute Affection (MAA) program for Infant and Young child feeding (IYCF)	Integrated disease surveillance program (IDSP)	National program for prevention of Cancer, Diabetes, Cardiovascular diseases and Stroke	Pradhan Mantri Swasthya Suraksha Yojana (PMSSY)
Universal Immunization Program (UIP)	Mid-day meal program	National Vector Borne Disease Control Program (NVBDCP)	National program for healthcare of elderly	
Mission Indradhanush/ Intensified Mission Indradhanush	National Iodine Deficiency Disorder Control Program	National AIDS control program (NACP)	National program for prevention and control of deafness	
Janani Suraksha Yojana	National program for prevention and control of fluorosis	National program on containment of anti-microbial resistance	National program for control of blindness and visual impairment	
Pradhan Mantri Surakshit Matritva Abhiyan	National Vitamin A Prophylaxis Program		National Oral Health Program	
Navjaat Shishu Suraksha Karyakram (NSSK)				

UNIVERSAL IMMUNIZATION PROGRAM

Key Features of UIP

- One of the largest public health programs with 2.9 crore pregnant women and 2.67 crore newborns as beneficiaries (Table 56.2).
- >90 lakh sessions planned every year
- Close to 27,000 cold chain points for storing and distributing vaccines

Objective of the program is to protect every child against deadly diseases preventable by vaccine by ensuring full immunization.

Supply Chain of Immunization

Cold chain consists of a series of storage and transport links, all of which are designed to keep the vaccine at the recommended temperature (+20°C to +80°C) from the point of manufacture until it reaches the target beneficiary (Fig. 56.2).

COMMUNICABLE DISEASES

National TB elimination program: RNTCP has been revised to NTEP with an aim to

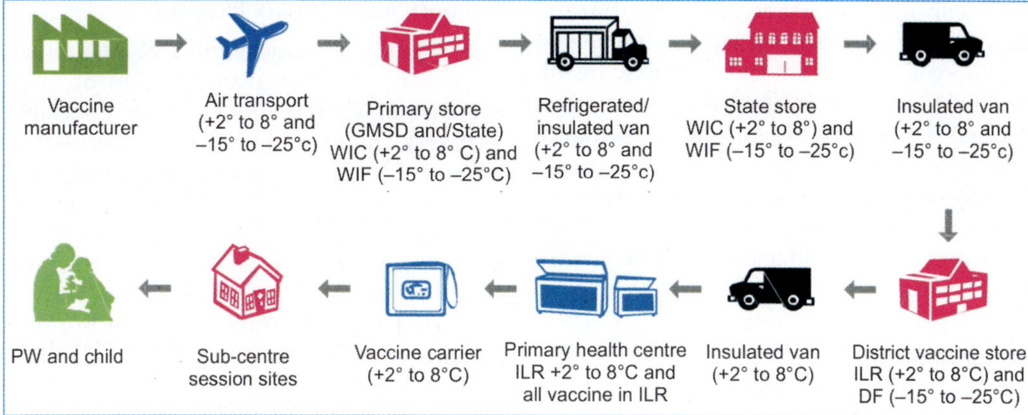

Fig. 56.2: Flow of vaccines from manufacturer till it reaches the beneficiary

Table 56.2: National Immunization schedule

Age	*Vaccines given*
Birth	BCG, OPV-0 dose, hepatitis B birth dose
6 Weeks	OPV-1, pentavalent-1, fIPV-1, Rota-1 & PCV-1
10 weeks	OPV-2, pentavalent-2 & Rota-2
14 weeks	OPV-3, pentavalent-3, fIPV-2, Rota-3 & PCV-2
9–12 months	MR-1, JE1, PCV-booster
16–24 months	MR-2, JE2, DPT-booster 1, OPV-booster
5–6 years	DPT-booster 2
10 years	Td
16 years	Td
Pregnant mother	Td1, Td2 or Td booster

OPV—Oral polio vaccine. OPV-0 dose can be given up to 15 days from birth (4 weeks before OPV-1), as minimum duration between 2 doses should be 4 weeks.

Hepatitis B birth dose should be given within 24 hr of birth; MR—measles rubella vaccine

DPT—diphtheria, pertussis and tetanus; JE—Japanese encephalitis vaccine-administered only in JE endemic districts; fIPV—Fractionated inactivated polio vaccine; PCV—pneumococcal conjugate vaccine-not available in all states. Td—tetanus and adult diphtheria toxoid.

eliminate TB by 2025, the 4 strategic pillars being "Detect-Treat-Prevent-Build".

Detect: Early detection ensures decreased risk of transmission and also detection of drug resistance. There has been ban on serology based testing for TB and mandatory notification of all confirmed TB cases through TB NIKSHAY portal.

Treat: Providing free daily fixed dose combinations with support of directly observed treatment (DOT) strategy. There is only one category for initiating treatment for drug sensitive cases which includes intensive phase of 2 months with 4 drugs which includes isoniazid, rifampicin, pyrazinamide and ethambutol and continuation phase of 4 months with 3 drugs that includes Isoniazid, rifampicin and ethambutol.

There are financial incentives for both TB notification and treatment completion for healthcare providers.

Prevent: BCG vaccination, isoniazid chemoprophylaxis for children <6 yr who were close contacts of confirmed TB case for 6 months, airborne infection control practices at healthcare facilities.

Build: TB elimination policies, empowering institutions and human resources will ensure building of a strong health system against TB.

Integrated Disease Surveillance Program (IDSP)

Was started to strengthen disease surveillance mechanisms for infectious diseases to detect and respond to outbreaks immediately. Surveillance data is collected at all levels of health system (mandatory for public health facilities) under 3 specified reporting forms, S, L and P forms. This IT enabled surveillance will identify early triggers (increase in cases of a specific type of disease or clustering of cases in one region) so as to handle it through trained Rapid respond teams (RRT) which are part of the program.

National Leprosy Eradication Program (NLEP)

As the country has reached elimination targets for leprosy, now the program aims to detect cases through active surveillance in the community through ASHA workers. Multi-drug therapy for paucibacillary and multibacillary cases, intensified health education and prevention of disability and medical rehabilitation services are the major activities.

National Vector-Borne Disease Control Program (NVBDCP)

This program is implemented for the prevention and control of 6 vector-borne diseases (VBD): Malaria, filariasis, kala-azar, dengue, Japanese encephalitis and chikungunya. The NVBDCP has a three-pronged strategy:

1. Disease management including early case detection and complete treatment, strengthening of referral services, epidemic preparedness and rapid response
2. Integrated vector management (IVM) including indoor residual spraying, insecticide treated bed-nets, use of larvivorous fishes, anti-larval measure in urban areas and source reduction
3. Supportive interventions such as behaviour change communication and public private partnerships, capacity building, operational research, web based information systems, vaccination against JE, monitoring and evaluation.

National AIDS Control Program

The NACP was launched in 1987 and aimed to prevent further transmission of HIV, decrease morbidity and mortality associated with HIV and to minimize its socio-economic impact. Preventive, curative and support services are provided with special care for high-risk groups such as CSW, MSM, IDU and bridge population under this program. Counselling and diagnostic services are provided via Integrated counselling and testing centres (ICTC). The NACP also includes prevention of parent to child transmission of HIV (PPTCT) and provides HIV/TB coordination for cross-referral, detection and treatment of TB in PLHIV. In order to monitor the trends of the infection, sentinel surveillance is carried out.

National Program on Containment of Anti-microbial Resistance

To tackle lack of availability of newer antibiotics and limit the spread of multi drug resistant bacteria, 20 anti-microbial resistance surveillance laboratories have been established in 18 states. National Centre for Disease Control (NCDC) has come out with National treatment guidelines on rational use of antimicrobials as well as National infection control guidelines for hospitals.

NATIONAL NUTRITION PROGRAMMES

There are two specific kinds of nutritional programmes:

1. Food Supply and Supplementation Programmes
   - Supplementary feeding program or Special Nutrition Program (SNP)
   - Mid-day Meal Program (MDM)
   - Provision of essential food-grains to poor households at subsidized rates through public distribution system (PDS)
   - Food for work program (FFW)
2. Vitamin and Mineral Supplementation Programmes

- Prophylaxis program against blindness due to vitamin A Deficiency
- Prophylaxis program to prevent nutritional anaemia in mothers and children.

Ministry of Women and Child Development has focused on the 'life-cycle approach' targeted at unmarried adolescent girls, pregnant women, mothers and children aged 0–6 years and brought out all the nutrition intervention programs under Umbrella ICDS. These programs will work to reduce the level of malnutrition, anaemia and low birth weight babies, ensure empowerment of adolescent girls and provide protection to the children.

Programs/schemes by Ministry of Women and Child Development under Umbrella ICDS

1. Anganwadi Services Scheme (formerly ICDS)
2. Pradhan Mantri Matru Vandana Yojana
3. National Creche Scheme
4. Scheme for Adolescent Girls
5. Child Protection Scheme
6. POSHAN Abhiyaan

POSHAN Abhiyaan

12 key themes of POSHAN Abhiyaan include:

1. ANC, diet, calcium, institutional delivery, etc.
2. Overall nutrition
3. Optimal breastfeeding
4. Complementary food and feeding
5. Full immunization and vitamin A supplementation
6. Growth monitoring and promotion
7. Anemia prevention in children, adolescent girls and women—diet, IFA, deworming
8. Food fortification and micronutrients
9. Diarrhoea management
10. Girls education, diet and right age at marriage
11. Hygiene, sanitation and safe drinking water
12. Early childhood care and education

Food safety regulations: Food Safety and Standards Authority of India (FSSAI) has been created for laying down scientific standards for articles of food and to regulate their manufacture, storage, distribution, sale and import to ensure availability of safe and wholesome food for human consumption.

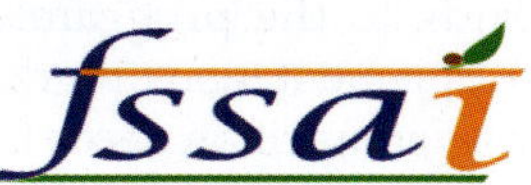

Logo for fortified foods: Any fortified food item available should have the logo with details of micronutrient fortified in the food item to be mentioned just below the logo.

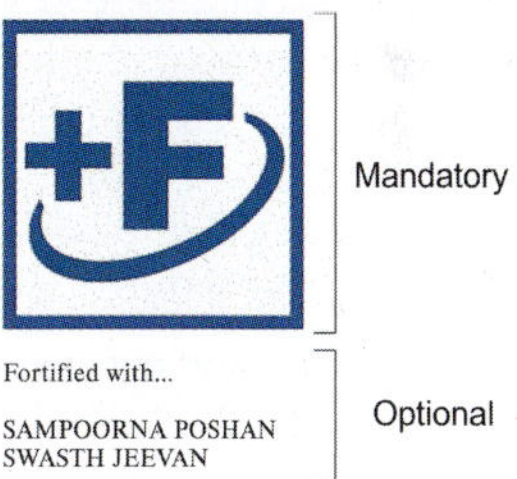

Anaemia Mukt Bharat (AMB): An intensified national iron plus initiative (I-NIPI)

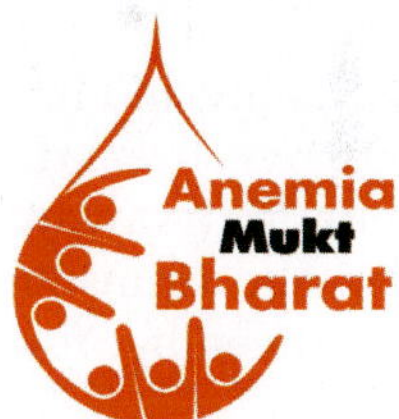

Dose of iron for pregnant and lactating women has been changed to 60 mg elemental iron for 180 days. In the programme currently, iron syrup is given to children aged 6 months to 5 yr and there are 3 coloured sugar-coated iron tablets available by age category: Pink tablets for children aged 6 to 9 years, Blue for adolescents under WIFS and Red for adult women in reproductive age group. Under WIFS programme, school teacher gives an adolescent one blue IFA tablet every week.

Periodic deworming (every 6 months) of school going children with Albendazole is one of the strategies of the initiative.

Mid-day meal program: It is a nutrition supplementation program for children studying from 1st to 10th standard and it combines nutrition with formal education. Both central and state government provide financial aids to the program. Like other nutrition supplementation programs, MDM is not adequate for nutrition needs for entire day of the child.

Prescribed provision of nutrition quantity is given below:

S.no.	Food items	Quantity	
		1st to 5th std	6th to 10th std
1	Food grains	100 g	150 g
2	Pulses	20 g	30 g
3	Vegetables	50 g	75 g
4	Edible oils	5 g	7.5 g
5	Salt	2 g	4 g

School principal/teacher updates number of children who have consumed the meal each day through mobile application.

Mother's absolute affection (MAA) program for IYCF: The program derives its name to signify the importance a mother should receive both at family and health facility for ensuring exclusive breastfeeding to her newborn. Community awareness through ASHA workers and counseling services to mother on breastfeeding, form part of this program.

National iodine deficiency disorder control program: To prevent the disorders resulting from deficiency of iodine, ensuring supply of iodine fortified salt which contains atleast 30 ppm of iodine at manufacturer level and 15 ppm at consumer level. Survey to assess magnitude of the problem, monitoring and health education activities to prevent iodine deficiency are other components of the program.

National program for prevention and control of Fluorosis: It aims to prevent and control Fluorosis in the country by focusing on community surveillance for cases, capacity building of staff, health education and public health interventions like defluoridation and comprehensive healthcare services for cases.

National vitamin A prophylaxis program—to prevent vitamin A deficiency a total of 9 doses of vitamin A will be given orally to children between 9 months to 5 years of age. First dose of 1 ml is given at 9 months followed by second dose of 2 ml at 18 months. Next 7 doses of 2 ml each are given at 6 monthly intervals. Treatment with Vitamin A for Xerophthalmia, Measles and children with severe acute malnutrition is also part of the program.

Zinc supplementation as part of diarrhea control program: Apart from the specific micronutrient programmes, to prevent recurrences of diarrheal episodes in children, zinc tablets are given along with Oral rehydration solution in children with acute diarrhea. 10 mg dispersible tablets are given for children aged 2 months to 6 months and 20 mg tablets for children above 6 months for a duration of 14 days.

NON-COMMUNICABLE DISEASES

National Program for Prevention and Control of Cancer, Diabetes, Cardiovascular diseases and Stroke (NPCDCS)

The program focuses on health promotion, capacity building and early diagnosis and management of these diseases with integration with the primary healthcare system. It provides massive health education and mass media involvement, opportunistic screening of individuals >30 years, referral facilities and establishment of NCD clinics at the CHC. This program is also linked with RBSK for prevention and control of rheumatic heart disease and, with NTEP for management of TB/diabetes co-morbidities. Screening services for early detection of cancers and strengthening tertiary centres for quality treatment and palliative care also fall within the purview of this program.

National Tobacco Control Program

This program was launched in order to facilitate the implementation of the tobacco control laws. The various components of this program are: Generation of public awareness, establishment of tobacco testing laboratories, research and training on alternate crops and livelihood for farmers growing tobacco, creation of tobacco control cells, training services and establishment of tobacco cessation facilities.

National Program for Healthcare of the Elderly (NPHCE)

The aim of this program is to provide specialized and comprehensive care to senior citizens at various levels of the healthcare delivery system as well as through outreach services. Preventive and promotive care, manpower development, IEC activities, establishment of rehabilitation centres at CHCs, geriatric units at district hospitals and department of geriatrics at super-specialized institutes are some of the strategies under the NPHCE.

National Mental Health Programme (NMHP)

The NMHP was launched in 1982 to ensure the availability of mental healthcare services for all. The strategies employed to achieve this are:

1. Integration of mental health with primary healthcare
2. Provision of tertiary care institutions for the treatment of mental disorders
3. Eradication of stigma associated with mentally ill patients and protecting their rights.

Under the district mental health program, counseling services at schools and colleges and like skills training, workplace stress management and suicide prevention services are provided.

[1] From Medical Council of India, *Competency based Undergraduate Curriculum for the Indian Medical Graduate*, 2018;1:136–144.

CHAPTER 57

Cancer Chemotherapy

> *Competency achievement:* The student should be able to:
>
> **PH 1.49** Describe mechanism of action, classes, side effects, indications and contraindications of anticancer drugs.[1]

Cancer is one of the major causes of death. Since the life expectency has increased in the present days, many more people live long enough to the age when they could develop cancer thereby further rising the incidence. The treatment of cancers, after so many years of research and experience, is still unsatisfactory due to certain special characteristics of the cancer cells—like capacity for uncontrolled proliferation, invasiveness, metastasis and dedifferentiation (loss of function because they are poorly differentiated) and such poorly differentiated cancer cells can multiply faster when compared to well-differentiated cancer cells. Moreover, the cancer cells are our own cells unlike microbes, which means that, drugs which destroy these cancer cells also can affect normal cells. The host defence mechanisms which help us in infections are not doing so in cancers because these cancer cells are also host cells. To further complicate the problem, the cancer cells can remain in a resting phase during which they are not sensitive to anticancer drugs but can start multiplying later resulting in recurrence. These features have made treatment of cancers quite difficult.

However, extensive research is being carried out on cancers. As a result, many of the cancers which would otherwise have been fatal, are now being cured.

Phases of Cell Cycle

In the multiplication process of a cancer cell, 4 phases are involved. The four phases of the cell cycle are G_1, S, G_2, and M (Fig. 57.1). G_1 is the presynthetic phase and the duration is variable. During the S phase, the synthesis of DNA occurs and hence the activity of replicating enzymes like DNA and RNA polymerases, topoisomerases, thymidine kinases and dihydrofolate reductases are maximum at this phase of 12 to 18 hr duration. G_2 is the postsynthetic phase (1 to 8 hr) and in the M phase (1 to 2 hr), mitosis takes place. The daughter cells may start dividing or may enter into a dormant phase called G_0. The knowledge of cell cycle may be used for staging and scheduling treatment because different drugs act at different stages of the cell cycle. However, some drugs are cell cycle non-specific (Table 57.1).

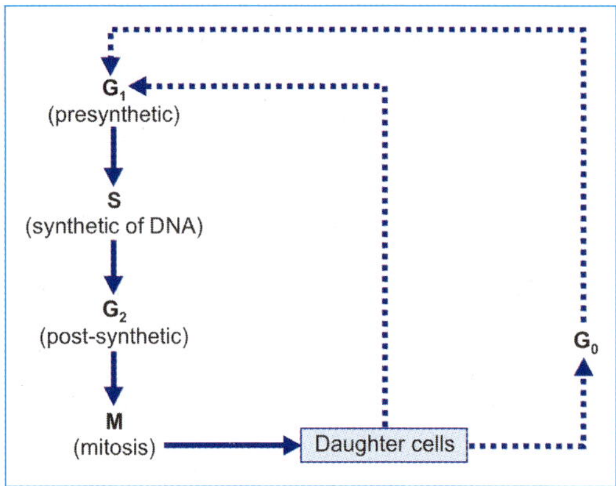

Fig. 57.1: Phases of cell cycle

Table 57.1: Cell cycle specific and non-specific drugs

Cell cycle specific drugs	*Cell cycle non-specific drugs*
S phase: Antimetabolites, doxorubicin, epipodophy–llotoxins	Alkylating agents Anticancer antibiotics
G_2 and M phases: Bleomycin	Cisplatin
M phase: Taxanes, vinca alkaloids.	Procarbazine, Camptothecins

COMMON ADVERSE EFFECTS TO ANTICANCER DRUGS

Since most anticancer drugs act on the rapidly multiplying cells, they are also toxic to the normal rapidly multiplying cells in the bone marrow, epithelial cells of skin and mucous membranes, lymphoid organs and gonads. Thus the common adverse effects are:

1. Bone marrow depression resulting in leukopenia, anaemia, thrombocytopenia and in higher doses—aplastic anaemia. In such patients, infections and bleeding are common.
2. *Other proliferating cells*
   - GIT—stomatitis, oesophagitis, glossitis and proctitis can be painful. Diarrhoea and ulcers along the gut are common.
   - Alopecia (loss of hair)—partial to total alopecia is seen following treatment with most anticancer drugs but it is reversible and the hair grows after the chemotherapy is completed.
   - Reduced spermatogenesis in men and amenorrhoea in women (due to damage to the germinal epithelium) can occur. For example, men treated with mechlorethamine for 6 months can become infertile.
3. *Immediate adverse effects:* Nausea and vomiting are very common with most cytotoxic drugs. They result from the stimulation of the CTZ and starts about 4 to 6 hr after treatment and may continue for 1 to 2 days. Prior treatment with powerful antiemetics is required (Table 57.2).
4. *Hyperuricaemia:* Rapid tumour cell lysis can result in an increased plasma uric acid levels and may lead to 'tumour lysis syndrome' and renal failure.
5. *Teratogenicity:* All cytotoxic drugs are teratogenic and are, therefore, contraindicated in pregnancy.
6. *Carcinogenicity:* Cytotoxic drugs themselves may cause secondary cancers, e.g. leukaemias may follow the treatment of Hodgkin's lymphoma.

Apart from the above, the adverse effects unique to some anticancer drugs are discussed under individual drugs and listed in Table 57.3. Measures to prevent adverse effects to anticancer drugs are mentioned in Table 57.2.

Table 57.2: Measures to prevent the adverse effects of anticancer drugs

Toxity	*Measures*
1. Nausea, vomiting	Antiemetics—ondansetron, granisetron, metoclopramide.
2. Hyperuricaemia	Allopurinol
3. Methotrexate toxicity	Folinic acid. Dose as per blood methotrexate levels.
4. Cystitis due to cyclophosphamide and ifosphamide	Mesna-IV; n-acetylcysteine—bladder wash; plenty of oral fluids.
5. Myelosuppression	Iron, blood transfusion
– Anaemia	Erythropoietin
– Leukopenia	G-CSF, GM-CSF
– Thrombocytopenia	Thrombopoietin
6. Nephrotoxicity due to cisplatin Xerostomia due to radiation	Amifostin

Drugs used in cancers may be classified as follows:

Classification

1. **Alkylating agents**	
• *Nitrogen mustards*	Mechlorethamine, cyclophosphamide, ifosfamide, chlorambucil, melphalan
• *Alkyl sulfonate*	Busulfan
• *Nitrosoureas*	Carmustine, streptozocin, bendamustine
• *Triazene*	Dacarbazine, temozolomide
• *Methylhydrazine*	Procarbazine
• *Ethylenimines*	Thio tepa, altretamine
• *Platinum analogs*	Cisplatin, carboplatin, oxaliplatin
2. **Antimetabolites**	
• *Folate antagonists*	Methotrexate (amethopterin), pemetrexed pralatrexate
• *Purine analogs*	Mercaptopurine, thioguanine, pentostatin, fludarabin, clofarabine, nelarabine, cladribine.
• *Pyrimidine analogs*	Fluorouracil, floxuridine, capecitabine, cytarabine (cytosine arabinoside) gemcitabine, azacytidine
3. **Natural and semisynthetic products**	
• *Anticancer antibiotics*	Actinomycin-D (Dactinomycin), daunorubicin, doxorubicin, bleomycin, mitomycin-C, mithramycin
• *Epipodophyllotoxins*	Etoposide, teniposide
• *Camptothecins*	Topotecan, irinotecan
• *Taxanes*	Paclitaxel, docetaxel
• *Vinca alkaloids*	Vincristine, vinblastine, vinorelbine
4. **Miscellaneous**	Hydroxyurea, l-asparaginase, tretinoin, imatinib, bortezomib, thalidomide, lenalidomide, mTOR inhibitors (temsirolimus, everolimus) monoclonal antibodies (rituximab, trastuzumab), vorinostat
5. **Hormones and their antagonists**	Glucocorticoids, androgens, antiandrogens, oestrogens, antioestrogens, progestins, aromatase inhibitors, 5 alpha reductase inhibitors, GnRH analogs
6. **Biological response modifiers**	Interferon alpha, interleukin 2, amifostine, haematopoietic growth factors

ALKYLATING AGENTS

Alkylating agents are drugs that alkylate (donate an alkyl group to) other molecules by covalent bonds. They also alkylate DNA, RNA and various enzymes and there is interstand cross-linking of DNA.

Actions

Alkylating agents exert

1. *Cytotoxic effects:* Alkylating agents destroy the rapidly multiplying cells—both cancer cells and normal host cells.
2. *Immunosuppressant effects:* Alkylating agents are good immunosuppressants for which they are used in rheumatoid arthritis and other autoimmune disorders.
3. *Radiomimetic effects:* The actions of alkylating agents resemble that of radiotherapy.

Mechanism of Action

On administration, alkylating agents form highly reactive derivatives (carbonium ions) which transfer alkyl groups to various cellular

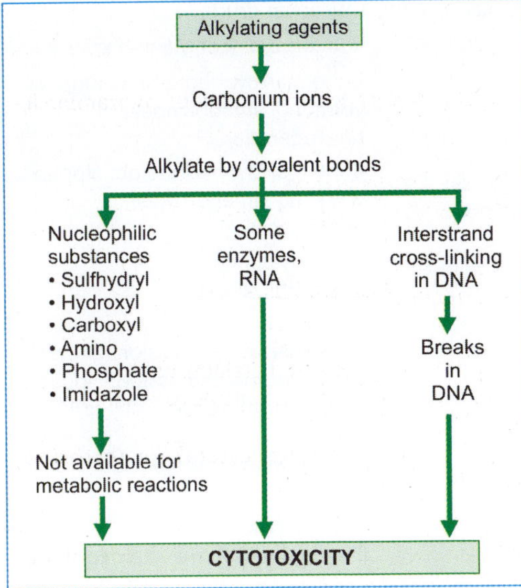

Fig. 57.2: Mechanism of action of alkylating agents

constituents like sulfhydryl, amino, hydroxyl, carboxyl, amine and phosphate groups and bind them with covalent bonds (Fig. 57.2). Thus such constituents are not available for normal metabolic reactions. They bind to one or both strands of DNA and also alkylate DNA which results in breakage of the DNA strand. They alkylate DNA at different sites, for example, at N7 position of guanine. Such alkylation leads to miscoding and abnormal base pairing or cross-linking, resulting in DNA strand breakages. Thus they produce cytotoxicity.

Resistance: The cells may acquire resistance to alkylating agents by one of the following ways:

i. Repair DNA lesions.
ii. Decreased transport of the drug into the cell.
iii. Increased production of enzymes which conjugate alkylating agents.

Nitrogen Mustards

Mechlorethamine: Mechlorethamine should be given only IV as it is a highly irritant compound. Adverse effects are those discussed under common adverse effects including bone marrow suppression, nausea, vomiting, diarrhoea, alopecia, gut ulcerations, amenorrhoea in women and reduced spermatogenesis in men. Since it is an irritant and a direct vesicant, it can cause severe pain and irritation at the site of injection. Mechlorethamine is not used currently and is now generally replaced by cyclophosphamide in MOPP regimen for Hodgkin's lymphoma.

Cyclophosphamide: Cyclophosphamide is a prodrug converted to the active metabolite aldophosphamide in the liver.

Aldophosphamide is inturn converted to phosphoramide mustard and acrolein. Phosphoramide is thought to be responsible for cytotoxic activity while acrolein causes adverse effects.

Cyclophosphamide is well absorbed on oral administration with **high bioavailability** and, therefore, it can be given orally or IV.

Cyclophosphamide is a commonly used alkylating agent. It also has immunosuppressant properties.

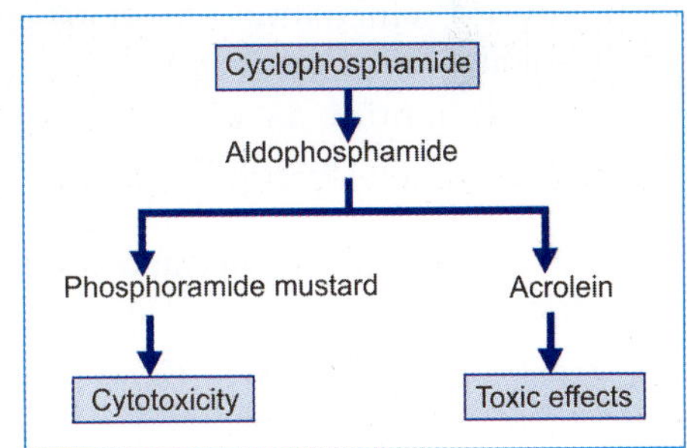

Adverse effects: Apart from common adverse effects to anticancer drugs, cyclophosphamide causes **cystitis** due to a metabolite **acrolein** (Tables 57.2 and 57.3). This can be prevented by giving IV Mesna, irrigating the bladder with acetylcysteine, and by giving large amounts of fluids. Mesna (sodium-2-mercaptoethane sulfonate) and acetylcysteine contain SH groups which bind the toxic metabolites and inactivate them.

Table 57.3: Specific adverse effects of some anticancer drugs

Drugs	*Specific adverse effects*	*Other prominent adverse effects*
Cyclophosphamide	Cystitis, stomatitis	Bone marrow depression, alopecia, vomiting, amenorrhoea, teratogenicity
Busulfan	Pulmonary fibrosis, stomatitis	Bone marrow depression, alopecia, vomiting, amenorrhoea, teratogenicity
Cisplatin	Ototoxicity	Renal dysfunction
Bleomycin	Pulmonary fibrosis, oedema of hands	Stomatitis, alopecia
Daunorubicin	Cardiotoxicity, red-coloured urine	Bone marrow depression, alopecia
Doxorubicin	Cardiotoxicity	Bone marrow depression, alopecia
Mithramycin (plicamycin)	Hepatotoxicity	Thrombocytopenia
Vincristine	Neurotoxicity, peripheral neuritis, mental depression	Muscle weakness, alopecia
Asparaginase	Pancreatitis, hepatotoxicity,	Allergic reactions
Mitotane	Dermatitis, mental depression	Diarrhoea

Uses

- Cyclophosphamide can be used in Hodgkin's lymphoma in place of mechlorethamine in MOPP regimen.
- In non-Hodgkin's lymphomas (NHL), it can be used with doxorubicin (hydroxy–daunomycin), vincristine (oncovin) and prednisolone (CHOP regimen).

  Cyclophosphamide is also useful in Burkitt's lymphoma in children, leukemias and myeloma.
- Cyclophosphamide is an immunosuppressive agent.

Dose: 2–3 mg/ kg/day oral. CYCLOXAN, ENDOXAN 50 mg tab 200, 500, 1000 mg inj

Ifosfamide, an analog of cyclophosphamide, has actions and toxicities similar to cyclophosphamide except that it is longer-acting. It causes cystitis like cyclophosphamide but it is less myelotoxic and less emetogenic than cyclophosphamide. Mesna is given with ifosfamide (1–2 g). Ifosfamide is used in sarcomas.

Chlorambucil is very effective against lymphoid malignancies. It was earlier the drug of choice in chronic lymphocytic leukaemia. Chlorambucil is also used in lymphomas. Alopecia, nausea and vomiting are milder than many other alkylating agents.

Dose: 4–10 mg daily.

Melphalan is given orally in multiple myeloma and in ovarian tumours. Its actions and toxicities are similar to other nitrogen mustards but alopecia, nausea and vomiting are comparatively milder.

Other Alkylating Agents

Busulfan, an alkyl sulfonate, has selective activity against cells of the myeloid series and was the drug of choice in chronic myeloid leukaemia—but now other drugs are preferred (Table 57.4). Busulfan can cause skin pigmentation, hyperuricaemia, gynaecomastia and pulmonary fibrosis.

Carmustine is effective in meningeal leukaemias and brain tumours because it crosses the blood–brain barrier. It causes profound bone marrow depression. It is also used in lymphomas and malignant melanoma.

Bendamustine is another alkylating agent which like other alkylating agents inhibits

DNA synthesis and causes cytotoxicity. It is found to be effective in chronic lymphocytic leukaemia, lymphomas, and multiple myeloma.

Streptozocin is an antibiotic. It is used in pancreatic islet cell tumours. It can cause nephrotoxicity apart from the other adverse effects common to most anticancer drugs.

Dacarbazine is useful in malignant melanoma, Hodgkin's lymphoma, soft tissue sarcomas and neuroblastoma. It is given parenterally but should be cautious because it may cause pain, if extravasated.

Adverse effects: Apart from nausea, vomiting and myelosuppression, it causes neurotoxicity, hepatotoxicity and flu-like syndrome.

Temozolomide is used in gliomas and melanoma. Photosensitivity and elevated values in liver function tests are noted apart from common adverse reactions. The active metabolite acts on all phases of the cell cycle. Timozolomide is completely absorbed on oral administration. Vomiting, myelosuppression, hepatotoxicity, neurotoxicity, flu-like syndrome and dermatological toxicity are common.

Procarbazine is effective orally in Hodgkin's lymphoma (MOPP regimen component) and in non-Hodgkin's lymphoma and brain tumours. It damages DNA and produces breakages and chromosomal damage. It also inhibits DNA, RNA and protein synthesis. This may make it carcinogenic. One of the metabolites is an MAO inhibitor and is responsible for related food and drug interactions.

Adverse effects are bone marrow suppression, nausea, vomiting, neurological and dermatological toxicity and behavioural disturbances.

Platinum Analogs

Cisplatin, carboplatin and oxaliplatin are platinum containing compounds. They get converted to the active form in the cell, inhibit DNA synthesis and cause cytotoxicity almost like alkylating agents. **Cisplatin** causes ototoxicity with tinnitus, loss of hearing and nephrotoxicity. To reduce nephrotoxic effects, cisplatin is given as slow in fusion with adequate hydration and a diuretic. Cisplatin is particularly **emitogenic** but vomiting is often well controlled with a 5-HT_3 antagonist like ondansetron. Though peripheral neuropathy and anaemia can occur, cisplatin is relatively less toxic to bone marrow.

Cisplatin is used in solid tumours like ovarian, testicular and bladder cancer and cancers of the head and neck**; particularly being useful in germs cell tumours.** **Carboplatin** is a less toxic derivative of cisplatin. Advantages over cisplatin are:

- Carboplatin is less nephrotoxic and does not require strict hydration unlike cisplatin
- Less toxic to gut—less vomiting
- Milder neurotoxicity
- Milder ototoxicity

For the above reasons, it is better tolerated and is often preferred in place of cisplatin. However, it is more bone marrow toxic.

Oxaliplatin in combination with flurouracil and leucovorine called FOLFOX regimen. Oxaliplatin is used in advanced colorectal cancer and in other cancers like ovarian and cervical cancers. However, it is neurotoxic (peripheral sensory neuropathy).

ANTIMETABOLITES

Folate Antagonists

Methotrexate (MTX) is a folic acid (FA) antagonist. It is a prodrug converted in the liver to its polyglutamates in the normal as well as tumour cells and the reaction is catalysed by the enzymes **folypolyglutamate synthase** (FPGS). Polyglutamates of methotrexate remain in the tumour cells. They are partly selective for tumour cells. Methotrexate binds to dihydrofolate reductase and prevents the formation of tetrahydrofolate (THF). This THF serves as a coenzyme essential in several reactions in DNA, RNA and protein synthesis (provides methyl groups). The deficiency

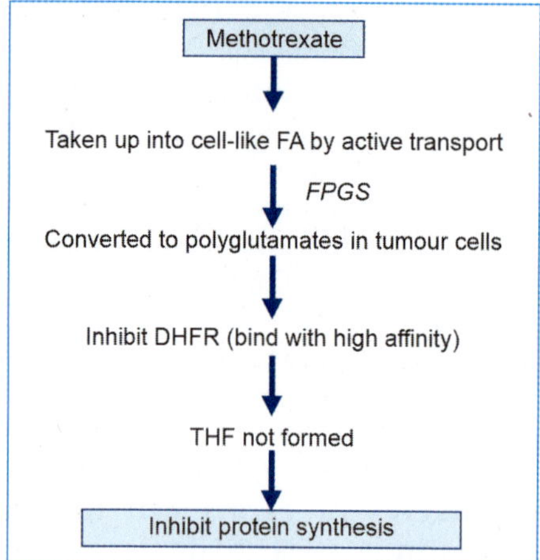

results in inhibition of DNA, RNA and protein synthesis. Thus rapidly multiplying cells are the most affected. Methotrexate is most effective on cells in the 'S' phase of the cell cycle. Resistance to methotrexate may be due to:

- Decreased drug transport
- Reduced formation of active metabolites.
- Increased synthesis of DHFR
- Altered DHFR with reduced affinity for methotrexate.

Actions

- *Cytotoxic actions:* Methotrexate mainly affects the bone marrow, skin and gastrointestinal mucosa and other rapidly dividing cells.
- It also has immunosuppressant and some anti-inflammatory properties.

Pharmacokinetics

Methotrexate is well absorbed when given orally with 50% protein binding. It can also be given parenterally (IM, IV, intrathecal). Higher doses should be given IV as absorption is erratic at such doses. It poorly crosses the BBB due to low lipid solubility. Methotrexate is taken up into the cells by the same active transport process as that of folic acid. It is metabolised in the liver to polyglutamates which are inhibitors of DHFR. Methotrexate is excreted largely by the kidneys—hence dose should be reduced in renal failure.

Adverse effects to methotrexate include the common adverse effects to most anticancer drugs—bone marrow suppression, nausea, vomiting, diarrhoea, alopecia and dermatitis.

Methotrexate can cause nephrotoxicity because the drug may be precipitated in the renal tubules and it is contraindicated in patients with renal impairment. Allergic pneumonitis can sometimes be fatal. When injected intrathecally, methotrexate can cause myelopathy and encephalopathy.

Methotrexate toxicity can be largely prevented by administering **folinic acid**. This folinic acid (also called leucovorin or citrovorum factor) gets converted to a form of THF that can be utilised by the cells. Folinic acid is more stable than THF, is the active coenzyme and does not require activation by DHFR. When high doses of methotrexate are needed, folinic acid **'rescue'** is recommended to avoid severe toxicity.

Drug Interactions

Salicylates, sulfonamides, penicillin, aspirin and probenecid inhibit the renal tubular secretion of methotrexate. Some of them also displace methotrexate from plasma protein binding sites.

Uses

1. *Choriocarcinoma:* Methotrexate is curative in choriocarcinoma treated early. Cure rates are >90%. 1 mg/kg/day is given alternately with leukovorin 0.1mg/kg/day 4 doses each. Such cycles are repeated depending on the response. In advanced cases, dactinomycin is added.
2. *ALL in children:* Methotrexate is used in high doses to induce remission in ALL and then maintenance doses are given.
3. *Other cancers:* Methotrexate is also tried as a component of multi-drug regimens in

lymphomas, breast cancer, bone sarcomas and soft tissue sarcomas.

4. *Psoriasis:* Methotrexate is given for 5 days (2.5 mg/day orally) with two days rest and such cycles are repeated in severe psoriasis.
5. *Rheumatoid arthritis:* Low dose methotrexate is used to induce remission in rheumatoid arthritis and psoriasis. The basis for the use of methotrexate in rheumatoid arthritis and psoriasis is its **immunosuppressant** property. Anti-inflammatory actions also help.

Pemetrexed is an antifolate drug activated in the cells to its polyglutamate form which inhibits DHFR. It is approved for use in mesothelioma and non-small cell lung cancer along with other drugs used in lung cancer.

Pralatrexate: Pralatrexate is a folate antagonist like methotrexate and shares the same mechanism of action and adverse effects. Folinic acid and vitamin B_{12} reduce toxicity to some extent. It is approved for the treatment of relapsed T cell lymphoma.

Ralitrexate: Ralitrexate is another folate antagonist undergoing trials.

Purine Analogs

6-Mercaptopurine, thioguanine, fludarabine, pentostatin and cladribine are purine analogs which act as **purine antagonists.** They are structurally similar to purines.

Mechanism of Action

Purine analogs enter the cells and get converted to active metabolites (triphosphates in most compounds) which are incorporated into DNA in place of regular purines (Key Box 57.1). They cause breakages in DNA strands and inhibit protein synthesis. Fludarabine triphosphate inhibits DNA polymerase while pentostatin inhibits adenosine deaminase.

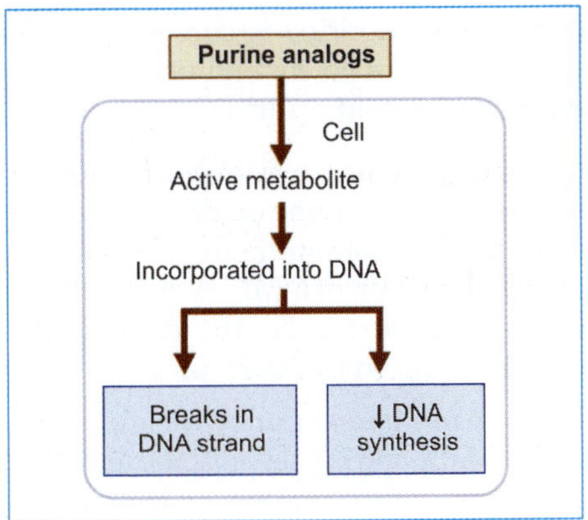

Mercaptopurine

Mercaptopurine (6-MP) is converted to an active metabolite which gets incorporated into the DNA and inhibits purine synthesis and thereby protein synthesis.

Mercaptopurine undergoes extensive first pass metabolism and oral bioavailability is 10–50%. It is metabolised by xanthine oxidase. **Adverse effects** include bone marrow depression which develops slowly after several weeks, anorexia, diarrhoea, nausea, vomiting, stomatitis, jaundice and dermatitis. Hyperuricaemia may be significant and would require treatment with allopurinol—dose of 6-MP should be reduced. Increased risk of squamous cell carcinoma of the skin and AML has been noted after prolonged use of 6-MP.

Uses: MP is used in acute leukaemias in children, choriocarcinoma and some solid

Key Box 57.1: Purine analogs

- Purine analogs get incorporated into DNA and inhibit protein synthesis.
- Mercaptopurine and thioguanine are used in acute leukaemias fludarabine and pentostatin in CLL and non-Hodgkin's lymphomas; cladribin is the drug of choice in hairy cell leukaemia.
- Purine analogs share the common adverse effects of anticancer drugs.
- Fludarabine and pentostatin combination can cause fatal lung toxicity.

tumours. Azathioprine is converted to 6MP in the cells and is a potent immunosuppressant used in rheumatoid arthritis.

Drug interaction: 6-Mercaptopurine is metabolised by xanthine oxidase. Allopurinol inhibits the enzyme xanthine oxidase and thus prolongs the action of 6-MP. When both drugs are given concurrently, the dose of 6-MP should be reduced by 50–75%.

Thioguanine is an analog of guanine, is effective orally and is used in acute leukaemias particularly acute granulocytic leukaemia.

Fludarabine, an analog of vidarabine (antiviral drug), is converted to an active triphosphate derivative which inhibits DNA polymerase. It is also incorporated into DNA and RNA, causes breakage and termination of the DNA chain and inhibits RNA function.

Adverse effects include nausea, vomiting, anorexia, weakness, fever, bone marrow depression, and neurotoxicity. Dose should be reduced in patients with renal dysfunction.

Fludarabine is used in the treatment of chronic lymphocytic leukaemia (CLL) and non-Hodgkin's lymphomas.

Pentostatin: Pentostatin obtained from ***Streptomyces antibioticus*** inhibits the enzyme adenosine deaminase. This results in accumulation of adenosine in the cells and other nucleotides which inhibit DNA synthesis.

Pentostatin can cause nausea, vomiting, diarrhoea, skin rashes and bone marrow suppression. Since pentostatin is largely excreted through the kidneys, dose should be reduced in renal failure.

Pentostatin is used intravenously in the treatment of hairy cell leukaemia, other chronic leukaemias and non-Hodgkin's lymphomas.

Cladribine: Cladribine is another purine analog. It gets activated intracellularly to cladribine triphosphate—which gets incorporated into DNA causing breakages in the DNA strands and also inhibits protein synthesis. Cladribine causes bone marrow suppression, nausea, vomiting, weakness and skin rashes.

Cladribine is given intravenously as a single 7 days course and is considered the drug of choice in hairly cell leukaemia. It is also useful in CLL, AML and some lymphomas.

Pyrimidine Analogs

Thymine and cytosine are the 2 pyrimidines present in the DNA. Pyrimidine analogs are converted to active metabolites which resemble natural nucleotides. They compete with natural nucleotides, are incorporated into DNA in place of natural nucleotides and inhibit DNA synthesis.

5-Fluorouracil

5-Fluorouracil (5-FU) is a pyrimidine analog. It is activated to a nucleotide metabolite which inhibits the enzyme thymidylate synthetase. Due to this, it inhibits the synthesis of thymine and thereby inhibits DNA synthesis. The active metabolites of 5-FU are also incorporated into DNA and RNA leading to inhibition of DNA and RNA synthesis.

Drugs which cause least/no bone marrow depression
- Hormones
- Vincristine
- Bleomycin
- L-asparaginase
- Cisplatin

Curable cancers
- Hodgkin's disease
- Choriocarcinoma
- Burkitt's lymphoma
- Testicular tumours
- Wilms' tumour
- Acute leukaemias in children
- Ewing's sarcoma

Tumours resistant to treatment
- Melanomas
- Pancreatic tumours
- Renal cancers
- Some lung cancers

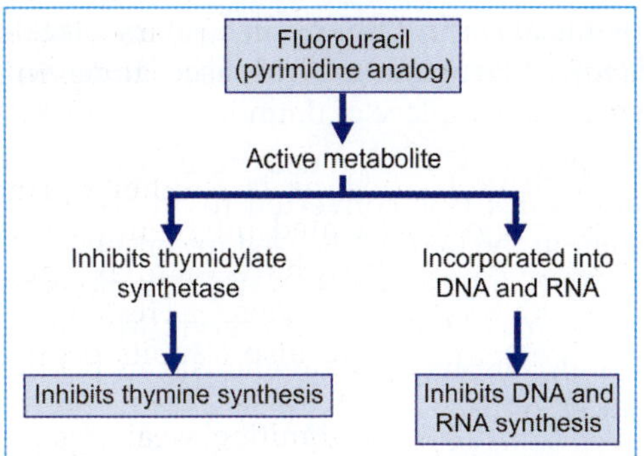

5-FU is given intravenously and has a short t½ of 10–20 min. Majority of the drugs is metabolised by an enzyme called **dihydropyrimidine dehydrogenase** (DPD). A small percentage of patients lack this enzyme—a pharmacogenetic variation and even therapeutic doses of 5-FU can result in significant toxicity.

Leucovorin potentiates the antitoxic effects of 5-FU and, therefore, can be administered along with it.

Uses

1. 5-FU is used in carcinoma of the stomach, colon, rectum, breast and ovaries.
2. Topical uses: Fluorouracil is available as an ointment for topical use in many precancerous (1%) and cancerous (5%) conditions:
   - Seborrhoeic keratosis
   - Warts (Verrica vulgaris)
   - Polyps
   - Benign skin tumours
   - Solar keratosis
   - Superficial basal cell carcinoma

Capecitabine is an orally effective prodrug which is converted to the active metabolite fluorouracil in the tumour cells. The conversion to fluorouracil is much more in the tumour cells (due to presence of a specific enzyme) than normal cells. This is, therefore, like achieving some drug targeting. Toxicity is milder than with fluorouracil. Nausea, vomiting and myelosuppression are milder. Capecitabine is used in breast cancer and colorectal cancer.

Cytosine arabinoside or cytarabine is the most effective agent in acute myeloblastic leukaemia. It enters the cells and is converted to an active metabolite. The active metabolite cytosine arabinoside triphosphate is incorporated into the DNA and inhibits DNA polymerase and thereby inhibits DNA synthesis.

It causes nausea, vomiting and bone marrow depression.

Cytarabine is used in acute leukaemias particularly myeloid leukaemia and in relapsed cases of acute lymphocytic leukaemia. It should be given by continuous IV infusion over 5–7 days.

Gemcitabine is a recently developed analog of cytarabine with mechanism of action similar to it. Gemcitabine is used in pancreatic, lung, cervical, bladder, ovarian and breast cancers. Adverse effects include myelosuppression, nausea, vomiting, thrombocytopenic purpura and nephrotoxicity.

NATURAL AND SEMISYNTHETIC PRODUCTS

Antibiotics

Actinomycin D: Actinomycin D is obtained from the fungus of Streptomyces species. It binds to DNA and forms a complex. It inhibits DNA-dependent RNA synthesis and also causes breaks in the DNA.

It is one of the most potent anticancer drugs and is given by intravenous injection. It is used in Wilms' tumour, rhabdomyosarcoma, choriocarcinoma and some soft tissue sarcomas. It is also used in Kaposi's sarcoma and Ewing's tumour. Dactinomycin is also an immunosuppressant and is used in renal transplants.

Toxic effects include myelosuppression, nausea, vomiting and dermatological manifestations. Extravasation of the drug can cause local pain.

Anthracycline Antibiotics

Daunorubicin and **doxorubicin** are anthracyclines. Epirubicin, idarubicin and mitoxantrone are other anthracycline analogs. They are converted to active metabolites which inhibit DNA synthesis.

Mechanism of Action of Anthracyclines

i. They form a complex with topoisomerase II and inhibit it.
ii. Bind to DNA and cause breakages in DNA.
iii. Lead to generation of free radicals which oxidize DNA strands.

They act on the 'S' phase of the cell cycle. Anthracyclines are given as IV infusion over 10–15 minutes. They are vesicants—cause blisters on the skin and, therefore, should be carefully injected to avoid extravasation. They are all metabolised by the liver and a dose reduction is required in presence of hepatic dysfunction.

Cardiotoxicity with hypotension, tachycardia, arrhythmias, cardiomyopathy and CCF is unique to both these drugs. Cardiomyopathy is of two types—an acute form with arrhythmias may be seen within 24 hr of administration. Pericarditis, myocarditis and pericardial effusion may follow. **Long-term toxicity** with CCF and myocardial damage may be seen **years after treatment** with anthracyclines. Children who receive anthracyclines may develop cardiotoxicity in adult life. Antioxidants offer significant protection against cardiotoxicity by anthracyclines. They also cause vomiting, stomatitis, alopecia and bone marrow depression. Both daunorubicin and doxorubicin may colour the **urine red**.

Daunorubicin is used in acute leukaemias while doxorubicin is useful in solid tumours and in acute leukaemias and non-Hodgkin's lymphomas.

Epirubicin, idarubicin and **mitoxantrone** are analogs of doxorubicin which are less cardiotoxic. Epirubicin is used in metastatic breast cancer and gastroesophageal cancer. Mitoxantrone is used in leukaemias, prostatic cancer and multiple sclerosis. **Valrubicin** is approved for intravesical therapy in urinary bladder cancer. Idarubicin may be used along with cytarabine in place of daunorubicin in AML.

Mitomycin C is obtained from *Streptomyces caespitosus;* it is converted to an alkylating agent in the body. It is used in cancers of the stomach, lungs, pancreas and squamous cell carcinoma of the anus and cervix. Mitomycin can also be used intravenously in bladder cancer.

Bleomycin

Bleomycin is obtained from *Streptomyces verticillus*. It binds with iron and generates free radicals and causes breakage in DNA strands. It has the advantages of the **unique mechanism of action** and is **less toxic to the bone marrow**—these are advantageous in combination regimens.

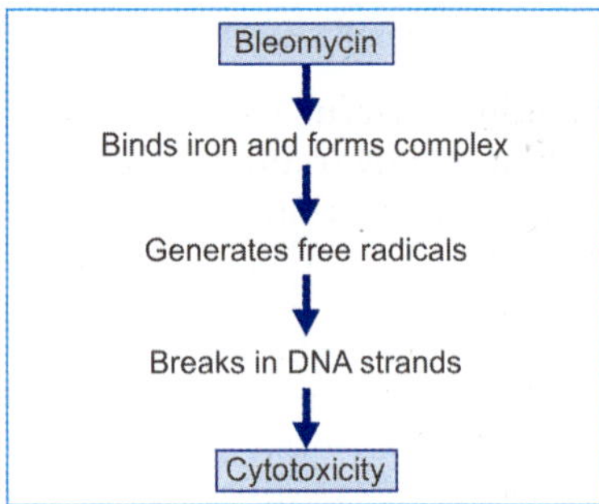

Adverse effects: Its most serious toxicity includes pulmonary fibrosis and cutaneous toxicity (dermagraphia—scleroderma-like changes) but does not cause significant bone marrow depression.

Uses: Bleomycin is used in solid tumours—testicular tumours, squamous cell carcinoma of the head, neck and oesophagus.

Epipodophyllotoxins

Podophyllotoxin is obtained from the root of the mandrake plant or May apple. Etoposide (VP-16) and teniposide (VM-26) are semisynthetic derivatives of podophyllotoxin. Etoposide is available for both oral and parenteral use.

Mechanism of action: Epipodophyllotoxins bind to topoisomerase II as well as to DNA and result in DNA strand breakages. The cells in S and G_2 phase of cell cycle are susceptible to these drugs.

Adverse effects include thrombophlebitis at the site of injection, nausea, alopecia, allergic reactions and myelosuppression.

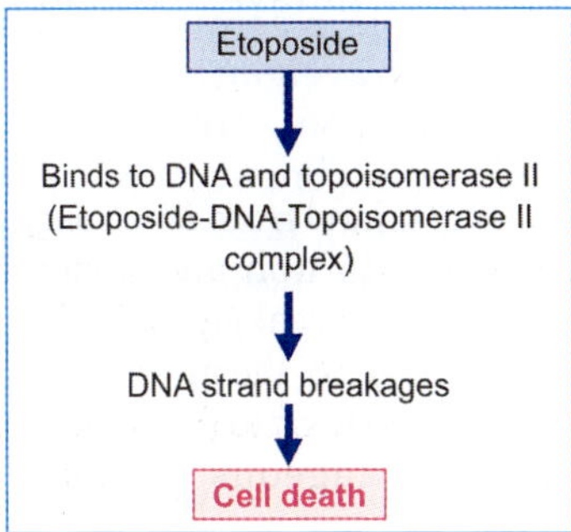

Uses

- Etoposide is useful in germ cell cancers (testicular and ovarian), lung and stomach cancers, leukaemias and lymphomas.
- Teniposide is used in acute lymphoblastic leukaemia.

Camptothecins

Camptothecins are obtained from the chinese tree *Camptotheca acuminata*. Camptothecin was the first anticancer agent in this group but was found to be too toxic. Its analogs, topotecan and irinotecan are less toxic and useful. They **inhibit topoisomerase** I resulting in DNA strand breakages leading to cell death. They act on the S phase of the cell cycle. Both are given intravenously.

Toxicity is mild and includes **diarrhoea** and reversible bone marrow suppression, nausea, weakness and skin rash. Irinotecan inhibits the enzyme acetylcholinesterase resulting in accumulation of acetylcholine causing excessive salivation, abdominal cramps, miosis, bradycardia and sweating which respond to treatment with atropine.

Uses

Topotecan is used in advanced ovarian cancer and lung cancer.

Irinotecan is a prodrug converted to its active metabolite in the liver. It is used in metastatic colorectal cancer. Diarrhoea can be significant and dehydration should be prevented.

Taxanes

Taxanes include **paclitaxel** and **docetaxel**. Paclitaxel is obtained from the bark of the Western yew tree. It binds to the beta-tubulin of microtubules and arrests mitosis—**mitotic spindle poison.**

Paclitaxel is given intravenously as an infusion over 3 hr and repeated every 3 weeks. It is metabolised by the liver microsomal enzymes and excreted through the gut. Drugs that induce and inhibit microsomal enzymes can alter the plasma levels of paclitaxel. Dose should be reduced in liver dysfunction. Adverse effects include myelosuppression, myalgia, allergic reactions, hypotension, arrhythmias and peripheral neuropathy. The vehicle used to administer paclitaxel can cause allergic reactions. Though the incidence of allergic reactions is low, it can be a cause for concern in some patients. Pretreatment with dexamethasone, diphenhydramine and an H_2 blocker is used to prevent the allergic response. An albumin bound formulation of paclitaxel is now available which is unlikely to cause allergic reactions and causes less neurotoxicity and myelosuppression.

Uses

Placlitaxel is useful in various solid tumours including breast cancers and ovarian cancers. It is also found to be effective in the cancers of ovary, head and neck, breast, oesophagus and lungs.

Paclitaxel is incorporated into drug eluting stents used for coronary angioplasty to prevent restenosis.

Docetaxel and cabazitaxel are similar in actions, toxicity and uses to paclitaxel. Cabazitaxel is useful in resistant prostatic cancers.

Vinca Alkaloids

Vincristine and **vinblastine** are vinca alkaloids obtained from the leaves of vinca rosea, the periwinkle plant. **Vinorelbine** is a semisynthetic derivative.

Mechanism of Action

Vinca alkaloids bind to microtubules in the mitotic apparatus and arrest cell division in metaphase. They are **spindle poisons.** They are cell cycle specific and act on the 'M' phase of the cell cycle.

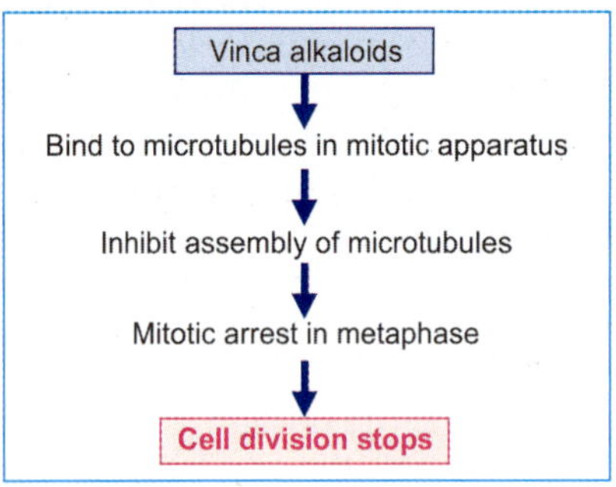

Though the structure and mechanism of action of vinca alkaloids are similar, they differ in toxicity and therapeutic uses.

Vinca alkaloids are metabolised in the liver by microsomal enzymes and are largely excreted through the gut.

Vincristine is neurotoxic while bone marrow depression is less. Peripheral neuropathy and mental depression can occur. Autonomic side effects, like constipation, could be profound and may need prophylactic laxatives. Urinary retension, orthostatic hypotension are reported. Other adverse effects include nausea, vomiting, alopecia and inappropriate secretion of ADH (SIADH). It is used in leukaemias, Hodgkin's lymphoma (MOPP regimen), non-Hodgkin's lymphoma, breast, lung and cervical tumours. It is also used in many paediatric solid tumours like Wilms' tumour, Ewing's sarcoma, brain tumour and rhabdomyosarcoma.

Vinblastine causes bone marrow depression, alopecia and vomiting. It is a vesicant and should be injected carefully. It is used with bleomycin and cisplatin (VBC) in testicular tumours; it is also useful in Hodgkin's and non-Hodgkin's lymphoma.

Vinorelbine is a semisynthetic vinca alkaloid used intravenously in lung cancers (non-small cell type), breast and ovarian cancers. It can cause bone marrow suppression, (granulocytopenia), nausea, vomiting and neurotoxicity (paraesthesias).

Other spindle poisons include ixabepilone and eribulin. They bind to beta tubulin on microtubules and inhibit its activity—act on M phase. Useful in drug resistant solid tumours including breast cancers.

MISCELLANEOUS

Hydroxyurea is an analogue of urea and acts by inhibiting the enzyme ribonucleotide reductase and thereby inhibits DNA synthesis. It acts on the 'S' phase of the cell cycle. It is orally effective, almost completely and rapidly absorbed. Adverse effects are myelosuppression, nausea, vomiting and skin pigmentation. Hydroxyurea is an useful drug in chronic myeloid leukaemia and is now considered the first-line drug in it.

L-asparaginase

The amino acid asparagine is synthesized by the normal cells but malignant cells are unable to synthesize asparagine and depend on the host for the supply. Asparaginase is an enzyme that converts asparagine to aspartic acid and deprives the malignant cells of asparagine supplies resulting in inhibition of protein synthesis.

Asparagine
↓ *Asparaginase*
Aspartic acid

For therapeutic purpose, it is obtained from *E. coli*. It is used in acute leukaemias. Hypersensitivity reactions are common as it is a foreign protein; it can cause haemorrhage due to inhibition of clotting factors; hepatotoxicity with raised serum transaminases and pancreatitis can occur. Inhibition of insulin synthesis may result in hyperglycaemia. It also causes nausea, vomiting and CNS depression. Bone marrow suppression and effects on GI epithelium are mild and it does not cause alopecia.

Protein Tyrosine Kinase Inhibitors

Imatinib, dasatinib and nilotinib act by inhibiting some selective tyrosine kinases (taking part in signal transduction) which are considered to be involved in the pathogenesis of chronic myeloid leukaemia.

Imatinib, dasatinib and nilotinib are almost completely absorbed when given orally, are metabolised by microsomal enzymes CYP3A4 and the metabolites are excreted through the gut. Other drugs metabolised by microsomal enzymes should be used cautiously to avoid drug interactions.

Adverse effects include skin rashes, nausea, vomiting, muscle cramps, oedema and elevated serum transaminases.

Uses

Imatinib is now the drug of choice in chronic myeloid leukaemia.

Imatinib resistant CML responds to dasatinib and nilotinib as they overcome imatinib resistance due to mutation.

Imatinib is also used in gastrointestinal tumors that express tyrosine kinase.

Dasatinib is effective in imatinib resistant cases of Philadelphia chromosome positive acute lymphoblastic leukaemia.

Gefitinib and **erlotinib** inhibit epidermal growth factor receptor (EGFR) tyrosine kinase. EGFR is overexpressed in several malignancies. Gefitinib is orally effective (250 mg/day) and metabolised by CYP3A4. Adverse effects include nausea, vomiting, anorexia, diarrhoea, pruritis and skin rashes. Gefitinib and erlotinib are approved for use in non-small cell lung cancer that has not responded to first-line drugs.

Sunitinib and sorafinib are tyrosine kinase inhibitors—they inhibit VEGF and are used in renal cell carcinoma and hepatocellular carcinoma and some GI tumours. Pazopanib is another VEGF inhibitor indicated in advanced renal cell carcinoma.

Bortezomib binds with high affinity to 26S proteosome and inhibits it, thereby promotes programmed cell death in neoplastic cells. Myelosuppression and peripheral neuropathy are dose limiting.

Bortezomib is used in refractory multiple myeloma.

Bosutinib: Another tyrosine kinase inhibitor is useful in CML resistant to other drugs.

Others

Thalidomide has made a comeback in medicine. It has been found to be useful in the treatment of **multiple myeloma**. The exact mechanism of action is not known but could be by stimulation of T cells and natural killer cells, inhibition of angiogenesis and tumour cell proliferation and modulation of haematopoietic stem cell differentiation. Sedation, constipation, peripheral neuropathy and carpel tunnel syndrome are the adverse effects. Thromboembolic events are rare.

Lenalidomide is a derivative of thalidomide which is more potent and safer than it. It is used in myeloma and relapsed NHL.

Monoclonal Antibodies

Cancer cells express several antigens which may be targetted by monoclonal antibodies. Many monoclonal antibodies are now available for treatment of lymphomas and solid tumours (Table 57.4). Some of the

Table 57.4: Some antigens, monoclonal antibodies and their indications in cancer

Monoclonal antibody	*Antigen*	*Indication*
Rituximab	CD20	Lymphoma, CLL
Alemtuzumab	CD52	Lymphoma, CLL
Trastuzumab	HER-2	Breast cancer
Cetuximab	EGFR	Colorectal, pancreatic, breast cancer
Bevacizumab	VEGF	Colorectal
Gemtuzumab	CD33	AML

monoclonal antibodies are combined with a radioactive isotope.

Rituximab targets antigen on the B cells causing lysis of the these cells. It targets the CD20 antigen on B cell and is found to be effective in B cell lymphomas and CLL. It has also been used as maintenance therapy to delay the progression. It is synergistic with chemotherapy in that rituximab sensitizes the lymphoma cells so that they are susceptible to the apoptotic effects of chemotherapy. It can cause infusion reactions and rarely dermatological toxicity.

Alemtuzumab binds to the CD52 antigen on B and T cells causing cell death in lymphomas and CLL. Since CD52 antigen is also expressed on normal neutrophils and lymphocytes, infections as expected can be quite serious, particularly if the patient is already immunosuppressed due to chemotherapy. Allergic reactions are common.

Trastuzumab is a humanised antibody against HER2 receptors. These HER2 receptors which belong to EGF family of receptors are overexpressed in breast cancer cells and are involved in resistance to chemotherapy. Trastuzumab can directly induce death of breast cancer cells. It may be used along with or following chemotherapy in (HER2 positive) breast cancers and stomach cancer. Allergic reactions and cardiac dysfunction have been reported.

Cetuximab, panitumumab: Epidermal growth factor receptor (EGFR or HER1) belongs to the family of growth factor receptors. Several epithelial cell cancers including colorectal cancer, breast, lung, kidney, prostate, pancreas, brain as well as head and neck cancers have shown an overexpression of these EGFR receptors. Cetuximab and panitumumab are monoclonal antibodies targeting the EGFR (it inhibits EGF binding and signalling) and are approved for the treatment of EGFR-positive metastatic colorectal cancer.

Bevacizumab: Vascular endothelial growth factor (VEGF) is an angiogenic growth factor which controls the growth of new blood vessels. These receptors are present in large numbers in the tumour. Bevacizumab is MAB that targets VEGF, prevents binding of VEGF to its receptors and thereby suppresses the tumour growth. Bevacizumab is approved as a first-line treatment for metastatic colorectal and lung cancer along with chemotherapy and in breast cancer and cervical cancers.

HORMONES IN CANCER CHEMOTHERAPY

Glucocorticoids

Due to their lympholytic action, glucocorticoids are used in acute leukaemias and lymphomas. Rapid clinical improvement is seen but duration can vary from 2 weeks to 9 months. They are used for initiation of therapy due to their rapid action.

Prednisolone or dexamethasone are commonly used.

Glucocorticoids are also of value in the following:

1. With radiation therapy to reduce radiation oedema.
2. In intracranial tumours to reduce cerebral oedema.
3. For symptomatic relief in critically ill patients.

Oestrogens are physiological antagonists of androgens. Hence they are useful in:

Prostatic carcinoma as it is an androgen-dependent tumour. **Fosfestrol** is a prodrug of oestrogen—gets converted to stilbestrol in prostatic tissue. It has another advantage that it attains high concentration in the prostate. Hence it is preferred in prostatic cancer.

Progestins are useful in the palliative management of endometrial carcinoma.

Androgens are used in the palliative treatment of breast cancer in postmenopausal women along with oophorectomy.

Hormone Antagonists

Aromatase Inhibitors

The enzyme aromatase catalyzes the conversion of androgens to oestrogens. Inhibitors of aromatase have been found to be effective in breast cancers. **Exemestane, anastrozole, and letrozole** are the aromatase inhibitors used.

Aminoglutethimide and trilastane inhibit the conversion of cholesterol to pregnenolone (the first step in corticosteroid synthesis) and thereby inhibit the synthesis of adrenocorticoids. Aminoglutethimide is useful in advanced breast cancers when cancer cells contain oestrogen receptors.

Octreotide, a somatostatin analog, is useful to reduce the secretion of growth hormone, insulin, glucagon and peptide hormones in carcinoid tumours and islet cell carcinomas of the pancreas.

Antioestrogens

Tamoxifen is an oestrogen receptor antagonist used in oestrogen receptor containing breast cancer (*see* page 482).

Fulvestrant is a SERD used in ER positive breast cancer. It downregulates the oestrogen receptors and is effective even in those resistant to tamoxifen.

GnRH Analogs

Long-term administration of leuprolide, goserelin and buserelin is useful in prostatic and breast cancers. They may be combined with tamoxifen in breast cancers.

Estramustine is a molecule containing both oestradiol and nitrogen mustard. It is useful in prostatic cancers which are not responding to oestrogens. Adverse effects are similar to that of oestrogen administration.

Antiandrogen: Flutamide and bicalutamide are used in prostatic cancer.

Radioactive Isotopes

Some radioactive isotopes can be used in the treatment of certain specific cancers.

Radiophosphorus P^{32} is used in polycythemia vera. It is taken up by the bone where it emits beta rays and has a half-life of about 14 days.

Strontium chloride emits beta rays and has a longer t½ in the bony metastases. It is used to alleviate pain in painful bony metastases.

Radioactive iodine I^{131} is used in the treatment of thyroid cancers (*see* page 465).

New Approaches in Cancer Chemotherapy

Immunotoxin: The interleukin receptor is expressed only on malignant lymphocytes (not on normal cells) and the immunotoxin is found to be effective in lymphomas. The **Immunotoxin, demileukin diftitox,** is a genetic recombination of interleukin 2 with diphtheria toxin to obtain an immunotoxin.

Hypertension, thromboembolic events and wound healing problems are noted.

Antibody Conjugates

Monoclonal antibody **gemtuzumab** is conjugated with an anticancer antibiotic (ozagamicin). The conjugate binds to CD 33 on the tumour cells, is taken up by the cells and causes breaks in DNA and finally cell death. It is approved for use in relapsed AML.

Radioimmunoconjugates form another approach to reach radioactive isotope into tumour cells using monoclonal antibodies. Several of them used to deliver isotopes to tumours have been developed—like arcitumab, capromab pendetide, nafetumomab, satumumab and tositumomab.

General Principles in the Treatment of Cancers

Chemotherapy in most cancers (except curable cancers) is generally palliative and suppressive. Because of the ability of cancers for recurrence, i.e. even if a few cells are spared during treatment, these cells can multiply and result in recurrence and regrowth of a tumour of earlier dimensions. To avoid this, it is essential to kill all the cancer cells during treatment—to achieve what is known as 'total cell kill'.

Chemotherapy is just one of the modes in the treatment of cancer. Other modes like radiotherapy and surgery are also employed to ensure 'total cell kill'. Combination of drugs is preferred for:

- Synergistic effect
- Reduced adverse effects and
- To prevent rapid development of resistance (Table 57.5).

Drugs which do not depress bone marrow are useful in combination regimens to avoid overlapping of adverse effects. With appropriate treatment, cure can now be achieved in a few cancers. Maintenance of good nutrition, treatment of anaemia, protection against infections, adequate relief of pain and anxiety and good emotional support—all go a long way in the appropriate management of these dreaded diseases (Table 57.6).

Table 57.5: Choice of drugs in some malignancies

Malignancy	*Preferred drugs*
Acute lymphatic leukaemia	Vincristine + prednisolone + L-asparaginase Maintenance—mercaptopurine/methotrexate, cyclophosphamide
Acute myeloid leukaemia	Cytosine arabinoside + daunorubicin
Chronic lymphatic leukaemia	Fludarabine/chlorambucil + prednisolone
Chronic myeloid leukaemia	Imatinib
Hodgkin's disease	*ABVD* A: Adriamycin (doxorubicin) B: Bleomycin V: Vinblastin D: Dacarbazine
Non-Hodgkin's lymphoma	Cyclophosphamide + Doxorubicin + Vincristine (oncovin) + Prednisolone (CHOP)*
Carcinoma of stomach	Fluorouracil + Cisplatin + Docetaxel
Carcinoma of colon	Fluorouracil + Irinotecan/oxaliplatin + Leucovorin
Multiple myeloma	CYBORD—cyclophosphamide +Bortezomib + Dexamethasone
Choriocarcinoma	Methotrexate
Carcinoma of testis	Etoposide + Bleomycin + Cisplatin
Osteogenic sarcoma	Methotrexate or doxorubicin, + Cisplatin
Wilms' tumour	Vincristine + Actinomycin-D after surgery
Carcinoma of the head and neck	Fluorouracil + Cisplatin
Carcinoma of lung	Cisplatin + Paclitaxel, Gemcitabine

**In CHOP, 'H' stands for doxorubicin formerly called hydroxydaunomycin. Earlier MOPP regimen with mechlorethamine, oncovin, procarbazine and prednisolone was used and is now replaced by CHOP.*

Table 57.6: Salient features of some commonly used anticancer drugs

Drugs	*MOA*	*Uses*	*Remarks*
Cyclophosphamide	Forms reactive derivatives, alkylates DNA and important groups → cytotoxicity	NHL, CLL, breast, ovarian cancer, soft tissue sarcoma, Wilms' tumour, rhabdomyosarcoma	Mesna—to avoid cystitis
Busulfan	Same as above	CML	Selective action on myeloid series
Methotrexate	Folate antagonist—MTX, polyglutamates decrease DHFR→inhibits protein synthesis	Choriocarcinoma, NHL, breast, bladder, head and neck cancer, osteogenic sarcoma	Folinic acid rescue
Mercaptopurine	Purine analog—incorporated into DNA and RNA—breaks in DNA, inhibits DNA synthesis	AML	DI with allopurinol
5-Fluorouracil	Pyrimidine analog—incorporated into DNA and RNA→inhibits DNA synthesis, inhibits TS.	Colorectal, anal, hepatocellular, gastric, breast, ovaries, head and neck cancers	Leucovorin potentiates antitoxic effects of 5-FU
Actinomycin-D	Inhibits DNA dependent RNA synthesis	Wilms' tumour, Ewing's tumour rhabdomyosarcoma, choriocarcinoma, Kaposi's and soft tissue sarcoma; immunosuppressant	Potent anticancer drug
Bleomycin	Bind iron, generates free radicals—breaks in DNA	Testicular tumours, head and neck cancer, HL and NHL	Suitable for combination regimens
Daunorubicin and doxorubicin	Bind DNA and inhibits topoisomerase II, generation of free radicals—breaks in DNA	Dauno: AML, ALL Doxo: Leukaemias, solid tumours, NHL	Cardiotoxicity
Etoposide	Inhibits topoisomerase II	NHL, gastric, lung cancer, germ cell tumours, leukaemias	Affect cells in S and G_2 phases
Topotecan,	Inhibits topoisomerase I	Lung and ovarian cancer	
irinotecan	—	Lung and colorectal cancer	Irinotecan inhibits acetylcholinesterase; Diarrhoea troublesome
Paclitaxel	Inhibits mitosis—mitotic spindle poison	Solid tumours	Myelosuppression and neurotoxicity
		Breast, lung, ovarian, head neck, oesophageal and prostate cancer	Used in drug eluting stents for angioplasty.
Vinblastine	Inhibits mitosis	HL, NHL, germ cell and breast cancer, Kaposi's sarcoma	Bone marrow toxic
Vincristine	Same as above	ALL, HL, NHL, Wilms' tumour rhabdomyosarcoma, neuroblastoma	Neurotoxic
Cisplatin	Active form inhibits DNA synthesis, forms DNA cross-links	Lung, breast, bladder, testis, ovarian, head and neck cancers	
Asparaginase	Converts aspargine to aspartic acid and deprives asparagine supply	ALL	Allergic reactions, haemorrhage

NHL: Non-Hodgkin's lymphoma
HL: Hodgkin's lymphoma
CLL: Chronic lymphocytic leukaemia
ALL: Acute lymphocytic leukaemia
TS: Thymidylate synthase
AML: Acute myeloid leukaemia
DI: Drug interactions

BIOLOGICAL RESPONSE MODIFIERS

Several agents are used to beneficially influence the patients' response to treatment and to overcome some adverse effects. These have also been termed biological response modifiers. They are as follows:

1. *Haematopoietic growth factors,* like erythropoietin and myeloid growth factors like GM-CSF, G-CSF, M-CSF and thrombopoietin (*see* page 448), are used to treat bone marrow suppression.
2. *Interferons* (*see* page 619), like interferon alpha, is used in hairy cell leukaemia, Kaposi's sarcoma and condylomata acuminata.
3. *Aldesleukin is recombinant interleukin 2*: It enhances cytotoxic activity of T cells, induces activity of natural killer cells and also induces interferon production. It is useful in inducing remission in renal cell carcinoma. Hypotension is the most troublesome side effect.
4. *Tretinoin* (all transretinoic acid) induces differentiation in leukaemic cells and the leukaemic promyelocytes loose their ability to proliferate. It is useful to induce remission in acute promyelocytic leukaemia.
5. *Amifostine* has been designed to offer selective cytoprotection to normal tissues from the effects of cytotoxic drugs. Amifostine activates an enzyme in the normal tissues which can inactivate the active form of cisplatin and radiation. It has also been shown to stimulate the bone marrow in some bone marrow disorders.

Resistance to Anticancer Drugs

Resistance to anticancer drugs may be primary or secondary. Resistance is primary when the cancer is not responsive to the drug at the first exposure itself. Secondary resistance is acquired during treatment with the drug and could be by the following mechanisms:

- The amount of the drug taken up into the cells may be decreased.
- Decreased accumulation of cytotoxic drugs in the tumour cells.
- Transport proteins like P-glycoprotein may expel the drug from the cell.
- Conversion of the drug to active metabolites may be reduced as most are prodrugs.
- Increased inactivation of the drug (e.g. cytarabine).
- Increased production of target enzyme (DHFA metabolites).
- Alternative metabolic pathway used by cancer cells as with antimetabolites.
- Altered target protein by genetic mutation, e.g. modified topoisomerases II.

Hence, it is important to treat cancers appropriately for successful chemotherapy.

[1] From Medical Council of India, *Competency based Undergraduate Curriculum for the Indian Medical Graduate*, 2018;1:136–144.

CHAPTER 58

Antiseptics and Disinfectants

Competency achievement: The student should be able to:

PH 1.62 Describe and discuss antiseptics and disinfectants.[1]

Disinfection is destruction of all pathogenic organisms but not spores. If spores are also killed, it is called *sterilization*. A **disinfectant** is used on ***inanimate objects***.

Antiseptic is an agent that destroys microorganisms and can be used on *living tissues*. The term ***germicide*** can be used for either drugs. Germicides are widely used in domestic products like soaps, toothpastes and after-shave lotions.

Mechanism of Action

Germicides may act by the following mechanisms:

1. Oxidation of bacterial protoplasm
2. Denaturation of bacterial proteins
3. Detergent like action
4. Competition with essential substrates for the important enzymes in the bacterial cell.

An ideal germicide should have a wide antibacterial spectrum, should be chemically stable, should have rapid action, non-irritating to the tissues, not interfere with wound healing activity even in presence of pus, exudates and tissue degradation products; it should not be absorbed into systemic circulation.

Factors that influence the activity of germicidal agents.

1. *Concentration of the drug and duration of contact:* In general, higher the concentration of the antiseptic, greater is its effect. However, alcohol is an exception to this and at 70% concentration maximum antiseptic effect is seen.
2. *Susceptibility of the organism:* Spores and viruses are resistant to many antiseptics.
3. *Temperature:* A rise in temperature will increase antiseptic activity.

Classification

1. *Acids*	Boric acid, benzoic acid
2. *Alcohols*	Ethanol, isopropyl alcohol
3. *Aldehydes*	Formaldehyde, glutaraldehyde
4. *Surfactants*	Soaps, benzalkonium, cetrimide, cetylpyridinium chloride, dequalinium chloride
5. *Phenol derivatives*	Phenol, cresol, resorcinal, chlorhexidine chloroxylenol, hexachlorophene
6. *Halogens*	Iodine, iodophors, chlorine, chloramines
7. *Oxidizing agents*	Hydrogen peroxide, Benzoyl peroxide potassium permanganate
8. *Dyes*	Gentian violet, methylene blue, brilliant green, acriflavine, proflavine
9. *Metallic salts*	Mercurial compounds, silver nitrate, zinc compounds

ACIDS

Boric acid and sodium borate (borax) have weak bacteriostatic and fungistatic activity. Aqueous solutions of boric acid are used for irrigating eyes, bladder, vagina and large wounds.

Benzoic acid is an antibacterial (below pH 5) and antifungal agent-used as a preservative in laboratory.

Salicylic acid has bacteriostatic, fungicidal and keratolytic properties. It is used as a dusting powder or 2% ointment for seborrhoeic dermatitis, warts and corns.

ALCOHOLS

Ethyl alcohol is employed as an antiseptic at 60–90% concentration. The antiseptic activity decreases above 90%. It rapidly denatures the bacterial proteins (*see* Chapter 20).

Disadvantages

1. It has poor activity against spores, some viruses and fungi.
2. Irritant causes burning when applied on open wounds
3. Alcohols are flammable—should be allowed to evaporate before using cautery or laser surgery.

Uses: Ethyl alcohol is used to clean the skin before injections and surgeries.

Isopropyl alcohol is more potent and more toxic than ethanol. It is used in 68–72% concentration as skin antiseptic.

ALDEHYDES

Formaldehyde is a gas at room temperature used for fumigation; the 40% aqueous solution is noncorrosive and has a broad antimicrobial spectrum. It has a pungent odour and is an irritant—highly irritating to respiratory mucous membranes and eyes. Formaldehyde is also a carcinogen and Occupational Safety and Health Administration (OSHA) has set standards to limit exposure of health care workers to formaldehyde.

Mechanism of action: Aldehydes act by alkylation of chemical groups in proteins and nucleic acids.

Uses

Formaldehyde gas is used for fumigation and for sterilizing instruments which cannot be moistened with solution. Formaldehyde 40% solution (100% formalin) in water is used for disinfection of surgical instruments and gloves; embalming and preservation of tissues. Fibreoptic endoscopies, respiratory therapy equipment, haemodialysers and dental handpieces which cannot withstand high temperatures of steam sterilisation are disinfected with formaldehyde.

Automatic circulating baths are used which increase penetration of aldehyde solution into the instruments and decrease operator exposure to the chemical. Its rapidity of action increases by making a solution in 70% propanol.

Glutaraldehyde is a dialdehyde used as a 2% solution. It is bactericidal, sporicidal, fungicidal and viricidal. pH should be between 7.4 and 8.5. It is less irritant than formaldehyde; has greater sporicidal activity; does not damage lenses and cementing material in endoscopes. Glutaraldehyde is superior to formaldehyde for sterilising rubber, plastic and metal appliances. Two per cent solution is used for local application in idiopathic hyperhidrosis of palms and soles.

SURFACTANTS

Surfactants are chemicals that lower the surface tension of solutions and are termed detergents. They may be anionic, cationic, ampholytic surfactants or polysorbates.

Anionic surfactants, e.g. soaps.

- They dissociate in aqueous solutions to form a large and complex anion which lowers the surface tension.
- Effective for gram-positive and acid-fast organisms.
- Microorganisms are enmeshed in the lather and washed away on rinsing.
- Anionic surfactants have a narrow spectrum; precipitate in hard water; cause drying of the skin.

Preparations

1. Potassium hydroxide or sodium hydroxide + vegetable oil.
2. Sodium lauryl sulphate—effective in hard water.

Cationic surfactants: For example, benzalkonium chloride, cetrimide, cetylpyridinium chloride, dequalinium chloride. Cationic surfactants dissociate into large cations.

They are:

- Active against gram-positive and gram-negative organisms (less active against spores, viruses and fungi)
- Most effective in neutral solution
- Non-irritating and safe
- Incompatible with anionic surfactants
- Absorbed by cotton and rubber
- One of the most commonly used germicidal agents.

Benzalkonium chloride has an aromatic odour and is soluble in water.

- 1:1000 solution for cleansing skin
- 1:2000 for mucous membranes and denuded skin
- 1:20,000 for irrigation of the bladder and urethra
- It is also used for (1:1000–4000) storing sterilised surgical instruments but instruments should be thoroughly washed before use.

Cetrimide 1% solution is used like above. It is also used as a cream. It is very effective for cleaning wounds. In combination with chlorhexidine is one of the most popular antiseptics.

Dose: CETAVLON 1% CETRIMIDE

Hibitane, Savlon is cetrimide 3% + chlorhexidine. Savlon causes irritation to the eyes and rarely skin. Allergic reactions can also occur. Hence Savlon should be wiped off the skin after application. Accidental exposure of the eyes to Savlon can cause intense burning, pain and abrasions of the cornea and conjunctiva. It should be immediately washed off followed by a few days of prednisolone eye drops to suppress inflammation.

Dequalinium chloride is used in gum paints and lozenges.

Cetylpyridinium chloride is used in mouthwashes and lozenges.

PHENOL DERIVATIVES

Phenol is one of the oldest antiseptics introduced by Lord Lister in 1867. It is bactericidal and fungicidal but has poor action against spores and viruses. It acts by denaturing the bacterial proteins. It also has a mild local anaesthetic action. Phenol rapidly penetrates even intact skin and mucous membrane. It is a protoplasmic poison.

Phenol is extremely irritant to exposed tissues (corrosive)—when swallowed, it burns buccal, oesophageal and gastric mucous membrane.

Uses: Phenol is used to disinfect urine, faeces, sputum of patients and is sometimes used as antipruritic because of its local anaesthetic action.

Cresol is methylphenol, which is as toxic as phenol but is more active. It is used as a **disinfectant for utensils and excreta**.

Lysol is cresol with soap solution. It has higher antiseptic activity and is an useful disinfectant for hospital and domestic use.

Chloroxylenol is a less toxic chlorinated phenol, effective against gram-positive and gram-negative organisms. Surgical dettol contains 1.4% of chloroxylenol for skin; 6.25% for instruments and 1 to 3% in antiseptic cream. Dettol liq. (13%); Obstetric cream (1.4%).

Hexachlorophene: This chlorinated phenol acts by inhibiting bacterial enzymes and causing lysis. It is effective mainly against gram-positive organisms and has weak action against gram-negative organisms. It is odourless and non-irritating to use on skin. It is used in soaps for surgical scrubbing, for cleaning the skin in obstetrics, carbuncles and seborrhoeic dermatitis. It may cause allergic reactions. It also reduces body odour by preventing bacterial decomposition of organic material and, therefore, is used as a deodorant. In USA, hexachlorophene was used to wash newborn babies which resulted in brain damage in such babies and, therefore, use of >3% hexachlorophene is banned.

Chlorhexidine is effective against gram-positive, gram-negative organisms and fungi. It is rapid acting and non-irritating.

SAVLON—Chlorhexidine + Cetrimide.

HALOGENS

Iodine is one of the oldest antiseptics. It has a broad-spectrum of activity, is a powerful bactericidal, sporicidal, fungicidal and viricidal agent. The activity is inhibited by organic material but enhanced by alcohol.

Disadvantages: It is irritating, painful, stains the area, and may delay wound healing. Rashes, fever and generalised skin eruptions may develop in some patients who are sensitive to iodine. Prolonged systemic use causes iodism.

Uses of Iodine

1. *Tincture iodine (I_2 in KI + alcohol)* is used to clean the skin before surgery. Iodine crystals are used to sterilize water for soaking vegetables and cleaning before use.
2. *Mandl's paint (compound iodide paint)* is used in the treatment of tonsillitis and pharyngitis.
3. *Iodine ointment* as fungicide in ringworm. Iodides have no antibacterial action.

Iodophors are soluble complexes of iodine with surfactants like detergents. The detergents serve as carriers and slowly release iodine, e.g. Povidone iodine–5% solution; Piodine—10% solution, Betadine 10% paint, 5% oint, cream.

Advantages

Iodophors are non-irritating, non-staining, water-soluble, less toxic and non-sensitizing to the skin.

Uses: Used for preoperative scrubbing, skin preparation, disinfection of instruments, as local antiseptic in boils, furunculosis, burns, ulcers, ringworm and in oral/vaginal moniliasis.

Chlorine is a potent germicide and is bactericidal against several gram-positive and gram-negative organisms in a very low concentration (0.1 PPM in 30 seconds). It also destroys protozoa and viruses. The antibacterial activity of chlorine is reduced in presence of organic matter since they bind chlorine and, therefore, need higher concentration of free chlorine. Chloramines are compounds that release chlorine slowly.

1. *Chlorinated lime* (bleaching powder) is obtained by the action of chlorine on lime. It is used for disinfection of water in swimming pools and water for drinking.
2. *Chloramine* is an organic chloride. The freshly prepared solution is used for mouthwash, irrigating the bladder and urethra.
3. *Eusol* is a solution of chlorinated lime with boric acid.

OXIDIZING AGENTS

Hydrogen peroxide is a colourless and odourless liquid. It liberates nascent oxygen when applied to tissues and then oxidizes bacteria and necrotic tissue. On application, there is effervescence and this helps in removing tissue debris, ear wax, etc. Hydrogen peroxide has poor penetrability and the action is of short duration. On keeping, it loses its potency. It is also a deodorant.

Uses

Hydrogen peroxide is used for cleansing wounds, abscesses and for irrigation. In dentistry, it is used to clean septic sockets and root canals and also as a mouthwash and deodorant gargle. It is used as ear drops while removing ear wax.

Potassium permanganate: It is an oxidizing agent and an astringent. The purple crystals are water-soluble. It acts by liberating oxygen which oxidizes bacterial protoplasm. Organic matter reduces its activity and the solution gets decolourised. It promotes rusting; concentrated solution is caustic and causes burns and blistering.

Uses

- 1:4000–1:10000 solution of potassium permanganate is used for gargling, irrigating cavities, urethra and wounds.
- For stomach wash in alkaloidal poisoning (except atropine and cocaine as these are not efficiently oxidized).
- 1% solution in mycotic infections like athletes foot.
- 5% solution as a styptic.
- Topically to oxidise venom in case of snake and scorpion bite.
- To purify well water.
- To disinfect vegetables and fruits.

DYES

Gentian violet (aniline dye, crystal violet or medicinal gentian violet) is effective against gram-positive organisms and fungi. Staining is the only disadvantage. It is a non-irritant and potent antiseptic. 0.5–1% solution is used topically on furunculosis, burns, boils, chronic ulcers, infected eczema, thrush, ringworm and mycotic infections of the skin and mucous membranes.

Brilliant green: Actions are similar to gentian violet. It is used as a 0.5–1% solution in the treatment of burns, impetigo and infected wounds like gentian violet.

Methylene blue is used systemically in cyanide poisoning as it converts methaemoglobin to haemoglobin.

Acriflavine and proflavine are acridine dyes active against gram-positive bacteria and gonococci (proflavine is better). They are non-irritant; efficacy is unaffected by organic matter but is increased in alkaline medium; 1:1000 solution is used in infected wounds and burns, 2% pessary in vaginitis and cervicitis.

Triple dye lotion contains gentian violet 0.25% + brilliant green 0.25% + acriflavine or proflavine 0.1%—it is used in burns dressing.

METALLIC SALTS

Silver compounds have antiseptic, astringent and caustic properties. Silver nitrate kills microbes rapidly and the action is prolonged due to slow release of silver ions from silver proteinate that is formed by an interaction with tissue proteins. The reduced silver gets deposited and stains the tissues black.

Silver nitrate is used for the prophylaxis of ophthalmia neonatorum.

Silver sulfadiazine is active against *Pseudomonas* and is used in burn wounds.

Colloidal silver compounds slowly release silver. They are non-corrosive, non-irritant, non-astringent and have better penetrability and used as nasal and eye drops.

Zinc salts like zinc oxide have astringent and mild antiseptic properties. Zinc oxide is used as an ointment or lotion in eczema, impetigo and psoriasis.

Mercury compounds act by inhibiting sulphydryl enzymes of bacteria. They are bacteriostatic and are poor antiseptics—not commonly used.

[1] From Medical Council of India, *Competency based Undergraduate Curriculum for the Indian Medical Graduate*, 2018;1:136–144.

Unit XIV

Immunopharmacology

Immunosuppressants, Management of Organ Transplant Rejection, Immunostimulants and Immunization

CHAPTER 59

Competency achievement: The student should be able to:

PH 1.50 Describe mechanisms of action, types, doses, side effects, indications and contraindications of immunomodulators and management of organ transplant rejection.[1]

The immune system is designed to protect the host from invasion by pathogenic organisms and disease. The components include—the innate and adaptive immune systems. Drugs influencing the immune system include immunosuppressants, immunostimulants and immunomodulators. Vaccines and antisera also act by stimulating or supplementing the immune system.

IMMUNOSUPPRESSANTS

Immunosuppressants are drugs which inhibit immunity. They may suppress cell-mediated or humoral immunity or both. It is necessary to suppress immune reaction in organ transplantation (to prevent graft rejection) and in autoimmune disorders.

Immunosuppressants are classified as:

Classification

1. **Calcineurin inhibitors**
   Cyclosporine, tacrolimus
2. **Antiproliferative drugs**
   Sirolimus, everolimus, mycophenolate mofetil
3. **Cytotoxic drugs**
   Azathioprine, methotrexate, cyclophosphamide, chlorambucil, leflunomide, teriflunomide.
4. **Glucocorticoids**
5. **Immunosuppressant antibodies**
   Muromonab CD3, antilymphocyte globulin, antithymocyte globulin, anti-Rh (D) immune globulin, adalimumab, infliximab, etanercept, basiliximab, daclizumab.
6. **Others**
   Hydroxychloroquine, thalidomide, lenalidomide, pomalidomide.

Calcineurin Inhibitors

Cyclosporine: Cyclosporine is a cyclic peptide antibiotic produced by a fungus *Beauveria nivea.*

Actions: Cyclosporine acts at an early stage, selectively inhibits T cell proliferation and suppresses cell-mediated immunity. It can be given orally and intravenously.

Mechanism of action

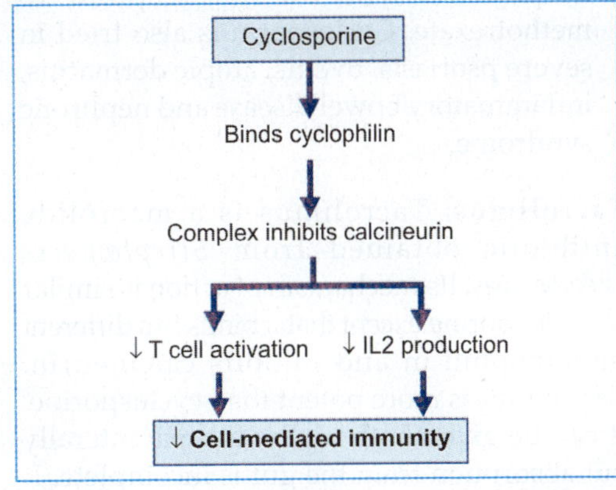

Cyclosporine binds to cyclophilin (an immunophilin) and this complex binds to and inhibits phosphatase calcineurin. This results in inhibition of T cell activation and IL-2 production. T cells do not respond to specific antigenic stimulation. Cyclosporine also suppresses the proliferation of cytoxic T cells.

Tacrolimus binds to another immunophilin and then the complex inhibits calcineurin.

Pharmacokinetics: Cyclosporine is effective by both oral and IV route. It is metabolised by microsomal enzymes cytochrome P450 in the liver. It can, therefore, interact with many drugs given concurrently.

Adverse effects include nephrotoxicity, hepatotoxicity, anorexia, gum hypertrophy and increased susceptibility to infections, hypertension, hyperglycaemia, hyperlipidaemia and hirsutism. An increased incidence of lymphoma and other cancers have been noted.

Uses

- In organ transplantation: Cyclosporine is very effective for the prophylaxis and treatment of graft rejection in organ transplantation surgeries—like kidney, liver, bone marrow and other transplants.
- Autoimmune disorders: Cyclosporine is also useful in some autoimmune disorders like rheumatoid arthritis as an alternative in patients who do not respond to methotrexate. Cyclosporin is also tried in severe psoriasis, uveitis, atopic dermatitis, inflammatory bowel disease and nephrotic syndrome.

Tacrolimus: Tacrolimus is a macrolide antibiotic obtained from *Streptomyces tsukubaensis*. Its mechanism of action is similar to cyclosporine except that it binds to a different immunophill in and inhibits calcineurin. Tacrolimus is more potent than cyclosporine. It can be given both orally and parenterally but absorption from the gut is incomplete. It is extensively bound to plasma proteins.

Adverse effects include nephrotoxicity, gastrointestinal disturbances, hypertension, hyperglycaemia, tremors and seizures.

Uses: For prevention of graft rejection in organ transplantation similar to cyclosporine.

Antiproliferative Drugs

Sirolimus: It is a macrocyclic lactone obtained from *Streptomyces hygroscopicus*, acts by inhibiting the activation of T cells.

Mechanism of action: Sirolimus inhibits the activation and proliferation of T cells. Sirolimus forms a complex with an immunophilin and the complex inhibits a protein kinase (mTOR) which is involved in cell growth and proliferation.

Sirolimus is given orally, rapidly absorbed and has a t½ of ~60 hr. It is metabolised by the same cytochrome enzyme (CYP3A4) as cyclosporine and tacrolimus—when used with these drugs the dose of sirolimus should be adjusted.

Toxicity includes hyperlipidaemia, gastrointestinal disturbances and an increased risk of infections and lymphomas.

Uses:

1. *Organ transplantation:* Sirolimus may be used alone or in combination with other drugs for the prophylaxis of organ transplant rejection. It may be used as an alternative to calcineurin inhibitors. Functioning of the kidney graft may be delayed because of its antiproliferative effects.
2. *Psoriasis:* Topical sirolimus is used.
3. *Choreoretinitis:* Sirolimus is used with cyclosporine
4. *Coronary stents:* Drug eluting stents use sirolimus (or paclitaxel). Sirolimus is incorporated into cardiac stents to inhibit local cell proliferation and to reduce restenosis.

Everolimus is similar to sirolimus with minor pharmacokinetic differences.

Mycophenolate mofetil (MMF), a prodrug, is converted to mycophenolic acid, which inhibits guanine nucleotide synthesis. B and T cells depend on this pathway for cell proliferation and thus mycophenolate selectively inhibits the proliferation and functions of lymphocytes. Mycophenolate mofetil is indicated as an adjunct to other immunosuppressive drugs in the prophylaxis of transplant rejection. MMF can be given both orally and intravenously.

Adverse effects include headache, gastro-intestinal disturbances, hypertension and bone marrow suppression.

Uses:

1. *Organ transplantation:* MMF may be used as an alternative to calcineurin to prevent graft rejection.
2. *Other uses:* MMF is also being tried in autoimmune diseases like rheumatoid arthritis, inflammatory bowel disease, lupus nephritis and psoriasis for its immunosuppressant properties.

Cytotoxic Drugs

Cytotoxic drugs, like azathioprine, cyclophosphamide and methotrexate, inhibit cell-mediated immunity (while cyclophosphamide predominantly suppresses humoral immunity). They are used in the prevention of graft rejection and in autoimmune disorders.

Azathioprine is a prodrug of mercaptopurine which is a purine analog. It is a cytotoxic immunosuppressive agent used in maintaining renal and other tissue transplants. It is also useful in SLE, glomerulonephritis, rheumatoid arthritis, Crohn's disease, multiple sclerosis and is being tried in idiopathic thrombocytopenic purpura and autoimmune haemolytic anaemia. Azathioprine is preferred to mercaptopurine because it is a better immunosuppressant, converted to mercaptopurine in the immune cells and also has a better bioavailability.

Cyclophosphamide and **methotrexate** are used for immunosuppressive properties. Pentostatin is also being now tried as an alternative to prevent graft rejection. Leflunomide is an orally effective prodrug. The active metabolite is an inhibitor of pyrimidine synthesis. It is used in rheumatoid arthritis and is also being studied for other autoimmune indications.

Glucocorticoids

Glucocorticoids have potent immunosuppressant activity and are used in the prevention of organ transplant rejection and in autoimmune disorders.

They may be used in combination with immunosuppressant drugs.

Immunosuppressant Antibodies

Muromonab CD3 is a monoclonal antibody to CD3 antigens on T lymphocytes. On intravenous administration, T cells disappear from the circulation within minutes. It is used with other immunosuppressants in organ transplantation. Fever, chills and pulmonary oedema may occur.

Antilymphocyte and antithymocyte antibodies: Antilymphocyte globulin (ALG) and antithymocyte globulin (ATG) are used to induce immunosuppression in solid organ transplants and bone marrow transplantation. They may be used along with cyclosporine to prepare the patient for transplantation by immunosuppression. Allergic reactions, particularly pain at the injection site, are common.

Infliximab is a monoclonal antibody and etanercept is a protein that blocks TNFα. Etanercept inhibits TNF-α mediated inflammation. They are useful in rheumatoid arthritis, Crohn's disease, ulcerative colitis and psoriatic arthritis. Adalimumab is an anti-TNF monoclonal antibody that brings remission in rheumatoid arthritis. Abatacept is a protein that blocks activation of T cells and is useful in rheumatoid arthritis.

Anti-IL-2 receptor antibodies, basiliximab and daclizumab, block the binding of interleukin-2 to the lympocytes and halt the immune process—used in organ transplantation.

Other monoclonal antibodies Efalizumab is used in psoriasis, omalizumab in bronchial asthma and abciximab to prevent platelet aggregation. Many others are under various stages of development.

Anti-Rh (D) immunoglobulin is human IgG with a high titer of antibodies to Rh(D) antigen of the red blood cell. When Rh negative mother delivers an Rh positive baby (or aborts), the Rh positive antigens from the red cells of the foetus enters into the maternal bloodstream. This sensitizes the mother to produce antibodies against Rh positive cells. In subsequent pregnancies, the maternal antibodies against Rh positive cells reach the foetus and may result in haemolytic disease of the newborn.

Injection of anti-Rh(D) immunoglobulin to the mother at the time of child birth (or after abortion) will bind the antigens on the RBCs of the baby which have entered the maternal circulation. This will prevent the formation of antibodies in the Rh negative mother against the Rh positive RBCs. Thus subsequent pregnancies would not be affected. The immunoglobulin should be given within 24–72 hours of child birth.

Dose: 300 μg intramuscularly.

Others

Hydroxychloroquine, an antimalarial drug like chloroquine, also has immunosuppressant and anti-inflammatory properties for which it is used in rheumatoid arthritis and SLE.

Thalidomide *see* immunostimulants.

MANAGEMENT OF ORGAN TRANSPLANT REJECTION

Organ transplantation is now seen as an option in several end stage organ failures. However, transplant rejection is the most common cause for transplant failure. Hence appropriate immuno suppression is needed for successful transplantation. Immunosuppression is associated with adverse effects like increased risk of infection and development of lymphomas.Three regimens used are:

- ***Induction regimen:*** Started before the transplant and continued for 2–12 weeks:
  Cyclosporine or Tacrolimus or Sirolimus + Prednisolone + MMF or Azathioprine

  Though 1-drug or 2-drug regimens may be used, 3-drug regimens provide better chances of graft survival.
- ***Maintenance regimen:*** 3 drug regimen
  Cyclosporine or Tacrolimus or Sirolimus + Prednisolone + Azathioprine + MMF

  Low doses are given for maintenance for a long-term. Here too, good results are seen with 3-drug regimen. Cyclophosphamide, chlorambucil, daclizumab/basiliximab are the 2nd line drugs.
- ***Anti-rejection regimen:*** A glucocorticoid like methylprednisolone for 3–5 days generally suppresses acute rejection episodes. Other drugs used for rescue therapy are muromonab CD3, MMF, tacrolimus and sirolimus.

IMMUNOSTIMULANTS

Immunostimulants and immunomodulators are drugs that modulate the immune response and can be used to increase the immune responsiveness of patients with immunodeficiency as in AIDS, chronic illness and cancers. This is still a developing field of pharmacology. The drugs currently used for this purpose are:

- BCG
- Cytokines
- Thalidomide
- Thymosin
- Levamisole
- Inosiplex
- Interferons
- Immunization

1. **BCG** vaccine, used in tuberculosis, has been tried in cancers and in COVID-19.

2. **Cytokines:** Interferons are cytokines with antiviral and immunomodulatory properties. Recombinant interferons α, β and γ are available for clinical use. They bind to specific receptors and bring about immune activation and increase host defences. There is an

increase in the number and activity of cytotoxic and helper T cells and killer cells. Interferons alpha and beta are mainly used for antiviral effects while interferon α for its immunomodulating actions.

Interferons are indicated in several tumours including malignant melanoma, hairy cell leukaemia, lymphomas, Kaposi's sarcoma, condylomata acuminata and in viral infections.

Other cytokines like IL-2, are being tried as adjuvants to vaccines. Cytokine inhibitors are also under investigation as immunomodulators.

3. **Thalidomide:** The teratogenic hypnotic of 1960s is now being tried in many clinical conditions. It has anti-inflammatory and immunomodulatory properties—inhibits angiogenesis, and enhances cell-mediated immunity by action on T cells. Thalidomide is used in multiple myeloma, lepra reactions and in lupus erythematosus. Adverse effects include teratogenicity, peripheral neuropathy, hypothyroidism and constipation. Because of the increased risk of deep vein thrombosis, an anticoagulant cover is needed. **Lenalidomide** and **pomalidomide** are similar to thalidomide.

4. **Thymosin** is synthesized in the thymus and purified from bovine and human thymus glands for therapeutic use. It induces the maturation of precursor T cells and is tried in hepatitis B and C.

5. **Levamisole:** Levamisole, used in helminthiasis, is found to enhance cell-mediated immunity in humans. It has also been tried in some cancers.

IMMUNIZATION

Competency achievement: The student should be able to:

PH 1.54 Describe vaccines and their uses.[2]

Vaccines and antisera are used for immunization against becterial and viral infections.

Vaccines stimulate the host immune system while antisera supplement and support the immune system with readymade antibodies.

Vaccines are suspensions of microorganisms (dead or live attenuated) which stimulate the immunological defence of the host by developing antibodies.

Toxoids: Bacterial exotoxins modified to remove toxicity but retain antigenicity are toxoids.

Antisera contain antibodies against a particular microorganism—they provide passive immunity. Antisera like tetanus antitoxin, gas gangrene, antitoxin, diphtheria and antirabies sera are obtained from sera of horses which are actively immunised against the specific organism. Sensitivity tests should be done before giving antisera. Allergic reactions may occur because of the animal source.

Immunoglobulins (Ig) are human gammaglobulins that carry the antibodies—like normal human gammaglobulin, tetanus Ig, rabies Ig, anti-diphtheria Ig and hepatitis-B Ig. Allergic reactions including serum sickness and anaphylaxis can occur with antisera, while it is uncommon with Igs.

Active immunisation is the administration of antigen to the host in order to induce antibody production. Vaccines are used for active immunisation. They impart active immunity, which takes sometime to develop and are, therefore, used prophylactically. The antibodies so developed destroy the specific microorganism when it enters the body. Some commonly used vaccines are given in Table 59.1. Vaccines for Japanese encephalitis, Kyasnur forest disease (KFD) and epidemic typhus are also available now.

Passive immunisation is imparting immunity to a host passively by the transfer of antibodies, e.g. antisera and immunoglobulins (Ig). This affords immediate protection because readymade antibodies are available.

Primary immunisation provides primary immunity and is usually given in children, e.g. DPT (triple antigen given to infants).

Classification of immunizing agents

	Bacterial	Viral	Rickettsial
1. Vaccines			
Live-attenuated vaccines	BCG Plague Typhoid (oral)	Oral polio Measles Mumps Rubella Influenza Yellow fever	Epidemic typhus
Inactivated or killed vaccines	Cholera Typhoid Pertussis Plague Meningococcal *H. influenzae* type b Pneumococcal	Rabies Polio Influenza Hepatitis B Japanese encephalitis KFD	
Toxoids	Diphtheria Tetanus		
2. Antisera and immunoglobulins			
Antisera	Diphtheria Tetanus Gas gangrene Botulism	Rabies	
Human Ig	Diphtheria Tetanus	Measles Varicella Mumps Hepatitis A Hepatitis B Rabies	***Others*** Rh (D)

Secondary immunisation: Secondary immunisation is done to reinforce the primary immunity by giving booster doses.

Vaccines in common use and their recommended schedules are given in Table 59.1. Preparations for passive immunisation are given in Tables 59.2 and 59.3.

Table 59.1: Vaccines in common use and their recommended schedules

Vaccine	*Type of agent*	*ROA*	*Primary immunisation*	*Booster*	*Indication*
Bacterial vaccines					
BCG	Live-attenuated	ID/SC	At birth	7 and 14 years	In all children
Cholera	Inactivated	SC/IM	Adults: Two doses 1 month apart	Every 6 months	People living in endemic areas
	Killed	Oral	2 doses 10–14 days apart		

Contd...

Table 59.1: Vaccines in common use and their recommended schedules *(Contd...)*

Vaccine	*Type of agent*	*ROA*	*Primary immunisation*	*Booster*	*Indication*
	Live-attenuated	Oral	Single dose		Risk of exposure
Diphtheria (TRIPLE ANTIGEN)	Toxoid	IM	6, 10, 14 weeks of age	18 months and at 4–6 years	For all children
Pertussis (TRIPLE ANTIGEN)	Inactivated	IM	6, 10, 14 weeks of age	18 months and at 4–6 years	For all children
Tetanus (TRIPLE ANTIGEN)	Toxoid	IM	6, 10, 14 weeks of age	18 months and at 4–6 years	For all children; *Adults:* Postexposure prophylaxis if >5 years has passed since last dose
Typhoid/ Parathyroid	Inactivated	SC	After 3 years at any age: Two doses 4 weeks apart	Every 3 years	Risk of exposure to typhoid fever
Typhoid (typhoral)	Live inactivated	Oral (capsules)	Above 6 years at any age: 3 doses on alternate days 1 hr before food	Every 3 years	Risk of exposure to typhoid fever All children >6 months
Typhoid conjugate vaccine	Conjugate	IM	Single dose	nil	
Meningococcal	Bacterial poly-saccharides	SC	One dose	–	1. Travellers to areas with meningococcal epidemics 2. Control of out-break in closed population
Plague	Inactivated	IM	One dose	–	In an epidemic
Haemophilus influenzae (type B)	Bacterial Polysaccharide	IM	One dose	–	1. For all children 2. Patients at risk
Pneumococcal	Bacterial Polysaccharides	SC	One dose	Every 3–5 years. If there is high risk of exposure	1. Travellers to areas with apidemics 2. Control of epidemics in closed population. 3. Military recruits
VIRAL VACCINES					
Poliomyelitis (OPV)	Live virus	Oral	6, 10 and 14 weeks of age	18 months; again at 4–6 years	For all children
Measles, Rubella (MR)	Live virus	SC	9 months	16–24 months	For all children

Contd..

Table 59.1: Vaccines in common use and their recommended schedules *(Contd...)*

Vaccine	*Type of agent*	*ROA*	*Primary immunisation*	*Booster*	*Indication*
Hepatitis A	Inactivated virus	IM	1 dose (2–4 weeks before trave-lling to endemic areas)	After 6–12 months	1. Travellers to endemic areas 2. Homosexual men 3. Persons at occupational risk
Hepatitis B	Inactive viral antigen	IM	At birth, 6, 10, 14 wks—UIP*, 0, 1, 6 months—adults	After 5 years but not routinely recommended	1. For all children 2. Persons at occupational risk 3. Haemophiliacs 4. Postexposure prophylaxis
Influenza (tetravalent) (influenza type A, type B, H1N1,H3N2)	Inactivated virus	IM	One dose	Yearly	High-risk people like elderly, pregnancy, asthmatics
Rabies (RABIPUR)	Inactivated virus	IM/ID	**Pre-exposure** 3 doses at days 0,7 and 21 **Postexposure** 5 doses IM at days 0, 3, 7, 14 and 28	After 1 year then at 2–5 years	1. Postexposure treatment 2. Pre-exposure prophylaxis in persons at risk for contact with rabies virus
Varicella	Live virus	SC	2 doses 4–8 weeks apart at 18 months	—	All children from 18 months to 13 years with no history of varicella infection
Yellow fever	Live virus	SC	1 dose	Every 10 years	1. Travellers to areas where yellow fever is seen 2. Laboratory per-sonnel at risk of exposure
Japanese encepahlitis	Killed Live	SC SC	2 doses 9 months	Before 1 year 16–24 months	Population at risk
Human papilloma-virus	Capsid protein	IM	3 doses 0, 2, 6 months	None	Females between 9 and 26 yr
Rotavirus	Live virus	Oral	3 doses 2, 4, 6 months 6, 10 and 14 wks in UIP	None	Infants 12–32 wk
Herpes zoster	Live virus	SC	1 dose	None	Adults >60 yr
Universal immunization program					
Polio (IPV)	Killed	ID	6 and 14 wk		All children
Liquid pentavalent vaccine (DPT Hep-B, HiB)	—	IM	6, 10, 14 wk		All children
Pneumococcal conjugate vaccine	Conjugate	IM	6 and 14 wk	9 months	All children

UIP*: Universal Immunization Program, ID–intradermal, SC–subcutaneous, IM–intramuscular, ROA–route of administration

Table 59.2: Passive immunisation

Preparation with source	*Dose and route*	*Indication*
Diphtheria antitoxin (horse)	IV or IM 20,000–1,20,000 IU	*Diphtheria* Clinical diphtheria—to be given immediately
Tetanus immunoglobulin (human)	IM Prophylaxis: 2500 IU Treatment: 3,000–6,000 IU	*Tetanus* Treatment and postexposure prophylaxis of unclean wounds in inadequately immunized persons
Tetanus antitoxin (ATS horse) (If tetanus Ig is not available)	IM/SC Prophylaxis 1500–3000 IU Treatment: 50,000–1,00,000 IU	*Tetanus* Treatment and postexposure prophylaxis of unclean wounds in inadequately immunised persons
Botulinum antitoxin	IM/IV 10,000 IU	Treatment and postexposure prophylaxis of botulism
Rabies immunoglobulin (human)	20 IU/kg; half the dose infiltrated around the wound; remaining given IM	*Rabies* Postexposure prophylaxis combined with rabies vaccine
Antirabies serum (ARS) (horse)	IM 40 IU/ kg	Used if rabies Ig is not available but is inferior to it
Gas gangrene antitoxin (AGS) (horse)	IM/SC/IV Prophylaxis: 10,000 IU Treatment: 30,000–75,000 IU	*Gas gangrene* Postexposure prophylaxis and treatment
Hepatitis B immunoglobulin (HBIG)	IM 0.06 ml/kg	Postexposure prophylaxis in nonimmune persons; Hepatitis B vaccine shall also be given.
Antisnake venom polyvalent (horse)	IV 20–30 ml to be given within 4 hr after the bite; additional doses may be required	Snake bite—cobra, vipers, krait
Human gammaglobulin		Gammaglobulin deficiency; prophylaxis of hepatitis A, measles, mumps, rubella
Anti-RhD Ig	IM 300 μg	To the Rh -ve mother after the birth of Rh +ve baby or after uncompleted pregnancy with Rh +ve father

Table 59.3: Conditions for which passive immunization is available

	Infections	*Others*
Botulism	Vaccinia	Snake bite
Diphtheria	Varicella	Black widow spider bite
Measles	Hepatitis A	Chronic lymphocytic leukaemia
Rabies	Hepatitis B	Idiopathic thrombocytopenic purpura
Rubella	Cytomegalovirus	Bone marrow transplantation
Tetanus	HIV-infected children	Anti-D (Rh) Ig
Respiratory syncytial virus		

[1–2] From Medical Council of India, *Competency based Undergraduate Curriculum for the Indian Medical Graduate*, 2018;1:136–144.

Unit XV

Toxicology

Heavy Metal Poisoning, Chelating Agents and Treatment of Common Poisoning, Common Stings and Bites

CHAPTER 60

Competency achievement: The student should be able to:
PH 1.53 Describe heavy metal poisoning and chelating agents.[1]

Heavy metals bind to and inactivate the functional groups (ligands) of essential tissue enzymes. By this they interfere with normal cell functions which require these ligands. Heavy metals cannot be metabolised in the body.

HEAVY METAL POISONING

Many heavy metals like lead, arsenic and mercury present in the soil and dust form major environmental pollutants. Toxicity due to heavy metals can result in prolonged morbidity and mortality

Lead

Lead is used in paints, add-on to petrol (now stopped), cosmetics, battery and also some traditional medicines. As lead is not degradable, it remains in dust and soil. Lead used in taps may be released slowly into drinking water.

Acute Lead Poisoning

Signs and symptoms: Nausea, vomiting, gastritis, muscle cramps, intestinal colic (lead colic) paraesthesiae, severe haemolytic anaemia and haemoglobunuria, convulsions, shock and death.

Treatment: Stomach wash and laxatives for removal of lead from the gut. Chelating agents like calcium disodium edetate 1 g in 250 ml saline infusion is given every 12 hours to chelate lead in the circulation. Diazepam may be needed to control convulsions.

Chronic Lead Poisoning

Long term exposure to even small amounts of lead can result in toxic effects particularly in children. Children who chew or suck lead toys or paint–coated articles may be poisoned. Occupational hazard in workers of paint and print industry has now reduced due to awareness and regulations.

Signs and symptoms

Low dose: Mild toxicity with abdominal discomfort and myalgia. Neurotoxicity with even the lowest level of lead can damage the developing brain resulting in reduced IQ, motor deficits and behavioural problems.

Moderate doses: Arthralgia, fatigue, abdominal pain, headache, anorexia, metallic taste and vomiting.

High doses can result in **lead encephalopathy** often associated with seizures and cognitive deficits. **Lead palsy** is neuromuscular deficits with wrist drop, foot drop and early neurodegeneration. Severe abdominal cramps **(lead colic)**, cardiotoxicity with hypertension, nephrotoxicity, immunosuppression, anemia and increased risk of cancers are noted.

Treatment: Further exposure stopped. Chelation with calcium disodium edetate 50 mg/kg and BAL 12 mg/kg/day should be started. Succimer may be used along with $CaNa_2$ edetate for better efficacy.

Mercury

Mercury is a liquid metal (also called liquid silver)—liquid in room temperature. Mercury compounds are used in therapeutics for their antibacterial property and was used in the treatment of syphilis. It is also used by dentists (amalgam). Vapors of mercury are released from volcanoes, burning petrol (fossil fuel) and also contaminate water when industrial waste is released into the rivers. Some scientific equipment like thermometer contains mercury and is also used in batteries.

Acute Mercury Poisoning

Symptoms: Gastric irritation, diarrhoea, metallic taste in the mouth, blurring of vision, dyspnoea and cough. Higher doses cause pulmonary edema, renal failure and convulsions.

Chronic poisoning: Coarse intentional tremors particularly hand tremors, abnormal gait, anorexia, nausea, metallic taste, colitis, inflammation of the gums, dementia, renal failure and psychotic disturbances. **Minimata disease** was identified in a place called minimata in Japan. Consuming large amounts of fish caught from Minimata bay lead to minimata disease which was due to organic mercury poisoning. The waste dumped by a fertilizer company into the sea had mercury which contaminated the fish.

Symptoms were mainly of the nervous system—with fever, ataxia, numbness in the hands and feet, neuropathies, speech disturbances and psychosis.

Treatment

1. BAL 100 mg IM every 4 hour for 48 h followed by every 8 hr for 7 days
2. Penicillamine 250 mg 4 times a day
3. Stomach wash should be given in acute poisoning. Activated charcoal, egg white or milk may be added to the stomach wash fluid for absorption

Arsenic

Salts of arsenic are a common cause of heavy metal poisoning. Arsenic gets absorbed through all route including oral, inhalational and skin and gets distributed to various tissues including bone and hair

Signs and symptoms: *Acute poisoning:* Fever, vomiting, abdominal pain, metallic taste, difficulty in swallowing, smells of garlic in breath, diarrhoea, renal failure, arrhythmias, convulsions and coma.

Chronic Poisoning

Mees' lines on finger nails, melanotic pigmentation on the skin, hyperkeratosis, anorxia, nausea, liver enlargement, jaundice, cirrhosis, kidney damage, anemia and neurological symptoms.

Treatment: Stomach wash, IV fluids, general supportive measures in acute poisoning. Chelation with BAL 3–5 mg/kg IM every 5 hours for 7–10 days depending on the severity of poisoning. Penicillamine 100 mg/kg/day in 4 divided doses for 5 days may be added. Chronic toxicity responds poorly to chelation haemodialysis may be needed to remove the metal. Chelating agents.

CHELATING AGENTS

Chelating agents or heavy metal antagonists bind the heavy metal ions and make them non-toxic. The chemical complex formed is called chelate (*Chele* = claw in Greek). The process of complex formation is **chelation**. The complex so formed is water-soluble and is eliminated by the kidneys.

Chelating agents are more effective in preventing the utilization of ligands than in reactivating them—hence, the earlier they are given, the better.

Calcium Disodium Edetate ($CaNa_2$ EDTA)

It chelates many divalent and trivalent metals like zinc, manganese, iron and lead. It is used in the treatment of lead poisoning. Given parenterally, lead deposits in the bone are mobilised, chelated and excreted through kidneys.

Adverse effects include nephrotoxicity, fatigue, fever, myalgia and dermatitis.

Uses: CaNa$_2$ EDTA is mainly used in lead poisoning. It can also be used in zinc, manganese and iron poisoning. Sodium edetate is used in severe hypercalcaemia.

Dimercaprol

Dimercaprol is a colourless, oily liquid developed by the British during World War II as an antidote to lewisite—an arsenical war gas. Hence it is also known as British Anti-lewisite or BAL. Dimercaprol chelates arsenic, mercury, lead and other heavy metals. It is given IM; appropriate plasma concentrations should be maintained.

Adverse effects are dose related and include hypertension, tachycardia, vomiting,

Table 60.1: Salient features of chelating agents

Chelating agent	*Uses*	*Toxicity*	*Remarks*
Calcium disodium edetate	Lead, zinc, manganese and iron poisoning	Nephrotoxicity, fatigue, fever, myalgia, dermatitis	Sodium edetate used in severe hypercalcaemia
Dimercaprol (BAL)	Arsenic, mercury and lead poisoning	Hypertension, tachycardia, vomiting, sweating, headache and burning sensation in the lips and mouth	Given IM; lewisite—an arsenical war gas; BAL developed during World War II
Unithiol	Lead and mercury poisoning	Allergic reactions	Analog of dimercaprol given orally and parenterally
Succimer	Acute and chronic arsenic poisoning, chronic lead and mercury poisoning	Anorexia, nausea, vomiting, diarrhoea and skin rashes	Analog of dimercaprol Given orally and IV
d-Penicillamine	1. Copper, mercury, lead poisoning 2. Wilson's disease—copper deposited in liver, brain causing degeneration 3. Rheumatoid arthritis 4. Cysteinuria forms soluble complexes and prevents formation of cysteine stones, promotes excretion of cysteine	Dermatitis, hypersensitivity reactions—patients allergic to penicillin may develop anaphylaxis; long-term uses causes renal, haematological and dermatological toxicities	Degraded product of penicillin
Desferrioxamine	Acute iron poisoning—Chronic iron poisoning as in thalassemia patients receiving repeated blood transfusions	Allergic reactions—rashes to anaphylaxis (rare), diarrhoea, muscle cramps and blurred vision. Urine turns orange-red	Source: *Streptomyces pilosus* given parenterally High affinity for iron Removes iron from haemosiderin, ferritin
Deferiprone and deferasirox	Thalassaemia major to chelate iron	Rashes, mild GI disturbances	Orally effective
Prussian blue	To reduce to biological half-life of radioactive cesium and thallium		Not absorbed, binds thallium and cesium, prevents their absorption, complex excreted through gut

sweating, headache and burning sensation in the lips and mouth.

Uses: Dimercaprol is used in arsenic and mercury poisoning; also used in lead poisoning with $CaNa_2$ EDTA.

Unithiol: Unithiol is a water-soluble analog of dimercaprol that can be given both orally and parenterally. It enhances the excretion of mercury, arsenic and lead. Adverse effects are mild and include allergic reactions. Unithiol may be used in mercury, lead and arsenic poisoning.

Succimer is a water-soluble analog of dimercaprol. It protects against acute arsenic poisoning and is also effective in lead and mercury poisoning. It can be given both orally and intravenously. Succimer is used in the treatment of chronic lead poisoning and in mercury and arsenic poisoning. Anorexia, nausea, vomiting, diarrhoea and skin rashes can occur.

d-Penicillamine

d-Penicillamine is prepared by degradation of penicillin but has no antibacterial activity. It chelates copper, mercury, zinc and lead. It is orally effective.

Adverse effects: Hypersensitivity reactions are fairly common. Patients allergic to penicillin may develop anaphylaxis; dermatitis may occur in some. On long-term use renal, haematological and dermatological toxicities can occur.

Uses

1. Treatment of copper, mercury and lead poisoning.
2. Wilson's disease (hepatolenticular degeneration)—copper is deposited in the liver and brain causing degeneration.
3. Rheumatoid arthritis (*see* page 172)
4. Cystinuria—penicillamine promotes excretion of cysteine by forming soluble complexes and prevents formation of cysteine stones.

Desferrioxamine

Desferrioxamine isolated from *Streptomyces pilosus,* chelates iron. It has a high affinity for iron, forms stable complexes and removes iron from haemosiderin and ferritin. It does not chelate the iron in haemoglobin and cytochromes. It is given parenterally.

Adverse effects: Allergic reactions range from rashes to anaphylaxis (rare), diarrhoea, muscle cramps and blurred vision. Urine turns orange-red.

Uses

1. *Acute iron poisoning:* Desferrioxamine is the drug of choice.
2. *Chronic iron poisoning* as in thalassaemia patients who receive repeated blood transfusion.

Deferiprone chelates iron and is orally effective. It is used in thalassaemia major to chelate iron as an alternative to desferrioxamine.

Deferasirox is an orally effective iron chelator. It has selectively high affinity for iron and is orally effective—well absorbed, binds iron and forms a complex which is excreted in the bile. It is used to treat iron overload that may be seen due to repeated blood transfusions in conditions like thalassaemia. Skin rashes and mild gastrointestinal disturbances can occur.

Poison information centres

Poison information centres are set up by WHO at New Delhi and Ahmedabad. They provide information through computer software INTOX. Regional centres are established at Chennai and Cochin – (software–POISONDEX). These centres may be contacted over the phone and email for information on treatment of poisoning. The information is available 24 × 7.

Prussian blue or ferric hexacyanoferrate is used commercially as a dark blue dye. Given orally it is not absorbed, binds some univalent cations like thallium and cesium prevent their absorption and the complex is excreted through the gut. Prussian blue is used to reduce the biological half-life of radioactive cesium and thallium.

TREATMENT OF COMMON POISONING

Competency achievement: The student should be able to:
PH 1.52 Describe management of common poisoning, insecticides, common sting and bites.[2]

Toxicology is the science that deals with the study of poisons, their source, properties, actions, detection and treatment of poisoning.

A **poison** may be defined as any substance, which if administered or comes in contact with a living being, produces ill-health, disease or death.

Every drug in a high dose can be poisonous. Poisoning could be accidental, suicidal or homicidal. Millions of poisoning cases are seen every year with several hundreds dying but several more are unreported. Mortality rate varies from country to country. In India, mortality due to poisoning is around 35% while in the United States of America it is 2%! When treated on time with appropriate drugs, considering the toxicokinetics and toxicodynamics, treatment of poisoning can be successful.

Sources

Venom, toxins and poisons may be originating from animals, microorganisms, plants or chemicals. Poisoning may be:

- *Acute:* A single large dose or multiple small doses repeated at short intervals result in acute poisoning. Onset of signs and symptoms are abrupt.
- *Chronic:* Small doses repeated over a long period result in chronic poisoning. Signs and symptoms appear gradually.

Symptoms and Signs

Acute poisoning can be rapidly fatal. Awareness of the symptoms of poisoning, mechanisms involved in death due to poisoning and early, appropriate treatment are all important to reduce the morbidity and mortality from poisoning. Clinical assessment for vital signs like respiration, heart rate, blood pressure, pupillary size, body temperature, neurological status and level of consciousness should be done. Generally, symptoms like hypotension and dehydration due to vomiting and diarrhoea are common; cardiac arrhythmias can occur particularly from drugs like digitalis, theophylline, amphetamines, ephedrine and some antiarrhythmic drugs. Bronchospasm and respiratory depression need immediate attention. In a comatose patient, airway obstruction and aspiration of stomach contents into the respiratory tract may result in death. CNS depressants can cause stupor and coma.

No time should be lost in identifying the exact poison. Treatment should be started immediately with supportive measures.

Steps in the treatment of poisoning include:

1. *Stop the source of poison:* The patient should be shifted away from the source of poison.
2. *Limit the absorption of poison:* This depends on the route of entry. If taken orally, vomiting may be induced or stomach wash may be given to prevent further absorption of the poison. Cathartics or bowel irrigation may also be tried. In case of poisoning through skin, e.g. by organophosphorus compounds, the clothing should be changed and the skin should be washed with soap and water.
3. *Supportive therapy:* Emergency stabilization of the cardiovascular and respiratory system is needed—ABC (**a**irway, **b**reathing, **c**irculation) of poisoning
   i. Airway should be cleared of any mucus or vomitus that may be present. Suction to clear the air passages may be needed and if required an endo-

Table 60.2: Some specific antidotes for drugs and chemicals

Agent causing toxicity	*Antidote*	*Dose*
1. Paracetamol	N-acetyl cysteine	Oral 140 mg/kg followed by 70 mg/kg every 4 hr, or IV 150 mg/kg infusion over 15 min repeated as required.
2. Morphine and other opioids	Naloxone	1–2 mg IV repeated every 10–15 minutes.
3. Heparin	Protamine Sulphate	1 mg IV for every 100 units of heparin.
4. Cyanide	Sodium nitrate + Sodium thiosulfate	10 ml of 3% solution IV 50 ml of 25% solution IV
5. Organophosphates	Atropine, Oximes	2 mg IV repeated every 10 minutes Pralidoxime 1 gram IV every 3–4 hr 3 doses
6. Theophylline, caffeine	Esmolol	25–50 µg/kg/min- IV
7. Atropine	Physostigmine	1–2 mg IV slowly (or SC) may be repeated if symptoms reappear
8. Curare and other non-depolarizing skeletal muscle relaxants	Neostigmine	2 mg IV repeated as required.
9. Copper	d-penicillamine	100 mg/kg/day orally in 4 divided doses for 3–7 days.
10. Iron	Desferrioxamine	15 mg/kg/hr IV (100 mg desferrioxamine binds 8.5 mg of iron)
11. Arsenic	Dimercaprol	Ist day 400–800 mg deep IM in divided doses; 2nd and 3rd day 200–400 mg; 4th day onwards 100–200 mg
12. Lead	Calcium disodium edetate	1 g in 250 ml saline infusion twice a day.
13. Streptokinase and other fibrinolytics	Epsilon amino caproic acid	5 g oral or IV followed by 1 g hrly till bleeding stops (Max 30 gm in 24 hr)
14. Insulin	Glucose	50 ml of 50% solution.
15. Digitalis	Digoxin specific antibody fragments	10 vials (DIGI FAB) emperic therapy or specific $\text{No. of vials} = \frac{\text{Total digoxin consumed}}{0.5}$
16. Methanol, ethylene glycol	Ethanol or Fomepizole	10% ethanol is given orally –0.7 mg/kg loading Dose: 0.15 ml/kg infusion. loading dose 15 mg/kg repeated every 12 hours.
17. Carbon monoxide	Oxygen	100% by high-flow non-rebreathing mask.
18. Nitrites	Methylene blue	0.1% solution slow IV in the dose of 1–2 mg/kg body weight.
19. Warfarin	Vitamin K_1 oxide, fresh blood	10 mg IM followed by 5 mg 4 hrly As required.
20. Benzodiazepines	Flumazenil	0.2 mg IV repeated as required (Max. 3 mg)
21. Iodine	Sodium thiosulphate	1–5%, solution orally

tracheal tube may be inserted. Patient should be put in lateral position.

ii. If breathing is depressed, artificial ventilation should be given. Oxygen may be needed.

iii. *Circulation:* Circulatory status should be assessed by pulse rate, blood pressure and urine output. Suitable IV fluids should be given. Generally 1 litre of normal saline with 1 litre of dextrose is injected in the first 24 hours. If hypotension is present, the foot end of the bed should be raised.

iv. If the patient is in coma, nothing should be given orally. Blood glucose should be estimated to rule out hypoglycaemic coma. In all comatose patients with signs of CNS depression, administration of ***'coma cock tail'*** is routinely recommended—it includes:

1. Naloxone – 2 mg
2. Thiamine – 100 mg
3. Dextrose – 50 ml of 50% solution

All are given intravenously.

These are given with the intention that if the poison is an opioid, naloxone overcomes the respiratory and CNS depression. Naloxone also overcomes the effects of opioids released in the body in pain; dextrose helps if the coma is due to hypoglycaemia. Thiamine helps to prevent Wernicke's encephalopathy in alcoholics.

4. *Specific therapy:* Specific antidotes, antivenoms and antitoxins should be used whenever available (Table 60.1). For some poisons, specific therapies may be available though they are not called antidotes. For example, ethanol in methanol poisoning, nitrites in cyanide poisoning. These can often be life saving.
5. *Other measures:* Forced diuresis, peritoneal dialysis, haemodialysis, haemoperfusion, exchange transfusion, and such similar procedures are carried out in certain cases of poisoning only if indicated. Excretion of acidic drugs like salicylates can be enhanced by **forced alkaline diuresis**—using frusemide, sodium bicarbonate and IV fluids. Excretion of basic drugs like amphetamines may be enhanced by **forced acid diuresis** using frusemide, ascorbic acid and IV fluids. However, these procedures may lead to volume overload and also expose the kidneys to a high dose of the toxin. Excretion of drugs like amphetamines, barbiturates, ethyl and methyl alcohol, phenytoin, salicylates, theophylline and lithium can be effectively carried out by **haemodialysis. Haemoperfusion** can be carried out in some poisons particularly the fat-soluble drugs.

GENERAL MANAGEMENT

1. **Gut decontamination:** Vomiting may be induced or stomach wash (gastric lavage) may be given to clear the stomach of the unabsorbed poison.

   a. *Emesis:* Vomiting can be induced with 20–30 ml of syrup of ipecac. It acts within 15 minutes. Alternatively freshly prepared mustard powder solution (1 teaspoon mustard powder in water) can be used. Vomiting may also be induced by mechanical stimulation of the pharynx with fingertips or by using strong salt solution (1 tablespoonful in half a glass of warm water) but both these are considered dangerous. Because salt solution can cause severe hypernatraemia, it is generally not recommended. However, salt solution is the most easily available household remedy and sometimes this could be time saving and, therefore, life saving. Moreover, most of the excess salt is lost in vomiting. Adequate fluid intake should be ensured. Induction of vomiting is helpful in clearing the poison which may be present in the stomach and also in duodenum.

   Vomiting should not be induced:

   - If the poison is a corrosive agent or a petroleum product
   - If the patient is unconscious

   b. *Stomach wash:* Washing the stomach with large amounts of water removes unabsorbed poison. Stomach wash can be carried out only in a conscious patient. Warm water or saline may be used for lavage. Cold lavage solutions can result in hypothermia. In alkaloidal poisons, tannic acid or potassium permanganate solution can be used. An orogastric tube of approximately ½ inch diameter and 150 cm in length may be employed. The patient is put in left lateral position and the tube inserted orally. Wash has to be carried out till the returning fluid becomes clear. Once this is achieved, a slurry of activated charcoal (1 g/kg) in water (10:1) is to be left in the stomach and the tube should be removed. The first returning fluid should be retained for chemical analysis.

There is some controversy regarding the time limit for stomach wash. Though generally stomach decontamination is recommended to be done up to 1 hour of poison ingestion, it is worth trying it up to days in all suitable cases because. (i) Poisons may be detected in the stomach even after 5–6 days of poisoning. (ii) certain poisons (some basic drugs) may diffuse into the stomach from blood vessels even when given intravenously. Hence, **it is worth giving a stomach wash in all suitable cases unless contraindicated.**

Contraindications:

i. Poisoning with corrosives (except carbolic acid)
ii. Petroleum products
iii. Foreign body ingestion
iv. Poisoning with convulsants

Activated charcoal is obtained by destructive distillation of wood and then treating it with an activating agent like steam, carbon dioxide, etc. Activated charcoal can adsorb (attract particles on to its surface) several drugs and thereby prevent their absorption. Activated charcoal has multiple microscopic pores which enhance its surface area (1000–2000 M^2/gram). This enables it to adsorb drugs and chemicals. It is administered as a solution of 4 parts of water mixed with one part of activated charcoal (dose 1 gram/kg body weight). It is a safe and useful measure except that it is unpalatable. In Western countries, a palatable preparation is available called ***medicoal***.

Activated charcoal is useful in several cases of poisoning including that of barbiturates, salicylates, paracetamol, antidepressants, phenytoin, carbamazepine, theophylline and many other organic and inorganic compounds. It is not effective in poisoning by heavy metals, alcohol and corrosives.

c. *Purgatives* Purgatives may help to speed up the excretion of drugs from the gut. If a purgative is needed, saline purgatives are generally used. Magnesium sulphate 20–30 g or sodium sulphate also 20–30 g may be given orally. Adequate fluid intake is needed.

Whole bowel irrigation with a balanced solution of polyethylene glycol and electrolytes may help in poisoning particularly due to sustained release preparations like that of iron.

2. **Management of respiratory failure:** To maintain a clear airway, the patient should be placed in a semiprone position, secretions should be aspirated regularly and tongue should be drawn forward. An oropharyngeal airway of suitable size may be inserted, if required. In comatose patients, airway can be kept clear with a cuffed endotracheal tube. Respiratory stimulants like doxapram or nikethamide may help some patients—but the benefit is not proved and, therefore, are not preferred. **Oxygen** may be given, if there is hypoxia or increased carbon dioxide (hypercapnoea) on blood gas analysis.

If profound respiratory depression is present, **mechanical ventilation** is needed. Pulmonary oedema and increased bronchial secretions may be caused by volatile irritant poisons and organophosphates. Pulmonary oedema should be relieved immediately as it can interfere with gaseous exchange. The patient should be in the sitting position. Secretions in the throat should be removed by suction. If there is cyanosis, oxygen (60–100%) may be administered using a facemask. Oxygen may be saturated with ethyl alcohol vapour by bubbling it through a bottle of alcohol. This causes collapse of the foam in the alveoli and allows better gas exchange. Intravenous frusemide (40 mg) relieves pulmonary oedema by shifting the blood from pulmonary to systemic circulation.

3. **Management of circulatory failure:** Hypotension-Foot end of the bed should be elevated. Plasma expanders like dextran or plasma itself may be needed in hypovolaemic shock. Vasopressors like dopamine (2–10 μg/kg), phenylephrine (5–20 μg/kg), methoxamine or mephentermine may be used intravenously in profound hypotension.
4. **Management of fluid and electrolyte imbalance**
   a. *Hyponatraemia* (plasma sodium <130 mEq/l) can cause salt and water retention, needs normal saline infusion.
   b. *Hypernatraemia* (plasma sodium >150 mEq/l):
      - A loop diuretic like frusemide.
      - Half normal saline helps to dilute plasma sodium levels.

   c. Hypokalaemia (plasma potassium <3.5 m Eq/l) can cause dangerous arrhythmias. Potassium chloride 4–6 mEq/l to a maximum of 40–80 mEq/day is administered orally in divided doses or as a **very slow** intravenous infusion. Potassium should never be pushed rapidly into the vein because it can cause cardiac arrest and sudden death.
   d. *Hyperkalemia* (plasma potassium >5.5 mEq/l): In mild hyperkalaemia, diuretics, like frusemide (1 mg/kg IV) and thiazides increase the excretion of potassium.

      Severe hyperkalaemia is a medical emergency. 10% calcium gluconate given slow IV minimizes membrane excitability. Dialysis is indicated in patients with chronic renal failure.
   e. *Hypocalcaemia* (plasma calcium <4 mEq/l)—10% calcium gluconate given IV raises the plasma calcium level.
5. **Metabolic acidosis:** Sodium bicarbonate 1–2 mEq/l IV over 30 minutes helps.
6. **Convulsions:** Diazepam 10 mg given slowly intravenously is the drug of choice. The same IV preparation of diazepam may be given rectally, if getting an IV line is difficult. Phenytoin 10 mg/kg IV or phenobarbitone 10 mg/kg are other alternatives. If seizures do not respond to these, a skeletal muscle relaxant (pancuronium) or IV anaesthetic thiopental sodium may be given.
7. **Antidotes:** An antidote is a substance which antagonizes and overcomes the effects of a poison. The right antidote used at the right time in right dose can reverse the effects of the corresponding poison and can be life saving. Unfortunately specific antidotes are available only for a few toxins. Therefore, in majority of the poisoning cases, treatment is only supportive and symptomatic.

Antidotes may be classified based on the mode of action into three groups as follows:

1. *Physical antidotes* act by reducing the adsorption of the poison, e.g. activated charcoal adsorbs alkaloids.
2. *Chemical antidotes* act by forming a complex with the poison, e.g. acetic acid reacts with alkalies. Potassium permangenate oxidizes compounds like barbiturates, phosphorus and alkalies; chelating agents bind heavy metals like lead, arsenic, copper, mercury, etc.
3. *Pharmacological antidotes:* These antidotes compete for binding to the same receptors

or sites where the toxin binds, e.g. naloxone for morphine, flumazenil for diazepam and atropine for organophosphorus poisoning.

Universal antidote consists of:

i. One part tannic acid (to precipitate alkaloids, glycosides and heavy metals)
ii. One part milk of magnesia (to neutralize acids)
iii. Two parts burnt toast (to adsorb alkaloid). This was earlier used with the hope of preventing absorption and overcoming the toxic effects of most of the poisons. We now know that actually ***it does not serve any purpose and is no more recommended.***

Insecticides (*see* Chapter 61: Pesticides).

TREATMENT OF COMMON STINGS AND BITES

Snakebite

There are more than 3000 species of snakes in the world of which about 216 are found in India. 52 types of the snakes in India are poisonous. All over the world snake bites are responsible for 30,000 to 40,000 deaths every year. In India, about 2 lakh people are bitten by snakes every year of which about 16,000 die. Vipers, cobras and kraits are the common poisonous snakes.

Signs and Symptoms

In all cases of snake bite, the patient is in great fear and is in a stage of neurogenic shock. The patient is in a semiconscious state with cold, clammy skin, feeble pulse, rapid and shallow breathing. Other symptoms vary according to the type of snake.

The signs and symptoms of systemic toxicity appear in about half an hour.

1. *Elapid bite* (cobra, krait, etc.—neurotoxic): *Local reactions* are pain, burning, swelling, discolouration of the site, oozing of blood-stained fluid are seen in 1–3 hours. Blisters and local necrosis may occur. Systemic effects include vomiting, headache, loss of consciousness, ptosis, ophthalmoplegia (eyes become fixed in central position) and convulsions followed by flaccid paralysis.
2. *Viper bite (haemotoxic):* Local reactions are prominent with swelling, discolouration, blister formation and bleeding from the site. Bleeding from the gums, haematuria, disseminated intravascular coagulation are seen.
3. *Sea snakes (hydrophids—myotoxic):* Local reactions are mild swelling and pain. Systemic myotoxic effects include muscle pain, stiffness; renal and hepatic necrosis.

Treatment

First aid

- Reassurance
- Immobilise the bitten part. Measures like local incision, suction, application of ice are all found to be ***harmful*** and no more recommended.

Supportive therapy: Blood pressure, respiration, and urine output are to be monitored. ECG and blood gas analysis are needed. Fresh blood transfusion may be needed to correct coagulation parameters. Analgesics like paracetamol for pain, prophylactic antibiotics as required and tetanus toxoid injection are to be given in all cases.

Specific therapy: Antisnake venom (ASV) is indicated in presence of signs of systemic envenomisation. Dose of antivenom varies.

- Mild envenomisation 3–5 vials
- Moderate envenomisation 5–10 vials
- Severe envenomisation 10–20 vials
- Infusion should be done after test dose.

Watch for reactions to ASV. Hypersensitivity reactions including anaphylaxis can occur. Clean the bite site with providone iodine.

Scorpion Sting

Scorpions belong to the class Arachnida with almost 100 species found in India. Scorpion venom is neurotoxic as well as cardiotoxic. Severity of symptoms depends on the quantum of venom injected.

Signs and Symptoms

- Local swelling, burning sensation and pain
- Vomiting, abdominal cramps, sweating, mydriasis
- Initial hypotension and bradycardia may be followed by hypertension, tachycardia and arrhythmias
- In more severe cases → convulsions and pulmonary oedema

Treatment

- The stung site should be immobilised and ice applied
- IV fluids should be started and oxygen may be required
- Hypo or hypertension may be treated with dopamine infusion or nifedipine/prazosin respectively
- Furosemide may be needed for pulmonary edema
- Antivenom for some species of scorpion is now available in India

Bee and Wasp Sting

Honey bees and wasps are commonly seen in India. Stings cause local pain and swelling and some may result in anaphylactoid reactions.

Placing ice at the sting site reduces pain. Antihistamines like chlorpheniramine or diphenhydramine and analgesics should be given. Glucocorticoids and oxygen for anaphylaxis and salbutamol for bronchospasm may be needed.

FOOD POISONING

Food poisoning can occur on consumption of food that is contaminated with micro-organisms, toxins or chemicals.

Nausea, vomiting, abdominal pain, fever, weakness and diarrhoea are the common symptoms of food poisoning. Other symptoms depend on the causative agent.

Causes for food poisoning

1. Micro-organisms
   - Bacteria

Table 60.3: Drugs used in food poisoning due to bacteria

Bacteria	*Incubation period*	*Mode of action*	*Treatment*
Staph. aureus	2–4 hours	• Enterotoxin	• Symptomatic
Shigella	1–3 days	• Enterotoxin+neurotoxin • Destruction of intestinal mucosa	• Ciprofloxacin
Salmonella	12 hours to 2 days (1 week in enteric fever)	• Destruction of intestinal mucosa	Ciprofloxacin Supportive measures
Bacillus cereus	3–8 hours	Enterotoxin	Symptomatic
Vibrio cholerae	Few hours to 5 days	Enterotoxin	Symptomatic—fluid and electrolyte replacement
Vibrio para-haemolyticus	6 hr 4 days	• Invasion of intestinal mucosa; • Enterotoxin	Symptomatic
Clostridium botulinum	6 hr 7 days	Neurotoxin	• Antitoxin, • Symptomatic
Campylobacter	1–8 days	• Enterotoxin, • Invasion of intestinal mucosa	Erythromycin
E. coli	1–3 days	• Enterotoxin • Invasion of intestinal mucosa	Ciprofloxacin

- Protozoa
- Viruses

2. Toxins—present in certain fish, plants and mushrooms.
3. Chemicals.

Food Poisoning due to Micro-organisms

Consumption of food contaminated with micro-organisms is the most common cause of food poisoning. The incubation period varies from a few (1–2) hours to a few days.

Bacteria: Several bacteria can cause food poisoning. *See* Table 60.3.

Virus: Viral gastroenteritis may be caused by rotavirus, parvovirus and adenovirus. Treatment is symptomatic.

Fungi: The spores of moulds grow on food and can release mycotoxin. These mycotoxins are heat stable. *Aspergillus flavens* can produce *aflatoxins, Penicillium islandicum* can produce islanditoxin.

Others: Protozoa like *Entamoeba histolytica* amoebiasis) and *Giardia lamblia* (giardiasis) are common causes of food poisoning. Metronidazole is the drug of choice in both.

Mushrooms: Of the large variety of mushrooms, only about 5% are poisonous. Consumption of such mushrooms can cause a variety of toxic effects depending on the toxin—they can cause cellular destruction, affect central or autonomic nervous system, gastrointestinal system or the kidney.

Treatment is symptomatic except when autonomic nervous system is involved. Inocybe, clitocybe and some species of amanita contain muscarine which stimulates the cholinergic muscarinic receptors. Symptoms include salivation, sweating, diarrhoea, constricted pupils, dyspnoea, bradycardia and hypotension. The specific antidote is atropine (1 mg IV repeated as required).

Chemicals: Contamination of food with chemicals like arsenic, mercury, antimony or insecticides in fruits and vegetables can cause poisoning. Monosodium glutamate is a food additive commonly used in chinese food. Dose more than 1 gram can cause troublesome symptoms including burning and numbness of face and neck, chest pain, headache, vomiting and vertigo. In children, convulsions can sometimes occur.

Treatment is supportive and symptomatic.

CARDIOPULMONARY RESUSCITATION (CPR)

Management of a collapsed patient requires early assessment and restoration of the circulation, airway and breathing (CAB) using basic life support (BLS) so that circulation is maintained until definite treatment with advanced life support can be administered.

Some important steps in CPR are:

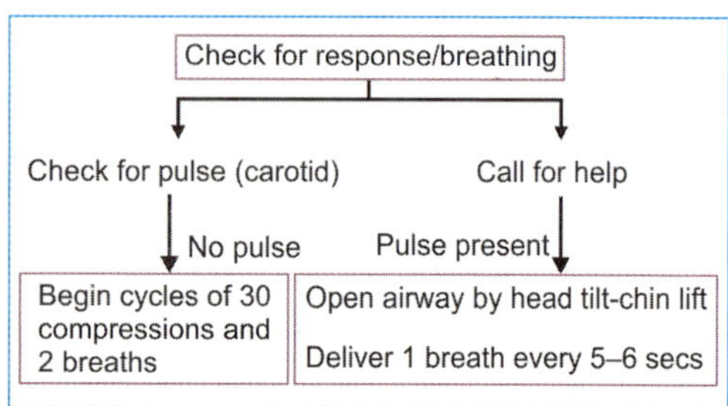

High quality CPR in an adult consists of:

- Rate at least 100/min.
- Compression depth at least 2 inches (5 cm).
- Allow complete chest recoil after each compression.
- Minimal interruptions in chest compressions.
- Avoidance of excessive ventilation.

[1–2] From Medical Council of India, *Competency based Undergraduate Curriculum for the Indian Medical Graduate*, 2018;1:136–144.

Occupational and Environmental Pesticides, Food Adulterants, Pollutants and Insect Repellents

CHAPTER 61

Competency achievement: The student should be able to:
PH 1.51 Describe occupational and environmental pesticides, food adulterants, pollutants and insect repellents.[1]

PESTICIDES

Pesticide is a compound which inhibits the growth of or kills pests. Pesticide could be used against insects, rodents, fungi, nematodes, ticks, mites, mollucs or weeds and herbs. They may be chemical or biological agents. Human beings may be exposed to pesticides as an occupational hazard, in the food consumed or from the environment. Pesticides are of 4 types:

1. **Organochlorines** like DDT, lindane, aldrin. Their degradation is very slow **(persistant pesticides)** and bioaccumulation occurs making them environmental pollutants. They also cause CNS toxicity and endocrine disturbances in man and animals.
2. **Organophosphates** like diazinon, dichlorvos, malathion, parathion. They are irreversible anticholinesterases—*see* page 116.
3. **Carbamates** like aldicarb, aminocarb, carbaryl, propoxur, pyrolan. They are reversible anticholinesterases—*see* page 114.
4. **Botanical pesticides** are of natural sources—**nicotine, rotenone,** and **pyrethrum**. **Nicotine** analogs (neonicotinoids) are agricultural pesticides and could have a role in bee colony collapse. **Rotenone** is obtained from *Derris elliptica* and other similar sources. Oral ingestion produces gastrointestinal irritation. Conjunctivitis, dermatitis, pharyngitis, and rhinitis can also occur. Treatment is symptomatic.

Pyrethrum obtained from Chrysanthamum consists of insecticidal esters which act on peripheral benzodiazepine receptors. CNS toxicity is common with them, manifesting as convulsions and tetanic paralysis.

Synthetic pyrethroids widely used as insect repellents in household as sprays, mosquito coils and mats. They are highly irritating to the eyes, skin, and respiratory tract. Spraying synthetic pyrethroids may cause cutaneous paresthesias in workers.The use of synthetic pyrethroids for insects on aircraft has caused respiratory and skin problems as well as some neurologic complaints in flight attendants and other aircraft workers. Severe occupational exposures to synthetic pyrethroids in China resulted in marked effects on the CNS, including convulsions. Treatment is symptomatic.

Herbicides

Herbicides are compounds used for the destruction of weeds. They are toxic to humans—can be fatal and can also cause environmental toxicity.

1. **Chlorophenoxy herbicides** are used for lawn weed control. Ingested in large doses can cause generalized muscle hypotonia. During environmental transformation, they generate a potent human carcinogen - dimethylnitrosamine.
2. **Glyphosate,** the most widely used herbicide in the world is absorbed through

the leaves and roots of plants. Glyphosate-resistant type of soybean and many corn crops are grown from patented seeds-genetically modified (GMO) crops. Glyphosate is an eye and skin irritant, can cause esophageal erosion, aspiration pneumonia and renal failure. Treatment is symptomatic.

3. **Paraquat** ingestion causes hematemesis, bloody stools and delayed effects include lung oedema, alveolitis and progressive fibrosis. Treatment is with oxygen and activated charcoal. Antioxidants acetyl-cysteine and salicylate, haemodialysis and haemoperfusion may help.

Rodenticides: Most of them are anti-coagulants like warfarin, bromadiolone, difethialone and brodifacoum. Some of them like zinc phosphide, bromethalin and strychnine have different mechanisms of action. Risk of ingestion by children and pets should be borne in mind.

FOOD ADULTERANTS

Food adulterants are poor quality substances added to food items for economic and technical benefits. Addition of these adulterants may:

1. Reduce the nutritional value
2. Be toxic or harmful
3. Cause allergies

Adulterants may be found in dairy products, cereals, pulses, grains, meat, vegetables, fruits, oils, beverages, etc.

Methods to Avoid Adulteration

1. Avoid dark colored, junk and processed foods.
2. Clean and store all the grains, pulses and other food products.

Table 61.1: Some examples of food adulterants

Food products	*Adulterant*	*Harmful effects*
Milk and curd	Water and starch powder	Stomach disorders
Ghee, cheese, butter	Mashed potatoes, Vanaspati and starch powder	Gastrointestinal disturbances
Grains	Dust, stones, straw, weed seeds, damaged grain, etc.	Liver disorders, other GI disorders
Pulses	Dyes, chemical and lead chromate	Stomach disorders
Coffee powder	Chicory, tamarind seeds powder	Diarrhoea
Tea	Artificial colouring agents	Liver disorders
Sugar	Chalk powder, washing soda, urea, etc.	Stomach disorders, kidney failure
Pepper	Dried papaya seeds and blackberries	Allergic reactions
Mustard seeds	Argemone seeds	GI disorders, colic
Edible oils	Mineral oil, karanja oil, castor oil, artificial colours	Gallbladder cancer, allergies, stroke, cardiac arrest, ↑ LDL cholesterol.
Turmeric powder	Pesticide residues, sawdust, chalk dust, dyes, arsenic, lead	Cancer and gastrointestinal disorders
Cumin seeds	Coloured grass seeds, sawdust and charcoal dust	Stomach disorders
Jam, juice and candies	Non-permitted dyes including metanil yellow and other artificial food dyes, colors and flavors	Gastritis. These dyes are highly carcinogenic
Jaggery	Washing soda, chalk powder	Vomiting
Honey	Molasses, dextrose, sugar and corn syrups	Stomach disorders
Fruits and vegetables	Chemical dyes, malachite green, calcium carbide, copper sulphate, oxytocin, saccharin, wax	Stomach disorders, vomiting, dyes used are highly carcinogenic

3. Wash fruits and vegetables thoroughly in running water before use
4. Check the seal before buying the food products like milk, oil and other pouches.
5. Products should have FSSAI label, license number, list of ingredients, manufacture and expiry date.

ENVIRONMENTAL POLLUTANTS

Environmental toxicology deals with the harmful effects of environmental pollutants **(air, soil, water pollutants)** on living organisms. The major contribution to air pollution is from industries and urbanization. Industrial chemicals, pesticides and chemicals used in food processing result in deleterious effects on living organisms including carcinogenicity. Man is also exposed to pesticides either during agricultural activities or while consuming such food. Chemicals like polychlorinated biphenyls (PCBs) enter the environment as industrial waste. These agents and their byproducts are highly carcinogenic. They enter human body mostly through food. For example, fish in Great Lakes of North America are toxic to eat due to accumulation of PCB in them. During the gas tragedy in Bhopal, India, acute exposure to methyl isocyanate, resulted in 4000 deaths and more than half a million injuries. In Minamata Bay, Japan, chronic exposure of methyl mercury resulted in Minimata disease.

Air Pollutants

Substances contributing to majority of air pollution are carbon monoxide (~ 52%), sulfur oxides, hydrocarbons, nitrogen oxides and their breakdown products.

Carbon monoxide (CO) is a byproduct of incomplete combustion.It binds to oxygen binding sites of hemoglobin to form carboxy Hb which is unable to transfer oxygen to tissues and leads to hypoxia.

Signs and symptoms: CO intoxication results in hypoxia resulting in:

1. Psychomotor impairment
2. Headache and tightness in the temporal area
3. Confusion and loss of visual acuity
4. Tachycardia, tachypnea, syncope
5. Coma, convulsions, shock, and respiratory failure.

Chronic exposure to low CO levels may lead to adverse cardiac effects, neurological, and emotional disturbances. Exposure of a pregnant woman to elevated CO levels may cause fetal death or serious birth defects.

Treatment: Patients to be removed from the source immediately. Respiration must be maintained and high flow oxygen should be administered. If respiratory failure is present, mechanical ventilation may be necessary.

Sulfur dioxide (SO_2) is an irritant gas generated by the combustion of sulfur-containing fossil fuels. Sulfurous acid is formed when SO_2 contacts moist membranes resulting in severe irritant effects on the eyes, mucous membranes, and skin.

Signs and symptoms: SO_2 intoxication results in irritation of the eyes, nose, and throat, reflex bronchoconstriction, and increased bronchial secretions. In asthmatic subjects, SO_2 evokes an acute asthmatic episode. In severe exposure, delayed-onset pulmonary oedema may be observed.

Nitrogen oxides (NO_2) is a brownish irritant gas sometimes associated with fires. Miners who are regularly exposed to diesel equipment exhaust are affected by NO_2 emissions with serious respiratory effects. Automobile emissions are the source of nitrogen oxides. Acute exposure causes irritation of the eyes and nose, cough, mucoid or frothy sputum production, dyspnea, and chest pain. NO_2 is a deep lung irritant, can produce pulmonary oedema in 1–2 hours and acute respiratory distress syndrome (ARDS). Inhalation interferes with the production of surfactant from the alveolar cells. Some patients develop nonallergic asthma or "twitchy airway" disease. It may result in bronchiolitis obliterans. Treatment is symptomatic.

Chemical Pollutants

Several halogenated compounds used in various industries have now been banned due to their toxic effects on the environment. **Fluorinated hydrocarbons** have been used in refrigerators, air conditioners and non-stick cookware but were harmful to the ozone layer and have been banned. **Perfluorinated compounds** like teflon have been used but are also not safe.

Asbestos use is now known to be associated with fibrosis of the lungs, lung cancer and other cancers. Hence use of asbestos in all forms has been banned in most countries.

Metals: Heavy metals like lead, mercury and arsenic cause poisoning (*see* page 705)

Carcinogens: Many environmental pollutants are carcinogens, some are genotoxic and others non-genotoxic. On exposure to a genotoxic carcinogen, development of cancer occurs in multiple steps. Nongenotoxic carcinogens act by enhancing steps leading to cancer or inhibiting protective processes. A chemopreventive agent acts by inhibiting steps leading to cancer or by increasing protective processes. Some carcinogens are as follows.

Compound	*Source*
Polycyclic hydrocarbons	Smoke, petrol and diesel smoke, burnt food
Aflatoxins	Groundnut, corn
Nitrosamines	Tobacco
Ethanol	Drinks
Estrogens	Drugs
Arsenic, asbestos	Environment, occupational

Chemoprevention: Drugs that interfere with the carcinogenic process to prevent cancer before it is diagnosed are termed *chemopreventive agents.*

Examples

- Curcumin (turmeric), aspirin in colorectal cancer
- Flavonoids in lung and pancreatic cancer
- Green tea polyphenols, chlorophyllins and oltipraz (antischistosomal drug) in hepatocellular cancer
- Alpha tocopheral (antioxidants) in prostatic cancer.

INSECT REPELLANTS

Insect repellents are used to repel mosquitoes, ticks, flies, and other biting insects. Repellents are not meant to kill insects, but to keep them away to prevent bites and the spread of disease.

The active ingredients in common insect repellants are DEET (N, N-diethyl-meta-toluamide), picaridin, IR3535 and oil of lemon eucalyptus. Oil of lemon eucalyptus and IR3535 are natural substances—called biopesticides. **Permethrin** is an effective repellent against mosquitoes and flies and can be used with a skin based repellent. They can be applied to human skin and some can be used on clothing as sprays, wipes or lotions. Prallethrin is a pyrethroid insecticide and 1.6% w/w liquid vaporizer is commonly used for the control of mosquitoes in the household. Biotransformation and bioaccumulation may be responsible for toxicity—therefore to be used cautiously as per instructions.

Some common adverse effects with insect repellants

Insect repellants	*Common adverse effects*
DEET	Eye, skin and respiratory irritation, gastritis, neurological effects, seizures
Picaridin	Skin and eye irritation, vomiting
IR3535 Oil of lemon eucalyptus }	Eye irritation

[1] From Medical Council of India, *Competency based Undergraduate Curriculum for the Indian Medical Graduate*, 2018;1:139–144.

Unit XVI

Miscellaneous Topics

CHAPTER 62

Dietary Supplements, Nutraceuticals, Vitamins, Herbal Medicines and Enzymes in Therapy

Competency achievement: The student should be able to:
PH 1.61 Describe and discuss dietary supplements and nutraceuticals.[1]

DIETARY SUPPLEMENTS AND NUTRACEUTICALS

Dietary supplements are given along with the diet as a pill, capsule, tablet or liquid. Dietary supplements are not meant to replace food but are to be used in addition to food for health maintenance. The supplements include vitamins, minerals, herbals, botanicals, amino acids, enzymes and also some substances that have not been proved as being essential but could be having a beneficial biological effect.

Examples:

- Vitamin D supplements in people who do not get sufficient exposure to ultraviolet light.
- Calcium supplements to reduce risk of osteoporotic fractures.
- Protein supplements in people recovering from chronic illness or injury.
- Amino acids individually or in combination. Taurine is a popular supplement claimed to improve sports performance.
- Glucosamine—used as a nutrient for cartilage in osteoarthritis of knee.
- Body building supplements like high protein drinks, branched chain amino acids, glutamine, arginine, essential fatty acids, and creatinine are used by those involved in body building, weight lifters and athletes to increase lean body mass.

NUTRACEUTICALS

A nutraceutical (also called bioceutical or superfood) is a pharmaceutical compound that could produce beneficial effects to the user. It is a food or fortified food product that supplements the diet and also assists in treating or preventing disease. The term "nutraceutical" was coined in 1989 by Stephen De Felice, founder and chairman of the Foundation for Innovation in Medicine.

Nutraceuticals based on their source:

- Plant—tomato, garlic
- Animal—shark liver oil, cod liver oil.
- Mineral—calcium, magnesium, phosphorus.
- Microorganism—bifido-bacterium, lacto-bacilli.

Compare and Contrast

Nutraceutical	*Pharmaceutical*
Nutraceutical is used to prevent diseases	Pharmaceutical is used for prevention and treatment of diseases
Referred to as health product	Referred to as drug.
No license is needed to sell	Requires a license from the regulatory body
No prescription is required for purchasing	Can be purchased only by prescription (except OTC drugs)

Uses: They may be used to improve health, delay the process of aging, prevent chronic disease, increase life expectancy or support the structure or function of the body.

Some Nutraceuticals

- Coenzyme Q10 or ubiquinone used as purified nutritional supplement is an antioxidant. It has been tried in hypertension, heart failure and IHD. An interesting application is in prevention of statin-induced myopathy. Coenzyme Q10 levels may be reduced on administration of statins which may have a role in myopathy
- *Flax seeds:* Prevent mammary, colon and rectal cancers. Reduces blood pressure in hypertensive patients, reduces risk of diabetes and coronary artery disease.
- *Spirulina* has an immunostimulant property, used in arthritis and for delaying aging process.
- *Bitter gourd* has a hypoglycemic effect. The extract of bitter gourd increases the rate of glycogen synthesis by 4–5 fold in liver.
- *Garlic* used in the treatment of hyperlipidemia
- *Turmeric (curcuminoids)* has antimicrobial and anti-inflammatory activity. Recent findings indicate that it also is an integrase enzyme inhibitor.
- *Tomato lycopenes* prevents prostate cancer.
- *Fenugreek* has a laxative, expectorant and demulcent property.

  Thus diet rich in nutraceuticals, along with regular exercise, stress reduction and maintenance of healthy body weight, will maximize health and reduce disease risk.

VITAMINS

Vitamins are organic compounds essential for normal metabolism in the body. They are supplied by the diet. A balanced diet supplies adequate amounts of vitamins to fulfill the daily requirement. The requirement is increased during periods of rapid growth, pregnancy and lactation. Vitamin deficiencies result in characteristic signs and symptoms.

Vitamins are grouped into fat-soluble and water-soluble vitamins (Table 62.1).

Fat-soluble Vitamins

Vitamin A

Vitamin A is present in the diet as retinol, dehydroretinol or as carotenoids. Carotenoids are pigments present in green yellow vegetables and fruits and are converted in the body to retinol.

Physiological functions: Vitamin A has an important role in dark adaptation. It is essential for the synthesis of rhodopsin, the photosensitive pigment of rods. Vitamin A is also essential for maintenance of the integrity of epithelial cells, for growth and cell-mediated immunity.

Signs and symptoms of deficiency: Xerophthalmia (dryness of eyes), Bitot's spots in the conjunctiva, night blindness, diarrhoea, dry and rough skin are seen in early stages. In the later stages, keratomalacia, perforation of the cornea, necrosis and blindness can occur.

Daily requirement 3000–5000 IU/day.

Uses: In the prophylaxis and treatment of vitamin A deficiency.

1. *Prophylaxis:* 3000–5000 IU/day in presence of increased requirement.
2. *Treatment:* 50,000–1,00,000 IU intramuscularly or orally for 1–3 days followed by oral supplementation.
3. *Acne:* Retinoic acid or synthetic analogs of vitamin A like tretinoin or isotretinoin are used.

Hypervitaminosis A: Since vitamin A is a fat-soluble vitamin, it accumulates in the body on prolonged administration. The symptoms are dry skin (hyperkeratosis), anorexia, fever, alopecia, anaemia, oedema, headache, skin ulcers and tenderness over the bones.

Table 62.1: Sources, recommended daily allowances and deficiency syndroms of various vitamins in the diet (for adults)

Vitamin	*Important dietary sources*	*Daily allowance*	*Deficiency symptoms*
Fat-soluble vitamins			
Vitamin A	Green leafy vegetables, carrots, mango, papaya, eggs, milk, butter, cheese, liver and fish liver oils	3000–4000 IU	Night blindness, xerophthalmia, hyperkeratosis of skin and epithelial tissues
Vitamin D	Liver, egg yolk, fish liver oils, milk, butter	200–400 IU	Rickets, osteomalacia
Vitamin E	Wheat germ, nuts, cereals, eggs, green leafy vegetables	10–15 mg	Not known
Vitamin K	Green leafy vegetables, liver, meat, cheese, egg yolk and tomatoes	50–100 mg	Hypoprothrombinaemia, haemorrhage
Water-soluble vitamins			
Vitamin B complex			
Thiamine (B_1)	Cereals, rice polishing, liver, egg yolk, pears, nuts, green leafy vegetables	1.2–1.4 mg	**Beriberi,** peripheral neuritis, anorexia
Riboflavin (B_2)	Milk, cereals, pulses, leafy vegetables, eggs, and meat.	1.5–2 mg	Stomatitis, glossitis, cheilosis, vascularisation of cornea.
Nicotinic acid (Niacin B_3)	Rice polishings, cereals, pulses, groundnut, liver, meat, fish	20 mg	**Pellagra** - diarrhoea, dermatitis, dementia; glossitis, stomatitis, delusions, confusion.
Pantothenic acid	Rice polishings, whole grains, meat, egg yolk, milk, peanuts	4–7 mg	Weakness, fatigue, burning sensation in the feet.
Pyridoxine (B_6)	Whole grains, pulses, cereals, green leafy vegetables, milk, liver, egg yolk	2 mg	Peripheral neuritis, glossitis, stomatitis
Biotin	Liver, nuts, egg yolk	0.1–0.2 mg	Not known; may cause dermatitis
Folic acid	Leafy vegetables, milk, liver, meat, cereals	100–200 μg	Megaloblastic anaemia, glossitis, GI disturbances
Vitamin B_{12}	Milk, egg yolk, liver, meat, fish	1–2 mg	Megaloblastic anaemia, demyelinating, neurological disorders of the spinal cord.
Vitamin C	Goose berry (amla), citrus fruits, green vegetable, tomatoes, germinating pulses, potatoes	50 mg	Scurvy—petechiae, bleeding gums, easy bruising, delayed wound healing, anaemia, weakness.

Vitamin D *see* page 521.
Vitamin K *see* page 315.

Vitamin E

Vitamin E or alpha tocopherol is present in wheat germ oil, rice germ oil and soya bean oil.

Physiological role: Vitamin E acts as an antioxidant. It prevents the damage due to free radicals in normal metabolic reactions. Vitamin E is essential for normal structure and function of the nervous system. It is also required to maintain the integrity of the biological membranes. Vitamin E deficiency in animals result in reproductive and haemopoietic system abnormalities, degenerative changes in the spinal cord and heart. Daily requirement is 10–15 mg.

Uses: Clinically vitamin E deficiency in human beings is not known. It has been tried in G6PD deficiency, sterility, menopausal syndrome and other conditions with no definite evidence of obvious benefit.

Water-soluble Vitamins

Vitamin B-complex

B-complex group of vitamins includes thiamine, riboflavin, nicotinic acid, pyridoxine, pantothenic acid, biotin and cyanocobalamin.

1. *Thiamine (Vitamin B_1, Aneurine)*

Sources and requirement: Table 62.1.

Physiological role: Thiamine is converted to thiamine pyrophosphate which acts as a coenzyme in carbohydrate metabolism.

Symptoms of deficiency: Thiamine deficiency produces *Beriberi.*

Dry beriberi is characterised by peripheral neuritis and muscular atrophy.

Wet beriberi: The characteristic features are dependent oedema and high output cardiac failure. Wernicke's encephalopathy and Korsakoff's psychosis are also thought to be due to thiamine deficiency.

Uses

1. *Pregnancy:* Prophylactically in presence of increased demand as in pregnancy, lactation and in infants.
2. *Beriberi:* 50 mg daily parenterally. Once the patient recovers, maintenance dose of 10 mg/day is given orally.
3. *Chronic alcoholics:* 50 mg daily.
4. *Empirical use:* Thiamine is tried in several neurological and cardiovascular disorders and morning sickness.

2. *Riboflavin (Vitamin B_2)*

Physiological function: Flavin mononucleotide (FMN) and flavin adenine dinucleotide (FAD) containing the active form of riboflavin are coenzymes in various oxidation–reduction reactions.

Symptoms of deficiency: Angular stomatitis, glossitis, seborrhoeic keratosis of the nose, ulcers in the mouth, dry skin, burning sensation in the plantar surface of the feet, vascularization of the cornea and alopecia.

Uses: Riboflavin is used for the prevention and treatment (2–10 mg) of riboflavin deficiency.

3. *Nicotinic Acid and Nicotinamide (Vitamin B_3)*

Nicotinic acid and nicotinamide are together known as *niacin.*

Physiological functions: Nicotinic acid is converted to nicotinamide. Nicotinamide adenine nucleotide (NAD) and its phosphate (NADP) are coenzymes involved in several oxidation–reduction reactions.

Nicotinic acid is also a lipid-lowering agent.

Symptoms of deficiency: Niacin deficiency results in pellagra characterised by dermatitis, diarrhoea and dementia. Other symptoms include: Pigmentation of the skin, stomatitis, glossitis, headache, insomnia, hallucinations, confusion and megaloblastic anaemia. Chronic alcoholics, people living on maize as the staple diet, patients with malabsorption and cirrhosis develop pellagra.

Uses

1. Prophylaxis and treatment of pellagra (50–500 mg).
2. Nicotinic acid is used in hyperlipoproteinaemia (*see* page 389).

4. *Pyridoxine (Vitamin B_6)*

Physiological functions: Pyridoxal phosphate is a coenzyme involved in the synthesis of several amino acids, biogenic amines and other compounds like GABA.

Symptoms of deficiency: Glossitis, peripheral neuritis, anaemia, dermatitis and low seizure threshold due to decreased GABA levels in the brain.

Uses

1. Prophylaxis and treatment of pyridoxine deficiency.
2. *INH-induced peripheral neuritis:* Pyridoxine is used both for prophylaxis and treatment.
3. Convulsions in infants due to pyridoxine deficiency.
4. *'Morning sickness' in pregnancy:* Pyridoxine may reduce vomiting by an unknown mechanism.

5. Pantothenic Acid

Physiological role: Pantothenic acid is converted to coenzyme A which is involved in several metabolic reactions. Pantothenic acid deficiency in human beings is not known. Experimentally induced deficiency results in fatigue and paraesthesia. Calcium pantothenate is a component of multivitamin preparations.

6. Biotin

Biotin is an organic acid found in liver, nuts, egg yolk and other foods. Biotin deficiency in humans is not known. Experimentally induced deficiency results in dermatitis, anorexia, alopecia and glossitis. Biotin is a coenzyme in several metabolic reactions. It is present in many multivitamin preparations. Avidin, a protein present in egg white prevents the absorption of biotin.

VITAMIN B_{12}, FOLIC ACID (*see* pages 446)

Vitamin C (Ascorbic acid)

Physiological role: Ascorbic acid is involved in several metabolic reactions including oxidation reduction reactions and in cellular respiration. It is essential for the integrity of connective tissue, for the development of cartilage, bone and teeth and for wound healing.

Symptoms of deficiency: Vitamin C deficiency results in scurvy characterised by connective tissue defects resulting in haemorrhages in subcutaneous tissues, petechiae, ecchymoses, impaired wound healing, tender bleeding gums, deformed teeth, brittle bones, anaemia and growth retardation.

Uses

1. Prevention of vitamin C deficiency—50–100 mg daily.
2. Scurvy—500–1000 mg daily.
3. Common cold—large doses (0.5–1.5 g) of vitamin C has been tried as a prophylactic against common cold with controversial benefits.
4. To acidify urine.

MINERALS

Minerals are natural compounds/elements. About 5% of human body is made up of minerals. Minerals are essential for the normal body functions. Some minerals are needed in large quantities while others are in small quantities (trace elements) (Table 62.2; Key Box 62.1).

Calcium (*see* page 519).

SODIUM

Distribution in the body: Sodium is mainly present in extracellular fluid and bone. It is present as a salt with chloride, phosphate, bicarbonate and lactase.

Metabolism: Sodium is excreted mainly by the kidneys. It is also lost in the sweat and in stools in patients with diarrhoea.

Absorption of sodium is increased both directly and indirectly by glucose. Absorption of glucose increases water absorption and sodium follows. Aldosterone enhances the sodium reabsorption by the kidneys. Sodium depletion increases plasma renin levels.

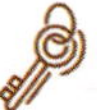

Key Box 62.1

Minerals needed in large quantities:
Calcium, sodium, potassium, magnesium, phosphorus, chloride, and sulphur.
Minerals needed in small quantities:
Iron, zinc, manganese, copper, iodine, fluoride, and cobalt.

Table 62.2: Salient features of minerals

Mineral and daily requirement	*Sources*	*Causes*	*Symptoms*
Sodium 5–15 g	Sodium chloride (salt) in diet	Hyponatremia: Excessive sweating, diarrhoea, burns, diuretics, starvation. Hypernatremia: Acute nephritis, aldosteronism, CCF, drugs like NSAIDs	Anorexia, lethargy, muscle cramps, hypotension and shock. Treat with IV normal saline Oedema ↑ blood pressure.
Magnesium 300 mg adults	Vegetables, grains, nuts, cocoa, fish, meat.	Severe diarrhoea, malab-sorption, diuretic therapy, hyperthyroidism, hyperparathyroidism, Aldosteronism, renal dysfunction	Neuromuscular irritability, tremors, nystagmus, difficulty in swallowing, cardiac disturbances, restlessness, altered behaviour and convulsions. Treatment is with magnesium sulphate
Zinc 10–100 mg	Vegetables, fruits, nuts, pulses, egg, milk, liver, meat	Dietary deficiency	Impaired wound healing, decreased acuity of taste and smell, alopecia, dermatitis and decreased growth in children.

Hyponatraemia

Causes: Excessive sweating, diarrhoea, burns, diuretics, starvation.

Signs and symptoms: Anorexia, lethargy, muscle cramps, hypotension and shock.

Treatment: Intravenous infusion of normal saline.

Hypernatraemia

Common causes: Acute nephritis, aldosteronism, CCF, drugs like NSAIDs.

Signs and symptoms: Oedema and increased blood pressure.

Treatment: Restricting dietary sodium intake, diuretics (frusemide) to promote sodium excretion in urine.

POTASSIUM

Potassium, a cation, is mainly present inside the cells. The total body content of potassium in an adult male is about 45 mEq/kg of which 70% is present in the muscles.

Sources: Coconut water, vegetables, fruits, nuts, meat and liver.

Daily requirement: 3–5 g in adults.

Physiological functions: Potassium is the chief cation in the cells (400 mg/dl) while plasma potassium is about 20 mg/ml. Potassium has an important role in regulating muscular activity, maintaining water and electrolyte balance and acid–base balance; potassium is also essential for neuronal activity (Table 62.3).

MAGNESIUM

Source: Vegetables, grains, nuts, cocoa, fish, meat.

Daily requirement: 300 mg in adults. Plasma magnesium levels — 1.8 to 2.4 mg/dl. The total body content of magnesium in an adult male is 20 to 30 g of which about 50 to 60% is present in bones and 25% in the muscles. Parathormone is essential for absorption of magnesium. It also helps in renal tubular reabsorption of magnesium.

Physiological Role

- Magnesium is a CNS depressant.
- Magnesium depresses neuromuscular transmission by inhibiting the release of

acetylcholine as well as antagonizing its depolarising activity at the motor end plate.

- Magnesium depresses the myocardium to some extent and also causes peripheral vasodilation resulting in flushing and hypotension.
- Magnesium is a cofactor in several enzyme mediated reactions.

Therapeutic Uses

1. *Magnesium deficiency:* Magnesium hydroxide is given orally in mild cases and magnesium sulphate is given slow IV. In severe deficiency, 5 ml of 50% magnesium is given slow IV.
2. *As antacids:* Magnesium hydroxide and magnesium trisilicate are used as antacids.
3. *Osmotic purgative:* Magnesium sulphate is used as osmotic purgative.
4. *As anticonvulsant:* Magnesium sulphate is used IV (or IM) to control seizures in toxaemia of pregnancy.
5. *Tocolytic:* IV magnesium sulphate may be used as an alternative to relax the uterus in preterm labour.
6. *Cardiac arrhythmias:* Magnesium chloride may be used in the treatment of arrhythmias that may follow myocardial infarction.
7. *In raised intracranial tension:* Rectal administration of magnesium sulphate solution may help to reduce intracranial tension.
8. *Topical:* 25–50% magnesium sulphate in glycerin (Mag sulf poultice) is used topically to relieve local oedema. Magnesium sulphate exerts osmotic effect (while glycerin is hygroscopic) and reduces local inflammation.

Deficiency: Magnesium deficiency may occur in severe diarrhoea, malabsorption, diuretic therapy, hyperthyroidism, hyperparathyroidism, aldosteronism and renal dysfunction. It is characterized by neuromuscular irritability, tremors, nystagmus, difficulty in swallowing, cardiac disturbances, restlessness, altered behaviour and convulsions. Treatment is with magnesium sulphate (or any other magnesium salt) 10 ml of 25% solution IM or slow IV.

Phosphorus (*see* page 520).

Iron (*see* page 443).

ZINC

Source: Vegetables, fruits, nuts, pulses, egg, milk, liver and meat.

Functions: Zinc is a cofactor of many enzymes like carbonic anhydrase, alkaline phosphatase.

Dificiency: Dificiency of zinc results in impaired wound healing, decreased acuity of taste and smell, alopecia, dermatitis and decreased growth in children.

Zinc is component of several multivitamin preparations.

MANGANESE

Manganese acts as cofactor for certain enzymes like decarboxylase. It also plays role in glycoprotein synthesis.

Sources: Cereals, nuts, whole grains, fruits and vegetables are rich in manganese. It is stored in the liver.

Deficiency symptoms are not known.

Misconceptions about the safety and efficacy of food supplements are very common. Wrong identification of the herbs and plants may interfere with their safety. Substandard products, impure or inadequately purified products with variations in potency are often seen. The belief that natural things are 'harmless' could add to unsafe use of these products. Hence adequate precautions are to be taken in prescribing dietary supplements. Dietary supplements do not generally undergo strict clinical trials. Unlike drugs, no government approval is required to make or sell a dietary supplement. However, the concerned regulatory body like FDA in USA and DCGI in India can decide that a dietary supplement is unsafe and can order removal from the market.

Table 62.3: Causes, clinical features and treatment of hypokalaemia and hyperkalaemia

Causes	*Clinical features*	*Treatment*
	Hypokalaemia	
• Dietary deficiency • Excessive loss in sweating, vomiting, diarrhoea • Diabetic ketoacidosis • Diuretic overdosage • Fanconi's syndrome • Nephrotic syndrome • Drug induced (ACE inhibitors, spironolactone) • Addison's disease	Fatigue, muscle weakness, mental confusion, thirst, hypotension, bradycardia, cardiac arrhythmias, renal impairment, neuro-muscular paralysis	Mild—oral potassium chloride Severe—KCl—**Slow** IV drip (rapid potassium infusion can cause sudden death due to cardiac arrest)
	Hyperkalaemia	
	Cardiac arrhythmias, skeletal muscle and respiratory paralysis, cardiac arrest	• ↑ urinary K^+ excretion by dialysis and diuretics (Frusemide + a thiazide) • Cation exchange resin, • Promoting K^+ shift into cells using plain insulin 5–10 units with 50 ml of 50% glucose IV over 5 min. • 10 ml of 10% calcium gluconate to prevent damage by K+ to the heart

HERBAL MEDICINES

Competency achievement: The student should be able to:
PH 1.59 Describe and discuss the herbal medicines.[1]

Herbal medicines include traditional medicines which use medicinal plant preparations for therapy. Traditional medicines have been mentioned in classical Indian texts—Rigveda, Atharvaveda, Charak Samhita and Sushruta Samhita. Pharmacotherapy under modern system of medicine differs from herbal medicine in that whole plants are used, it is claimed that the effect of the whole herb is greater than the summed effects of its components and toxicity is reduced (described as "buffering"). In modern system, purified molecules are used. **Safety of herbal medicines** is a great concern because:

1. There are no well-defined purification steps in the production of herbal products. Hence, quality variation is common from one lot to another.
2. Self medication and simultaneous use of modern medicine may result in **herb-drug interactions**.
3. Some of them contain mercury, lead, arsenic, corticosteroids or poisonous organic substances in harmful amounts. Hepatic failure, renal failure and even death following ingestion of herbal medicines have been reported. Several women developed renal fibrosis after taking Chinese herbs prescribed by a slimming clinic. When medicinal plant materials are stored improperly, *Aspergillus flavus* may grow which produces aflatoxin—a mycotoxin.

Some examples of herbal medicines

Echinacea: *Echinacea purpurea* has shown immune modulation, anti-inflammatory, antibacterial, antifungal, antiviral, and antioxidant effects in *in vitro* studies. It has been used in respiratory tract infections, UTI and vaginal fungal infections. Adverse effects with oral commercial formulations are unpleasant taste, gastrointestinal upset, allergic reactions. Echinacea should be avoided in immunodeficiency and auto-immune disorders.

Garlic (*Allium sativum*): Raw garlic contains allicin (responsible for the odor) but aged garlic extract contains water-soluble organosulfur compounds and is odor-free. The pharmacologic activity of garlic is due to organosulfur compounds. *In vitro*, allicin inhibits HMG-CoA reductase, is active against some bacteria, fungi (*Candida albicans*), protozoa (*Entamoeba histolytica*), some viruses and also exhibits antioxidant effects. Clinical trials have shown lipid lowering effects, antiplatelet effects (possibly through inhibition of thromboxane synthesis or stimulation of nitric oxide synthesis) following garlic ingestion and is also studied for anticancer effects. Patients using anticoagulants, antiplatelets and NSAIDs should use garlic cautiously as it has antiplatelet activity. Garlic may reduce the bioavailability of saquinavir.

Ginko: *Ginkgo biloba* extract prepared from the leaves of the ginkgo tree contains flavone glycosides and terpenoids. Ginkgo has been shown to increase blood flow, reduce blood viscosity, and promote vasodilation, thus improving tissue perfusion. Increase in endogenous nitric oxide effects, antagonism of platelet-activating factor, antioxidant and radical-scavenging properties are noted. Ginkgo has shown significant benefits in dementia. Adverse effects include nausea, headache, stomach upset, diarrhoea, allergy, anxiety, insomnia and bleeding. It should be avoided with antiplatelet drugs, anticoagulants and in seizure disorders.

Ginseng is derived from *Panax ginseng*, and *P. quinquefolius* contains ginsenosides. Reported beneficial effects include modulation of immune function, antioxidant activity, anti-inflammatory effects, antistress activity, analgesia, vasoregulatory effects (increased endothelial nitric oxide), cardioprotective activity, antiplatelet activity; improved glucose homeostasis and anticancer properties. Ginseng is also claimed to help improve physical and mental performance. Investigational use: Common cold prevention, lowering blood glucose, cancer prevention, and reducing cancer-related fatigue. Adverse effects include vaginal bleeding, mastalgia, insomnia, nervousness and hypertension. Patients receiving phenelzine, lithium, neuroleptics, warfarin and immunosuppressants should avoid ginseng.

St. John's Wort or *Hypericum perforatum*/ hypericum, is claimed to be useful in the treatment of depression. *In vitro* studies have shown inhibition of reuptake of serotonin, norepinephrine, and dopamine in nerve terminals. Investigational uses: Depression, premenstrual dysphoric disorder, climacteric complaints, somatoform disorders, and anxiety. Adverse effects are photosensitization, mild gastrointestinal symptoms, fatigue, sedation, restlessness, dizziness, headache, and dry mouth. Drug interactions can occur with antidepressants, digoxin, hormonal contraceptives, cyclosporine, HIV protease and non-nucleoside reverse transcriptase inhibitors, warfarin, irinotecan, theophylline, and anticonvulsants.

***Rauwolfia serpentina* (Sarpagandha)** contains reserpine. It is used as an antipsychotic and antihypertensive (*see* page 242)

Forskolin (Mainmool, *Coleus forskoli Briq)* directly stimulates adenylate cyclase and cyclic AMP and is an inotrope

***Boswellia serrata* (Sallaki)**—Boswelic acid inhibits 5-lipooxygenase and leukotreine B4 resulting in anti-inflammatory and anti-complement effects.

***Albizzia lebek* (Shirish)**—prevents mast cell degranulation, similar to sodium cromoglycate.

***Withania somnifera* (Ashwagandha)** is a GABA-A receptor agonist.

***Picrorhiza kurua* (Katuka)** has anti-oxidant effects like tocopherol, and also influences the glutathion metabolism in liver and brain.

Use of herbal medicines in jaundice, presumably viral hepatitis, has been known in India since long ago. Four herbal medicines that have been found to be promising in the treatment of viral hepatitis are: (i) Silymarin (ii) Extracts of *Picrorhiza kurroa*, ('Kutaki') (iii) Extract of some plants of the genus Phyllanthus and (iv) Glycyrrhizin.

Liv 52 an ayurvedic preparation contains extracts of several plants and is reported to improve serum enzyme values in liver dysfunction and is widely used in these patients.

ENZYMES IN THERAPY

Enzymes are proteins produced by the living cells. They catalyse several biochemical reactions. Some substances act with specific enzymes and are called coenzymes. Enzymes used in therapeutics (Table 62.4) are:

1. Mammalian enzymes: Hyaluronidase, trypsin, chymotrypsin, alpha chymotrypsin, pancreatic dornase.

2. Bacterial enzymes: Streptokinase, streptodornase, collagenase, serratiopeptidase, L-asparaginase.

3. Plant enzymes: Papain (papase).

Mammalian Enzymes

Hyaluronidase is obtained from mammalian testes. It depolymerizes hyaluronic acid of connective tissue. Given subcutaneously, it increases the tissue permeability and enhances the rate of absorption of subcutaneously administered fluids and drugs.

Hyaluronidase can produce allergic reactions. It should not be injected around an infected site to avoid the spread of infection.

FACIDASE 1500 IU inj

Uses

1. Hyaluronidase is used for hypodermoclysis in infants and children in whom, large volumes of fluids are given subcutaneously.
2. To hasten resorption of fluids and blood in haematoma.
3. Along with local anaesthetics—to increase the effectiveness of local anaesthesia.
4. Radiography: Hyaluronidase enhances absorption of the radio-opaque substances.

Trypsin is obtained from bovine pancreas. It is a proteolytic enzyme which directly hydrolyses natural proteins. It digests dead tissue, bacteria and debris. Trypsin may be used topically, sublingually or intramuscularly. Allergic reactions can occur.

Uses

1. Trypsin (freshly prepared solution) is used topically for debridement of necrotic tissues.
2. Used topically for liquefaction of coagulated blood and exudates.
3. Trypsin-containing gelatin capsules are inserted into sinuses and fistulae that cannot be adequately irrigated.
4. It can also be used for irrigation of nasal cavities.
5. Used sublingually for thrombophlebitis, deep contusions and skin ulcers.

Chymotrypsin is an endopeptidase obtained from bovine pancreas. Like trypsin, it hydrolyses natural proteins. It is used in several skin conditions including abscesses and ulcers and postoperatively to reduce inflammation and oedema. It is also used following tooth extraction and tooth impaction.

CHYMIN FORTE, CHYMAROL FORTE (chymotrypsin + trypsin) 1 lakh unit cap

Alpha chymotrypsin: It has proteolytic activity like chymotrypsin. It is used in cataract operations to dissolve the suspensory ligament of the lens (enzymatic zonulolysis). This makes it easy to remove the lens.

Pancreatic dornase is a deoxyribonuclease. It acts extracellularly and makes the secretions thin by degrading deoxyribonucleoprotein. It is obtained from pancreas of cattle and is used as an aerosol. It can cause allergic reactions. See mucolytics (*see* page 408).

Bacterial Enzymes

Streptokinase obtained from beta haemolytic streptococci causes fibrinolysis (*see* page 395).

Streptodornase is a group of proteolytic enzymes which catalyse depolymerization of

Table 62.4: Salient features of enzymes in therapy

Enzymes	*Source and route*	*Actions and ADR*	*Uses*
Mammalian enzymes			
Hyaluronidase	Mammalian testes	Depolymerises connective tissue, ↑ tissue permeability	Hypodermoclysis, for faster resorption of fluids and blood in haematoma, to ↑ effectiveness of LA, In radiography as radio-opaque substance
	Topical, SC, IM Intra-articular	Allergic reactions, avoid injection around infected wound to avoid spread of infection	To promote absorption of drugs
Trypsin chymotrypsin	Bovine pancreas Oral, topical	Proleolytic, hydrolyses natural proteins, dead tissue, bacteria Allergic reactions	• Topically for debridement of necrotic tissues, for liquefaction of coagulated blood and exudates • Irrigation of sinuses, fistulae and nasal cavity • SL for thrombophlebitis, deep contusions and skin ulcers • To ↓ inflammation and oedema—skin conditions, like abcesses, ulcers, postoperatively, after tooth extraction
Alpha chymotrypsin	Bovine pancreas Oral, parenteral	Acts extracellularly-proteolytic Allergic reactions	Cataract surgery to dissolve suspensory ligaments (zonulolysis) during lens removal
Pancreatic dornase	From cattle pancreas Aerosol	Secretions become thin Allergic reactions	Mucolytic
Bacterial enzymes			
Streptokinase Streptodornase	Streptococci Parenteral	Proteolytic enzyme lysis of nucleoproteins in dead cells and pus Contraindicated in bleeding Should not be used around infected area	Fibrinolytic Topically to liquefy clotted blood, pus and clear debris in chronic ulcers
Collagenase	*Clostridium histolyticum*	Proteolytic	Topical debridement of dermal ulcers and burns To promote growth of granulation tissue
Serratiopeptidase	Serratia species Oral	Proteolytic enzyme Anti-inflammatory activity	To relieve inflammatory oedema in soft tissues Adjuvant in inflammatory conditions like RA, osteoarthritis, sinusitis Pulmonary TB to facilitate expectoration
Plant enzymes Papain	Fruit of *Carica papaya*	Proteolytic activity	Topically for debriding wound surfaces

nucleoproteins like deoxyribonucleic acid that are present in dead cells of the pus. Thus streptodornase liquifies viscous and purulent material. It has no effect on living cells.

Streptokinase and streptodornase are used in combination both topically and for instillation into body cavities.

Adverse effects: Allergic reactions may occur. Streptokinase and streptodornase are contra-indicated in presence of bleeding. They should not be used around a local infected area.

Streptokinase and streptodornase are used topically to liquify clotted blood, pus and to clear the debris in chronic ulcers, osteomyelitis and other wounds and lesions.

Collagenase obtained from *Clostridium histolyticum* is used topically for the debridement of dermal ulcers and burns. It also promotes the growth of granulation tissue.

Serratiopeptidase is a proteolytic enzyme obtained from the serratia species.

It is administered orally to relieve inflammatory oedema in the soft tissues. It is claimed to digest necrotic tissue, exudates and clots which are cleared faster from the site of trauma. However, adequate evidence to prove its efficacy is currently not available.

Serratiopeptidase is tried as an adjuvant in a wide variety of conditions associated with inflammation like rheumatoid arthritis, osteoarthritis, cervical spondylosis, ankylosing spondylitis, fractures and other musculoskeletal disorders; sinusitis, otitis, bronchitis, bronchial asthma and pulmonary tuberculosis to facilitate expectoration; subconjunctival haemorrhage and hyphaema; Postoperative patients, traumatic injury, following tonsillectomy, episiotomy, perineal laceration; dental infections, pericoronitis and alveolar abscess.

LYSER FORTE, PEPDOL 10 mg tab, SERATAB 5, 10, 20 mg

L-asparaginase is obtained from *E.coli* cultures for commercial use (*see* page 678).

Plant Enzymes

Papain is obtained from the unripe fruit of *Carica papaya*. It is a proteolytic enzyme used topically for debriding wound surfaces.

[1] From Medical Council of India, *Competency based Undergraduate Curriculum for the Indian Medical Graduate*, 2018;1:136–144.

Drug Administration in Special Situations: Pregnancy, Lactation, Paediatrics, Geriatrics, Renal and Hepatic Diseases

CHAPTER 63

Competency achievement: The student should be able to:

PH 1.56 Describe basic aspects of geriatric and pediatric pharmacology.[1]

DRUGS IN PREGNANCY

Great caution is required in the use of drugs in a pregnant lady for the safety of both the mother and the foetus. There are certain physiological changes during pregnancy. Such changes could alter the pharmacokinetics and to some extent the pharmacodynamics of certain drugs administered during pregnancy. Moreover, most drugs cross the placenta and reach the foetus which is exposed to both the therapeutic and toxic effects of drugs. Gastric emptying time is prolonged and gut motility is reduced due to raised progesterone levels. Hence, absorption of drugs is delayed. The total body water and thereby the plasma volume is increased by 30% during pregnancy leading to hemodilution. Hence the volume of distribution of drugs that largely remain in the vascular compartment increases because of the increased body fluid volume. Progesterone induces enzymes in the liver. Hence, drugs may get metabolized faster. Due to the increase in the renal blood flow, drugs are excreted faster, e.g. aminoglycosides. Hence dose of some drugs needs to be increased to compensate for all the above pharmacokinetic changes in pregnancy.

However, for several diseases, there could be one or two drugs that are known to be safe in pregnancy. For example, methyldopa in hypertension, chloroquine in malaria. The doctor should be aware of it or refer to such a list before prescribing in pregnancy. Studies on teratogenicity are limited because of the ethical constraints in conducting such research. Hence drugs should be generally avoided during pregnancy and if required, be used cautiously, balancing the risk verses benefit in both the mother and the child.

Transfer of Drugs Across Placenta

Lipid-soluble, unionized drugs readily cross the placenta and attain a high concentration in the foetus. Drugs of low molecular weight can easily cross the placenta while larger molecules like heparin cannot cross and hence is the preferred anticoagulant in pregnancy. However, the placenta has some transporter proteins which can carry larger molecules across it. On the other hand, we now also know of some **P-glycoprotein transporters** which transport certain drugs back into the maternal circulation and thereby protect the foetus. For example, (i) antiretroviral drugs like protease inhibitors attain low concentration in the foetus and thus may not be reliable in the prevention of vertical HIV transmission from the mother to the foetus, (ii) antidiabetic drug glyburide attains very low concentration in the foetal blood.

Total body water increases during pregnancy—therefore, there is an increase in the volume of distribution of poorly lipid-soluble drugs as they largely remain in the vascular compartment. Drugs which are largely bound to plasma proteins poorly cross the placental barrier but if drugs are highly lipid-soluble, the effect of protein binding in transfer across placenta is insignificant.

Placenta is capable of metabolizing some drugs like barbiturates. On the other hand, the placenta may convert some drugs to toxic metabolites. Placenta is also the route of drug elimination for the foetus. In pregnancy, hepatic microsomal enzymes are induced (thought to be the effect of progesterone). Hence drugs metabolized by these enzymes may be degraded faster. However, it is not of much clinical significance.

Due to increase in renal blood flow (and thereby GFR), the rate of elimination of drugs by kidneys significantly increases in pregnancy. Hence the dose of some such drugs needs to be increased. Example: Cefuroxime, ampicillin, phenytoin, carbamazepine.

Effect of Drugs on the Foetus

Since most drugs cross placenta and reach the foetus, the foetus is at the risk of harmful effects of drugs. Several drugs are teratogenic. The harmful effects depend on the drug and the period of gestation. Drug categories (*see* page 64, Table 4.1). Teratogenicity (*see* page 63).

DRUG PRESCRIPTION AND LACTATION

Most drugs are excreted into the breast milk. However, the quantity excreted is so small that they do not attain adequate concentration in the plasma of the baby. Hence, most drugs taken in therapeutic doses by the mother will not harm the infant. However, there are some exceptions.

The following facts should be noted in using drugs during lactation:

1. Breastfeeding is vital for the health of the child. It supplies the necessary nutrients and immunoglobulins to the neonate which protect it from several diseases. The mother should be educated regarding its importance.
2. Suckling is the stimulus for prolactin and oxytocin secretion and, therefore, for milk production and ejection.
3. Most lipid-soluble drugs are readily secreted in the milk. Drugs reach milk mostly by passive diffusion.
4. Highly protein bound drugs are not secreted into the milk in significant amounts since only the unbound fraction can reach the milk.
5. Some drugs, like metronidazole, may change the taste of milk (bitter) though it is otherwise a safe drug during lactation.
6. Most sedative hypnotics attain good concentration in the milk to produce drowsiness in the child.
7. Antibiotics like penicillins, erythromycin, antimalarials like chloroquine, most anti-epileptics and beta blockers may be safely used in lactating women.
8. Tetracyclines (risk of teeth, discolouration) opioids (dependence), lithium (low renal clearance in infant), anticancer drugs, antithyroid drugs, radioactive substances, immunosuppressants, ergotamine (ergotism) and ephedrine (CNS stimulation) are some of the drugs **contraindicated** in lactating women.

PAEDIATRIC PHARMACOLOGY

Our knowledge of pharmacokinetics and pharmacodynamics in paediatric age group is largely inadequate because of the constraints in conducting studies in this age group. Moreover, children are more susceptible to adverse effects of drugs. Hence utmost caution is required in prescribing drugs in children.

Pharmacokinetics

Though the pharmacokinetics of drugs in children largely resemble that in adults, there are certain minor differences. They should be kept in mind while prescribing drugs for this age group of patients.

Absorption

Certain physiological changes occur in the gastrointestinal function during the first few days of life.

They are:

- Gastric acidity is low in premature infants and neonates. Hence acid-labile drugs, like penicillin, attain a better bioavailability while weakly acidic drugs, like phenobarbitone, attain lower plasma concentrations (need acid for absorption).
- Gastric acid secretion gradually increases and would need several hours after birth (3–4 days in premature). Hence oral administration of drugs which are to be metabolised by gastric acid should be avoided in the first 2–3 days in a preterm infant.
- Gastric emptying is slow—hence drugs that are mostly absorbed from the stomach are absorbed better.
- Intestinal motility is slow and unpredictable; therefore, the amount of drug absorbed may be more, resulting in toxicity.
- Absorption from the skin is faster because skin as a barrier is yet to be fully developed in infants. For example, salicylic acid ointment application can produce salicylism in neonates.
- In premature infants, absorption following intramuscular injection is erratic due to small muscle mass and reduced blood flow to the periphery. There is a risk of large amount of the drug being absorbed in a short period, if the blood flow improves and could result in toxicity (example—anticonvulsants). However, in older children, absorption from intramuscular injection is satisfactory and largely reliable.
- The secretion of bile acids and lipase is low in the newborn because of which there may be reduction in the absorption of lipid-soluble drugs.

Distribution

In premature babies and infants, the extracellular fluid volume is much larger than in the adult, while the body fat is much lower—in premature infants, it is 1–2%, full-term infants 15%, higher in children around one year of age ~30% and in adults it is around 18%. Hence water-soluble drugs with low protein binding which remain mostly in ECF compartment need to be given in much lower doses in premature children. Dosage calculation should be based on the surface area because this is closer to the dosage calculation based on the ECF volume, and is more appropriate in them as compared to the total body weight.

Plasma Protein Binding

The concentration of plasma proteins are lower in prematures and infants because:

a. Liver is immature to synthesize them
b. A large fraction of albumin is bound by bilirubin.

Hence, the free drug levels of extensively protein bound drugs, like warfarin, increase and may result in toxicity. *Other examples:* Lignocaine, diazepam, ampicillin.

Several drugs which bind to albumin may compete with and displace bilirubin (bound to albumin) which may be dangerous in neonates having jaundice. On the other hand, raised bilirubin (as in physiological jaundice) may displace drugs bound to albumin (e.g. phenytoin) resulting in toxicity.

The permeability of the BBB is higher in infants because it is poorly formed and many drugs can cross the BBB and attain higher concentration in the brain and CSF. Because of the higher uptake of morphine in the brain in infants, it should not be used up to 6 months of age to avoid respiratory depression.

Metabolism

The rate of drug metabolism is relatively slower in infants. The reason for slow metabolism is that some of the metabolizing enzymes like hydroxylases, esterases and conjugases are poorly developed (especially glucuronide conjugation). As a result, plasma half-life of several drugs get prolonged and can result in toxicity

Some of the notable examples are as follows:

- Drugs like salicylates and nalidixic acid are poorly metabolized due to inadequately developed glucuronide conjugation.
- Only a small dose of paracetamol is metabolized by glucuronidation. However, this is to some extent compensated by sulphate conjugation.
- Chloramphenicol can cause gray-baby syndrome in the newborn due to its poor metabolism in them, once again by poor glucuronidation.
- Diazepam has a longer half-life in premature babies (40–120 hr) as against 20–80 hr in adults. This is due to inadequate phase I hydroxylation.
- Succinylcholine has a longer duration of action due to poorly formed plasma esterases.
- Local anaesthetics of the ester group also act longer due to the same reason.
- Pivampicillin is not very effective in infants since its hydrolysis to the active metabolite ampicillin (formed by hydrolysis) does not take place adequately in them.
- It takes about 5 months to 5 years of age for phase I reactions to attain adult levels while phase II reactions reach adult values much earlier, i.e. by 3 to 6 months of age. Premature babies require a little more longer time.
- If the pregnant mother was receiving an enzyme inducer like phenobarbitone, then it could cause enzyme induction in the foetus too. This could result in faster metabolism of such drugs metabolized by microsomal enzymes causing lower plasma drug levels than expected.

Excretion

The excretory mechanisms, particularly the kidneys are not fully functional in the neonates. Hence their capacity to excrete drugs is also much lower compared to adults. All renal processes including GFR, renal tubular secretion, tubular reabsorption and even renal blood flow are much lower compared to adult values. For example, GFR is only 30–40% of the adult values in the neonates. Tubular secretion is only 20%. Hence renal clearance of drugs is much lower. Examples: Penicillin (clearance 1/5th that of adults) aminoglycosides, digoxin, ceftazidime, diazepam are slowly cleared in neonates. Phenytoin has a t½ of 80 hr in neonates while it is 12–18 hr in adults.

Therefore, because of the less efficient excretory mechanisms, the neonates, the premature and the infants require drugs in much lower doses and for much lesser duration particularly the drugs that depend on kidneys for elimination.

Pharmacodynamics

There is not much of variation in the response to drugs in neonates compared to adults with a few exceptions. Several drugs are teratogenic, e.g. tetracyclines, phenytoin.

- Drugs that inhibit PG synthesis (indomethacin) can promote rapid closure of ductus arteriosus.
- Administration of PGs can delay the closure of ductus arteriosus. This effect can be made use of in Fallot's tetralogy.
- Neonates are more prone for dehydration and acidosis and drugs that could precipitate these should be used carefully, e.g. diuretics, aspirin.
- Use of aspirin in children with influenza or chickenpox may increase the risk of Reye's syndrome in them.

Drug Administration in Children

Administration of drugs requires special care in children particularly in neonates and infants. Special drug formulations are available for use in children. Use of tablets is inconvenient and injections are resisted because they are painful. The preferred formulations are liquids like suspensions, drops and elixirs. The parents should be instructed on the proper use of drug formulations in children. Drug use is further complicated by rejection, spitting out and also vomiting particularly in infants. In the process, the drug may be partly or fully lost and the question of repeating the dose arises.

Proper measurement of the liquids using calibrated measuring cups ensures appropriate dosing to a large extent.

Suspensions need to be shaken well before use because the actual drug may accumulate at the bottom of the bottle. This results in inadequate initial doses and higher doses towards later days of treatment which could result in toxicity. Convenient dosage forms and dosing schedules go a long way in improving compliance.

Calculations of dose should be based on body weight and parents should be educated on the importance of the right dosing.

The formulae for calculating paediatric dose are:

$$\text{Dose} = \frac{\text{Adult dose} \times \text{Age (years)}}{\text{Age} + 12}$$

Clarkís formula:

$$\text{Dose} = \frac{\text{Adult dose} \times \text{Weight (kg)}}{70}$$

GERIATRIC PHARMACOLOGY

People above the age of '65' years are called the 'elderly'. Though the age considered is 65 years, it is just arbitrary and infact, by 5th decade many of the age-related problems start. In women, it could be even earlier because, the onset of menopause itself may mark the beginning of such health problems. Hence, geriatric medicine has emerged as a speciality by itself.

The population of the elderly is constantly increasing and could result in a major change in the population structure. The increase in life expectancy consequent to better health services and growth of medical science have contributed to a rise in the number of the elderly.

In general, elderly are considered to be two to three times at a higher risk of developing an adverse drug reaction. Elderly are more prone to adverse reactions for the following reasons.

1. The pattern of drug use in the elderly—it is estimated that >80% of people above 65 years suffer from one or more chronic diseases and consume 40% of all drugs. Thus elderly tend to have multiple diseases requiring multiple drugs.

   Polypharmacy is excessive and unnecessary use of multiple drugs. Each drug may result in some adverse effect. More drugs are given to treat these adverse drug reactions, e.g. antacids are given to treat gastritis induced by NSAIDs. Use of multiple drugs can also result in drug interactions. Polypharmacy would result in decreased compliance and increased financial burden to the patient.
2. Altered response to drugs in the elderly.
3. Older patients often have visual, auditory and cognitive impairment which could lead to errors in drug intake.

Table 63.1: Some age-related physiological changes which could influence pharmacokinetics

Pharmacokinetic changes	*Potential effect*
↓ Blood supply to oral mucosa	↓ Absorption by sublingual route
Delayed gastric emptying	Impaired absorption
↓ Splanchnic blood flow	↓ Presystemic elimination
↓ Lean body mass, body water	↓ Distribution volume
↓ Serum albumin	↑ Free drug concentration
↓ Mixed function oxidases	↓ Hepatic metabolism
↓ GFR, tubular function	↓ Renal clearance

4. Elderly are generally physically weaker section. They are also psychologically and emotionally helpless and down. These make them more susceptible for adverse effects. Age-related changes—there could be certain pharmacokinetic and pharmacodynamic changes in the elderly which also make them more susceptible to adverse drug effects.

PHARMACOKINETIC CHANGES

Drug Absorption

Several functional changes could be seen in old age like a decrease in gastric acid production, blood flow to the gut, gastrointestinal motility and mucosal absorbing area. There is also an alteration in the gastric pH which may affect ionization and solubility of the drugs. However, these changes may not have significant effects on the absorption of drugs. It could be because some of the changes counter each other. For example, factors that decrease absorption, like decreased blood flow, may be opposed by decreased GI motility which allows drugs to remain longer in the gut. Some drugs have increased bioavailability in the elderly. A decrease in first pass metabolism may increase the bioavailability of drugs like propranolol, levodopa, nifedipine and morphine. Absorption of drugs by sublingual route may be reduced due to decrease in the blood supply to the oral mucosa. Absorption of drugs may be slower and somewhat less complete in the elderly.

Distribution

Depending on the properties of the drug, the following changes can influence the drug distribution:

- Changes in the body composition due to older age can modify drug distribution.
- Changes such as decrease in total body water, body weight, lean body mass and plasma protein concentration and increase in percentage of body fat are common in the elderly.
- Drugs that are extensively bound to plasma proteins will now have more free fraction to act and can produce a greater response. (because of decreased plasma proteins).
- Water-soluble drugs, like morphine, will have a higher concentration in the body because they are distributed in a smaller volume of body water.
- Lipid-soluble drugs have a larger volume of distribution, they are distributed in a larger volume of fat and, therefore, have a longer half-life. Increased body fat acts as a reservoir for such lipid-soluble drugs and can also result is problems related to drug storage—there could be accumulation of the drugs in the fatty tissue and thereby prolonged action. All these changes could put the elderly at a higher risk of toxicity from drugs. Hence, these problems should be anticipated and necessary dosage adjustments should be done.

Metabolism

Since liver is the primary site for drug metabolism, age-related changes in liver function can affect the process of biotransformation. In the elderly, the drug metabolizing capacity of the liver decreases because of the decrease in the liver size, amount of blood flow and hepatic enzyme activity. Many drugs are metabolized more slowly and drugs would remain active for longer periods of time compared to young adults. Moreover, the oxidative pathways are inhibited. Hence drugs metabolized by oxidation like piroxicam, diazepam, ibuprofen and phenytoin have a longer half-life in the geriatric age group.

Excretion

The kidneys are the primary organs of drug excretion from the body. The renal function is depressed in the elderly because of a decline in renal blood flow, renal mass and function of renal tubules. As a result, there is a decrease in

GFR, tubular secretion and a consequent reduction in excretion of drugs. Studies have shown drug excretion to be reduced by 35–50% due to decrease in GFR. Thus age-related changes in the renal function can result in a significant reduction in drug excretion leading to accumulation of drugs and their metabolites in the body. The half-lives of the drugs get longer, and their clearance diminishes. Thus reduced renal function should be taken into account whenever drugs are prescribed in the elderly. The overall effects of the pharmacokinetic changes associated with aging are that drugs remain active in the body for longer periods thereby prolonging their effects as well as adverse effects. For example, half-life of certain drugs, like diazepam, may be increased by as much as four times in the elderly. However, the extent of age-related pharmacokinetic changes vary from person-to-person. Thus drug dosages should be adjusted and adverse drug reactions minimized after considering all the above factors.

PHARMACODYNAMIC CHANGES

Age-related alterations in the physiological functions can influence the systemic response to various drugs. Factors like decreased function of the smooth muscles of the viscera, decreased baroreceptor sensitivity, impaired postural control, altered thermoregulatory responses and a reduced cognitive function can all influence the response to a drug.

The receptor function may also be blunted, i.e. the affinity and binding of the drug to the receptor and the cellular functions may be altered in some tissues due to aging. However, the extent of variations depends on the extent of changes in the physiological functions.

Other factors that influence response in the elderly include presence of multiple diseases, poor diet and poor general health.

Adverse Reactions in the Elderly

As discussed earlier, elderly are more prone to adverse effects. The adverse effects which are more common in the elderly and need special caution include—postural hypotension, dizziness, sedation, urinary retention, constipation, depression, dehydration, confusion, extrapyramidal symptoms, fatigue and weakness.

Postural hypotension: Causes dizziness and syncope because of reduced blood supply to the brain. This could result in falls and fractures, cerebral and cardiac infarcts. The older subjects have comparatively less physical activity and lower cardiovascular function—all these factors can increase the chances of postural hypotension in the elderly. Any additional impairment of these mechanisms by drugs would make them even more susceptible to postural hypotension.

Dizziness: Drug-induced dizziness is common in the elderly. Drugs that produce sedation, altered vestibular function, antihypertensives and even some analgesics can cause dizziness. Orthostatic hypotension also results in dizziness and dizziness also increases the risk of falling due to imbalance. Hence, it is necessary to be watchful in the elderly for this adverse effect.

Sedation and confusion: Several drugs produce sedation and confusion as side effects. Elderly people may also be on hypnotics as many of them may have insomnia. Such sedation may often result in confusion and disorientation.

Fatigue and weakness: Most geriatric subjects have a weaker muscle mass and many are already debilitated. Drugs that produce muscle weakness like skeletal muscle relaxants, drugs like β-blockers which reduce heart rate and cardiac output; diuretics causing dehydration, decreased cardiac output and hyponatraemia and oral antidiabetics producing hypoglycaemia can all result in worsening of fatigue and weakness.

Depression: Several drugs can cause depression as an adverse effect and elderly are more susceptible to drug-induced depression.

Dehydration: It is a common problem in the elderly. They are more susceptible to this particular side effect due to age-related physiological changes like decrease in lean body mass, increase in fat, and reduced capacity of the kidney to concentrate urine. Symptoms of dehydration include altered sensorium, dizziness, lethargy, confusion and weakness which are all vague and may be misinterpreted for other geriatric problems. Dehydration may also be due to drugs like diuretics, digoxin, vasodilators and laxatives. Dehydration would result in volume depletion, which in turn may reduce cardiac output. It also causes weakness and fatigue.

Criteria for Safe Prescribing in the Elderly

Guidelines are available for safe prescribing in the elderly, *viz* Beers criteria, START and STOPP criteria.

Beers Criteria

These serve as guidelines for good prescription practice in the elderly, particularly when multiple drugs are used. They help to avoid drug interactions and adverse drug reactions.

START: Screening Tool to Alert doctor to the Right Treatment.

STOPP: Screening Tool in Older persons for Potentially inappropriate Prescriptions.

The START/STOPP criteria may also be used to guide clinicians in appropriate and safe use of drugs in the elderly.

ADMINISTRATION OF DRUGS IN RENAL DISEASES

Kidney is the primary excretory organ and most drugs are eliminated through it. Kidney also concentrates many drugs in it, therefore, kidney is itself exposed to large concentrations of drugs. Several drugs are almost totally excreted through the kidneys and in renal impairment their plasma levels rise and such drugs accumulate. However, the extent depends on the drug and the degree of renal dysfunction.

Absolute caution is required in the administration of drugs in presence of renal diseases particularly those drugs that are excreted largely through the kidneys. Dose of several drugs needs adjustment in presence of renal dysfunction—has been mentioned in the respective chapters. Also, constant monitoring of renal function is needed as the maintenance dose of drugs may need to be altered depending on the renal function. Nomograms are now available for reference. In patients undergoing dialysis, some drugs are easily dialysable and should be administered after dialysis. Treatment with drugs of low safety margin may require additional caution.

The following guidelines may be followed.

1. Use only drugs that are absolutely needed.
2. Avoid nephrotoxic drugs.
3. In a group of drugs, select a drug that is not nephrotoxic, if possible.
4. Dose of several drugs need to be reduced while many drugs may have to be avoided in patients in renal dysfunction. Dose of the drugs should be adjusted with the help of a nomogram.
5. Duration of treatment should be restricted as far as possible.
6. Therapeutic drug monitoring may be done wherever required.
7. Serum creatinine may be used as an important parameter to gauge the extent of renal impairment.
8. Corrected dose =

$$\text{Normal dose} \times \frac{\text{Patient's creatinine clearance}}{\text{Normal creatinine clearance (100 ml / min)}}$$

Cockroft Gault formula for creatinine clearance

$$\text{(CL) cr men} = \frac{(140 - \text{age in yr})(\text{weight in kg})}{72 \times \text{Scr}}$$

(CL) cr women = male value × 0.85

(CL) cr—creatinine clearance

Scr—serum creatinine

List of some drugs that require dosage adjustment in renal impairment

Ibuprofen	Cotrimoxazole
Piroxicam	Ceftazidime
Diclofenac	Cefotaxime
Indomethacin	Imipenem
Aminoglycosides	Ciprofloxacin
Vancomycin	Amphotericin
Teicoplanin	Chloroquine
Enalapril	Pyrazinamide
Captopril	Acyclovir
Perindopril	Azathioprine
Atenolol	Sotalol
Metoprolol	Propranolol
Digoxin	Phenobarbitone
Beta blockers	Morphine
Pethidine	

Some nephrotoxic drugs

Ciprofloxacin	Cyclosporine
NSAIDs	Aminoglycosides
Sulfonamides	Amphotericin B
Acyclovir	Methoxyflurane
Cytotoxic agents	Outdated tetracyclines

DRUG ADMINISTRATION IN LIVER DISEASES

Presence of liver diseases largely influences pharmacokinetics and to some extent pharmacodynamics. Some of the drugs (e.g. paracetamol) may be activated to toxic metabolites in the liver. Some drugs are exclusively metabolized in the liver while some are partly metabolized and others are excreted unchanged. Presence of liver diseases raises the plasma levels of many drugs.

Liver diseases may reduce hepatic blood flow, cause hepatocellular damage and dysfunction, reduce the production of albumin and raise the bilirubin levels.

Several drugs may themselves be hepatotoxic. This may worsen pre-existing liver diseases.

The extent to which hepatic dysfunction influences the metabolism depends on:

1. The degree of liver dysfunction—higher the dysfunction greater the impact.
2. The drug itself, i.e. the extent to which the drug depends on the liver for metabolism.

In presence of liver disease

Some drugs that need dose reduction	*Some drugs to be avoided*
Propranolol	Pethidine
Pentazocine	Chloramphenicol
Lignocaine	Aspirin
INH	Theophylline
Diazepam	
Vancomycin	
Heparin	
Phenobarbitone	
Warfarin	
Cyclophosphamide	

Prodrugs depend on hepatic activation. Some drugs undergo extensive first pass metabolism and some drugs undergo high hepatic clearance, e.g. propranolol, morphine, lignocaine. Plasma levels of such drugs are grossly affected by liver dysfunction. Many drugs undergo low hepatic clearance and they are only partly metabolised by the liver, e.g. paracetamol, phenytoin, chloramphenicol, warfarin.

Hepatic extraction ratio is the fraction of the drug removed from the blood during single transit through the liver.

$$\text{Hepatic extraction} = \frac{\text{Hepatic clearance}}{\text{Hepatic blood flow}}$$

Raised liver enzymes may be used as a guide to assess the hepatic impairment though they do not exactly point to the pathology.

GENE THERAPY

Gene therapy is the replacement of defective gene by the insertion of a normal, functional gene. It is the genetic modification of cells for the prevention or treatment of a disease. Gene transfer may be done to replace a missing or defective gene or provide extra-copies of a normally expressed gene.

Vectors

Gene transfer requires vectors to deliver the DNA material. An ideal vector should be safe and effective in inserting the therapeutic gene into the target cells.

- *Physical vectors:* DNA is complexed with substances like lipids and administered.
- *Chemical vectors:* Liposomes are used to carry genes into the cells.
- *Biological vectors:* The most important biological vectors are viral vectors—viruses invade cells and use the metabolic processes of these host cells for replication. This property of viruses helps to deliver the gene—adenoviruses and retroviruses are used.

Therapeutic Applications

Gene therapy is at present a developing area. Though originally it was seen as a remedy only for inherited single gene defects, gene therapy has now been found to be useful in several acquired disorders too. The principle applications are in single gene defects like thalassaemia, cystic fibrosis and haemoglobinopathies and in the treatment of cancer, cardiovascular diseases, atherosclerosis, immunodeficiency disorders—particularly AIDS; anaemia, Alzheimer's disease and many infectious diseases. Some examples are:

1. *Growth hormone deficiency:* Growth hormone gene is transferred to myoblasts and these are implanted in patients.
2. *Familial hypercholesterolemia:* LDL receptor gene is introduced into liver cells.
3. *Cancer*
    - Introducing genes which make the malignant cells sensitive to drugs.
    - Inactivating the expression of oncogenes.
    - Introducing genes that attach to cancer cells and make them susceptible to host defence cells.
    - Introducing genes to healthy cells to protect them from cytotoxic drugs.
4. *HIV infections*
    - Introducing genes coding for CD4 cells that could inactivate HIV before entering the cell itself.
    - Introducing genes that enhance immunity against HIV.
5. *Diabetes mellitus:* Introducing insulin gene into the liver which can produce insulin.
6. *Coronary atherosclerosis:* Prevention of restenosis and ischaemia in coronary vessels by genes which inhibit the growth of vascular endothelial cells.
7. *Blood*
    - *Sickle cell anaemia* introducing sickle cell inhibitor gene.
    - *Haemophilia*—introducing factor VIII gene.

[1] From Medical Council of India, *Competency based Undergraduate Curriculum for the Indian Medical Graduate*, 2018;1:136–144.

CHAPTER 64

Drugs used in Skin Disorders

Competency achievement: The student should be able to:
PH 1.57 Describe drugs used in skin disorders.[1]

For actions on the skin and mucous membrane, drugs are largely used topically. Occasionally, some drugs may be used systemically for effects on the skin.

Drugs used topically may be intended for actions on the surface of the skin and mucous membrane or on the layers of the skin and sometimes meant to be absorbed through the skin. Certain properties of the drugs are important for them to be effective topically. The drug should be highly lipid-soluble and have a low molecular mass. An adequate concentration gradient should be present for the drug to be absorbed. Adequate hydration of the skin increases penetration. Presence of inflammation, thin skin and occlusive dressing enhance absorption. In children, absorption through the skin is greater because of their thinner skin.

Some drugs used for their effects on the skin and mucous membrane are as follows.

KERATOLYTICS

Keratolytics are drugs that dissolve the intercellular cement substance and cause peeling of the superficial layers of the skin. They are used in hyperkeratotic conditions of the skin like warts, cones, calluses and even severe xerosis. **Salicylic acid** (10–20%), **lactic acid, urea, sulfur** and **propylene glycol** may be used as keratolytic agents. **Propylene glycol** may be used alone (40–70%) or with salicylic acid. Propylene glycol is a good keratolytic, poorly absorbed from the skin and the absorbed portion is metabolised by the liver. It also has hygroscopic properties and acts as a humectant. Propylene glycol is used in hyperkeratotic conditions of palm and sole, ichthyosis, hypertrophic lichen planus and psoriasis. Testing for allergic reactions prior to the therapeutic application of propylene glycol is recommended. **Urea** also has keratolytic (20%) and humectant (2–20%) effects similar to propylene glycol and is used for similar indications as propylene glycol. **Podophyllum resin**—obtained from the mandrake plant or May apple is used in condylomata acuminata. It is applied topically (25%) to the wart for 2–6 hr depending on the ability of the patient to tolerate the preparation. **Benzyl peroxide** 5–10% is used as cream/lotion for its keratolytic effects in acne.

SUNSCREENS

Sunscreens are agents that protect the skin from the effects of the UV rays. UV rays are of three types: depending on the wavelength - UVA (320–400 nm), UVB (290–320 nm) and UVC (100–290 nm). The effects of UVA are largely responsible for photoaging and phototoxicity. UVB causes sun burns and tanning. UVC the most dangerous of the three is held back by the ozone layer of the atmosphere. UV rays can cause skin cancer by damaging the DNA. Sunscreens can act by:

i. *Reflection of UV rays:* These are opaque substances that block or reflect the UV rays—also called physical sunscreens or sunshades, e.g. titanium dioxide, calamine, zinc oxide, heavy petroleum jelly.

ii. *Absorption of UV rays* and thereby prevent their effects on the skin, e.g. PABA and its derivatives, cinnamates, salicylates, benzophenones (oxybenzone) and avobenzene.

The activity of sunscreens is measured by the unit—**sun protection factor** (SPF) which gives an idea about the efficacy of sunscreens. Sunscreens include:

- **UVA sunscreens**—avobenzene, oxybenzene, titanium dioxide, zinc oxide, ecamsule.
- **UVB sunscreens**—PABA derivatives, cinnamates, salicylates (octyl salicylate).

ANTIMICROBIALS

Antibacterials, antifungals and antiviral drugs used on the skin and mucous membrane are described in the respective chapters. Antibacterial agents are used topically for the prevention and treatment of infection in wounds. Bacitracin, gramicidin, polymyxin, mupirocin, neomycin and the newer agent retapamulin are used exclusively topically for skin infections.

Retapamulin is a semisynthetic compound effective in the treatment of uncomplicated skin infections due to streptococci and staphylococci. Used as 1% ointment retapamulin can occasionally cause local irritation. **Gramicidin** is a peptide effective against aerobic and anaerobic cocci and some bacilli including streptococci, staphylococci, gonococci, meningococci, tetanus and diphtheria bacilli. Gramicidin is used in combination with other antibacterials for skin infections. Erythromycin, clindamycin, gentamicin, sulphacetamide and metronidazole are also available for topical use.

Topical antifungal drugs clotrimazole, miconazole, cyclopirox olamine, naftifine, terbinafine, butanafine, tolnaftate are all used topically for superficial fungal infections of the skin. Griseofulvin is given orally for dermatophyte infections.

Topical antiviral drugs (*see* Chapter 52): Acyclovir, penciclovir, valacyclovir, famciclovir, docosonal trifluoridine are used topically for herpes infections.

GLUCOCORTICOIDS

Glucocorticoids are one of the most commonly used drugs in dermatology. A variety of preparations with mild to strong potency are available for topical use and also for use by other routes of administration. For detailed pharmacology, *see* Chapter 38.

DRUGS USED IN ACNE

Acne is a common skin disorder in adolescents. The production of sebum is increased in adolescents due to androgenic activity and this is associated with hyperkeratinization and excessive desquamation of the epithelial cells of the hair follicle leading to blockade of the follicular opening. This results in comedones (black and white heads). The bacteria present in the hair follicles, *Propionibacterium acnes*, break the lipids in the sebum to form irritating free fatty acids which evoke local inflammation resulting in the formation of papules, nodules or pustules. The pustules may heal with scarring or hyperpigmentation. Drugs used in the treatment of acne are:

Antibacterials

Antibacterials include clindamycin (1% gel), erythromycin as a 2% lotion and ointment and metronidazole (0.75% cream).

Benzyl peroxide is converted to benzoic acid in the skin which has antibacterial, comedolytic and keratolytic actions. Available as 2.5–10% cream/gel, it is applied once daily, the frequency depending on the patient's ability to tolerate the irritation. It can cause local stinging sensation and redness.

PERSOL, PERNOX 2.5%, 5% gel.

Azelaic acid obtained from *Pityrosporum ovale* inhibits many aerobic and anaerobic microorganisms on topical application. It is also used in melasma. It is available as 10 and 20% cream.

AZIDERM 10, 20% cream.

Systemic antibiotics are not commonly used for acne. However, low doses of tetracycline (250 mg BD), doxycycline (100 mg OD) or erythromycin (500 mg BD) has been used for 4–8 wks when multiple infected acne are present.

Retinoids

Retinol, tretinoin, isotretinoin, retinoic acid, adepalene, tazarotene are effective in the treatment of acne. Retinoids are derivatives of retinol and act on retinoic acid receptors.

Tretinoin used topically reduces hyperkeratinization, is a comedolytic and decreases pigmentation and also prevents the formation of comedones. It is used as a 0.025% lotion, cream or gel. The response is slow—given for 4–6 wks and if the patient responds, it may be continued for another 8–12 wks. More prolonged use should be avoided. Tretinoin may also be used for the treatment of photoaged skin.

EUDYNA 0.05% cream.

Adapalene is also used topically as 0.1% gel and may be combined with benzoyl peroxide.

ADAPEN 0.1% gel.

Isotretinoin is given orally 0.5 mg/kg/day for 4 weeks and continued for the next 8–12 wks, if response is encouraging. It is used only in severe acne that is unresponsive to topical drugs.

IRET 200 mg tab.

All retinoids can cause dryness of the skin and itching. Oral retinoids can cause conjunctivitis and a rise in intracranial tension and plasma lipids. All retinoids are **highly teratogenic**.

DRUGS USED IN PSORIASIS

Psoriasis is a chronic skin disorder of autoimmune aetiology characterised by inflammatory, thickened patches or lesions. The erythematous plaques of varying shapes and sizes are covered with silvery scales and may be localised to involve other areas including the scalp, finger nails and sometimes the joints (psoriatic arthritis). An exacerbation may be triggered by bacterial infections, stress and drugs. Drugs are used to control the symptoms and prolonged treatment is required—may be used topically or systemically.

A. *Topical therapy*
   - In mild lesions, emollients, keratolytics, retinoids and glucocorticoids are used topically.
   - Emollients like soft paraffin, hydrate and soften the skin.
   - Keratolytics like salicylic acid (2–10%), propylene glycol, urea, formalin and lactic acid may be used in combination with coal tar, dithranol and/or glucocorticoids.
   - Dithranol, a systemic compound inhibits the mitotic activity of the cells in the skin. It may be applied topically (after testing for allergy) on lesions except on face.
   - The topical retinoid used in psoriasis is tazarotene (0.5–1% gel). Tazarotene may be combined with a topical glucocorticoid.
   - Crude coaltar of different concentrations is available and may be used as a greasy vehicle or as shampoo along with salicylic acid for topical use.

B. *Systemic therapy:* A small percentage of patients may require systemic therapy but is more toxic, more expensive and requires constant monitoring.

Retinoids

Etretinate, a vitamin A analog, is given orally (0.5–1 mg/kg/day) along with phototherapy in psoriasis. Because of the risk of teratogenicity, pregnancy as well as blood donation should be ruled out before starting therapy and pregnancy should be avoided during and for 3 years after the treatment with retinoids is completed.

Acitretin, a metabolite of etretinate, is an oral retinoid effective in psoriasis particularly in severe forms but is now withdrawn from the market in some countries.

Calcipotriol

Calcipotriol, a derivative of vitamin D, is applied topically in plaque type psoriasis while it inhibits the proliferation of epidural keratinocytes; applied as 0.005% ointment for 6–8 wks either alone or with a glucocorticoid. It can cause irritation. Phototherapy may be combined with vitamin D therapy.

Immunosuppressants

Tacrolimus, an immunosuppressant, has been found to be effective in psoriasis and is given orally.

Mycophenolate mofetil is also useful in psoriasis and other immunologically mediated skin conditions. It is well tolerated and has been used in the dose of 1–2 g/day.

Cyclosporine inhibits interleukin-2 production and is used in severe refractory psoriasis.

Antiproliferative Drugs

Methotrexate inhibits T cell expansion and suppresses immunocompetent cells in the skin and is effective in moderate to severe chronic plaque psoriasis. It may be used along with other drugs like biological agents and phototherapy in psoriasis. Started with 5 mg/wk the dose may be increased gradually to 20–30 mg/wk, if needed. Methotrexate must never be combined with NSAIDs as they compete with protein binding, increase plasma levels of methotrexate and can cause fatal bone marrow suppression. **Azathioprine** may be used in place of methotrexate.

Biological Agents

Since psoriasis is an immunologically mediated disorder, several biological agents have been found to be effective and are currently tried in moderate to severe psoriasis.

Alefacept is a recombinant human fusion protein that binds to T cells and blocks its activation. Given 15 mg IM/week for 12 wks and then extended, if required, it induces long remissions in psoriasis.

Etanercept, a fusion protein is a TNF receptor antagonist binds to TNF alpha and inhibits its action. It is beneficial in psoriasis and psoriatic arthritis.

Infliximab, a monoclonal antibody, binds to TNF alpha and inhibits the binding of TNF alpha to its receptors and is being studied for use in psoriasis.

Efalizumab binds to T cells and interferes with its activation and migration in the skin and vascular endothelial cells. It is given SC 1 mg/kg once a week for 12–24 wks in moderate to severe psoriasis.

Glucocorticoids

Glucocorticoids may be needed systemically only in severe cases of psoriasis.

Phototherapy or Psoralen Ultraviolet A (PUVA) Therapy

This therapy is used in severely ill psoriatic patients. Psoralen (methoxasalen trioxasalaen) is given orally followed by exposure to UVA therapy after 1–2 hours. Such treatment is repeated on alternate days and continued for 2 wks. Psoralens are photosensitizing drugs and interfere with DNA synthesis in the epithelial cells. Their use is associated with the risk of skin cancers and cataract and is, therefore, restricted only to severe disease.

[1] From Medical Council of India, *Competency based Undergraduate Curriculum for the Indian Medical Graduate*, 2018;1:136–144.

CHAPTER 65

Drugs used in Ocular Diseases

Competency achievement: The student should be able to:

PH 1.58 Describe drugs used in ocular disorders.[1]

Drugs used for their effects on the eye are generally administered by local route. Ocular routes are:

- Topical
- Subconjunctival
- Subtenon
- Retrobulbar injection

} most commonly used for anterior segment infections

- Intraocular injection—for iritis, uveitis, endophthalmitis
- Intravitreal injection—for retinitis, endophthalmitis

Topical—Drugs administered topically dissolve in the tears and may get absorbed across the cornea (transcorneal) or conjunctiva (transconjunctival). Higher the concentration of the drug in the tear film, better is the absorption. Part of the drug may get absorbed systemically across the nasal mucosa as it gets drained through the nasolacrimal duct. Other routes are used in more specific situations.

Drugs used locally in the eye are:

1. Antimicrobials—antibacterials, anti fungal, anti viral
2. NSAIDs—diclofenac, ketorolac, flurbiprofen
3. Glucocorticoids
4. Antihistamines and mast cell stabilizers
5. Immunosuppressants
6. Miotics and Mydriatics
7. Artificial tears

1. **Antimicrobials** used on the eye are: Fluoroquinolones like ciprofloxacin, moxifloxacin, levofloxacin, gatifloxacin, ofloxacin

Sulphacetamide, chloramphenical, erythromycin and bacitracin

Infections of the eye like conjunctivitis, iritis, keratitis, infection of the lacrimal sac, endophthalmitis and panophthalmitis are generally of bacterial origin. Topical antibiotics are used in most of them. Endophthalmitis and panophthalmitis are treated with intravitreal and systemic antibiotics.

Antiviral drugs—are used in many ocular viral infections.

Viral keratitis by herpes simplex, varicella zoster → topical trifluridine/ganciclovir

Herpes zoster ophthalmicus → systemic acyclovir, valacyclovir, famciclovir.

Viral retinitis—CMV, herpes simplex, VZV, adenovirus → parenteral antiviral drugs; alternative → intravitrial ganciclovir.

Antifungal drugs—incidence of fungal keratitis and infections of other structures of the eye have now increased in immunocompromised patients. Use of contact lens and trauma are other predisposing factors for fungal keratitis.

Some of the antifungal drugs used on the eye are:

- Topical amphotericin—0.1–0.5% drops, subconjunctival—1 mg, intravitreal—5 mg
- Miconazole 5–10 mg subconjunctival
- Natamycin 5%

Other antifungal drugs like fluconazole and ketoconazole are given orally.

2. **NSAIDS.** Suspensions or eye drops of NSAIDs are available for topical use like diclofenac, ketorolac, flurbiprofen and nepafenac. They are used to suppress the inflammation and reduce pain including postoperative pain and trauma pain.
3. **Glucocorticoids.** Many of the glucocorticoids are available for topical use on the eye like dexamethasone, betamethasone, prednisolone and hydrocortisone. Ocular inflammatory conditions and allergy respond well to topical steroids.
4. **Antihistamines and mast cell stabilizers.** Antihistamines like pheniramine, antazoline, azelastine and levocabastine are available as eye drops for allergies of the eye. Mast cell stabilizers like cromolyn sodium, nedocromil, olopatadine and ketotifen are also useful in vernal ketarrah and allergic conjunctivitis.
5. **Immunosuppressants** like cyclosporine are used topically to treat chronic dry eye.
6. **Artificial tears**—tear substitutes consists of hypotonic or isotonic solutions of electrolytes, viscosity increasing agents like polyethylene glycol, carboxymethyl cellulose and glycerine along with some preservatives.
7. **Miotics**—drugs that constrict the pupil like pilocarpine, acetylcholine (muscarine agonists) and physostigmine (anticholinesterase) are used in glaucoma, iritis and acute uveitis.
8. **Mydriatics** are drugs that cause dilatation of the pupil. Examples: antimuscarinics like atropine, homatropine, cyclopentolate, and tropicamide. Some of them also cause spasm of accommodation or cycloplegia. Alpha agonists like phenylephrine are sympathomimetics which produce mydriasis without cycloplegia. Mydriatics are used for:
   1. Testing of refraction
   2. Fundoscopic examination of the eye
   3. Providing rest to the iris
   4. Alternatively with miotics to break the adhesions between the iris and the lens.

[1] From Medical Council of India, *Competency based Undergraduate Curriculum for the Indian Medical Graduate*, 2018;1:136–144.

CHAPTER 66

Important Drug Interactions

Interacting drugs	Consequence	Pharmacological basis
1. β-blockers + hydralazine/frusemide	↑ β-blocking effect	↓ metabolism of propranolol
2. β-blockers + insulin	i. β-blockers mask palpitation, the most important warning symptom of hypoglycaemia ii. They prolong recovery from hypoglycaemia	• Blockade of cardiac β receptors • Block hepatic glycogenolysis mediated by β_2 receptors; homoeostatic mechanisms are blocked
3. Propranolol + verapamil	May cause heart block resulting in cardiac arrest	Both drugs depress conducting tissues of the heart and have negative inotropic effects
4. Calcium channel blockers + phenytoin/rifampicin	↓ effects of CCBs	Both increase metabolism of CCBs by enzyme induction
5. Digoxin + hydrochlorothiazide	Digoxin toxicity	Thiazides cause hypokalaemia which in turn aggravates digoxin toxicity
6. Digoxin + antacids/ sucralfate/metoclopramide	↓ bioavailability of digoxin	Reduce absorption of digoxin
7. Bile acid-binding resins + frusemide/thiazides/ thyroid hormones	↓ bioavailability of latter drugs	BAB resins bind and prevent absorption of orally administered drugs
8. Anticoagulants + phenylbutazone	Anticoagulant toxicity	Inhibit anticoagulant metabolism
9. Warfarin + aspirin	i. ↑ Anticoagulant toxicity ii. Bleeding from aspirin-induced peptic ulcer	• Aspirin displaces warfarin from binding sites • Inhibition of platelet aggregation by aspirin potentiates anticoagulant effect • Aspirin-induced gastric erosion and ulcers may bleed more due to anticoagulant effects
10. Alcohol + disulfiram cephalosporins, metronidazole, sulfonylureas)	Antabuse reaction	Disulfiram inhibits aldehyde dehydrogenase resulting in accumulation of acetaldehyde
11. Alcohol + CNS depressants like opioids/antidepressants	Profound CNS depression	CNS depressant effect gets added up
12. Carbamazepine + haloperidol/oral contra-ceptives/corticosteroids	Decreased efficacy of interacting drugs	Carbamazepine is an enzyme inducer—increases metabolism of interacting drugs
13. Carbamazepine + cimetidine/erythromycin/ INH/ketoconazole	Decreased carbamazepine metabolism	Inhibition of drug metabolising enzymes by interacting drugs

Interacting drugs	Consequence	Pharmacological basis
14. Phenytoin + carbamazepine	Decreased effects of both	Phenytoin and carbamazepine increase each other's metabolism
15. Phenytoin + chloramphenicol/cimetidine/warfarin	Phenytoin toxicity	The interacting drugs inhibit phenytoin metabolism
16. Phenytoin + steroids/ doxycycline/theophylline	Phenytoin increases metabolism of interacting drugs	Phenytoin is an enzyme inducer
17. Barbiturates + CCBs/corticosteroids/ketoconazole/ estrogen/chloramphenicol/ tricyclic antidepressants	Decreased efficacy of interacting drugs	Barbiturates are enzyme inducers. They increase the metabolism of other drugs metabolised by microsomal enzymes
18. TCA + carbamazapine/ rifampicin	Increased metabolism of antidepressants	Carbamazepine and rifampicin are enzyme inducers
19. TCA + SSRIs (e.g. fluoxetine)	↓ metabolism of antidepressants	SSRIs inhibit metabolising enzymes
20. TCA + MAO inhibitors	Hypertensive crisis	Uninhibited action of catecholamines due to inhibition of MAO
21. Levodopa + phenothiazines	↓ antiparkinsonian effect	Phenothiazines block DA receptors
22. Levodopa + pyridoxine	↓ antiparkinsonian effect	Pyridoxine increases peripheral decarboxylation of levodopa
23. Lithium + diuretics	Lithium toxicity	Decreased excretion of lithium
24. NSAIDs + frusemide	Blunting of diuretic effect	PG inhibition may result in salt and water retention
25. Aspirin + warfarin/ phenytoin/ sulfonylureas	Toxicity of co-administered drugs	Aspirin displaces these drugs from protein binding sites
26. Quinolone antibiotics + sucralfate/antacids	↓ Bioavailability	Reduced gastrointestinal absorption of quinolones
27. Quinolones + theophylline/caffeine	Toxicity due to theophylline/caffeine	Quinolones inhibit the metabolism of theophylline/caffeine
28. Chloramphenicol + phenytoin/sulfonylureas	Toxicity due to phenytoin/sulfonylureas	Chloramphenicol decreases metabolism of these drugs
29. Rifampicin + oestrogens/ corticosteroids/sulfonylureas/ theophylline	Therapeutic failure of drugs added	Rifampicin is an enzyme inducer
30. Antacids + quinolones/ salicylates/tetracycline	↓ Bioavailability	Antacids may adsorb drugs and reduce their absorption
31. Antacids + sucralfate	Therapeutic failure of sucralfate	Sucralfate acts in acidic pH while antacids make the gastric pH alkaline
32. Allopurinol + 6-mercaptopurine/azathioprine	6-mercaptopurine toxicity	Allopurinol inhibits xanthine oxidase which metabolises 6-MP
33. Piperazine citrate + pyrantel pamoate	Therapeutic failure	Piperazine causes hyperpolarization while pyrantel causes depolarization. They antagonise each other's effects
34. Glucocorticoids + erythromycin/ ketoconazole/cyclosporine/isoniazid	↑ Plasma levels of glucocorticoids	Decreased metabolism of glucocorticoids
35. Glucocorticoids + phenobarbitone/ other enzyme inducers	↓ Plasma levels of glucocorticoids	Increased rate of metabolism of glucocorticoids
36. Dabigatran/apixaban/rivaroxaban	↑ anticoagulant effect	↓ elimination of anticoagulants
37. Verapamil + cyclosporine/ tacrolimus/sildenafil	↑ levels of calcineurin inhibitors	Verapamil inhibits CYP3A enzyme

Bibliography

1. Bertram G Katzung, Basic and Clinical Pharmacology 14th Edition, McGraw-Hill education Lange 2018.
2. Brayfield, Alison, Martindale: The Complete Drug Reference 39th edition. Pharmaceutical press 2017.
3. Harrison's Principles of Internal Medicine, 20th Edition, McGraw-Hill International edition 2018.
4. Health programmes/Wellness.National health portal: Government of India. Available from : https://www.nhp.gov.in/healthprogramme/national-health-programmes. (accessed on 27 April 2020)
5. Hiralal Konar, Dutta's Textbook of Gynaecology 7th edition, 2016.
6. HL Sharma, KK Sharma, Principles of Pharmacology 3rd edition. Paras Publishing 2017.
7. James Ritter, Rod Flower, Graeme Henderson, Yoon Kong Loke, David MacEwan, Humphrey Rang-Rang & Dale's Pharmacology 9th edition Elsevier Churchill Livingstone: International edition 2019.
8. Karen Whalen (editors: Sangeetha Sharma, Thirumurthy Velpandian)-Lippincott Illustrated Reviews: Pharmacology South Asian Edition 2018-Wolters Kluwer publishers.
9. KD Tripathi Essentials of Medical Pharmacology, 8th edition, Jaypee Brothers: New Delhi, 2018.
10. Kellerman MD, Rakel MD. Conn's Current therapy 1st edition, Elsevier 2019.
11. Laurence Brunton, Bjorn Knollmann, Randa Hilal-Dandan, Goodman and Gilman's: The Pharmacological Basis of Therapeutics, 13th edition. McGraw-Hill: New York, 2017.
12. Laurence L Brunton, Randa Hilal-Dandan, BJörn C. KNOLLMANN, Goodman and Gilman's. The Pharmacological Basis of Therapeutics 13th edition, 2017.
13. Morris Brown, Pankaj Sharma, Fraz Mir, Peter Bennett, Clinical Pharmacology, 12th Edition, Elsevier Churchill Livingstone: London 2018.
14. Park's Text Book of Preventive & Social Medicine 25th edition. Bhanot Publishers, Jabalapur, 2019.
15. Parson's Diseases of the eye, 23rd edition 2019.
16. Satoskar RS, Nirmala Rege, Bhandarkar SD, Raakhi K Tripathi, Pharmacology and Pharmacotherapeutics 25th edition 2017.
17. Seth SD, Seth V. Textbook of Pharmacology, 3rd edition 2009.
18. Anemia Mukt Bharat. Available from: https://anemiamuktbharat.info/ (accessed on 27 April 2020)
19. During revision of this textbook, several research and review articles from journals of pharmacology and medicine, WHO and other international guidelines and many textbooks have been referred.
20. National programme on Anti-microbial resistance containment. National Center for disease control. MoHFW: Government of India. Available from: https://ncdc.gov.in/index1.php?lang=1&level=2&sublinkid=384&lid=344 (accessed on 27 April 2020)
21. Page CP, Curtis MJ, et al. Integrated Pharmacology, 3rd edition Mosby, London 2006.
22. Pradhan Mantri Bhartiya Janaushadi Pariyojana. National Portal of India. Available from: https://www.india.gov.in/spotlight/pradhan-mantri-bhartiya-janaushadhi-pariyojana ((accessed on 27 April 2020).
23. Umbrella ICDS. Department of Women and Child Development: Government of India. Available from: https://wcd.nic.in/schemes-listing/2404 (accessed on 27 April 2020)
24. HYPERLINK "http://www.ncbi.nlm.nih.gov/pubmed/26998708"Qato DM, Wilder J, Schumm LP, et al: Changes in prescription and over-the-counter medication and dietary supplement use among older adults in the United States, 2005 vs 2011. JAMA Intern Med 176(4):473-82, 2016. doi: 10.1001/jamainternmed.2015.8581.

25. Drug therapy in the elderly: Nobel; HYPERLINK "https://www.ncbi.nlm.nih.gov/pubmed/14577060" Metabolism. 2003 Oct;52(10 Suppl 2):27–30.
26. Gurwitz JH, Field TS, et al. Incidence and preventability of Adverse drug events among older persons in the ambulatory care setting. JAMA, 2003;289 (9):1107.
27. Williams CM. Using medications appropriately in older adults. Am Fam Physician 2002;66(10):1917.
28. HYPERLINK "https://www.hindawi.com/69287236/" Paul AF. Jansen and HYPERLINK "https://www.hindawi.com/93693185/" Jacobus RBJ. Brouwers Clinical Pharmacology in Old Persons Volume 2012, Article ID 723678, 17 page http://dx.doi.org/10.6064/2012/723678
29. https://www.sciencedirect.com/topics/biochemistry-genetics-and-molecular-biology/dietary-supplement
30. HYPERLINK "http://www.who.int>areas>QualityAssurancePharmVol2" www.who.int>areas>QualityAssurancePharmVol2
31. HYPERLINK "https://www.ncbi.nlm.nih.gov/pmc/articles/PMC4336979/"Int J Prev Med. 2014 Dec; 5(12): 1487>1499./)
32. HYPERLINK "https://www.pharmaceutical-journal.com/PJ,-July-2000/385.issue" The Pharmaceutical Journal 8 JUL 20000
33. https://www.ncbi.nlm.nih.gov/pmc/articles/PMC4152533
34. https://www.tribalcafe.com/site/tribal-juice-bar-menu-2/supplements-superfoods

Index

E